Volume 2

FRACTURES

IN ADULTS

EDITED BY

Charles A. Rockwood, Jr., M.D.

Professor and Chairman, Department of Orthopaedics, The University of Texas Health Science Center at San Antonio, San Antonio, Texas

AND

David P. Green, M.D.

Clinical Professor, Department of Orthopaedics; and Consultant, Hand Surgery Service, The University of Texas Health Science Center at San Antonio, San Antonio, Texas

WITH 31 CONTRIBUTORS

Volume 2

FRACTURES
IN ADULTS

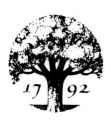

J.B. Lippincott Company
PHILADELPHIA / London / Mexico City / New York
St. Louis / São Paulo / Sydney

Sponsoring Editor:
  Sanford Robinson
Manuscript Editor:
  Delois Patterson
Indexer:
  Tony Greenberg, M.D.
Art Director:
  Maria S. Karkucinski
Designer:
  Ronald Dorfman

Production Supervisor:
  N. Carol Kerr
Production Coordinator:
  George V. Gordon
Compositor:
  Monotype Composition Company
Printer/Binder:
  Halliday Lithograph

The authors and publisher have exerted every effort to ensure that drug selection and dosage set forth in this text are in accord with current recommendations and practice at the time of publication. However, in view of ongoing research, changes in government regulations, and the constant flow of information relating to drug therapy and drug reactions, the reader is urged to check the package insert for each drug for any change in indications and dosage and for added warnings and precautions. This is particularly important when the recommended agent is a new or infrequently employed drug.

2nd Edition

1   3   5   6   4   2

Library of Congress Cataloging in Publication Data
Main entry under title:

Fractures in adults.

  Rev. ed. of: Fractures. [1975]
  Bibliography.
  Includes index.
  1. Fractures. 2. Dislocations. I. Rockwood,
Charles A. II. Green, David P. III. Fractures.
[DNLM: 1. Dislocations. 2. Fractures. WE 175 F7982]
RD101.F739 1984   617'.15   84-847
ISBN 0-397-50623-6 (set)

Contributors

Bijan Ahmadi, M.D.
Formerly, Assistant Professor, Orthopaedic Surgery, University of Louisville, Louisville, Kentucky

Lewis D. Anderson, M.D.
Professor and Chairman, Department of Orthopaedic Surgery, University of Southern Alabama College of Medicine, Mobile, Alabama

Thomas D. Brower, M.D.
Professor and Chairman, Division of Orthopaedic Surgery, University of Kentucky College of Medicine, Lexington, Kentucky

Michael W. Chapman, M.D.
Professor and Chairman, Department of Orthopaedic Surgery, University of California, Davis School of Medicine, Davis, California

Bernd F. Claudi, M.D.
Chief of Traumatology Division, Technical University, Munich

Richard L. Cruess, M.D.
Dean, Faculty of Medicine, McGill University; Professor of Surgery, McGill University; Senior Orthopaedic Surgeon, Royal Victoria Hospital and Shriners Hospital for Crippled Children, Montreal, Quebec

Jesse C. DeLee, M.D.
Associate Professor, Department of Orthopaedics, The University of Texas Health Science Center at San Antonio, San Antonio, Texas

James H. Dobyns, M.D.
Clinical Professor of Orthopaedic Surgery, Mayo Medical School; Consultant in Orthopaedic Surgery and Surgery of the Hand, Mayo Clinic, Rochester, Minnesota

Charles H. Epps, Jr., M.D.
Professor and Chief, Division of Orthopaedic Surgery, Howard University College of Medicine, Washington, D.C.

C. McCollister Evarts, M.D.
Dorris N. Carlson Professor of Orthopaedics; Chairman, Department of Orthopaedics, University of Rochester School of Medicine and Dentistry; Orthopaedic Surgeon-in-Chief, Strong Memorial Hospital, Rochester, New York

David P. Green, M.D.
Clinical Professor, Department of Orthopaedics; Consultant, Hand Surgery Service, The University of Texas Health Science Center at San Antonio, San Antonio, Texas

Charles F. Gregory, M.D. (deceased)
Formerly, W. B. Carrell-Scottish Rite Professor and Chairman, Division of Orthopaedic Surgery, The University of Texas Health Science Center at Dallas, Dallas, Texas

Sigvard T. Hansen, Jr., M.D.
Professor and Chairman of Orthopaedic Surgery, University of Washington School of Medicine, Seattle, Washington

v

James W. Harkess, M.D., Ch.B.
Orthopaedic Surgeon, Jewish Hospital; Formerly, Kosair Professor, University of Louisville, Louisville, Kentucky

James D. Heckman, M.D.
Associate Professor and Deputy Chairman, Department of Orthopaedics, The University of Texas Health Science Center at San Antonio, San Antonio, Texas

Mason Hohl, M.D.
Associate Clinical Professor of Orthopaedic Surgery, University of California at Los Angeles School of Medicine; Consultant in Orthopaedics, Wadsworth Veterans Administration Facility, West Los Angeles, California

Donald C. Jones, M.D.
Orthopaedic Consultant and Womens' Sports Team Physician, Athletic Department, University of Oregon, Eugene, Oregon

William J. Kane, M.D., Ph.D.
Professor of Orthopaedic Surgery, Northwestern University Medical School; Attending Orthopaedic Surgeon, Northwestern Memorial Hospital and Children's Memorial Hospital, Chicago, Illinois

Herbert Kaufer, M.D.
Professor of Orthopaedic Surgery, University of Michigan Medical Center, Ann Arbor, Michigan

Thomas F. Kling, M.D.
Assistant Professor of Surgery, Section of Orthopaedic Surgery, University of Michigan Medical Center, Ann Arbor, Michigan

Robert L. Larson, M.D.
Clinical Assistant Professor of Surgery, Division of Orthopaedics and Rehabilitation, School of Medicine, Oregon Health Sciences University, Portland, Oregon; Orthopaedic Consultant, University of Oregon Athletic Department; Director of Athletic Medicine, University of Oregon, Eugene, Oregon

Robert E. Leach, M.D.
Professor and Chairman, Department of Orthopaedic Surgery, Boston University Medical School, Boston, Massachusetts

Ronald L. Linscheid, M.D.
Professor of Orthopaedic Surgery, Mayo Medical School; Consultant on Orthopaedic Surgery and Surgery of the Hand, Mayo Clinic, Rochester, Minnesota

Philip J. Mayer, M.D.
Head, Spine Surgery, Department of Orthopaedics, Marshfield Clinic, Marshfield, Wisconsin

Vert Mooney, M.D.
Professor and Chairman, Division of Orthopaedic Surgery, The University of Texas Health Science Center at Dallas, Dallas, Texas

Charles S. Neer II, M.D.
Professor of Clinical Orthopaedic Surgery, Columbia University College of Physicians and Surgeons; Attending Orthopaedic Surgeon and Chief of Adult Orthopaedic Service, New York Orthopaedic Hospital, Columbia-Presbyterian Medical Center, New York, New York

William C. Ramsey, M.D.
Orthopaedic Surgeon, Jewish Hospital, Louisville, Kentucky

Charles A. Rockwood, Jr., M.D.
Professor and Chairman, Department of Orthopaedics, The University of Texas Health Science Center at San Antonio, San Antonio, Texas

Spencer A. Rowland, M.D.
Associate Clinical Professor, Department of Orthopaedics; Consultant, Hand Surgery Service, The University of Texas Health Science Center at San Antonio; Consultant in Hand Surgery, Brooke Army Medical Center, San Antonio, Texas

Dempsey S. Springfield, M.D.
Associate Professor, Department of Orthopaedic Surgery; Chief of Orthopaedic Oncology, University of Florida College of Medicine, Gainesville, Florida

E. Shannon Stauffer, M.D.
Professor and Chairman, Department of Orthopaedic Surgery and Rehabilitation, Southern Illinois University School of Medicine, Springfield, Illinois

Kaye E. Wilkins, M.D.
Clinical Associate Professor, Department of Orthopaedics, The University of Texas Health Science Center at San Antonio, San Antonio, Texas

Frank C. Wilson, M.D.
Professor and Chairman, Division of Orthopaedics, University of North Carolina School of Medicine, Chapel Hill, North Carolina

Contents

Volume 1

Volume 2

18   Fractures and Dislocations of the Ankle
Frank C. Wilson   **1665**

19   Fractures and Dislocations of the Foot
James D. Heckman   **1703**

Index

Volume 2

FRACTURES

IN ADULTS

Fractures and Dislocations of the Spine

E. Shannon Stauffer
Herbert Kaufer
Thomas F. Kling

Part I: THE CERVICAL SPINE

E. Shannon Stauffer

HISTORICAL REVIEW

The diagnosis of a broken neck has carried an ominous prognosis since antiquity. When accompanied by spinal cord damage, death all too often is the outcome and, indeed, is anticipated by many surgeons. In the writing of the ancient Egyptians, as recorded in the Edwin Smith papers, traumatic quadriplegia was considered "a condition not to be treated."[14] From Hippocrates' time, the tragic sequela of the unstable fracture has been recognized, and many ingenious frames have been used to prevent or correct the resulting gibbus deformity.[53]

The early history of treatment is bleak. There was no hope of reversing spinal cord paralysis secondary to cord injury. There was no hope of stabilizing the unstable spine or preventing the metabolic complications that soon took the life of the paralytic. Paul of Aegina (625 to 690 A.D.) noted that if the spinal laminae were splintered by a direct blow, these laminae could be removed to decompress the injured spinal cord. Thus the first laminectomy of record. Nearly a millenium later, at the dawn of modern surgery, Ambroise Paré (1510 to 1590) paraphrased the Edwin Smith papers saying, "By symptoms of numbness and palsy of the arms and the urine and excrement coming against their will and knowledge, you may foretell that death is at hand for reason that the spinal marrow is hurt. Having made such a prognostique, you may make an incision and take forth the splinters of the broken vertebra in cases where the neural arch was injured, which are driven in and press the spinal marrow and nerves thereof."[14] The desperation philosophy of Paré remains today in the minds of many surgeons, who believe that the prognosis of recovery of neurologic loss is so poor and the patient so likely to die; therefore, what further harm can be done by laminectomy?

This negativism has no place in modern understanding of patients with fractures and dislocations of the cervical spine, with or without spinal cord injury.

The indications for laminectomy seen by both Paul of Aegina and Paré were direct damage to the spinal cord by spicules of fractured laminae driven into it. This type of injury may have been prevalent a thousand years ago, secondary to sword, mace, and other blunt-instrument trauma. Direct blunt injury fracturing the lamina is a rare cause of spinal cord injury in our modern mechanized age. By far the great majority of spinal cord injuries are due to fracture-dislocation disruption of the osseous and ligamentous components of the spine, secondary to axial load forces on the cervical spine. The exact type of resultant injury depends on the flexed, extended, tilted, or rotated position of the spine at the time of impact (Figs. 12-1 and 12-2). Routine laminectomy, even after 100 years, has yet to be proved beneficial in the management of the closed fracture or dislocation of the cervical spine, except in very rare instances involving incomplete spinal cord syndromes that demonstrate progressive deterioration.[16]

Indiscriminate use of wide laminectomy has led to a worse condition in many patients.[8,16] Among the disastrous effects of the usual wide laminectomy are increasing neurologic loss at the time of surgery and increasing late instability with progressive gibbus formation and late neurologic deterioration. Today, we are able to accurately diagnose the injury with x-rays and to reduce and stabilize the fractured spine, either by closed methods of traction and manipulation or by open surgical procedures. We are able to stabilize the unstable spine with external fixation with the halo body jacket or internal stabilization with the anterior or posterior approach. We are also able to prevent the progressive gibbus deformity from occurring due to late instability. Finally, we are able to prevent the metabolic complications that in years past soon claimed the life of many patients with a fractured spine. Promising new research is on the horizon, which may enable us to prevent the catastrophic, overwhelming permanent loss of sensory and motor power of traumatic quadriplegia.[73,75,121] We are as yet unable to reverse established paralysis in complete spinal cord lesions by any surgical or medical means. Our treatment consists of providing the best conditions for recovery from incomplete cord injury and root injury, preventing further neurologic damage in the unstable area, achieving stable bone and ligament healing in satisfactory position, preventing metabolic complications from being fatal, mobilizing the patient early, and rehabilitating to provide maximum functional independence with the remaining muscle power available to the quadriplegic patient.

ANATOMY

To understand the mechanism of injury and methods of treatment, a review of certain points of anatomy is necessary. The cervical spine consists of the seven vertebrae of the axial skeleton closest to the skull. These vertebrae are unique in structure and function. The first two, C1 and C2, are specifically designed for flexion, extension, and rotary

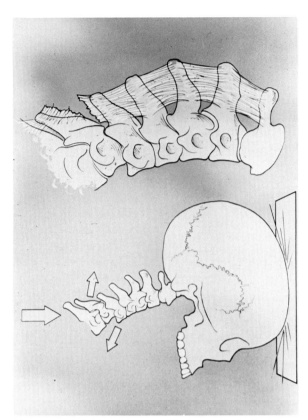

Fig. 12-1. Axial load force with the neck in flexion causing tearing of the posterior ligaments and dislocation.

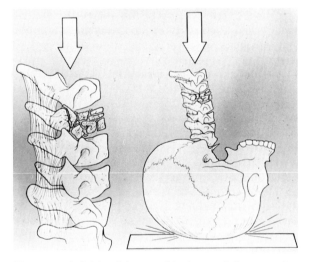

Fig. 12-2. Axial load force with the neck in neutral causing a comminuted burst fracture.

motion. The first cervical vertebra has no central body. The portion of the center of C1 sclerotome develops as the superior projection of the C2 vertebral body, the odontoid. The C1 vertebra is a ring of bone (Fig. 12-3) with large lateral masses that provide the only two weight-bearing articulations between the skull and the vertebral column. The superior articulation of C1 is concave anteroposteriorly to provide flexion and extension of the occipital condyle. The inferior articulations are concave mediolaterally to provide rotation on the C2 facet articulation.

The anterior tubercle of the C1 vertebra is quite thin and held adjacent to the odontoid by the transverse ligament posterior to the odontoid. This limits the amount of rotation and anteroposterior excursion of C1 on C2. The posterior element of C1 is a thin, bony ring, which completes the neural arch. The ring of C1 is quite thin just posterior to the facet joints. This is due to a depression in the superior aspect of the ring to allow the vertebral artery to pass between the ring of C1 and the occiput after it emerges from the foramen transversarium of C1 without danger of being pinched. Fractures of the C1 vertebra frequently occur in this thin area.

The second cervical vertebra (Fig. 12-4) is designed to provide rotation at its superior articulation with C1, and limited flexion, tilt, and rotation at its inferior articulation with C3. The body of C2 is the largest of the cervical vertebrae. The superior articulations are on the lateral masses. They are adjacent to the body. The superior projection of the odontoid is stabilized to the C1 ring by the transverse and alar ligaments. The lateral masses of C2 have an aperture for accepting the transversing vertebral artery. The posterior articulations at the intervertebral facet joints are true arthrodial joints.

The C3 through C7 vertebrae (Fig. 12-5) all have a similar appearance. They are structured to provide limited flexion, extension, tilt, and rotation, as well as stability to support the head. The vertebral bodies have a superior cortical surface concave laterally and convex anteroposteriorly. This configuration allows flexion, extension, and lateral tilt by gliding motion of the facets. The bodies of the vertebrae articulate by the intervertebral disks, which are contained by the annulus fibrosis and the anterior and posterior longitudinal ligaments. The lateral aspect of the vertebral body has a superior projection (the uncinate process). As the disks become degenerative, these projections approximate with the bodies of the next vertebrae above. The result

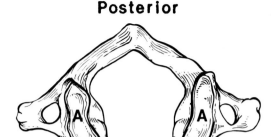

Posterior

Anterior

Fig. 12-3. Superior view of the first cervical vertebra (atlas). The superior articular facets (*A*) provide support and flexion-extension motion of the occiput.

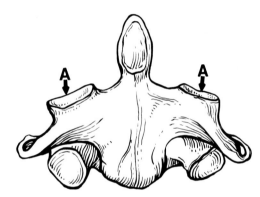

Fig. 12-4. The second cervical vertebra (axis) superior articular facets (*A*) provide rotatory motion of C1 and C2.

is the degenerative joint changes called the joints of Luschka[72] (uncovertebral).

The inferior cortical surface of the vertebral body is convex on an anteroposterior projection, providing an inferior projecting beak on the front of the vertebral body. The vertebral foramen in the lateral masses contains the vertebral artery, which transverses C6 through C1, bypassing the empty foramen in C7. Behind the vertebral artery is a groove in the superior aspect of the lateral mass to allow egress of the nerve roots from the spinal canal. Directly posterior to the nerve root canal lie the facet joints.

The facet joints are in a coronal plane at a 45° angle to the horizontal. The gliding motion allows flexion, extension, and lateral tilt. Due to the 45° incline, lateral tilt is accompanied by rotation, and conversely any rotation of the spine between C3

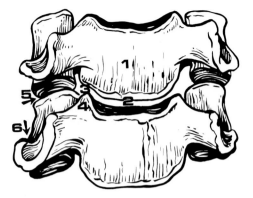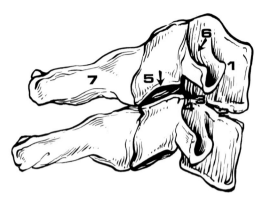

Fig. 12-5. Anterior (*left*) and lateral (*right*) views of the mid-cervical vertebrae (C4 and C5). (*1*) Vertebral body, (*2*) disk, (*3*) uncovertebral joint, (*4*) uncinate process, (*5*) facet joint, (*6*) nerve root canal, (*7*) spinous process.

and C7 must be accompanied by lateral tilt in the same direction. The laminae of the cervical spine progress from a very heavy lamina at C2 with a large spinous process for cervical extensor muscle insertion to the small, thin laminae of C3, C4, and C5 in the hollow of the lordotic curvature. The spinous processes of C3, 4, and 5 are bifid and designed especially for attachment of muscle insertion. The laminae and spinous processes of C6 and C7 become progressively heavier and larger and approach the appearance and size of the thoracic dorsal elements. The disks between the bodies of the vertebrae consist of the nucleus pulposus and the surrounding dense annulus fibrosis. This minimally movable joint limits the motion available at each level of the cervical spine. The posterior interspinous and supraspinous ligaments insert on the spinous processes and limit flexion.

TOPOGRAPHICAL ANATOMY

Certain surface landmarks can be used to identify structures in the cervical spine. Posteriorly, the prominent spinous process of C2 is palpable beneath the prominence of the occiput. The posterior ring of C1 is not palpable. The spinous processes of C3, C4, and C5 are usually not palpable owing to overlying muscle. The spinous process of C7 is palpable at the base of the neck. The most prominent spinous process is the first thoracic vertebra.

Anteriorly, through the open mouth, the tubercle of C1 and the anterior portion of the body of C2 can be palpated through the anesthetized posterior pharyngeal mucosa. At the level of the cricothyroid membrane, the prominent carotid tubercle (Chas-

saignac's tubercle) can be palpated on the lateral mass of the C6 vertebra. This is directly lateral to the C5-C6 disk space.

NEUROANATOMY

The spinal cord and its meningeal covering is a caudal continuation of the brain, extending from the foramen magnum through the spinal canal to the upper lumbar area. In the cervical area, the spinal cord and its dural contents occupy approximately 50% of the spinal canal. At each intervertebral disk space, the ventral and dorsal rootlets join to form a nerve root that exits the spinal canal through the neural foramen. There are seven cervical vertebrae and eight cervical nerve roots on each side. The C1 nerve root exits in the canal between the occiput and the C1 vertebral ring. C2 exits between the C1 and C2 vertebrae, and so on, down to the C8 nerve root, which exits between the C7 and T1 vertebrae. The cervical nerve roots proceed almost directly laterally from the spinal cord and exit through the foramen above the body for which they are named. For example, the C6 nerve root exits through the foramen between the C5 and C6 vertebral bodies.

The spinal cord and intraspinous portions of the nerve roots are contained in the tough dura mater. Between the cord and the dura in the subarachnoid space is a fluid shock absorber that completely surrounds the spinal cord. This cerebrospinal fluid circulates from the subarachnoid space in the brain to communicate with the subarachnoid space around the spinal cord. The spinal cord is also cushioned by the epidural fat in the space between the dura and the neural arch of the vertebra. The spinal cord in the cervical area consists of a large, central gray matter, containing motor cells, which innervate the muscles of the neck and upper extremity. The central gray matter also consists of the internuncial fibers, which transmit impulses from the sensory dorsal roots to reflex synapses and the long tracts to the thalamus. The more peripheral white matter contains the long tracts for carrying sensation and motor impulses to and from the trunk and lower extremities. Therefore the lower motor neuron fibers to the arms emanate in the cervical portion of the cord and the upper motor neuron fibers to the lower extremities traverse the cervical portion of the cord.

DIAGNOSIS

HISTORY

Fracture or dislocation of the cervical spine should be suspected in all cases in which a patient complains of pain in the neck area following an injury. A careful history is recorded regarding the nature of the accident. Was the patient thrown from the vehicle? Did he strike his head? At the time of the accident, were there any signs of paralysis? If quadriplegic paralysis was noted, were there any clues that the patient was able to move his hands or feet for a short time following the injury and then lost that ability? This is very important for diagnosis and prognosis of the neurologic injury. Was the patient knocked unconscious at the time of the accident? Are there any previous episodes of cervical spine disease, such as previous injuries, previous paralysis, or weakness, spondylosis, or history of seizures? Has he had any previous x-ray examination? The most common causes of injuries to the neck are: motor vehicle collisions, diving into shallow water, and gunshot wounds to the neck.

PHYSICAL SIGNS

The physical examination is, of course, the most important aspect of the entire work-up. Inability to move the neck or pain on motion requires careful immobilization of the head and neck until adequate physical and x-ray examinations are performed. Of course, any obvious weakness, numbness, or paralysis of the arms, hands, or feet warrants a presumptive diagnosis of cervical spinal cord injury until proved otherwise.

GENERAL PHYSICAL EXAMINATION

The patient should be lying flat on his back with the neck immobilized with sandbags or cervical halter traction.

Observation. Lacerations or abrasions on the scalp, face, neck, or shoulder are clues that help to verify the mechanism of injury and draw attention to the neck, cervical spinal cord, shoulder, and brachial plexus. All voluntary motion of the arms, hands, legs, feet, fingers, and toes should be observed and recorded. Sustained penile erection indicates severe cervical spinal cord injury. Observe the attitude of the patient's head and whether he has limitation of his spontaneous, voluntary movements from side to side. Ask the patient to move his head gently from side to side; observe whether the motions are equal; and question the patient about pain on motion.

Palpation. Without moving the patient, the examiner palpates for areas of tenderness over the head or the back of the neck, as well as for any step-off or local hematoma secondary to ligament disruption or dislocation.

Survey of Vital Signs in the Quadriplegic Patient. General examination of vital signs demonstrates low blood pressure secondary to spinal cord shock with decreased vascular tone associated with absence of reflexes below the level of the cord injury. Quadriplegia provides a temporary generalized sympathectomy effect on the trunk and lower extremities. Blood pressure is frequently 90/50 in the traumatic quadriplegic. This should not be confused with hemorrhagic shock due to blood loss, as the specific treatment is quite different. Blood loss needs to be replaced, whereas excessive fluids will not raise the blood pressure in neurogenic shock and may cause serious fluid overload to the kidneys, lungs, and heart. Pulse rate is usually not elevated and is within normal limits (70 to 90 beats a minute).

Associated Injuries. Associated injuries (*e.g.,* rib fracture, intra-abdominal injury, and fractures of extremity long bones) should be sought as well. If a paralysis with loss of sensation is present, all bones and joints of the paralyzed extremities must be carefully palpated for swelling, crepitus, instability, or other signs of fracture or ligament injury. If there is any suspicion of intra-abdominal bleeding, a peritoneal lavage is carried out.

NEUROLOGIC EXAMINATION

Sensory Examination. The neurologic sensory examination should be done with a pinwheel and very light pressure. Identify sharp and dull discrimination of the face (cranial nerve 5); then examine the cervical nerves serially. Documentation of intact sharp-dull sensation of cervical nerves (Fig. 12-6) is performed by examining the back of the scalp (C2), over the anterior aspect of the neck (C3), laterally and inferiorly over the clavicles down to the second rib interspace (C4), over the lateral deltoid area of the arm (C5), over the radial aspect of the forearm, thumb, index, and middle finger (C6), over the ring and small fingers (C7) and the ulnar border of the hand and forearm (C8), the medial side of the upper arm (T1), and the anterior chest wall above the nipple line (T2). At the level at which hypesthesia is encountered, work backward with the pinwheel from anesthetic area to sensitive area and draw the sensation line on the skin with a marker. This indicates the level of cord lesion or the area of involved root loss if the cord is intact and the root has been injured. When the level of sensation is established, the sensory dermatomes of the rest of the trunk and lower extremities must be examined carefully for signs of sacral sparing in the apparent complete cord injury. If any sharp-dull discrimination sensation is found distal to the injury, the injury is classified as an incomplete lesion, and the patient may recover.

Of primary significance is the examination of the sacrally innervated skin: the perianal, anal, scrotal, or labial skin, and the plantar surface of the toes. Perianal sensation may be the only sign to indicate an incomplete lesion, and it is frequently missed owing to the failure of the examiner to search for it. It is easily accomplished with the patient on his back, by gently abducting the legs and examining the perineal skin with the pinwheel or pin. Sharp-dull discrimination indicates preservation of lateral spinal cord columns, and recovery of muscle function is quite likely.

Sharp-dull discrimination testing is followed by a similar examination for the presence or absence of light touch (anterior column), deep pressure, vibration and position sense (posterior column).

Motor Examination. Following the sensory examination, with marking of the sensory level on the skin and documentation in the medical chart (Fig. 12-7), the presumptive determination of a root or cord lesion is made. Also, the diagnosis of a complete or incomplete syndrome is documented. A careful motor function test is then carried out by

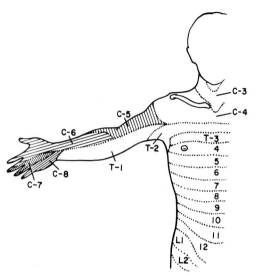

Fig. 12-6. Sensory dermatomes of cervical nerves, including all overlap, document lowest functioning nerve root in a traumatic complete quadriplegia.

sequential nerve root levels. Survival of people with cervical spine lesions and quadriplegia proximal to the C4 level is rare, owing to the sudden paralysis of all respiratory muscles, which causes death at the scene of the accident. If the patient is found breathing with diaphragm motion, he will also have an active trapezius and sternocleidomastoid contraction control. This documents C4-nerve-root-level function. Voluntary activity of the deltoid and biceps documents intactness of the C5 level. Voluntary contraction of the extensor carpi radialis longus or -brevis documents function of the C6 level. Voluntary contraction of the pronator teres or flexor carpi radialis or triceps or finger extensors documents function at the C7 level. Voluntary flexor digitorum sublimi or profundi documents function at the C8 level, and intrinsic function documents T1.

Following documentation of the lowermost functioning muscles and thus, establishment of a functional level, the rest of the body must be examined for any evidence of voluntary muscle function indicating corticospinal tract sparing. Specifically, the toe flexors, toe extensors, and rectal sphincter must be tested. As in the case of sacral sensory sparing, sacral motor sparing (consisting of voluntary control of the sphincter or toe flexor muscles) may be the only evidence of an incomplete motor quadriplegia.

When examining for toe flexor control, do not touch the toes, but ask the patient to move the toes of either foot. Do not be confused by the "flexor withdrawal reflex," which is commonly present after complete cervical cord transection. The patient must be able voluntarily to contract the toes of one foot, individually and independently, before it can be classified as true voluntary control.

Rectal Examination. The rectal examination verifies the impressions gained by the sensory and motor examinations and is the most important part of the evaluation. This clinches the diagnosis of complete lesion.

Rectal Sensation. Inability of the patient to feel the pin prick on the anal skin or the gloved finger in the rectum confirms a complete sensory lesion.

Rectal Motor Examination. If the sphincter does not contract voluntarily about the gloved finger and there are no other signs of voluntary motor power below the upper extremities, complete motor paralysis is confirmed.

Reflexes. A squeeze on the glans penis, tap on the clitoris, or a tug on the urethral catheter causing a stimulation of the trigone of the bladder causes a reflex contraction of the anal sphincter about the gloved finger—the bulbocavernosus reflex. If this reflex is absent and the sphincter is flaccid, the patient may still be in spinal shock (absence of all spinal reflex activity below the cord lesion). If spinal shock is present, a permanent complete lesion cannot be diagnosed with certainty. However, complete spinal shock usually lasts less than 24 hours, and the bulbocavernosus reflex will return within that time. If there is no voluntary sensory or voluntary motor sparing and the bulbocavernosus reflex is present, the patient is out of spinal shock, and the complete cord lesion is confirmed. With this confirmation one may expect no functional recovery of muscles distal to the upper extremity in the future regardless of treatment. With very few exceptions, the bulbocavernosus will have returned within 24 hours, and a diagnosis can be confirmed and subsequent treatment can be based on this predictable prognosis of a complete lesion.

SPINAL FLUID DYNAMICS

Beyond the physical examination, there are no physical procedures that correlate consistently with the diagnosis and prognosis. The relevance of spinal fluid dynamics in the diagnosis and prognosis has not been confirmed. According to Comarr and

Kaufman,[28] as would be expected, the more severe injuries, those with complete spinal cord lesions, demonstrate a higher percentage of block of spinal fluid manometrics. A greater percentage of incomplete lesions, those with less spinal cord damage, have a higher percentage of normal cerebrospinal fluid manometrics. It does not necessarily follow, however, that patients with complete spinal cord injury always have a complete block or that patients with the incomplete syndrome always have normal manometrics.

The Queckenstedt test is performed with the patient on his side. A spinal puncture with an 18-gauge spinal needle is performed at the low lumbar area. Cerebrospinal fluid pressure is measured with the manometer. The pulse should rise and fall with the heartbeat. Respiration also causes a general pressure level to rise and fall. A Valsalva maneuver should cause a pressure rise secondary to an increase in abdominal venous pressure. The purpose of the Queckenstedt test is to determine the flow of spinal fluid in the subarachnoid space at the area of the cord injury. If there is a free flow of fluid past the injured area, increased pressure in the cranium is reflected by increased rise in the manometer with a lumbar puncture. Therefore if pressure is placed over both jugular veins (by manual squeezing of the neck), the patient should feel his head "get full" as the arterial input to the brain continues, and the venous outflow is obstructed. A normal Queckenstedt test is then recorded by a rapid rise in cerebrospinal fluid pressure in the lumbar manometer. If the pressure does not rise with jugular compression, this indicates a block of cerebrospinal fluid dynamics between the cerebral ventricles and the lumbar puncture site. This test, along with the cerebrospinal fluid protein, which also rises with a chronic complete or partial block, is an important diagnostic test for tumor, abscess, or herniated disk. It is of questionable value in the evaluation of the fracture or dislocation of the cervical spine, and worthless in the complete lesion, but it should be part of the work-up of the patient with an incomplete lesion who fails to make progressive recovery. A negative test, as evidenced by a free rise and fall of fluid with jugular compression, indicates that there is no extrinsic pressure on the spinal cord. A false-negative test may occur if a partial block is present but there is enough fluid circulation around the block to transmit fluid at the same rate that it passes through the needle used for lumbar puncture. The positive test (*i.e.,* no rise and fall with jugular compression), that follows acute fractures and dislocations indicates a

A

Spine Fracture Study

Surgeon's Name _____

Patient _____ Age _____ Gender _____ Occupation _____ MR# _____

Injury level _____ Incomplete   Quad.   Frankel _____ Cause _____

Complete   Para.

Date of injury _____ Date of adm. _____ Date of surgery _____ Date disch. home _____

Other Injuries or Complications _____

Treatment _____
(Days bedrest, type brace or cast)   (Surgery, instruments used, levels fused, graft)

Comments _____

TRAUMA MOTOR INDEX

2yr	1yr	6mo	3mo	1mo	1wk	init.	Date LEFT	Muscles		Date RIGHT	init.	1wk	1mo	3mo	6mo	1yr	2yr
							0/+	Diaphragm	C-4	0/+							
							0-5	BICEPS	C-5	0-5							
							0-5	WRIST EXT	C-6	0-5							
							0-5	TRICEPS	C-7	0-5							
							0-5	FLEX PROF	C-8	0-5							
							0-5	INTRINSIC	T-1	0-5							
							0/+	Intercost	2-9	0/+							
							0/+	Abdominal	10-12	0/+							
							0-5	ILIOPSOAS	L-2	0-5							
							0-5	QUADRICEP	L-3	0-5							
							0-5	TIB ANTER	L-4	0-5							
							0-5	EX HALLIC	L-5	0-5							
							0-5	GASTROC	S-1	0-5							
							0/+	Blad sph	S-2	0/+							
							0/+	Anal sph	S-3	0/+							
							0/+	B-C reflex		0/+							
							50	TOTAL		50							

BILATERAL TOTAL   100

FRANKEL CLASS (A-E)

INCOMPLETE SYNDROME
(ant, cent, B.S., mx
conus, cauda)

ADAPTED FROM AUSTIN

Sacral Sparing

	CERV.	Jefferson	Hangman	Odontoid	Facet Dx	Body Comp	Burst	Other
	T–L	Comp	Slice	Burst (ant body)	Burst (post body)	Chance	Dislocation	Other

X-Ray Evaluation

Date							
X-Ray Evaluation	init.	1wk	1mo	3mo	6mo	1yr	2yr
KYPHOS ANGLE-degree							
ANTERIOR DISP-mm							
LAT SCOLIOSIS ANGLE-degree							
LAT DISPLACEMENT-mm							
MYELOGRAM % BLOCK							
TOMOGRAMS % BLOCK							
C.A.T. SCAN % BLOCK							

N. I. A.

Sensation: ☐ ▨ ▧

NORMAL ☐

IMPAIRED ▨

ABSENT ▧

Rectal Tone ⊞ 0

B.C. Reflex ⊞ 0

Summary (treatment, results, complications)

3 mo   6 mo   1 yr

Total hosp. days _____

B

Date	TRAUMA MOTOR INDEX		Date
LEFT	MUSCLES		RIGHT
0+	Diaphragm	C-4	0+
0-5	Biceps	C-5	0-5
0-5	Wrist ext	C-6	0-5
0-5	Triceps	C-7	0-5
0-5	Flex Prof	C-8	0-5
0-5	Intrinsic	T-1	0-5
0+	Intercost	2-9	0+
0+	Abdominal	10-12	0+
0-5	Iliopsoas	L-2	0-5
0-5	Quadricep	L-3	0-5
0-5	Tib anter	L-4	0-5
0-5	Ex hallic	L-5	0-5
0-5	Gastroc	S-1	0-5
0+	Blad sph	S-2	0+
0+	Anal sph	S-3	0+
0+	B-C reflex		0+
50	TOTAL		50
	BILATERAL TOTAL		100

◀ **Fig. 12-7.** (*A*) Flow sheet to document fracture type, initial neurologic function, and progress during continued care. (Southern Illinois University; Stauffer, E. S.: Cervical Spine Trauma, Section 24. *In* Orthopaedic Knowledge Update I: Home Study Syllabus, pp. 199–208. Chicago, A.A.O.S., 1984.) (*B*) Trauma motor index used by the author.

block of cerebrospinal fluid dynamics. It is due to the intrinsic cord edema and has no significance in deciding the course of treatment.

RADIOGRAPHIC SIGNS

When a neck injury is suspected, a lateral film of the cervical spine should be taken without moving the patient from the original emergency room stretcher. The entire spine from the occiput to C7 must be visualized. Fracture dislocations of C6 on C7 and C7 on T1 are often missed in the original x-ray because of inadequate exposure. The lower part of the cervical spine is often obscured by a shadow of the shoulders elevated by muscle spasm (Fig. 12-8A). It may be necessary to stabilize the head with a canvas traction halter and hold down on the arms gently to visualize the entire C7 vertebra (Fig. 12-8B). If no fracture or dislocation is seen at the fifth or the sixth cervical vertebra but the seventh vertebra cannot be seen, intravenous diazepam may be given to relax the shoulder elevators completely. The level of the neurologic injury as determined by clinical examination provides a clue to the level where a fracture or dislocation may be suspected. The swimmer's view in which one arm is abducted 180°, the other arm pulled down along the side, and the beam directed at a 60-° oblique angle, may be necessary to reveal the C7-T1 articulation (Fig. 12-9). This view is often difficult to evaluate, owing to overlap of the bony structures, such as the humeri, scapulae, and ribs. If an adequate lateral x-ray reveals no fracture or dislocation, then a complete x-ray examination, including anteroposterior, open-mouth, and oblique projections is performed. In supervising the exposure of the oblique films, it is important to rotate the patient's entire body 45° in order to get a complete oblique view of the entire cervical spine. It is not satisfactory simply to rotate the supine patient's head 45° to one side. If all views are negative for fracture, dislocation, or subluxation, and there is still some concern about a possible ligamentous injury, a "stretch test"[117] should be done by applying a 20 pound distraction force by way of cervical halter traction in the supine position. Any widening of the posterior interspinous processes on the lateral x-ray will identify occult ligamentous ruptures and potential instability. The retropharyngeal soft tissue space must be evaluated for swelling as evidence of an occult fracture if the bony architecture appears normal. The prevertebral fascia anterior to the C2–3 vertebrae is very thin and should not exceed 3 mm anterior to the body of C3. Anterior to C4 and C5 the soft tissue shadow includes the perilaryngeal muscles and esophagus. The thickness varies from 8 mm to 10 mm and is less reliable as a measurement of soft tissue swelling. Laminagraphy may be necessary to detect lateral mass, pedicle, and laminar fractures, if there are significant clinical findings but essentially negative x-rays (Fig. 12-10). These latter studies are rarely performed as emergency measures, since undisplaced fractures of the posterior neural ring do not modify early treatment.

MYELOGRAPHY

Myelography may be of value in incomplete spinal cord injuries, to pinpoint an area of segmental

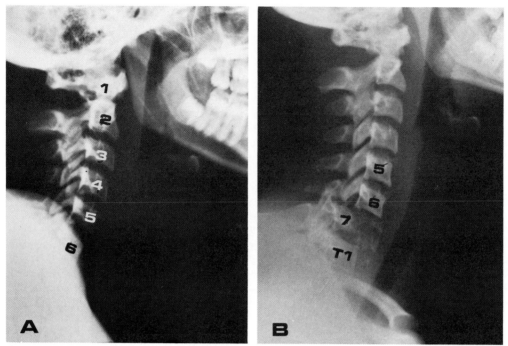

Fig. 12-8. Lateral x-ray of the cervical spine. (*A*) Initial emergency room x-ray is "negative for fracture." C7 was not visualized. (*B*) Traction on the shoulders reveals a fracture-dislocation of C6 and C7.

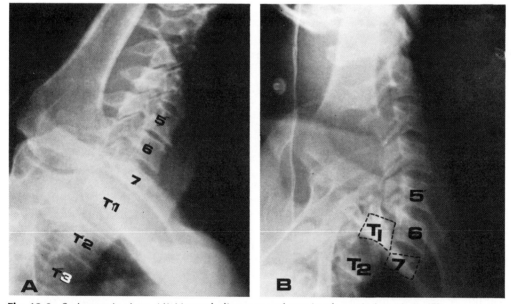

Fig. 12-9. Swimmer's view. (*A*) Normal alignment of cervicothoracic junction. (*B*) Severe fracture-dislocation of C7 on T1.

spinal cord compression. However, this is not recommended during the period soon after injury because of (1) the manipulation necessary for an adequate myelographic examination with the patient prone in the head-down position, (2) the possibility of further irritation to the already compromised neural tissue with swelling and vascular engorgement at the injury site, and (3) the possible reaction of Pantopaque with the mixture of cerebrospinal fluid and blood, which may irritate the injured tissue even more. Myelographic findings in the period early after injury will not modify the treatment. If the patient has an incomplete lesion, he has a good chance of making further recovery. This cannot be improved by early surgery, and the patient may be made worse. If the patient has a complete neurologic lesion secondary to closed fracture or dislocation, he most likely will demonstrate a block on the myelogram, owing to intrinsic edema of the cord, and surgical decompression by laminectomy on the basis of a myelographic block is not correlated with neurologic improvement in complete injuries. Frequently, repeat x-rays made after laminectomy show that the myelographic intradural block persists. Water soluble agents (metrizamide) may be injected in small amounts through a lateral C1–2 dural puncture with the patient in the tilted, head up position. This technique will demonstrate those patients with a block of the subarachnoid space. The value of this finding in the early postinjury state as an aid in management has yet to be determined. Therefore, the myelogram should be delayed and reserved for those patients with incomplete lesions who fail to show progressive improvement, and in whom there is an indication that the lesion may be due to persistent neural pressure not manifest on the ordinary x-rays. The injuries amenable to surgery that are most likely to be found by myelographic examination are retropulsion of the disk or comminuted fragments of the vertebral body injuring or putting pressure on the spinal cord, producing an anterior cord syndrome.

COMPUTED TOMOGRAPHY

Increasing experience with computed tomography (CT scan) indicates that this diagnostic technique opens new vistas in the accurate diagnosis of "hidden" fractures and specific localization of bone fragments. The earlier scanners demonstrated the value of axial tomograms in identifying fractures of the upper and lower cervical spine, areas which are difficult to visualize on standard x-rays. Suspicion of fractures of the ring of C1 (Fig. 12-11)

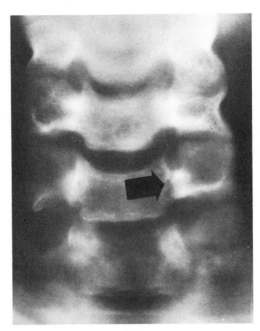

Fig. 12-10. An anteroposterior laminagram shows a fracture of the lateral mass of cervical vertebra (arrow).

and C7 are quickly identified without the multiple radiation exposure and patient manipulation required by conventional tomography. The newer scanners have the capability to reconstruct images in the sagittal and coronal planes (Fig. 12-12).

These three-dimensional images—axial, sagittal, and coronal—provide a much clearer description of fractures and encroachment on the spinal canal. The effect that more accurate diagnosis provided by the CT scan will have on treatment has yet to be determined. There is no statistical correlation as yet relating the degree of fracture and canal compromise with neurologic deficit or recovery. Only further documentation of data will provide rational treatment guidelines.

LABORATORY EXAMINATION

Laboratory work-up consists of hemoglobin and hematocrit, baseline total protein, blood urea nitrogen, (BUN), and blood gas determinations, and measurement of the vital capacity and of urine output. Before any surgical procedures are initiated, the hemoglobin should be at least 10 grams%; hematocrit, at least 30%; blood gases, within normal range; and vital capacity, 1000 ml of air. If the vital capacity is less than 1000 ml of air or 20% of predicted normal, a preoperative tracheostomy may be indicated. In any case, the tracheostomy set should be in readiness after the operation, and mechanical respirator assist—tank iron lung or Bennett volume respirator—must be available.

THE SPINAL CORD LESION

The early examination is of primary importance to accurately determine if there is an injury to the spinal cord or to the cervical nerve roots. If the patient has no cord or root injury, it is unlikely that he will have progressive neurologic loss if the spine is maintained in a reduced position by skeletal traction. If he has neurologic injury complicating his spinal fracture or dislocation, it is of primary importance to document whether this is a complete transverse cord lesion or an incomplete lesion. Accurate diagnosis can be made within the first 24 to 48 hours in almost all cases. This gives the surgeon a realistic prognosis and permits a more intelligent choice from among the available treatment regimens.

CLASSIFICATION OF NEUROLOGIC INJURY

ROOT INJURY

A nerve root may be damaged at the neural foramen by a fractured or dislocated facet or a fracture of the uncinate process of the vertebral body. These are essentially peripheral nerve lesions and are expected to recover, at least partially. Root avulsion rarely occurs, except in a classic brachial plexus injury with a distraction force on the shoulder.

INCOMPLETE SPINAL CORD LESIONS

Partial loss of cord function may be determined by the presence, although altered, of voluntary muscle power or sensory preservation distal to the cord injury. The pattern of preserved sensory and motor function differentiates the various incomplete cord lesion syndromes. Each syndrome has a specific prognosis for the probability of recovery. In general, any sparing distal to the injury constitutes an incomplete lesion, and recovery, varying from minimal to full, is possible. The greater the motor and sensory sparing, and the more rapid the recovery during the first several days, the better the prognosis for full recovery.

Brown-Séquard Syndrome. An injury limited to either lateral half of the spinal cord produces ipsilateral muscle paralysis and contralateral hypesthesia to pain and temperature. This syn-

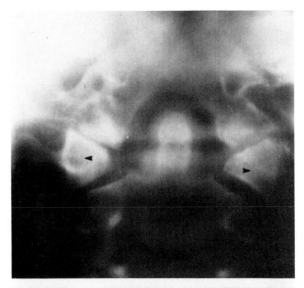
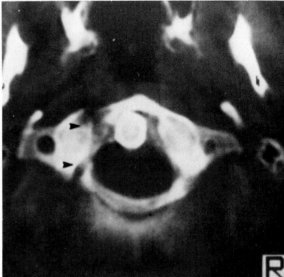

Fig. 12-11. (*Top*) An open-mouth tomogram of a fracture of the ring of C1. (*Bottom*) CT scan of a fracture of the ring of C1 (anterior and posterior to facet at *arrows*).

drome has a good prognosis for partial recovery, and most patients regain bowel and bladder control and the ability to walk.[17]

Central Cord Syndrome.[87,90] Central cord syndrome is the most common incomplete cord syndrome. It is usually associated with an extension injury to an osteoarthritic spine in a middle-aged person. X-ray examination may reveal no fracture or dislocation; however, the patient demonstrates

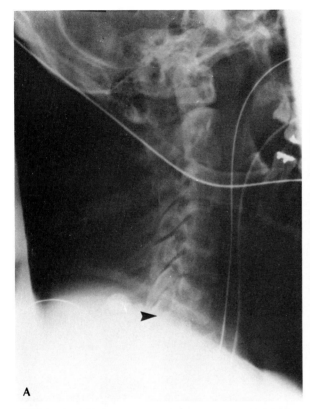

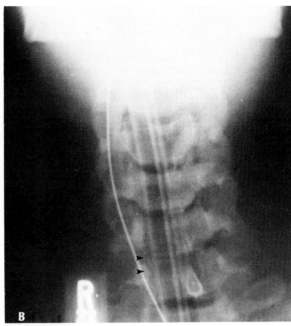

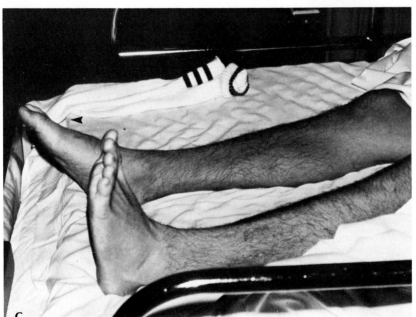

Fig. 12-12. (*A*) Lateral x-ray of the cervical spine of a 20-year-old man with multi-system trauma. C7 not adequately visualized. (*B*) Anteroposterior x-ray reveals indistinct C6-7 disk space and mild compression of the right side of the right body of C7. (*C*) Physical examination demonstrated paralysis of the right leg and numbness of the left leg.

(*Continues on p. 1000.*)

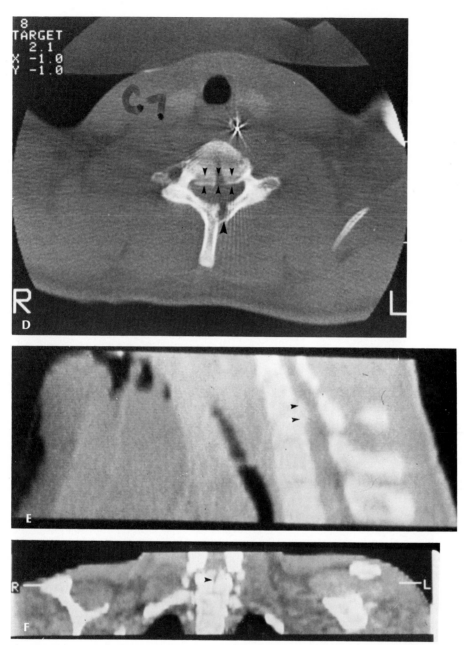

Fig. 12-12. (*Continued*). (*D*) CT scan reveals fracture of the body of C7 with bone fragments impinging into the spinal canal and a fracture of the left lamina. (*E*) A sagittal reconstruction demonstrating fragments of the C7 vertebral body impinging into the spinal canal. (*F*) Coronal reconstruction demonstrating sagittal split fracture in the body of C7.

almost complete, flaccid quadriplegia. Impact damage to the central gray matter, produced by the pincer effect of the osteophytes anteriorly and the infolded ligamentum flavum posteriorly, produces severe flaccid lower-motor-neuron paralysis of the fingers, hands, and arms. Damage to the central portion of the corticospinal and spinothalamic long tracts in the white matter produces upper-motor-neuron spastic paralysis of the trunk and lower extremities. The sacral tracts are positioned on the periphery of the cord and are usually spared from injury. The patient demonstrates gross quadriplegia, but careful examination reveals sacral sparing manifested by perianal sharp-dull sensation and an early return of sphincter control. Prognosis for this syndrome is fair. The patient can be expected to have progressive return of motor and sensory power to the lower extremities and trunk, but he will have poor recovery of hand function, owing to irreversible central gray matter destruction. He is likely to regain bowel and bladder control and to walk with a spastic gait, but paralysis of the hands will probably be permanent.[17]

Anterior Cord Syndrome.[85] The anterior cord syndrome is manifested by complete motor paralysis and sensory anesthesia, with the exception of dorsal column sparing providing deep pressure and proprioception as the only retained sensation of the trunk and lower extremities. Prognosis is good if recovery is evident and progressive during the first 24 hours. After 24 hours have elapsed and no sign of sacral pain or temperature sensation sparing is present, prognosis for further functional recovery is poor.[17] Most patients with permanent complete motor paralysis and only vague deep-pressure sensory sparing fall in this incomplete syndrome.

Posterior Cord Syndrome.[17] The posterior cord syndrome consists of the loss of deep pressure, deep pain, and proprioceptive sensation only. The patient has full voluntary motor power and pain and temperature sensation throughout the body. Therefore he will walk with a slapping gait similar to that of tabes dorsalis. This incomplete spinal cord injury syndrome is rare.

COMPLETE SPINAL CORD INJURY

Complete anesthesia and complete absense of voluntary motor power distal to the level of injury on the first examination suggests complete spinal cord injury. Prior to making a diagnosis of a complete spinal cord injury, sacral sparing must be examined for specifically. If the patient has immediate paralysis and no signs of sacral sparing, he is then considered to have a complete cord lesion.[52] As soon as spinal shock is over (as heralded by the return of the bulbocavernosus reflex), a definite diagnosis of complete lesion can be made. The bulbocavernosus reflex is elicited while the gloved finger is still in the rectum (see p. 993). This reflex is mediated through the spinal cord reflex centers

and indicates that reflex activity has returned to the distal spinal cord segment and that spinal shock is over. This bulbocavernosus reflex usually recovers within the first 24 hours and precedes the return of deep tendon reflexes by many weeks. With a positive bulbocavernosus reflex and complete paralysis and anesthesia, a definite prognosis can be made: the patient will not recover functional motor power to the lower extremities. There may be progressive return of nerve root function in the cervical nerve roots, with recovery of wrist and hand muscle function, but this must not be confused with regeneration or recovery of spinal cord function. Early determination of a diagnosis and prognosis allows one to make a more intelligent choice of treatment techniques suited to individual patients and their families.

CLASSIFICATION OF FRACTURES AND DISLOCATIONS

At the present time, patients who suffer sudden, traumatic disruption of the cervical spine are frequently diagnosed in a general category as "fracture-dislocation" of the cervical spine without attempt to further refine the diagnosis into a workable anatomical description on which treatment—specifically reduction and immobilization—can be based. The fracture or dislocation must be recognized and described accurately. An accurate anatomical diagnosis will provide an understanding of the mechansim of injury and allow an intelligent decision on the type of treatment.

DISLOCATIONS

Since each intervertebral articulation consists of at least three joints—the disk and the paired posterior facet joints—each joint must be described accurately. The same definitions for normal flexion and extension (Fig. 12-13 *left*), excursion, subluxation, dislocation, and associated fracture are used in the cervical spinal joints as in other joints of the body. In subluxation the joint surfaces are in an abnormal position but articular surfaces are still in partial contact. If the articular surfaces are completely out of normal position and the articular surfaces do not touch, the joint is dislocated. With a complete unilateral facet dislocation, the interbody disk joint shows subluxation of approximately 25% (Fig. 12-13 *center*). With complete bilateral facet dislocation (the so-called locked facets) the interbody subluxation must be displaced anteriorly at least 50% (Fig. 12-13 *right*).

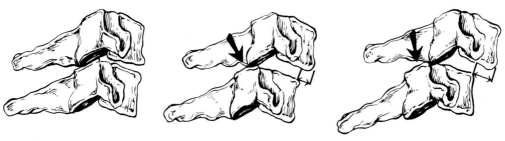

Fig. 12-13. Diagram of an intervertebral dislocation. (*Left*) Normal flexion range of motion of the facet and disk space. (*Center*) The vertebral body displaced 25% forward indicates fracture or subluxation of one facet (*arrow*). (*Right*) Fifty percent forward displacement of the interbody disk indicates bilateral facet dislocation (*arrow*).

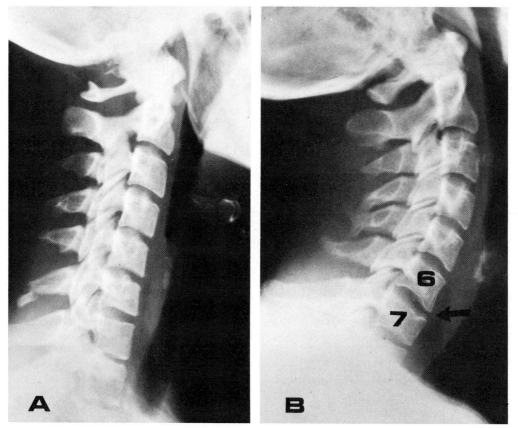

Fig. 12-14. Stable fractures not associated with neurologic damage. (*A*) Clay shoveler's fracture (spinous process C6). (*B*) Compression fracture of the cervical body (C7) with no ligamentous disruption.

FRACTURES

Fractures may occur as isolated bony injuries or a part of a complex injury associated with the dislocation. Fractures of the articular facet result from rotary flexion forces. If the rotation component is greater than the flexion component, the facet joint will fracture rather than dislocate. Fractures through the pedicles (floating pedicles) are grossly unstable and are often misdiagnosed as bilateral facet dislocation. Fractures of the lamina without associated joint disruption are usually secondary to hyperextension forces. Fractures of the spinous processes are a result of strenuous muscle contraction causing avulsion of the insertion of the muscle in the spinous process (clay shoveler's fracture)[51] or direct blows (Fig. 12-14A).

MECHANISMS OF INJURY

Excessive forces applied to the neck in any direction may disrupt the bony and ligamentous complex of the cervical spine and cause fracture, dislocation, or both (Table 12-1).

FORWARD FLEXION FORCES WITHOUT AXIAL LOAD OR ROTATION

The flexion excursion of the facet joints and the disks is limited by the posterior ligamentous complex and the anterior and posterior longitudinal ligaments. The energy of a pure flexion force is expended on a compression fracture of the cancellous cervical vertebral body (Fig. 12-14B). Since there is no tearing of the ligamentous complex posteriorly and no dislocation of the joints, these are stable fractures. Rarely are these injuries associated with neurologic loss or late instability.

FLEXION-ROTATION FORCES

The addition of rotation to flexion places unequal stresses on the posterior interspinous ligaments and facet joint capsules. This causes a disruption of the facet capsule, allowing a unilateral facet dislocation. If the unilateral facet is locked in a dislocated position, the intervertebral disk joint is also subluxated anteriorly. If the rotation-flexion forces are carried farther, the opposite facet joint capsule will also be torn, and the facet will dislocate, producing a bilateral locked facet dislocation. This causes further anterior subluxation of the intervertebral disk joint. Dislocations of the facets may be accompanied by fracture of the facet, fractures of the lamina, or fractures of the vertebral body. The anterior longitudinal ligament is usually the only ligamentous structure that remains intact. This, with the anterior annulus fibrosus and the longus coli muscles, is the main stabilizing structure of the cervical spine at the dislocated level. Neurologic injury associated with dislocation is quite variable. The patient may have no neurologic loss; there may be minimal isolated motor and sensory loss from nerve root compression at the neural foramen of the injured level; or the patient may suffer an incomplete or complete quadriplegia secondary to spinal cord damage. These patients with neurologic

Table 12–1. Classification of Fractures and Dislocations of the Cervical Spine

Lesion	Mechanism of Injury
Fracture of arch of C1	Axial load on top of the head

Dislocation of C1 on C2
  a. Anterior
  b. With fracture of odontoid
  c. Posterior
  d. Rotatory
	
	Flexion of head with laceration of transverse ligament
	Flexion of head
	Sudden extension of head
	Rotation of head

Fracture of pedicles of C2 with subluxation of body of C2 on C3 (Hangman's fracture)	Axial load with head extended

Dislocation of midcervical spine:
  Facet joints dislocated
  Disk joint in forward subluxation
	Flexion rotation of neck

Compression fracture of vertebral body without comminution	Flexion
Comminuted vertebral body fracture with posterior subluxation	Axial load, such as diving into shallow pool and hitting the head on the bottom
Lateral mass fractures	Lateral flexion
Lamina fracture with avulsion of anterior superior chip of vertebral body	Extension
Spinous process fracture	Avulsion by spine extensor and scapular elevator muscles (clay shoveler's)
Gunshot wound	Gunshot wound

loss associated with dislocations tend to have a higher incidence of incomplete spinal cord injuries than those patients with comminuted vertebral body fractures secondary to axial load compression. The latter have a higher incidence of complete spinal cord injuries.

AXIAL LOAD COMPRESSION

Axial load forces, as from striking the head on a solid object in a diving position, exert tremendous longitudinal compressive force on the midcervical spine, regardless of whether the head is flexed or extended. This force results in an explosion comminuted fracture of the vertebral body, usually C5, being caught between the pincer motion of C4 and C6 (Fig. 12-15). The C5 vertebral body is disrupted, the anterior one fourth displaced anteriorly (resembling a teardrop,[88] and the posterior three fourths is split sagittally and displaced posterolaterally in both directions. The posterior inferior margin of the vertebral body is frequently fractured and pushed into the spinal canal. The inferior disk between C5 and C6 is also frequently expelled posteriorly into the spinal canal. The dorsal elements are usually not fractured but are displaced posteriorly with such force that the facet capsules are disrupted and there is posterior subluxation of the vertebral body into the spinal canal. The posterior ligamentous complex of interspinous ligaments usually remains intact and provides the only remaining stability at the injured area. Severe neurologic loss, consisting of complete spinal cord damage resulting in quadriplegia or complete motor paralysis secondary to anterior spinal cord syndrome with only deep pressure sensation remaining intact, is quite frequent with this injury.

EXTENSION FORCES

The dorsal elements of the cervical spine are well designed to limit hyperextension motion, and the facet joints lock in extension as the laminae and spinous processes approach each other. The tough anterior and posterior longitudinal ligaments prevent distraction of the vertebral bodies anteriorly. Forces exceeding the normal extension range of the facet joint cause the joints to lock in extension, and as the laminae and spinous processes abut, the force is expended either in fracture of the dorsal element by compression or in avulsion of the superior margin of the vertebral body by the anterior longitudinal ligament and annulus fibrosus, or both[21] (Fig. 12-16). The spinal cord may be

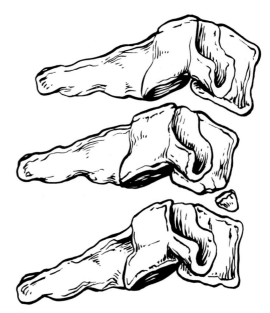

Fig. 12-15. Diagram of a comminuted fracture of a vertebral body secondary to axial load forces causing comminution of the body and separation of the spinous processes.

caught between the lamina and ligamentum flavum posteriorly and the bulge of the disk anteriorly and suffer severe damage, especially if there is an element of osteophytosis or hypertrophic bone spurring of the vertebral bodies (Fig. 12-17). The patient may suffer a complete spinal cord injury or a severe central cord syndrome injury without remarkable fracture or dislocation being evident on x-rays.

LATERAL FLEXION

Compression or distraction forces caused by lateral flexion may cause lateral mass fractures of the pedicles, vertebral foramina, or facet joints (Fig. 12-18). These rarely cause injury to the spinal cord but may cause a Brown-Séquard syndrome or nerve root entrapment syndromes. These are stable injuries.

GUNSHOT WOUNDS

Low-velocity missile wounds are increasing in frequency as a cause of cervical spine and spinal cord injuries. High-velocity missiles, such as military weapons and large game hunting rifles, usually cause complete spinal cord injuries when striking the mid-cervical spine due to the impact of the

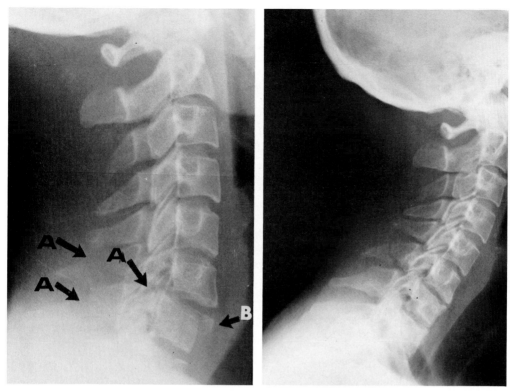

Fig. 12-16. X-ray of an extension injury. (*Left*) Fracture of the dorsal elements and avulsion of the anterosuperior portion of the vertebral body. (*Right*) The fracture is reduced and healed in the flexed position.

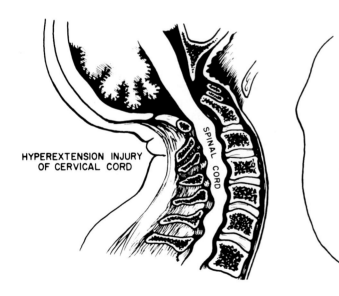

HYPEREXTENSION INJURY
OF CERVICAL CORD

SPINAL CORD

Fig. 12-17. Hyperextension injury to the cervical spinal cord without fracture or dislocation.

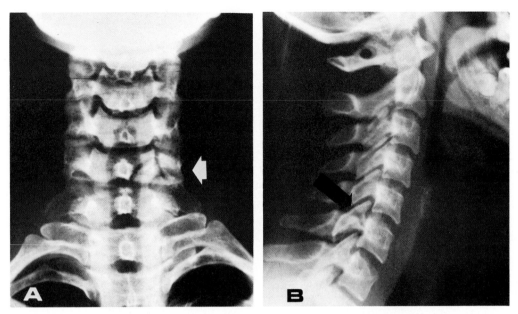

Fig. 12-18. (*A*) An anteroposterior x-ray of a fracture of the lateral mass of C6. (*B*) Lateral view demonstrates the fracture extending through the pedicle and the facet.

bullet against the bony element. These frequently cause gross instability, due to destruction of vertebral elements (Fig. 12-19). Missiles with low muzzle velocity, such as many hand guns and .22-caliber rifles, strike the osseous elements with less impact and produce a higher percentage of incomplete spinal cord injuries. Low-velocity missiles rarely cause sufficient destruction to produce instability. (For a more complete discussion of high- and low-velocity missile wounds, see Chapter 1).

TREATMENT—GENERAL CONSIDERATIONS

REDUCTION WITH TRACTION

As with the treatment of any fracture or dislocation, it is equally imperative in the cervical spine to realign the bony fragments and reduce the joint dislocation. Urgency of reduction is dictated by neurologic loss. If the patient has no neurologic loss, there is no urgency. The patient may be maintained in skeletal traction with cranial tongs. If the dislocation is not easily reducible with longitudinal traction, he may be taken to the operating room for an open reduction on an elective basis. If the dislocation is reduced easily, he may be maintained in skeletal traction for as long as 12 weeks to allow spontaneous bony union. If the patient has a neurologic loss, the spine should be reduced as quickly as practical. The most widely accepted method of treatment is skeletal traction with cranial tongs, as first described by Crutchfield in 1933 (Fig. 12-20).[30] These have been modified and improved on by Vinke,[112] Barton,[11] and others. The Gardner-Wells tongs (Fig. 12-21) are currently used in many spinal trauma centers due to the simplicity of design and ease of application. No special tools are required. The tongs are inserted under local anesthesia with no drilling or cutting of bone necessary. The cranial halo (Fig. 12-22) developed by Perry and Nickel[68] offers the best method of multi-plane control of the head and cervical spine to produce traction and allow relaxation of the muscle spasm. Traction may be required over several hours to dislodge dislocated facets and realign the spine. It requires 10 pounds of traction to overcome the weight of the head and approximately 5 pounds of traction for each interspace, with a maximum of 35 to 40 pounds for dislocations of the C6-C7 interspace. Additional weight above this level will not be more effective in overcoming muscle spasm, and if the spine does not reduce with this amount of weight combined with muscle relaxant medication and sedation, the problem is most likely a mechanical bony block. Further weight does not improve the reduction, but traction from a different direction is indicated, usually increasing flexion with slight rotation, to unlock the locked

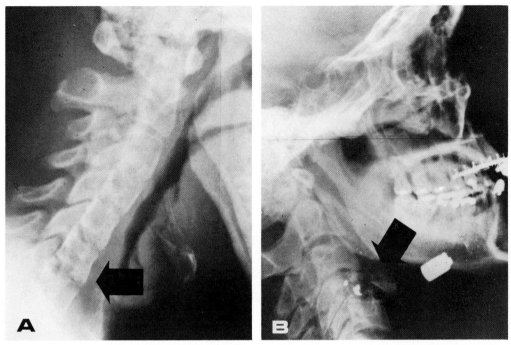

Fig. 12-19. Gunshot wounds of the cervical spine. (*A*) Low-velocity missile through the disk of C6 and C7. The spine is stable. (*B*) A high-velocity missile caused complete destruction of the C4 body. The spine is unstable.

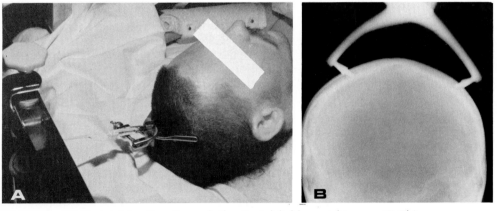

Fig. 12-20. (*A*) Skeletal traction through the Crutchfield cranial tongs. (*B*) This x-ray shows placement of the Crutchfield tongs through the outer table of the skull.

facet. Careful manual reduction of the dislocation under x-ray control may be attempted with either analgesic sedation or general anesthesia. Several series using this method of reduction in patients with and without neurologic deficit have been reported with success in spinal injury centers in South Africa and Australia.[22] Manual manipulation has not been widely used in the United States.

METHODS OF TREATMENT

In choosing a method of treatment for the fracture or dislocation of the cervical spine, it is imperative to understand the natural healing process of the various injuries and to be able to make a prognosis as to the success rate of open or closed treatment in each of the injuries. If the spine can be realigned

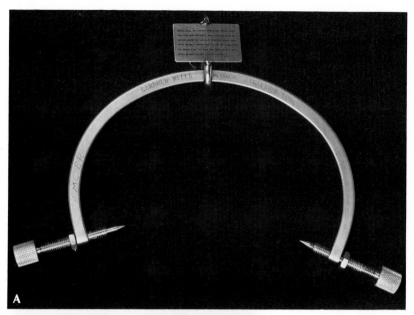

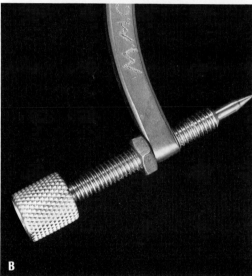

Fig. 12-21. The Gardner-Wells tongs for cervical traction. (*A*) Full view. (*B*) Close-up.

by closed skeletal traction, three courses of subsequent treatment are open. The first is continuous traction in the supine position until the bone and ligament injuries have healed; the second is immobilization of the spine in the reduced position with a halo and plaster or plastic body jacket (Fig. 12-23); and the third is operative stabilization.

In order to select the appropriate method of treatment, it is important to understand the type and degree of neurologic injury and its significance. Incomplete spinal cord injuries may make marked recovery, in spite of failure to gain anatomical

realignment. Immediate complete spinal cord injuries that remain complete for 24 hours cannot be expected to show neurologic recovery, regardless of the adequacy of alignment of the spine. Therefore, if the dislocation cannot be reduced with traction in the first several hours and if neurologic loss persists, the patient should be prepared for open reduction. In the operating room under preoperative sedation, gentle manual traction with slight flexion and rotation manipulation under image-intensifier, x-ray control may achieve closed reduction of the dislocated facets. If this is not successful, a general anesthetic is administered. Lateral x-rays should always be taken following endotracheal intubation. The muscle-relaxing effects of the succinylcholine or curare may have achieved reduction during intubation. If this fails, the patient should have an open reduction with internal fixation with 20-gauge wire and fusion with segmental bone grafting. (Techniques are discussed under treatment considerations of specific dislocations.)

FACTORS THAT INFLUENCE THE CHOICE OF TREATMENT

In dealing with patients with severe spinal cord injuries associated with paralysis, one must be aware of the metabolic complications that occur in a recumbent paralyzed patient. A person with no neurologic loss can tolerate the 8 to 12 weeks of bed rest necessary to allow healing of fractures and dislocations without serious difficulty. However,

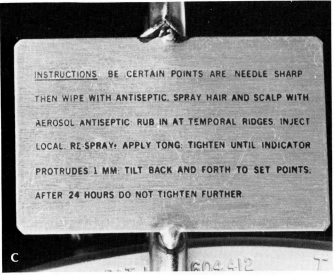

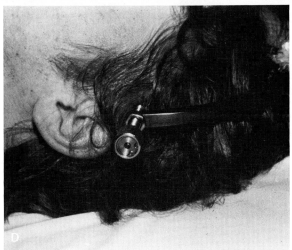

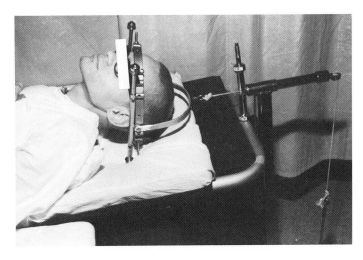

Fig. 12-21. (*Continued*). (*C*) Instructions with tongs. (*D*) Tongs in place.

Fig. 12-22. A patient in halo-cranial traction.

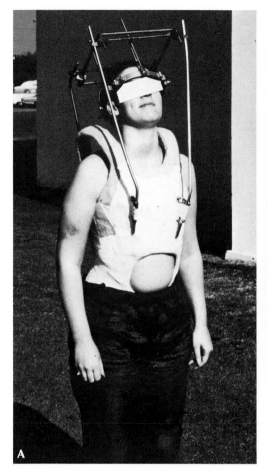

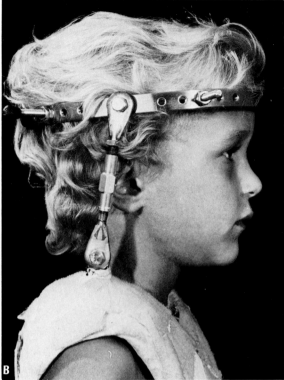

Fig. 12-23. (A) Ambulatory treatment of reduced dislocation in a halo-body jacket. (B) Low-profile halo attached to the plaster body jacket with adjustable turnbuckles. (C) The plastic body jacket used with the halo in quadriplegic patients.

the patient with a severe spinal cord injury tolerates the recumbent position poorly. In general, the greater the neurologic deficit, the greater the effort should be to move the patient into the upright position early. During the first 2 weeks, the mortality of patients with complete cervical spinal cord injury is quite high. The mortality is not due to fracture of the neck or injury to the spinal cord *per se*, but to the metabolic complications of the respiratory, cardiovascular, and gastrointestinal tracts.

Complications Associated with Early Care of the Quadriplegic

1. Respiratory insufficiency with atelectasis and pneumonia.
2. Pressure ulceration of the skin over bony prominences.
3. Gastrointestinal bleeding from hemorrhagic gastritis.
4. Urinary retention with bladder distention and calculus formation.
5. Joint contractural deformity.
6. Skeletal osteoporosis.
7. Psychologic withdrawal.

Gastrointestinal Complications

Following the initial evaluation and determination of the vertebral and spinal cord injury, a nasogastric tube should be passed into the stomach. This is prophylaxis against gastrointestinal ileus that is likely to occur and against regurgitation and aspiration of gastric content. Gastric bleeding from diffuse hemorrhagic gastritis is a common early complication. This occurs as early as the second day after injury and is usually self-limiting when treated with gastric ice water lavage, Maalox, and parasympathomimetic drugs. The cause is unknown. It is usually too early to be ascribed to steroids, which may be used in treatment of the spinal cord injury. Occasionally, however, a gastric ulcer occurs, which perforates into the peritoneal cavity. Any indication of gastric mucosa hemor-

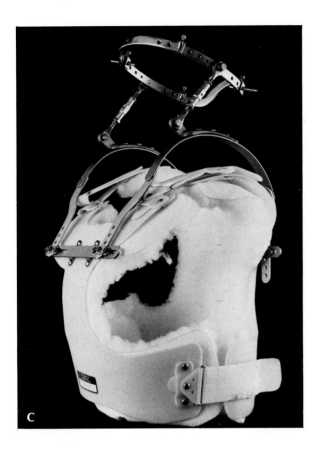

C

rhage, as evidenced through the Levine tube, must be treated vigorously and early.

Urologic Complications

A urethral catheter is placed in the bladder for the first 24 hours to monitor urinary output. The catheter should be taped up on the abdomen to prevent a penoscrotal fistula. During the first 24 to 48 hours the patient has low blood pressure and demonstrates a generalized sympathectomy-type picture. The urine output is usually low, and therefore intravenous and oral fluids should be restricted during the first 24 to 48 hours. When urinary diuresis occurs at 36 to 48 hours, oral and intravenous fluids can be administered accordingly. The paralyzed bladder should then be treated with intermittent catheterization.

Skin Care

It is imperative to institute a turning program early. Due to the anesthesia of the skin, the patient must be turned in bed or on the special turning frame every 2 hours, around the clock, without fail. It is usually more convenient and safer to treat the patient in traction in a regular bed, turning from the supine to the side-lying position every 2 hours. Special turning frames have two disadvantages. First, they allow the patient to lie in only two positions, flat on his back or flat on his abdomen, thereby increasing the possibility of pressure ulceration of the skin over the bony prominences, especially the sacrum. The second disadvantage is the safety factor; the patient may have his position of traction changed during turning on a frame, or even fall out of the frame. Circle frame beds are probably specifically contraindicated for fracture dislocations of the spine, because the mechanics of traction change markedly with each rotation through the standing position. Owing to their restricted vital capacity (see below), patients with acute traumatic quadriplegia tolerate the prone position poorly. The vital capacity is further decreased, and the patient often has a feeling of suffocation.

Pulmonary Complications

It must be remembered that the acute quadriplegic patient is breathing only with his diaphragm. His intercostal and abdominal muscles are paralyzed, and his vital capacity is approximately 25% of the predicted normal. He cannot forcibly exhale; he cannot cough to clear his pulmonary secretions; and he cannot sigh. Therefore his secretions accumulate in the lungs; atelectasis develops, and then pneumonia. This frequently causes the patient's early demise.

A vigorous program of preventive pulmonary therapy must be instituted immediately. Intermittent positive-pressure respiration several times daily to maintain full expansion of the lungs with proper humidification is essential. Mechanical respirator assistance must be available and should be used at the first signs of respiratory fatigue. Tracheostomy must be used if secretions cannot be cleared by nasal or oral suctioning. Occasionally bronchoscopy with a fiberoptic bronchoscope is necessary to remove retained inspissated bronchial plugs and allow adequate ventilation.

During the first week, patients also frequently develop pulmonary edema and congestive right heart failure secondary to excessive intravenous fluid overload. During the first several days—when the sympathetic tone of the vascular tree is diminished—the blood pressure is low, the intravascular space expands, and the urinary output is low. Several days after the injury, when the sympathetic tone returns, the excess fluid is forced out of the cardiovascular tree, and pulmonary edema with right-sided cardiac failure may occur. Silent thrombophlebitis with pulmonary embolism may confuse and confound the already existing pulmonary complications. It is important to remember that the usual signs of pain with thrombophlebitis are lacking in the anesthetic extremity.

These early, serious metabolic complications, together with long-range problems of protracted bed rest (such as osteoporosis of the skeleton with hypercalciuria, muscle atrophy of the remaining actively functioning muscles, and negative nitrogen balance) plus pressure ulceration of the skin from inadequate positioning and turning, all influence the choice of the early method of treatment. Will the patient benefit most by skeletal traction in bed, or early mobilization by halo and plaster cast, or surgical stabilization?

HALO BODY CASTS

Rigid immobilization of the cervical spine may be afforded by a halo attached to a plaster or plastic body jacket cast.[68] Longitudinal traction with a cranial halo affords control and positioning in cervical flexion, extension, tilt, and rotation, as well as longitudinal distraction forces.

APPLICATION OF THE HALO

The application of a cranial halo requires two people and is best done by three. The patient is placed supine on a treatment table, operating room table, or stretcher. One person supports the head, just over the end of the stretcher. The cervical spine and occiput are supported by sandbags on the end of the stretcher. The patient's head is then prepared by washing the hair in the area where the halo is to be applied with a surgical prep solution, such as pHisoHex or Betadine. It is usually not necessary to cut the hair. The halo pins are applied through the wet hair into the skin. (A small area in the immediate area of pin insertion may be cut and shaved, if desired.) The second person holds the sterilized halo in the correct position around the skull. The halo must be held low, just above the eyebrows, almost touching the tops of the ears to insure that the halo will encircle the skull below the area of greatest diameter. That is necessary to prevent superior slippage during traction. The third person then injects local Xylocaine (1%) into the four areas selected for pin insertion. If possible, all four halo pins should be placed in the hairline, to prevent the dimpled scar that results from the halo pin in the forehead skin. The third person screws the four sterilized halo pins through the appropriate holes in the halo and into the anesthetized skin

(no stab wounds are necessary). All four pins are placed through the skin and alternately tightened to maintain the halo equidistant from the skull circumferentially. The pins are advanced through the scalp into the outer table of the cranium by tightening opposite pins simultaneously (left front and right rear, and right front and left rear), with a torque screwdriver, to 5 pounds resistance. Lock nuts are then placed over the pins to secure their position in the halo. The sharp points of the specifically designed halo pins permit fixation into the outer table of the skull, and the broad shoulders of the halo pins prevents penetration of the pin through the outer table.

When the halo is secure, traction up to 50 to 60 pounds may be applied without difficulty. The halo pins should be tightened to 5 pounds torque screwdriver resistance daily for 1 week. The patient in halo traction should be examined daily for asymmetry of extraocular movement and the presence of nystagmus. An early sign of excessive distraction forces is abducens nerve palsy causing nystagmus and unequal extraocular motion.

APPLICATION OF THE BODY JACKET

Either immediately following application of the halo or after a period of longitudinal traction and recumbency, the body jacket can be attached to secure rigid fixation of the cervical spine and allow ambulation or wheelchair mobilization in the upright position. A plaster body jacket is applied in a conventional manner. It may be applied on a special frame (such as Goldthwaite irons) or on a conventional fracture table. The body jacket is carefully molded over the iliac crests, to distribute pressure on the soft tissue rather than the bony iliac crest. It extends to the pubis and over the iliac crests halfway to the greater trochanters. This provides adequate fixation to the pelvis and allows flexion of the hips for sitting. The halo is then attached to the body cast with the outrigger overhead attachment. The halo and the outrigger, originally developed to control paralytic scoliosis, is being modified. The current design, as described by Anderson and Bradford,[6] consists of a single lateral upright attachment from the shoulder of the cast to the halo. (Fig. 12-23B illustrates a low profile halo with adjustable turnbuckle).

PLASTIC HALO VESTS

There are several varieties of plastic body jackets for halo stabilization (Fig. 12-23C). These are particularly useful for the management of quadriplegic patients and elderly patients. The light weight decreases the encumbrance to mobility, the design allows frequent auscultation and x-ray examination of the chest, and the jacket may be adjustable to changing contours of the patient's body. The plastic jacket has a significant disadvantage in dealing with young, neurologically normal patients on an outpatient basis. They can adjust, loosen, and even disengage the straps, buckles, and screws and may compromise the deduction and stability obtained with the halo jacket. Therefore, I prefer the plaster jacket halo (Fig. 12-23B) for younger patients and the plastic jacket for older patients with upper cervical fractures, such as odontoid fractures, and patients with severe quadriplegia.

After the patient is in the upright position, x-rays are then obtained to insure adequate positioning of the reduction. The halo may be adjusted, if necessary, to improve the position of the reduction of the fracture or dislocation.

CERVICAL ORTHOSES

A cervical orthosis is used to protect the stability of the healing spine following stable soft tissue injuries and postoperative fusions. Johnson and associates[57] found that conventional orthoses limit cervical motion approximately 45%, while the halo limits normal cervical motion approximately 75%. There is little difference in the effectiveness of the currently used orthoses. We currently use the plastizote-kydex cervical immobilizer for postoperative patients (Fig. 12-24 *left*) and a similar cervical thoracic immobilizer (Fig. 12-24 *right*) if the patient has a tracheostomy or requires lower cervical stabilization.

TREATMENT OF SPECIFIC DISLOCATIONS

OCCIPUT-C1 DISLOCATION

The mechanism of injury of the occiput-C1 dislocation is a violent, twisting force of the head that tears all the ligamentous connections between the occiput and the C1 vertebra.[38] These injuries are very unstable and nearly always fatal, due to high spinal cord injury. If the patient survives, traction is contraindicated, due to the gross instability. Rigid immobilization is imperative. The use of a halo

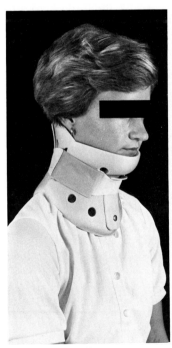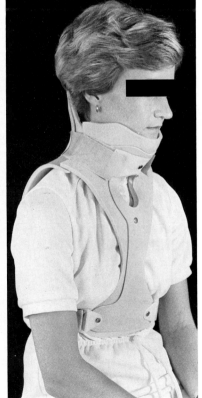

Fig. 12-24. (*Left*) Postoperative plastizote-kydex cervical orthosis. (*Right*) Cervicothoracic orthosis with tracheostomy aperture.

attached to a plaster body jacket is preferred. If the reduction is not exactly accurate, the head can be positioned into more flexion or extension by adjusting the halo attachment. With the patient in the halo body jacket apparatus, exposure for pos-

terior surgery is facilitated. Patients with this injury should be treated with early posterior bone graft stabilization from the occiput to C2 and then maintained in the halo body jacket until fusion is mature (Fig. 12-25).

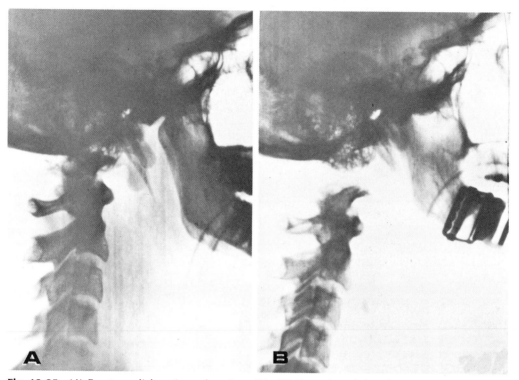

Fig. 12-25. (*A*) Fracture-dislocation of occiput-C1. (*B*) Gross instability demonstrated by traction.

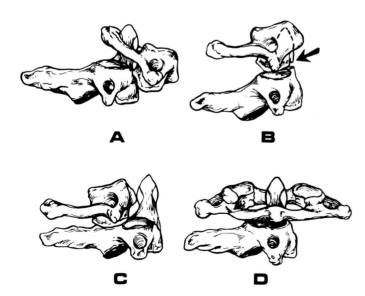

Fig. 12-26. Diagram of C1-C2 dislocation. (*A*) Forward dislocation of C1 with rupture of the transverse ligament (usually fatal). (*B*) Forward subluxation of C1 with fracture of the odontoid. (*C*) Posterior dislocation of C1, slipping posteriorly over the odontoid. (*D*) Rotary subluxation.

C1-C2 DISLOCATION

C1 may be dislocated from the articular facets of C2 by one of four mechanisms (Fig. 12-26).

ANTERIOR DISLOCATION WITH RUPTURE OF THE TRANSVERSE LIGAMENT

The atlas dens interval should not exceed 3 or 4 mm. A distance of 5 mm or more indicates an accompanying decrease of the space available for the spinal cord between the dens and the posterior ring of C1. If the cord space is less than 10 mm, the patients frequently demonstrate pathologic long tract signs of increased reflexes, weakness, paresthesias, and may develop progressive quadriparesis.

Anterior dislocation with rupture of the transverse ligament is more likely to be fatal, due to the intact odontoid causing a high injury to the spinal cord. If the patient survives, this condition should be treated by immobilization with the head in extension, with an early elective posterior C1-C2 fusion. Healing of the ligaments cannot be relied on to provide adequate stability, and the chronically unstable C1-C2 dislocation is potentially lethal.

ANTERIOR DISLOCATION WITH FRACTURE THROUGH THE BASE OF THE ODONTOID

Dislocation associated with fracture of the odontoid is less likely to be associated with severe neurologic damage and may be treated by immobilization with the odontoid in the reduced position until union occurs. Reducing the odontoid fracture with halo traction in extension followed by application of the halo cast is preferred. However, application of a Minerva cast is adequate to maintain position. If, however, there appears to be chronic instability 12 to 16 weeks after injury as manifested by displacement on gentle active flexion and extension lateral x-rays or by increasing sclerosis about the margins, posterior fusion should be advised to prevent persistent instability due to the ununited odontoid fracture (see p. 1022).

POSTERIOR C1-C2 DISLOCATION

The mechanism of this injury is sudden extension of the head, usually by a blow on the submental area. The anterior portion of the atlas is lifted over the top of the odontoid and settles posterior to the odontoid. This rare lesion is treated by longitudinal traction, followed by gentle extension and flexion manipulation under x-ray control, to effect reduction of the ring of the C1 over the top of the odontoid into its normal position. Since the transverse ligament is not disrupted in this injury, it can be treated by immobilization in a halo body jacket or Minerva plaster jacket for 6 to 8 weeks. This should be protected by a brace for an additional 8 weeks, and 12 to 16 weeks after injury flexion-extension x-rays should be taken. If there is abnormal motion or pain at the site, a C1-C2 fusion should be performed.

ROTARY SUBLUXATION

Rotary subluxation of C1 on C2 occurs when excessive rotary force on the head causes one inferior facet of C1 to slip anterior to the superior facet of C2 and become fixed in this position. The patient has marked limitation of motion toward the subluxated side and pain when attempting to rotate the head beyond neutral.

X-ray findings demonstrate asymmetry of the odontoid-lateral mass of C1 space on the open-mouth anteroposterior view. This asymmetry remains consistent as one attempts to rotate the head from one side to the other. (Figs. 12-27 and 12-28)

Lateral x-rays may demonstrate the C1 inferior facet positioned anterior to the C2 superior facet in severe cases (Fig. 12-29). Treatment consists of skull traction, preferably with a halo, to allow longitudinal forces to be placed at the C1-2 interspace. When the fixed rotary subluxation has reduced, immobilization in the halo in the reduced

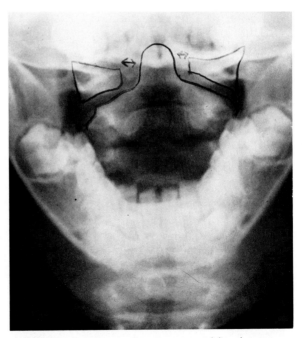

Fig. 12-27. Open-mouth tomogram of fixed rotary subluxation of C1-C2.

position for 6 weeks is followed by removal of the body jacket and application of a cervical orthosis to allow institution of motion. If the fixed rotary subluxation recurs, a posterior C1-2 fusion should be performed.[42,124]

DISLOCATIONS FROM C3 TO C7

Dislocations of the facet and intervertebral disk areas in this area are due to flexion-rotation forces with rupture of the posterior ligament complex. These forces are generated by the kinetic energy of the patient's body flying through space and coming to a sudden stop as the head strikes a stationary object, such as an automobile windshield, with the head in flexion. The momentum of the body causes a buckling deformity to occur at the mid-cervical spine. The ligaments rupture and the facets and disks dislocate.

RADIOGRAPHIC SIGNS

Due to superimposition of the facet joints on the lateral x-ray, dislocation of a single facet may go unrecognized. The clue to a facet disruption, either fracture or dislocation, is the alignment of the posterior aspect of the vertebral bodies. While each vertebral body may be expected normally to move forward 2 mm to 3 mm with respect to the inferior adjacent vertebral body on a flexion film, any forward displacement of a single vertebral body on the one below in a neutral position x-ray indicates a fracture or dislocation of one posterior facet joint. Oblique films are imperative to visualize the facet

joints. Unilateral facet dislocation or fracture allows forward vertebral body subluxation up to 25% of the anteroposterior dimension of the disk space (Fig. 12-30). Bilateral dislocated locked facets produce at least 50% forward subluxation of the intervertebral disk space. A true lateral projection x-ray readily demonstrates bilateral locked facets (Fig. 12-31). On the anteroposterior projection, facet dislocation may be suggested by the single-level widening of the interspinous processes, a slight deviation in the alignment of the spinous processes, and a widening of the intervertebral disk space at the joint of Luschka (Fig. 12-32).

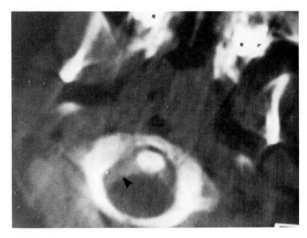

Fig. 12-28. A CT scan of rotary lateral subluxation of C1-C2.

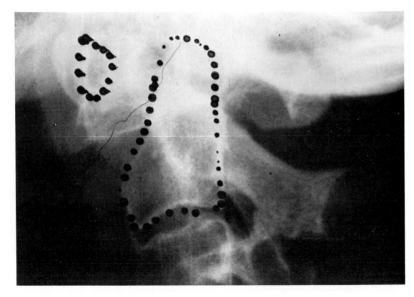

Fig. 12-29. A lateral x-ray of rotary dislocation of C1-C2.

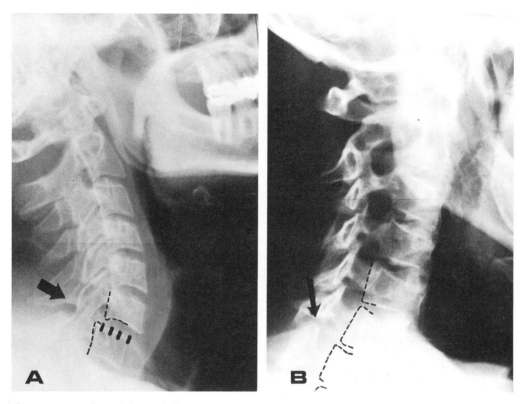

Fig. 12-30. Unilateral facet dislocation. (*A*) Lateral view shows forward subluxation of vertebral bodies, 25%. (*B*) Oblique view shows dislocation of facet, C6 and C7.

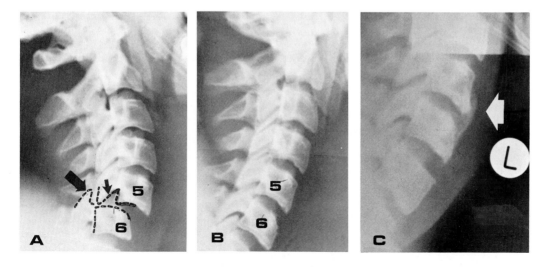

Fig. 12-31. Dislocation with bilateral locked facets. (*A*) Anterior subluxation with 50% vertebral body displacement. (*B*) Reduced and held in extension. (*C*) Healed with anterior spontaneous ankylosis.

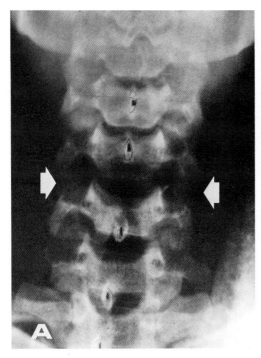 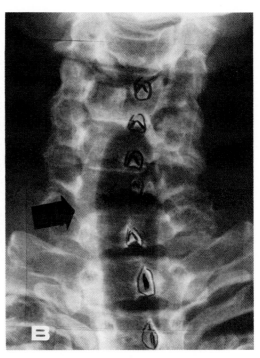

Fig. 12-32. Anteroposterior x-rays of dislocations. (*A*) Bilateral dislocation; increased width between spinous processes and open disk space. (*B*) Unilateral dislocation; malalignment of spinous processes and opening of joint of Luschka unilaterally.

TREATMENT

The goals of treatment of a dislocation are (1) to reduce the dislocation to provide a pain-free, straight, stable spine, with a normal range of motion, and (2) to relieve any constricting pressure from the spinal cord as soon as possible if there is cord or nerve root damage paralysis.

Treatment consists of application of skull tongs or a cranial halo with immediate traction of 20 pounds. If reduction is not easily accomplished by 35 or 40 pounds of longitudinal traction within several hours, increasing the weight above this level rarely achieves reduction, and the lateral x-rays must be reviewed carefully for a mechanical block to reduction. This is usually due to locked facet joint dislocation, which cannot be distracted due to the remaining competent anterior longitudinal ligament. Under x-ray control, this mechanical block may be overcome with traction in the longitudinal direction, gradually moving the head up into flexion and then back into extension. If this is successful in reducing the facet dislocation, the patient can then be placed in a body jacket with the neck held in extension for a total of 12 weeks

to allow adequate healing of the posterior ligament complex. This in itself, however, cannot be relied on for adequate stability; subligamentous ossification usually occurs beneath the anterior longitudinal ligament and provides a spontaneous interbody ankylosis (Fig. 12-33). Failure of spontaneous ankylosis at 12 to 16 weeks is an indication for a posterior spinous process wiring and fusion (Fig. 12-34).

If, however, reduction of a dislocation is not successful within several hours, the patient should be taken to the operating room, and under preoperative muscle-relaxing sedation while the patient is awake, gentle flexion and extension manipulation of the head by the halo may be performed. If this is successful, the patient may be placed in a plaster body jacket to which the halo is fixed, thereby holding the head and neck in the reduced position. If this does not succeed in accomplishing adequate reduction of the facet joints, then open reduction and internal fixation with wire, and bone graft fusion, should be performed. This internal fixation eliminates the need for the halo body jacket, and the postoperative immobilization then

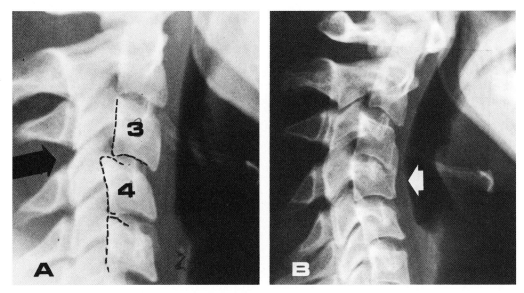

Fig. 12-33. (*A*) Unilateral facet dislocation, C3 on C4. (*B*) Healed with anterior spontaneous ankylosis.

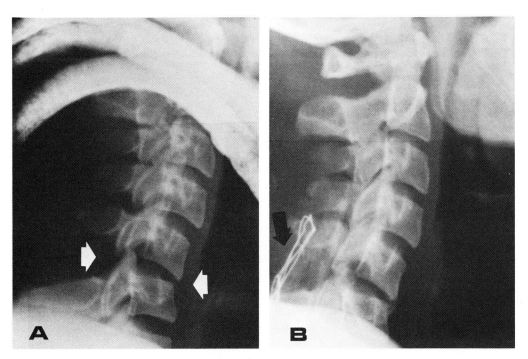

Fig. 12-34. Dislocation treated in traction. (*A*) Three months after injury insufficient anterior ankylosis and posterior ligamentous healing for stability. (*B*) Six weeks after posterior fusion *in situ* there was a meager attempt at anterior spontaneous ankylosis.

consists of a cervical brace, full time for 6 weeks, and then in daytime only for an additional 6 weeks (for a total of 12 weeks). During this time the patient may be ambulatory is he is neurologically normal; if paralyzed, he is started on a rehabilitation program. The posterior approach to the spinous process, lamina, and facet joints is preferred over the anterior cervical approach to the vertebral body, because it allows direct visualization of the dislocated facet joints and disrupted posterior structures. A more accurate reduction of the dislocated facets and rigid fixation in the reduced position can be performed by the posterior approach (Fig. 12-35). The anterior approach requires removal of the anterior longitudinal ligament, the annulus, and the intervertebral disk, which increases the instability of the cervical spine. It is more difficult to disengage the locked facets by manipulation of the vertebral bodies, and once reduced, the facets cannot be held firmly in the reduced position. Dislocations treated by anterior cancellous bone graft frequently displace and allow the deformity to recur (Fig. 12-36).[25,102] Posterior reduction and fusion allow the anterior ligament to remain in place as a checkrein, which, together with rigid fixation of the laminae and spinous processes with wire posteriorly, provides stability for early mobilization of the patient.

Reduction may also be accomplished by skeletal traction through cranial tongs (Crutchfield, Vinke, Gardner-Wells). An alternative method of treatment following reduction by traction is 8 to 12 weeks of continuous maintenance traction by the skeletal tongs in the recumbent position. The patient may be treated in bed or on a turning frame until spontaneous anterior interbody ankylosis occurs or until 3 months have elapsed and ligamentous stability is demonstrated by flexion and extension x-rays. The advantages of this treatment are that it does not require the use of the halo or body cast or a surgical procedure. The disadvantages are the prolonged hospitalization required and the complications of bed rest. The neurologically normal patient may develop muscle atrophy, joint stiffness, and disturbing psychological symptoms after confinement to one room for a prolonged period of time. In the paralyzed patient there is the added danger of pressure sores, pulmonary atelectasis, and urinary tract calculi. Continuous traction can be used if there is a contraindication to the halo jacket technique or open reduction; however, most patients will not choose traction as the method of treatment. The incidence of chronic instability

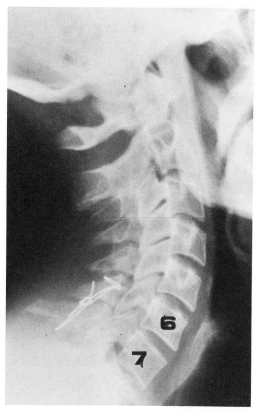

Fig. 12-35. Postoperative film following open reduction and interspinous process wiring of a facet dislocation.

following continuous closed traction has been estimated at 5% to 7% by Cheshire.[23]

The third alternative method of treatment is early elective surgical posterior stabilization after successful reduction by closed method.[44] The disadvantage of this method is that it requires an anesthesia and a surgical procedure in the prone position. The advantage is early mobilization, within several days following surgery, in a cervical brace instead of prolonged bed rest or a halo plaster jacket. This allows early discharge from the hospital and more secure fixation without the necessity of immobilizing the entire spine and head. Early fixation and fusion also virtually eliminates the possibility of late instability requiring a late surgical fusion or further damage to the injured area in a future accident.

AUTHOR'S PREFERRED METHOD OF TREATMENT

My preferred treatment of most cervical vertebral dislocations uncomplicated by fractures consists of

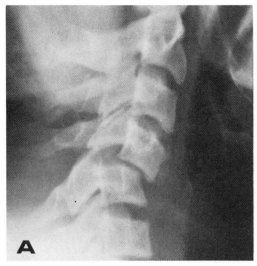
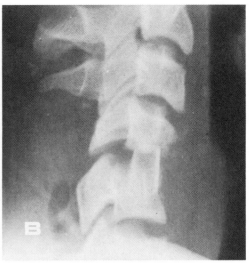

Fig. 12-36. Dislocation treated by anterior fusion. (*A*) Bilateral facet dislocation. (*B*) Anterior removal of the disk and contiguous intervertebral body surfaces leads to increased instability (*and in this case, increased neurologic loss requiring laminectomy*). Acute dislocations should *not* be treated with anterior discectomy and fusion.

application of a cranial halo, traction, reduction of the dislocation, and immobilization of the neck in a halo body cast. Open reduction and fusion is necessary only for those cases that cannot be reduced by closed methods or those that demonstrate persistent instability on flexion-extension x-rays 3 months after injury. Open reduction should be performed from a posterior approach.

TREATMENT OF SPECIFIC FRACTURES

Fractures of the cervical spine may be stable or unstable and may or may not be associated with spinal cord damage. Accurate diagnosis of specific fractures and understanding of the mechanism of injury will allow a more accurate determination of stability and characterization of the neurologic loss.

Compression fractures of the vertebral body without dislocation of the posterior facets or the intervertebral disk joint and without comminution of the body are stable and heal without instability. One must be careful in evaluating the integrity of the posterior ligaments in patients with seemingly simple compression fracture. If there is any widening of the interspinous process space[115] or separation of the spinous processes by the stretch test,[117] progressive instability with anterior displacement may occur: Spinous process avulsion fractures, fractures of the lateral mass, and most low-velocity gunshot wound fractures are also stable. These injuries are treated with a cervical orthosis and early exercise program.

C1 FRACTURE—JEFFERSON'S FRACTURE

The mechanism of this injury is an axial load on top of the head with the patient's body stationary.[56] This causes centrifugal forces on the ring of the atlas, and fractures occur anterior and posterior to the lateral facet joints (Fig. 12-37). These fractures do not cause encroachment of the neurologic canal, and they rarely have associated neurologic loss.

Diagnosis may be difficult on plain x-rays. The anteroposterior open-mouth view demonstrates lateral shift of the C1 lateral masses in relationship to the occipital condyles and the C2 superior facets. The ring of C1 must break in at least two places if fracture occurs, since it is a solid bony ring. Anteroposterior tomograms demonstrate the lateral shift (see Fig. 12-10A) and CT scans of C1 identify the fractures (see Fig. 12-10B). Serial CT scans document healing of the fractures. Retroaural pain and numbness of the posterior scalp may persist due to irritation or scarring of the C2 nerve root as it exits between the C1 ring and C2. Initial treatment consists of cranial skeletal traction (tongs

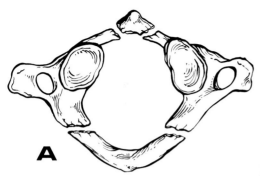

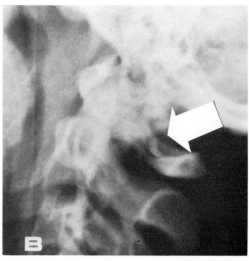

Fig. 12-37. (*A*) Diagram and (*B*) lateral x-ray of a fracture of the posterior ring of C1 (Jefferson's fracture).

or halo) until muscle spasm diminishes and pain subsides. Then the patient can be treated in a halo-plaster cast for 6 to 8 weeks, followed by a cervical brace for 6 to 8 weeks. Four months after the injury, if there is no displacement on gentle flexion and extension films and the patient has no pain on motion of the neck, bracing may be discontinued.

AUTHOR'S PREFERRED METHOD OF TREATMENT

I prefer to immobilize the fracture with a halo plaster jacket for 8 weeks followed by a cervical orthosis support for 8 weeks. At 4 months, range of motion exercises should begin.

FRACTURES OF THE ODONTOID

Anderson and D'Alonzo have classified fractures of the odontoid into three groups.[5] Group I is avulsion fractures of the tip of the odontoid. Since these fractures are above the restraining area of the transverse ligaments, they are usually stable, rarely displaced significantly, and generally heal with immobilization. Group II fractures are fractures through the isthmus or waist of the odontoid, superior to the body of C2 (Fig. 12-38). These fractures have a 50% success rate for healing with immobilization. Fractures in young people (under 40 years old) and undisplaced fractures have a 60% to 80% healing rate. Fractures in older people (over 50 years old) and displaced more than 4 mm have a 20% to 40% healing rate. Therefore, fractures displaced more than 4 mm in patients over 50 years old have the least percentage of healing with immobilization. Group III fractures are fractures

extending down into the body of C2. These heal in a very high percentage of cases with immobilization. It is not clear if a halo body jacket is necessary to obtain healing in type I and type III fractures. I prefer to treat type I fractures with a cervical orthosis, undisplaced type III fractures with a cervical orthosis, and displaced type III fractures with a halo body jacket. I treat all type II fractures with a halo body jacket for 12 weeks. Stability is then assessed by x-ray criteria in the anteroposterior open-mouth projection and polytomography, as well as the clinical criteria of pain with neck motion. Flexion and extension films are also taken to identify any instability in the fracture area. If one of these three signs is present, the patient should have his treatment continued in a cervical orthosis and monitored at monthly intervals. If two of the signs (persistent fracture line on x-ray, motion on flexion-extension films, or pain on motion) are present, then the patient should have a posterior C1-2 arthrodesis performed (Fig. 12-39). It appears that many older patients fail to achieve bony union, but develop a functional fibrous ankylosis that is stable and pain-free. If severe spinal cord damage occurs with this fracture, the injuries are almost always fatal, owing to respiratory paralysis at this high level of the spinal cord.

FRACTURES THROUGH THE PEDICLE OF C2— TRAUMATIC SPONDYLOLISTHESIS (HANGMAN'S FRACTURE)

The fracture through the pedicle of C2 is termed the *Hangman's fracture* because it was the ideal lesion inflicted in a judicial hanging. A displaced

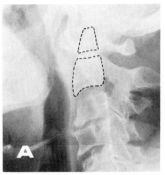
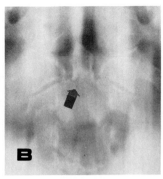
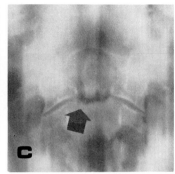

Fig. 12-38. Fracture through the base of the odontoid. (*A*) The lateral x-ray shows mild displacement of the fracture. (*B*) Anteroposterior laminagram shows the fracture through the base of the odontoid. (*C*) Delayed union is demonstrated by a laminagram taken 3 months later.

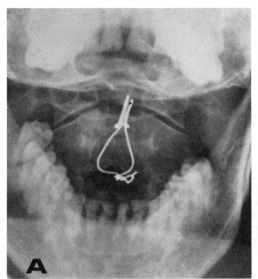
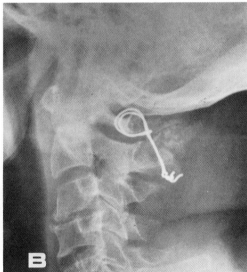

Fig. 12-39. (*A*) Anteroposterior and (*B*) lateral views of delayed union of an odontoid fracture treated by posterior C1-C2 fusion.

fracture at the C2 level, caused by sudden extension forces, produces sudden death by respiratory paralysis instead of a slow death by strangulation. When seen clinically, this lesion most commonly results from sudden deceleration vehicular accidents produced by an axial load as the head strikes the windshield in the extended position. A better name for this injury is traumatic spondylolisthesis of C2 on C3. I treat this fracture with immobilization using a halo body jacket. These fractures unite well if immobilized in a halo body cast, even in a displaced position (Fig. 12-40). Since the mechanism of injury is distraction-extension forces, it is difficult to improve the position of the head with

the halo. The halo cast must remain on until evidence of union occurs, which requires 10 to 12 weeks. If nonunion or instability persists, it may be treated with a posterior C1-2 wire stabilization and fusion. However, an anterior C2-3 fusion provides the necessary stability without compromising the rotation range of motion of the C1-C2 articulation (Fig. 12-41).[19]

COMMINUTED (TEARDROP) BODY FRACTURES

This devastating, complex injury is very unstable.[88] It is caused by an axial compression force associated

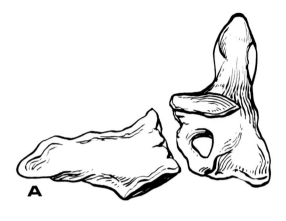

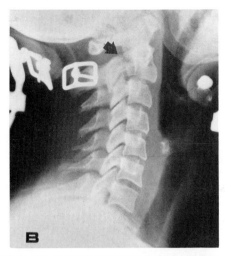

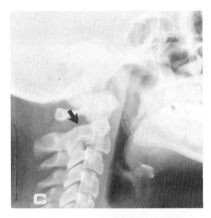

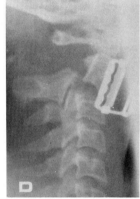

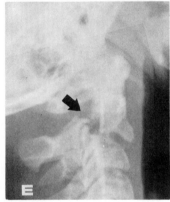

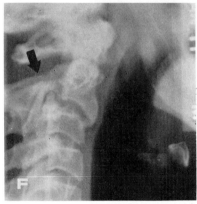

Fig. 12-40. Fracture through the pedicles of C2 (Hangman's fracture). (*A*) Diagram of the fracture. (*B*) This fracture was minimally displaced and it was treated with a brace. (*C*) The fracture healed by primary bony union. (*D*) A grossly displaced Hangman's fracture. (*E*) This fracture was treated by ambulatory treatment with a halo body cast. (*F*) Solid bony union following 4 months in halo body jacket.

with flexion of the midcervical spine (Fig. 12-42). The most frequent cause of injury is a diving accident (Fig. 12-43); the head strikes a solid object, such as the bottom of a swimming pool, a rock in a lake, or the sand in the surf. The head may be in flexion or extension at the occiput-C1 junction at the time of impact. This injury has a very high

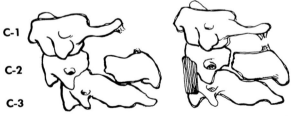

Fig. 12-41. Anterior fusion for rare delayed union of traumatic spondylolisthesis of C2-C3.

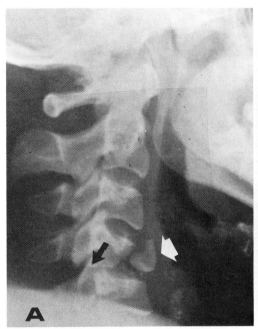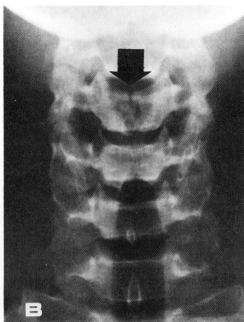

Fig. 12-42. A comminuted body fracture. (*A*) The lateral view shows a coronal fracture. (*B*) The anteroposterior x-ray shows a sagittal fracture.

incidence of severe cord damage with complete motor and sensory paralysis. The vertebral body is fragmented and pushed back into the spinal canal, causing sudden impact to the spinal cord. The bony fragments can be reduced by longitudinal traction, which realigns the spinal column and removes the bony fragments from the spinal canal (Fig. 12-44). There is a high incidence of late instability, due to lack of anterior subligamentous new bone formation and loss of structural stability of the vertebral body (Fig. 12-45).

Due to complete lack of anterior structural stability, treatment of a comminuted vertebral body fracture requires continuous traction until bony union occurs. Progressive redisplacement or persistent instability may cause increasing neurologic symptoms from irritation of cord and nerve roots. The halo and body jacket may not be adequate to maintain sufficient distraction at the injured area to prevent displacement. If the patient has no neurologic loss, he may be maintained in traction in bed for 8 to 12 weeks, followed by cervical bracing when the patient assumes the upright position for an additional 4 to 8 weeks, or he may be treated with an anterior surgical stabilization. If there is no redisplacement and no motion on flexion-extension films at 4 months, the patient may be removed from the brace, and an active

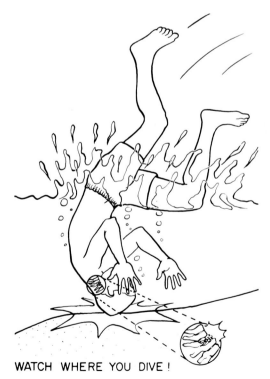

WATCH WHERE YOU DIVE !

Fig. 12-43. The mechanism of injury causing a comminuted body fracture.

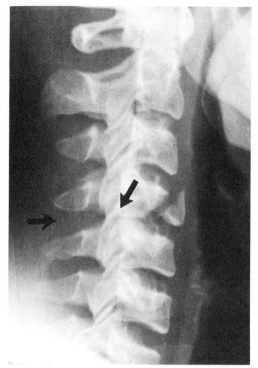

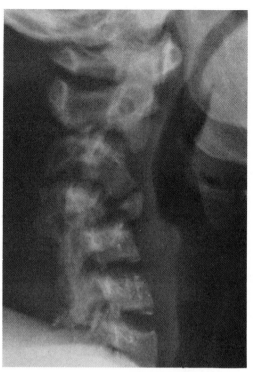

Fig. 12-44. A comminuted body fracture of C4. Longitudinal traction reduces the posterior subluxation into the spinal canal.

Fig. 12-45. Late instability due to poor spontaneous anterior ankylosis following injury.

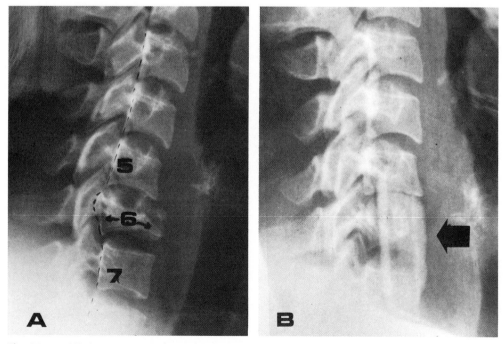

Fig. 12-46. (*A*) A comminuted interbody fracture. (*B*) The fracture was treated with interbody fibular graft stabilization.

exercise program may be instituted. Follow-up x-rays, however, must be taken at 6 months and 1 year, to confirm continued stability. If there is redisplacement or instability on flexion-extension films at 4 months, the patient should then have an anterior fusion with excision of the comminuted vertebral body and a fusion from the normal vertebral body above the fracture of the normal vertebral body below the fracture (*e.g.*, a C4-C6 fusion for a C5 fracture).

If the patient has complete neurologic loss that persists for 24 hours with no sign of incomplete sparing, he may still be treated with continual traction in the recumbent position, but the surgeon must be prepared to deal with the complications of prolonged bed rest in the paralytic. An alternate method of treatment for this comminuted vertebral body fracture in the quadriplegic patient is early anterior debridement of the comminuted fracture fragments and internal stabilization with a cortical strut bone graft, such as the fibula, replacing the comminuted vertebral body[8] (Fig. 12-46). This affords internal fixation of the cervical spine in the reduced position and allows early mobilization of the patient to a wheelchair and institution of a rehabilitation program (Figs. 12-47 and 12-48).

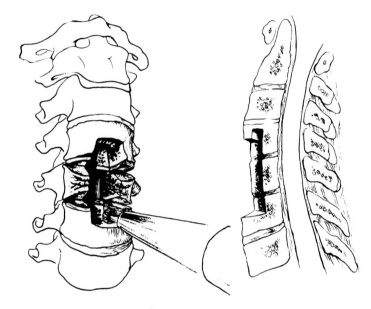

Fig. 12-47. Diagram of anterior debridement of a comminuted body fracture. (*Left*) Removal of the center portion of the comminuted body and contiguous disks exposes the posterior longitudinal ligament. (*Right*) A lateral view shows superior notching in a normal vertebra above the fracture.

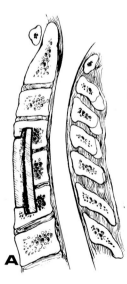
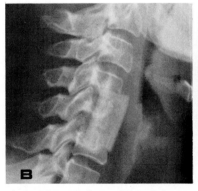
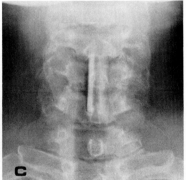

Fig. 12-48. Undercutting of the superior and inferior vertebrae and placement of fibula for stability. (*A*) Diagram of the graft. (*B*) Lateral and (*C*) anteroposterior x-rays show the fibular graft in position.

Some surgeons believe that early operative fusion improves the recovery of nerve root function at the fracture site; however, there is no evidence that any surgical procedure improves recovery of cord function in the complete quadriplegic. Posterior fusion is an acceptable method of immobilizing the injured area, but it does not offer the ability to remove the comminuted vertebral body fragments and the disrupted disks, or the ability to achieve the same internal stability as with an anterior cortical strut graft.

AUTHOR'S PREFERRED METHOD OF TREATMENT

I treat the stable burst fracture (no posterior fracture or ligamentous rupture or comminution of the vertebral body into the neural canal) in the neurologically normal patient with a halo body jacket for 8 weeks. I treat the unstable burst fracture in the quadriplegic with anterior strut stabilization. The patient with an unstable fracture and a normal neurologic examination is treated with halo traction for 6 weeks followed by an *in situ* fusion if x-ray evidence of healing is not present. Early anterior fusion in the neurologically normal patient may be indicated if the advantages outweigh the risks.

INDICATIONS FOR LAMINECTOMY

Laminectomy is rarely indicated in the treatment of patients with closed injury of the cervical spine. The indications and goals of the procedure should be outlined clearly prior to surgery. The trauma sustained by the spinal cord with a fracture or dislocation occurs at the instant of impact. It has been clearly shown by Ducker,[33] Albin and White,[2,3] Osterholm and Mathews,[73] and others[32] that within several hours punctate hemorrhages occur in the gray matter that coalesce to form large hemorrhagic areas. These areas produce irreversible changes within 4 hours that proceed to cystic destruction of the spinal cord. Animal experiments have not been able to report a decrease in the neurologic sequelae of the experimentally injured animal by removal of the dorsal elements, with or without opening the dura. The intramedullary edema cannot be decompressed by removal of the posterior structures. There are no documented clinical studies that indicate that results of treatment of closed spinal injuries with complete spinal cord lesion by laminectomy are superior to those achieved by nonoperative methods.

DEFINITE INDICATIONS FOR LAMINECTOMY

There is one candidate for a laminectomy on which almost all surgeons agree. This is the patient with an incomplete neurologic syndrome who is becoming progressively worse.[86] This patient has functioning neurons that are losing function. This condition may be due to an epidural hematoma, which causes progressive compression and neurologic loss. It is a rare condition in the cervical spine. It must be specifically sought, however, in the patient with Marie-Strümpell arthritis who fractures through his bamboo spine and has a slowly progressive neurologic loss. This patient may have an epidural hematoma that may be relieved, thereby preventing progressive destruction of the cord secondary to pressure.[16] Patients with complete lesion quadriplegia frequently have an ascending neurologic loss of one or two root levels over several days, secondary to ascending edema. This can be expected to recover gradually over the ensuing several days, and it is not to be considered in the same context as an incomplete lesion which is progressing. It is therefore not considered an indication for laminectomy.

Removal of the posterior elements compounds the problems of instability, especially in the comminuted teardrop vertebral body fracture with anterior stability already destroyed. There are several series, including those of Bailey and Kingsley,[9] and Bohlman,[16] that demonstrate the disastrous results of further destabilization of the already traumatized spine and increasing neurologic deficit in the severely paralyzed patient following such operation.

RELATIVE INDICATIONS FOR LAMINECTOMY

There are other relative indications as described by Schneider[86] that are not universally accepted as beneficial in the treatment of patients with immediate traumatic quadriplegia. These relative indications include the following:

Queckenstedt Test. A complete block of the cerebrospinal fluid in the subarachnoid space by jugular vein compression is not confirmatory, because a patient may have significant pressure on the spinal cord and still allow enough fluid to flow through a small-gauge needle into the lumbar space to produce a negative test. A positive test indicating a complete block is usually due to intrinsic cord edema, which does not respond to laminectomy alone.

The Presence of Bone Fragments in the Spinal Canal. On rare occasions a patient demonstrating an incomplete injury may have bone fragments in the spinal canal that are compressing the dura. Any damage these bone fragments may have caused to the spinal cord happened at the time of impact, and their continued presence is of little significance in the neurologic outcome.

Acute Anterior Spinal Injury Syndrome.[85] The presence of deep-pressure and proprioceptive sensation is a relative indication for laminectomy and section of the dentates. Schneider believes that if the patient fails to improve, this syndrome is an indication for a laminectomy and section of the dentate ligaments. However, others, among them Cloward,[26] believe that if decompression is indeed indicated, anterior debridement of bone fragments and disk would be preferable.

Psychologic Reasons. A frequent indication for laminectomy is the psychologic effect on patient and family—the satisfaction of knowing that the cord was looked at and that everything that could possibly be done has been done for this catastrophic injury with a dismal prognosis. Most surgeons, however, feel that the potential damage to be done with an unnecessary operation cannot be justified as a psychologic salve for the patient and family, and there are no data that indicate it is neurophysiologically helpful.

CONTRAINDICATIONS TO LAMINECTOMY

There are several specific contraindications to laminectomy and they are as follows:

1. *The acute central cervical spinal cord syndrome,* which frequently accompanies extension injuries in middle-aged patients with hypertrophic osteoarthritis. This has been described by Schneider.[87] The prognosis for spontaneous progressive cord recovery is good, and the patient will not be helped by a laminectomy.
2. *Metabolic complications,* especially pulmonary, which would increase the risks of anesthesia
3. *Other severe injuries requiring priority surgery (i.e.,* gunshot wounds of the chest or abdomen)

THE AUTHOR'S INDICATION FOR LAMINECTOMY

I believe that the only absolute indication for laminectomy is a patient with an incomplete neu-rologic lesion and a documented progressive neurologic deficit getting worse under observation.

INDICATIONS FOR EARLY SPINAL SURGERY

Other indications for early surgery on injuries to the cervical spinal cord include the following:

1. *Open fractures or gunshot wounds* to the cervical spine. Early debridement should be performed to prevent persistent draining, sinus tracts, and cerebrospinal fluid fistulas.
2. *Open reduction of irreducible locked facets* has been mentioned during the treatment of dislocations.
3. *Foraminotomy of a compressed root of* a persistent unilateral facet dislocation is indicated for persistent weakness and hypesthesia over the root distribution.

SURGICAL ANATOMY

Posterior approaches to the cervical spine are relatively safe with the patient in the prone position. The patient should be in traction with the neck in neutral alignment. The spinous processes of C2 and C7 can be palpated through the skin. Beneath the white median raphe will be found the spinous processes with their central muscle insertions. By careful subperiosteal dissection, the paraspinous extensor muscles can be stripped from the spinous processes, laminae, and lateral edge of the facet joints with safety, up to the level of the C1-C2 articulation. The cervical laminae overlap sufficiently so that there is little danger of dropping between the laminae and causing spinal cord injury if a wide elevator is used. Osteotomes, gouges, and mallets must not be used to remove the cervical laminae or facets. A small rongeur can be used safely to remove portions of fractured laminae and facets. A high-speed air drill is good for decorticating the laminae and facets in preparation for fusion.

The occiput-C1 articulation requires special comment. The posterior ring of C1 is quite thin and hidden deep between the prominences of the occiput and the large C2 spinous process. Careful dissection from below exposes the posterior ring of the C1 vertebra and the thin membrane that covers the dura between C1 and the occiput. The posterior ring of C1 must be carefully exposed subperiosteally and no wider than 2.0 cm from the midline bilaterally, as the C1 and C2 vertebral nerve roots exit behind the facet joints. Moreover, the vertebral artery courses through the vertebral foramen of C1 and loops posteriorly into the foramen magnum, and a wide dissection of the C1 posterior arch endangers the vertebral artery.

SURGICAL ANATOMY OF THE ANTERIOR CERVICAL SPINE EXPOSURE

A transverse skin incision is preferred by the author, as described by Southwick and Robinson.[97] This allows adequate mobilization of the skin to expose the vertebrae from C2 to C7, and has a better cosmetic result than a longitudinal incision. The incision should be centered over the vertebral body or disk that is to be removed. Comparison of surface anatomy of the thyroid cartilage and cricoid cartilage with their positions on the lateral x-ray will indicate the proper level of the skin incision. The platysma is transected in line with the skin incision. Beneath the platysma the midcervical fascia is identified, the sternocleidomastoid muscle is retracted laterally, exposing the carotid sheath at its medial edge. The carotid sheath is also retracted laterally. The thyroid, larynx, trachea, and esophagus are retracted medially as a group. Beneath the visceral fascia, the loose areolar prevertebral fascia is divided by blunt, gloved-finger dissection. Several veins and motor nerves to the strap muscles cross this area and may be transected. If the dissection is carried up to the level of C3, the superior thyroid artery and superior laryngeal nerves are identified and carefully retracted superiorly. (Injury to the superior laryngeal nerve results in loss of the ability to sing high notes and to talk with a falsetto voice.) In the inferior aspect of the incision at the level of the C6-C7 intervertebral space will be found the omohyoid muscle. This can usually be retracted inferiorly out of the field; however, division of the muscle may be necessary, and it leads to no functional disability. The middle thyroid vein may be ligated without concern after first confirming that there is no aberrant recurrent laryngeal nerve accompanying the vessel. The anterior surface of the vertebra is identified by palpation of the prominences of the intervertebral disk space and its surrounding annulus fibrosus. The glistening anterior longitudinal ligament is flanked on each side by the longus coli muscles. Beneath the longus coli muscles laterally on both sides Chassaignac's tubercle can be palpated on the sixth cervical transverse process to confirm the level of the C5-C6 interspace. Palpation over the longus coli muscle must be gentle, to avoid injury to the sympathetic chain, which travels deep to its surface. The ver-

tebral bodies are supplied with a nutrient artery at the midpoint of each body. Therefore, as the longus coli muscles are stripped from the vertebral body subperiosteally, each nutrient artery must be cauterized with electrocautery to prevent backflow from the vertebral body. The longus coli muscles can be safely reflected laterally to the uncinate process. At this point, lateral dissection should be stopped. The central portion of the vertebral body, the disk, and joints of Luschka are exposed. Any further exposure may jeopardize the sympathetic chain, or an instrument that drops inadvertently between the transverse processes may damage the vertebral artery.

SPINAL INJURY CENTERS

Ideally, patients who have significant neurologic loss should be transferred to a center for specialized care of spinal injuries as soon as possible.[99,103] Preferably, this should be within 24 hours of the injury. At the present time, each region of the United States has a federally funded civilian spinal injury treatment center. These centers are available 24 hours per day for consultation and transfer. The Veterans Administration also has designated centers for care of spinal injured veterans.

Improper early handling may impair recovery of neurologic loss and may actually increase the neurologic deficit. Newer methods of early treatment now under investigation may reduce the neurologic sequelae if they are instituted within several hours of injury. At a special center, realistic goals are established regarding the patient's spinal fracture, healing, and the prognosis of the neurologic deficit syndrome. Treatment is aimed at early mobilization with prevention of metabolic complications and rehabilitation for functional activity within the limits of the paralysis. An entire paramedical professional team is necessary to establish and initiate the treatment program. The nursing, physical therapy, occupational therapy, and vocational goals are established for functional independence. Psychologic difficulties are anticipated, and the entire team assists the family with psychologic readjustment. Life expectancy of the person with a spinal injury is greatly improved if he is transferred early to a special treatment center. The early complications and common causes of death are prevented with early prophylactic measures, especially the respiratory complications of atelectasis, pneumonia, and skin complications of pressure ulcers.

Training in the diagnostic and management of

musculoskeletal injuries, as well as rehabilitation of physically disabled people, places the orthopaedic surgeon in a unique position to manage the diagnosis, early spine surgery, rehabilitation, late reconstructive surgery, and follow-up care of spinal injured patients.

REHABILITATION AND LONG-TERM CARE

UROLOGIC MANAGEMENT OF THE PARALYZED BLADDER

Initially, a urinary retention catheter should be placed in the bladder for 24 to 48 hours to monitor urinary output and fluid replacement. This catheter should be withdrawn at 48 hours and an intermittent catheterization program should be started to develop automatic reflex emptying of the bladder. Persons with traumatic quadriplegia have an "upper-motor-neuron bladder" that is controlled by the reflexes through the conus medullaris at the distal end of the spinal cord. Automatic reflex emptying of the bladder is the anticipated goal. If intermittent catheterization technique is not available, bladder range-of-motion-exercises are performed by clamping the catheter tube for 50 minutes and opening it for 10 minutes every hour during the day to allow the bladder to distend and drain at regular intervals and to develop a reflex emptying pattern. Urologic consultation should be obtained early, as well as baseline intravenous urograms. If reflex emptying with residual bladder urine volumes of less than 100 cc does not occur within 6 to 9 months, urologic procedures, such as external sphincterotomy or bladder neck resection, may be necessary to achieve a balanced bladder. All possible attempts should be made to remove the catheter and have catheter-free, reflex emptying of the bladder. Urinary diversion through ileal loops and cutaneous ureterostomies have not proved them to be superior to drainage by reflex emptying, and they are not recommended in routine care of patients with spinal injuries at this time.

The rehabilitation nurse, occupational therapist, medical social worker, orthotist, and psychologist form the core of the rehabilitation team. Under the direction of the orthopaedic surgeon, each performs an initial evaluation of the patient's injury, disability, remaining available function, and the preinjury lifestyle. Each then formulates a treatment plan of methods to achieve realistic goals and the estimated time necessary to achieve these goals.

These are reviewed by the orthopaedic surgeon and implemented as spinal stability allows. Rapid mobilization and aggressive rehabilitation allow early discharge from the hospital at maximum physical function.

NURSING GOALS

The education of the patient is the primary concern of the nursing staff. In the period immediately after injury, the nursing staff is responsible for prevention of pressure ulcerations of the skin. It is the nurse's responsibility to turn and position the patient every 2 hours and to inspect his skin frequently for areas of persistent redness. The patient must not be allowed to develop pressure sores. He is taught this as soon as possible, and the family is taught turning and positioning procedures to prevent pressure ulcers. The only sure method of preventing pressure ulcers is strict nursing care and gradual shifting of responsibility for the skin care to the patient and the family. Special beds, mattresses, and pads are not reliable to prevent pressure sores. Sleeping in the prone position with a pillow bridging bony prominences is the most reliable method of preventing ulcers, and the patient must be taught to sleep prone as soon as neck stability allows.

FAMILY EDUCATION

Acceptance by the patient and family of the paralysis and a new way of life requires careful discussion by the nursing staff and the psychologist as well as the physician. These discussions continue for the entire course of the hospitalization and outpatient visits. The family must be taught care of the catheter or the external urinary collecting device, how to catheterize a patient should a urinary retention emergency arise, and also how to recognize the danger signs of urinary tract infection and sympathetic dysreflexia.

BOWEL PROGRAM

Reflex emptying of the bowels with suppository stimulation is the goal of bowel training. Every second or third day the bowel reflex is stimulated by insertion of a glycerine or Dulcolax suppository, with digital stimulation if necessary. Patients should not be given large-volume enemas, as this routine destroys the bowel reflex. Stool softeners and mild laxatives may be necessary on occasion.

BEDS

A conventional hospital bed and pillow are preferred for quadriplegic patients (Fig. 12-49). Special fluid beds and air mattresses have the specific disadvantage of relying on pumps, valves, and fluid or airtight systems that may leak. These outweigh the possible advantages. There are no special mattresses or beds developed as yet that can prevent pressure ulcers. Turning frames have a distinct disadvantage of allowing only two positions, supine and prone. Patients are very apprehensive lying in a prone position, owing to the decreased vital capacity. Therefore they spend most of the time on their backs. For this reason a high percentage of patients treated on turning frames develop sacral pressure ulcers. Patients can be treated in cervical traction in a conventional bed and moved gently every 2 hours from the supine to the right- or left-side-lying position, propped up with pillows. Circle frame beds should not be used for patients with fractures of the cervical spine. The mechanics of traction and distraction are altered as the patient is turned 180° from the supine to the upright to the prone position and then back through the upright to the supine position. Pressure ulcers develop on the sacrum from lying immobile too long in the supine position, and on the bottoms of the heels, if the patient is left in the semi-standing position more than 2 hours.

A side-to-side rotating bed has been used in several spinal centers to help prevent the complications of pressure sores and pulmonary atelectasis in the early postinjury phase (Fig. 12-50). It appears to be effective during the first week following injury. As soon as the spine is stabilized in traction and the lungs are clear, the patient should be moved to a regular bed to start rehabilitation education and training.

PHYSICAL THERAPY

The physical therapist assesses the patient's sensory and motor power and evaluates him for spasticity. Realistic goals of bed-to-wheelchair transfer activities (Fig. 12-51), wheelchair propulsion, and am-

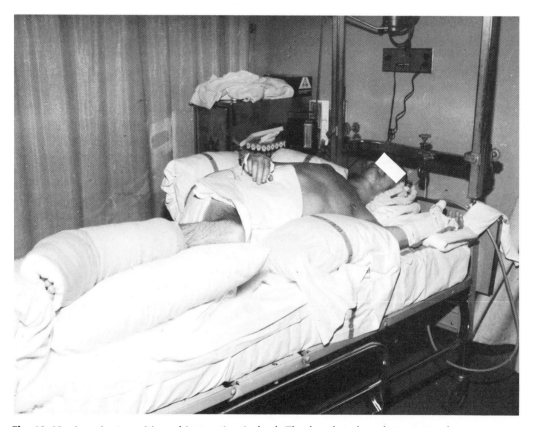

Fig. 12-49. A patient positioned in traction in bed. The head and neck are turned as a unit each time the patient is log-rolled in bed. Note reciprocal flexion and extension of the arms and legs with positioning hand splints.

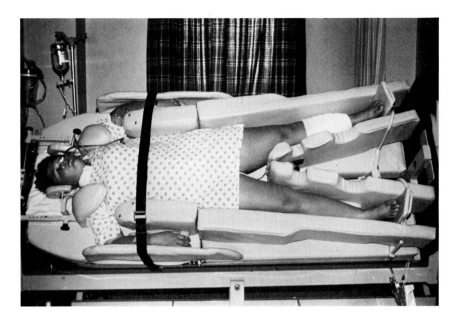

Fig. 12-50. A side-to-side rotating bed may be used during the first week following injury to help prevent pressure sores and pulmonary atelectasis and pneumonia.

bulation for the incompletely injured patient are designated by the physical therapist. The specific wheelchair prescription for the appropriate level of disability is of utmost importance. Lower extremity bracing prescriptions for the incompletely injured patient should be as small and light as possible. The patient with a complete cord lesion and function to the C6 level has voluntary control of deltoids, biceps, wrist extensors, and pectoral muscles. He can be taught independent transfer from bed to wheelchair and independent propulsion of his wheelchair with plasticized rim or quad pegs on the handrims, and he can be taught to dress himself. Complete lesion quadriplegics with function to C7 and C8 have more motor power of the wrist and hand muscles and are more likely to be independent with dressing and wheelchair propulsion for transfer activities. The patient with function only to C5 has no wrist extensors. Therefore he is not capable of performing independent transfer, wheelchair propulsion, or dressing. He will always require assistance in these activities. In some instances improvement of upper extremity function can be provided with tendon transfers. These have been described by Lipscomb and associates,[62] Zancolli,[128] and Moberg.[67]

OCCUPATIONAL THERAPY

The occupational therapist evaluates the function, motor power, and sensory sparing, as well as spasticity and contractures in the upper extremity. Prehension pinch is required for activities of daily living, such as personal hygiene and dressing. A wrist-driven prehension wrist-hand orthosis powered by wrist extensor muscles gives a patient with a C6 or C7 functional level a functional pinch (Fig. 12-52). Special prehension orthoses are required for patients with a functional level of C5 (no muscles to activate hand or wrist), along with mobile arm supports to provide upper extremity function (Fig. 12-53). Automobile driving with hand controls and specialized adaptive equipment is a realistic goal for strong C6 and C7 quadriplegic patients who have strong deltoids and biceps, pectoralis major, and wrist extensor muscles. Without this minimal muscle power, automobile driving is not a realistic goal. Community living skills—getting about in the wheelchair, shopping, keeping house—and vocational skills are evaluated, and training is instituted by the occupational therapist. Psychological counselling of the patient and the family facilitate the psychologic adaptations the patient must go through to cope with his disability. Counselling in sexual rehabilitation is of utmost importance to these patients, most of whom are young, otherwise healthy men. Group discussions of common difficulties encountered in their adjustment to a new way of life help the patient and the family to cope. Families require group discussions to explore the problems of reintegration of the person with spinal injuries into the community. Vocational rehabilitation must begin prior to discharge from the hospital. The patient is evaluated and advised about occupations that can be performed from the wheelchair.

Control of urinary sepsis and other metabolic

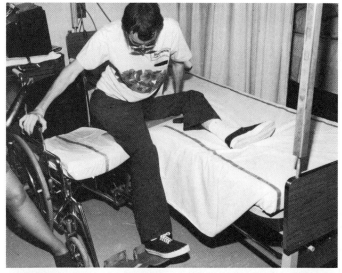

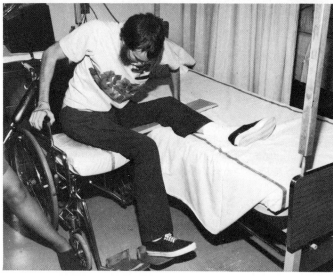

Fig. 12-51. The transfer of a quadriplegic patient from bed to wheelchair.

complications by modern medical treatment ensures the quadriplegic patient a much greater life expectancy than was ever possible several years ago. With the increase of violent accidents in our mechanized society and with improved medical care, the size of this patient group will continue to increase. At the present time they require expert medical care to prevent complications. In the future, hopefully, techniques will be developed for prevention and care of spinal paralysis.

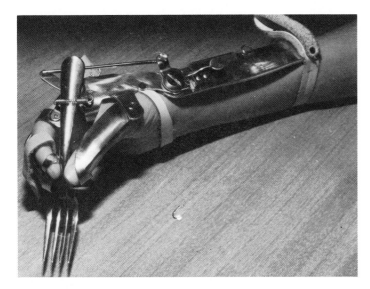

Fig. 12-52. A wrist-driven prehension orthosis.

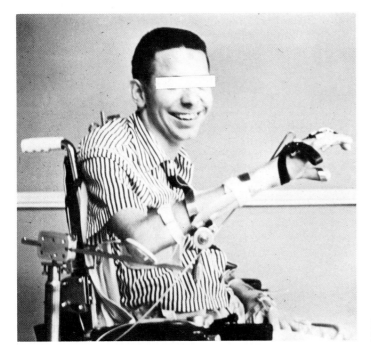

Fig. 12-53. A mobile arm support and electric hand splint.

Part II: THE THORACOLUMBAR SPINE

Herbert Kaufer

Thomas F. Kling

Injury in the thoracolumbar region is both common and highly variable. Severity of the injury can range from a rather subtle muscle strain or ligament sprain to an overt and obvious fracture-dislocation with total and permanent paraplegia. From a public health point of view, the isolated soft tissue injuries (sprain, strain, disk derangement) are the most important, because they are much more common than fracture or dislocation, and an apparently trivial soft tissue injury can cause severe and prolonged disability. However, the isolated soft tissue injuries defy precise definition and cannot be objectively quantitated. For these reasons, thoracolumbar injuries that cannot be demonstrated by objective findings or x-rays are excluded from further discussion.

Post-traumatic spinal deformity and its relation to paraplegia has been recognized since antiquity. Prior to routine use of x-rays most physicians and laymen believed that almost all spine fractures were paralyzing and rapidly fatal. It is now clear that no more than 5% of spine fractures are associated with neurologic deficit.[220] The remaining 95% are simple skeletal injuries associated with relatively brief disability and excellent long-term prognosis.[144,241,250] Unfortunately, most laymen and some physicians still equate "a broken back" with a major disaster.

Hipprocrates recognized that these injuries need not be associated with neurologic deficit. He described several methods of forceful manipulative reduction of the deformity. His detailed description of reduction techniques included both longitudinal traction and direct pressure over the prominence of the deformity. This combination of forces remains the cornerstone of most modern methods for correction of spinal deformity, traumatic or atraumatic.

The thoracolumbar junction marks an abrupt transition between stiff and mobile segments, as does the lumbosacral junction.[184] The lumbar spine is the second most mobile region of the spine. If force applied to the torso is sufficient to produce motion beyond the physiologic range, the lumbar spine, because of its location between less mobile and more stable regions of the spine, is highly susceptible to fracture or dislocation.[171,193,217] Therefore, in spite of massive architecture and rugged construction, the great majority of spine fractures occur in the lumbar and distal thoracic regions of the spine.[220] The region from T12 to L2 accounts for more than 50% of all vertebral body fractures,[208,220,241] and approximately 40% of all spinal cord injuries are at the T12-L1 level.[220]

Motion in the thoracolumbar region of the spine has six degrees of freedom (flexion, extension, right lateral bending, left lateral bending, right torsion, and left torsion). One might expect to see an equal number of disruptions due to stress in each of these directions. However, the vast majority of lumbar and thoracic fractures are the result of hyperflexion.[174,217,241] When faced with a situation of impending trauma the victim, by reflex, adopts a posture of flexion to protect the face, abdomen, and genitalia. As the victim is prepositioned in flexion, forces applied to the torso produce further flexion rather than motion in any other direction. The preponderance of flexion fractures of the spine should not, therefore, be considered evidence of spinal deficiency in withstanding flexion stress.

ANATOMY

GENERAL OSSEOUS AND ARTICULAR CHARACTERISTICS

The thoracolumbar spine has well-developed anteroposterior curves, lordotic in the lumbar region and kyphotic in the thoracic region. Normally there is no significant lateral curve, although many spines do show a very slight, probably physiologic, lateral thoracic curve, convex to the right with an apex at T8.[220] There are usually 12 osseous segments in the thoracic region and five in the lumbar region. There is a progressive increase in size of osseous segments from cranial to caudal within the thoracic and lumbar regions. Each intervertebral disk of the thoracic and lumbar spine is larger and thicker than the one above, except for the lumbosacral disk which, while larger in cross section than the L4-L5 disk, is usually thinner (Fig. 12-54). This is especially true if there is a fault of segmentation at the lumbosacral junction (as there is in 15% of cases).[189] By itself, a thin lumbosacral disk should seldom be considered a sign of acute traumatic significance. Each osseous segment is, in general, ring-shaped (Fig. 12-55), with a large central vertebral foramen, the spinal canal, which perforates the bone from top to bottom and surrounds the dural tube and its contents. The osseous segment is arbitrarily but logically divided by the spinal canal into anterior and posterior portions. The anterior portion consists of the vertebral body, the largest single structural component of each segment, which articulates with its caudal and cranial neighbors through intervertebral disks, forming a synchondrosis.

Each intervertebral disk consists of an avascular gelatinous nucleus bordered above and below by the cartilaginous vertebral end-plate and peripherally by the annulus fibrosis, which has very secure fibrous attachments to the vertebral body margins.[177] The annulus is reinforced by a broad and very substantial anterior longitudinal ligament and by a much narrower and weaker posterior longitudinal ligament.[177,247] The anterior portion of the spine is well suited for bearing vertical compressive loads and permits considerable motion around all three spatial axes, while at the same time limiting translation.[243]

The gelatinous nucleus enclosed within a fibrocartilage annulus is an excellent elastic shock absorber.[217,243] Also, when under compression the vertebral end-plates deform, forcing blood out of the cancellous bone through multiple vascular foramina, which results in load damping quite similar to that of an automobile shock absorber. If compressive loads are large enough, the end-plate deformation increases, ultimately resulting in fracture,[214,226] which allows the nucleus to invade the body, producing a "traumatic Schmorl's node."[220] The vertebral end-plate always fails prior to annulus rupture in the normal spine (at a load of approximately 230 kg).[214] Rupture of nuclear material through the annulus occurs only in an abnormal disk.[162]

The posterior portion of the spinal ring, the neural arch, consists of paired pedicles, paired laminae, and a midline spinous process. The paired superior articular processes project superiorly from the superior margin of the neural arch at the junction of the pedicles and laminae. The articular surfaces of the superior facets face posteriorly in the thoracic region (see Fig. 12-55), posteriorly and medially in the lumbar region (Fig. 12-56). The inferior articular processes project downward from the inferior border of the neural arch at the junction of the pedicles and laminae. The articular surfaces of the inferior facets face anteriorly in the thoracic region, anteriorly and laterally in the lumbar region. The transverse processes arise between the superior and inferior facets at the junction of the pedicle and lamina and project laterally and posteriorly in the thoracic region, and laterally in the lumbar region.[177]

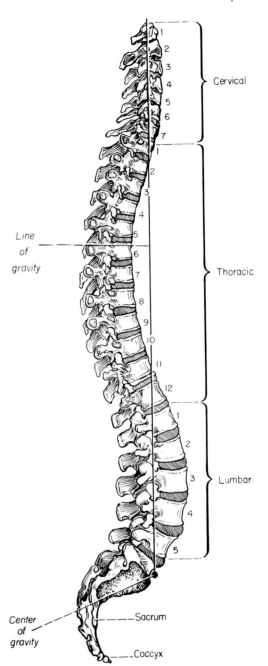

Fig. 12-54. Lateral view of the vertebral column showing its curves and their relationship to a plumb line through the center of gravity of the body. (Woodburne, R. T.: Essentials of Human Anatomy. New York, Oxford University Press, 1957.)

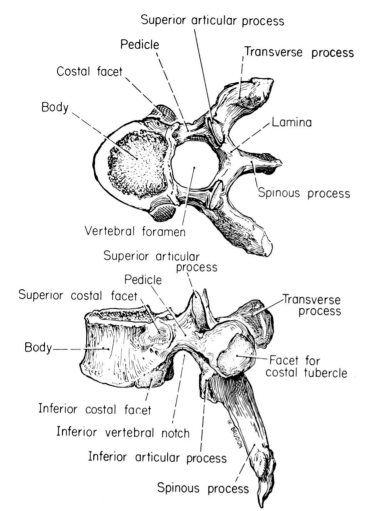

Superior articular process

Pedicle

Transverse process

Costal facet

Body

Lamina

Spinous process

Vertebral foramen

Superior articular process

Pedicle

Superior costal facet

Transverse process

Body

Facet for costal tubercle

Inferior costal facet

Inferior vertebral notch

Inferior articular process

Spinous process

Fig. 12-55. A typical thoracic vertebra, superior and lateral view. (Woodburne, R. T.: Essentials of Human Anatomy. New York, Oxford University Press, 1957.)

The articular facets form true synovial joints with substantial capsules. The neural arches are further bound together by the highly elastic ligamentum flavum, which runs between laminae. The interspinous ligament runs from the inferior border of a spinous process to the superior border of the next most caudal spinous process. It runs the entire length of the spinous process from the junction of the two laminae to the tip of the spinous process (Fig. 12-57). The most superficial portion of the interspinous ligament forms a more or less discrete band called the supraspinous ligament, which runs from the tip of one spinous process to the tip of another. The intertransverse ligaments run between adjacent transverse processes and are best developed in the lumbar region. The intervertebral foramen is a space between pedicles of adjacent vertebrae. It is bordered anteriorly by the vertebral body and disk, and posteriorly by the articular facets. Through this foramen passes the spinal nerve with its dural sleeve and accompanying arteries and veins.[247]

The neural arch and vertebral body form a ring of bone that protects the dura and its contents. The neural arch, with its associated processes, capsules, and ligaments, limits and controls the extent and direction of motion at each level. By modulating the excursion of intersegmental motion, the neural arch is largely responsible for spinal stability.[193,242,243]

In all articulations, there is an inverse relationship between mobility and stability. Those joints with the greatest mobility are potentially the least stable. Normally the thoracolumbar spine is capable of moving around all three spatial axes (Fig. 12-58). The excursion of intersegmental motion in each

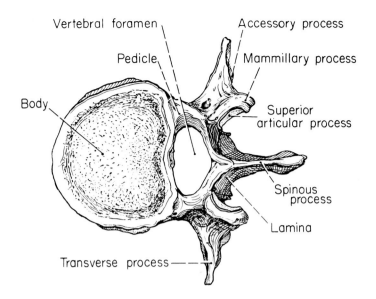

Vertebral foramen
Accessory process
Pedicle
Mammillary process
Body
Superior articular process
Spinous process
Lamina
Transverse process

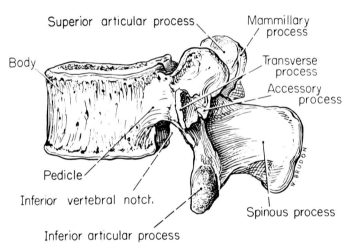

Superior articular process
Mammillary process
Body
Transverse process
Accessory process
Pedicle
Inferior vertebral notch
Spinous process
Inferior articular process

Fig. 12-56. A mid-lumbar vertebra, superior and lateral view. (Woodburne, R. T.: Essentials of Human Anatomy. New York, Oxford University Press, 1957.)

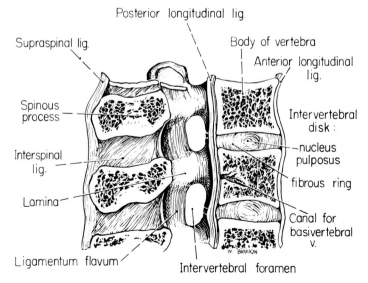

Posterior longitudinal lig.
Supraspinal lig.
Body of vertebra
Anterior longitudinal lig.
Spinous process
Intervertebral disk:
  nucleus pulposus
Interspinal lig.
fibrous ring
Lamina
Canal for basivertebral v.
Ligamentum flavum
Intervertebral foramen

Fig. 12-57. A median section of the mid-lumbar vertebral column to show the ligaments, disk, and intervertebral foramina. (Woodburne, R. T.: Essentials of Human Anatomy. New York, Oxford University Press, 1957.)

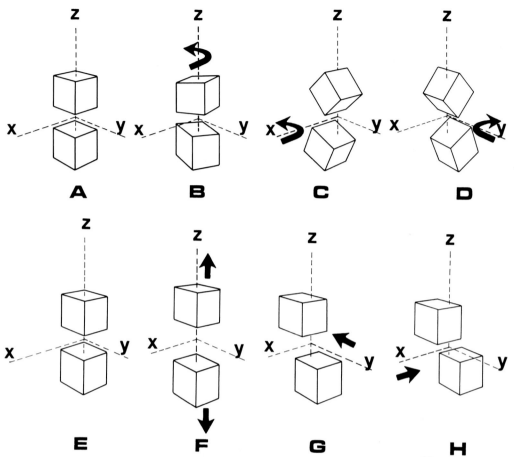

Fig. 12-58. Spatial relationship of two bodies, relative to the conventional x, y, and z-axes of three-dimensional space. (*A*) Angular (rotation) motion may occur around each of the three axes. (*B*) Angular motion around the z axis (torsion). (*C*) Angular motion around the x axis (flexion-extension). (*D*) Angular motion around the y axis (lateral bending). (*E*) Nonangular (translation) motion may occur along each of the three axes. (*F*) Nonangular motion along the z axis (distraction, compression). (*G*) Nonangular motion along the y axis (anteroposterior shear). (*H*) Nonangular motion along the x axis (lateral shear).

direction varies, depending on the segmental level and the characteristics of the person's connective tissue.[167,171] However, translation (nonangular displacement) does not occur to any appreciable degree in an intact thoracolumbar spine. Since motion between segments is a normal characteristic of the spine, demonstration of motion at an injured area is not necessarily an indication of abnormal stability. Instability is defined as increased motion in a normal direction or any motion in an abnormal direction.

SPECIAL CHARACTERISTICS OF THE THORACIC SPINE

Ribs are certainly the most obvious anatomical feature of the thoracic spine. (Fig. 12-59) A pair

of ribs articulates with each thoracic vertebra. Each rib has two articular facets. The head of each rib articulates with the vertebral body at the level of the intervertebral disk. The vertebral side of the costovertebral joint consists of the disk and two small facets (demi-facets), one on each vertebral body adjacent to that disk. Since ribs have a caudal slope, their second facet, at the tubercle of the rib, articulates with the anterior tip of the transverse process (costotransverse joint) of the vertebra, which is caudal to the disk with which the head of that rib articulates.[247]

The configuration of the thoracic cage permits the ribs to function as stabilizing outriggers, markedly restricting lateral bending, flexion, and extension of the thoracic spine. However, the generally

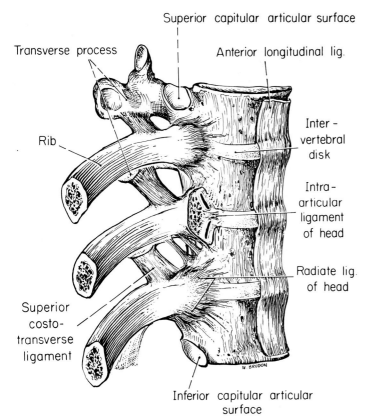

Superior capitular articular surface

Transverse process

Anterior longitudinal lig.

Rib

Inter-vertebral disk

Intra-articular ligament of head

Radiate lig. of head

Superior costo-transverse ligament

Inferior capitular articular surface

Fig. 12-59. An anterolateral view of the midthoracic spine to illustrate the costovertebral and costotransverse joints and ligaments. (Woodburne, R. T.: Essentials of Human Anatomy. New York, Oxford University Press, 1957.)

parallel arrangement of the ribs offers comparatively little restriction to torsion.[193,243] The thoracic articular facets lie in the frontal plane and allow relatively free motion around all three spatial axes.

Laminae in the thoracic region are well developed and so wide that they overlap one another, much like shingles on a roof.[177] The interlaminar ligaments are, therefore, quite short and limit the rotation and bending excursion of the thoracic spine markedly.[242] Overlapping spinous processes and comparatively short interspinous and supraspinous ligaments also contribute to this effect. The net effect of these specialized structures is a relatively immobile thoracic spine. Thoracic intervertebral disks are thinner than the disks of any other mobile area of the spine,[177] so that the potential for thoracic spine motion is minimal, even without the limiting effects of ribs and posterior processes. Rotation is the freest motion. Seventy percent of thoracolumbar rotation occurs within the thoracic region.[167]

The 11th and, to a greater extent, the 12th thoracic vertebrae are transitional, in that they have many lumbar characteristics such as shorter, more horizontal spinous processes, articular facets de-

viated toward the sagittal plane, and no costotransverse articulation. The diminutive 11th and 12th ribs are further evidence of the transitional nature of these segments.[247]

SPECIAL CHARACTERISTICS OF THE LUMBAR SPINE

The most obvious anatomical features of the lumbar spine are the very large vertebral bodies and posterior processes, by far the most massive of any region of the spine. Because the thickest intervertebral disks are found in the lumbar region, there is potential for a large arc of motion around all three spatial axes. The spinous processes are thicker, more horizontal, and more widely separated than those in the thoracic spine. The laminae are relatively narrower and do not overlap.[177] There is an interlaminar distance of 1 cm to 2 cm. As a consequence of much longer interlaminar, interspinous, and supraspinous ligaments, the neural arch of the lumbar spine permits freer motion than the neural arch of the thoracic spine.

The articulating surfaces of the lumbar articular facets lie close to the sagittal plane. This arrangement allows a wide arc of flexion-extension, limits lateral bending moderately, and limits rotation markedly. The inferior articular facets of L5 lie in the frontal plane; therefore, greater rotation is allowed at the lumbosacral junction than elsewhere within the lumbar spine.[162] L5 has features showing transition to the sacral type, including a lumbosacral disk that is thinner than the disk above.[249]

DURA

The dural tube and its contents (spinal cord, nerve roots, cauda equina) lie within the spinal canal. A dural sleeve surrounds each spinal nerve and accompanies it through the intervertebral foramen. The root sleeves have a fairly firm connective-tissue attachment to the walls of the intervertebral foramen. These attachments constitute the major anchoring support for the spinal dural tube.[247] The

dural sac tapers to its end, usually at the second sacral segment. The filum terminale, a fibrous band, extends from the caudal end of the dural sac and attaches to periosteum of the coccyx. It serves as a caudal anchor for the dural tube.

SPINAL CORD AND ROOTS

The spinal cord usually terminates at the level of the intervertebral disk between L1 and L2 (Fig. 12-60).[247] In general, the cord decreases in size as it descends through the thoracolumbar region. There is, however, a localized enlargment that usually lies between the upper border of T10 and the lower border of T12. This enlargment gives rise to the nerves of the lower extremities and includes cord levels L2 through S4.[177,247]

The smallest part of the thoracic spinal cord

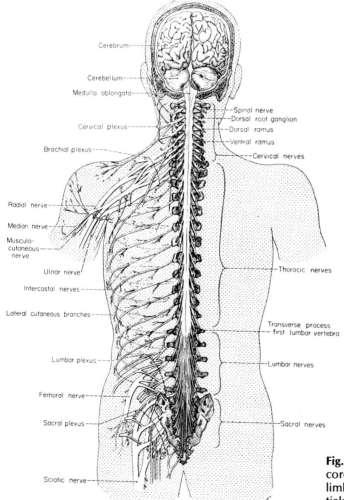

Fig. 12-60. Posterior view of the spinal cord, cauda equina, spinal nerves, and limb plexuses. (Woodburne, R. T.: Essentials of Human Anatomy. New York, Oxford University Press, 1957.)

measures 8.0 mm wide and 6.5 mm anteroposteriorly.[159] At the largest part of its lumbosacral enlargment (located between T10 and T12) it is 9.6 mm wide and 8.0 mm anteroposteriorly. The average dimensions of the thoracic vertebral spinal canal are 17.2 mm wide and 16.8 mm anteroposteriorly.[159] The cord, therefore, occupies a little less than half of the available space.

Caudad to the first lumbar vertebra, there is no spinal cord.[182] The roots of the cauda equina are the only neural content of the spinal canal. As the canal descends, it contains progressively fewer nerves, as one pair of spinal nerves exits at each intervertebral level. Because the average dimensions of the lumbar vertebral spinal canal are 23.4 mm wide and 17.4 mm anteroposteriorly, the lumbar region has quite a bit of free space available within the spinal canal relative to other regions.[159] For this reason, fractures or dislocations in the lumbar spine usually require more displacement than their counterparts in the thoracic spine in order to produce nerve damage.[168,173,181,184]

Within the spinal canal, the sensory and motor roots of the spinal nerves remain separate (Fig. 12-61). The sensory root (dorsal) ganglion is located near the vertebral foramen through which that root passes.[184] The preganglionic sensory root fiber synapses are in the ganglion. Postganglionic sensory root fibers that leave the ganglion fuse with the motor root almost immediately to form the spinal nerve, which exits from the intervertebral foramen. Motor roots are the axons of the anterior horn cells and are actually peripheral nerves all the way from their spinal cord origin to their terminus at the motor end-plate. However, the sensory root is not a peripheral nerve until it exits from the dorsal root ganglion. That portion of the sensory root that runs from the cord to the ganglion is actually a fiber of the central nervous system and has the very limited repair potential characteristic of the cord. Neurologic deficit due to damage of motor roots (including, of course, damage to the motor component of the cauda equina) has the comparatively favorable prognosis of a peripheral nerve injury.[181]

Neurologic deficit due to skeletal disruption at or above T10 is due almost entirely to cord damage. Between T10 and L1, neurologic deficit is usually due to both cord and root damage, the proportion of root damage increasing with progressively more caudal skeletal levels. Below L1, neurologic deficit is due entirely to root damage (see Fig. 12-61).[168,182,184]

Traumatic loss of cord function may recover if the injury is a reversible anatomical lesion (edema or mild hemorrhage), or if the disturbance is physi-

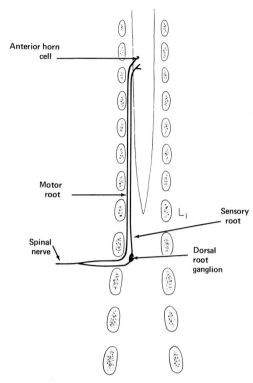

Fig. 12-61. Schematic representation of the thoracolumbar spine showing the relationship of a motor root, sensory root, sensory root ganglion, and spinal cord to the vertebral pedicles.

ologic without an anatomical lesion (e.g., concussion).[181] However, loss of function due to major anatomical disruption of the spinal cord (division of axones or destruction of cells) has little or no chance for recovery, owing to the minimal repair potential of the adult central nervous system. Since immediate and complete loss of neurologic function following trauma is usually a sign of major anatomical disruption of the cord, it is axiomatic that such patients have no potential for neurologic recovery, regardless of their treatment.[168,175,199,201] However, if the neurologic deficit is due to cauda equina (root) damage, then the portion of the deficit due to damage of motor fibers may recover, even if the axons are crushed or divided, so long as the fibrous perineurium of the fasciculi remains intact.[169,181] This is not true of the sensory components of the cauda equina, because regeneration does not occur if the lesion is located proximal to the peripheral nerve cell of origin, the dorsal root ganglion cell.[182]

These neurologic details and the abundant space available in the lumbar spinal canal account for the generally more favorable neurologic prognosis for injuries in the lumbar spine as compared to those in the thoracic spine.

BLOOD SUPPLY

One would expect that a structure as important as the spinal cord would have an abundant blood supply with multiple anastomoses. The blood supply of the cord is, however, surprisingly precarious.[247] The arterial supply consists of two posterior spinal arteries and a single anterior artery.

The two posterior spinal arteries originate from branches of the posterior inferior cerebellar arteries and run the length of the spinal cord. Lying on its posterior surface, they supply the posterior third and peripheral lateral portions of the cord. The anterior spinal artery originates from a fusion of branches from the vertebral artery and runs the length of the spinal cord, lying in its anterior longitudinal fissure. It supplies the anterior two thirds and central portion of the cord. These arteries are quite small, even at their origin. They are supplemented along the length of the cord by eight anterior and 12 posterior medullary feeder vessels that reinforce the longitudinal anterior and posterior spinal arteries.[152] Anastomoses between anterior and posterior spinal arteries are sparse, especially in the midthoracic cord.[177,247]

In the thoracic and lumbar regions of the spine, spinal branches of the intercostal and lumbar segmental arteries pass through their respective intervertebral foramina and divide into posterior and anterior radicular branches. They supply extraspinal structures and also contribute to the posterior and anterior spinal arteries.[152] These spinal branches are not constant and do not enter the cord at every segmental level. They are especially sparse in the area between T4 and T9, the "critical zone of the spinal cord" where it is most vulnerable to ischemic insult.[152] The segmental arteries are interconnected from level to level at the lateral borders of the vertebral segments, which allows division of segmental arteries anterior to the spinal column with relatively little risk of cord infarct. An abundant segmental contribution usually enters at upper thoracic levels, most often at T4.[152,153] Additional significant anastomosing vessels contribute to spinal artery flow at or near the thoracolumbar junction, entering most often at the T11 level on the left side.[185] The segmental anterior radicular branch entering at this level is frequently called the great radiculomedullary artery, or the artery of Adamkiewicz. This artery has received considerable attention, because neurologic syndromes have been identified that may be due to interference with its flow.[185,223] However, ligation of the artery of Adamkiewicz does not always produce a neurologic deficit and, conversely, its preservation does not assure preservation of neurologic function. It is, therefore, wise to preserve each contributing segmental artery so far as is surgically possible.

The conus medullaris blood supply is supplemented by a communicating vessel on each side that connects the anterior and posterior spinal arteries and are reinforced by sacral medullary vessels, branches of the lateral sacral arteries, which accompany the roots of the cauda equina to the terminal portion of the spinal cord.

Within the substance of the spinal cord, the branches of the anterior and posterior spinal arteries are end arteries without anastomoses between their respective capillary beds. Each terminal branch is responsible for perfusion of a specific zone of the spinal cord. While some overlap of zones is present, anastomoses between zones are not.

PATHOGENESIS OF NEUROLOGIC DEFICIT

Neurologic deficit secondary to thoracolumbar fractures or dislocation may be produced by several distinct mechanisms, including displacement of fracture fragments or intervertebral disc, distortion of the spinal canal due to segmental displacement, penetration by foreign bodies, and/or interruption of the vascular supply.

Distortion of the spinal canal due to segmental displacement is by far the most common mechanism for production of neurologic deficit.[175,183,239] Displacement may be angular or translational. Angular displacements are the most common but, fortunately, they are relatively benign because, although they distort the contour of the dural tube, they cause relatively little invasion of intradural space (Fig. 12-62). This explains the low incidence of neurologic deficit secondary to hyperflexion injuries, even with marked wedge deformity of a vertebral body. Neurologic deficit due to angular displacement is seen only with very severe deformity and is due to dural contents being stretched over the convexity of the displaced vertebral bodies.[137] The site of neural compression is anterior over the convexity of the deformed spine as shown in Figure 12-62. In such a case, laminectomy alone cannot relieve anterior compression due to angular displacement.[136,137] One would have to excise a portion of the vertebral body anterior to the dura

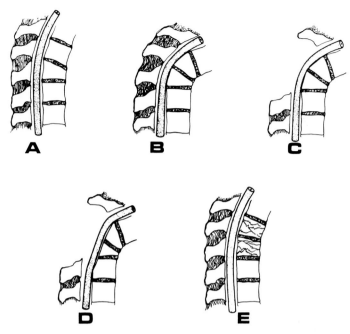

Fig. 12-62. Schematic representation of neural compression due to angular spinal displacement and the effect of various methods of decompression. (*A*) Moderate angular deformity due to an anterior wedge fracture of a vertebral body produces minimal distortion of the spinal canal and no dural compression. (*B*) Severe angular deformity due to an anterior wedge fracture of more than one vertebral body may cause neural compression as a result of neural stretching over the convexity of the deformed vertebral bodies. (*C*) Laminectomy, even at multiple levels, does nothing to relieve anterior neural compression produced by a severe angular deformity. (*D*) Decompression can be achieved if laminectomy is combined with an excision of the posterior vertebral bodies. This procedure produces marked spinal instability. (*E*) Decompression can be achieved by a reduction which reduces the bony prominence and relieves anterior dural compression. This procedure does not impair spinal stability.

in order to achieve decompression. This would be technically difficult and potentially hazardous because it would impair the stability of the spine. Experimental studies have definitely shown that spinal instability leads to progressive neural deficit.[156,157] Reduction of the deformity is the simplest, safest, and most effective means of eliminating the compressing bony prominence. However, if neurologic deficit were to increase over time due to progressive deformity, then anterior decompression and posterior stabilization may be necessary.[137]

Horizontal translation displacement (see Fig. 12-58),[138] although relatively less common than angular displacement, is far more likely to produce neural deficit because even small displacements can diminish the area of the spinal canal markedly.[136] However, vertical translation is comparatively benign,[225] because it does not alter the contour or area of the spinal canal. Translational displacement is definite evidence of instability with all of its progressive deformity and neural implications. Laminectomy for dural decompression due to angular displacement is futile, but is relatively more effective in reducing dural compression due to horizontal translation. However, compression due to translation is relieved most effectively by reduction (Fig. 12-63)[136,229] and laminectomy in this situation is very likely to increase the spinal instability and could, therefore, contribute to an increase in the neural deficit.

Neural compression due to displaced fragments is relatively uncommon.[224] It may be seen in fractures with comminution of the posterior cortex of the body (Fig. 12-64), or with displaced fragments of the neural arch. Rarely is it due to a retropulsed intervertebral disk, but disk fragments may encroach on the dural sac along with fragments of the vertebral body.[224] In these situations there may be little or no angular or translational displacement of spinal segments. Reduction can succeed in replacing the displaced fragments,[239] but it is an unreliable means of relieving neural pressure. Decompression in these situations is best achieved by direct operative removal or replacement of the displaced fragments. Decompression of the dura secondary to posterior displacement of fragments of the body or disk may best be accomplished by an anterior surgical approach to the injured spine.[138,180,187,249] Transthoracic approaches to the thoracic spine, a retroperitoneal approach to the lumbar spine, and a combined thoracoabdominal approach to the thoracolumbar spine (T10-L2) are most applicable.[137,*,245] While providing anterior decompression, these procedures are likely to significantly increase the spine's instability. It is, therefore, wise to do a posterior approach at the same time or a subsequent procedure to improve stability with appropriate internal fixation.[160,227] A costo-

* Leatherman, K.: Personal communication, 1982.

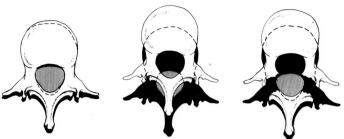

Fig. 12-63. A schematic superior view of two lumbar vertebrae, showing a cross section of the spinal canal (after Böhler). (*Left*) There is an ample cross-sectional area within the
spinal canal (*shaded region*) when the vertebrae are well
aligned. (*Center*) Nearly total loss of the cross-sectional area
of the spinal canal is produced by a moderate degree of
translational displacement. (*Right*) Removal of the posterior
neural arch (*laminectomy*) can effectively restore the cross-
sectional area of the spinal canal in a spine with the type of
displacement illustrated in the *center* diagram.

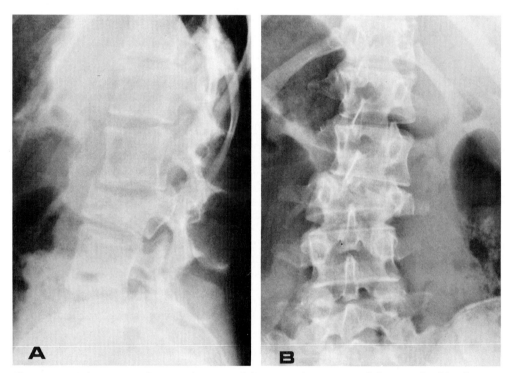

Fig. 12-64. A fracture with comminution of the posterior cortex of the vertebral body
associated with partial paraplegia due to a displaced fragment. Lateral wedge fractures are rarely this severe and are seldom associated with neural deficit. (*A*) Lateral
view, showing posterior fragments of the vertebral body protruding into the spinal
canal. The neural arch is intact. (*B*) Anteroposterior view of the same patient,
showing a severe lateral wedge deformity of the vertebral body.

transversectomy approach to the anterior portion of the spinal canal combined with a posterior exposure for insertion of internal fixation devices through the same skin incision may be used to accomplish both anterior decompression and posterior stabilization at a single procedure.[156]

In spite of the technical problems inherent in operations on a severely injured patient in the region of a large retropleural or retroperitoneal hematoma, anterior approaches to the thoracolumbar spine have been shown to provide excellent exposure, which facilitates effective decompression of the dura, thus contributing to preservation of neural function.[137,156] Surgical management of these patients is facilitated by high quality anesthetic support, a thorough understanding of spinal-cord-injured patients, and familiarity with anterior approaches to the spine. Although a few cases of remarkable recovery of neural function have been observed, it has not been proved that the decompression was responsible for the recovery. Instances of considerable recovery have also been observed in patients in whom no decompressive procedure was performed.[146,169] However, at the present time, combined anterior decompression and posterior stabilization are most promising.

Neural damage from vascular impairment is extremely rare in thoracolumbar fractures.[224] When present it is due to interruption of the arterial supply to the cord from lumbar and lower intercostal arteries (the great radiculomedullary artery of Adamkiewicz).[223] A circulatory basis for neural dysfunction should be strongly suspected if the level of neurologic deficit is cephalad to the level of the skeletal disruption. If neurologic deficit secondary to thoracolumbar fracture is not on a circulatory basis, the sensory and motor level is always either at or (more often) caudad to the level of the skeletal disruption.[182] Although it is rare, it is important to recognize paraplegia due to circulatory disturbances, because these cases represent a neural infarct and have a totally dismal prognosis for neural recovery.[224]

Neurologic deficit due to a penetrating foreign body, usually a missile, is unfortunately becoming more common even in civilian practice. Although fractures are frequent in these injuries, the fracture is usually a minor component of the total injury and the spine is seldom unstable (Fig. 12-65). Treatment of these injuries is essentially the treatment of open wounds of the spinal cord or dura.[221] Treatment should include debridement, hemostasis, closure as indicated, and antibiotics. Usually the fracture can be ignored.[168] In a study of gunshot

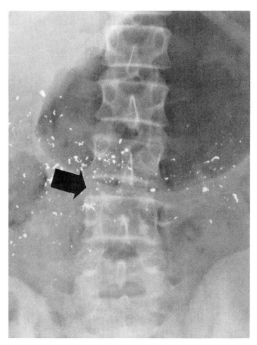

Fig. 12-65. A gunshot wound of the lumbar spine. Unilateral facet damage (*arrow*) between L3 and L4 is the only evidence of fracture. Paraplegia was immediate, total, and permanent.

wounds of the spine, laminectomy has been shown to be of no neurologic benefit and is complicated by increased instability in 6% of cases and a cerebrospinal fluid fistula or infection in 10% of cases.[231]

SPINAL STABILITY

Stability and instability are familiar terms often applied to fractures and dislocations. A fracture or dislocation whose fragments are not likely to move during the healing process is generally considered to be stable. An unstable fracture or dislocation is one whose fragments will probably shift their relative positions prior to final healing. It is well known that a wedge fracture of the vertebral body often shows progression of deformity prior to final union (Fig. 12-66).[218,220] Nevertheless, these fractures are generally considered stable. Clearly the terms "stable" and "unstable" are used in a special sense when applied to injuries of the spine.

A spinal fracture or dislocation is considered unstable if, during the healing phase, its fragments are capable of displacement that might produce

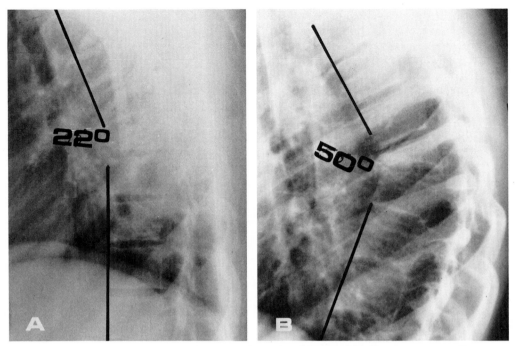

Fig. 12-66. (*A*) An anterior wedge fracture of T7. The degree of kyphos measures 22°. The patient was treated with an extension brace. (*B*) Four months later there was marked progression of the wedging. The degree of kyphos then measured 50°. There was no further progression.

nerve damage. An unstable spine has the potential to produce a neural deficit where none existed initially or to cause an increase in a previously incomplete neural deficit. Such instability may be either acute or chronic.

A spine is acutely unstable if it is capable of neurologically threatening displacement at the injured level during the period early after the injury. Although both angular and translational displacements are capable of producing neural damage, transverse translation, anteroposterior or lateral, is by far the most hazardous because a relatively small displacement may greatly reduce the space available for neural structures within the spinal canal (see Fig. 12-63).[136] As healing progresses, either by bone or by scar, translational mobility becomes progressively less and, after several weeks, it is no longer sufficient to threaten neural function. Since only marked degrees of angular displacement are capable of producing neural deficit secondary to distortion of the spinal canal (see Fig. 12-62), it is quite rare for neural deficit to occur in the early period after injury as a result of pure angular deformity. Translational mobility is rarely a feature of thoracolumbar fractures, but it is present to some

degree in all dislocations. Therefore, thoracolumbar fractures seldom exhibit acute instability, but all thoracolumbar dislocations and fracture-dislocations are examples of acute spinal instability.[184,208,229,241]

A spine is chronically unstable if it is capable of progressive deformity that may continue for months or years. As time passes and deformity increases, angulation becomes an increasing threat to neural function and may produce neurologic deficit years after the acute trauma (Fig. 12-67).[207] Chronic instability is seen in both fractures and dislocations of the thoracolumbar spine.[218]

Because of therapeutic and prognostic implications, it is desirable to identify the unstable spine injury. The direct approach to a determination of spinal stability would require an attempt to displace the injured segments (*i.e.,* flexion and extension x-rays) and observation of the direction and degree of displacement that occurs. Obviously such a procedure is too hazardous to be practical.

If one considers the spine as two structural columns,[187,243] it is possible to identify those injuries with the potential for acute (*i.e.,* transverse translational) instability. The anterior structural column

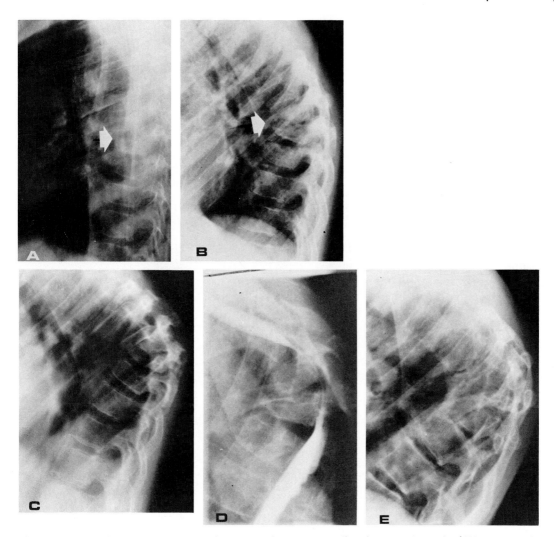

Fig. 12-67. (*A*) This patient sustained a minimal anterior wedge fracture (*arrow*) of T6. He was neurologically negative. A "prophylactic" laminectomy of T6 was performed. (*B*) Three months later there was definite progression of the flexion deformity. (*C*) One year after injury, the flexion deformity was severe. The patient had developed lower extremity clonus. (*D*) A myelogram made at that time shows an almost complete block. (*E*) An attempt at correction and anterior interbody fusion succeeded in halting progression of the kyphos. He has a persistent partial paraplegia and lower extremity clonus.

consists of the vertebral bodies and discs. The posterior structural column consists of the neural arch, associated processes, and ligaments. Acute instability (potential for transverse translational displacement) is possible only if both structural columns are disrupted (Fig. 12-68). If any degree of transverse translation can be observed, acute instability is certainly present (Fig. 12-69).

Chronic instability is more difficult to predict; it may occur with damage to only one of the two structural columns, but it is more likely if both columns are damaged.[218,229] Skeletal immaturity and laminectomy are especially likely to contribute to chronic instability (see Fig. 12-67).[138,194,247] Fortunately only a marked degree of angular displacement is likely to produce neurologic sequelae. Therefore, the ability to predict chronic instability is somewhat less important. One need only observe

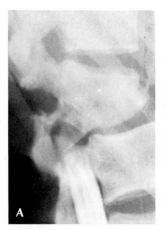
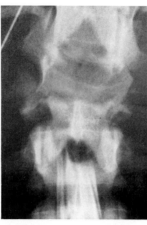
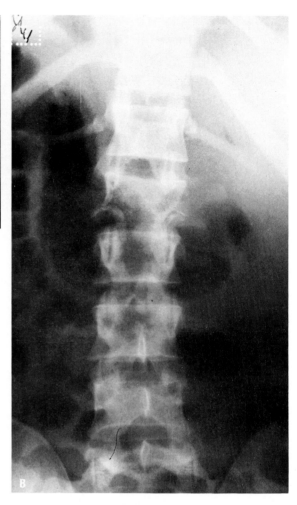

Fig. 12-68. Fracture of L1 with nearly complete neurologic deficit. (*A*) Preoperative myelogram showing a complete block, neural arch comminution, and vertebral body fractures. (*B*) Anteroposterior x-ray following total laminectomy of L1 and L2.

the patient over a period of time. The chronically unstable spine will identify itself by a gradual increase in angular deformity. Appropriate definitive therapy may be safely delayed until chronic instability has been thus confirmed. Surgical correction of a severe fixed spinal deformity is far more difficult than stabilization of a potentially unstable minimally deformed spine.[138,143,180] One must, therefore, guard against the insidious progression of deformity to a degree that is difficult to correct. In clinical situations where careful close monitoring of progressive deformity is difficult, it may be preferable to perform an early surgical stabilization on the suspicion of potential chronic instability rather than run the risk of allowing a severe and, perhaps, uncorrectable deformity to occur (see Fig. 12-67).[138,180]

PATHOMECHANICS OF SKELETAL DAMAGE

Thoracolumbar injuries are the result of either direct or indirect trauma. Those due to direct trauma are located at the point where traumatic force was applied. Direct trauma produces significant fracture or dislocation less often than indirect trauma. Fractures due to direct trauma are the product of direct blows from missiles, knives, clubs, or the like. The injured spine is rarely unstable, but neurologic deficit is relatively common, since the injuries are frequently complicated by open wounds of the dura, nerve roots, and spinal cord.[231] Neural deficit in these cases is the result of a penetrating foreign body or displaced fragments of bone (see Fig. 12-64). The associated fractures are seldom un-

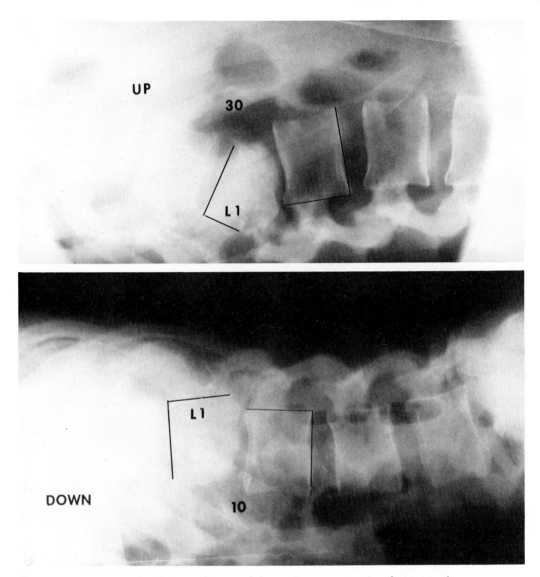

Fig. 12-68 (*Continued*). (C) Lateral x-ray of the patient on a turning frame, positioned face up and face down, demonstrating marked angular and translational displacement with change in position on the turning frame. This severe degree of instability is the result of traumatic disruption of both the anterior and posterior structural columns of the spine and was probably enhanced by a total laminectomy at two levels.

stable and seldom require treatment beyond basic wound care and pain control.[231]

Thoracolumbar fractures or dislocations due to indirect trauma characteristically occur at some distance from the points where the traumatizing force was applied. While instability and neurologic deficit are relatively uncommon, thoracolumbar

injuries due to indirect trauma are far more frequent than those due to direct trauma. Therefore, they account for most cases of neural deficit, at least in civilian practice. Injuries due to indirect trauma are the result of excessive load, muscular violence, motion beyond physiologic limits, or motion in a direction in which the spine does not normally

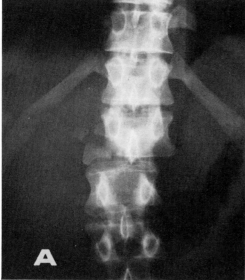
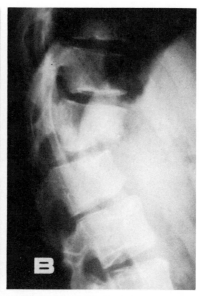
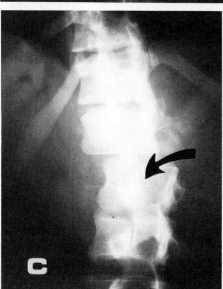

Fig. 12-69. In a typical fracture-dislocation produced by a combination of flexion and torsion, the anterior and posterior structural columns of this spine have been disrupted, and it is unstable. (*A*) Anteroposterior projection shows an oblique fracture line and lateral displacement as evidence of torsion. (*B*) Lateral projection shows an anterior wedge deformity of the vertebral body as evidence of flexion. Note the transverse translational displacement between L1 and L2. (*C*) An oblique projection shows the facet dislocation (*arrow*) particularly well.

bend. Any catalogue of traumatic pathomechanics must include hyperflexion, hyperextension, excessive lateral bending, excessive rotation, compression, distraction, shear fore and aft, and lateral shear.

ANGULAR STRESS

FLEXION

Flexion fractures are the most common of all failure patterns. They are most frequent at the thoracolumbar junction (Fig. 12-70), a region of transition between stiff and mobile areas of the spine.[174,175,208,241]

Flexion injuries are seen (but less frequently) at the lumbosacral junction, another region of transition between stiff and mobile spinal regions. If the flexing force is applied to the posterior thorax, as is the case when falling rocks land on a stooping miner, then the thoracolumbar junction is the most likely site of fracture.[208] If the flexing force is applied to the posterior pelvis, as happens when a patient falls from a height and lands on his buttocks, the lumbosacral junction is a likely site of fracture.[144]

Although no human joint has a fixed axis of rotation, the flexion axis of the thoracic and lumbar segments is always quite close to the center of the

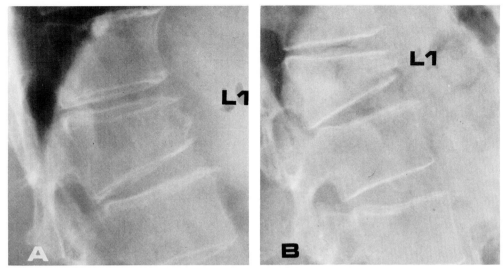

Fig. 12-70. (*A*) A typical flexion fracture characterized by an anterior wedge deformity of the body of L1. The fracture involves the anterior cortex of the body. The posterior cortex of the body and the neural arch are intact. The spinal canal has not been compromised. This spine is stable. (*B*) Two months later there has been a slight but definite increase in the degree of wedging. A small amount of progression of angular deformity is common but is of no functional or neurologic significance.

intervertebral disk.[208,243] In the thoracic region the distance between the flexion axis and the tip of the spinous process is three times greater than the distance between the axis and the anterior margin of the vertebral body. In the lumbar region, this ratio is 4:1. Therefore, when exposed to flexion stress, the anterior portion of the vertebral body experiences a compressive load that is three or four times greater than the tensile load experienced by the spinous process and supraspinous ligament (Fig. 12-71).[243] For this reason, hyperflexion produces a wedge-shaped fracture deformity of the vertebral body but it never results in posterior element avulsion or ligament rupture.[208,243] Greater flexion produces greater crushing, but it cannot produce a combination of wedge fracture of the vertebral body and rupture of the posterior ligaments. Crushing of the anterior body allows energy dissipation and damping of peak loads so that tensile stress sufficient to cause posterior ligament rupture cannot be generated by flexion alone.[243] Since flexion injures only the anterior structural column of the spine, flexion injuries do not exhibit acute instability and are generally neurologically benign.[144,208,210,241] The vertebral body fracture seldom involves the posterior cortex of the body. However, a very severe flexion injury may produce comminution of the posterior cortex of the vertebral body and cause neurologic loss due to posterior displace-

ment of vertebral body fragments. Chronic instability sufficient to cause neurologic loss as a result of progressive angular displacement is occasionally seen following a flexion fracture.[207]

EXTENSION

Hyperextension is an extremely common and important cause of cervical fractures and dislocations. However, in the thoracolumbar spine extension fractures are quite rare. When they do occur, they are most frequently seen in the mid-lumbar region. One may occasionally see an avulsion fracture of the anterior portion of the vertebral body or a fracture through the pars interarticularis (true traumatic spondylolysis).[232,239] Traumatic spondylolysis is now recognized to be a relatively frequent problem in female gymnasts, broad-jumpers, and football players at interior line positions.[164,179] Repeated forced lumbar extension is a common feature of these athletic activities, and is the probable cause of spondylolysis in these athletes. The lesion may progress to spondylolisthesis, especially in skeletally immature children and adolescents.[179] Except for the true traumatic spondylolysis with spondylolisthesis, extension injuries are stable and tend to do well regardless of treatment. They usually heal by bone, and neurologic deficit is extremely uncommon.

LATERAL BENDING

Excessive lateral bending produces asymmetrical loading of the vertebral body and may result in a lateral wedge fracture (see Fig. 12-64), which is basically quite similar to the anterior wedge fracture produced by hyperflexion.[208] Lateral bending fractures are relatively uncommon, but when they occur they are most often in the mid-lumbar region. They are basically stable and seldom associated with neural deficit and they require no treatment beyond control of symptoms.

ROTATION

The vast majority of rotational thoracolumbar fractures occur between T10 and L1.[193] The first through the tenth thoracic vertebrae articulate with ribs in a way that increases their resistance to torsion. The lumbar spine has an inherently high torsional stiffness due, in large part, to the orientation of its facets. Due to its transitional characteristics, the region between T10 and L1 has relatively great rotational mobility. Therefore, it is especially susceptible to those fractures in which torsion plays an important role.[243] While a fracture due to rotation alone is quite rare (Fig. 12-72), a combination of rotation and flexion is the most common cause of dislocation and fracture-dislocation in the thoracolumbar spine (see Fig. 12-69).[173,208,241] When the spine is exposed to combined rotation and flexion, the flexion component may produce a wedge fracture of the vertebral body, but flexion alone cannot cause disruption of the neural arch or posterior ligament structures because too little posterior tension is generated. If there is simultaneous rotation, neural arch tension may be increased to the point of structural failure.[217,243]

An anteroposterior x-ray often shows an oblique fracture of the vertebral body with lateral displacement as evidence of torsional stress. A wedge fracture of the vertebral body (best seen in the lateral projection) is clear evidence of the role played by flexion. (see Fig. 12-69) The "slice" fracture-dislocation, which Holdsworth[173,174] has emphasized as an especially unstable spinal injury, is a variant of the rotation-flexion injury, the result of relatively more rotation and relatively less flexion.

Although flexion and torsion are angular motions, their combination may yield a transverse translational displacement if there has been significant disruption of both structural columns. Neural deficit due to spinal instability is seen in 60% to 70% of all thoracolumbar dislocations and fracture-dislocations.[184,208,229,241]

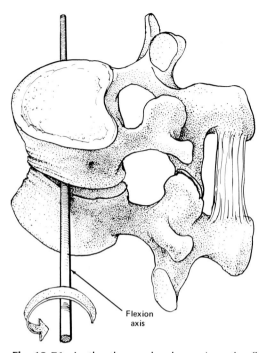

Fig. 12-71. In the thoracolumbar spine, the flexion axis passes through the nucleus of the disk. The distance from the flexion axis to the tip of the spinous process is three to four times greater than the distance from the axis to the anterior margin of the vertebral body. With hyperflexion the anterior body receives a compressive load which is three to four times greater than the tensile load placed on the supraspinous ligament. Therefore, an anterior body fracture occurs prior to posterior ligament rupture. Larger forces produce more wedging. As the anterior body deformation progresses, energy is dissipated so that posterior ligament rupture does not occur with pure flexion. (Smith, W. S., and Kaufer, H.: Patterns and mechanisms of Lumbar Injuries Associated with Lap Seat Belts. J. Bone Joint Surg., **51A**:239–254, 1969.)

The more unstable the spine, the more likely it is that spontaneous reduction will occur when the patient is placed in a supine position. Due to spontaneous reduction, a dangerously unstable spine may show little or no displacement in the x-rays.[173,184] It is, therefore, extremely important to recognize the potential for acute instability by analyzing the extent of damage to the two structural columns of the spine with an adequate x-ray evaluation. A thorough knowledge of unstable fracture patterns will allow the surgeon to identify those injuries that are potentially dangerous and which may benefit from effective stabilization.

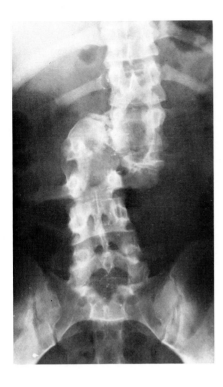 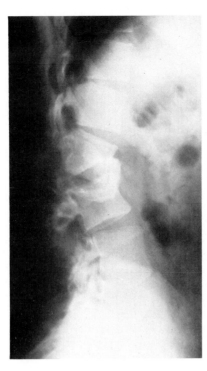

Fig. 12-72. Anteroposterior and lateral x-rays of a pure torsional fracture of the lumbar spine with an oblique fracture extending from L1–L2 and complete lateral displacement. Whether in a long bone or in the spine, an oblique fracture line at approximately a 45° angle to the long axis of the bone and side-to-side displacement of the fragment are the hallmarks of a torsional fracture. The spine has healed in this position. The patient is neurologically normal and back symptoms are minimal.

Rotational trauma also plays a dominant role in production of the common posterolateral disk herniation and secondary sciatica.[162] Although it is often assumed that herniation of disk material through the annulus is due to compressive force, studies by Brown[139] and Virgin[236] show that this is not the case. Excellent biomechanical studies by Farfan strongly suggest that rotation is primarily responsible for this lesion.[162]

NONANGULAR STRESS

SHEAR

Following severe trauma, marked translational displacement of spinal segments may be seen. The spine in Figure 12-73 shows no posterior ligament disruption and no side-to-side displacement or rotational displacement of the injured segments. Since there is neither a wedge fracture of the vertebral body nor angular displacement, there is no evidence of flexion. This gross dislocation cannot, therefore, be explained by the usual rotation plus flexion mechanism. It is the result of transverse shear and is highly unstable. As in other cases of marked transverse translation, neurologic deficit, after a shearing fracture, is very common.[149] However, there is some hope for neural sparing. For example, the patient shown in Figure 12-73 was neurolog-

ically negative. In the majority of anterioposterior shear fractures, the cranial segments are displaced anterior to the caudal segments as in figure 12-73. These fractures occur most often in the mid- and upper lumbar spine. An important subtype of the anteroposterior shear fracture was described by De Oliveira in 1978.[149] In this fracture, the caudal segments are displaced anterior to the cranial segments (Fig. 12-74). Almost all have some degree of neurologic deficit. Unlike the more common variety of shear fractures with anterior displacement of the cranial segments in which open reduction is usually successful, complete reduction of shear fractures with anterior displacement of the caudal segments by either open or closed techniques is virtually impossible and has not been reported.[149]

Treatment of shear injuries must correct the instability in order to avoid progressive neurologic loss and enhance the possibility of neural recovery. In all cases of translational instability, the goals of acute fracture management are restoration of spinal alignment and stability.[175,184,199,244]

COMPRESSION

Although they are quite different, the compression fracture and flexion fracture are often confused. Compression fractures are the result of excessive vertical load without flexion, rotation, or lateral

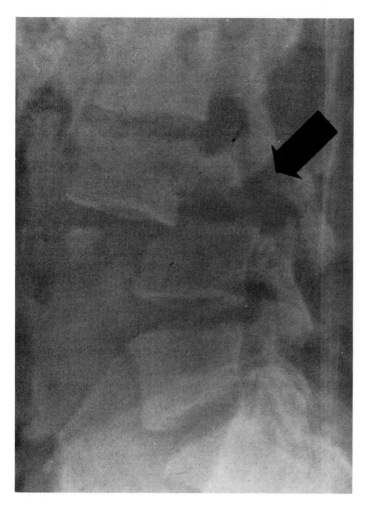

Fig. 12-73. Severe transverse translational displacement due to anteroposterior shear. There is no residual evidence of either torsion or flexion. Note the grossly displaced fracture through the pars interarticularis of L3. This is a true traumatic spondylolysis. The patient was neurologically negative. He has performed his own laminectomy.

bending.[17] They are most common in the mid-lumbar region. An effective crash restraint system, such as a lap belt combined with shoulder harness, restricts angular displacement of the spine during stress. Such a system favors production of compression fractures, which are often seen in race car drivers and in pilots who have used an ejection seat. Load secondary to muscle contraction alone may produce compression fracture, especially in osteoporotic bone.[148]

Due to its very high water content, an intact nucleus is not compressible under load.[217] Its behavior is characteristically hydraulic. However, the adjacent cancellous bone is readily deformable and, if loaded sufficiently, it will fracture centrally, producing an imprint of the adjacent noncompressible, spherical nucleus (Fig. 12-75). Significant damage is limited to the anterior structural column of the spine. The compression fracture is, therefore,

stable and rarely associated with neural deficit. The familiar Schmorl's node[220] (protrusion of the nuclear material through the vertebral end plate) is an expression of the compression fracture mechanism. However, protrusion of nuclear material through the annulus of a normal intervertebral disk is never the result of compression alone.[139,236]

Although the typical compression fracture of a vertebral body is produced by invasion of the cranial disk, a comparable fracture may be produced by invasion of the caudal disk. If a vertebral body is invaded by both of its adjacent disks, a highly characteristic biconcave profile is produced. The familiar "codfish" spine, sometimes seen in advanced cases of osteoporosis, is a clear example of bone deformation due to chronic compressive stress (Fig. 12-76). When subjected to extreme compressive loads, the spherical depression of the superior and inferior vertebral end-plates may be joined by

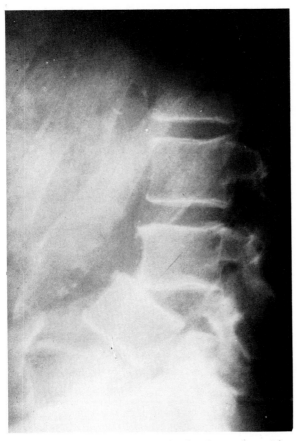

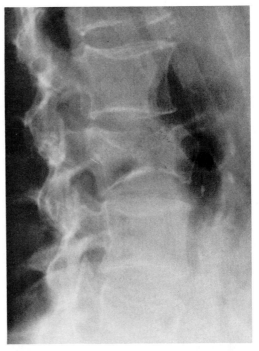

Fig. 12-75. Lateral projection of a compression fracture of L3. The center of the vertebral body is distorted more than the anterior or posterior margins. Note the circular profile of the deformed superior and inferior vertebral end plates produced by an intact disk nucleus. The comminuted anterior body has been displaced anteriorly. The spinal canal is not distorted. The neural arch is intact. This spine is stable. Compression fractures frequently occur at multiple levels.

Fig. 12-74. Shear fracture of the lumbar spine with marked anterior displacement of L4 and L5.

a vertical fracture line as the invading nuclei split the vertebral body in two (Fig. 12-77). The fracture configuration thus produced is the "burst" fracture, described so well by Holdsworth (Fig. 12-78).[173] Like other compression injuries, the burst fracture is stable but, in severe cases of burst fracture, the posterior portion of the fractured vertebral body may be displaced posteriorly into the spinal canal. Neurologic deficit in these cases is due to the displaced fragment and does not indicate spinal instability.

A compressive load acting parallel to the long axis of the spine will produce a compression fracture if it passes directly through the center of the nucleus (Fig. 12-79). If the compression vector of the load passes anterior to the nucleus, the spine will be forced into flexion and a flexion fracture is likely to occur.[243] Because of the normal thoracic kyphosis and the lumbar lordosis, a compressive load is more

likely to produce a flexion fracture in the thoracic spine and an extension fracture of the lumbar spine (Fig. 12-79). A typical compression fracture (see Figs. 12-75 and 12-77) occurs only if the resultant compression vector passes through, or very close to, the center of the nucleus.[243] If large compressive loads are applied to a spine with degenerated and extensively fibrosed intervertebral discs, the resulting fracture will be a uniform flattening of the involved vertebral body rather than the spherical depression that is produced by a healthy nucleus pulposus.[217]

DISTRACTION

Distraction or tension fractures of the thoracolumbar spine are most common between L1 and L4 (Fig. 12-80).[225] These injuries are uncommon, but are frequently seen in patients who were wearing a lap seat belt at the time of injury.[216,225] Since there

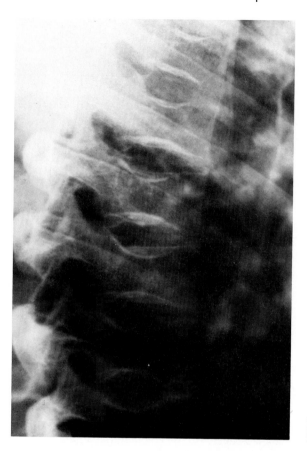

Fig. 12-76. Multiple central depressions of vertebral bodies in an osteoporotic spine ("codfish spine").

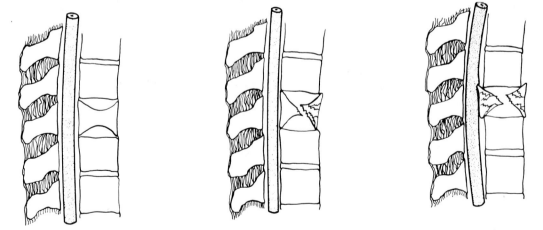

Fig. 12-77. Progressive degrees of compression fracture. (*Left*) Severe compression fracture showing the biconcave profile produced by the adjacent disks. (*Center*) A more severe degree of fracture. A vertical fracture has joined the deformed concave end plates. The anterior body fragment is comminuted and displaced anteriorly. (*Right*) A more severe degree of compression fracture. The posterior body fragment is now comminuted and displaced posteriorly into the spinal canal. Neural damage may occur. The neural arch is intact. This spine is stable.

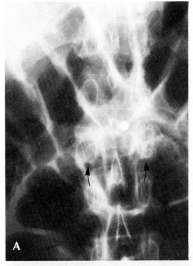

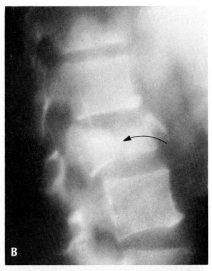

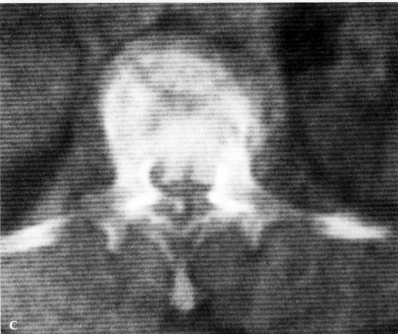

Fig. 12-78. Burst fracture of L2 due to excessive compression load. (*A*) Anteroposterior x-ray showing compression of the body of L2 and interpedicular widening (*arrows*). There is no increase in the interspinous distance. (*B*) Lateral x-ray shows a spherical depression of both the superior and inferior end-plates. There is a vertical fracture line (*arrow*) through the center of the vertebral body. Note posterior displacement of vertebral body substance into the spinal canal. (*C*) Transverse CT scan of a section of L2. Note the stellate configuration of the fracture through the vertebral body with centripetal displacement of fragments including posterior displacement nearly occluding the spinal canal. (Courtesy of E. Shannon Stauffer, M.D., Springfield, Illinois.)

is no vertebral body wedging, no torsional displacement, and no transverse displacement, neither flexion, torsion, nor shear could have produced these spinal disruptions. The x-rays suggest that these spines were literally pulled apart (Fig. 12-80).

When the wearer of a lap-type seat belt is subjected to sudden deceleration, his body is flexed over the restraining belt. In this situation, the point of contact between the belt and the abdominal wall becomes the axis around which flexion occurs (Fig.

12-81). All portions of the spinal column are posterior to the flexion axis. Therefore, the entire vertebral body is exposed to tensile stress as well as the neural arch.

Fractures and dislocations of the lumbar spine associated with a lap seat belt may occur through soft tissue only, through bone only, or through both. Because of the known tendency for bone to be avulsed when ligaments are subjected to tension, the "all bone" variety of lumbar seat belt injury is especially good evidence of failure due to tensile stress (Fig. 12-82). This fracture, first described by C. Q. Chance, is extremely rare, except in patients who wear a lap seat belt at the time of injury.[142,184,225]

Distraction (seat belt) injuries are usually neurologically benign. Although the typical distraction pattern shows considerable longitudinal translation, the type of displacement most likely to cause neural damage (severe angular displacement or significant transverse translational displacement) is notably absent. Neural damage due to spinal instability is seen in less than 5% of patients with the tension pattern of failure.[225]

However, due to destruction of both structural columns of the spine (see Fig. 12-80), a distraction dislocation or fracture-dislocation is acutely unstable and has the potential for significant transverse translational displacement and subsequent neurologic damage. Treatment must, therefore, control instability and maintain alignment of the spine in order to avoid progressive neurologic loss.[187,225,244]

In sharp contrast to the instability of distraction dislocations, distraction fractures (Chance fractures) are stable.[142,181,225] Although the Chance fracture damages both structural columns of the spine, there is minimal damage to the major ligaments (see Fig. 12-82). The injury consists of a

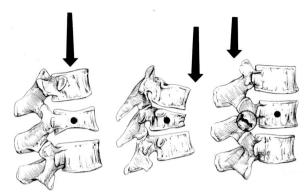

Fig. 12-79. The effect of compression loads on the spine. (*Left*) If the compression vector of the load passes through or near the flexion axis, then a central depression-"compression" fracture of the vertebral body may occur. The load produces neither flexion nor extension. (*Center*) If the compression vector or the load passes anterior to the flexion axis, the spine will be forced into flexion and an anterior wedge, "flexion" fracture may occur. Due to the normal thoracic kyphosis, this is more likely to occur in the mid-thoracic spine. (*Right*) If the compression vector of the load passes posterior to the flexion axis of the spine, the spine will be forced into extension and a neural arch fracture, true traumatic spondylolysis, may occur. Due to the normal lumbar lordosis, this is more likely to occur in the mid-lumbar spine.

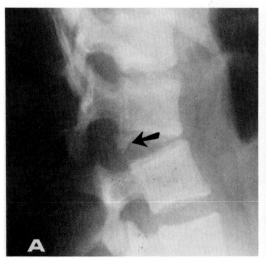
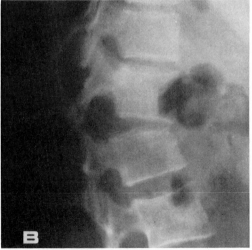

Fig. 12-80. Distraction fracture-dislocations of L1 on L2 occurring in a mother (*A*) and daughter (*B*) when they were involved in a deceleration-type of automobile crash. Both were wearing lap seat belts. Posterior structural column disruption is indicated by the neural arch separation and facet dislocations. The widened disk space is evidence of disruption of the anterior structural column. These spines are unstable. The displacement that occurred is mostly longitudinal translation. The posterior body fragment (*A, arrow*) is characteristic of an avulsion fracture. These spines were literally pulled apart. (Smith, W. S., and Kaufer, H.: Patterns and Mechanisms of Lumbar Injuries Associated with Lap Seat Belts. J. Bone Joint Surg., **51A:** 239–254, 1969.)

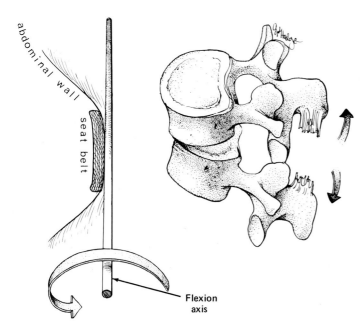

Flexion axis

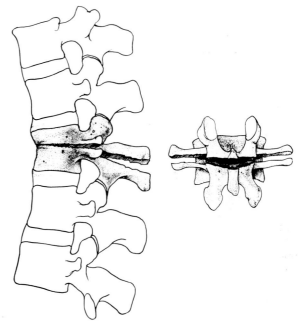

Fig. 12-81. Abnormal lumbar mechanics occur during deceleration in a person wearing a lap belt. The flexion axis passes through the point of contact between the belt and the abdominal wall. All portions of the spine are posterior to this axis and are subjected to tensile stress. (Smith, W. S., and Kaufer, H.: Patterns and Mechanisms of Lumbar Injuries Associated with Lap Seat Belts. J. Bone Joint Surg., **51A:**239–254, 1969.)

transverse, noncomminuted fracture of the vertebral body and neural arch.[142] In spite of definite disruption of both structural columns of the spine, interdigitation of irregularities on the opposing fracture surfaces accounts for the Chance fracture's resistance to transverse translational displacement. The typical Chance fracture is, therefore, quite stable, nonprogressive, and heals rapidly by bone.[142,181,216,225]

VIOLENT MUSCLE FORCES

Fracture of a lumbar transverse process is the most common thoracolumbar fracture due to muscle force alone. Transverse process fractures are most often multiple (Fig. 12-83). The spine is seldom unstable, but nonunion of the transverse process fracture is common. In spite of this, the prognosis is excellent.[239] Relief of symptoms is the only requirement of treatment.

In contrast to the cervical spine, avulsion fracture of a spinous process is quite uncommon in the lumbar and thoracic spine.[136,239]

Occasionally a compression or flexion fracture of the vertebral body may be the result of muscle violence alone.[239] If there is significant osteoporosis, these fractures are more likely. Vertebral body fracture due to muscle force alone is more common in the thoracic than in the lumbar spine.[148] Spine fractures secondary to convulsion—whether natural or iatrogenic (*e.g.*, shock therapy for psychosis)—tend to occur in the upper half of the thoracic region.[136,148,239]

Fig. 12-82. The "all bone" variety of lumbar distraction injury. (Smith, W. S., and Kaufer, H.: Patterns and Mechanisms of Lumbar Injuries Associated with Lap Seat Belts. J. Bone Joint Surg., **51A:**239–254,1969.)

DIAGNOSIS

HISTORY

Most patients with a thoracolumbar fracture give a clear history of a sudden violent episode of trauma followed by severe and persistent localized back-ache. The back pain is relieved when the patient lies recumbent and is exacerbated when the patient is moving, bearing weight, or coughing. A description of the accident may supply enough information to direct attention to a specific area, which is especially useful if the patient is unconscious. For example, if a patient wearing a lap seat belt is involved in a head-on automobile collision, special attention should be directed to the mid- and upper lumbar regions. If the patient was injured as the result of a cave-in, special attention should be directed to the thoracolumbar junction. The examiner should be immediately alerted to the possibility of a thoracolumbar spine injury if the patient complains of impaired sensation or decreased motor function of one or both lower extremities.

Sometimes the history describes a traumatic event that seems quite trivial, such as a violent sneeze or stooping to lift a very light object. Fractures due to apparently trivial trauma usually occur in osteoporotic or otherwise abnormal bone and should alert one to the possibility of a pathologic fracture. Fractures resulting from this type of trauma are flexion or compression fractures and are almost always stable and seldom associated with neurologic loss. However, they are true fractures and are sometimes associated with severe and prolonged backache.

PHYSICAL SIGNS

If thoracolumbar injury is suspected, the patient should be examined in the position in which he is first seen. If the spinal injury is grossly unstable, displacement may occur as the patient is being positioned for physical examination. This can significantly increase his neural damage. The physician should resist the temptation to place the patient in the conventional supine position for physical examination. An adequate screening physical examination can be performed with the patient in a lateral or prone position. Determination of blood pressure, pulse, respiration, assessment of the airway, and evaluation of gross hemorrhage certainly claim first priority. Attention may then be turned to evaluating the suspected thoracolumbar spine injury.

An adequate evaluation cannot be performed if the patient is clothed. Clothing must be removed so that the entire area of interest is available for unhampered palpation and visual inspection. In order to avoid displacement of an unstable spine, it is usually safest to cut off the clothing. Suitable

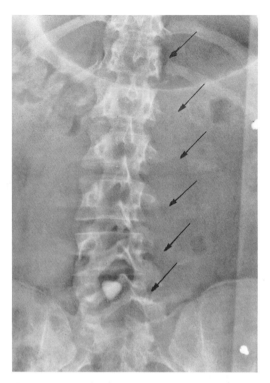

Fig. 12-83. Multiple transverse process fractures (*arrows*) with marked displacement. The retained myelographic dye is from a diagnostic procedure that antedated this injury.

draping will meet the demands of modesty and preserve the patient's dignity.

The entire trunk should be inspected for contusions, abrasions, or other cutaneous evidence of trauma. Swelling, mass, ecchymosis, or distortion of the expected thoracic kyphosis and lumbar lordosis are obviously significant. The thoracolumbar region should be palpated carefully, especially the posterior midline. The spinous processes should be in a straight line, at regular intervals, with no step-off or interspinous gap.

Physical examination of patients who have sustained a thoracolumbar fracture is often very unimpressive. Flexion and compression injuries, which account for the majority of thoracolumbar fractures, have skeletal damage limited to the vertebral body and, therefore, show no posterior mass, misalignment, or localized tenderness. However, these patients usually show paravertebral muscle guarding, limitation of spine motion, diffuse paraspinous tenderness, and tenderness to percussion along the posterior midline. Some exhibit tenderness on deep abdominal palpation. Spines with more severe injury exhibit a local gibbus at the level of injury

(Fig. 12-84).[136,208] If there has been a significant neural arch injury, one may identify posterior swelling, sharply localized tenderness, a palpable interspinous gap, or a step-off. These findings are highly suggestive of acute spinal instability.[136,208] A spine with these signs should be considered acutely unstable until proved otherwise.

One should always look for cutaneous contusions and abrasions. A contusion over the scapula suggests a flexion-plus-rotation injury and should direct attention to a possible fracture-dislocation at the thoracolumbar junction. A transverse, lower abdominal seat belt contusion (Fig. 12-85) would strongly suggest the possibility of a seat belt (distraction) fracture. Seat belt contusions are present in 80% of patients with a seat belt fracture, but absence of contusion at the initial examination is not a source of reassurance because cutaneous evidence of the contusion may not appear until 48 to 72 hours after injury.[184]

A careful peripheral neurologic examination is essential in all cases of suspected vertebral fracture.[168,221] A record of the initial *and* serial examinations of spinal cord injured patients is critical in documenting the level of the initial injury and in following progression of any neurological deficit (Fig. 12-86). The Spinal Cord Injury form provides such a record and should become a *permanent* part of the patients's chart. Using such a tabular form makes leaving out critical parts of the examination (*i.e.,* perianal sensation) less likely. Its use as a document when patients are transferred is invaluable. One must survey voluntary control and grade the strength of all lower extremity and trunk muscles. Elevation and separation of the costal margins with deep inspiration indicates intact in-

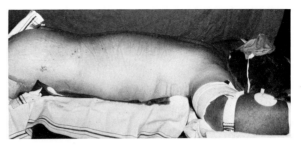

Fig. 12-84. Thoracolumbar kyphus in a patient with post-traumatic fracture-dislocation at the thoracolumbar junction.

tercostal muscles. Abdominal bulging when coughing is attempted suggests abdominal paralysis. Cephalad migration of the umbilicus with an attempted cough indicates lower abdominal muscle paralysis. Discrete voluntary control of toe flexors and extensors is especially important because intact toe flexors and extensor function may be the only clinical sign that a neurologic lesion is incomplete. Discrete toe function can be of enormous prognostic significance. Unfortunately, determination of voluntary control of toe flexors and extensors, and much of the rest of a complete motor examination, are often neglected in an emergency room examination.

All deep tendon reflexes, abdominal cutaneous reflexes, the cremasteric reflex, and the bulbocavernosus reflex should be tested. A digital rectal examination allows one to judge anal sphincter tone while testing for the bulbocavernosus reflex. Paralyzed muscles with an intact deep tendon reflex usually indicate a spinal cord or upper motor neuron lesion, while muscle paralysis with an

(*Text continues on p. 1066.*)

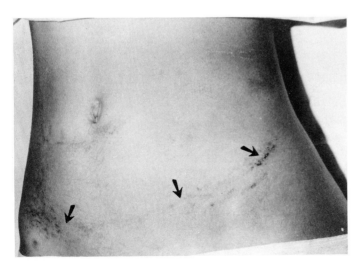

Fig. 12-85. A characteristic seat-belt contusion (*arrows*) traversing the lower abdomen from one anterior superior iliac spine to the other. (Smith, W. S., and Kaufer, H.: Patterns and Mechanisms of Lumbar Injuries Associated with Lap Seat Belts. J. Bone Joint Surg., **51A**:239–254, 1969.)

IN-PATIENT NOTES
Neurological Exam Flow-Sheet

SPINAL CORD INJURY RECORD OF EXAMINATION

(When to fill out: Admission daily X3)

Date:

DATE & TIME OF INJURY _____

LOCATION	DATE	SERVICE
Reg. No.		Class
		Name
		Address

			Examiner:									
			Date/Time:									
				R	L	R	L	R	L	R	L	R	L

†MOTOR			R	L	R	L	R	L	R	L	R	L
Shoulder	Deltoid	C5										
Elbow	Flex.	C5,C6										
	Ext.	C7										
Wrist	Ext.	C6										
	Flex.	C7										
Fingers	Flex.	C8,T1										
	Ext.	C7,C8										
	Abd. (intrinsics)	T1										
Trunk	Up Abdom.	T5-T10										
	Low Abdom.	T10-T12										
Hip	Flex.	L1.2.3										
	Abd.	L4,5										
Knee	Ext.	L3,4										
	Flex. (med. Ham.)	L4,5										
	Flex. (lat. Ham.)	L5,S1										
Ankle	Dorsiflex (Ant.Tib.)	L4,5										
	Plan, Flex. (Gastroc.)	S1										
Foot	Ev. (PL,PB)	S1										
Hallux	Ext. (EHL)	L5										
Toes	Flex. (FDL)	S1										
Rectal Tone												
††REFLEXES:	Biceps	C5										
	Brachioradialis	C6										
	Triceps	C7										
	Knee jerk	L2,3,4										
	Ankle jerk	S1										
	Bulbocavernosus	S2,3,4										
	Anal wink	S2,3,4										
	Cremasteric	T12										
	Plantar	UMN										

†MOTOR GRADING KEY:

5	100%	N	Normal:	Complete ROM against gravity with full resistance.
4	75%	G	Good:	Complete ROM against gravity with some resistance.
3	50%	F	Fair:	Complete ROM against gravity only.
2	25%	P	Poor:	Complete ROM with gravity eliminated.
1	10%	T	Trace:	Evidence of slight contractility with no joint motion.
0	0%	0	Zero:	No evidence of contractility.

S - Spasm   If spasm, contracture, or injury limit ROM,
C - Contracture   place S, C, or I after the grade of a movement
I - Injury   incomplete for this reason.

††REFLEX GRADING KEY:

0 - No activity
1 - decreased activity
2 - Normal activity
3 - Hyperactive
4 - Clonus

II-2042289   THE UNIVERSITY OF MICHIGAN—UNIVERSITY HOSPITAL   (flip up and over)

Start writing here:

Examiner:										
Date/Time:										
	R	L	R	L	R	L	R	L	R	L

SENSATION (Indicate Last Normal Level)

Pin prick										
Light touch										
Warm										
Cold										
*Deep pain: heel cord										
*Vibration MM/RS**										
*Position sense: fingers										
toes										

*Record N = Normal, I = Impaired, A = Absent
**MM/RS = Medial Malleolus/Radial Styloid

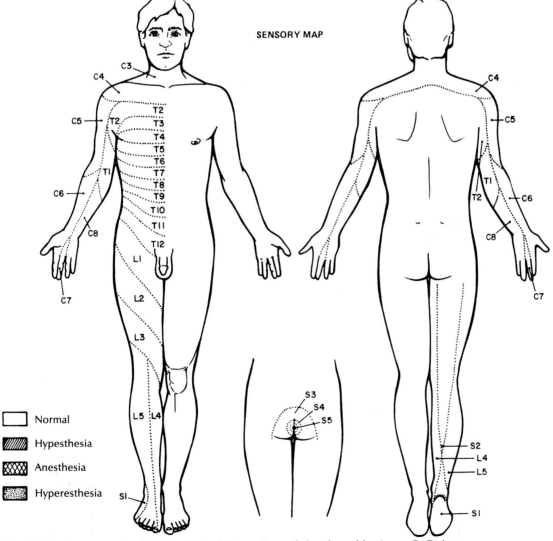

SENSORY MAP

Normal
Hypesthesia
Anesthesia
Hyperesthesia

◀ **Fig. 12-86.** An example of a Spinal Cord Injury Record developed by Jesse C. DeLee, M.D., of the University of Texas Medical School at San Antonio.

absent deep tendon reflex generally indicates a lower motor neuron (cauda equina) lesion with a comparatively favorable prognosis. However, in the period immediately after injury, absence of a deep tendon reflex is not a reliable basis for differentiating between upper and lower motor neuron damage because the reflex may be inhibited by post-traumatic spinal shock.[182] Post-traumatic spinal shock is a temporary state of total absence of all spinal reflex activity distal to a spinal cord injury. Absence of spinal reflexes due to this common phenomenon seldom lasts more than 24 hours (see the section on spinal shock). Return of the bulbocavernosus reflex is a reliable sign that the period of post-traumatic spinal shock has passed[169] (see p. 993).

Sensory testing, because of its highly subjective nature, is often inconsistent and sometimes misleading. Sensory testing should, however, always be done, especially in the perianal area, because many cord levels are represented in this relatively small cutaneous area. Preservation of a small area of cutaneous sensation in this region may be the only evidence that an apparent complete lesion is actually an incomplete lesion with a much more favorable prognosis. The minimal sensory examination should include sharp-dull discrimination with a needle, light touch, and deep pain, as well as motion and position sense of the toes bilaterally.

RADIOGRAPHIC SIGNS

Anteroposterior and lateral projections are the minimal radiographic views required in any case of suspected thoracolumbar fracture or dislocation.[218] By careful positioning of the plate and tube it is usually possible to safely obtain these views as well as oblique projections, even with the most unstable spine.[184] Laminagrams may be very helpful in clarifying obscure situations,[221,224] but they need not be a part of all, or even most, spine injury evaluations. When laminagraphy is indicated, anteroposterior projections are usually less informative than the lateral projection. The x-rays should be scrutinized for evidence of communication or displacement of the posterior cortex of the vertebral body, transverse translation displacement, or disruption of the posterior neural arch, since these are the features of an unstable or neurologically threatening spinal injury. Flexion-extension and lateral bending films are potentially hazardous at the initial emergency examination and should not be performed unless the physical examination and standard films have convinced you that the spine is stable.

CT scans can be of great value in demonstrating the details of the fracture and the relation of displaced fragments to the neural canal (Fig. 12-87).[211] The addition of metrizamide into the epidural space allows CT scans to define precisely the relation of both bone and soft tissue fragments to the dural tube and demonstrate the space available for the spinal cord and its roots.[151,211] One must recognize, however, that demonstration of a fragment or fragments within the spinal canal is not an indication for their removal unless neurologic signs due to the displaced fragments are present.

Myelography provides excellent visualization of the dural tube, but a myelogram is of little practical value for evaluating most thoracolumbar fractures.[168,175,184] Although some surgeons believe that a myelographic block is an indication for surgical decompression,[231] neural damage is better evaluated by a clinical neurologic examination.[182] Holdsworth and Hardy[175] have observed that myelography is not an aid in deciding about the need for decompression because they have seen cases of complete block without neurologic deficit and, conversely, complete neurologic deficit without a block. In most cases, the myelogram is not needed for localization, because the location of neural damage is clearly indicated by the location of the fracture, which is readily apparent on standard x-rays of the spine.

A myelogram is clearly indicated only for those patients with post-traumatic neurologic deficit who have no apparent skeletal damage or in patients whose neurologic deficit does not correlate with the level of skeletal damage.[168,182] Other specialized x-ray techniques, such as angiography, magnification, and subtraction, have not yet earned a place in the clinical evaluation of an acute spine injury.

DIFFERENTIAL DIAGNOSIS

Post-traumatic fracture or dislocation of the thoracolumbar spine is seldom a diagnostic problem. However, some congenital and some acquired conditions can mimic the x-ray appearance of these injuries.

A diminutive lumbar rib may be mistaken for a transverse process fracture (Fig. 12-88). This congenital variant is almost always limited to the first lumbar segment and may be bilateral.[140,189] The rib and transverse process have a smooth, rounded contour. Close inspection may reveal a well-developed costotransverse articulation. By contrast, a true traumatic transverse process fracture (see Fig.

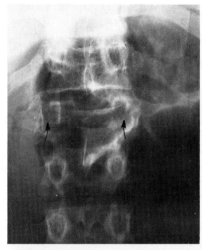
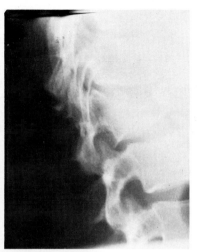
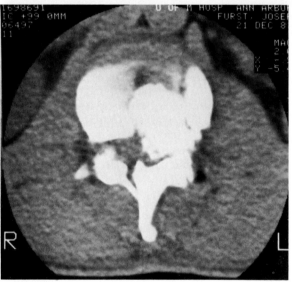

Fig. 12-87. (*Top*) Injury of L1 with comminuted fracture of the neural arch and interpedicular widening. Interpedicular widening (*arrows*) is commonly associated with lacerations of the dura and division of nerve roots[194] as was the case in this patient. (*Bottom*) CT scan of L1 showing nearly complete obliteration of the spinal canal by displaced fragments of the vertebral body on the left side. Findings at surgery confirmed a laceration of the dura and complete division of all roots of the cauda equina to the left of the midline with complete neurologic deficit on the left and neurologic sparing on the right.

12-83) is usually multiple, occurs at lower lumbar levels, and is almost always unilateral. The fracture surfaces have a jagged appearance.

Congenital kyphosis,[246] particularly when associated with total or partial absence of a vertebral body, closely resembles the x-ray appearance of an anterior wedge vertebral body fracture (Fig. 12-89). More severe degrees of deformity can mimic a fracture-dislocation. The tendency for these anomalies to occur at the thoracolumbar junction makes it even more likely for them to be confused with a post-traumatic deformity. Differentiation between traumatic and congenital deformity may have to depend on details of the history because, in some cases, there is no certain way to make the distinction by radiographic criteria.

The somewhat more common lateral hemivertebra[140,196] can be confused with a lateral bending vertebral body fracture. However, the congenital anomaly is usually associated with unilateral absence of a pedicle. This is never seen in lateral wedge fractures of the vertebral body.

Juvenile vertebral apophysitis (Scheuermann's disease) and mild forms of spondylolepiphyseal dysplasia may be confused with anterior wedge fractures of the thoracic vertebral bodies.[140] These conditions can usually be distinguished from post-traumatic deformity because, unlike trauma, the wedging deformity is usually present at several levels and is associated with marked narrowing of the intervening discs.

Spondylolisthesis[140,246] associated with spondy-

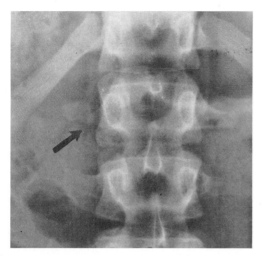

Fig. 12-88. Unilateral lumbar rib (*arrow*).

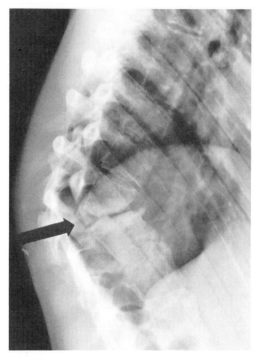

Fig. 12-89. Congenital thoracolumbar kyphos. Note the hypoplastic vertebral body (*arrow*) at the apex.

lolysis is seldom the result of a single traumatic episode. It is almost always located at L5 and may or may not be associated with backache. The roentgenographic appearance of the pars interarticularis defect is smooth and does not suggest an acute fracture. Spondylolysis due to repeated hy-

perextension strain in some young athletes is more likely to have the sharp edge, jagged fracture line appearance of an acute fracture. True traumatic spondylolysis, due to a single episode of trauma, is very rare.[232] It tends to occur at mid- or upper lumbar levels and may heal by bone if recognized promptly and treated adequately (see Figs. 12-96 and 12-97). The pars defect shows the jagged irregularity characteristic of acute fractures. A radionucleotide bone scan can be of great value in differentiating developmental pars interarticulars defects from those due to recent trauma. A "cold" scan strongly suggests that the pars defect is old rather than of relatively recent traumatic origin.

LABORATORY EXAMINATION

Because most thoracolumbar fractures follow an episode of significant trauma, the laboratory workup should include a survey of vital functions. Urinalysis, hematocrit, and white count determinations are definitely indicated, as well as an x-ray of the chest. Most patients should have an electrocardiogram (EKG) to detect cardiac contusion and to serve as a baseline for the patient with coronary artery disease. The electromyogram (EMG) is of little value and is seldom indicated in the period early after injury. Other laboratory studies may be indicated by specific circumstances in a given patient.

TREATMENT

Stimulated by the fact that a crooked back is the universal stigma of a cripple and guided by the principle that function depends on structure, physicians since antiquity have struggled to restore anatomical alignment to the traumatically deformed spine. Davis,[147] Böhler,[136] and Watson-Jones[239] have been among the most vocal advocates of manipulative reduction for post-traumatic spinal deformity. They claim improved posture, decreased symptoms, better neurologic recovery, and less stiffness as benefits of reduction. Their hyperextension techniques are quite effective for closed reduction of flexion and compression fractures of the lower thoracic and lumbar spine. However, flexion injuries above T9 can seldom be reduced (and even less often maintained) by hyperextension techniques.[135,212,241] Recognizing that upper thoracic flexion deformity seldom responds to closed reduction, Böhler[135] believed so strongly in the benefits of reduction that he advocated open reduction of these injuries through a transthoracic approach. However, many other surgeons believe that reduction is neither necessary nor desirable.[168,173,174,208,241]

On the basis of his wide experience as consulting surgeon to The British Miners' Welfare Commission, Nicoll,[208] in a classic paper published in 1949, challenged the virtue of reduction for all patients. He pointed out that even in the lower thoracic and lumbar regions, complete reduction is not consistently accomplished and such reduction as is achieved is seldom maintained.[229] His observation of lack of correlation between reduction and long-term symptoms or function was even more important.

Nicoll[208] even suggests a negative correlation, since the best functional results (based on a fracture patient's ability to return to mining underground) were observed in patients in whom reduction had not been attempted. These patients were treated with a brief period of rest followed by graduated exercises of increasing difficulty. They returned to light work within 12 weeks of injury. Nearly 25 years later, in a study of over 6000 stable fractures of the thoracolumbar spine, Young again noted this probable negative correlation.[250] He observed the worst symptomatic and functional results in patients who had received the most vigorous treatment.

In patients with residual symptoms after a stable fracture of the thoracolumbar spine, low back pain is the rule.[208,213] Pain at the level of the fracture is less frequent. Nicoll[208] attributed this to associated soft tissue damage involving the paravertebral muscles and ligaments. It is likely that an increased lumbosacral lordosis, necessary to compensate for the fracture deformity, also contributes to the frequency and severity of lumbosacral symptoms.[136,240] The advocates of reduction contend that less compensatory lordosis is necessary if the fracture has been reduced.[136,239,244,249] Therefore, patients whose fractures have been reduced should have less discomfort. However, patients treated by reduction and 4 to 6 months of immobilization in extension (which is necessary to maintain the reduction) tend to have more pain and more stiffness than similar patients treated by early mobilization without reduction.[208,250] It is clear that prolonged immobilization of uninjured segments in a nonphysiologic position more than cancels the expected benefits of reduction. For this reason, extreme hyperextension, a position necessary for maintenance of reduction, should be avoided if at all possible. It is logical to hope that open reduction with effective internal fixation will prove capable of providing the advantages of reduction and avoiding the disadvantages of prolonged external immobilization. Recent experience with segmental spinal stabilization is very encouraging and suggests that, in most cases, internal fixation can be so secure and reliable that no external supports are necessary.[163]

STABLE FRACTURES WITHOUT NEURAL DEFICIT

Stable fractures without neural deficit include almost all anterior wedge, lateral wedge, and central compression fractures of the vertebral body in which there is no fracture of the posterior cortex of the vertebral body and no disruption of the posterior neural arch or related ligaments. All isolated fractures of the transverse and spinous processes are also in this group. It must be stressed that, owing to spontaneous reduction of a dislocation or failure to visualize a neural arch fracture,[168,173,174] a thoracolumbar injury may be far more severe than the x-ray indicates. The converse is never true; skeletal damage is never less severe than the x-rays indicate. Even with this reservation, stable fractures without neural deficit account for the vast majority of thoracolumbar fractures.[183,184,220,241] Pain at the level of injury is the patient's major initial problem.

After the initial diagnostic work-up (described above) the patient is placed at bed rest on a bed that does not allow the mattress to sag. Most modern hospital beds are adequate. Sitting is not permitted, and the head of the bed should not be raised more than 20° or 30°, even for meals. The patient should be encouraged to roll from side to side.

Pain may be severe. Adequate analgesics should be administered liberally, unless contraindicated by an associated condition, such as a head injury. Because of an associated ileus, injectable analgesics may be necessary.

Transient ileus and gastric dilitation due to retroperitoneal hemorrhage is extremely common. The patient should, therefore, be given a liquid diet and observed carefully. If ileus develops, all oral feedings should be stopped. Nasogastric suction and intravenous fluids may be necessary. Ileus may not develop until 24 hours after injury, and it seldom lasts longer than 3 to 5 days.

Patients with thoracolumbar vertebral body fractures and retroperitoneal hemorrhage have an increased risk of thromboembolic complications. They should be protected against these complications by elevation of the foot of the bed, active ankle motion, and elastic stockings. If additional factors are present that increase the patient's susceptibility to thromboembolic complications (such as gross obesity, a history of previous deep venous thrombosis, or cardiac arrhythmia) systemic anticoagulants should be given. If the first dose of anticoagulant is delayed until 12 hours after injury, excessive bleeding at the fracture site can usually be avoided.

As soon as the discomfort comes under control, usually in 2 to 5 days, the patient is permitted to sit. Ambulation, initially with assistance, is started shortly thereafter. The patient is instructed in exercises that strengthen spinal extensor muscles. Exercises that encourage spine flexion, such as sit-ups, are not allowed. The patient will progress rapidly to more advanced functional levels. Discharge from the hospital is dictated by the individual patient's symptoms and activity tolerance and skill at the activities of daily living. Activities of daily living are an important discharge prerequisite, especially for the disabled, for the elderly, and for those who live alone.

Return to work is a complex and highly individual matter. It is as dependent on the patient's motivation and the type of work as it is dependent on the nature of the injury and the treatment. Some well-motivated persons with suitable jobs who are quickly recovering may return to work within 2 weeks.

EXTERNAL SPINE SUPPORTS

Most external spine supports (brace, corset, harness) are of questionable value. While it is true that a well-constructed, well-fitted brace can limit the extremes of spinal motion, excellent studies have shown that no external device is capable of truly immobilizing the spine.[192,210,238] In fact, in some persons a spine support may, paradoxically, increase electromyographic activity of spinal muscles and increase spine motion, particularly at the lumbosacral joint.[192,198,210,238] Although it has been shown that abdominal compression by a brace can decrease spinal compression loads significantly, it is doubtful that abdominal compression of sufficient magnitude is achieved by conventional spine supports.[197,200,238] However, many patients do expect to be given a supporting garment of some sort and often seem to derive benefit (perhaps psychologic) from these devices. A reinforced corset type of brace is relatively inexpensive, not confining, and entirely suitable for use on a stable spine injury. Most patients say that they are comfortable and feel more

secure when wearing the corset. They are, of course, permitted to remove the brace for sleep and personal hygiene.

If the spinal deformity is severe (loss of more than 50% of vertebral body height), a more substantial spine support is justified because severe injuries are more likely to demonstrate progressive deformity[218] and may actually represent a spontaneously reduced unstable injury.[173,208] The Jewett three-point spine extension brace is popular for this purpose. However, if the Jewett brace is fitted well and adjusted properly, it forces the lumbar spine into marked extension, which is awkward and uncomfortable and carries with it all the disadvantages of immobilization in a strained position. If the Jewett brace is adjusted for greater comfort, it becomes ineffective. Therefore, we prefer to use a well-molded plaster jacket, which has the added advantage of being relatively resistant to modification by the patient.

The cast is best applied with the patient supine, supported on Goldthwaite irons (Fig. 12-90). The cast should extend from the symphysis pubis to the manubrium. The lumbar spine is held in a physiologic degree of lordosis. No effort is made to achieve reduction. The cast is a protective positioning device intended to prevent progressive deformity and protect against instability.[208] Ambulation and extension exercises in the cast are encouraged. The cast is used for 12 to 16 weeks and then replaced by a reinforced corset, which is used for an additional 2 months. A molded polypropylene thoracolumbar orthosis is an acceptable alternative for a body cast (Fig. 12-91). It is capable of spine immobilization as effective as a cast. Advantages of the plastic orthosis compared to a cast are greater patient acceptance and ease of removal for inspection of skin and for personal hygiene. Disadvantages are increased cost and time delay for fabrication; the plastic orthosis is also more likely to be modified or removed by the patient contrary to the physician's recommendation. When a plastic orthosis is used, the time for treatment and activities during treatment are the same as for a plaster cast.

RESIDUAL SYMPTOMS AND DEFORMITY

Approximately 25% of patients with stable thoracolumbar fractures have no residual symptoms. Fifty-five percent of patients report mild discomfort but no disability, and 20% report symptoms severe enough to produce some degree of disability.[250]

The degree of deformity associated with flexion fractures at the thoracolumbar junction tends to

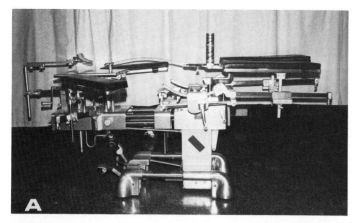

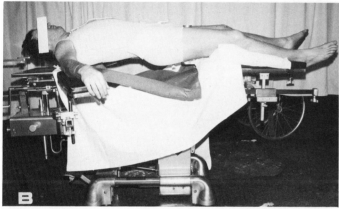

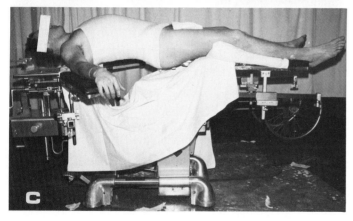

Fig. 12-90. Application of a plaster cast for thoracolumbar fractures. (*A*) A fracture table with Goldthwait irons adjusted for a gentle arc. (*B*) The patient in position for plaster. Padding is placed over the pubis, sternum, and iliac crests. (*C*) The completed cast extends from manubrium to pubis. Ample anterior groin cut-out permits sufficient hip flexion to allow sitting with comfort. Hyperlordosis should be avoided.

progress somewhat during healing and patients with these fractures are more likely to have pain at the lumbosacral junction than at the site of injury (probably due to the increased lumbar lordosis necessary to compensate for post fracture kyphus). For these reasons, some surgeons have recommended internal fixation for flexion fracture of T12 or L1 if the anterior compression of the vertebral body is 30% to 50% or more of the original height of the vertebral body.

It is said that internal fixation will prevent progression of the fracture deformity and, hopefully, decrease associated lumbosacral pain. However, progression of fracture deformity, when it occurs, is rarely severe and no data are available to demonstrate that decreased fracture kyphus is associated

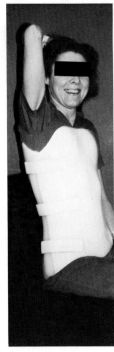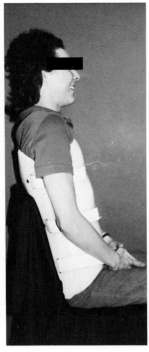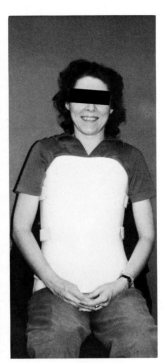

Fig. 12-91. A 28-year-old woman, 2 weeks following fracture-dislocation of T11 with immediate and complete paraplegia at that level, was treated by immediate open reduction and Harrington rod fixation. Postoperative rehabilitation activities in an upright position started on the fifth postoperative day. The patient is shown here on the 15th postoperative day, sitting independently with security and comfort. (*Left*) The oblique view shows the polypropylene molded jacket with anterior and posterior shells joined by lateral Velcro fasteners. Generous anterior thigh cut-outs permit sitting with 90° of hip flexion. Generous axillary cut-outs permit unrestricted upper extremity function. (*Center*) The lateral view shows close molding to trunk contours. (*Right*) The anterior view. Ease of removal facilitates skin inspection and hygiene.

with decreased lumbosacral pain. In fact, past studies have shown that there is *no* correlation between kyphus and the degree of disability.[208,213,250] At the present time, in the absence of neurologic deficit, the only undeniable benefit of reduction and internal fixation for severe flexion fractures at the thoracolumbar junction is cosmetic. Indications for such a procedure are, therefore, very limited.

AUTHORS' PREFERRED TREATMENT FOR STABLE FRACTURE WITHOUT NEUROLOGIC DEFICIT

If the vertical height of the fractured body has been decreased by 30% or less, the patient is fitted with a reinforced corset type of thoracolumbar spinal orthosis and progressive ambulation is started as soon as associated ileus and other injuries have been resolved. For the first 3 months after injury the orthosis is used whenever the patient is upright. The patient is encouraged to do spine extensor strengthening exercises while wearing the orthosis.

If the height of the fractured vertebra has been decreased by 50% or more, a plaster jacket is applied in the supine position using Goldthwaite irons, holding the spine in a neutral position (see Fig. 12-90). The cast is applied as soon as the ileus has resolved and the status of associated injuries has been clarified. The cast extends from the pubis to the manubrial notch with sufficient groin cut-outs to permit hip flexion to at least 90° without compression of the anterior thigh. After the cast has been applied, spine extension exercises are started.

The cast is maintained for 12 to 16 weeks. It is

then removed and replaced with a reinforced corset type of thoracolumbar spinal orthosis, which is maintained for an additional 3 months. Spine extensor muscle strengthening exercises are continued throughout the period of immobilization.

A plastic thoracolumbar orthosis is used instead of a cast only in patients who are certain to cooperate with the treatment regimen (plaster casts are much more resistant to patient modification) in whom the plastic orthosis fabrication delay presents no problem. Postoperative care must include close follow-up with periodic evaluation by x-ray to detect significant progression so that appropriate remedial action may be taken it if occurs.

STABLE FRACTURES WITH NEURAL DEFICIT

Neural damage in this group of patients is due to displaced fragments rather than instability of spinal segments. Patients with injury to the spinal cord resulting in immediate and total loss of neurologic function which persists for 48 hours, in the presence of an intact bulbocavernosus reflex, have no chance for neural recovery.[168,169,181,199,221] The neurologic examination should be very careful and very thorough to be certain that the deficit is, in fact, complete.[168,169,221,224] In these patients, treatment efforts should be directed to the patient's prompt rehabilitation as a paraplegic.[168,169] Efforts at decompression will be fruitless. The fracture should be managed as described for stable injuries without neural deficit, except that plaster casts should be used with great care or not at all[168] because of the danger of pressure sores in paraplegics. A molded plastic orthosis with appropriate padding should be used in these cases because ease of removal for skin inspection is especially important for patients with trunk anesthesia. When available, well-made plastic orthoses are, therefore, preferable to plaster casts for paraplegic patients in whom external spine support is necessary.

Exotic therapeutic measures, such as spinal cord cooling[130,134,155,186] and myelotomy, have succeeded in limiting neurologic deficit due to reversible lesions in laboratory situations. However, to be effective, these surgical treatments must be administered within 4 hours of injury. The logistics of patient transportation and operating room preparation are such that this time limit can almost never be met. Therefore, the potential benefits of cord cooling will never be available to a significant number of patients. Large doses of systemic steroids administered within 4 hours of injury are also effective in reducing permanent neural deficit due

to a reversible lesion.[134,155] This treatment can be administered without the delay inherent in procedures requiring operating room facilities and, unless there is a specific contraindication, all patients with neural deficit secondary to spinal trauma should receive large doses of intravenous steroids as soon as possible.[222,224] Dexamethosone, 4 mg to 6 mg every 6 hours, is the drug of choice because it is the most potent of the anti-inflammatory steroids.[155,222,224]

If injury to the spinal cord produces an incomplete neural deficit, it is more likely that the neural dysfunction is reversible.[168,169,181,187,224,233] Therefore, there may be some benefit from decompression, especially if the spine is stable. If a definite displaced fragment is producing dural compression, CT scans with metrizamide contrast material is especially useful for making this determination (see Fig. 12-87). However, Guttmann[168,169] states that laminectomy is not indicated, even with incomplete neural deficit, because it delays rehabilitation and is seldom beneficial. Carey,[141] Morgan,[196] and others go even further, stating that laminectomy is actually harmful and is sometimes followed by an increase in neural deficit. Kelly,[187] Whitesides,[244] and Leatherman[249] believe the deleterious effects of laminectomy are due to conversion of stable injuries into unstable ones as a result of surgical disruption of the posterior ligament complex. It is in this situation that anterior decompression is most attractive. Anterior decompression has been shown to be an effective technique for relief of dural compression, which facilitates neurologic recovery of incomplete lesions.[137,138,151,180] Even in late cases, decompression of the cord is sometimes followed by dramatic improvement in neurologic function.[137,138,180]

The direct anterior thoracoabdominal approach, either transpleural or retroperitoneal, is used most often but some surgeons have found a lateral rachotomy approach to be useful for anterior thoracolumbar decompression.[138,180] Whichever approach is used, stabilization by posterior instrumentation at the same or a subsequent operative procedure is usually indicated. If anterior decompression is attempted by a posterior approach, great care must be exercised to avoid rendering the spine unstable.[187] When adequate exposure requires destruction of the posterior ligament complex, every effort should be made to restore posterior stability with internal fixation. Stability can sometimes be obtained with the Meurig-Williams type of spine plate[175] applied to both sides of the spinous processes and extending at least two seg-

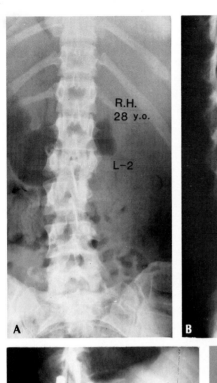

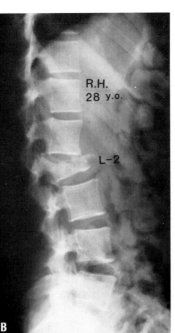

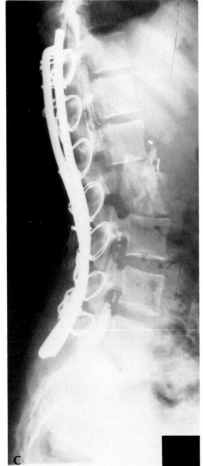

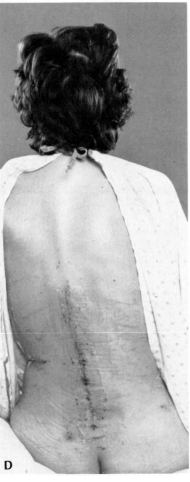

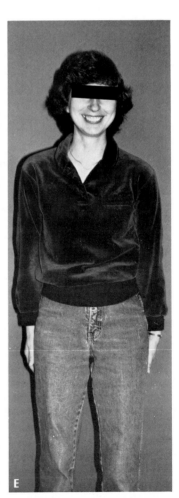

ments cephalad and two segments caudad to the unstable level. Meurig-Williams plates are of historical interest, but are no longer widely used. Harrington rods are currently preferred for spine stabilization in this situation.[151,180,244,249] If there has been an extensive laminectomy of several segments, it may be impossible to achieve stability immediately, even with Harrington rods. A transverse process fusion does nothing to enhance spine stability until bone union occurs. It is in this situation that segmental spinal stabilization recently popularized by Luque is most attractive.[163,*] If restoration of immediate posterior stability is impossible, prolonged immobilization on a turning frame is necessary, but of uncertain effectiveness (see Fig. 12-68). In this situation the circle frame is specifically contraindicated because each turning cycle imposes a weight-bearing load on the unstable spine. A side-to-side turning frame is preferable. However, a highly unstable spine (see Fig. 12-68) is capable of dangerous angulation and translation during turning even with careful turning frame techniques.

Complete or incomplete neural deficit due to cauda equina damage is far more likely to recover than deficit due to spinal cord damage.[150,168,169,182] These injuries should be approached with optimism. If decompression of a cauda equina injury associated with a stable fracture is attempted, one must exercise the same caution against rendering the spine unstable as has previously been mentioned in the discussion of decompression of the spinal cord.

Cauda equina or cord decompression is indicated most clearly if there is a progressing neurologic deficit and displaced fragments invading the spinal

canal (see Fig. 12-87).[151,168,221,234] A decompressive operative procedure is never indicated for neurologically negative patients with a stable thoracolumbar injury, regardless of the size or apparent location of the displaced fragments.[168,169]

AUTHORS' PREFERRED TREATMENT FOR STABLE FRACTURES WITH NEUROLOGIC DEFICIT

If the patient's neurologic deficit is immediate and complete, a well-molded and well-padded plastic orthosis (see Fig. 12-91) is used and the patient's rehabilitation as a paraplegic is started as soon as the status of associated injuries is clear.

If the patient's neurologic deficit is incomplete or if its onset was delayed and if a compressive lesion has been demonstrated either by myelogram or CT scan, then early surgical intervention is preferred. Systemic Decadron is administered immediately in a dose of 4 to 6 mg every 6 hours for 3 days and then rapidly tapered over the subsequent 4 days. The operation is performed with the aid of somatosensory evoked potentials (SEPs) to monitor spinal cord function during the procedure.

If the site of neural compression is anterior, a transthoracic approach is preferred for thoracic lesions, a combined thoracolumbar approach for lesions at the thoracolumbar junction, and a retroperitoneal approach for lumbar lesions. Anterior decompression is accomplished by removal of fractured vertebral body and disk fragments from the spinal canal. The intervertebral disks on either side of the fractured body should be excised and an interbody fusion is performed using either autogenous rib or iliac crest or a combination of the two for supplemental bone graft.

Posterior segmental spinal stabilization (Luque) is performed approximately 1 week later (see Fig. 12-92). Between procedures, the patient is nursed

---

* Luque, E.: Personal communication, 1982.

◄ **Fig. 12-92.** A 28-year-old woman with a hyperflexion fracture of L2 producing an incomplete neurologic deficit at that level. (A) Anteroposterior x-ray shows fracture deformity at L2. Note interpedicular widening, which is frequently associated with traumatic tears of the dura and transection of cauda equina roots.[195] (B) Lateral x-ray demonstrating the severe hyperflexion fracture of L2 with considerable retropulsion of vertebral body material into the spinal canal. Note that kyphus deformity contributes to decreased spinal canal capacity. (C) Operative treatment included anterior corpectomy of L2 with a tricortical iliac crest graft spanning L1 through L3. This procedure was followed by posterior segmental spinal stabilization and fusion extending three levels above and below the fracture. Normal sagittal curves were restored and maintained by appropriate bends in the rods. (D) At 5 days postoperative the patient sits independently without external supports. Her rehabilitation mobilization begins at this time. (E) At 3 months postoperative, the patient stands and walks independently. Neurologic recovery is complete. Spinal stability has been maintained by posterior segmental spinal stabilization. No brace or cast was used.

on a side-to-side turning frame. Posterior segmental spinal stabilization should extend at least three segments above and two segments below the level of fracture. If the site of compression is posterior or if it is both posterior and anterior as, for example, a displaced fracture of the neural arch and the vertebral body, then a posterior approach is performed with relief of the compressive lesion by partial laminectomy if necessary. Frequently, however, decompression can be achieved by removing fragments and debris through the fracture site without any additional laminectomy.

Internal fixation by the segmental spinal stabilization technique is performed at the same procedure. Here again, segmental spinal stabilization rods should extend at least three segments above and two segments below the level of fracture. An anterior site of compression can often be relieved by removal of fragments through the fracture or laminectomy defect prior to application of the segmental spinal stabilization rods. During the first week, following satisfactory posterior segmental spinal stabilization, mobilization of the patient is started without a cast or brace (see Fig. 12-91 and 12-92).

UNSTABLE FRACTURES WITH OR WITHOUT NEURAL DEFICIT

Unstable fractures with or without neural deficit include all dislocations and fracture-dislocations of the thoracolumbar spine, but they account for no more than 10% of thoracolumbar injuries.[184,220] Neural deficit due to instability is present in 50% to 60% of these cases.[184,208,229,241] If an unstable spine is suspected, the patient should be placed on a side-to-side turning frame. There is no need to transfer the patient to an x-ray table. A complete radiographic work-up can be performed while the patient is on the frame.[184] If there is a neural deficit, intravenous dexamethasone should be administered at once, unless there is a specific contraindication.[155,222,224] Laminectomy should be avoided because it is a relatively ineffective[133,136] method for decompression and is sometimes harmful.[141,196]

In a displaced, unstable spine, the dural tube may be compressed posteriorly by the lamina and anteriorly by the vertebral body (Fig. 12-93). Laminectomy can relieve posterior compression, but it cannot relieve anterior compression.[136] If the vertebral body prominence is excised in order to complete the dural decompression, then spinal instability is exacerbated.[136,244] The dura can be decompressed most effectively by reduction, which

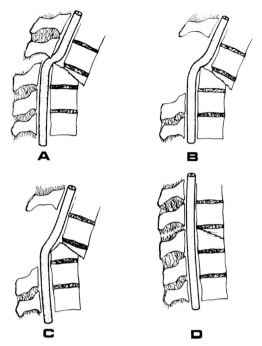

Fig. 12-93. (*A*) A fracture-dislocation with transverse translational displacement can compress the dura anteriorly as well as posteriorly. (*B*) Laminectomy can relieve the posterior compression but may not relieve the anterior compression. (*C*) Laminectomy in addition to excision of the posterior vertebral body prominence can relieve both sites of compression but instability will be markedly increased. (*D*) Reduction and restoration of the spinal canal relieves both sites of compression and enhances spinal stability.

relieves the anterior as well as the posterior site of compression.[136,151] The large diameter of the spinal canal in relation to the relatively small volume of its neural contents assures that decompression by reduction is truly effective, especially in the lumbar spine. Furthermore, reduction definitely enhances stability by allowing the dislocated neural arch processes to reengage,[175,184] thereby affording protection to uninjured neural structures.

Reduction is the treatment of choice for unstable spines with incomplete neural deficit because it is the best method for decompression.[136,184] Reduction is the treatment of choice for unstable spines with complete neural deficit because it often restores stability and permits prompt rehabilitation activities.[151,178,180] Finally, reduction is also the treatment of choice for unstable spines without neural deficit because reduction improves spinal stability,[175,184] thereby offering protection against the development of neural deficit, a complication that has been observed in patients whose unstable spines were not reduced (Fig. 12-94).[184,185,229]

Increased neural deficit has been observed frequently following attempts at closed reduction of unstable thoracolumbar injuries.[219] We, therefore, prefer open reduction because damage to neural structures can be avoided if these structures are under direct vision during the reduction maneuver.[184] The operation should be performed on the turning frame so that accidental, uncontrolled reduction during transfer to the operating table is avoided.

The possibility of an increase in neurologic deficit as a complication of spinal surgery has long been a major concern. Although the precise incidence of this complication is not known, occasional increase of neurologic deficit as a result of either open or closed procedures on the traumatized spine has been documented.[184,196,219] It would, therefore, be desirable to have a reliable method for monitoring spinal cord function during operative procedures so that neurologic dysfunction can be identified as soon as it occurs and, perhaps, be reversed. In recent years, two promising techniques have emerged. They are intraoperative monitoring of neural electrical activity and the intraoperative "wake-up" test.

During the late 1970s, spinal cord monitoring has come into its own and several techniques have been developed.[204] All employ stimulation of a peripheral nerve or the spinal cord through a spinous process electrode, either caudal or cephalad to an existing or potential spinal cord lesion. Transmission of the impulse across the lesion is recorded either from the cord or the contralateral cerebral cortex. The process is analogous to peripheral nerve conduction studies.

At present, three systems are in use for spinal cord monitoring. The first is somatosensory cortical evoked potential.[159,206,209] This system repeatedly stimulates a peripheral nerve, such as the posterior tibial, peroneal, ulnar, or median with a mild electrical stimulus. The summated cortical response is recorded from the scalp. Latency, amplitude, and wave form in the first 100 milliseconds are parameters of spinal cord conduction. The second is somatosensory spinal evoked potentials. In this system, the stimulus is the same, but recordings are taken directly from the spinal cord, by a spinous process electrode place above the lesion. The third method is spinal-spinal evoked potentials.[209] In this method, both the stimulus and the recording are directly from the spine, which is exposed during

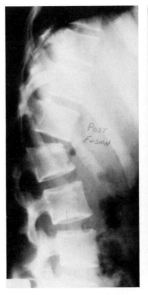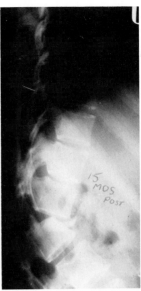

Fig. 12-94. (*Left*) Fracture-dislocation of L1 on L2 without neurologic deficit. A posterior fusion was performed *in situ* without an attempt at reduction and without internal fixation. (*Right*) Fifteen months following the arthrodesis procedure. Deformity has progressed, arthrodesis has not occurred, and a lower extremity motor deficit has appeared.

surgery. Spinal-spinal stimulation and recording systems can be used to study both efferent and afferent transmission. They also have the advantage of greater sensitivity and speed. Weighted against these advantages are the disadvantages of the spinal-spinal evoked potential system, which are its invasiveness, the relatively short time that electrodes can be left *in situ* for postoperative recording, and the possibility of electrode migration.

From clinical and laboratory studies, there is a body of evidence that indicates that cerebral SEPs are mediated primarily by the dorsal column-medial lemniscal system.[166,176] Division of the cervical spinothalamic tract has been shown to have no significant effect on SEP characteristics,[190,203] but division of the dorsal columns all but abolish the SEP.[145] Therefore, SEP abnormalities are most likely to be associated with impairment of joint position and vibration sense. Despite this, Nash and others have evidence that more than the function of the dorsal columns can be evaluated by spinal cord monitoring techniques.[206]

In thoracic and lumbar spine trauma, spinal cord monitoring can be used for several purposes. First, and perhaps most important, monitoring can detect evidence of impending dysfunction of the spinal cord during surgery.[205,206,228] If recognized before irreversible damage has occurred, appropriate measures may be taken to reverse the process. Spinal cord monitoring can also determine if procedures such as decompression or stabilization of an incomplete spinal cord injury produce improvement in cord transmission. Correlation of intraoperative changes with the subsequent clinical course may help to prove whether surgery contributes to neurologic recovery. Although spinal cord monitoring has no well-established norms, each patient can serve as his own control. The precise parameters for predicting impending neurologic dysfunction have not been worked out, but available data indicate that a reduction in peak amplitude of more than 50% or increased latency (delay in transmission) are significant, especially if these changes fail to improve within 10 to 15 minutes. Nash[206] found that patients who showed decreased amplitude and increased latency or loss of a SEP response during surgery had an increased neurologic loss at the end of the procedure. He has noted that, if the rod was promptly removed, patients with depressed SEP after Harrington instrumentation for scoliosis correction had no neurologic loss. Spiezholz[228] found that, in patients with incomplete spinal cord lesions, if the SEP remained at its control level during decompression or stabilization surgery no increase in neurologic deficit was noted after operation. Therefore, when operating on patients with thoracic or lumbar spine trauma, spinal cord monitoring can provide a continuous display of spinal cord function and can add an extra measure of safety.

A satisfactory intraoperative SEP assures the surgeon that the spinal cord has not sustained added damage. The presence of a favorable intraoperative SEP change is usually associated with some degree of subsequent clinical recovery. However, this correlation has not been consistent.[154] Interpretation of the results of spinal cord monitoring remains uncertain. We do not know which components of the SEP are the most reliable predictors of neurologic functional change.

Spinal cord function can also be monitored with the "wake-up" test, which was popularized by Vauzelle and Stagnara and is in wide clinical use in scoliosis surgery.[235] The "wake-up" test of Stagnara is simple and safe. Cases have been reported in which the test was positive, leading to reduction of the correction or the removal of instrumentation with subsequent return of preoperative neurologic function.[170,237] Although the Stagnara test does not require special equipment, drawbacks limiting its usefulness in trauma are that only a limited number of tests can be done on one case and the test monitors motor function only. The results can be equivocal and the technique is difficult to apply in patients with incomplete neurologic lesions.

To fully exploit the decompressive, stabilizing, and rehabilitative virtues of a reduction, the operation should be performed early—certainly within 12 hours of injury—unless an associated injury claims treatment priority or definitely contraindicates an operative procedure.[175] If facets are locked and prevent reduction, partial resection of the locked facets permits reduction without sacrifice of stability after reduction. Total facet resection should be avoided. Internal fixation should be used whenever possible to enhance stability[143,151,180,184] and avoid the need for prolonged postoperative recumbency.[175]

If the bony structure of the posterior neural arch is intact, a simple wire loop surrounding adjacent spinous processes is adequate (Fig. 12-95).[184] Reduction of the dislocated facets eliminates translational instability by allowing the dislocated posterior articular facets to reengage, thereby providing a bony obstacle to transverse translation. Resistance to transverse translational displacement is provided by intact, reduced articular facets, and not by the wire. The wire loop functions simply as a prosthetic ligament, restoring the tethering function of the posterior ligament complex.[174,175] Weiss springs function in the same way.[240] They impart stability by maintaining reduction of intact articular processes and posterior neural arch structures. The elasticity of the spring allows maintenance of stability in selected cases without a cast or brace. Springs have the added advantage of quick and easy insertion with minimal dissection.

However, if there is an extensive posterior fracture, or if the neural arch has been separated from the vertebral body, then reduction does little to increase stability, and a posterior wire loop or Weiss springs are inadequate (Fig. 12-96).[175,187*,244] In these cases, stability must be provided by the internal fixation device itself. Therefore, more substantial internal fixation, such as Meurig-Williams plates (Fig. 12-97), Harrington rods (Fig. 12-98), or Luque rods (Fig. 12-99; see also Fig. 12-92) may be necessary. Either distraction or compression rods may be used. Bilateral compression rods have been shown to produce the most stable postfixation construction if used to stabilize a thoracolumbar "slice" fracture-dislocation in which the posterior neural arch disruption is totally or predominantly

---

* Stauffer, E.S.: Personal communication, 1982.

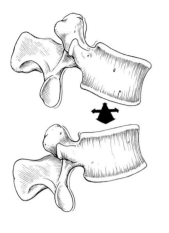

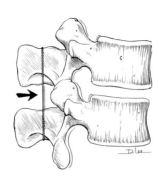

Fig. 12-95. (*Left*) Disruption of the intervertebral disk and dislocation of the posterior facets destroy both structural columns of the spine. Transverse translational displacement can now occur. The spine is grossly unstable. (*Right*) After reduction of the posterior facets, the articular processes interdigitate and effectively resist translational displacement. The wire loop (*arrow*) simply maintains the reduction. It is the reduction that produces stability.

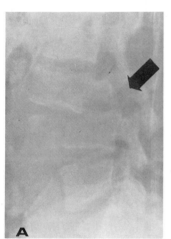

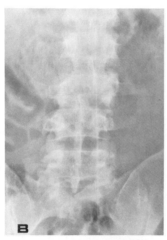

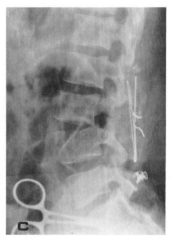

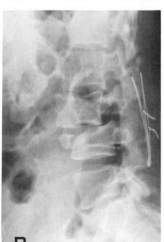

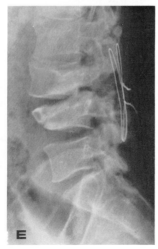

Fig. 12-96. A severe fracture-dislocation with a widely displaced bilateral pars interarticularis fracture. The patient is neurologically negative. (This is the same patient as in Fig. 12-73). (*B*) The anteroposterior view. (*C*) Total laminectomy, open reduction, wire fixation, and autogenous bone graft were performed. (*D*) Dislocation promptly recurred. Without the stabilizing effect of an intact neural arch, the wire loop is inadequate. (*E*) Four years later, deformity has progressed. Fusion has not occurred; the patient complains of pain at the level of injury.

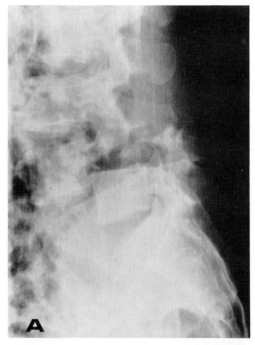

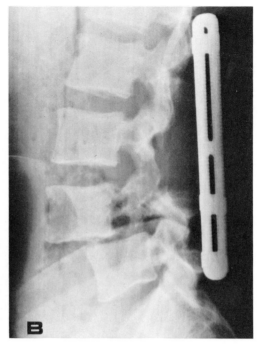

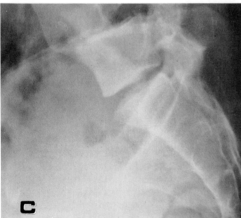

Fig. 12-97. (*A*) A total dislocation of L4 on L5. There is a widely displaced bilateral pars interarticularis fracture (true traumatic spondylolysis). The patient is neurologically negative. (*B*) In spite of immediate open reduction, total laminectomy, posterior plating, and autogenous grafting, recurrent dislocation promptly developed. (*C*) Stability and symptom control were ultimately achieved with an anterior interbody fusion.

ligamentous.[230] If the neural arch disruption includes a significant fracture of lamina or facets, especially if the neural arch fracture involves more than one segment, then compression rods become much less effective and potentially dangerous because compression will simply crowd the neural arch fragments together, potentially adding to dural tube compromise without appreciably enhancing spine stability. If there are neural arch fractures or a prior laminectomy, then distraction rods are preferable to compression rods.[202,215,230] Distraction rods effectively reduce flexion deformity by exerting a posteriorly directed force on the upper and lower hooks and an anteriorly directed force on the posterior prominence of the gibbus.

The Harrington distraction rod's three-point bending force mechanism for reduction of deformity can be appreciably enhanced by appropriate bends in a square end rod or by use of appropriate-size polyethylene sleeves placed over the rod at the gibbus prominence.[151,158] Unfortunately, while enhancing the reduction effectiveness of distraction rods, these maneuvers increase hook loads and contribute to loss of fixation as a result of hook "cut-out," particularly of the upper hook. Experimental studies have shown that upper hook loads

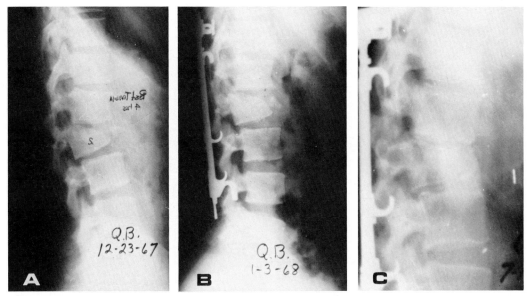

Fig. 12-98. (*A*) Fracture-dislocation of L1 on L2. The patient is paraplegic. (*B*) Early reduction was accomplished and maintained with Harrington rods. (Note distraction rod on one side, compression rod on the other.) (*C*) A later anterior decompression and interbody fusion were performed. Stability has been maintained. The patient made a nearly complete neurologic recovery. (Courtesy of Kenton Leatherman, M.D., Louisville, Kentucky)

are decreased proportional to the number of segments spanned by the rod.[202,215,230] It is therefore recommended that, if used for reduction of a flexion deformity, the upper hook of the distraction rod should be at least three segments above the level of the traumatic disruption.[215] Correction of the flexion deformity combined with distraction can effectively disimpact vertebral body fragments, thereby contributing to a complete reduction and dural tube decompression.[151,180] Effective external immobilization, either cast or brace, should also be used to protect the instrumented spine until union has occurred.

With distraction rods, stability is achieved by lengthening the anterior portion of the spine, thereby generating tensile loads in the anterior longitudinal ligament. Postoperative spinal stability is the result of a dynamic balance of compressive loads in the rods and tensile loads in the anterior longitudinal ligaments.[132] If the anterior longitudinal ligament is torn, lengthening of the distraction rod will simply separate the injured spinal segments (Fig. 12-100) and stability may never be achieved.[132] Excessive lengthening of the injured spine should be avoided because it may contribute to neurologic deficit and may also contribute to failure of fusion. If disruption of the anterior longitudinal ligament is suspected, one should consider either segmental spinal stabilization[163,*] or use of a compression rod on one side and a distraction rod on the other.[249]

Although intuition would lead one to expect that the combination of compression and distraction rods will produce a troublesome lateral curve, this is not the case.[243,249] Leatherman[249] believes stability is best achieved with a compression rod on one side of the spine and a distraction rod on the other and that this combination should be used more often. However, in some cases even substantial devices that span multiple segments may be inadequate to consistently maintain complete reduction (see Fig. 12-97).

In contrast to the nearly universal spontaneous anterior fusion observed by Holdsworth[175] and Nicoll[208] in their cases of thoracolumbar fracture-dislocation, American surgeons find that spontaneous anterior fusion is not reliable.[184,218] It is likely that reduction of the deformity is responsible for our lower frequency of spontaneous fusion.[210] Since spontaneous anterior fusion frequently fails to occur if the deformity has been reduced,[184] a posterior or posterolateral fusion with autogenous graft should be performed at the time of open reduction and internal fixation. A secure posterior fusion ensures

---

* Luque, E.: Personal communication, 1980.

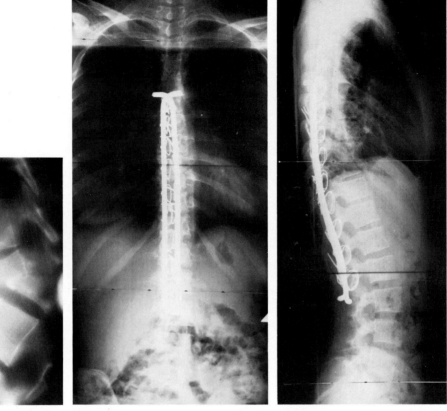

Fig. 12-99. An 18-year-old woman sustained a complete fracture-dislocation of T10 with immediate and complete paraplegia. Open reduction and internal fixation were performed on the day of injury. At exploration, extensive fractures were found involving the lamina of T9, T10, and T11. Luque instrumentation was extended to include three intact laminae above and below the region of fracture. Secure internal fixation permitted immediate unrestricted rehabilitation activities with no external trunk supports. (*Left*) Lateral laminogram shows completely displaced fracture-dislocation of T10 with obliteration of the spinal canal. (*Center*) Anteroposterior x-ray shows bilateral Luque rods extending from T6 through L2, restoring excellent alignment and stability of the thoracolumbar spine. Note the C-shaped contour of the rods that protects against proximal or distal rod migration. (*Right*) Lateral x-ray demonstrates the contoured Luque rods, which reestablish thoracic kyphus and lumbar lordosis. Note that the spinal canal has been restored.

maintenance of reduction and decreases pain at the fracture site.[184,187,244,249]

If Meurig-Williams plates, Harrington rods, or Luque rods are used, the fusion must include all segments spanned by the fixation device.[173,175,249] However, these devices should be used only if a wire loop is certain to be ineffective. Fusion of four or more segments in Nicoll's[208] patients with plate fixation was certainly a factor in limiting spinal mobility and subsequent disability.[184]

After open reduction, internal fixation, and fusion have been accomplished, the patient remains on the turning frame. If stability was achieved at the operating table, a cast is applied as described for stable fractures 2 weeks after the operation and progressive ambulation is started along with extension exercises. If stability was not achieved at the operation, the patient should remain on the frame for 6 weeks before cast application and ambulation.

The same schedule is followed for paralyzed patients, except that a cast is not used if there is anesthesia over the iliac crests and pubis.[168] A well-padded brace is used for these patients.

Internal fixation of unstable thoracolumbar fractures and dislocations secure enough to allow immediate postoperative mobilization of the patient without any cast or brace is desirable, especially in patients with neurologic deficit because of the pressure ulceration problem in these patients and because of cast or brace interference with rehabilitation procedures. Our recent experience with segmental spinal stabilization, a procedure pioneered and popularized by Eduardo Luque[163,*] of Mexico, has demonstrated that this technique is capable of reliably providing internal fixation so secure that immediate mobilization is possible without any external support and with no loss of reduction or stability (see Fig. 12-99).

One rod is wired to the lamina on each side of the spinous process. The rods should extend at least three segments above and two segments below the level of injury. The wires pass through the spinal canal, completely surrounding the lamina. Two wires are used at each level, except for the end vertebrae, where four wires are used because stress is greatest at the end vertebra. The rods can be bent prior to insertion in order to completely correct traumatic deformity and recreate normal thoracic kyphosis and lumbar lordosis. After the rods have been secured, a bilateral facet arthrodesis extending out to the transverse processes is performed and augmented with iliac bone graft. Postoperative management uses a standard hospital bed and no brace or cast. The patient is allowed to sit on the second or third postoperative day and, depending on other injuries, unrestricted rehabilitation activities are initiated by the end of the first postoperative week. If an anterior decompression has been performed, posterior segmental spinal stabilization can provide fixation so secure that immediate mobilization including ambulation is possible with no external support (see Fig. 12-92).

Our experience with twenty paraplegic thoracolumbar fracture patients treated with segmental spinal stabilization has been very satisfactory. There has been no increase in neurologic deficit, no loss of reduction or fixation, and no cast or brace was used. Our favorable experience with this technique has been duplicated by others.[163]

Problems associated with segmental spinal stabilization include difficulty maintaining spinal distraction, and an increased operative time. Increased neurologic deficit is a possibility and transient postoperative nerve root pain has been observed.[163] Because of these problems, great care must be exercised when placing the wires, especially at

* Luque, E.: Personal communication, 1980.

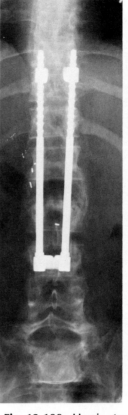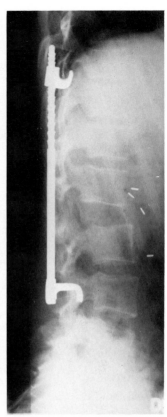

Fig. 12-100. Harrington distraction rod fixation of a patient who had traumatic disruption of the anterior longitudinal ligament, resulting in excessive lengthening of the spine at the level of injury. The patient has a complete neurological deficit. Although satisfactory arthrodesis ultimately occurred in this patient, excessive lengthening of an injured spine is likely to favor a failure of fusion and may contribute to neurologic deficit.

levels cephlad to the injury. Patients without neurologic deficit in whom a postoperative cast or brace can be used with relative safety are probably better managed by the Harrington rod technique.

AUTHORS' PREFERRED TREATMENT FOR
UNSTABLE FRACTURES WITHOUT
NEUROLOGIC DEFICIT

Unstable fractures without neurologic deficit are best treated by early (within the first 12 to 24 hours) open reduction, internal fixation, and fusion. The operation is performed with the aid of SEPs for spinal cord monitoring. At the time of open reduction, the dura can be inspected and protected from damage during the reduction maneuver. If the facets are locked, reduction is facil-

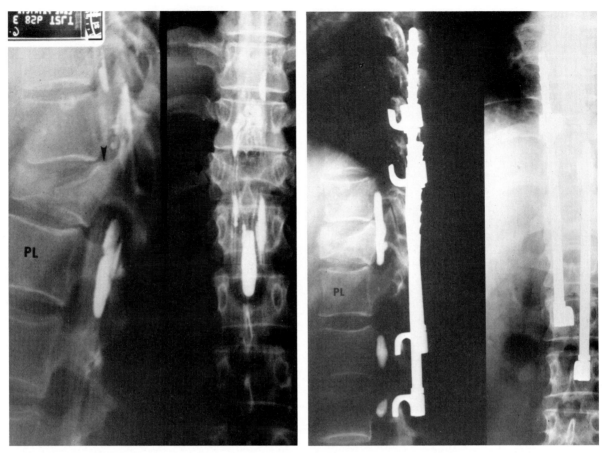

Fig. 12-101. A 28-year-old woman with a flexion-compression fracture of T12. She has weakness and paresthesias of both lower extremities and impaired sphincter control. (*Left*) Preoperative myelogram shows posterior displacement of the fractured vertebral body causing a large defect in the dye column. (*Right*) At 1-year postoperative, note the bend in the Harrington distraction rod that aided complete reduction of the fracture deformity. Residual myelographic dye shows that there is no longer any distortion of the anterior spinal canal. Staggered distraction rods and hook placement help to protect against hook cut-out.

itated by excision of the superior portion of the superior facets of the segment below the level of dislocation. Total facetectomy should be avoided because it will compromise postreduction stability of the spine.

If the bony substance of the posterior neural arch is intact, (posterior disruption is predominantly ligamentous), then a simple wire loop provides adequate internal fixation. The wire loop is placed beneath the spinous process of the segment below the level of dislocation and passes through the base of the spinous process of the segment above the level of dislocation. The wire loop serves as a prosthetic ligament, preventing separation of the two neural arches. Stability of the spine is provided by maintenance of a normal relationship between the neural arches on either side of the dislocation.

If the exploration reveals a significant fracture of the posterior neural arch or if a pedicle fracture has separated the neural arch from the vertebral body, then a wire loop is not adequate. These fractures are best treated by open reduction and internal fixation with two Harrington distraction rods extending at least three segments above and two segments below the level of dislocation (Fig. 12-101).

If there is *severe* spinal instability with disruption of the anterior longitudinal ligament, the distraction rods may simply separate the injured segments of the spine and may not produce adequate stability (see Fig. 12-100). If this is suspected and confirmed by an intraoperative x-ray examination, then the distraction rods should be removed and replaced with a compression rod on one side of the spinous processes and a distraction rod on the other. The compression rod should be applied first. To distribute the hook loads more widely, it is desirable *not* to have the hooks of the two distraction rods on the same vertebral segment (see Fig. 12-101). This is especially important at the level of the cephalic hook since cephalic hook "cut out" is far more frequent than caudal hook "cut out." Prior to reduction, articular cartilage is resected from the dislocated facets. Following reduction and internal fixation, the posterior neural arch is decorticated and autogenous iliac bone obtained from one post-iliac crest is placed over the decorticated neural arches as supplementary bone graft. It is usually not necessary to extend the fusion out onto the transverse processes. The fusion should extend the entire length of the fixation device. The wound is closed in routine fashion and the patient is nursed postoperatively on a side-to-side turning frame.

Approximately 5 to 7 days postoperatively, a plaster cast is applied as described in the section "Stable Fractures Without Neurologic Deficit."

AUTHORS' PREFERRED TREATMENT FOR UNSTABLE SPINE FRACTURES WITH NEUROLOGIC DEFICIT

Systemic Decadron is administered immediately to all patients with neurologic deficit in a dose of 4–6 mg every 6 hours for 3 days and then rapidly tapered over the subsequent 4 days. Early open reduction and internal fixation and fusion is preferred in patients with incomplete neurologic deficit in order to protect neural elements from trauma due to spinal instability in the early postinjury phase.

In patients with immediate and complete neurologic deficit, early open reduction, internal fixation, and fusion are desirable to permit early and uninhibited rehabilitation activities (see Fig. 12-99). This is of value to patients with partial neurologic deficit as well. The operation is performed with the aid of SEPs for spinal cord monitoring. To avoid the problems inherent in casts or braces, when used for patients with impaired sensation, we have preferred segmental spinal stabilization in patients with neurologic deficit (see Figs. 12-92 and 12-99).

The rod is fixed to the lamina, on one side of the spine cephalic to the traumatic disruption, and on the other side of the spine, it is fixed to the lamina of segments caudal to the traumatic disruption. Reduction is accomplished by manually reducing the free ends of the partially fixed rods to the underlying neural arches and completing the fixation by sequentially tightening the wire loops. A controlled and complete reduction of deformity can be accomplished in this way.

Following fixation of the rods, the exposed spinous processes and lamina are decorticated and the facet joints are excised. The fusion is augmented by autogenous iliac bone graft obtained from one posterior crest. If a laminectomy has been done, the fusion is extended out onto the transverse processes at the laminectomy level. The wound is closed in the conventional way and postoperative rehabilitation activities are started without cast or brace during the first postoperative week (see Fig. 12-99).

COMPLICATIONS

Progressive deformity (chronic instability) is often a complication of unstable injuries in which fusion fails to develop.[187,208,218] Progressive deformity may have only cosmetic significance, but it may be associated with pain at the deformity[184,213] or in the compensatory curves. In rare instances, the deformity may progress to grotesque proportions and produce neurologic deficit. Progression of this degree is more likely in children and after laminectomy.[138,244,248]

Kilfoyle[188] has reported seven cases of collapsing paralytic curve of the lumbar spine associated with paraplegia. Although this complication is most likely in children, it may be seen in adults, especially those with a thoracic level of neural deficit. The curve eventually becomes fixed and can compromise balance.[188] An extensive lumbar fusion may be necessary to control it.

Pain is, by far, the most common long-term problem of patients who have had a thoracolumbar fracture.[169,248,250] The degree of pain varies and the overall figures are similar to those given for stable fractures without neural deficit (see p. 1070). Pain following a stable injury is most often at the lumbosacral junction. Symptoms following unstable fractures are more often at the level of injury.[184,241,248] Pain at the fracture site can often be relieved by a successful arthrodesis.[184] Pain at the lumbosacral junction is difficult to manage and is seldom relieved by arthrodesis. A lumbosacral support may be helpful.

REFERENCES

The Cervical Spine

1. Abbott, K. H., and Hale, N.: Cervical Trapeze. An Apparatus for Ambulatory Treatment of Fractures of the Cervical Spine. J. Neurosurg., **10**:436–437, 1953.
2. Albin, M. S.; White, R. J.; Acosta-Rua, G.; and Yashon, D.: Study of Functional Recovery Produced by Delayed Localized Cooling after Spinal Cord Injury in Primates. J. Neurosurg., **29**:113–120, 1968.
3. Albin, M. S.; White, R. J.; Yashon, D.; and Harris, L. S.: Effects of Localized Cooling on Spinal Cord Trauma. J. Trauma, **9**:1000–1008, 1969.
4. Allen, A. R.: Surgery of Experimental Lesion of Spinal Cord Equivalent to Crush Injury of Fracture Dislocation of Spinal Column. A Preliminary Report. J.A.M.A., **57**:878–880, 1911.
5. Anderson, L. D., and D'Alonzo, R. T.: Fractures of the Odontoid Process of the Axis. J. Bone Joint Surg., **56A**:1663–1674, 1974.
6. Anderson, S., and Bradford, D. S.: Lo-profile Halo. Clin. Orthop., **103**:72–74, 1974.
7. Apuzzo, M. L.; Heiden, J. S.; Weiss, M. H.; Ackerson, T. T.; Harvey, J. P.; and Kurze, T.: Acute Fractures of the Odontoid Process. An Analysis of 45 Cases. J. Neurosurg., **48**(1):85–91, 1978.
8. Bailey, R. W., and Badgley, C. E.: Stabilization of the Cervical Spine by Anterior Fusion. J. Bone Joint Surg., **42A**:565–594, 1960.
9. Bailey, R. W., and Kingsley, T. C.: Dislocation of Cervical Spine following Laminectomy. J. Bone Joint Surg., **51A**:1029, 1969.
10. Barnes, R.: Paraplegia in Cervical Spine Injuries. J. Bone Joint Surg., **30B**:234–244, 1948.
11. Barton, L. G.: The Reduction of Fracture-Dislocations of the Cervical Vertebrae by Skeletal Traction. Surg. Gynecol. Obstet., **67**:94–96, 1938.
12. Bedbrook, G. M.: Spinal Injuries with Tetraplegia and Paraplegia. J. Bone Joint Surg., **61B**:267–284, 1979.
13. Bellamy, R.; Pitts, F. W.; and Stauffer, E. S.: Respiratory Complications in Traumatic Quadriplegia. Analysis of 20 Years Experience. J. Neurosurg., **39**:596–600, 1973.
14. Bick, E. M.: Source Book of Orthopedics. Baltimore, Williams & Wilkins, 1948.
15. Böhler, J.: Fractures of the Odontoid Process. J. Trauma, **5**:386–391, 1965.
16. Bohlman, H. H.: Acute Fractures and Dislocations of the Cervical Spine. An Analysis of Three Hundred Hospitalized Patients and Review of the Literature. J. Bone Joint Surg., **61A**:1119–1142, 1979.
17. Bosch, A.; Stauffer, E. S.; and Nickel, V. L.: Incomplete Traumatic Quadriplegia: A Ten-Year Review. J.A.M.A., **216**:473–478, 1971.
18. Braakman, R., and Pennig, L.: Injuries of the Cervical Spine. Amsterdam, Exerpta Medica, 1971.
19. Brashear, R., Jr.; Venters, G.; and Preston, E. T.: Fractures of the Neural Arch of the Axis. A Report of Twenty-Nine Cases. J. Bone Joint Surg., **57A**:879–887, 1975.
20. Brooks, A. L., and Jenkins, E. B.: Atlanto-axial Arthrodesis by the Wedge Compression Method. J. Bone Joint Surg., **60A**:279–284, 1978.
21. Burke, D. C.: Hyperextension Injuries of the Spine. J. Bone Joint Surg., **53B**:3–12, 1971.
22. Burke, D. C., and Berryman, D.: The Place of Closed Manipulation in the Management of Flexion-Rotation Dislocations of the Cervical Spine. J. Bone Joint Surg., **53B**:165–182, 1971.
23. Cheshire, D. J. E.: The Stability of the Cervical Spine following the Conservative Treatment of Fractures and Fracture-Dislocations. Paraplegia, **7**:193–203, 1969.
24. Cloward, R. B.: Treatment of Acute Fractures and Fracture-Dislocations of the Cervical Spine by Vertical-Body Fusion. A Report of Eleven Cases. J. Neurosurg., **18**:201–209, 1961.
25. Cloward, R. B.: Surgical Treatment of Dislocations and Compression Fractures of the Cervical Spine by the Anterior Approach. Proceedings of the Seventeenth Annual Clinical Spinal Cord Injury Conference, IB, 11-15:26, September and October, 1969. Washington, D. C., Veterans Administration, 1970.
26. Cloward, R.B.: Skull Traction for Cervical Spine Injury: Should It Be Abandoned? J.A.M.A., **226**:1008, 1973.
27. Comarr, A. E.: Neurogenic Bladder. Paraplegia, **2**:125–131, 1964.
28. Comarr, A. E., and Kaufmann, A. A.: A Survey of the Neurological Results of 858 Spinal Cord Injuries: A Comparison of Patients Treated with and without Laminectomy. J. Neurosurg., **13**:95–106, 1956.
29. Crutchfield, W. G.: Skeletal Traction for Dislocation of the Cervical Spine. Report of a Case. South. Surg., **2**:156–159, 1933.
30. Crutchfield, W. G.: Further Observations on the Treatment of Fracture-Dislocations of the Cervical Spine with Skeletal Traction. Surg. Gynecol. Obstet., **63**:513–517, 1936.
31. Crutchfield, W. G.: Treatment of Injuries of the Cervical Spine. J. Bone Joint Surg., **20**:696–704, 1938.
32. Dohrmann, G. J.; Wagner, F. C., Jr.; and Bucy, P. C.: The Microvasculature in Transitory Traumatic Paraplegia: An Electron Microscopic Study in the Monkey. J. Neurosurg., **35**:263–271, 1971.
33. Ducker, T. B.; Kindt, G. W.; and Kempe, L. G.: Pathological Findings in Acute Experimental Spinal Cord Trauma. J. Neurosurg., **35**:700–708, 1971.
34. Durbin, F. C.: Fracture-Dislocations of the Cervical Spine. J. Bone Joint Surg., **39B**:23–38, 1957.
35. Eismont, F. J., and Bohlman, H. H.: Posterior Atlanto-occipital Dislocation with Fractures of the Atlas and Odontoid Process. J. Bone Joint Surg., **60A**:397–399, 1978.
36. Eismont, F. J., and Bohlman, H. H.: Posterior Methyl Methacrylate Fixation for Cervical Trauma. Spine, **6**:347–353, 1981.
37. Effendi, B.; Roy, D.; Cornish, B.; Dussault, R. G.; and Laurin, C. A.: Fractures of the Ring of the Axis. A Classification Based on the Analysis of 131 Cases. J. Bone Joint Surg., **63B**:319–327, 1981.
38. Evarts, C. M.: Traumatic Occipito-atlantal dislocation. J. Bone Joint Surg., **52A**:1653–1660, 1970.

39. Eyering, E. J.; Murray, W. R.; Inman, V. T.; and Boldery, E.: Simultaneous Anterior and Posterior Approach to the Cervical Spine. Reduction and Fixation of an Old Fracture-Dislocation with Cord Compromise. J. Bone Joint Surg., **46A**:833–836, 1964.

40. Fielding, J. W.: Cineroentgenography of the Normal Cervical Spine. J. Bone Joint Surg., **39A**:1280–1288, 1957.

41. Fielding, J. W., and Hawkins, R. J.: Atlanto-axial Rotary Fixation (Fixed Rotary Subluxation of the Atlantoaxial Joint). J. Bone Joint Surg., **59A**:37–44, 1977.

42. Fielding, J. W.; Hawkins, R. J.; and Ratzan, S. A.: Spine Fusion for Atlanto-axial Instability. J. Bone Joint Surg., **58A**:400–407, 1976.

43. Forsyth, H. F.: Extension Injuries of the Cervical Spine. J. Bone Joint Surg., **46A**:1792–1797, 1964.

44. Forsyth, H. F.; Alexander, E., Jr.; and Underdal, R.: The Advantages of Early Spine Fusion in the Treatment of Fracture-Dislocation of the Cervical Spine. J. Bone Joint Surg., **41A**:17–36, 1959.

45. Francis, W. R.; Fielding, J. W.; Hawkins, R. J.; Pepin, J.; and Hensinger, R.: Traumatic Spondylolisthesis of the Axis. J. Bone Joint Surg., **63B**:313–318, 1981.

46. Frankel, H. L.; Hancock, G. H.; Melzak, J.; Michaelis, L. S.; Ungar, G. H.; Vernon, J. D. S.; and Walsh, J. J.: The Value of Postural Reduction in the Initial Management of Closed Injuries of the Spine with Paraplegia and Tetraplegia. Paraplegia, **7**:179–192, 1969.

47. Freehafer, A. A., and Mast, W. A.: Transfer of the Brachioradialis to Improve Wrist Extension in High Spinal-Cord Injury. J. Bone Joint Surg., **49A**:648–652, 1967.

48. Griswold, D. M.; Albright, J. A.; Schiffman, E.; Johnson, R.; and Southwick, W.: Atlanto-axial Fusion for Instability. J. Bone Joint Surg., **60A**:285–292, 1978.

49. Guttman, L.: Early Management of the Paraplegic. Symposium on Spinal Injuries. J. R. Coll. Surg., **8**:249, 1963.

50. Guttman, L.: Spinal Cord Injuries: Comprehensive Management and Research. London, Blackwell, 1973.

51. Hall, R. D. M.: Clay-Shoveler's Fracture. J. Bone Joint Surg., **22**:63–75, 1940.

52. Holdsworth, F.: Fractures, Dislocations, and Fracture-Dislocations of the Spine. J. Bone Joint Surg., **52A**:1534–1551, 1970.

53. Howorth, B., and Petrie, J. G.: Injuries of the Spine. Baltimore, Williams & Wilkins, 1964.

54. Jackson, H.: The Diagnosis of Minimal Atlanto-axial Subluxation. Br. J. Radiol., **23**:672–674, 1950.

55. Jacobs, B.: Cervical Fractures and Dislocations (C3-7). Clin. Orthop., **109**:18–32, 1975.

56. Jefferson, G.: Fracture of Atlas Vertebra: Report of Four Cases, and a Review of Those Previously Recorded. Br. J. Surg., **7**:407–422, 1920.

57. Johnson, R. M.; Hart, D. L.; Simmons, E. F.; Ramsby, G. R.; and Southwick, W. O.: Cervical Orthoses. A Study Comparing their Effectiveness in Restricting Cervical Motion in Normal Subjects. J. Bone Joint Surg., **59**:332–339, 1977.

58. Kahn, E. A.: On Spinal Cord Injuries. J. Bone Joint Surg., **41A**:6–11, 1959.

59. Koch, R. A., and Nickel, V. L.: The Halo Vest: An Evaluation of Motion and Forces across the Neck. Spine, **3**(2):103–107, 1978.

60. Kostuik, J. P.: Indications for the Use of the Halo Immobilization. Clin. Orthop., **154**:46–50, 1981.

61. Lipscomb, P. R.: Cervico-occipital Fusion for Congenital and Post-traumatic Anomalies of the Atlas and Axis. J. Bone Joint Surg., **39A**:1289–1301, 1957.

62. Lipscomb, P. R.; Elkins, E. C.; and Henderson, E. D.: Tendon Transfers to Restore Function of Hands in Tetraplegia, Especially after Fracture Dislocation of Sixth Cervical Vertebra on the Seventh. J. Bone Joint Surg., **40A**:1071–1080, 1958.

63. Lucas, J. T., and Ducker, T. B.: Motor Classification of Spinal Cord Injuries with Mobility, Morbidity, and Recovery Indices. Am. Surg., **45**:151–158, March, 1979.

64. MacNab, I.: Acceleration Injuries of Cervical Spine. J. Bone Joint Surg., **46A**:1797–1799, 1964.

65. Meirowsky, A. M.: Penetrating Wounds of the Spinal Canal. Problems of Paraplegia and Notes on Autonomic Hyperreflexia and Sympathetic Blockade. Clin. Orthop., **27**:90–106, 1963.

66. Merrill, V.: Atlas of Roentgenographic Positions, Vol. 1, 3rd ed. St. Louis, C. V. Mosby, 1967.

67. Moberg, E.: Surgical treatment for Absent Single-hand Grip and Elbow Extension in Quadriplegia. J. Bone Joint Surg., **57A**:196–206, 1975.

68. Nickel, V. L.; Perry, J.; Garrett, A.; and Heppenstall, M.: The Halo: A Spinal Skeletal Traction Fixation Device. J. Bone Joint Surg., **50A**:1400–1409, 1968.

69. Norton, W. L.: Fractures and Dislocations of the Cervical Spine. J. Bone Joint Surg., **44A**:115–139, 1962.

70. Nurick, S.; Russell, J. A.; and Deck, M. D. F.: Cystic Degeneration of the Spinal Cord following Spinal Cord Injury. Brain, **93**:211–222, 1970.

71. O'Brien, J. J.; Butterfield, W. L.; and Gossling, H. R.: Jefferson Fracture with Disruption of the Transverse Ligament. A Case Report. Clin. Orthop., **126**:135–138, 1977.

72. Orofino, C.; Sherman, M. S.; and Schechter, D.: Luschka's Joint—A Degenerative Phenomenon. J. Bone Joint Surg., **42A**:853–858, 1960.

73. Osterholm, J. L., and Mathews, G. J.: Treatment of Severe Spinal Cord Injuries by Biochemical Norepinephrine Manipulation. Surg. Forum, **22**:415–417, 1971.

74. Pepin, J. W., and Hawkins, R. J.: Traumatic Spondylolisthesis of the Axis: Hangman's Fracture. Clin. Orthop., **157**:133–138, 1981.

75. Perlman, S. G.: Spinal Cord Injury: A Review of Experimental Implications for Clinical Prognosis and Treatment. Arch. Phys. Med. Rehab., **55**:81–87, 1974.

76. Petrie, J. G.: Flexion Injuries of the Cervical Spine. J. Bone Joint Surg., **46A**:1800–1806, 1964.

77. Pitts, F. W., and Stauffer, E. S.: Spinal Injuries in the Multiple Injury Patient. Orthop. Clin. North Am., **1**:137–149, 1970.

78. Queckenstedt, M. E.: Zur Diagnose der rukenmarks Kompression. Dtsch. Z. Nerv., **55**:316, 1916.

79. Rogers, W. A.: Treatment of Fracture Dislocation of the Cervical Spine. J. Bone Joint Surg., **24**:245–258, 1942.

80. Rogers, W. A.: Fractures and Dislocations of Cervical

Spine: An End-result Study. J. Bone Joint Surg., **39A:**341–376, 1957.

81. Ruge, D.: Spinal Cord Injuries. Springfield, Illinois, Charles C Thomas, 1969.

82. Schlicke, L. H., and Callahan, R. A.: A Rational Approach to Burst Fractures of the Atlas. Clin. Orthop., **154:**18–21, 1981.

83. Schweigel, J. F.: Halo-thoracic Brace Management of Odontoid Fractures. Spine, **4**(3):192–194, 1979.

84. Schneider, R. C.: A Syndrome in Acute Cervical Injuries for which Early Operation is Indicated. J. Neurosurg., **8:**360–367, 1951.

85. Schneider, R. C.: The Syndrome of Acute Anterior Cervical Spinal Cord Injury. J. Neurosurg., **12:**95–122, 1955.

86. Schneider, R. C.: Trauma to the Spine and Spinal Cord. *In* Correlative Neurosurgery, p. 597. Springfield, Illinois, Charles C. Thomas, 1971.

87. Schneider, R. C.; Cherry, G.; and Pantek, H.: The Syndrome of Acute Central Cervical Spinal Cord Injury with Special Reference to the Mechanisms Involved in Hyperextension Injuries of the Cervical Spine. J. Neurosurg., **11:**546–577, 1954.

88. Schneider, R. C., and Kahn, E. A.: Chronic Neurological Sequelae of Acute Trauma to the Spine and Spinal Cord. Part I. The Significance of the Acute Flexion or "Teardrop" Fracture-Dislocation of the Cervical Spine. J. Bone Joint Surg., **38A:**985–997, 1956.

89. Schneider, R. C.; Livingston, K. E.; Cave, A. J. E.; and Hamilton, G.: "Hangman's Fracture" of the Cervical Spine. J. Neurosurg., **22:**141–154, 1965.

90. Schneider, R. C.; Thompson, J. M.; and Bebin, J.: The Syndrome of Acute Central Cervical Spinal Cord Injury. J. Neurol. Neurosurg. Psychiatry, **21:**216–227, 1958.

91. Segal, D; Whitelaw, G. P.; Gumbs, V.; and Pick, R. Y.: Tension Band Fixation of Acute Cervical Spine Fractures. Clin. Orthop. **159:**211–222, 1981.

92. Shields, C. L., Jr., and Stauffer, E. S.: Late Instability in Cervical Spine Fractures Secondary to Laminectomy. Clin. Orthop., **119:**144–147, 1976.

93. Sim, F. H.; Svien, H. J.; Bickel, W. H.; and Janes, J. M.: Swan-Neck Deformity following Extensive Cervical Laminectomy. A Review of Twenty-One Cases. J. Bone Joint Surg., **56A:**564–580, 1974.

94. Smith, G. W., and Robinson, R. A.: The Treatment of Certain Cervical Spine Disorders by Anterior Removal of The Intervertebral Disk and Interbody Fusion. J. Bone Joint Surg., **40A:**607–624, 1958.

95. Southwick, W. O.: Management of Fractures of the Dens (Odontoid Process). J. Bone Joint Surg., **62A:**482–486, 1980.

96. Southwick, W. O., and Keggi, K.: The Normal Cervical Spine. J. Bone Joint Surg., **46A:**1767–1777, 1964.

97. Southwick, W. O., and Robinson, R. A.: Surgical Approaches to the Vertebral Bodies in the Cervical and Lumbar Regions. J. Bone Joint Surg., **39A:**631–644, 1957.

98. Spence, K. F., Jr.; Decker, S.; and Sell, K. W.: Bursting Atlantal Fracture Associated with Rupture of the Transverse Ligament. J. Bone Joint Surg., **52A:**543–549, 1970.

99. Stauffer, E. S.: Orthopedic Care of Fracture Dislocations of the Cervical Spine. Proceedings of the Seventeenth V. A. Clinical Spinal Cord Injury Conference, September and October, 1969. Washington, Veterans Administration, 1970.

100. Stauffer, E. S.: Orthotics for Spinal Cord Injuries. Clin. Orthop., **102:**92–99, 1974.

101. Stauffer, E. S., and Smith, T. K.: Complications Associated with the Use of the Circular Electrical Turning Frame. J. Bone Joint Surg., **57A:**711–713, 1975.

102. Stauffer, E. S., and Kelly, E. G.: Fracture Dislocations of the Cervical Spine: Instability and Recurrent Deformity following Treatment by Anterior Interbody Fusion. J. Bone Joint Surg., **59A:**45–48, 1977.

103. Stauffer, E. S.; Wilcox, N. E.; Nickel, V. L.; and Erickson, E. R.: Interdisciplinary Clinical, Educational and Research Aspects of a Regional Center for the Rehabilitation of a Spinal Cord Injured Person: A Final Report, Funded by a Social and Rehabilitation Service Grant #RD, 2114M-68-C2, 1969.

104. Stone, W. A.; Beach, T. P.; and Hamelberg, W.: Succinylcholine—Danger in the Spinal Cord Injured Patient. Anesthesiol, **32:**168–169, 1970.

105. Stryker, H.: A Device for Turning the Frame Patient. J.A.M.A., **113:**1731–1732, 1939.

106. Suwanwela, C.; Alexander, E., Jr.; and Davis, C. H., Jr.: Prognosis in Spinal Cord Injury, with Special Reference to Patients with Motor Paralysis and Sensory Preservation. J. Neurosurg., **19:**220–227, 1962.

107. Tarlov, I. M., and Klinger, H.: Spinal Cord Compression Studies. II. Time Limits for Recovery after Acute Compression in Dogs. Arch. Neurol. Psychiatry, **71:**271–290, 1954.

108. Taylor, A. R.: The Mechanism of Injury to the Spinal Cord in the Neck without Damage to the Vertebra Column. J. Bone Joint Surg., **33B:**543–547, 1951.

109. Thompson, H.: The "Halo" Traction Apparatus. A Method of External Splinting of the Cervical Spine after Injury. J. Bone Joint Surg., **44B:**655–661, 1962.

110. Verbiest, H.: Anterior Operative Approach in Cases of Spinal Cord Compression by Old Irreducible Displacement or Fresh Fracture of Cervical Spine. J. Neurosurg., **19:**389–400, 1962.

111. Verbiest, H.: Anterolateral Operations for Fractures and Dislocations in the Middle and Lower Parts of the Cervical Spine. Report of a Series of Forty-Seven Cases. J. Bone Joint Surg., **51A:**1489–1530, 1969.

112. Vinke, T. H.: A Skull Fracture Apparatus. J. Bone Joint Surg., **30A:**522–524, 1948.

113. Wanamaker, G. T.: Spinal Cord Injuries. A Review of the Early Treatment in 300 Consecutive Cases during the Korean Conflict. J. Neurosurg., **11:**517–524, 1954.

114. Watson-Jones, R.: Fractures and Joint Injuries, 4th ed. Edinburgh, E. & S. Livingstone, 1955.

115. Webb, J. K.; Broughton, T.; McSweeney, T.; and Park, W. M.: Hidden Flexion Injury of the Cervical Spine. J. Bone Joint Surg., **58B:**322–327, 1976.

116. Wharton, G. W., and Morgan, T. H.: Ankylosis in the Paralyzed Patient. J. Bone Joint Surg., **52A:**105–112, 1970.

117. White, A. A.; Johnson, R. M.; Panjabi, M. M.; and Southwick, W. O.: Biomechanical Analysis of Clinic Sta-

bility in the Cervical Spine. Clin. Orthop., **109**:85–96, 1975.

118. White, A. A., and Panjabi, M. M.: Clinical Biomechanics of the Spine. J. B. Lippincott Company, Philadelphia, 1978, pp. 143–151.

119. White, A. A.; Southwick, W. O.; and Panjabi, M. M.: Clinical Instability of the Lower Cervical Spine. A Review of Past and Current Concepts. Spine, **1**:15–27, 1976.

120. White, J. C.: Injuries to the Cervical Cord. Fundamental Factors in Treatment and Rehabilitation (Editorial). J. Bone Joint Surg., **41A**:11–15, 1959.

121. White, R. J.; Albin, M. S.; Harris, L. S.; and Yashon, D.: Spinal Cord Injury: Sequential Morphology and Hypothermic Stabilization. Surg. Forum, **20**:432–434, 1969.

122. Whitehill, R.; Reger, S. I.; Weatherup, N.; Werthmuller, C.; Bruce, J.; Gates, P.; and Rollins, G.: Posterior Cervical Spine Fusions: A Biomechanical Analysis of their Immediate Stability. Transactions of the 27th Annual Meeting of the Orthopaedic Research Society. **6**:199, 1981.

123. Whitley, J. E., and Forsyth, H. F.: A Classification of Cervical Spine Injuries. Am. J. R., **83**:633–644, 1960.

124. Wilson, J. N.: Providing Automatic Grasp by Flexor Tenodesis. J. Bone Joint Surg., **38A**:1019–1024, 1956.

125. Wood-Jones, F.: The Ideal Lesion Produced by Judicial Hanging. Lancet, **1**:53, 1913.

126. Wortzman, G., and Dewar, F. P.: Rotary Fixation of the Atlantoaxial Joint: Rotational Atlantoaxial Subluxation. Radiology, **90**:479–487, 1968.

127. Yashon, D.; Jane, J. A.; and White, R. J.: Prognosis and Management of Spinal Cord and Cauda Equina Bullet Injuries in Sixty-Five Civilians. J. Neurosurg., **32**:163–170, 1970.

128. Zancolli, E.: Structural and Dynamic Bases of Hand Surgery. Philadelphia, J. B. Lippincott, 1968.

The Thoracolumbar Spine

129. Aebey, C.: Die Altersverschiedenheithen der menschlichen Wirbelsaule. Arch. Anat. Physiol. Entwcklngsgesch., **1**:77–138, 1879.

130. Albin, M. S.; White, R. J.; Acosta-Rua, G.; and Yashon, D.: Study of Functional Recovery Produced by Delayed Localized Cooling after Spinal Cord Injury in Primates. J. Neurosurg., **29**:113–120, 1968.

131. Alffram, P., and Lindberg, L.: External Counting of ⁸⁵SR in Vertebral Fractures. J. Bone Joint Surg., **50A**:563–569, 1968.

132. Anden, U.; Lake, A.; and Nordwall, A.: The Role of The Anterior Longitudinal Ligament in Harrington Rod Fixation of Unstable Thoracolumbar Spine Fractures. Spine, **5**:23–25, 1980.

133. Benassy, J.; Blanchard, J.; and Lecog, P.: Neurologic Recovery Rate in Para- and Tetraplegia. Paraplegia, **4**:239–263, 1967.

134. Black, P., and Markowitz, R. S.: Experimental Spinal Cord Injury in Monkeys: Comparison of Steroids and Local Hypothermia. Surg. Forum, **22**:409–411, 1971.

135. Böhler, L.: Operative Treatment of Fractures of the Dorsal and Lumbar Spine. J. Trauma, **10**:1119–1122, 1970.

136. Böhler, L.: The Treatment of Fractures, 5th ed. Vol. 1. New York, Grune & Stratton, 1956.

137. Bohlman, H. H., and Eismont, F. J.: Surgical Techniques of Anterior Decompression and Fusion for Spinal Cord Injuries. Clin. Orthop., **154**:57–67, 1981.

138. Bradford, D. S.; Akbarnia, B. A.; Winter, R. B.; and Seljoskog, E. L.: Surgical Stabilization of Fracture and Fracture Dislocations of the Thoracic Spine. Spine, **2**:185–196, 1977.

139. Brown, T.; Hansen, R. J.; and Yorra, A. J.: Some Mechanical Tests on the Lumbosacral Spine with Particular Reference to the Intervertebral Discs. J. Bone Joint Surg., **39A**:1135–1164, 1957.

140. Caffey, J.: Pediatric X-Ray Diagnosis, 6th ed. Vol. 2. Chicago, Year Book Medical Publishers, 1972.

141. Carey, P. D.: Neurosurgery and Paraplegia. Rehabilitation, **31**:27–29, 1965.

142. Chance, C. Q.: Note on a Type of Flexion Fracture of the Spine. Br. J. Radiol., **21**:452–453, 1948.

143. Convery, F. R.; Minteer, M. A.; Smith, R. W.; and Emerson, S. M.: Fracture-Dislocations of the Dorsal-Lumbar Spine: Acute Operative Stabilization by Harrington Instrumentation, Spine, **3**:160–166, 1978.

144. Creech, P.: Falls from Coconut Trees. East Afr. Med. J., **41**:63–68, 1964.

145. Cusick, J. F.; Myklebust, J. D.; and Larson, S. J.: Spinal Cord Evaluation by Cortical Evoked Response. Arch. Neurol., **36**:140–143, 1979.

146. Davies, W. E.; Morris, J. H.; and Hill, V.: An Analysis of Conservative (Non-Surgical) Management of Thoracolumbar Fractures and Fracture-Dislocations with Neural Damage. J. Bone Joint Surg., **62A**:1324–1328, 1980.

147. Davis, L.: Treatment of Spinal Cord Injuries. Arch. Surg., **49**:488–495, 1954.

148. Davis, P. R., and Rowland, H. A. K.: Vertebral Fractures in West Africans Suffering from Tetanus. A Clinical and Osteological Study. J. Bone Joint Surg., **47B**:61–71, 1965.

149. De Oliveira, J. C.: A New Type of Fracture-Dislocation of the Thoracolumbar Spine. J. Bone Joint Surg., **60A**:481–488, 1978.

150. Dewey, P., and Browne, P.S.H.: Fracture-Dislocation of the Lumbo-sacral Spine with Cauda Equina Lesion. J. Bone Joint Surg., **50B**:635–638, 1968.

151. Dickson, J. H.; Harrington, P. R.; and Wendell, D. E.: Results of Reduction and Stabilization of the Severely Fractured Thoracic and Lumbar Spine. J. Bone Joint Surg., **60A**:799–805, 1978.

152. Dommisse, G. F.: The Blood Supply of the Spinal Cord. A Critical Vascular Zone in Spinal Surgery. J. Bone Joint Surg., **56B**:225–235, 1974.

153. Doppman, J. S.; DiChiro, G.; and Ommaya, A. K.: Selective Arteriography of the Spinal Cord. St. Louis, Warren H. Green, 1969.

154. Dorsman, L. J.; Perkash, I.; Bosley, T.M.; and Cumins, K.L.: Use of Evoked Clinical Potentials to Evaluate Spinal Somatosensory Function in Patients with Traumatic and Surgical Myelopathies. J. Neurosurg., **52**:654–660, 1980.

155. Ducker, T. B., and Hamit, H. F.: Experimental Treatment

of Acute Spinal Cord Injury. J. Neurosurg., **30**:693–697, 1969.

156. Ducker, T. B.; Salcman, M.; Lucas, J. T.; Garrison, W. B.; and Perot, P.: Experimental Spinal Cord Trauma. II. Blood Flow, Tissue Oxygen, Evoked Potentials in Both Paretic and Plegic Monkeys. Surg. Neurol., **20**:64–69, 1978.

157. Ducker, T. B.; Salcman, M.; Perot, P.; and Ballantine, D.: Experimental Spinal Cord Trauma. I. Correlation of Blood Flow, Tissue Oxygen and Neurologic Status in the Dog. Surg. Neurol., **10**:60–63, 1978.

158. Edwards, C. C.; DeSilva, J. B.; and Levine, A. M.: Spinal Rod Sleeve. In Thoracic and Lumbar Spine Injury. Early Clinical Results. Presented at the A.A.O.S. meeting, New Orleans, Louisiana, 1982.

159. Elliot, H. C.: Cross Sectional Diameters and Areas of the Human Spinal Cord. Anat. Rec., **93**:287–293, 1945.

160. Engler, G. L.; Spielholz, N. L.; Bernhard, W. N.; Danziger, F.; Merkin, H.; and Wolfe, T.: Somatosensory Evoked Potentials During Harrington Instrumentation for Scoliosis. J. Bone Joint Surg., **60A**:528–532, 1978.

161. Erickson, D. L.; Leider, L. L., Jr.; and Brown, W. E.: One Stage Decompression—Stabilization for Thoracolumbar Fractures. Spine, **2**:53–56, 1977.

162. Farfan, H. F.; Cossette, J. W.; Robertson, G. H.; Wells, R. V.; and Kraus, H.: The Effects of Torsion on the Lumbar Intervertebral Joints: The Role of Torsion in the Production of Disc Degeneration. J. Bone Joint Surg., **52A**:468–497, 1970.

163. Ferguson, R.; Allen, B. L.; and Seay, G. B.: The Evolution of Segmental Spinal Instrumentation. In The Treatment of Unstable Thoracolumbar Spine Fractures. Presented at the A.A.O.S. meeting, New Orleans, Louisiana, 1982.

164. Ferguson, R. J.: Low Back Pain in College Football Linemen. J. Bone Joint Surg., **56A**:1300, 1974.

165. Flesch, J. R.; Leider, L. L.; Erickson, D. L.; Chou, S. N.; and Bradford, D. S.: Harrington Instrumentation and Spine Fusion for Unstable Fractures and Fracture-Dislocation of the Thoracic and Lumbar Spine. J. Bone Joint Surg., **59A**:143–153, 1977.

166. Giblin, D. R.: Somatosensory Evoked Potentials in Healthy Subjects and in Patients with Lesions of the Nervous System. Ann. N.Y. Acad. Sci., **112**:93–142, 1964.

167. Gregersen, G. G., and Lucas, D. B.: An In vivo Study of the Axial Rotation of the Human Thoracolumbar Spine. J. Bone Joint Surg., **49A**:247–262, 1967.

168. Guttmann, L.: Surgical Aspects of the Treatment of Traumatic Paraplegia J. Bone Joint Surg., **31B**:399–403, 1949.

169. Guttmann, L.: Spinal Cord Injuries: Comprehensive Management and Research. Oxford, Blackwell, 1976.

170. Hall, J. E.; Levine, C. R.; and Sudhir, K. G.: Intraoperative Awakening to Monitor Spinal Cord Function During Harrington Instrumentation and Spine Fusion. J. Bone Joint Surg., **60A**:533–536, 1978.

171. Hansen, S. T.; Taylor, T. K. F.; and Honet, J. C.: Management Problems in Fractures of the Ankylosed Thoracic Spine [Abstr.]. J. Bone Joint Surg., **50A**:1060–1061, 1968.

172. Hirsch, C., and Sonnerup, L.: Macroscopic Rheology in Collagen Material. J. Biomech., **1**:13–18, 1968.

173. Holdsworth, F. W.: Fractures, Dislocations, and Fracture-Dislocations of the Spine. J. Bone Joint Surg., **45B**:6–20, 1963.

174. Holdsworth, F. W.: Review Article. Fractures, Dislocations and Fracture-Dislocations of the Spine. J. Bone Joint Surg., **52A**:1534–1551, 1970.

175. Holdsworth, F. W., and Hardy, A.: Early Treatment of Paraplegia from Fractures of the Thoracolumbar Spine. J. Bone Joint Surg., **35B**:540–550, 1953.

176. Holliday, A. M.: Changes in the Form of Cerebral Evoked Response in Man Associated with Various Lesions of the Nervous System, Electroenceph. Clin. Neurophysiol., (Suppl.) **26**:178–192, 1967.

177. Hollinshead, W. H.: Anatomy for Surgeons: The Back and Limbs, Vol. 3. New York, Paul Hoeber, 1958.

178. Howland, W. J.; Curry, J. L.; and Buffington, C. G.: Fulcrum Fractures of the Lumbar Spine. J.A.M.A., **193**:240–241, 1965.

179. Jackson, D. W.; Wiltse, L. L.; and Cirincione, R. J.: Spondylolysis in the Female Gymnast. Clin. Orthop., **117**:68–73, 1976.

180. Jacobs, R. R.; Asher, M. A.; and Snider, R. K.: Thoracolumbar Spinal Injuries: A Comparative Study of Recumbent and Operative Treatment in 100 Patients. Spine, **5**:463–477, 1980.

181. Kahn, E. A.: Editorial on Spinal Cord Injuries. J. Bone Joint Surg., **41A**:6–11, 1959.

182. Kahn, E. A.; Crosby, E. C.; Schneider, R. C.; and Taren, J. A.: Correlative Neurosurgery. Springfield, Illinois, Charles C Thomas, 1969.

183. Kallio, E.: Injuries of the Thoracolumbar Spine with Paraplegia. Acta Orthop Scand., [Suppl. 60]: 1963.

184. Kaufer, H., and Hayes, J. T.: Lumbar Fracture-Dislocation. A Study of 21 Cases. J. Bone Joint Surg., **48A**:712–730, 1966.

185. Keim, H. A., and Hilal, S. K.: Spinal Angiography in Scoliosis Patients. J. Bone Joint Surg., **53A**:904–912, 1971.

186. Kelly, D. L., Jr.; Lassiter, K. R. L.; Calogero, J. A.; and Alexander, E., Jr.: Effects of Local Hypothermia and Tissue. Oxygen Studies in Experimental Paraplegia. J. Neurosurg., **33**:554–563, 1970.

187. Kelly, R. P., and Whitesides, T. E., Jr.: Treatment of Lumbodorsal Fracture-Dislocations. Ann. Surg., **167**:705–717, 1968.

188. Kilfoyle, R. M.; Foley, J. J.; and Norton, P. L.: Spine and Pelvic Deformity in Childhood and Adolescent Paraplegia. A Study of 104 Cases. J. Bone Joint Surg., **47A**:659–682, 1965.

189. Kohler, A.: Borderlands of the Normal and Early Pathologic in Skeletal Roentgenology, 2nd ed. New York, Grune & Stratton, 1961.

190. Larson, S. J.; Sances, A., Jr.; and Christenson, T. C.: Evoked Somatosensory Potentials in Man. Arch. Neurol., **15**:88–93, 1966.

191. Lewis, J. and McKibbin, B.: The Treatment of Unstable Fracture-Dislocations of the Thoraco-Lumbar Spine Accompanied by Paraplegia. J. Bone Joint Surg., **56B**:603–612, 1974.

192. Lumsden, R. M., and Morris, J. M.: An In vivo Study of

Axial Rotation and Immobilization at the Lumbosacral Joint. J. Bone Joint Surg., **50A:**1591–1602, 1968.

193. Markolf, K. L.: Deformation of the Thoracolumbar Intervertebral Joints in Response to External Loads. A Biomechanical Study Using Autopsy Material. J. Bone Joint Surg., **54A:**511–533, 1972.

194. Mayfield, J. K.; Erkkila, J. C.; and Winter, R. B.: Spinal Deformity Subsequent to Acquired Childhood Spinal Cord Injury. J. Bone Joint Surg., **63A:**1401–1411, 1981.

195. Miller, C. A.; Dewey, R. C.; and Hunt, W. E.: Impaction of the Lumbar Vertebrae with Dural Tear. J. Neurosurg., **53:**765–771, 1980.

196. Morgan, T. H.; Wharton, G. W.; and Austin, G. N.: The Results of Laminectomy in Patients with Incomplete Spinal Cord Injuries. Paraplegia, **9:**14–23, 1971.

197. Morris, J. M.: Biomechanics of the Spine. Arch. Surg., **107:**418–423, 1973.

198. Morris, J. M.; Lucas, D. B.; and Bresler, B.: Role of the Trunk in Stability of the Spine. J. Bone Joint Surg., **43A:**327–351, 1961.

199. Munro, D.: The Role of Fusion or Wiring in the Treatment of Acute Traumatic Instability of the Spine. Paraplegia, **3:**97–111, 1961.

200. Nachemson, A., and Morris, J.: In-vivo Measurements of Intradiscal Pressure. J. Bone Joint Surg., **46A:**1077–1092, 1964.

201. Naffziger, H. C.: The Neurological Aspects of Injuries to the Spine. J. Bone Joint Surg., **20:**444–448, 1938.

202. Nagel, D. A.; Koogle, T. A.; Piziali, R. L.; and Perkash, I.: Stability of the Upper Lumbar Spine Following Progressive Disruptions and the Application of Individual Intenal and External Fixation Devices. J. Bone Joint Surg., **63A:**62–70, 1981.

203. Namerow, N. S.: Somatosensory Evoked Responses Following Cervical Cordotomy. Bull. Los Angeles Neurol. Soc., **34:**184–188, 1969.

204. Nash, C. L. (ed.): Proceedings: Clinical Application of Spinal Cord Monitoring for Operative Treatment of Spinal Diseases. Cincinnati, Case Western Reserve University Press, 1978.

205. Nash, C. L., and Brown, R. H.: The Intraoperative Monitoring of Spinal Cord Function: Its Growth and Current Status. Orthop. Clin. North Am. **4:**919–926, 1979.

206. Nash, C. L., Jr.; Lorig, A.; Schatzinger, M. L. A.; and Brown, R. H.: Spinal Cord Monitoring During Operative Treatment of the Spine. Clin. Orthop., **126:**100–105, 1977.

207. Nash, C. L., Jr.; Schatzinger, L. H.; Brown, R. H.; Brodkey, J.: The Unstable Stable Thoracic Compression Fracture: Its Problems and the Use of Spinal Cord Monitoring in the Evaluation of Treatment. Spine, **2:**261–265, 1977.

208. Nicoll, E. A.: Fractures of the Dorso-lumbar Spine. J. Bone Joint Surg., **31B:**376–394, 1949.

209. Nordwall, A.; Valencia, P.; Harada, Y.; Axelgaard, J.; McNeal, D.; Brown, J. C.; and Nickel, V.: Spinal Cord Monitoring Using Spinal Evoked Potential. Presented at the 12th Annual Meeting of the Scoliosis Research Society, 1977.

210. Norton, P. L., and Brown, T.: The Immobilizing Efficiency of Back Braces. J. Bone Joint Surg., **39A:**111–139, 1957.

211. Nykamp, P. W.; Levy, J. M.; Christensen, F.; Dunn, R.; and Hubbard, J.: Computed Tomography for a Bursting Fracture of the Lumbar Spine. J. Bone Joint Surg., **60A:**1108–1109, 1978.

212. Olsson, O.: Fractures of the Upper Thoracic and Cervical Vertebral Bodies. Acta. Chir. Scand., **102:**87–92, 1951.

213. Osebold, W. R.; Weinstein, S. L.; and Sprague, B. L.: Thoracolumbar Spine Fractures: Results of Treatment. Spine, **6:**13–34, 1981.

214. Pennal, G.: Stress Studies of the Lumbar Spine [Abstr.]. J. Bone Joint Surg., **48B:**180, 1966.

215. Purcell, G. A.; Markolf, K. L.; and Dawson, E. G.: Twelfth Thoracic-First Lumbar Vertebral Mechanical Stability of Fractures After Harrington-Rod Instrumentation. J. Bone Joint Surg., **63A:**71–78, 1981.

216. Rennie, W., and Mitchell, N.: Flexion Distraction Fractures of the Thoracolumbar Spine. J. Bone Joint Surg., **55A:**386–390, 1973.

217. Roaf, R.: A Study of the Mechanics of Spinal Injuries. J. Bone Joint Surg., **42B:**810–823, 1960.

218. Roberts, J. B., and Curtiss, P. H., Jr.: Stability of the Thoracic and Lumbar Spine in Traumatic Paraplegia following Fracture or Fracture-Dislocation. J. Bone Joint Surg., **52A:**1115–1130, 1970.

219. Rogers, W. A.: Cord Injury during Reduction of Thoracic and Lumbar Vertebral-Body Fracture and Dislocation. J. Bone Joint Surg., **20:**689–695, 1938.

220. Schmorl, G., and Junghanns, H.: The Human Spine in Health and Disease. New York, Grune & Stratton, 1971.

221. Schneider, R. C.: Surgical Indications and Contra-indications in Spine and Spinal Cord Trauma. Clin. Neurosurg., **8:**157–184, 1962.

222. Schneider, R. C.: Head and Neck Injuries in Football. Baltimore, Williams & Wilkins, 1973.

223. Schneider, R. C., and Crosby, E.: Vascular Insufficiency. Neurology, **9:**649–656, 1959.

224. Schneider, R. C.; Crosby, E. C.; Russo, R. H.; and Gosch, H. H.: Traumatic Spinal Cord Syndromes and their Management. Clin. Neurosurg., **20:**424–492, 1973.

225. Smith, W. S., and Kaufer, H.: Patterns and Mechanisms of Lumbar Injuries Associated with Lap Seat Belts. J. Bone Joint Surg., **51A:**239–254, 1969.

226. Sonoda, T.: Studies on the Strength for Compression, Tension and Torsion of the Vertebral Column. J. Kyoto Pref. Med. Univ., **71:**659–662, 1962.

227. Spencer, D. L., and DeWald, R. L.: Simultaneous Anterior and Posterior Surgical Approach to the Thoracic and Lumbar Spine. Spine, **4:**29–36, 1979.

228. Spielholz, N. I.; Benjamin, M. V.; Engler, G. L.; and Ransohoff, J.: Somatosensory Evoked Potentials During Decompression and Stabilization of the Spine, Methods and Findings. Spine, **4:**500–505, 1979.

229. Stanger, J. K.: Fracture-Dislocation of the Thoracolumbar Spine. With Special Reference to Reduction by Open and Closed Operations. J. Bone Joint Surg., **29:**107–118, 1947.

230. Stauffer, E. S., and Neil, J. L.: Biomechanical Analysis of Structural Stability of Internal Fixation in Fractures of the Thoracolumbar Spine. Clin. Orthop., **112:**159–164, 1975.

231. Stauffer, E. S.; Wood, W.; and Kelly, E. G.: Gunshot Wounds of the Spine: The Effects of Laminectomy. J. Bone Joint Surg., **61A**:389–392, 1979.

232. Sullivan, C. R., and Beckwell, W. H.: Problems of Traumatic Spondylolysis. Am. J. Surg., **100**:698–708, 1960.

233. Tarlov, I. M.: Spinal Cord Compression: Mechanism of Paralysis and Treatment. Springfield, Illinois, Charles C Thomas, 1957.

234. Taylor, R. G., and Ceave, J. R. N.: Injuries to the Cervical Spine. Proc. R. Soc. Med., **5**:1053, 1962.

235. Vauzelle, C.; Stagnara, P.; and Jouvinroux, P.: Functional Monitoring of Spinal Cord Activity During Spinal Surgery. Clin. Orthop., **93**:173–178, 1973.

236. Virgin, W. J.: Experimental Investigations into the Physical Properties of the Intervertebral Disc. J. Bone Joint Surg., **33B**:607–611, 1951.

237. Waldman, J.; Kaufer, H.; Hensinger, R. N.; Callaghan, M. D.; and Leiding, K. G.: "Wake Up" Technique to Avoid Neurologic Sequelae During Harrington Rod Procedures. A Case Report. Anes. Anal., **56**:733–735, 1977.

238. Waters, R. L., and Morris, J. M.: Effect of Spinal Supports on the Electrical Activity of Muscles of the Trunk. J. Bone Joint Surg., **52A**:51–60, 1970.

239. Watson-Jones, R.: Fractures and Joint Injuries, 4th ed., Vol. 2. Baltimore, Williams & Wilkins, 1955.

240. Weiss, M.: Dynamic Spine Alloplasty (Spring-Loading Corrective Devices) After Fracture and Spinal Cord Injury. Clin. Orthop., **112**:150–158, 1975.

241. Westerborn, A., and Olsson, O.: Mechanics, Treatment and Prognosis of Fracture of the Dorso-lumbar Spine. Acta Chir. Scand., **102**:59–83, 1951.

242. White, A. A., III, and Hirsch, C.: The Significance of the Vertebral Posterior Elements in the Mechanics of the Thoracic Spine. Clin. Orthop., **81**:2–14, 1971.

243. White, A. A., and Panjabi, M. M.: Clinical Biomechanics of the Spine. Philadelphia, J. B. Lippincott, 1978.

244. Whitesides, T. E.; Kelley, R. P.; and Howland, S. C.: The Treatment of Lumbodorsal Fracture-Dislocations [Abstr.]. J. Bone Joint Surg., **52A**:1267, 1970.

245. Whiteside, T. E.: Traumatic Kyphosis of the Thoracolumbar Spine. Clin. Orthop., **128**:78–92, 1977.

246. Winter, R. B.; Moe, J. H.; and Wang, J. F.: Congenital Kyphosis. Its Natural History and Treatment as Observed in a Study of 130 Patients. J. Bone Joint Surg., **55A**:223–256, 1973.

247. Woodburne, R. T.: Essentials of Human Anatomy. New York, Oxford University Press, 1957.

248. Yasuoka, S.; Peterson, H. A.; and MacCarty, C. S.: The Incidence of Spinal Deformity and Instability After Multiple Level Laminectomy: Its Difference in Children and Adults. Presented at the 16th annual meeting of the Scoliosis Research Society, Montreal, 1981.

249. Yocum, T. D.; Leatherman, K. D.; and Brower, T. D.: The Early Rod Fixation in Treatment of Fracture-Dislocations of the Spine [Exhibit]. J. Bone Joint Surg., **52A**:1257, 1970.

250. Young, M. H.: Long-term Consequences of Stable Fractures of the Thoracic and Lumbar Vertebral Bodies. J. Bone Joint Surg., **55B**:295–300, 1973.

13

Fractures of the Pelvis *William J. Kane*

In the last decade a number of advances in the management of fractures of the pelvis have been introduced, and in the ensuing years there have been numerous reports dedicated to defining the indications and benefits of these newer diagnostic and therapeutic modalities. Three of the innovations are computed tomography of the pelvis, the somewhat broader acceptance of the concept of arteriography and arterial embolization for the management of hemorrhage associated with fractures of the pelvis, and the wider use of fixation devices—both external and internal—in the stabilization of pelvic fractures.

To be sure, these have not been the only contributions to the treatment of patients with pelvic fractures; indeed, it may very well be that the most important development of the last decade with respect to pelvic fractures is the change in attitude of the literature and, more important, of the treating surgeons to adopt an anticipatory rather than reactionary management program. By this I mean that authors and their readers are trying to more actively define the extent of the hard and soft tissue trauma associated with fractures of the pelvis, rather than to passively allow the fractures and their sequelae to reveal themselves in a gradual unfolding.

The advantages of such a management program have been highlighted by the recognition of the lethality of open pelvic fractures, by the investigation and treatment of lower urinary tract injuries, by the need for adequate intra-abdominal diagnostic procedures, as well as by the use of computed

tomography (CT) scans, arterial angiography and embolization, and fixation of fractures to achieve early mobilization. These advances are affecting patient care in a very positive fashion. That there has been a distinct alteration in the concepts of traumatologists treating patients with severe disruptions of the pelvis resulting in a more optimistic prognosis and a more active management regimen seems undeniable.

Fractures of the pelvis constitute one out of every 1000 surgical admissions[475] and 3% of all skeletal fractures.[500] Pelvic fractures are challenging and fascinating not only because of the effect they have on the musculoskeletal system but also because of the consequences on the soft viscera contained within the pelvis. "Fractures of the pelvis are secondary only to those of the skull in terms of interest, mortality, and other complications."[87] The pelvic fracture "may be the least important of the multiple injuries sustained"[462] in a trauma, and be of "less consequence than the mischief occasioned by the force which produced it,"[119] but the overriding concern in managing a fracture of the pelvis is to maintain a vigilance and awareness of the complications associated with fractures of the pelvis.

McLaughlin[275] put it best, I believe, when he stated that "in general, fractures of the pelvis should not be considered as specialized orthopaedic problems or even as fracture problems. They are problems for a physician who will not permit himself to be diverted from considering the possibilities of lethal visceral damage by the presence of broken bones, no matter how spectacular these may appear; one who will discipline himself to maintain a broad surgical horizon and who will not hesitate to call for help when it is required. . . . It is when the physician allows his attention to be diverted from the possibility of concomitant visceral injuries by some obvious fracture that the results so often are devastating.''

Conway[89] also emphasized that, although visceral complications attendant on pelvic fractures are relatively infrequent, a sense of complacency should not be allowed to develop. He reported four instances of genitourinary injury in 56 cases. Gilmour[155] reported nine cases of bladder rupture in 81 cases, and Colp and Findlay,[85] in a series of 35 consecutive cases, found three instances of ruptured bladder and two with ruptured urethra. Wakeley,[489] in a series of 100 cases, noted visceral complications in 11. Rankin,[377] however, reported a much lower incidence of visceral injury with pelvic fractures, finding only ten instances of bladder or urethra rupture in 449 cases. In this series there were 41 deaths.

The important message here, however, is not a statistical one; it is one of the necessity for alertness, perception, and concern. These are the factors that caused the mortality rate for pelvic fractures (reported to be 87% prior to 1890) to drop to about 50% from 1890 to 1905, to about 40% from 1905 to 1916,[370] to 10% to 30% around 1939,[502] and finally to 5% to 20% in the recent literature.[87,141,181,194,254,350] The advent of more specific diagnostic tools, the widespread availability of whole blood and volume expanders, the possibility of direct and early surgical intervention when indicated, and the continued assessment and analysis of therapies in clinical and experimental environments have contributed in a major way to the improved prognosis and decreased mortality rates for fractures of the pelvis.

The role of the automobile as the most common cause of pelvic fractures became apparent in reviews from industrialized nations as early as the mid-1930s.[377] Since then, the car has been responsible for most fractures of the pelvis in virtually every age group except those over 60 years, in whom falls in the home represent the major cause of pelvic fractures (followed by vehicular accidents).[145,181] Traffic accidents are responsible for about two thirds of all pelvic fractures, and pedestrians are more frequently injured than are the occupants of vehicles. About one fourth are due to minor falls, primarily in older persons, and about one tenth are due to industrial accidents and major falls.

ANATOMY

The pelvic girdle consists of two innominate bones that articulate anteriorly with each other at the symphysis pubis and posteriorly with the sacrum, which in turn articulates inferiorly with the coccyx. Each innominate bone is made up of the ilium, ischium, and pubis, all of which contribute to the formation of the acetabulum. The coccyx articulates at the inferior edge of the sacrum and provides some additional posterior protection to the abdominal and pelvic viscera found within the pelvic cavity. The pelvis is anatomically and functionally divided into two portions by an oblique plane passing through the upper symphysis pubis, the iliopectineal and arcuate lines, and the promontory of the sacrum. These boundaries form the pelvic inlet. Above the pelvic inlet is the upper or false pelvis, a cone-shaped structure that is actually a part of the abdomen, and below the pelvic inlet is the lower or true pelvis. In the erect position the plane of the pelvic inlet forms an angle of approximately 55° with a horizontal. The posterior surface of the symphysis faces upwards and backward, and the pelvic surface of the sacrum faces downward and forward.[287] The true pelvis contains the organs of reproduction, and through it pass portions of the urinary and digestive systems and major vessels and nerves to the lower extremities. The major function of the pelvis—in addition to protection—is the support of the spine in both sitting and erect postures. In the erect posture the weight-bearing forces are transmitted from the upper femora to the acetabula and then through thick rings of the ilia called the arcuate lines, which curve superiorly and posteriorly to the sacroiliac joints and then into the spinal column through the sacrum. This is the femorosacral arch. In the sitting position, the weight is borne through the sacroiliac joints into the ilia and then down to ischial tuberosities, forming the ischiosacral arch. These two main arches are augmented by two subsidiary (or tie) arches that join the extremities of the main ones. One, made up of the bodies of the pubic bones and their horizontal rami, connects the femorosacral arch; the other, made up of the ischial rami and inferior pubic rami, connects the ends of the ischiosacral arch (Figs. 13-1 and 13-2). There is a complex system of bony trabeculae in the pelvic bones corresponding to the lines of force.[221] When traumatized, the tie arches give first, then the main arches. The areas most susceptible to interruption are the pubic symphysis, the pubic rami, and the areas just lateral to the sacroiliac joints.[40,500]

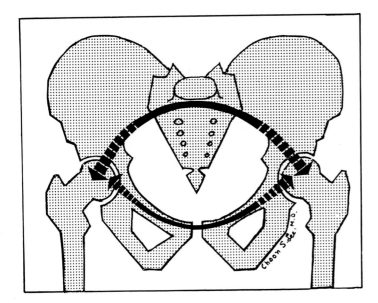

Fig. 13-1. In the erect position, weight-bearing forces are transmitted from the upper femora to the acetabula and then through thick rings of the ilia, called the arcuate lines, which curve superiorly and posteriorly to the sacroiliac joints and then into the spinal column through the sacrum. This forms the femorosacral arch. This main arch is augmented by a subsidiary tie arch that joins the extremities of the femorosacral arch. The subsidiary arch is composed of the bodies of the pubic bones and their horizontal rami.

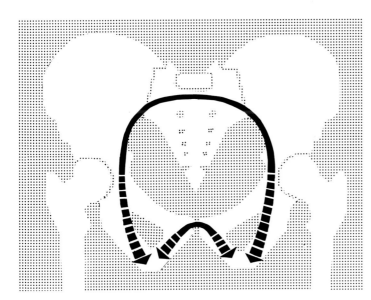

Fig. 13-2. In the sitting position the weight-bearing forces are transmitted from the ischial tuberosities through the ilia and into the sacroiliac joints. This forms the ischiosacral arch. This main arch is augmented by a subsidiary tie arch that joins the extremities of the main arch. It is composed of the bodies of the pubic bones, the inferior pubic rami, and the ischial rami.

Since the joints of the pelvic ring (*i.e.,* the sacroiliac, the symphysis pubis, and the sacrococcygeal joint) are virtually immobile, there is little need for muscles to act across these joints. However, the pelvis is the origin for a number of muscles that are used to provide locomotion through the hips and knees, and it provides attachments that are used to maintain posture through the musculature of the torso.

In common with many other flat bones, the pelvic bones are a significant source of hematopoietic marrow in the adult and a locus for the storage of minerals, including calcium, phosphorus, and sodium.

The pelvis is thus a protective cage for the lower abdominal viscera and a weight bearer between the trunk and lower limbs, and many structures either lie within, pass through, or are attached to its surfaces. This has been expressed somewhat poetically by Howell[196]: "Within its borders are housed a portion of the urinary and intestinal systems and the female genitalia; through its foramina pass the great nerve trunks and blood vessels, while beneath its arches, pass all mankind, with few exceptions, the most notable Julius Caesar.''

BONES

The innominate bone, which is also called the hip bone or the os coxae, is made up in childhood of three separate bones that fuse in adult life at the acetabulum. These parts are the ilium, the ischium, and the pubis. The ilium forms the superior third of the acetabulum, the pubis the anterior third, and the ischium the posteroinferior third (Fig. 13-3).

The ilium is a fan-shaped bone composed of a body and a wing. The cephalad edge of the wing, called the iliac crest, runs subcutaneously from the anterior superior iliac spine superiorly and posteriorly in a curving fashion to the posterior superior iliac spine. The remainder of the bone is covered by muscles, medially by the origins of the iliacus, the quadratus lumborum, and the erector spinae (iliocostalis lumborum) as well as the transversus abdominis. Laterally, the ilium serves as origin for the three gluteii muscles as well as the tensor fasciae latae, sartorius, straight and reflected heads of the rectus femoris, and the piriformis. In addition, it also serves as the attachment for the latissimus dorsi and the internal and external obliquus abdominis. The posterior superior iliac spines are level with the midpoint of the sacroiliac joints as well as the second sacral vertebra, while the posterior inferior iliac spines are level with the third sacral vertebra. The sacral surface of the ilium, which is in the posterosuperior portion of the fan-shaped portion of the ilium, is divided into two unequal sections. The posterior and superior portion, which is called the iliac tuberosity, is very rough and serves for the attachment of the dorsal and interosseous sacroiliac ligaments. Inferior and anterior to this more or less oval region lies an auricular-shaped region that is covered with cartilage and serves as the lateral surface of the sacroiliac joint. Posterior to the auricular surface is the posterior inferior iliac spine, the posterior and inferior continuation of the iliac crest. Beneath the auricular surface lies the greater sciatic notch. The inner surface of the ilium is divided by the iliopectineal line into the large, smooth, concave upper surface called the iliac fossa and the small roughened posterior portion that articulates with the sacrum.

The pubis is an angular bone that consists of a blunted apex, called the body, and a superior ramus, which forms the superior border of the obturator foramen and which runs horizontally and posteriorly to the acetabulum. The body of the pubis articulates through the symphysis pubis with the opposite pubis, and it gives rise to the inferior ramus, which is directed posteriorly and laterally to articulate with the ischium and forms the inferior boundary of the obturator foramen. The inferior ramus of the pubis and the ramus of the ischium form the conjoint ramus, and the conjoint rami of both sides form the pubic arch. Beneath the symphysis pubis the inferior pubic ramus serves as origin for the levator ani, the deep transverse

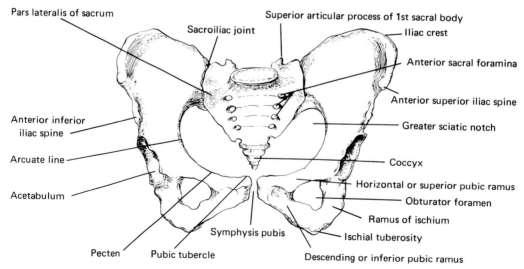

Fig. 13-3. The anatomical features seen in a routine anteroposterior view of the pelvis.

perineus, and sphincter urethrae, as well as the adductor longus, adductor brevis, gracilis, and portions of the obturator externus, obturator internus, and adductor magnus. The superior ramus gives origin to the pectineus and is also the insertion of the rectus abdominis. The symphysis pubis also serves as the medial attachment of the inguinal ligament, which is also attached at the anterior superior iliac spine.

The ischium is an irregular semilunar-shaped bone consisting of a body superiorly that participates in the formation of the acetabulum, a posteriorly and inferiorly directed tuberosity, and a thinner, anterior ramus directed medially, which articulates with the inferior pubic ramus. On the posterior border of the body of the ischium is the ischial spine, which forms the lateral portion of the inferior border of the greater sciatic notch and the superior border of the lesser sciatic notch, which is bounded at its inferior portion by the ischial tuberosity. The ischial spine gives rise medially to the coccygeus and the levator ani and laterally to the superior gemellus. Its extreme posterior surface gives rise to the sacrospinous ligament, which forms the medial portion of the inferior border of the greater sciatic foramen.

The ischial tuberosity is a rough protuberance palpable just lateral to the anus. Laterally, the ischial tuberosity gives rise to the semimembranosus, semitendinosus, and biceps, as well as the quadratus femoris and a portion of the adductor magnus. Medially, it gives rise to the ischiocavernosus. Portions of the obturator externus and obturator internus arise from the body, the tuberosity, and the ramus of the ischium. The sacrotuberous ligament arises from the tuberosity of the ischium and forms the medial border of both the lesser sciatic foramen and the greater sciatic foramen. This ligament attaches to the posterior surfaces of the lower three sacral vertebrae as well as a posterior portion of the iliac crests in the region of the two posterior iliac spines. The sacrotuberous and the sacrospinous ligaments, which attach to the lateral border of the lower part of the sacrum and to the coccyx, brace the pelvis against rotation of the sacrum between the two hip bones. The weight of the body on the upper end of the sacrum tends to force it downward and forward so that the coccygeal end would move upward and backward were it not for these two ligaments.

The sacrum is a large irregular truncated pyramid with six surfaces. It is formed of five fused vertebrae that diminish in size in the caudad direction. The base, the upper aspect of the first sacral vertebra, is tilted forward in the erect position at an angle of approximately 30° to 40°. The posterior surface is a slightly convex, roughened surface formed from the spinous processes of the four cephalad vertebrae into a median sacral crest, which is deficient caudally, creating a dorsally located sacral hiatus. The gently concave anterior surface consists of the fused bodies of the sacral vertebrae, and transverse lines indicate that the regions of the fusion can be noted on the anterior surface. This anterior surface of the sacrum forms the posterior wall of the pelvis. On both the anterior and dorsal surfaces, there are four sets of sacral foramina opposite each other that connect medially with the sacral portion of the vertebral canal. Through the dorsal sacral foramina emerge the posterior primary rami of the spinal nerves, while the anterior primary rami emerge through the anterior sacral foramina and later converge to form the sacral plexus. The large lateral mass of the sacrum, called the pars lateralis, is formed by union of the lateral extremities of the lateral processes of the upper three sacral vertebrae and articulates on each side with the articular portion of the ilium. Despite what could be anticipated teleologically of the sacroiliac joints, the posterior dimension of the sacrum is not wider than the anterior dimension; consequently, the body weight pressing down on the sacrum does not increase the stability as one might expect, extrapolating from the keystone principle in the arch. Rather, the two lateral surfaces of the sacrum, which articulate with the ilia, are suspended by the extremely strong and heavy posterior sacroiliac ligaments.

The superior surface of the sacrum articulates with the inferior surface of the last lumbar vertebra by an intervertebral disc, and two superior articular processes articulate via synovial joints with the inferior articular processes of the last lumbar vertebra. The superior anterior margin of the first sacral vertebra projects forward in a sharp lip called the promontory of the sacrum. The inferior surface of the sacrum articulates with the superior surface of the coccyx. The apex of the sacrum is directed downward and articulates with the body of the first coccygeal vertebra by a fibrocartilaginous disc.

The coccyx consists of four or five fused vertebral bodies that are quite rudimentary and are attached to the inferior sacral surface by ligaments. The proximal segment is web-shaped and toward midlife it becomes fused with the sacrum.[212] The last three or four segments are usually fused together and angulated forward to some degree. Four important muscles attach to the coccyx.[256] They are the gluteus maximus posteriorly, the coccygeus anteriorly, the sphincter ani to the anterior tip, and the levator ani to the posterior tip. Johnson[212] stated that in men the high position of the coccyx in close proximity to the tuberosities of the ischia make it less vulnerable to trauma.

In the female pelvis, to accommodate its normal reproductive functions the iliac wings are more vertical, the symphysis is wider, the lesser pelvis is wider and more shallow, the pubic arch is wider, and the sacrum is broader and less curved. An oval pelvic opening more adapted overall to the process of parturition is the result (Figs. 13-4 and 13-5).

Hollinshead[189] noted the abundant vascular supply of the innominate bone as evidenced by its numerous vascular foramina, and this fact is well recognized by surgeons who remove portions of the ilium for bone grafting or who osteotomize the innominate bone for reconstruction. This supply comes from virtually all of the neighboring smaller arterial branches, including the deep iliac circumflex, iliolumbar, obturator, superior and inferior gluteal as well as the medial and lateral femoral circumflex arteries.[189] This rich vascular supply has a significance that is frequently unrecognized but will be touched on in the management of hemorrhage associated with pelvic fractures.

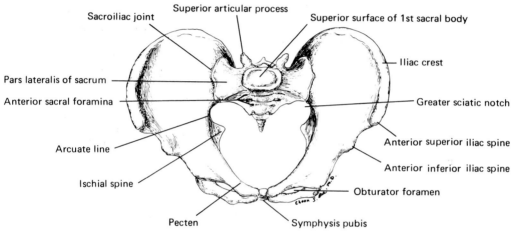

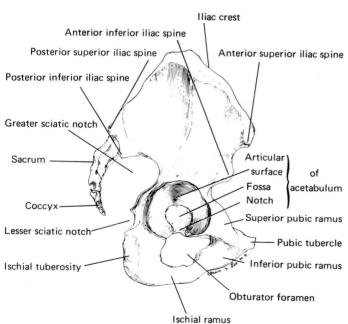

Fig. 13-4. (*Top*) "Inlet" and (*left*) lateral views of a typical male pelvis demonstrating that it is generally heavier and more conical than the female pelvis. The iliac bones are less flared, the muscle attachments are more strongly marked, and the pubic arch is more angular in shape, representing an aperture of 70° to 75°. The sacrosciatic notch is narrower, and the distance between the lower border of the sacrum and the ischial spine is smaller than in the female pelvis. Relatively speaking, the distance between the anterosuperior iliac spines is somewhat less in the male, as are all diameters of the pelvic cavity.

JOINTS AND LIGAMENTS

The posterior lumbosacral joints consist of diarthrodial gliding joints, which are located between the articular processes of the last lumbar vertebra and the sacrum. They are true diarthroses—they have joint cavities, capsules, and articular surfaces covered with hyaline cartilage. Although the superior interlumbar joints are sagittal, the lumbosacral joints are oblique to both the sagittal and coronal planes in order to prevent forward slipping of the fifth lumbar vertebra on the sacrum. The joint between the body of the fifth lumbar vertebra and the body of the first sacral vertebra is an amphiarthrosis because of the thick intervening fibrocartilaginous intervertebral disk. Sacrolumbar ligaments and iliolumbar ligaments attach to the lateral extremities of the transverse processes of the most distal lumbar vertebrae, reducing the amount of rotation that can take place at the joints and also limiting the amount of forward motion of the lower lumbar vertebrae on the sacrum.[103]

The sacrococcygeal joint is an amphiarthrosis with a thin intervertebral disk. The anterior sacrococcygeal ligament is a continuation of the anterior longitudinal ligament of the vertebral column, while the deep portion of the posterior sacrococcygeal ligament is a continuation of the posterior longitudinal ligament of the vertebral column, and the superficial portion is a continuation of the supraspinous and interspinous ligaments.

The sacroiliac joint is usually classified as a gliding diarthrodial joint, but other authors classify the joint as an amphiarthrosis because of the presence of fibrous bands that cross the true joint cavity and that sometimes completely obliterate the joint space.[44,415] Of considerable additional stabilizing benefit, despite their reversed taper, is the fact that the surfaces of the sacroiliac joints are not smooth but are rather undulating concavoconvex in shape, and there is a "small but effective shelf which is formed anteriorly by the iliac component of the sacroiliac joint."[117] The major structures that resist descent and forward rotation of the sacrum are the strong interosseous sacroiliac ligaments, which are posterior and superior to the articular surfaces (Fig. 13-6).[117] As the sacrum is broader above than it is below, it is wedge-shaped; being suspended by ligaments, the heavier the weight it is bearing the more tightly it is held. Kapandji[221] calls it a "self-locking system." The dorsal sacroiliac ligaments assist in stabilizing the sacrum, while the sacrotuberous and sacrospinous ligaments prevent posterior rotation of the lower portion of the sac-

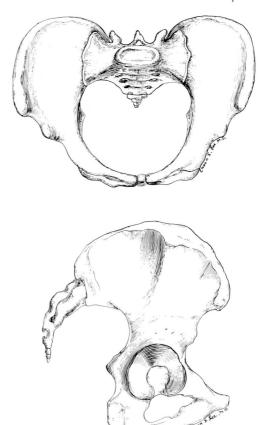

Fig. 13-5. (*Top*) "Inlet" and (*bottom*) lateral views of the female pelvis reveal anatomical differences for the accommodation of normal reproductive functions. The symphysis pubis is wider, the lesser pelvis is wider and more shallow, the pubic arch is wider, and the sacrum is broader and less curved. The female pelvis is, generally speaking, lighter, lower, and more circular than the pelvis of the male. The muscle attachments are less strongly marked, the pubic arch presents an aperture of 90° to 100° in the female. The sacrosciatic notch is broader, and the distance between the lower border of the sacrum and the ischial spine is wider than in the male pelvis.

rum.[445,502,503] The anterior sacroiliac ligaments are thin and weak and really serve only as a joint capsule to separate the joint cavity from the pelvic cavity (Fig. 13-7). Unless the tie-beam of the pubis is intact, Dommisse[118] stated, "the sacroiliac joints must and do separate or widen in front. The separation of the two pubic bones leads to wider spacing of the iliac bones so that the sacrum, being less tightly held, can move forward. The anterior

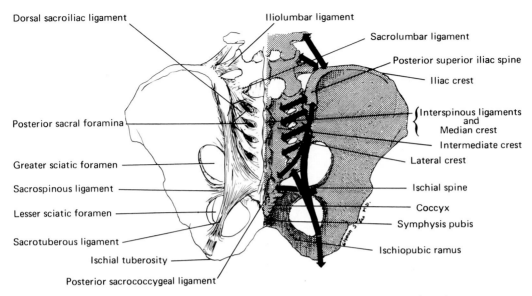

Dorsal sacroiliac ligament

Iliolumbar ligament

Sacrolumbar ligament

Posterior superior iliac spine

Iliac crest

Interspinous ligaments and Median crest

Intermediate crest

Lateral crest

Ischial spine

Coccyx

Symphysis pubis

Ischiopubic ramus

Posterior sacral foramina

Greater sciatic foramen

Sacrospinous ligament

Lesser sciatic foramen

Sacrotuberous ligament

Ischial tuberosity

Posterior sacrococcygeal ligament

Fig. 13-6. The chief bracing ligaments of the sacroiliac joint are the strong dorsal sacroiliac ligaments which resist descent and forward rotation of the sacrum. The sacrotuberous and sacrospinous ligaments prevent posterior rotation of the lower portion of the sacrum. Sacrolumbar and iliolumbar ligaments attached to the lateral extremities of the transverse processes of the lowermost lumbar vertebrae reduce the amount of rotation that can take place at the joints and also limit the amount of forward motion of the lower lumbar vertebrae forward on the sacrum. The greater sciatic foramen is separated from the lesser sciatic foramen by the sacrospinous ligament. The sacrotuberous ligament forms the medial border of both the greater sciatic foramen and the lesser sciatic foramen.

(sacroiliac) ligaments are too thin to offer any resistance to this diastasis." Peltier,[350] among others, disputed the claim, stating, "Weight-bearing is not impaired in patients with deficiency of the anterior pelvic ring due to congenital defects associated with extrophy of the bladder or after resection of this portion of the ring for tumors or osteomyelitis." Sullivan[462] showed x-rays of two laborers who had had surgery that completely removed the tie arches for osteomyelitis, but left the iliac bones and sacrum; each returned to work without sacroiliac symptoms or instability. "One must assume that the sacroiliac, sacrotuberous, and sacrospinous ligaments are perfectly adequate to support the ordinary stresses imposed on the pelvis without its tie arch.[462] Resolution of this apparent difficulty may lie in the fact that adult men who lose the mobility of their sacroiliac joints are less in need of the anterior tie arch, but women, especially in the child-bearing age, might be less able to tolerate the stress of the sacroiliac joints without the anterior tie arch. Mobility of the sacroiliac joints is described as very slight at the most, consisting of a gliding vertical movement with slight

anteroposterior movement. With the exception of the pubertal and pregnant female, the mobility in the joint tends to diminish as age increases, as does the articular cartilage. It usually disappears in men about the fourth decade and in women usually toward the end of the fifth decade.[44,117,140,415]

The symphysis pubis is an amphiarthrosis in which the bodies of the two pubic bones are united by a fibrocartilaginous disk. The superficial fibers of the upper border of the disk are blended with the superior pubic ligament and those of the lower border with the arcuate pubic ligament. The pubic fibrocartilage may be solid, but frequently there is a narrow fissure. This has been interpreted as a degenerative change frequently accelerated by pregnancy.[144]

As a result of the increased mobility of all the pelvic joints in conjunction with pregnancy and parturition, there is an increased susceptibility that the woman may be traumatized near delivery by unusually wide disruptions of the symphysis and the sacroiliac joints. Baijal reported on this and hypothesized that it may be for the same reason that the abnormal degree of laxity facilitates re-

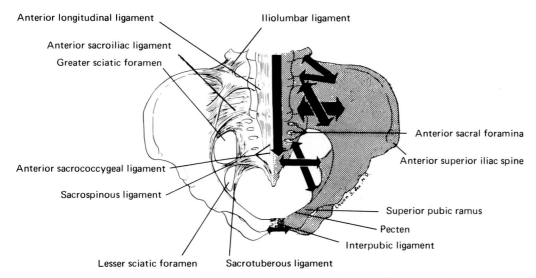

Anterior longitudinal ligament

Anterior sacroiliac ligament

Greater sciatic foramen

Iliolumbar ligament

Anterior sacral foramina

Anterior superior iliac spine

Anterior sacrococcygeal ligament

Sacrospinous ligament

Superior pubic ramus

Pecten

Interpubic ligament

Lesser sciatic foramen

Sacrotuberous ligament

Fig. 13-7. The anterior sacroiliac ligaments are thin and weak and really serve only as a joint capsule to separate the joint cavity from the pelvic cavity. The anterior sacrococcygeal ligament is a continuation of the anterior longitudinal ligament of the vertebral column.

duction of the disruption, a maneuver "which is often technically difficult in the non-pregnant patient."[16] In 1905 Goldthwait and Osgood noted the relaxation of pelvic articulations associated with pregnancy; the relaxation was most marked in the symphysis and less so in the sacroiliac joints. This mobility, while slight, was reported almost universally in pregnant women and it was "always absent in non-pregnant women."[162]

Dommisse stressed the importance of the anterior interpubic ligament, stating that it dwarfs in strength the superior and inferior interpubic ligaments, which are really just extensions of the greater anterior ligament. He compared the histologic appearance of the interpubic ligament, which shows dense interwoven collagen fibers, with that of the Achilles tendon, and he ascribed the reason for the great strength of this ligament to the great demand made on it. The interpubic ligament assures the integrity of a tie mechanism linking the halves of an arch of which the sacrum forms the summit and the arcuate lines of the ilia, the haunches.

Dommisse maintained that in addition to a central arch formed on each side by the sacrum there are two additional arches formed by the lateral wall of the pelvis between the acetabulum and the anterior superior iliac spine and by the iliotibial tract with the gluteus medius and minimus down to their femoral attachments. These latter arches flank the central arch. "An arcade structure thus exists perfect for carrying the load that the trunk imposes upon it."[117]

Anatomically, the acetabulum may be divided into thirds, which in fact correlate well with the clinical division of the acetabulum into the inner wall, the superior dome, and the posterior acetabulum, formed, respectively, by the pubic, iliac, and ischial portions of the acetabulum.

The iliac portion of the acetabulum is the chief weight-bearing area of the joint and is consequently more important in the joint. The posterior third of the joint provides greater stability for the joint, and the bone here formed by the ischium is thick. The inner wall of the acetabulum is made up of the pubis and is quite thin and much more easily fractured. The acetabulum is directed not only laterally but also forward and downward. The inferior portion of its wall is deficient; this gap is called the acetabular notch, which is in turn bridged by the transverse ligament, a fibrous band that completes the rim. The floor of the acetabulum above the notch shows a depression called the acetabular fossa. The pubis forms about 20% of the acetabulum, the ischium about 45%, and the ilium about 35%.[103,400]

BLOOD VESSELS

The abdominal aorta divides into two common iliac arteries at the level of the fourth lumbar vertebra, a little to the left of the median plane. At the level of the sacroiliac joint, each artery that has passed downward and laterally divides into the external and internal iliac branches.

The external iliac artery passes underneath the midpoint of the inguinal ligament, where it becomes the femoral artery. Posteriorly, the fascia of the iliacus and psoas major muscles lie behind the artery. The two named branches of considerable size rising from the external iliac artery are (1) the inferior epigastric, which runs cephalad on the posterior abdominal wall, eventually penetrating the substance of the rectus muscle where it anastomoses with the superior epigastric artery and the lower posterior intercostal arteries, and (2) the deep circumflex iliac, which runs laterally upward to the anterior superior iliac spine on the iliacus, eventually supplying the transversus abdominis and anastomosing with branches of the iliolumbar artery.

The internal iliac artery, also known as the hypogastric, supplies the major portion of the pelvis and divides opposite the sacroiliac joint at the level of the lumbosacral disk, ending near the upper border of the greater sciatic notch in two divisions, anterior and posterior. The posterior division is made up of the iliolumbar, lateral sacral, and superior gluteal vessels. The superior gluteal vessel appears to be vulnerable to a shearing force because of the acute angulation of the vessel as it passes out of the pelvis.[302] Also, it is short and has very little muscle to protect it, and thus may be exposed to direct trauma from the sharp, jagged fragments of comminuted fractures. Leaving the pelvis through the upper part of the greater sciatic foramen, it passes above the piriformis muscle and then enters the gluteal region, where it divides under cover of the gluteus maximus into superficial and deep branches.

The iliolumbar artery runs out of the true pelvis toward the iliac fossa, where it anastomoses with the previously described deep circumflex iliac. The lateral sacral arteries, superior and inferior, run downward and medially, supplying the sacrum and, by perforating both the superior and posterior sacral foramina, supplying the muscles on the back of the sacrum and anastomosing with branches of the superior and inferior gluteal arteries.

The branches of the anterior division of the internal iliac can be characterized as either parietal or visceral. The parietal branches are the obturator, internal pudendal, and inferior gluteal. The obturator artery runs forward and downward along the side wall of the true pelvis to the obturator fora-

men, through which it passes ending almost immediately on the distal side of the obturator foramen by dividing into anterior and posterior terminal branches. The internal pudendal, arising in common with the inferior gluteal artery, runs caudad and posteriorly to the lower part of the greater sciatic foramen, leaving the pelvis below the piriformis. It lies on the ischial spine under cover of the gluteus maximus and next passes through the lesser sciatic foramen and enters the perineum, in the anterior part of which it ends by dividing into the deep and dorsal arteries of the penis or the clitoris. The inferior gluteal artery passes posterolaterally with the internal pudendal vessel and exits the pelvis through the lower part of the greater sciatic foramen to enter the gluteal region just below the piriformis, passing distally into the proximal part of the thigh.

The visceral branches of the anterior division of the internal iliac are the umbilical, superior vesical, middle rectal, and either the inferior vesical in the male or the uterine-vaginal in the female. The umbilical artery is the remaining portion of the major vessel from the placenta during fetal life, and from it arises the superior vesical artery, which passes medially to the upper part of the urinary bladder. The middle rectal artery runs medially and is distributed to the rectum as well as to the prostate, the seminal vesicle, and the vas deferens. It anastomoses with its contralateral branch and with the inferior vesical from which it sometimes arises. The inferior vesical artery runs medially on the upper surface of the levator ani to the lower part of the bladder, branching through the seminal vesicles, the vas deferens, and the lower part of the ureter and prostate. The vaginal artery runs downward and medially on the floor of the pelvis to the side of the vagina and divides into numerous branches that ramify on its anterior and posterior walls. The corresponding branches of opposite sides anastomose and form the anterior and posterior longitudinal vessels, which are the so-called azygos arteries. They also anastomose above with the vaginal branches of the uterine arteries and below with the perineal branches of the internal pudendal. The uterine artery, which arises either separately or in common with the vaginal or middle rectal artery, runs medially and slightly forward on the upper surfaces of the levator ani to the lower border of the broad ligament, where it passes medially and arches above the ureter to the side of the neck of the uterus, ending as an ovarian branch at the superior margin of the uterus.[103]

The rich anastomotic network of the pelvic

arterial system and its accompanying venous system have a significance that will be dealt with later in the section dealing with hemorrhage.

NERVES

The nerves involved in pelvic fractures are derived from the lumbar plexus and the sacral plexus.

The lumbar plexus is formed by the anterior primary rami of the first three lumbar nerves and a part of the fourth, with the addition (in 50% of the cases) of a small branch from the subcostal nerve. The muscular branches to the quadratus lumborum and the psoas muscles and the iliohypogastric are rarely, if ever, involved directly in fractures of the pelvis. The ilioinguinal nerve appears at the lateral border of the psoas and continues forward deep to the aponeurosis of the external obliquus just above the inguinal ligament and comes to lie in the inguinal canal. This supplies motor branches to the abdominal wall, along which it passes, and sensory branches to the skin and fascia over the symphysis pubis, the medial proximal thigh, and the superior portion of the scrotum, and root and dorsum of the penis in the male and the mons pubis and labium major in the female. The genitofemoral nerve also appears on the posterior abdominal wall, piercing the psoas fascia and extending along the lateral side of the common and external iliac arteries down to the inguinal ligament. The genital branch supplies the external pudenda of the male and the female. The femoral branch passes beneath the inguinal ligament lying on the lateral side of the femoral artery and subserves the superior portion of the anterior region of the thigh. The lateral cutaneous nerve of the thigh crosses the iliacus muscle and enters the thigh behind the lateral end of the inguinal ligament and supplies the lateral portion of the thigh. The obturator nerve arises in the substance of the psoas major and lies along the lateral aspect of the internal iliac vessels. It then passes below the pelvic brim in contact with the upper part of the obturator internus to the obturator groove of the obturator foramen, through which it reaches the thigh, where it supplies the muscles on the medial aspect. The femoral nerve passes obliquely through the psoas major muscle and runs downward in the groove between the psoas and the iliacus, to enter the thigh behind the inguinal ligament lateral to the femoral sheath and femoral vessels. Virtually all of the branches of the femoral nerve are extrapelvic in their distribution and innervation.

The sacral plexus is formed by the anterior primary rami of the part of the fourth lumbar nerve, the fifth lumbar, the upper three sacral, and a part of the fourth sacral nerve. It lies on the dorsal wall of the pelvis between the piriformis muscle and its fascia, and interior to it lie the internal iliac vessels, the ureter, the pelvic colon on the left, and a portion of the ileum on the right. The nerves that form this plexus converge toward the inferior portion of the greater sciatic foramen, where the broad triangular neural band forms the sciatic nerve as it exits the greater sciatic foramen below the piriformis muscle. In addition to the sciatic nerve, the sacral plexus gives rise to numerous smaller nerves, some of which arise from the front of it and some from the back. The anterior branches consist of the nerve to the quadratus femoris and inferior gemellus, the nerve to the obturator internus and superior gemellus, the pelvic splanchnic nerves, and the pudendal nerves. The posterior branches on the muscular twigs to the piriformis and to the coccygeus and levator ani, the superior gluteal nerve, the inferior gluteal nerve, the posterior cutaneous nerve of the thigh, the perforating cutaneous nerve, and the perineal branch of S4.[103]

THE LOWER URINARY TRACT

The bladder lies behind the symphysis pubis and two pubic bones (Fig. 13-8). Prather[368] noted that the bladder of an infant or child is an abdominal organ and does not attain its pelvic position until adulthood, meaning that a proportionately greater portion of the child's bladder is covered by peritoneum. In the adult, the peritoneum is reflected from the anterior abdominal wall over the bladder dome and down to the bladder base posteriorly. If the bladder is empty, peritoneum extends to the symphysis, but if distended, the bladder rises above the symphysis, lies in contact with the abdominal wall, and can be entered extraperitoneally (Fig. 13-9).

The bladder neck, from which the urethra proceeds, is attached to the pelvis both through its continuity with the urethra and by certain ligaments of the bladder. In men the neck of the bladder is in close contact with the prostate gland, which surrounds the proximal portion of the urethra. In women the neck of the bladder is in more direct contact with the pubococcygeal portions of the levator ani muscles, on which it rests. Posterior to the bladder in the woman are the upper vagina, cervix, and uterus, and posterior to the bladder in men are the seminal vesicles. Posterior to these structures is the rectum. The lateral ligaments of the bladder, made up of the neurovascular pedicle

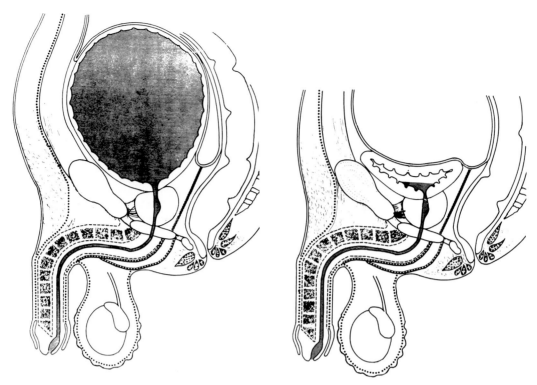

Fig. 13-8. Sagittal sections of the male pelvis showing the relationship of the full and empty bladder. As the bladder fills, it displaces the peritoneal reflection from the anterior wall of the abdomen and moves cephalad into the peritoneal cavity. The empty bladder is almost entirely retropublic (*right*). It is important to note in the full bladder (*left*) that it rises above the symphysis pubis, lies in contact with the abdominal wall, and can be entered extraperitoneally.

of the bladder (and in men, of the vas deferens) and covered by connective tissue that is continuous with the sheaths about the lower bladder, attach the bladder to the levator ani. In addition, the bladder is anchored to the posterior surface of the two pubic bones by way of the pubovesical ligaments in the female and in the male by way of the puboprostatic ligaments, which actually attach to the sheath of the prostate and indirectly to the bladder through the continuity of the sheaths of the bladder and the prostate. These bladder ligaments form the floor of the space of Retzius, which is anterior to the bladder and posterior to the pubis.

The male urethra is conceptually divided into three portions. The pelvic portion of the urethra in the male is about 2 cm long and passes vertically downward surrounded by the prostate; it is called the posterior urethra or, more precisely, the prostatic urethra. Below the apex of the prostate the urethra passes through the urogenital diaphragm, the floor of the pelvis, and it is called the membra-

nous urethra. The male urogenital diaphragm consists of two layers of fascia enclosing the transverse perineal muscles, the bulbourethral glands, and the urethral sphincter. Both the fascia and the muscles are attached laterally to the ischiopubic rami. Above the diaphragm lie the pubococcygeus portions of the levator ani, which pass from the pubis and around the urethra and the dorsal vein of the penis. The urogenital diaphragm is quite prominent in men, being 1 cm to 1.5 cm thick. The membranous portion of the urethra ends by passing through the inferior urogenital diaphragmatic fascia and entering the corpus spongiosum of the penis. This portion is therefore called either the cavernous, or spongy, or anterior portion of the urethra. Its first portion is called the bulbous urethra.

In women the urethra is 3 cm to 5 cm long and is fixed both by its attachment along its entire length to the anterior vaginal wall and its penetration of the pelvic floor, including the urogenital diaphragm. In women, however, the diaphragm is

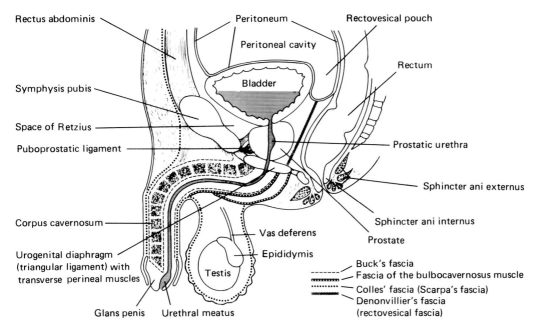

Rectus abdominis
Peritoneum
Rectovesical pouch
Peritoneal cavity
Rectum
Bladder
Symphysis pubis
Space of Retzius
Prostatic urethra
Puboprostatic ligament
Sphincter ani externus
Sphincter ani internus
Corpus cavernosum
Vas deferens
Prostate
Epididymis
Urogenital diaphragm
(triangular ligament) with
transverse perineal muscles
Testis
Buck's fascia
Fascia of the bulbocavernosus muscle
Colles' fascia (Scarpa's fascia)
Denonvillier's fascia
(rectovesical fascia)
Glans penis   Urethral meatus

Fig. 13-9. Sagittal section anatomy of the lower pelvis and male genitalia. The male urethra is divided into three portions: the prostatic urethra as it passes through the prostate, the membranous urethra as it passes through the urogenital diaphragm (triangular ligament), and the anterior or cavernous urethra, which is surrounded by the corpus spongiosum of the penis. The first portion of the anterior urethra is called the *bulbous urethra.*

not so well developed, for the deep transverse perineal muscle is as a rule quite poorly developed and the diaphragm is perforated not only by the urethra but also by the vagina, which almost splits it into halves. Consequently, the female urethra, because of its shortness, the absence of the prostate, and the greater mobility of the female urogenital diaphragm, is less subject to injuries associated with pelvic fractures.

The extravasation of urine resulting from ruptures of the urethra or of the bladder obviously depends on the anatomical location of the ruptures. In most instances of urinary extravasation in association with pelvic fractures, the extravasation is above the urogenital diaphragm and consequently is intrapelvic. Intrapelvic extravasation can be subdivided according to whether the peritoneal cavity has been entered or not. Consequently, there can be intraperitoneal extravastions subsequent to bladder-dome rupture, and there can be extraperitoneal extravasations subsequent to bladder neck rupture or rupture of the urethra posterior to the urogenital diaphragm. In the latter instance the extravasation can be described as either perivesical, if the urine dissects in the retroperitoneal space about the bladder and the anterior wall of the rectum, or

prevesical, when the urine is confined to spaces anterior to the bladder.

It is the prostatomembranous portion of the urethra that is most apt to be ruptured by external violence causing associated pelvic fractures.[474] If the rupture is below the urogenital diaphragm, it allows extravasation of urine into the superficial perineal compartment, the scrotum, and eventually onto the abdominal wall, but rarely into the thighs because of the fusion of Colles' fascia to the conjoined rami.[140]

Rupture of the spongy urethra anterior to the urogenital diaphragm leads to extravasation of urine within the corpus spongiosum, but if Buck's fascia, which envelops the corpus spongiosum, is ruptured, then the extravasation of urine and blood can be spread throughout the superficial area of the scrotum and extend to the abdominal wall between the superficial fascia and the fascia covering the abdominal wall musculature[101]

THE LOWER GASTROINTESTINAL TRACT

The portions of the gastrointestinal tract within the confines of the pelvis include a small portion of the descending colon, the pelvic colon, the rectum, and the anus.

The descending colon, which begins at the left flexure of the colon, curves downward and medially to the iliac crest and then further distally in the iliac fossa lying in front of the iliacus muscle. Slightly above the inguinal ligament, it turns medially over the left psoas major, ending at its medial border by dipping into the true pelvis and becoming the pelvic colon.

The pelvic colon begins at the medial border of the left psoas muscle and ends at the level of the third sacral vertebra. It is covered with peritoneum and has a well-developed mesentery which permits considerable mobility. It ordinarily descends first into the true pelvis and then crosses from left to right and bends backward, returning along the posterior wall of the pelvis toward the median plane, where it turns distally and passes into the rectum.

The rectum is that portion of the gastrointestinal tract between the pelvic colon and the anal canal. It has only a partial covering of peritoneum and no mesentery. It begins at the level of the third sacral vertebra and ends at a point 3.8 cm in front of and slightly below the tip of the coccyx. It first descends along the front of the sacrum and coccyx and then rests for about 3.8 cm on the posterior part of the pelvic floor formed by the union of the two levatores ani, and finally it bends abruptly backward and downward, becoming the anal canal.

A narrow interval exists between the medial borders of the levatores ani, through which the lower end of the bowel passes. The anal canal is only 2.5 cm to 3.8 cm long, and it ends at the anus. Its direction is downward and backward. It is separated posteriorly from the coccyx by the anococcygeus body, which is a mass of mixed fibrous and muscle tissue. Anteriorly, it lies close behind the perineal body and the bulb of the penis in men, and a sound in the urethra can be easily felt by the finger introduced into the anal canal, particularly in thin individuals. In women it is separated from the vagina by the perineal body.[103]

CLINICAL EXAMINATION

The examination of the patient with a fractured pelvis begins with a history (as does every examination insofar as the physician is able to obtain reliable information). The history pertinent to a work-up of a pelvic fracture includes timing and description of the trauma, subsequent care, and present complaints. Information about recent fluid intake, voiding, and present state of bladder sensation provide data about urological damage. The same is true of the gastrointestinal tract with respect to the interval since food was last eaten, for this bears, at times, on the choice of anesthesia. The point in the women's menstrual cycle affects the significance attached to blood in the vagina, and a knowledge of whether the patient is pregnant may also affect later decisions. A quick general physical examination should precede a more circumscribed examination of the pelvis, as does treatment obviously undertaken for life-threatening problems involving the airway, cardiac action, shock, and external hemorrhage.

The patient with a pelvic fracture frequently is unconscious and presents with a number of injuries which, as previously noted, could obscure the diagnosis and delay initiation of appropriate management. Fracture of the pelvis should be assumed to be present in all victims of serious accidents and especially those with multiple injuries.[335]

On completion of the basic resuscitative maneuvers, the patient who is suspected of having a pelvic fracture should be examined for the presence or absence of intra-abdominal injury. This will include an examination of the urinary tract (see p. 1180). In the majority of instances, however, the pelvic fracture, even if it is minor, will be the chief presenting complaint.[377] Pain and tenderness are most commonly present, followed by difficulty in walking, abdominal tenderness, and crepitus. Perineal and pelvic swelling, ecchymoses (Fig. 13-10), lacerations, deformity, and tenderness should be sought as well as irregularity of the pubic symphysis. The iliac crests, the pubic rami, and the ischial rami should be palpated, since they are relatively subcutaneous. Additionally, the sacroiliac joints should be examined as well as the posterior surfaces of the sacrum and coccyx.

Three simple maneuvers should be performed carefully on any patient suspected of a pelvic fracture: (1) Exert posterior pressure on the iliac crests of the supine patient in such a fashion that, if a fracture is present, the pain will be noted at the fracture site as the pelvic ring is opened. (2) Compress the pelvic ring in a side-to-side direction by pressure and compression on the iliac rings in a lateral-to-medial direction. (3) Direct downward pressure on the symphysis pubis. This will cause pain and springiness if the anterior pelvic ring is broken. In the course of this examination range of motion of the hips should also be determined.

Milch[300] described three eponymic physical signs seen in conjunction with fractures of the pelvis. A large hematoma that becomes superficial above the inguinal ligament or in the scrotum is referred to as Destot's sign. In lateral compression fractures the distance from the greater trochanter to the pubic spine is diminished on the affected side (Roux's sign). On rectal examination the bony prominence or a large hematoma can be palpated, and there is definite tenderness along the lines of the fracture (Earle's sign).

Following an examination of the abdomen and the pelvis for local signs of disruption of the lower urological tract, the first step in a urological work-up is a urethrogram or a urethral catheterization[301] if there is no evidence that the patient has spontaneously voided microscopically clear urine following the trauma. Later, more revealing x-ray studies can be performed based on preliminary studies and the need for and feasibility of subsequent studies.

RADIOGRAPHIC FINDINGS

Because an accurate physical diagnosis is difficult or impossible in a patient obtunded because of head trauma or who has severe or multiple lower extremity injuries, such patients should have an x-ray of the pelvis. Many physicians dealing with busy trauma services believe, as I do, that every patient who has sustained a fracture of a major long bone in the lower extremity as the result of trauma should have an x-ray of the pelvis. It is also my opinion that the unconscious patient who has sustained multiple injuries should routinely be given the benefit of a pelvic x-ray.

Film studies will begin with a plain anteroposterior view (Fig. 13-11), and subsequent studies should be requested based on what is known and what needs to be known, depending on the preceding studies. This requires the physician to be present for the x-ray studies of the patient with serious or multiple injuries and the patient with suspected major fractures of the pelvis. There is little to advocate a "routine" series of films for the pelvic fracture patient; usually they are too little or too much, and unless a physician is with the patient to emphasize by his presence the urgency of the patient's condition, there is little reason to suspect that the patient's x-ray studies will be expedited. Conversely, a physician in attendance, monitoring both the patient's condition and the x-ray positioning does, in fact, catalyze the entire process. Based on his interpretation of baseline films, he may order oblique views of the pelvis in two different perpendicular planes—transverse and

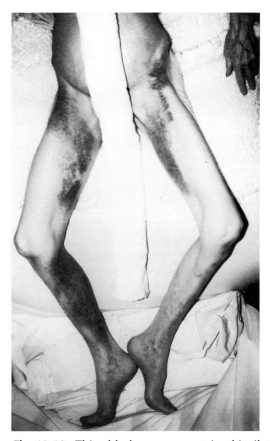

Fig. 13-10. This elderly woman sustained ipsilateral superior and inferior pubic rami fractures, which were undisplaced, in a fall at her home. These extensive ecchymoses developed approximately 3 days after the trauma. Note the extension of the ecchymoses to the supramalleolar region in the right lower extremity. The patient was up and about for approximately 48 hours following the trauma before she sought medical attention.

sagittal. Internal and external rotation views of the pelvis with a posteriorly directed x-ray beam can reveal displacements that other views do not (Figs. 13-12 and 13-13).[121,216] Dunn and Morris[121] stated that two other views helpful for detecting displacement of fragments are an x-ray made with the beam in the sagittal plane directed 25° caudal to the pelvis (the inlet view), which reveals the amount of internal or external rotational deformity or the amount of medial displacement, and a view with the tube angled 35° cephalad, by which rotational deformity in the coronal plane is defined (Figs. 13-14 and 13-15). Some clinicians rely heavily on stereo films, but I have not availed myself frequently of this technique. Tomography or CT scans are

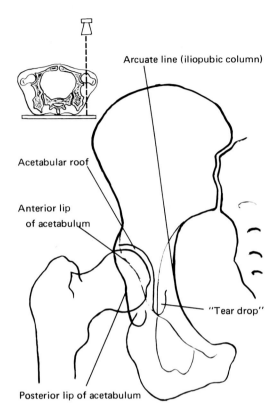

Arcuate line (iliopubic column)

Acetabular roof

Anterior lip
of acetabulum

"Tear drop"

Posterior lip of acetabulum

Fig. 13-11. An anteroposterior x-ray view of the right hemipelvis. The arcuate line is made up of the iliopubic column. The teardrop, or the "radiographic U," is composed medially of the flat, parasagittal surface of the ilium and laterally of the inferior and anterior portions of the acetabular fossa. The lateral portion of the teardrop continues on into the acetabular roof. The inset shows the view of the x-ray beam as it passes through a cross section of the supine pelvic region. (After Judet, R.; Judet, J.; and Letournel, E.: Fractures of the Acetabulum: Classification and Surgical Approaches for Open Reduction. J. Bone Joint Surg., **46A:**1615–1646, 1964.)

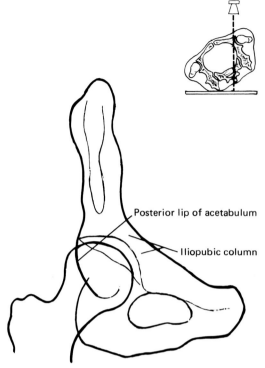

Posterior lip of acetabulum

Iliopubic column

Fig. 13-12. An internal oblique x-ray view of the right hemipelvis. The entire iliopubic column is shown in profile, the wing of the ilium is viewed on edge, and the posterior lip of the acetabulum is more clearly identified. The inset shows the x-ray beam passing through a cross section of the pelvic region with the patient rotated approximately 45° *away from* the affected side. (After Judet, R.; Judet, J.; and Letournel, E.: Fractures of the Acetabulum: Classification and Surgical Approaches for Open Reduction. J. Bone Joint Surg., **46A:**1615–1646, 1964.)

additional radiographic studies that have proved their value in many complicated fractures as well as in fractures where the disruption has been difficult to identify and assess (Fig. 13-16).

McLaughlin[275] noted that the pubic rami form a rigid bony circle, as does the pelvic ring, and as long as either is broken in only one place, displacement cannot occur. Likewise, the converse is true; if displacement is present, then the pelvis must be disrupted in a second place. If displacement of pubic fragments is seen, it still may be difficult to identify the second break, and it is for this reason that additional views are necessary. As a rule there

will be a disruption or minor subluxation of the ipsilateral sacroiliac joint.

Through these initial phases as well as later ones, the comfort and the safety of the patient may be jeopardized by ill-advised, time-consuming, and crepitus-producing maneuvers that add little or nothing to what is known about the patient's condition. Unnecessary movements of the pelvic fragments cause additional damage and aggravate the problems associated with blood loss; clots are disturbed, tamponade may be lost, and impacted stable fractures may be rendered unstable. Of necessity the initiation of treatment frequently precedes the completion of all diagnostic studies; intravenous replacement of blood, stanching of external hemorrhage, and so on need not wait on the final and complete answer to all of the diagnostic questions posed by a patient with multiple injuries.

As diagnoses are revealed, treatment is started, contingent on a general priority system that exists for all patients and a specific priority system that can be created for each patient.

Outline for the Management of a Patient with a Fracture of the Pelvis

I. Early resuscitation
   A. Maintain a clear airway and relieve hypoxia.
   B. Control serious hemorrhage and relieve hypotension. Give Ringer's lactate solution while awaiting arrival of blood. The transfusion can be guided by monitoring central venous pressure and hourly urinary output.

II. History
   A. Note the time and characteristics of the trauma.
   B. Note the time the patient last passed urine. If he has not voided, urge him not to void.
   C. Note the time and amount of food and drink taken prior to the injury. An empty viscus (*e.g.*, gastrointestinal tract, bladder) rarely ruptures.
   D. Determine whether a woman is pregnant or menstruating.
   E. Note the symptoms of associated injury (*e.g.*, other sites of pain, loss of consciousness).

III. Examination
   A. General
      1. Record the pulse, blood pressure, respiration, and adequacy of airway. Chart these signs regularly.
      2. Rapidly survey all potential sites of injury. Remove all clothing and examine front and back, head, spine, thorax, abdomen, pelvis, and limbs.
   B. Local
      1. Inspect the perineum for lacerations, ecchymoses, swelling, and deformity.
      2. Determine the instability of the pelvic rim by palpating the symphysis pubis and rami, and compressing and distracting the wings of the ilium.
      3. Perform a rectal examination to search for a rectal laceration, and to feel a displaced prostate in case of ruptured urethra or tenderness over a fracture line.

IV. Investigations
   A. Radiologic (Routine)
      1. Plain films of pelvis, abdomen, chest and other regions of suspected injury
   B. Radiologic (Special)
      1. Plain films of pelvis in internal and external rotation, as well as inlet and outlet views
      2. CT scan of pelvis
      3. Arteriography and venography
   C. Urologic Studies

      1. Urethrogram as indicated
      2. Catheterization
      3. Retrograde cystogram and post-washout film of bladder.
      4. Intravenous pyelogram, cystoscopy, and retrograde pyelography when indicated
   D. Diagnostic Peritoneal Lavage

V. Treatment
   A. Operative, for ruptured abdominal or pelvic viscera, and rarely for hemorrhage.
   B. Nonoperative to reduce and stabilize pelvic fractures. This includes skeletal traction, pelvic slings, and plaster spicas.
   C. Operative to reduce and stabilize pelvic fractures. This includes open reduction with internal or external fixation, and closed reduction with internal or external fixation.
   D. Transcatheter embolization for hemorrhage.

After Conolly, W. B., and Hedberg, E. A.: Observations on Fractures of the Pelvis. J. Trauma, 9:104–111, 1969.

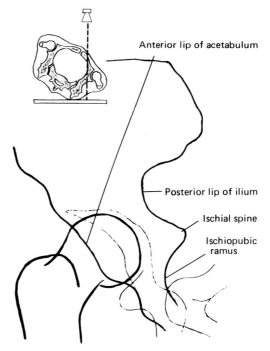

Fig. 13-13. External rotation x-ray view of the right hemipelvis. Medially the posterior lip of the ilium, as it forms the greater sciatic notch, is brought into profile. More inferiorly the ischial spine is seen in profile, and it blends into the medial surface of the ischiopubic ramus. The anterior lip of the acetabulum is brought into profile. The inset shows the x-ray beam passing through a cross section of the pelvic region, with the patient rotated approximately 45° *toward* the affected side. (After Judet, R.; Judet, J.; and Letournel, E.: Fractures of the Acetabulum: Classification and Surgical Approaches for Open Reduction. J. Bone Joint Surg., **46A:**1615–1646, 1964.)

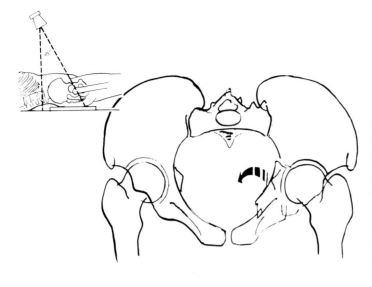

Fig. 13-14. "Inlet view of the pelvis. With the x-ray beam tilted 25° caudad in the sagittal plane, the x-ray reveals the amount of internal or external rotational deformity of the fracture components or the amount of medial displacement. The inset shows the direction of the x-ray beam through the supine patient's pelvis. (After Dunn, W., and Morris, H. D.: Fractures and Dislocations of the Pelvis. J. Bone Joint Surg., **50A:**1639, 1968.)

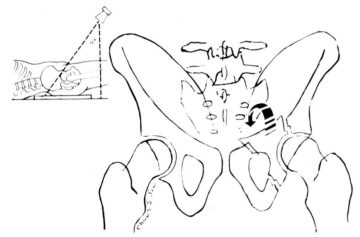

Fig. 13-15. "Tilt" view of the pelvis. With the x-ray beam tilted 35° cephalad in the sagittal plane, an amount necessary to significantly reduce normal pelvic inclination as seen on a straightforward anteroposterior view, the x-ray reveals the amount of rotation present in the anteroposterior plane. The inset shows the direction of the x-ray beam through the supine patient's pelvis. (After Dunn, W., and Morris, H. D.: Fractures and Dislocations of the Pelvis. J. Bone Joint Surg., **50A:**1639, 1968.)

CLASSIFICATION

Classifying fractures of the pelvis is not merely an academic exercise but has important clinical ramifications with respect to diagnosis and treatment. There are a number of classifications of fractures of the pelvis that I believe should be presented. Each can serve a purpose.

Conolly and Hedberg[87] have classified fractures of the pelvis as major if they involve the line of weight transmission from the spine to the acetabulum or if they involve the rami on both sides of the symphysis pubis. The remaining fractures of the pelvis are classified as minor. The "major fracture" category includes fractures of the acetabulum, fractures of the hemipelvis (Malgaigne), bilateral fractures of the pubic rami, symphysis

pubis separations, and fractures of the sacrum. The "minor fracture" category includes unilateral fractures of the pubic rami, isolated fractures of the ilium, and avulsion fractures of the pelvis. In reviewing 200 cases of fracture of the pelvis, Conolly and Hedberg found that 109 were major fractures, and 28 of these patients died. This simple classification has an obvious prognostic impact.

Watson-Jones[495] divided fractures and dislocations of the pelvis into three groups: (1) avulsion fractures from muscular violence; (2) fractures and dislocations of the pelvic ring from crushing injuries; (3) injuries of the sacrum and coccyx. Apparently Watson-Jones recognized that categories 1 and 3 contained only a small portion of the total number of pelvic fractures and that lumping all the rest into the second group did little to classify the

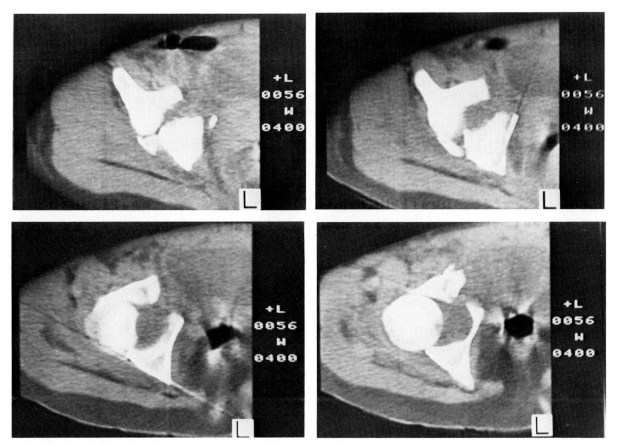

Fig. 13-16. CT scans of a Malgaigne fracture of the pelvis with an associated comminuted fracture of the acetabulum provided further essential information that facilitated open reduction and internal fixation. The patient was a 28-year-old woman driver of a vehicle that struck a tree.

majority of pelvic fractures. He further subdivided category 2 into (A) isolated injuries of the ilium and sacroiliac subluxation, and (B) combined injuries of the pelvic ring, including combined injuries of the pubic segment of the pelvic ring and combined injuries of the iliac and the pubic segments of the pelvic ring.

Huittinen and Slätis[201] emphasized the close relationship between the direction and site of impact and the resulting injury. Lateral impact was well recognized as a cause of pubic rami fracture,[508,515] but its effect on injuries in the sacroiliac region was less well understood until more recently.[438] These authors relied on stability as a key determination in their classification and cautioned that even though the anterior third of the pelvis is not weight bearing, fractures of the pubic rami or pubic separation should not be neglected as they pointed to a posterior injury in 21% of the unilateral anterior fractures and 61% of the bilateral anterior fractures.

On the basis of the trauma mechanism, the supporting function of the pelvis, and clinical frequency Huittinen and Slatis formulated this classification of pelvic fractures: (1) isolated fractures of the pubic rami; (2) double vertical fractures of the pelvis; (3) fractures involving the hip joint; (4) isolated fractures of the pelvic rim; and (5) crushed pelvis. While stability is a minor determinant it seems not to be used in any orderly fashion (*e.g.,* types 2 and 5 are unstable, type 3 can be stable or unstable, and types 1 and 4 are stable). The classification is largely based on clinical frequency, which seems to be a less useful determinant than stability.

Looser and Crombie[262] categorized pelvic fractures sustained in violent trauma into two groups excluding elderly patients, whose fractures tended to be isolated and without attendant soft tissue trauma. Group I comprised patients who had pure anterior fractures, either single or multiple; they were localized to the ischium, pubis, acetabulum, and pubic symphysis. Group II comprised patients with posterior fractures involving sacrum, ilium, and sacroiliac joints. Looser and Crombie noted that these patients almost invariably had anterior fractures as well. This classification, while admittedly limited to violent traumatic pelvic fractures, fails to be all-inclusive, lends little in the way of prognostic significance (group I patients' average length of stay was 23.8 days—with a range of 1 to 145 days—and group II patients' average stay was 35.1 days—with a range of 1 to 148 days), and fails to provide a basis of understanding of the kinetic forces and the fracture: "There was no real correlation between the method of injury and the location of fractures."[262]

Pennal, Tile, Waddell and Garside[354] take a different view of the role of forces and the types of pelvic disruption, and they characterize pelvic disruption according to force along one of the three axes of the pelvis: (1) anteroposterior compression; (2) lateral compression, with or without rotation; and (3) vertical shear. Nevertheless, they too note that "in each of the three major forces, the anterior lesion may be through the symphysis pubis or through the pubic rami. The posterior lesion may be through the sacrum, through the sacroiliac joint with a marginal fracture of the ilium, or through the ilium itself. Also, and this must be stressed, the anteroposterior compression and lateral compression fractures may be associated with a stable or unstable hemipelvis; by definition, the vertical shear fractures are all grossly unstable. The degree of instability indicated best by the disruption and posterior displacement at the sacroiliac area is of extreme importance as a prognostic indicator for the general resuscitation of the patient."[354] It is clear that this classification refers only to disruptions of the pelvis where there would be two or more breaks in the pelvic ring, and as they emphasize by referring to the work of Gertzbein and Chenoweth,[152] even undisplaced pubic rami fractures may be associated with unrecognized posterior damage.

Monahan and Taylor[305] used a classification based on whether the pubic symphysis was subluxated or dislocated (group 1), whether the sacroiliac joints were subluxated or dislocated (group 2), or whether a combination existed (group 3). This classification fails to include all the possible types of pelvic fracture and offers no prognostic significance.

Trunkey and co-workers[478] have classified a series of 173 pelvic fracture patients into three groups. Type I, the comminuted or crush injuries, include three or more major components (rami, ilium, acetabulum, sacrum), are often unstable, and consist of combinations of type II fractures. Type II fractures, the unstable injuries, require immobilization or traction to reduce hemorrhage or to maintain the weight-bearing portions in position, and include diametric fractures with cranial displacement of the hemipelvis, the undisplaced diametric fractures, the open book or sprung pelvis, and acetabular fractures. Type III fractures, which are stable and require immobilization only for symptomatic relief, include isolated fractures and pubic rami fractures. This classification proceeds from the worst to the best in terms of violence and prognosis, and includes in the type II grouping acetabular fractures, which require a separate classification and which in many instances are completely stable.[71] The classification of Trunkey and co-workers does recognize the use of the presence and absence of stability as a major determinant of prognosis.

The Trunkey classification system, excepting what I believe is its retrograde numeration, is closest to the classification system used in this chapter, that of Key and Conwell,[231] which is logical, all-encompassing, easily applied, and progressive (in the sense that the fracture types are graded according to their increasing complexity). This classification has prognostic significance and has been used for over three decades:

I. Fractures of individual bones without a break in the continuity of the pelvic ring
  A. Avulsion fractures
    1. Anterior superior iliac spine
    2. Anterior inferior iliac spine
    3. Ischial tuberosity
  B. Fracture of the pubis or ischium
  C. Fracture of the wing of the ilium (Duverney)
  D. Fracture of the sacrum
  E. Fracture or dislocation of the coccyx
II. Single break in the pelvic ring
  A. Fracture of two ipsilateral rami
  B. Fracture near, or subluxation of, the symphysis pubis
  C. Fracture near, or subluxation of, the sacroiliac joint
III. Double breaks in the pelvic ring
  A. Double vertical fractures or dislocation of the pubis (straddle fractures)
  B. Double vertical fractures or dislocations of the pelvis (Malgaigne)
  C. Severe multiple fractures
IV. Fractures of the acetabulum
  A. Undisplaced (discussed in this chapter)
  B. Displaced (discussed in Chapter 14)

RELATIVE INCIDENCE

The relative incidence of fractures of the pelvic bones has been best analyzed in Rankin's series,[377] in which the left pubic rami were most frequently fractured (163 of 449 cases) and the superior ramus was fractured more frequently than the inferior ramus. The right pubic bone, fractured in 149 cases, was second in frequency, and again the superior ramus was more frequently involved than the inferior one. The combined total for fractures of the pubic bone was 312 of 449, or 69%. The right ilium was fractured in 95 cases, the left ilium in 89, the right ischium in 70, and the left ischium in 72. The left acetabulum was fractured 41 times, and the right 32 times. The sacrum was fractured 37 times; the coccyx 58 times. Of the pubic bone fractures, Rankin encountered a fracture of a single ramus more often than multiple-ramus fractures. Next in frequency were two rami on one side and then two rami, one on each side, followed by four rami, and then by three rami. Of the ischium, a single ramus was first; two rami, one on each side, second; and two rami on the same side, third. There was an upward displacement of one half of the innominate bone (the Malgaigne fracture) in only ten cases, or 2.2%.

Another excellent series that has been analyzed with respect to fracture incidence in accordance with the classification of Key and Conwell is the study done by Eid.[125] Most of the 186 patients had fractures resulting from motor vehicle accident trauma (80.7%) or a fall from a height (16.1%). The remainder of the fractures were mostly due to compression between two pieces of machinery (2.7%). Type I fractures occurred in 24.2% of patients, with fractures of a single pubic ramus (15.0%) or a fracture of the iliac wing (5.4%) accounting for most of the instances. Fractures with a single break of the pelvic ring (Type II fractures) occurred in 17.7% of patients, with fractures of the ipsilateral rami being responsible for the majority (11.8%). Type III fractures were almost equally divided, with double vertical fractures or dislocations of the pubis, or both, accounting for 11.8% of injuries, Malgaigne fractures for 11.8%, and severe multiple crush injuries accounting for 10.8%.

At this point in the chapter it might be beneficial to repeat the advice of Harrison McLaughlin,[275] who warned that there were three main pitfalls in the management of the injured pelvis, and of these "the most common and catastrophic is to treat an obvious fracture and overlook some associated visceral injury until the penalties of infection or hemorrhage have taken their toll. A second common pitfall is to overtreat a stable pelvic fracture, and the third is to treat an unstable fracture without recognizing its potentialities for producing permanent disability or anatomical deformity."

FRACTURES OF INDIVIDUAL BONES WITHOUT A BREAK IN THE PELVIC RING (TYPE I FRACTURES)

Fractures of individual bones without a break in the continuity of the pelvic ring are often seen. They occur as approximately one third of all pelvic fractures[231] and are subdivided into (1) avulsion fractures (Fig. 13-17), (2) fractures of a single ramus about the obturator foramen, (3) fractures of the iliac wing, (4) fractures of the sacrum, and

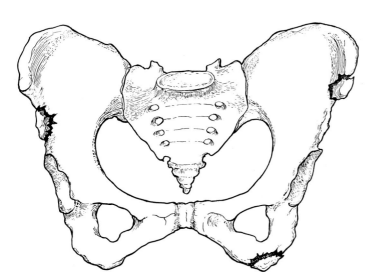

Fig. 13-17. Avulsion fractures. This illustration demonstrates a left anterior-superior iliac spine avulsion, a right anterior-inferior iliac spine avulsion, and a left ischial tuberosity avulsion.

(5) fractures of the coccyx. With the exception of coccygeal fractures, which are noted for their delayed healing,[496] due to the many muscles that are constantly moving the coccyx, the rest of these fractures are recognized for their stability and for their ready healing.

AVULSION FRACTURE OF THE ANTERIOR SUPERIOR ILIAC SPINE

Forcible contraction of the sartorius muscle may avulse the anterior superior iliac spine with slight distal displacement of the fragment, because the fascia lata and the lateral portion of the inguinal ligament[392,402] prevent more than a mild displacement (Fig. 13-18).[275] Until 1935 there had been fewer than 50 cases reported in the literature, and the majority of the patients were athletic males under 16 or 17 years old, the age at which the epiphysis of the iliac crest unites to the ilium. Clinical findings with fracture of the anterior superior iliac spine are local pain, swelling, tenderness, and pain on attempts to flex or abduct the thigh on the affected side.

Incomplete avulsion of a portion of the iliac epiphysis by sudden, severe contraction of the abdominal muscles has also been reported with similar clinical findings.[161] Metzmaker and Pappas[294] have reported a series of 18 avulsion fractures of the pelvis in teen-aged athletes with the following incidence: anterior superior iliac spine, nine; ischium, five; anterior inferior iliac spine, two; and iliac crest, two. These authors emphasize the problems they experienced in making a differential diagnosis when the patients recalled no clearly described traumatic incident. However, osteomyelitis and Ewing's sarcoma are primarily intramedullary lesions with intramedullary destruction and adjacent periosteal reaction, whereas the avulsion fracture does not affect intramedullary trabecular patterns.

The treatment of choice is bedrest with flexion and abduction of the hip with pillows or a splint. Key and Conwell[231] have noted that sitting with the thighs abducted is the ideal position, and the patient may be allowed to sit up as soon as he wishes. Although spica cast immobilization has been used, it is not necessary, because while the avulsed fragment usually unites at a slightly lower level, it results in no functional impairment. The patient may be up and about in 4 or 5 weeks, depending on the presence of symptoms. Robertson[392] has reported replacing the fragment under direct vision and maintaining the reduction by internal

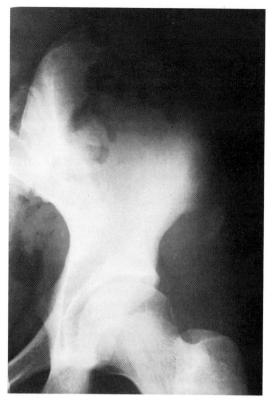

Fig. 13-18. Avulsion of the anterior-superior iliac spine and anterior portion of the iliac apophysis in a 16-year-old boy.

fixation, and he has also treated the avulsion fractures by means of a spica cast applied with the hip flexed and adducted and the knee flexed. This spica cast was used for 1 month's time, followed by crutches for 3 weeks. Since operation offers little benefit in terms of reduced disability or hastened recovery, there seems to be little reason to subject the patient to operative intervention in view of the fact that complete functional recovery is usually present after about 2 months when the nonoperative approach is used. Return to full competition was achieved in virtually all patients in 4 months' time.[294]

AVULSION FRACTURE OF THE ANTERIOR INFERIOR ILIAC SPINE

Avulsion of the anterior inferior iliac spine is much less common than avulsion of the anterior superior iliac spine, but it does occur as a result of forceful contraction of the straight head of the rectus femoris, which originates from this spine (Figs. 13-17, and 13-19 to 13-21). Köhler[237] is believed to have recorded the first incident of anterior inferior iliac spine avulsion. Weitzner[504] maintained that because of the later ossification of the anterior superior iliac spine as well as because of the greater stresses placed on it, there is a marked discrepancy in the incidence of avulsions of these iliac spines, in the ratio of 50 anterior superior iliac spine avulsions to one or two anterior inferior iliac spine avulsions. Both Watson-Jones[496] and Weitzner[504] reported it in rugby and football players, who kick the ball great distances. At the moment of kicking the ball, sharp pain is felt in the groin, ambulation is difficult, if not impossible, and active flexion of the hip is found to be painful and limited. X-rays show downward displacement of a fragment of the anterior inferior iliac spine. The intact reflected head of rectus femoris prevents marked displacement.[275] Watson-Jones noted that the fracture should be distinguished from the epiphyseal line of a separate ossicle of bone (os acetabuli), which may develop normally in this region (see Figs. 13-14 to 13-16). Ideal treatment includes recumbency for 2 to 3 weeks with the hip flexed, as symptoms indicate.

Irving[207] has reported exostosis formation after traumatic avulsion of the anterior inferior iliac spine in two cases. In his article he explicitly contrasts the exostoses in his cases with cases of myositis ossificans in the same area.

AVULSION FRACTURE OF THE ISCHIAL TUBEROSITY

Avulsion of the ischial apophysis is reported relatively infrequently[1,28,80,229,299] and is most often

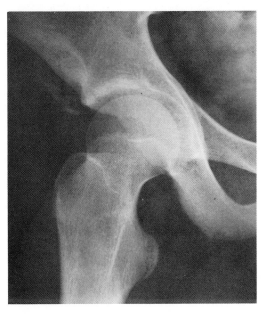

Fig. 13-19. Avulsion of the right anterior-inferior iliac spine in a 13-year-old girl.

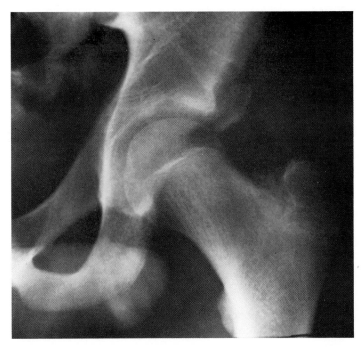

Fig. 13-20. Avulsion of the left anterior-inferior iliac spine in a 16-year-old boy.

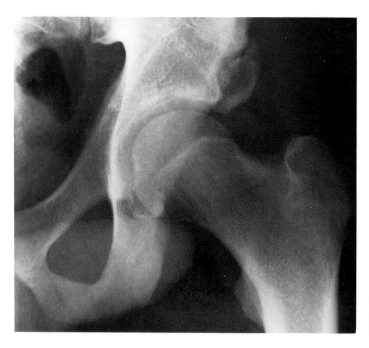

Fig. 13-21. The appearance of the avulsion of the left anterior-inferior iliac spine shown in Figure 13-20, 15 weeks after injury.

sustained during the strenuous motions required by vigorous activities such as hurdling, pole-vaulting, and acrobatic dancing. The avulsion of the ischial apophysis is most commonly seen in youths whose apophyses are not united. The ischial apophysis develops from a separate ossification center and does not unite with the body of the ischium until between the 20th and 25th years.[299] In fact, it is one of the last to unite with the bony skeleton. The apophysis is pulled downward, forward, and outward due to the action of the hamstrings, which are subjected to excessive strain while they are taut (Figs. 13-17 and 13-22 to 13-25). The sacrotuberous ligament is the primary antagonistic force to such displacement; it resists downward and outward detachment.

Symptoms may present acutely, while on the other hand chronic symptoms prior to the diagnosis are not unusual.[394] Patients complain about pain when moving or sitting and have tenderness with pressure over the involved tuberosity. Flexion of the thigh with the knee in extension increases pain, while with the knee flexed and the hamstrings relaxed this does not occur. On rectal examination the tuberosity is tender, and pressure on the sacrosciatic ligament causes traction on the fragment and arouses exquisite pain.

Watson-Jones stated quite definitely that there is no need at all for surgical intervention,[496] and Kelley[229] agreed that open reduction was no longer

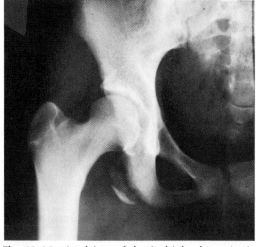

Fig. 13-22. Avulsion of the ischial tuberosity in a 16-year-old girl.

recommended and that eventual recovery could be anticipated with conservative care. On bedrest the thigh should be placed in extension and external rotation with slight abduction. Frequently, recovery by conservative treatment culminates with considerable new bone formation; if pain and disability persist, it may be necessary to excise the bone and cartilage comprising the apophysis and the associated exuberant callus.[394] Rogge and Romano[394] stated that the patient should be placed in the

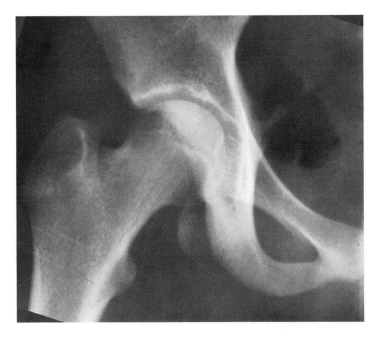

Fig. 13-23. Avulsion of the ischial tuberosity in a 13-year-old girl.

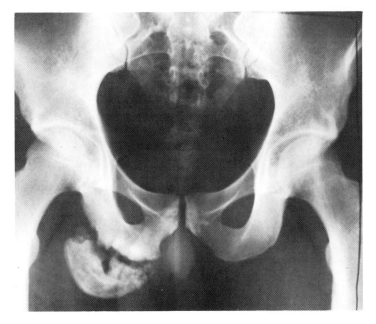

Fig. 13-24. An avulsion of the right ischial tuberosity shows considerable new bone formation 3 weeks after injury.

prone position and the incision should curve from the posterior border of the greater trochanter to the midline of the thigh, paralleling the gluteal crease. The incision will permit reflection of the gluteus maximus muscle near its insertion and avoid injury to the posterior femoral cutaneous nerve.

FRACTURES OF A SINGLE RAMUS OF THE PUBIS OR ISCHIUM

An isolated fracture of only one ramus around the obturator foramen, whether it be of the pubis or of the ischium, is a very stable fracture that cannot be displaced, because the obturator foramen is a rigid bony circle (Figs. 13-26 to 13-28).[275]

The series by Rankin[256] provides the best insight into the frequency of this fracture. He reports in his series of 449 cases of pelvic fractures that the pubic bone was fractured 312 times and the ischium 142 times. A fracture of a single pubic ramus was encountered more often than concomitant fractures of two or more rami; a single ischial ramus was involved most commonly. Other authors[87,121,143,495] seem to confirm this distribution, but uniformity of classification of pelvic fractures is lacking in these series, and it is difficult to get an exact picture of the distribution of particular types of pelvic fractures.

The single ramus fracture is commonly seen in the elderly age groups, in whom falls in the home are the most frequent cause of pelvic fractures.[145,181] In this age group it is frequently necessary to make an important distinction between a fracture of the pelvis and an undisplaced or impacted fracture of the neck of the femur, but the finding of tenderness over the pubic bone may make the diagnosis apparent. One may easily overlook a fracture of the pubic ramus if, in evaluating a suspected injury to the hip, only an inadequate exposure showing just the hip joint and acetabulum is obtained. A torus fracture may be sustained at the ischiopubic junction, and if symptoms persist, repeat angled x-rays must be obtained.

FRACTURES OF THE BODY OF THE ISCHIUM

In addition to avulsion fractures of the ischial tuberosity (see above), there is a different type of isolated fracture of the ischium. This second type of fracture is the result of violent external injury, causing a fracture of the ischial body or tuberosity (Fig. 13-29).

Key and Conwell[231] noted that this fracture of the tuberosity is a very rare injury that may result from a fall in the sitting position. Stimson[458] ob-

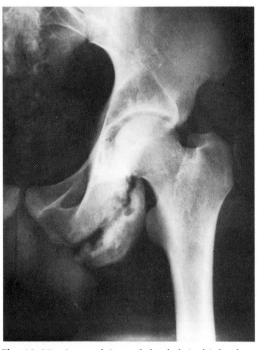

Fig. 13-25. An avulsion of the left ischial tuberosity shows considerable new bone formation 8 weeks after injury.

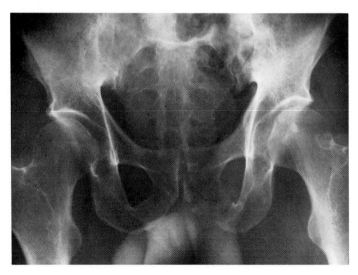

Fig. 13-26. A fracture of the left inferior pubic ramus was sustained in a fall by a middle-aged construction worker.

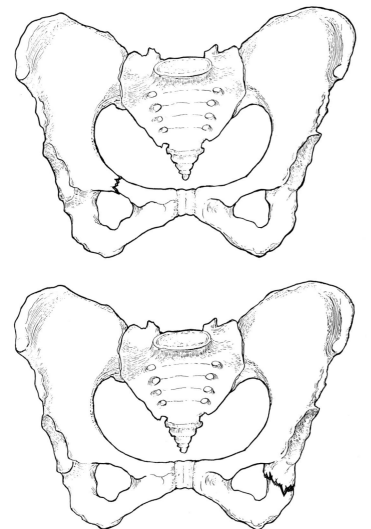

Fig. 13-27. A fracture of the right superior pubic ramus.

Fig. 13-28. A fracture of the ischial ramus.

served that it is one of the rarest fractures of the pelvis. In Milch's[299] review of the fracture, he noted that isolated fractures of the ischium are rare and that Malgaigne appeared to be the only author who had discussed these fractures at some length, although Malgaigne[280] too lacked personal experience with this type of fracture.

One of the cases that Malgaigne commented on was that of a woman who 2 years before had sustained a double vertical fracture of the pelvis with subsequent narrowing of the pelvic outlet. During a forceps delivery necessitated by the results of her injury, the ischium was broken. The five other cases on which Malgaigne commented were all the result of severe external violence: long falls, gunshot wounds, or mine explosions.

The diagnosis may be deduced from the history and the presence of local pain and tenderness when tension is put on the hamstrings. It should be confirmed by radiography, however.

Treatment of fractures of the tuberosity or body of the ischium consists simply of bed rest until the patient is symptom-free, usually in 4 to 6 weeks. Sitting may often by painful for some time after the fracture, and pneumatic cushions are useful when such a complication presents.

STRESS FRACTURES OF THE PUBIS OR ISCHIUM

Stress fractures of the pelvis are uncommon but have been reported[195] to occur during the last

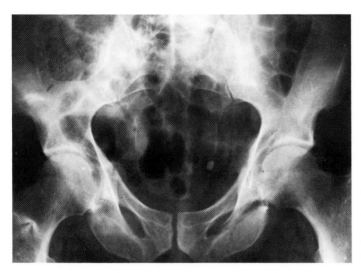

Fig. 13-29. A 53-year-old man sustained a comminuted fracture of the body of the ischium with a large butterfly fragment extending into the inferior pubic ramus. Incidentally, a fracture of the right acetabulum without displacement also appears on this film.

trimester of pregnancy, causing so much pain and tenderness that the expectant mother could not walk or stand. Follow-up x-rays revealed healing with very little callus production, which would be compatible with a fatigue fracture.

Selakovich and Love[420] reported five cases of stress fractures of the inferior pubic ramus. These were seen in recruits undergoing rigorous military training. The authors hypothesized that the condition was due to an unusual pull and strain of the adductors and hamstring muscle groups on the inferior pubic ramus. Pain is moderate to severe in the region of the ischial tuberosity and inferior ramus of the pubis and is aggravated by motion and stress. The patient walks with a limp, and deep pressure may be necessary to elicit the pain that differentiates the condition from ischiogluteal bursitis. These authors noted that the pain in a stress fracture usually persists, gradually diminishing over a period of 4 to 6 weeks, while pain in a traumatic fracture of the same region disappears in 1 to 2 weeks, and they stressed the pitfall of overdiagnosing a stress fracture as a tumor. At the other extreme, however, Godfrey[160] demonstrated a case of avulsion of the anterior inferior iliac spine which was first diagnosed as an athletic injury but which subsequently revealed itself as a chondrosarcoma.

Treasure[476] in 1963 reported on two women, aged 55 and 65, in whom fractures of the inferior pubic ramus were found without any previous history of injury. At first it was thought that these lesions were stress fractures, but finally it was decided that dietary osteomalacia led to spontaneous fractures of the pelvis.

Stress fractures heal regardless of treatment, which is usually only symptomatic. Bed rest, analgesics, and relief from full weight bearing by means of crutches are all that is needed. Garcia[145] noted that prolonged traction or immobilization is not only unnecessary in the elderly but also unwise. Because the elderly can tolerate a considerable amount of deformity without a significant change in their functional capacity, there is no reason for them to run the risks of prolonged bedrest, and resumption of normal activities is encouraged.

FRACTURES OF THE ILIAC WING

Isolated fractures of the iliac wing, first reported by Duverney,[122] are not uncommon fractures of the pelvis. Peltier[350] found they represented 6% in his series. They are due to direct violence, usually lateral compression forces. The fracture fragments are quite variable, but usually displacement is minimal, since muscle attachments tend to replace the fragment as lateral pull is applied to the lateral surfaces of the ilium (Figs. 13-30 and 13-31). The history of a lateral compression injury or severe direct trauma in association with pain, swelling, and tenderness over the iliac wing should alert the surgeon to the possibility of a pelvic wing fracture. While the iliac wing is richly supplied with blood vessels, the fractures of this bone are frequently "hinged" through the body of the ilium, and the superior wing is folded over medially at the time of impact and moves back to a more normal position as a result of the muscle pull. The relative lack of displacement of the fragment usually indicates that the patient is not ordinarily subjected to severe hemorrhage from laceration of named arteries within

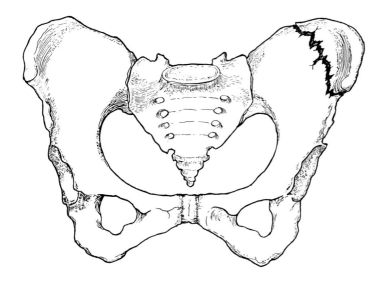

Fig. 13-30. A fracture of the left iliac wing (Duverney's fracture).

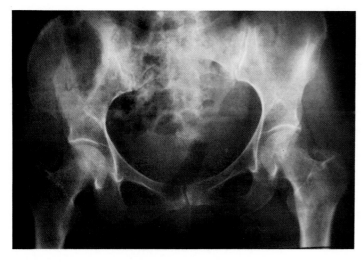

Fig. 13-31. A fracture of the right iliac wing (Duverney's fracture) was sustained by a 32-year-old woman pedestrian. It extends from just above the right anterior-inferior iliac spine to the superior margin of the right sacroiliac joint. The fracture line roughly parallels the iliac crest.

the pelvis, and consequently surgical shock is ordinarily not a prominent feature, nor does the patient appear to be severely injured. The presence of the hip abductors on the iliac wing insures that attempts at walking are quite painful, and a positive Trendelenburg is present, as well as pain over the superior region of the hip. Lateral compression of the iliac wings may demonstrate false motion. Key and Conwell pointed out that if the anterior superior spine is displaced upward, as in Duverney's fracture, the distance between the anterior superior wing and the internal malleolus is increased. Routine anteroposterior x-rays are usually sufficient to establish the diagnosis.

Iliac wing fractures are routinely treated with bed rest on a firm mattress. It has been stated[231] that during the early stages of management of this fracture a wide adhesive strapping of the pelvis below the iliac crests may provide symptomatic relief. Later, the adhesive swathe can be removed and a light canvas belt 3 inches wide can be fitted. I have not used these straps; the benefit from these devices is purely symptomatic, but weight bearing on the affected side should be postponed until hip abduction is painless.

Displaced fragments are not amenable to reduction, but the slight displacements that do persist seem to have little effect on function.

If iliac fractures involve the acetabulum, certainly every emphasis should be given to directing one's attention to that aspect of the fractured pelvis. Ordinarily, the possibility of lower abdominal tract injury subsequent to iliac wing fracture is uncommon, but delays between the injury and the manifestation of abdominal visceral injuries is not unusual, and abdominal rigidity, lower quadrant tenderness, and ileus are almost routine findings in these patients.[350] The ileus can be managed by nasogastric suction and parenteral fluids.

FRACTURES OF THE SACRUM

Isolated transverse fractures of the sacrum are usually due to direct trauma from behind with slight anterior angular displacement due to the fracture force and to the pull of muscles (Figs. 13-32 to 13-34). Furey[143] reported that isolated fractures of the sacrum were seen in 8% of his series, but this figure was two to three times higher than comparable percentages in other series. In Noland and Conwell's[324] 1930 series, there were only three cases of fractures of the sacrum in association with 125 cases of pelvic fractures, for an incidence of 2.4%. Conolly and Hedberg[87] reported only seven fractures of the sacrum in association with 200 fractures of the pelvis in their series.

Byrnes and associates[55] reported two cases of isolated sacral fracture and stressed its relative rarity, a fact further supported by Faruzzi,[132] who quotes Ghilardi and Ettore as finding an incidence of six cases in 7000. Fountain and associates[139] made the diagnosis of transverse sacral fracture in six patients, four of whom were admitted directly to their emergency room, in a group of 184 pelvic fracture patients; their study yielded an incidence rate of approximately 2.2%.

The diagnosis of a transverse fracture of the sacrum is made on the basis of a history of injury with pain, swelling, bruising, and tenderness over the back of the sacrum and tenderness over the front of the sacrum on rectal examination. Bimanual and alternating pressure between a finger placed inside the rectum and another finger placed on the posterior surface of the sacrum will elicit pain and demonstrate false motion. Bucknill and Blackburne[50] found associated transverse process fractures and abnormal neurologic function distally in three patients.

In the group reported by Fountain and associates,[139] all patients initially had evidence of urinary retention, decrease in anal tone, or both. Diagnostic confirmation was assisted by tomography. All of their group had neurologic deficits involving the bowel or bladder and various other potential complications subsequent to transverse sacral fractures such as impotence, perineal hypesthesia, rectal laceration, and cerebrospinal fluid leakage. It is true that sacral fractures occasionally have marked forward displacement with injury to the lower sacral nerves bilaterally and resultant disturbance of the anal sphincter, sensation in the perineal region, and sphincter control of the bladder and urethra with impairment of urinary control and sexual activity. However, more commonly, as Bonnin[37] noted (see p. 1196), the neurologic injury seen with sacral fractures is usually of the higher sacral roots and does not involve the bowel or bladder.

These fractures may be difficult to detect on the x-ray and may go undiagnosed. The fracture line tends to be roughly transverse at about the level of the lower end of the sacroiliac joints, and the lower fragment may be displaced forward into the pelvis. Close study of the sacral body, the wings of the sacrum, and more particularly the sacral fora-

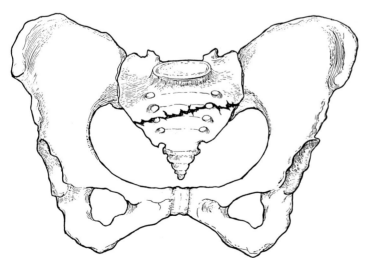

Fig. 13-32. A transverse fracture of the sacrum.

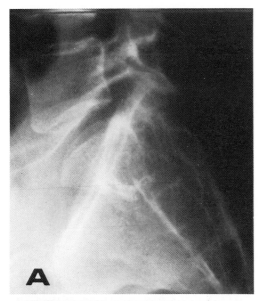

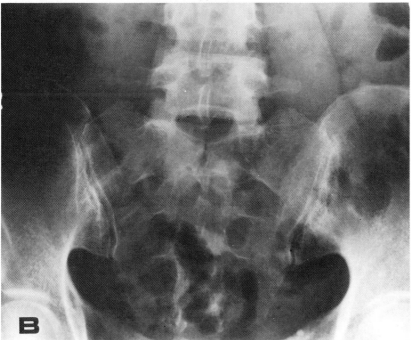

Fig. 13-33. (A) Lateral view of the fractured sacrum reveals anterior displacement of S1 on S2 in a 52-year-old woman automobile passenger. (B) Anteroposterior view of the sacrum of the same patient. The fracture line begins at the left inferior sacroiliac junction extending medially and superiorly into the second left sacral foramen, then cephalad into the first left sacral foramen, then transversely into the first right sacral foramen, and then laterally to end at the superior margin of the right sacroiliac joint. It is extremely difficult to visualize.

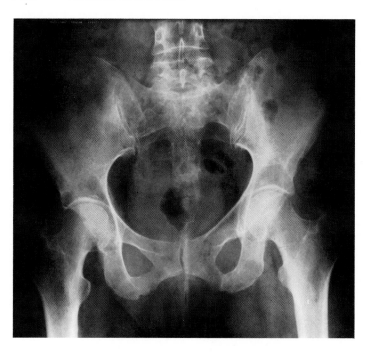

Fig. 13-34. An anteroposterior view of the sacrum in a 42-year-old nurse who fell in an airline terminal. Past history revealed earlier sacral trauma, and anteroposterior views demonstrate asymmetry of the pars lateralis of the opposite sides. The sacral foramina also are asymmetrical.

mina gives clues leading to the discovery of many of the more obscure fractures. Buckling of one edge of a single sacral foramen, similar to that seen in the periosteal bulge of a torus fracture of the radius, has proved to be of great value in locating some of the fainter lines of fracture.[143] Medelman[292] found no appreciable degree of displacement of the sacral fractures, except in two of the cases, and he explained this by the fact that the fractures were usually not complete. Medelman found in the majority of cases that the fractures could be detected on x-rays extending through the bone only between the adjacent anterior sacral foramina and then back completely through the longitudinal extent of the sacrum. In fact, a sharp angulation rather than the normal smooth outline of the upper margins of one foramen or of adjacent foramina is the only sign that the fracture is present in some of the cases. Because of the relative thinness of the cortical bone of the sacrum, and the fact that the cortex can be visualized on profile on anteroposterior views only at the upper margins of the foramina, accounts for the difficulty of visualizing such disturbances on x-rays.[292] With displacement, a lateral x-ray shows the fracture, but the anteroposterior x-ray must be in exact alignment to show the fracture site. Some[50] advocate oblique views to help determine the extent of forward dislocation.

For the linear fractures or undisplaced fractures,

bed rest for 3 to 5 weeks, with or without a sacral canvas band, is all that is necessary. Later, the application of heat and massage and adhesive cross-strapping of the buttock for weakness of the lower back may help. I strongly advise against attempts at manual reduction of displaced fragments using a finger in the rectum to obtain the reduction. Whenever manual reposition through the rectum is being attempted, a laceration of the wall of the rectum can occur, converting a closed fracture into a seriously contaminated compound fracture involving the retroperitoneal space. An inflated rubber ring may be necessary later to provide for comfortable sitting.[142,149,231]

Fountain and associates[139] concluded that transverse sacral fractures uncomplicated by neurologic deficits should be managed conservatively, as should those in which the neurologic deficit is improving. If a neurologic lesion compromises bowel, bladder, or sexual function, then a posterior sacral laminectomy and decompression should be considered.

Fractures of the sacrum are more common in massive crush injuries of the pelvis than they are as isolated entities.

FRACTURES OF THE COCCYX

Most coccygeal fractures occur in women, probably on account of the breadth of the female pelvis and the more exposed position of the coccyx. They are generally caused by falls in the sitting position,[149] but fractures of the coccyx may also occur during obstetrical and gynecologic maneuvers.[301] Symptoms are local pain on sitting as well as on defecation due to spasm of the surrounding anococcygeal muscles. Pain is exquisite, and tenderness is sharply localized over the coccyx. In recent injury, swelling and ecchymosis may be found over the lower sacral region, and there may be prominence of the sacrococcygeal junction as well as tenderness localized in this area. Because the lower fibers of the gluteus maximus are attached to the coccyx, arising from the sitting position will also cause pain over the coccyx, as well as straining at stool as a result of increased tension on the levator ani. Palpation, externally and rectally, is most important.

Lewin[256] relied almost completely for his diagnosis on a bidigital rectal examination with the patient in the lateral Sims' position. If abnormal mobility at the coccygeal articulation and accompanying sensitivity and tenderness are present, then the diagnosis is made. Lewin doubted that x-rays often revealed much in the way of demonstrable pathology, but Johnson[212] stated that x-ray examination was of definite value. Johnson advocated a straight anteroposterior view as well as a lateral with sharp flexion of the thighs (Fig. 13-35).

Bedrest for a week or so is usually sufficient to alleviate the majority of symptoms. Tight cross-strapping of the buttocks lessens pain in some patients, but in others it aggravates it. Again, the patient should sit on an inflated rubber ring. Many patients find that sitting on one buttock and turning approximately 30° to 45° to one side is sufficient to eliminate pain and the discomfort of sitting squarely on both ischial tuberosities. In the same fashion, slouching in a chair with the body weight on the posterior surface of the sacrum rather than across the more inferior portions of the buttock and the coccyx reduces symptoms. Some patients prefer a hard surface, allowing the ischia alone to bear the body weight. Sitz baths help relieve muscle spasm, and stool softeners should be provided so that constipation does not aggravate the symptoms. Closed manipulation can be attempted. This procedure, however, is usually doomed to failure, as the muscle pull causes recurrence of the displacement. The patient should be warned that the period of healing can be prolonged, owing to the muscle forces continually in play. If severe disability due to pain persists after heat and bed rest, the patient need not necessarily be labeled a hysteric or psy-

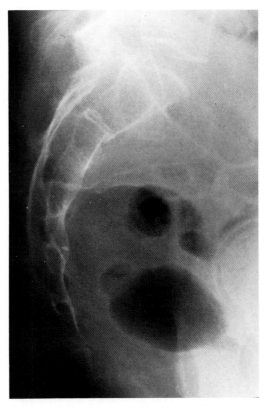

Fig. 13-35. External examination of the coccyx as well as rectal examination revealed exquisite tenderness of the coccyx in the patient shown in Figure 13-34. Faintly visible on this lateral x-ray is the anterior angulation of the distal segments of the coccyx. Note also angulation secondary to old trauma in the upper portion of the sacrum.

choneurotic. Watson-Jones strongly stated that coccygectomy should be considered for those patients who have severe disability following a coccygeal fracture.[496]

Surgical removal of the coccyx is best accomplished through a slightly curved paramedian incision that extends from the sacrococcygeal junction distally. The sacrococcygeal joint is identified and disarticulated; the proximal coccyx is grasped with a towel clip; and dissection is carried on distally, close to the bony fragment. The sharp distal margin of the sacrum should be bevelled with a thin narrow chisel so that no prominence remains. The pelvic diaphragm is repaired by reanchoring the structures stripped from the coccyx, and the gluteus maximus is then reattached to the posterior sacral fibrous aponeurosis.[212,256]

SINGLE BREAKS IN THE PELVIC RING (TYPE II FRACTURES)

Single breaks in the pelvic ring generally occur in close proximity to either the symphysis pubis or the sacroiliac joint, where, owing to the slight mobility of these two joints, it is possible that a single break in the pelvic ring can take place. If the pelvic ring were a truly rigid ring, single breaks could not happen any more than one can break a crisp pretzel ring or a Lifesaver™ candy in one spot. While it is this very minimal motion that allows a single fracture to occur in the pelvic ring, it is rigid enough, for all practical purposes, to be bound by the statement that little or no displacement can occur, so long as it is disrupted at a single level.[137,495] Of perhaps greater clinical significance is the fact that the converse is also valid; if displacement is present, then there must be a second disruption elsewhere in the pelvic ring. As McLaughlin[275] pointed out, it is common to see displaced pubic fractures without detecting the second break in the ring, and, as a rule, the second plane of injury is a partial disruption of the ipsilateral sacroiliac joint.

Recently, Gertzbein and Chenoweth[152] documented six middle-aged and elderly patients who presented with solitary pelvic fractures, usually after a minor fall (5 of 6 patients). By bone scanning, they demonstrated that the apparently isolated injuries were associated with disruptions elsewhere within the ring, most commonly at the sacroiliac joint. Additional patient studies and animal experiments further validate the concept that these seemingly isolated fractures are actually relatively stable, type III fractures.[73] Poigenfurst[360] states that no disturbance in the dorsal pelvic region is expected if the symphyseal diastasis is less than 15 mm, or if there is a break of a single ramus about the obturator foramen. This observation is not merely academic, since it determines to a large extent the manner in which these fractures are treated. Included in this category are the fractures of two rami ipsilaterally, the fractures near, or subluxations of, the symphysis pubis, and the fractures near, or subluxations of, the sacroiliac joint. By definition these fractures are extremely stable, but it cannot be concluded that they are not associated with soft tissue injuries. At the moment of impact the break in the pelvic ring could perforate a viscus, or merely the inertial force could interrupt visceral integrity. In one large series,[121] two thirds of the patients sustained stable fractures of the pelvic ring, and one of every four in this group had major associated soft tissue injuries of the pelvic contents. Seventy-seven percent had fractures of one or more rami, 15% had iliac wing fractures, and 8% had fractures of the sacrum.[121]

The mechanism by which these fractures occur is generally direct trauma from a blow or a crushing injury, but indirect trauma via forces transmitted through the femur can also cause them. The amount of force determines the number of pelvic components involved and, consequently, also determines the stability. This runs the gamut from a class I fracture without pelvic ring involvement to a class III fracture with pelvic disruption, and marked instability. If the force is exerted in an anteroposterior direction with a portion of the pelvis fixed, the portion that responds to the force tends to first open up anteriorly with a fracture of the anterior ring through ipsilateral rami or through a slight symphyseal separation. If the force is directed in a posteroanterior direction, the disruption is at or near the sacroiliac joint, with slight separation at the symphysis. If a lateral compression force occurs, the fractures of the anterior ring tend to "close" or override rather than "open" or separate, as seen in the anteroposterior causation.

FRACTURE OF TWO RAMI IPSILATERALLY

The mechanism of the fracture also provides clinical findings that assist in making the diagnosis, for local signs of injury such as bruises or lacerations define the direction of the force. Lateral compression on the iliac crests demonstrates false motion as well as pain and tenderness at the fracture sites, where palpation may reveal subcutaneous discontinuity and tenderness in conjunction with subcutaneous ecchymoses and hematoma. The Faber test is markedly positive. (With the patient supine the heel of one foot is put on the patella of the contralateral extended limb and the hip to be tested is Flexed, ABducted, and Externally Rotated vigorously; hence the acronym, Faber test. The production of pain is a positive sign.) Unilateral fractures of both pubic rami represent one of the most common varieties of pelvic fracture,[87] and because of their inherent stability and lack of displacement they can be treated with recumbency for a few weeks, and during this period the patient can be treated symptomatically with no need for special positioning—neither favoring one position nor avoiding another—nor is any immobilization necessary (Figs. 13-36 to 13-40).

If slight displacement has occurred with separation, then a pelvic sling with bilateral Buck's traction may be used after the method of Noland

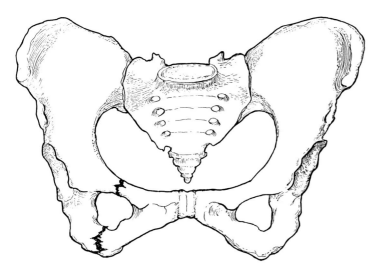

Fig. 13-36. Fractures of the right superior and inferior pubic rami.

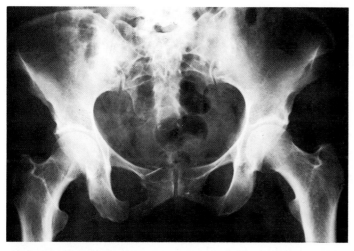

Fig. 13-37. Fractures of two rami ipsilaterally. The fracture of the right superior pubic ramus is at the junction of the ramus and the body of the pubis. The right inferior pubic ramus is fractured at the ischiopubic junction. This 55-year-old woman was a pedestrian struck by an automobile.

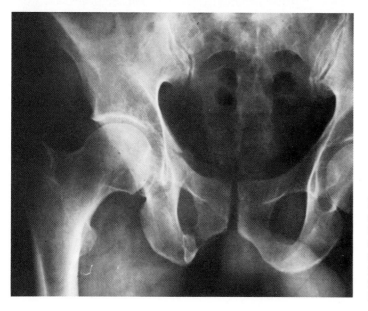

Fig. 13-38. Fractures of two rami ipsilaterally. This 59-year-old male pedestrian sustained a fracture of his inferior pubic ramus at its junction with the body of the pubis and a fracture of the superior pubic ramus farther laterally as it joins the ilium in the formation of the iliopectineal line, also known as the arcuate line.

1127

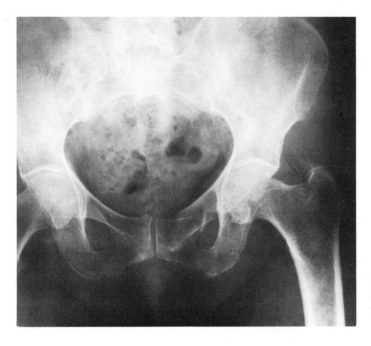

Fig. 13-39. Fractures of two rami ipsilaterally. This 71-year-old woman sustained fractures of the superior and inferior pubic rami in a fall at her home.

and Conwell.[324] Bilateral lower extremity skin traction is advised, as it relieves muscle spasm and the patient's discomfort.[231] Depending on the degree of patient discomfort and the amount of disruption, the sling, if used, is discontinued in about 4 to 6 weeks, and followed by the use of a pelvic belt, followed by progressive ambulation as tolerated by the patient. Pick[358] has written that he allows weight bearing from the start if the patient can do active straight leg raising. If the fracture is less severe with no displacement, then bedrest alone is all that is required, and the patient can proceed in his convalescence at a more rapid pace. Return to normal activity will occur in 10 to 16 weeks.

FRACTURE NEAR, OR SUBLUXATION OF, THE SYMPHYSIS PUBIS

An isolated fracture near (Fig. 13-41), or subluxation of, the symphysis pubis is a rare injury,[87] but if due to major trauma it may present with genitourinary tract injury in a high percentage of cases. Sever[426] maintained that sacroiliac separation goes hand in hand with pubic separation. Taylor[466] agreed with this, if the pubic separation was severe, but he stated that a subluxation or dislocation of the symphysis pubis may occur alone. Berg[26] reports on 24 cases occurring in cowboys who had been riding a bucking horse. In the 15 persons who were thrown into the fork of the saddle, there were no

internal visceral injuries; however, in the nine persons who landed on the saddle horn, eight had severe pelvic disruption, and there were three cases of bladder rupture, three cases of membranous urethral rupture, and two cases of anterior rectal wall tears. There was one case with a urethral tear as well. The injury has also been reported in falls from the mechanical bulls in "country-western" saloons.*

It is generally stated that these dislocations are produced by direct anteroposterior violence, but Taylor,[466] through his investigation of cases seen at the Sheffield Royal Infirmary, demonstrated that such was not the case and that indirect violence is a responsible factor. Taylor stated that the normal degree of movement at the symphysis pubis is 0.5 mm in men and 1.5 mm in women, and any separation in excess of this must be regarded as either subluxation or dislocation. Taylor recorded 73 pelvic fractures and found seven cases of dislocation or subluxation of the symphysis pubis alone. The symphysis pubis may show subluxation in either a sagittal or coronal plane. Dislocations of the joint may occur in three directions—the articulating surfaces may overlap in the midline, or one articulating surface may be above and behind its opposite number, or below and in front of it. The dislocation may occur in a vertical direction,

* Selby, D. K.: Personal communication, 1981.

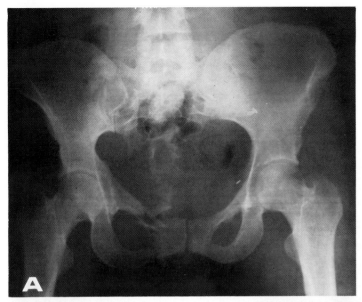

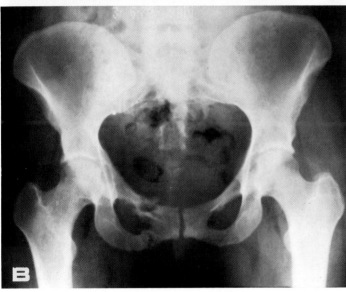

Fig. 13-40. (*A*) A comminuted fracture of the superior pubic ramus and a fracture of the inferior pubic ramus at its junction with the body of the pubis. (*B*) A film taken 4 months later reveals healing of both the superior and inferior pubic rami.

and the articulating surfaces of the dislocated side may be displaced laterally from the sound side. The susceptibility of the ligamentous structures of the symphysis pubis to the relaxing estrogenic hormones just prior to parturition is a factor in some of these injuries.

Wishner and Mayer[521] described five cases of postpartum separation of the symphysis pubis associated with pain localized in the region of the pubic arch and a waddling gait due to posterior displacement of the hip joints. I have seen two patients who sustained painful pubic symphysis separations in association with pregnancy—with impending delivery in one instance and after recent delivery in the other. The expectant mother in her third trimester sustained a slight twisting fall and was incapacitated by severe symphyseal pain that relented on bed rest prolonged for 2 weeks after delivery. Subsequent films failed to show a stress fracture. The second patient, 3 weeks postpartum, had a painful symphysis pubis which clicked audibly with each step.

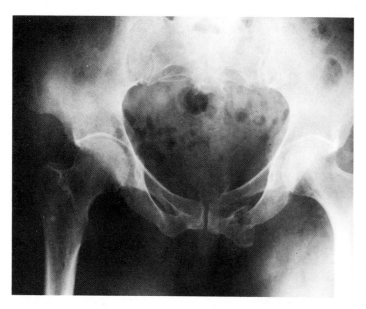

Fig. 13-41. An oblique fracture through the superior portion of the body of the pubis also involves a fracture of the inferior pubic ramus just lateral to the junction with the body of the pubis.

Taylor[466] found his patients routinely severely shocked with subnormal temperatures and pulse rates at or above 100. The patients lie on their backs with both legs externally rotated, more so on the affected side. Active movement is limited, and pain is produced by anteroposterior and lateral compression of the pelvis. Local pain over the symphysis pubis is severe, and displacement of the joint is easily palpable. Pain can also be felt over the sacroiliac joint if the latter is subluxated. Taylor remarked on the absence of bruising over either the symphysis pubis or the sacroiliac joint.

Treatment of these disruptions is quite similar to that of fractures of the ipsilateral rami, although it may be necessary (since these are "opening"-type pelvic injuries) to use greater lateral compression forces to allow for a stable repair. In my opinion these separations or fractures demand careful and regular x-ray observation in order that a late disruption of the sacroiliac joint does not go unrecognized. I agree with the opinion that the anterior tie-arch is not nearly so essential as is the integrity of the weight-bearing posterior arch, which involves the sacroiliac joint.[350] Chronic post-traumatic sacroiliac arthritis is a much more symptomatic problem than a symphyseal disruption.

Postpartum, the patient can be given a 3-inch wide circumferential strap that runs below her iliac crests and above her trochanters. She should be advised to return to bed rest in the full lateral position and to keep lateral compression on the symphysis. The pregnant patient can only avail herself of lateral recumbency.

FRACTURE NEAR, OR SUBLUXATION OF, THE SACROILIAC JOINT

Isolated fractures near, or separations of, the sacroiliac joint with little or no displacement are rare[495] and are most often the result of direct trauma (Figs. 13-42 and 13-43). Bonnin[37] noted that the long auricular-shaped facet of the sacroiliac articulation extends from the level of the upper margin of the first sacral foramen to the upper margin of the third. The first and second anterior and posterior sacral foramina thus weaken considerably that part of the bone that connects the lateral mass of the sacrum with the body of the bone, and they provide the most readily broken link in the solid connections between the ilium and the vertebral column. From this weak spot, fractures of the sacrum caused by direct violence are prone to start and spread, and it follows that any fracture of the sacrum caused by violence transmitted through the sacroiliac joints affects this area more than any other in the sacrum.

Isolated breaks of the posterior part of the pelvic ring are quite rare, because in nearly every instance in which the posterior ring is broken there is also a fracture through the relatively weak anterior portion of the ring. However, in the rare instance when direct severe trauma occurs from behind, or behind and laterally, the anterior ring may remain intact. The history of severe trauma to the posterior portion of the pelvis as well as pain and tenderness in the vicinity of the sacroiliac joint should lead one to suspect a fracture near the sacroiliac joint. Compression of the pelvis in either the anteropos-

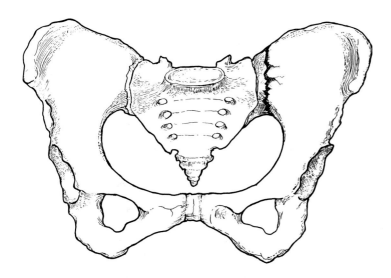

Fig. 13-42. A fracture next to the sacroiliac joint through the body of the ilium.

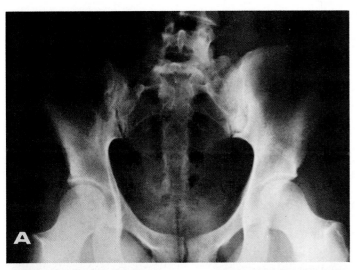

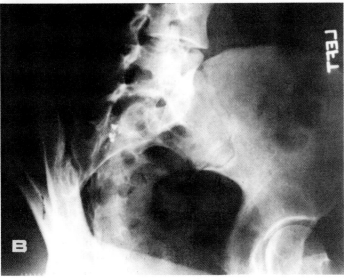

Fig. 13-43. (*A*) Unusual finding within the sacroiliac joint. This 24-year-old woman was referred for evaluation of a 2-year history of low back pain that followed a minor fall. The ossicle seen in the left sacroiliac joint, perhaps deserving the name *os sacroilii*, was interpreted as a congenital anomaly. Note the abnormal lumbosacral take-off giving rise to a mild left lumbar scoliosis.
(*B*) Eleven months after myelography, discography, and chemical disk dissolution had failed to provide relief, oblique films show subsidence of the previously more noticeable sclerotic rim about the ossicle. The patient responded quickly but temporarily to sacroiliac steroid injections; gradually symptoms subsided. The question remains whether this is an osteochondral fracture from the ilium or an os sacroilii.

1131

terior or lateral direction elicits pain in the posterior pelvis. The Faber test also causes pain at the affected region, and straight leg raising is painful. The typical displacement is one of the ilium pushed slightly backward and toward the midline. The posterior superior iliac spine is therefore more superficial than the corresponding bony prominence on the opposite side, and it lies nearer to the spinous processes. The ilium overlaps the shadow of the sacrum to an abnormal degree and is unduly close to the midline.

Treatment of these unusual fractures or separations should be symptomatic and prophylactic; relief of patient discomfort and prevention of further disruption of the posterior ring injury can be accomplished by bed rest, the use of a pelvic sling or pelvic belt, and the cautious, well-monitored institution of graduated activities leading to a return to normal in 10 to 16 weeks. Watson-Jones reduced the disruption in the same way as for complete disruptions of the pelvis by rotating the ilium forward and immobilizing the joint in plaster for 3 months. If imperfect reduction occurs and traumatic arthritis develops, the fusion according to Smith-Peterson and Rogers[444] can be performed.

In the management of these apparently stable disruptions, I have stressed vigilance and a deliberate pace as far as returning to weight bearing is concerned, but for the elderly, a more rapid rehabilitation is indicated. Garcia[145] advised that, while most pelvic fractures of the elderly are minimally displaced, these patients can tolerate considerable osseous deformity without compromising their functional result, and that prolonged immobilization or traction is unwise if the functional result is not significantly improved. This is true even for the sacroiliac joint, because of the diminished requirements for extended weight bearing in patients of this age group.

DOUBLE BREAKS IN THE PELVIC RING (TYPE III FRACTURES)

Whereas the distinction between types I and II in the classification of pelvic fractures is straightforward (it depends on whether or not the pelvic ring is involved), I have already alluded to the fact that single breaks in the pelvic ring are often, in fact, double breaks without displacement. For this reason the distinction between type II and type III fractures is less obvious. Some fractures are quite obviously type IIIs, and they, because of massive disruption of the pelvic ring, are recognizably un-

stable. Stability or lack of it is, in fact, the criterion for classifying a fracture as type II or type III. If there is significant displacement of major pelvic fragments, it can be assumed that the fracture is unstable and may be categorized as a type III fracture.

Type III fractures include (1) the double vertical fractures or dislocations of the pubis—the straddle fracture, (2) the double vertical fractures or dislocations of the pelvis—the Malgaigne fracture, and (3) the severe multiple fractures of the pelvis.

The incidence of these unstable fractures appears to be half that of stable fractures of the pelvic ring.[121] They are frequently associated with crushing industrial or mining accidents, falls from heights, and vehicular trauma, and because of the forces involved, the pelvic fracture is usually associated with other fractures or internal injuries.

DOUBLE VERTICAL FRACTURE OR DISLOCATION OF THE PUBIS

Straddle fractures involving bilateral components of the anterior tie arch of the pubis (Figs. 13-44 to 13-47) accounted for about one third of the unstable fractures in the Dunn-Morris series[121] or about one ninth of the entire series. Conolly and Hedberg[87] reported a 17% incidence of this type of pelvic fracture and noted that one of every three patients with this fracture had associated major lower urinary tract damage. Trafford[474,475] stated that urethral rupture is most likely to occur in this fracture in which both a stretching and shearing force are exerted on the organ. Peltier[350] reported this type in 20% of his entire series; the highest incidence of injuries was to the abdominal viscera (38%), and the mortality rate was 19%. He categorized them as "the most dangerous of all pelvic fractures because of the high incidence of injuries to the abdominal viscera and the serious extent of the local hemorrhage into the pelvic region."

The injury may be sustained in a fall straddling a hard object that fractures the pubic arch, or it can be caused by lateral compression of the pelvis.[495] Because the fracture does not involve the main weight-bearing arch or affect the length of the lower extremities, care is chiefly symptomatic and directed against aggravating any displacement of the fragments. This may be achieved simply by bed rest in recumbency or in the semi-sitting posture to relax the medial thigh muscles and the anterior abdominal muscles. If lateral compression was a causative factor, the lateral decubitus position is contraindicated. To a large extent, however, the

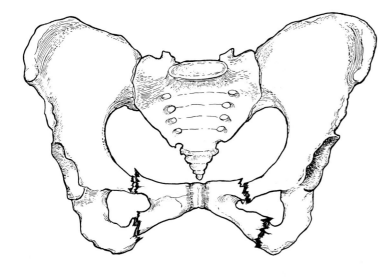

Fig. 13-44. Bilateral fractures of the superior and inferior pubic rami, also called straddle fractures, frequently result from falls.

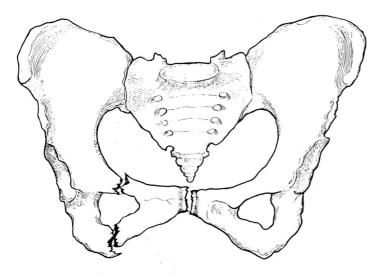

Fig. 13-45. Double vertical fracture-dislocation of the pubis. A variant of the straddle fracture is that of both ipsilateral rami in conjunction with a symphyseal separation.

patient's symptoms will modify the position he chooses and a comfortable position will be a good one for his injury.

DOUBLE VERTICAL FRACTURES OR DISLOCATIONS OF THE PELVIS (MALGAIGNE FRACTURES)

Dislocations and fracture-dislocations of the pelvis are commonly referred to as Malgaigne fractures (Figs. 13-48 to 13-61). Strictly speaking, if one refers to the original description, the term should be reserved for the fractured pelvis in which the anterior fracture is in the superior and inferior rami of the pubis separating the body of this bone from the ilium and ischium, and the posterior fracture or dislocation is always behind the acetabular cavity, generally in the ilium (more rarely the sacrum) or a sacroiliac dislocation. Holdsworth's[187] series showed that sacroiliac dislocation is about twice as common as a para-articular fracture.

Malgaigne,[280] in his *Treatise on Fractures*, described a complex of multiple fractures of the pelvis that he felt merited special attention:

> It is a combination of two vertical fractures, separating at one side of the pelvis a middle fragment comprising the hip-joint; according as this fragment is carried upward or inward, the femur follows its movements, and hence result in changes in the length and direction of the limb which have often misled practitioners. Of these two fractures the

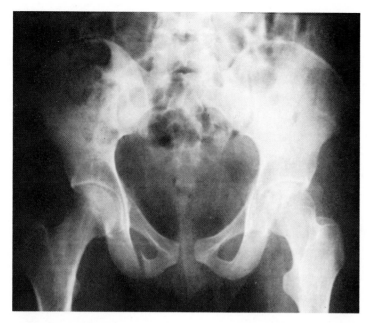

Fig. 13-46. Double vertical fractures of the pubis. This patient has fractures of the right superior and inferior rami as well as a dislocation of the symphysis pubis. Coincidentally, there is an undisplaced fracture of the left acetabulum. Were it not for the acetabular component, this fracture could have been managed according to symptomatic goals. Because of the acetabular element and the potential for late loss of reduction, the patient was treated with a prolonged period of no weight bearing.

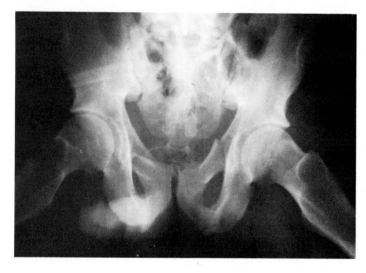

Fig. 13-47. Double vertical fractures of the pubis. This 32-year-old man was subjected to lateral compression forces across his pelvis, and sustained a fracture of the left inferior ramus at the ischiopubic junction, an oblique fracture of the right superior pubic ramus, a segmental fracture of the left superior pubic ramus, and a fracture of the left inferior ramus at the ischiopubic junction. There is slight diminution of the normal transverse diameter of the pelvis and, consequently, side-to-side compression dressings or slings were contraindicated for this patient.

anterior is almost constantly seated in the horizontal and descending rami of the pubis, separating this bone from the ilium and ischium; the posterior is always back of the cotyloid cavity, and generally in the ilium; once, however, it was seen by Richerand in the sacrum. Lastly, instead of a fracture, we may have here a separation of the sacroiliac symphysis.

Malgaigne described the features of the fracture as pain, contusion and swelling, and diminished motion of the lower extremity. Sometimes the middle fragment is movable and has associated crepitus, but Malgaigne felt that the most conclusive

information could be derived from the displacements, which are of two kinds. The most common is a cephalad displacement of the middle fragment that gives rise to an apparent shortening of the lower extremity of about 1.3 cm. The other type of displacement consists in various inclinations of the middle fragment; the anterior border of the middle fragment can be depressed into the pelvis while the posterior border projects outward. In such an instance the rotation occurs on an axis parallel with the longitudinal axis of the torso. Another type of displacement occurs when the

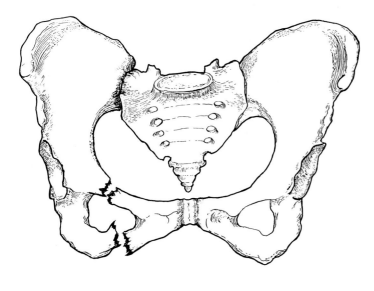

Fig. 13-48. Double vertical fracture-dislocation of the pelvis. This Malgaigne fracture consists of pubic ramus fractures and an ipsilateral sacroiliac dislocation.

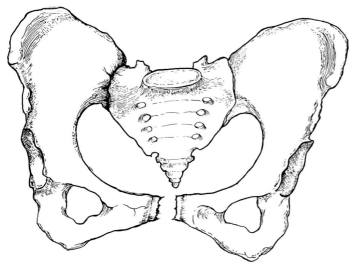

Fig. 14-49. This Malgaigne fracture consists of a symphyseal dislocation and a right sacroiliac dislocation.

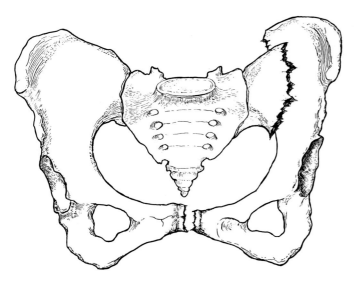

Fig. 13-50. This Malgaigne fracture consists of a symphyseal dislocation and fracture of the ilium.

1135

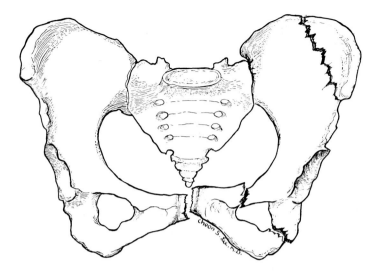

Fig. 13-51. This Malgaigne fracture consists of a symphyseal separation, left superior and left inferior rami, a left sacroiliac dislocation with cephalad displacement of the intervening fragment, and a fracture of the wing of the ilium (Duverney's fracture).

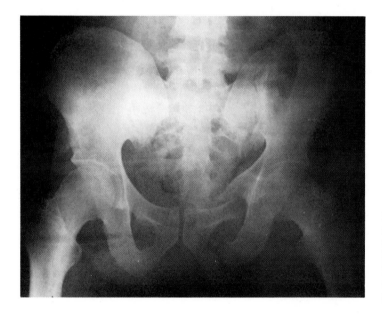

Fig. 13-52. This typical Malgaigne fracture consists of fractures of the left superior and inferior rami and a fracture of the left ilium with cephalad displacement of the intervening fragment. This is the original double vertical fracture according to Malgaigne's classic description.

lower portion of the middle fragment is driven into the pelvis while the superior portion is rotated outward, the rotation taking place on a more or less anteroposterior axis. This type of displacement tends to widen the superior strait of the pelvis and to diminish the inferior strait.

Malgaigne noted that the diagnosis is easy when a portion of the middle fragment can be palpated. (Bear in mind that he was dealing with these fractures before the advent of the x-ray.) He stated that this lesion may be confounded with a fracture

of the femoral neck, because the causative injury and the physical findings (i.e. shortening of the limb, eversion of the foot, and crepitation elicited by pushing up the femur or by pressing on the greater trochanter) are similar in both conditions. The methodical measurement of the limb, by which one can learn not only that the shortening is not in the thigh but that the anterior superior iliac spine is more cephalad than usual, safeguards against this error. The diagnosis is confirmed by seeking the signs of anterior fracture by examining

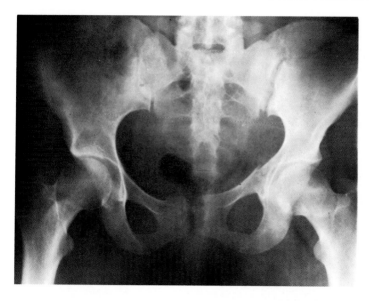

Fig. 13-53. This Malgaigne fracture consists of a symphyseal subluxation, fractures of the left superior and inferior rami, and a dislocation of the left sacroiliac joint. In addition, there is a fracture through the posterior wing of the ilium.

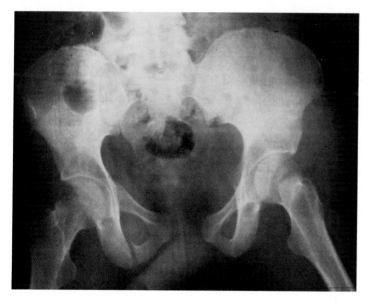

Fig. 13-54. This patient sustained a diastasis of the symphysis pubis and a dislocation of the left sacroiliac joint with cephalad displacement of the left hemipelvis. The presence of the right superior and inferior pubic rami can also be noted. This represents a Malgaigne fracture, since the major elements necessary for a Malgaigne fracture are present; bilateral vertical dislocations or fractures with cephalad displacement of the intervening fragment. In this instance the right pubic rami fractures do not contribute to the Malgaigne fracture, nor do they, in conjunction with the left sacroiliac fracture, constitute a "buckethandle" fracture, because the disruption of the symphysis pubis intervenes between the right pubic rami fractures and the left sacroiliac dislocation.

the perineum and fold of the groin, and the signs of posterior fracture by examining back of the trochanter. Any of the displacements alluded to may be detected by the finger introduced into the vagina or rectum.[284]

Some authors of major articles on pelvic fractures and dislocations[117,121,187,495] have chosen not to use the eponym or even make reference to Malgaigne's description. This has led to confusion as well, for, if these major contibutors do not mention him, then the reader may reasonably question the value

of his early contribution. Perhaps the eponym is avoided because it means different things to different people.

The terminology of "Malgaigne fractures" has been complicated by the fact that modern authors,[231,350,358] (benefiting from the availability of x-rays) include under this umbrella term those fractures in which the anterior and posterior halves of the pelvis are simultaneously involved. This includes dislocation of the symphysis pubis as well as fractures of both pubic rami with any one of the

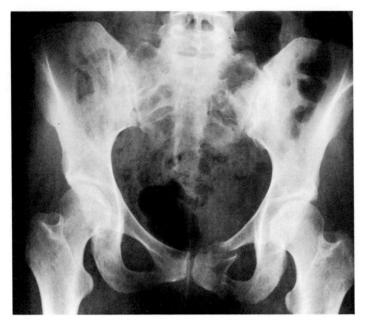

Fig. 13-55. This Malgaigne fracture consists of left pubic rami fractures and a left sacroiliac subluxation. There is also cephalad displacement of the major portion of the left hemipelvis. This fracture, were it not for the obvious sacroiliac subluxation, might have been considered a simpler fracture, that is, a fracture near the symphysis pubis, constituting a single break in the pelvic ring. The subluxation of the sacroiliac joint adds an element of instability that should be recognized by the treating physician.

previously mentioned posterior disruptions. While the purist might quibble that the name, "Malgaigne fracture," must be reserved for those pelvic disruptions that have superior and inferior pubic rami fractures, it might be more practical and useful to consider in the category of Malgaigne fractures all pubic fractures of both the superior and inferior rami, or a pubic symphyseal dislocation in conjunction with an ipsilateral posterior disruption consisting either of a sacral fracture, an iliac fracture, or a sacroiliac dislocation. In conjunction with these combined anterior and posterior disruptions, another element is the potential for displacement of the middle fragment containing the hip joint. The displacement may be cephalad translation, rotation in a transverse plane with the symphysis spread, rotation in a coronal plane with either the superior or inferior strait narrowed, or rotation in the sagittal plane with the hemipelvis more commonly tipped posteriorly.

Some authors,[121,187] shunning the eponym, have resorted to what I believe is unproductive overcategorization, using, in one instance a category for sacroiliac joint dislocations and a separate category for fracture of the ilium or sacrum adjacent to the sacroiliac joint. In one instance,[121] categories were created for "vertical shear", "pelvic dislocation", "lateral compression", and the rare "bucket-handle" fracture, where the rami are fractured contra-

laterally from the posterior disruption, which is located on the side of the impact.

Other authors[244,257,414,472] have emphasized the posterior disruptions of the pelvis to the point where the titles of their articles are partially misleading: "Complete Anterior Dislocation of the Sacro-Iliac Joint," "Bilateral Sacroiliac Joint Dislocation with Intrapelvic Protrusion of the Intact Lumbosacral Spine and Sacrum," "Traumatic Sacroiliac Disruptions," and so forth. In each instance an associated anterior pelvic fracture or dislocated symphysis means that the problem is a "Malgaigne Fracture", and not simply a sacroiliac dislocation. I believe the term, "Malgaigne fracture", can be useful if it is used to denote a disruption of the pelvis both anteriorly and posteriorly with real or potential displacement of the intervening fragment.

INCIDENCE

Watson-Jones[495] reported that Malgaigne fractures constituted 12% of pelvic fractures in his series, but he excluded a number of other fractures included in other series, thereby raising the proportion of the Malgaigne variety. He also pointed out that many less severe fractures may not be referred to orthopaedists. Fifteen of his 18 patients had dislocation of the symphysis, 14 had sacroiliac dislocation.

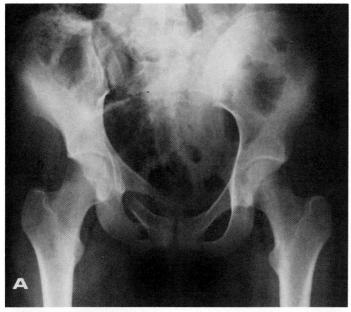

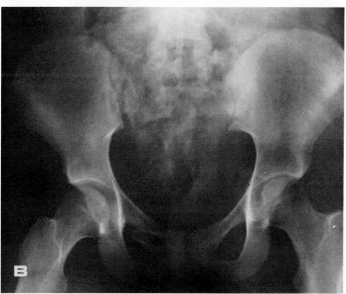

Fig. 13-56. (*A*) This Malgaigne fracture consists of right superior and inferior pubic rami and right sacral fractures as well as left sacral fractures. Coincidentally, there are fractures of the transverse processes of L4 and L5 on the left side. (*B*) This film taken 48 hours later further defines the posterior disruption of the sacrum and the sacroiliac joints bilaterally. Repeat films are often essential in the clarification of the diagnosis of pelvic fractures.

Peltier[350] reported an incidence of Malgaigne fractures as 7% of all pelvic fractures, and he indicated that the incidence appeared to be rising in his series. Later, Dunn and Morris[121] reported an incidence of 20% in their series, and these fractures represented two thirds of all unstable fractures. Conolly and Hedberg[87] reported an incidence just over 10%, and they found the Malgaigne fracture of the hemipelvis has the highest morbidity and mortality of any category. Of 21 patients, 18 had associated fracture, 16 had severe intrapelvic hemorrhage, 11 had central nervous system injuries, 7 had urinary tract damage, 7 had abdonimal complications, 5 had intrathoracic injuries, and 17 of the 21 died.

Holdsworth[187] did not support such dire projections. His series of 50 fracture-dislocations of the pelvis had four cases of major urinary tract damage,

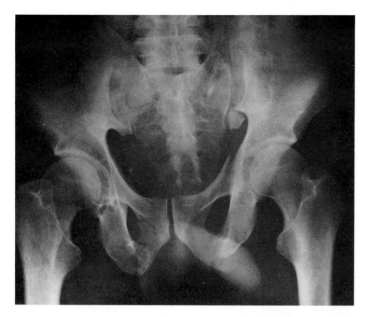

Fig. 13-57. This Malgaigne fracture consists of left superior and inferior pubic rami and left iliac fractures in conjunction with cephalad displacement of the intervening fragment. Coincidental fractures include a fracture of the left posterior inferior iliac spine and comminuted fractures of the right superior pubic ramus and right inferior pubic ramus at their junctions with the body of the pubis.

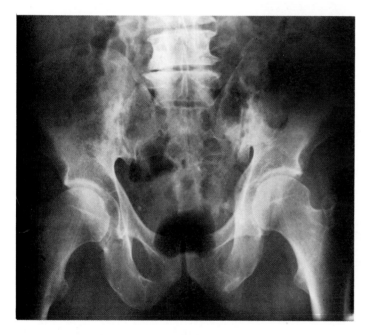

Fig. 13-58. A 15-year follow-up on the fractures seen in Figure 13-57. The patient was asymptomatic in the region of the anterior pelvic fractures but had intermittent low-grade complaints relative to his left parasacral fracture. These symptoms did not warrant surgical intervention such as fusion of the left sacroiliac joint.

eight cases of hemorrhage, and six deaths (a mortality rate of 12% compared to Conolly and Hedberg's 81%). Conwell in a discussion of Holdsworth's paper estimated that in his series of over 400 cases of fractures of the pelvis about one fourth involved fractures and fracture-dislocations of the sacroiliac joint. He also reported these injuries to be severe, quite the contrary of Holdsworth.

MECHANISM OF INJURY

The mechanism of this injury has been discussed and disputed. Malgaigne indicated that the double vertical fracture of the pelvis could be sustained by lateral compressive forces, by anteroposterior compressive forces, and by indirect forces caused by falls on the lower extremity from a height. Taylor[466]

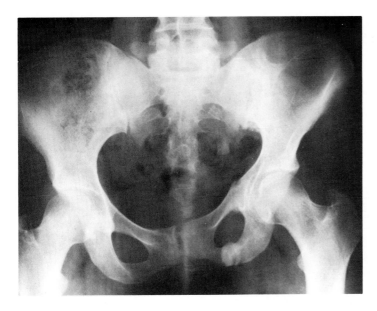

Fig. 13-59. This Malgaigne fracture was seen 8 months after injury with healing of the left pubic rami and left iliac fractures. There was slight persistent cephalad displacement of the intervening fragment, but the patient was asymptomatic and there was no disability associated with the slight functional leg length discrepancy.

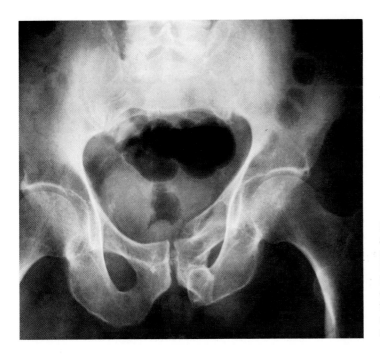

Fig. 13-60. This 62-year-old miner sustained a Malgaigne fracture approximately 4 years prior to this film. The left iliac fracture healed satisfactorily, as did the left pubic rami fractures, but the left sacroiliac dislocation gave rise to chronic disabling symptoms that led to a left sacroiliac fusion. Fusion of the joint brought about amelioration of symptoms.

believed the injury is sustained by indirect violence when the lower limb in hyperextension and hyperabduction acts as a long lever to dislocate the pelvis. He postulated that the hindquarter, which contains the mobile hip joint, moves as a solid piece, because there are certain "locked positions" of the hip joint, especially in extension and abduction. Beyond a certain limit these movements are prevented by the interlocking of the joint surfaces and the strength of the surrounding ligaments. In a same manner, muscles that pass over the pubic bone struts to the femoral shaft exert powerful leverage whenever hyperextension or hyperabduction is applied. This leverage is further exaggerated if the muscles are in spasm. Holdsworth, however, supported the view that the injury is the result of

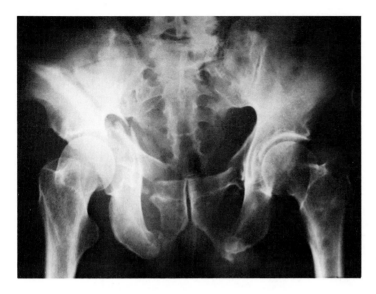

Fig. 13-61. Double vertical fractures of the pelvis. This 51-year-old man sustained a "buckethandle" fracture involving the right superior and inferior pubic rami and the left ilium. The rami are fractured contralaterally from the posterior disruption, which is located on the side of the impact.

severe direct violence, either as an anteroposterior thrust or a torsion injury where the sacrum was fixed and one ilium was forced back by direct anteroposterior force, opening the pelvis like a book. Dommisse[117] classified the etiologic violence as either transmitted or direct compression. In the former instance, the femur is neither adducted nor abducted and is flexed at less than a right angle. The acetabulum resists the force, and the interpubic ligaments and the anterior sacroiliac ligaments are torn; or the ligaments hold, and an anterior pubic, sacral, or iliac fracture occurs. Dommisse claimed that direct-compression fractures may be side-to-side, front-to-back, or transmitted through an ischial tuberosity as in a fall from a height. Watson-Jones[495] ascribed the combined injuries of the pelvis to forcible compression in the anteroposterior axis. It is my belief that most of these injuries are due to direct violence in an anteroposterior direction but that on occasion the violence may be transmitted or may be due to side-to-side compression.

Fractures of the anterior and posterior rings on opposite sides, bucket-handle fractures,[121] are due to oblique forces directed in an anteroposterior direction. The ischiopubic rami are fractured on the side opposite impact, and the hemipelvis on the side of impact may be rotated and displaced upward and inward.

One of the largest series of Malgaigne fractures, that of Slatis and Huittenen,[439] reviewed 163 patients with double vertical fractures of the pelvis. They found that the anterior injuries comprised pubic fractures and separation of the symphysis in

a ratio of 5:1, whereas injuries to the posterior pelvic ring were confined to the sacrum and the sacroiliac regions in a ratio of 3:2. Gross pelvic disruption occurred in 18% of their cases. Eleven patients died (a mortality rate of 6.7%) and 98% of the remaining patients resumed their work within 1 year. Of considerable interest is the fact that there were a number of late sequelae recorded, including obliquity of the pelivs, impaired gait, disabling low back pain, and signs of persistent nerve damage in the lumbosacral plexus.

Müller-Farber and Müller[318] reviewed 693 patients with pelvic fractures over a 15-year period. Two hundred and forty-one cases (34.8%) had pelvic fractures that did not affect the stability of the pelvic ring. These included unilateral and nondisplaced bilateral fractures of the pubic rami (category I). The unstable fractures were of two types. Category II comprised the so-called isolated dislocation of the symphysis, and the unilateral or bilateral fractures of the pubic rami combined with dislocation of the symphysis. The unstable pelvic ring fractures—category III—comprised all ruptures of the posterior weight-bearing area of the pelvic ring. Two hundred and seventy patients (39%) had category II fractures and 182 patients (26%) had category III fractures. In this series the category I fractures were treated with recumbency only and with early mobilization. Category II fractures were commonly treated in recumbency with a pelvic sling for 12 weeks. Most of the category III fractures were treated conservatively with recumbency in a pelvic sling but some 15 fractures were treated surgically by plating, bone grafting, plating and bone grafting, or by external fixation. As a result of their study, these authors believed that conservative treatment is the prevailing method of choice, but if pelvic stability cannot be achieved by conservative means the secondary surgical treatment of internal or external fixation should be performed.

DIAGNOSIS

The diagnosis of a Malgaigne fracture of the pelvis is facilitated by the signs and symptoms of a severe pelvic injury in conjunction with deformity and the apparent shortening of the leg. Subcutaneous deformity, crepitus, tenderness on compression, and a discrepancy in the umbilicus-medial malleolus lengths of the two limbs without a discrepancy in the anterior superior iliac spine-medial malleolus lengths of the two limbs are additional useful signs. Despite subcutaneous swelling, it may be possible to determine that the anterior iliac crest is displaced and mobile. X-ray examination confirms the diagnosis.

Less obvious Malgaigne disruptions must be suspected, according to Poigenfurst[360] if (1) a symphysis disruption exists with diastasis of more than 15 mm, (2) a symphysis disruption occurs with overlapping of the pubis, (3) a symphysis disruption and at least unilateral fractures of both pelvic rami are present independent of the size of the diastasis, or (4) bilateral breaks of both pelvic rami are present.

METHODS OF TREATMENT

While it is not always possible to arrive at a clear-cut explanation of the etiology in Malgaigne fractures, it is more important that the mode of treatment for the pelvic disruption be planned according to the direction of the displacement (which can be determined by careful analysis of the x-rays).

Malgaigne stated that the first step in treatment is to determine the exact relations of the fragments, and, if there is any shortening, to provide traction to the leg. He stressed that the fragment must go into place properly and be as completely reduced as possible until consolidation is accomplished in about 45 to 50 days. He counteracted the tendency to shorten with an inclined plane and the two thighs fastened together so as to make them less mobile:

"... the feet fixed to the footboard, and the body confined by a loop placed beneath the axillae. Against the other displacements, I know of nothing more efficacious

than a very firm body-bandage, or what is better, a wide girdle buckled around the pelvis above the trochanters, with compresses to push the iliac crests inward if this be necessary; while a broad pad between the thighs, and a handkerchief fastening the knees together, would have the effect of carrying the two ischiatic tuberosities outward.[280]

Astley Cooper[92] was an early advocate of the sling method of managing pelvic fractures. Noland and Conwell[325] modified the sling with a wooden spreader bar (to alter the side-to-side compressive force) and added longitudinal traction on the legs (Fig. 13-62). Key and Conwell[231] advised that the leg of the affected side be reduced by heavy longitudinal traction, or, if that was unsuccessful, by a manipulation under general anesthesia if the patient's condition allowed. Holm[191] showed that dual pelvic traction slings can also be used advantageously, especially in symphyseal diastasis, or laterally displaced hemipelvis, or total pelvic disruption with lateral spread. Separate slings over the trochanters and the iliac crests allow variation in the traction forces according to the weight and lateral displacement of each sling. The separate slings facilitate nursing care, Holm said, because they may be separated or moved independently without seriously jeopardizing immobilization.

Watson-Jones[495] maintained that these combined injuries of the iliac and pubic segments of the pelvic ring are produced mainly by anteroposterior compression and that the displacement is due to rotation around the longitudinal axis and possibly cranial translation of the middle fragment. He believed that reduction required traction to the limb of the affected side to reduce the cranial displacement followed by pelvic slings and girdles to maintain the reduction and prevent further separation of the major fragments. Watson-Jones believed the key to successful reduction is the position of lateral recumbency. He likened the dislocated pelvis to a partly opened bivalve shell (e.g., an oyster or a mussel). When it is laid on a hinge at the back, gravity keeps the two halves apart, but laid on one side, the two halves close. Similarly, if the patient with the dislocated pelvis lies on one side, the two halves of the pelvis fall together.

This premise of Watson-Jones leads naturally to his method of postural reduction in which the patient is placed on his uninjured side on a plaster table in the full lateral position. X-ray examination determines whether the bones are well reduced, and if not, manipulation can be tried, using pressure over the crest of the ilium, pushing it downward and forward toward the normal half of the pelvis.

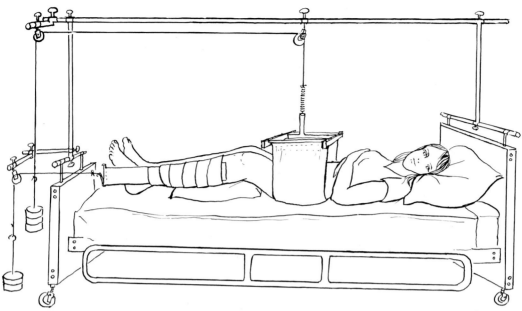

Fig. 13-62. If cephalad displacement of a double vertical fracture-dislocation of the pelvis has not taken place, longitudinal traction through Buck's traction can be used to prevent displacement; attention should be directed at ensuring that sufficient skin area is used with the traction apparatus and that excess weight is not applied to the Buck's traction. If cephalad displacement of the intervening fragment has occurred in a Malgaigne fracture, skeletal traction must be used. Reduction of the cephalad displacement of the intervening fragment must take place before the pelvic sling is used, otherwise the pelvic sling will tend to prevent reduction of the intervening fragment. (After Key, J. A., and Conwell, H. E.: J.A.M.A., **94**:174, 1930.)

When x-ray examination reveals good reduction, a double plaster spica is applied from the distal thighs to the costal margins over the well-padded iliac and trochanteric prominences (Fig. 13-63). Watson-Jones encouraged his patients to lie on one side throughout the entire period of recumbency and reapplied the plaster spica if it became loose after 4 or 5 weeks. He continued his immobilization for 3 months and throughout this period of immobilization, used physiotherapy to prevent stiffening of the knee joints and to maintain quadriceps strength.

Holdsworth[187] believed that only two methods are really rational: (1) the Watson-Jones method of lateral recumbency or plaster, and (2) the leg traction and pelvic hammock method. Holdsworth concluded that lateral recumbency and plaster was theoretically sound but difficult in practice. He used the sling method exclusively, with a firm canvas sling that extended from above the iliac crest to below the greater trochanters. Suspension cords of the sling criss-crossed the patient, raising him off the bed. The hips were placed in flexion with the limbs on Braun frames, and if there was cephalad displacement of the hemipelvis, skeletal traction was applied to the affected limb. It must be emphasized that distal skeletal traction should be applied before the pelvic sling is used, in order that the lateral displacement might be taken advantage of in reduction of the cephalad displacement. Once the cephalad displacement is reduced, the pelvic sling can be used. If rotational displacement is also present, manipulation may be necessary, and the patient will probably require a general anesthetic before he is rolled onto his normal side for reduction of the rotated fragment.

The degree of compression by the pelvic sling can be adjusted by altering the obliquity of the traction ropes and the weights applied; x-rays should be taken frequently during the first days after reduction. Reduction is maintained for 12 weeks, but after 6 weeks, traction weights can be removed and the leg exercises begun. Weight bearing is postponed until 12 weeks have passed. In

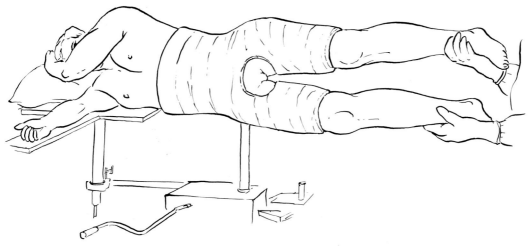

Fig. 13-63. Bilateral pelvic spica applied in lateral recumbency according to the method of Watson-Jones. X-ray examination is performed before the application of the plaster cast to determine if the bones are well reduced. If they are not, manipulation can be tried, using pressure over the crests of the affected ilium, pushing it downward and forward toward the normal half of the pelvis on which the patient is lying in a full lateral position. When x-ray reveals good reduction, a double plaster spica extending from the distal thighs to the costal margins is applied over the well-padded iliac and trochanteric prominences. (After Watson-Jones, R.: Dislocations and Fracture-Dislocations of the Pelvis. Br. J. Surg., **25:**773–781, 1938.)

one series[121] in which two patients were permitted to ambulate at 5½ weeks, partial redisplacement resulted, and both had residual disability due to chronic sacroiliac pain. Holdsworth noted that, while in his 50 cases end results were good, the prognosis of dislocations of the sacroiliac joint was not as good as in the case of fractures near that joint. He noted that while all patients complained of pain in the pubis at first, the symptoms eventually disappeared; but even in the best cases there was often aching in the back after prolonged effort. In sacroiliac dislocations this pain was severe. His patients often had marked limitation of straight leg raising on the affected side. Because of the frequency of persistent sacroiliac pain after dislocation of the joint, Holdsworth advised consideration of early sacroiliac fusion, especially in those patients with severe localized pain that persisted for 1 to 2 years after injury. He hypothesized that the anterior sacroiliac ligaments were torn from the front of the sacrum and ilium and curled within the joint preventing true restoration of position and allowing an unsound ankylosis to develop.

Bucholz[48] has recently confirmed Holdsworth's surmise[187] in an elegant and detailed post-mortem evaluation of 150 consecutive multiple-trauma victims in which 47 (31%) had pelvic injuries. Anatomic reduction of the posterior fracture-dislocation in the Malgaigne fractures by external manipulation was impossible in the majority of the cadavers because of either ligamentous or osseous interposition in the sacroiliac joint, or because of triplane displacement of the hemipelvis. Bucholz also demonstrated three types of pelvic ring disruption under the general heading of a Malgaigne fracture-dislocation: (1) group I (14 cadavers) showed only anterior injury radiologically but on dissection all had either a nondisplaced vertical fracture of the sacrum or slight tearing of the anterior sacroiliac ligament; (2) group II (5 cadavers) revealed that in addition to a recognized anterior pelvic ring injury there was also radiologic evidence of partial sacroiliac joint disruption with complete tearing or avulsion of the anterior sacroiliac ligament with sparing of the posterior sacroiliac ligaments; (3) group III (11 cadavers) showed complete disruption of all sacroiliac ligaments allowing triplane displacement of the hemipelvis, usually cephalad, posteriorly and externally rotated. Reduction of the posterior displacements were attempted in all cadavers. Group I cadavers were essentially nondisplaced and showed little tendency to displace with axial or posteriorly directed loading. Two group II injuries were ordinarily reducible by lateral compression but three were not because of infolding of the anterior sacroiliac ligament or interposition of sacral avulsion fracture fragments into the joint. Reduction by traction and external manipulation of group III injuries was impossible in all 11 cadavers because of ligamentous and osseous tissue interposition in the sacroiliac joint. Moreover, the concavoconvex undulations of the apposing surfaces were not sufficiently prominent to provide stability even when the interposing tissue had been removed and reduction achieved. These findings have major implications for the advocates of fixation devices, whether internal or external. While Key and Conwell[231] stated that good position of the pelvic fragments was not always necessary for good functional results, the dramatic example they showed to illustrate this point did not have a sacroiliac dislocation, and the patient's fractures of the sacrum and ilium had healed, providing a solid posterior weight-bearing arch.

Others,[107,520] however, reporting on patients with traumatic symphyseal diastasis and consequently with a posterior pelvic disruption, usually at the sacroiliac joint, have echoed Key and Conwell.[231] While accurate reduction by traction, sling, or spica cast has been usually considered essential, it was the finding in one series of 25 patients with severe symphysis pubis diastasis that even when nonoperative treatment had to be abandoned because of the need to mobilize the patient for pulmonary care, there was no patient with residual symphysis pain, and only three of 25 patients had significant residual low back pain. Day concluded that operative intervention for symphysis diastasis is unnecessary and that many patients with pulmonary problems who are mobilized early can have subsequent satisfactory closure of the diastasis since closure of the diastasis can progress even while the patient is ambulatory. Overall, Day found that significant residual low back pain and disability from a symphysis diastasis were infrequent.[107]

Almost identical conclusions were drawn by Winter and Marsh[520] from a study of 30 patients with significant separations of the symphysis pubis. They found that neither accurate reduction, prolonged bed rest, nor the patient's age correlated with the final functional status. Mild sacroiliac pain was present in six of the 30 patients but it was not severe; only one took an occasional aspirin. Chronic pain at the symphysis pubis was not noted to be a problem, and only one patient of the 30 failed to return to work because of pelvic pain being the reason. The authors advocated bedrest and a pelvic sling or snug-fitting corset until the pain subsided,

allowing progressive ambulation with crutches within the pain tolerance. It would appear that all of the patients treated in this fashion were patients who would have been categorized as having either group I or group II injuries according to Bucholz's classification system,[48] for it is unreasonable to anticipate that patients with wide diastasis of the symphysis pubis with an associated *complete* disruption of the posterior sacroiliac ligament complex would have achieved such satisfactory results; in other series of more severe Malgaigne fractures the end results have been much less gratifying.

In a study of 53 patients with Malgaigne fractures, Semba and co-workers[422] reported that 26 (49%) had sacral fractures, 24 (45%) had disruption of the sacroiliac joint, and 5 (9%) had fractures of the ilium. Two patients (4%) had bilateral posterior involvement, and 23 (43%) of the patients had cephalad dislocation of the hemipelvis; there was more than 1 cm displacement occurring in 13 of the cases (25%). In thirty patients who were followed for more than 2 years after injury, late complications included 8 (27%) with low back pain of extreme or disabling severity, 9 (31%) with gait disturbance, 11 (37%) with lower extremity paresthesias, and 2 (7%) with fecal incontinence. These authors found a direct correlation between the presence of disabling and severe pain and the amount of posterior and anterior pelvic ring displacements. This retrospective study revealed that most patients had been treated with traction (Buck's traction in 5 patients; skeletal traction in 20 patients), although a few were treated with the external fixator. They concluded that anatomical reduction of the hemipelvis and anatomical configuration is essential for prevention of late sequelae.

Tile and Pennal[469,470] manage anteroposterior fractures with an intact posterior complex by reduction of the diastasis and maintenance using sling, spica, or external fixator. Lateral compression fractures may require reduction under anesthetic followed by skeletal traction or an external fixator. Vertical shear fractures, easily reducible, are maintained only with difficulty, usually by internal or external fixation to achieve compression posteriorly.

Broomhead[45] reported a case of dislocation of the sacroiliac joint together with fracture of the pubic ramus and widening of the symphysis pubis that responded to Hoke well-leg traction. In this method, a spica is applied from the foot of the sound side to the costal margin and then down almost to the knee of the affected side. A low femoral Steinmann pin is inserted and by means of two straps and a rack-and-pinion apparatus attached to a Thomas ring inserted into the pantaloon on the affected side, the traction then can be transmitted effectively to the affected hemipelvis.

Jahss[208] implemented the lever principle by means of heavily padded long-leg casts united by turnbuckles that could, depending on the forces used, apply either medial compression or lateral distraction to the pelvic fragments (Fig. 13-64). Jahss listed the advantages of his treatment as excellent realignment of the fracture, restoration of normal inlet and outlet measurements, immediate relief of pain, ability of the patient to sit, avoidance of soiling, and the elimination of the need for anesthetic. Subsequently Jahss found that unless one turnbuckle was placed approximately on the anteromedial surface of the cast and one on the posteromedial surface, a great deal of leverage was lost, as the limbs tended to go into external rotation (Fig. 13-64). To combat this, the two turnbuckle positions were devised with the posterior turnbuckle being used as a derotator. Lacking turnbuckles, a block of wood and a webbed strap can achieve similar results,[435] as can the Roger Anderson well-leg traction splint.[211]

External and Internal Fixation

There have been few advances in the management of pelvic fractures more dramatic than the introduction and dissemination of concepts of external and internal fixation of complex pelvic fractures. The obvious disadvantages of prolonged conservative management of complicated pelvic fractures includes prolonged bed rest, increased susceptibility to thromboembolic phenomena, decubiti, renal calculi, psychosocial deprivation, and the not inconsiderable likelihood of loss of reduction with subsequent malunion or chronic subluxation. To overcome these problems, there have been various attempts at fixation of the pelvis.

As mobility of the patient is inversely related to the stability of the fractures, it is the goal of these fixation devices to achieve sufficient stability that the patient's mobility might be enhanced, thereby reducing the period of prolonged bed rest and also enhancing cardiopulmonary function. Another benefit of fixation is early control of osseous bleeding.

Whiston[511] described the use of crossed stainless steel pins in five patients, indicating that this technique had not previously been described in the literature; he did give credit to Levine[255] for describing the use of a curved metal plate to fix a fracture of the iliac fossa and acknowledged the

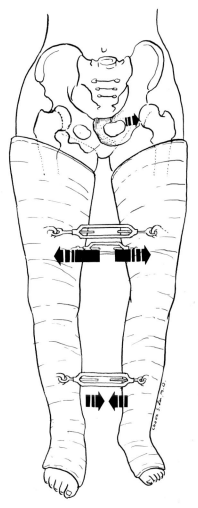

Fig. 13-64. Jahss' method of treatment of pelvic fractures. Using the lever principle by means of heavily padded long-leg casts united by turnbuckles, one distally and two proximally, Jahss could apply either medial compression or lateral distraction of pelvic fragments. Jahss obtained excellent reduction of fractures, restoring normal inlet and outlet measurements. The method relieved pain, promoted personal hygiene by virtue of the patient's being able to sit, and eliminated the need for general anesthesia. In the illustration shown, lateral distraction forces are being used to overcome overriding of the symphysis pubis. (After Jahss, S. A.: Injuries Involving the Ilium. A New Treatment. J. Bone Joint Surg., **17:**338–346, 1935.)

"Stader splint" as a forerunner of today's external fixation devices. Subsequent to Whiston's report there have been sporadic reports of the use of iliac crest hooks,[8,158] iliac crest wires, or femoral, pubic, and iliac crest pins by percutaneous methods followed by the use of external fixation or traction forces.[38,131,224,252,315,440]

Letournel[252] has indicated that he has used external fixation in conjunction with Judet since 1962. Carabalona[62] and Bonnel[35] studied the use of the external fixator of Hoffmann, and determined that two groups of three pins should be inserted between the two cortices of the iliac crests behind the anterior superior iliac spines. The reduction and fixation of the frame is effected by two compression rods completing a parallelogram; these authors had good results in all seven cases of severe pubic diastasis.

Slatis and Karaharju[440,441] used three pins as well in each wing of the ilium, but connected them with a trapezoidal frame constructed at 70° to the longitudinal axis of the body, more or less in the direction of the sacroiliac joints. Karaharju and Slatis[224] found that displacements of the hemipelvis were more easily reduced than juxta-articular fractures but were more apt to redislocate with respect to disruptions of the posterior pelvis. After the application of the compression frame, the patients were allowed to turn freely in bed or to be turned by the nursing staff and to half sit. Three weeks after the application of the frame, the patients were allowed out of bed and were encouraged to bear 30 kg to 40 kg of weight on the affected leg while using crutches. In all instances the frame was removed six weeks after application.

Slatis and Karaharju[441] reported on their experiences with the trapezoid frame in their first 22 patients, all of whom had sustained a Malgaigne fracture. Using general anesthesia and the image intensifier while the patient was on a conventional operating table, they achieved reduction by traction and manipulation. If it was necessary, any locked rotation of the hemipelvis was corrected by dislodging the hemipelvis by hyperextension and external rotation and then reducing the disengaged hemipelvis under x-ray control. Reduction of longitudinal fractures of the sacrum was often difficult but retention was relatively easily accomplished once compression had been applied; with dislocations of the sacroiliac joint, reductions were usually easily accomplished but retention was often difficult to maintain. Weight bearing was begun 3 weeks following the accident and the frame removed 6 weeks after the injury. At follow-up the reduction was rated as excellent in 15 patients, fair in five patients, and poor in two patients. The authors found that better results were obtained in patients who had been subjected to repositioning maneuvers within 2 days after the injury had been

sustained. In late follow-up, only two of the 22 patients subjected to the use of the trapezoid compression frame had impaired gait and only one had disabling back pain.

In a previous series reported by Slatis and Huittinen,[439] in unilateral double vertical fractures and dislocations the trapezoid compression frame provided sufficient stability as indicated by laboratory testing procedures. The authors allowed patients with such fractures who had been appropriately reduced and stabilized to start immediate weight bearing. They found, however, that in bilateral double vertical fractures the external fixation device served mainly in retention for the displaced pelvic halves, and they could not allow the patient out of bed until 3 weeks after the accident. They still advocate recumbency for 4 to 6 weeks for patients with bilateral double vertical fractures, the shorter time for patients with fractures through the sacrum or ilium and the longer time for dislocations of the sacroiliac joints. Overall, Slatis and Huittinen were gratified by the achievements of the external compression fixation device, particularly in comparison with the reports of conventional treatment, which showed a high incidence of impaired gait and persistent back pain. Earlier studies in patients with double vertical fractures showed significant long-term sequelae. Monahan and Taylor,[305] in 1975, reported impaired gait in 41% of patients and persistent back pain in 52%, while Slatis and Huittinen,[439] in 1972, reported impaired gait in 32% and persistent back pain in 17%.

The method of inserting the half pins can be either under direct visualization or by use of a jig that facilitates the closed insertion of the half pins. In the open method the patient is under general anesthetic and is in the supine position. An anterior iliac crest incision is performed and the dissection carried down to the anterior iliac crest so that the inner and outer tables of the iliac crest can be observed during the insertion of three groups of half pins in the anterior and three pins into the anterior-inferior iliac crest. This is done bilaterally, and, then, the Hoffmann apparatus is used while a ball joint is attached to each cluster of three pins and a straight rod is employed to bridge the ball joints on each side. Two articulation couplings are then added to each of the straight rods. Additional rods are used to give added strength to the external fixation device. Reduction of anterior pubic separations by means of the pin clusters and the attached rods is easily achieved in most instances but the reduction should be observed under direct x-ray visualization (Fig. 13-65).

Closure is routinely achieved around each of the

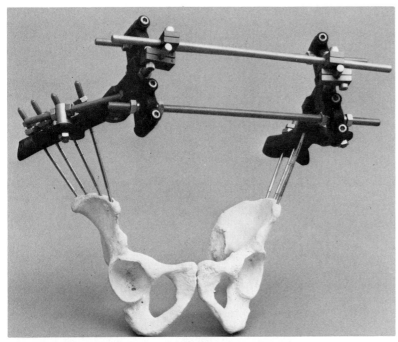

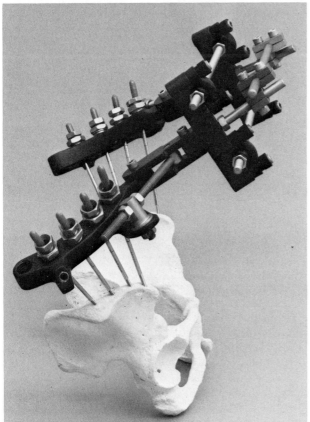

Fig. 13-65. External fixator using a cluster of four pins. (Courtesy of Richards Manufacturing Co.)

pin clusters and the reduction is checked radiographically. The patient is encouraged to get into a chair as soon as is possible considering the presence of other associated injuries. Skin care is limited to simply the use of daily hydrogen peroxide cleansing, and under ordinary circumstances the patient is left in the frame for approximately 6 weeks.

The external fixation devices have been effective in achieving rigidity anteriorly, but clinical and biomechanical tests have shown that they do not adequately provide posterior stability if there has been significant disruption in the posterior pelvic ring. For such situations the use of transpelvic pins inserted with the use of a directional jig from the anterior-inferior iliac spine to the posterior-inferior iliac spine is advocated. These pins are then attached using anterior and posterior quadrilateral frames. It is recognized that the presence of an anterior as well as a posterior external fixation device demands a higher degree of technical proficiency and also complicates nursing care. Such an arrangement, however, is necessary because it has been demonstrated that unstable posterior disruptions cannot be adequately managed even for bed-chair transfer exclusively depending on the anterior external fixation devices.

An alternative means of fixing the posterior disruptions has been sought; in general this has led to application of internal fixation devices with cancellous screws crossing the sacroiliac joint. In 1960 Dommisse[117] wired screws together that had been affixed to the opposite sides of the symphysis pubis, and in 1973 Sharp[427] designed a special plate to hold the reapproximated symphysis together. In 1978 Jenkins and Young[210] advocated the closed reduction of sacroiliac joints and the open fixation of the associated disruption of the symphysis pubis by means of a suitable AO dynamic compression plate (DCP) that had been fashioned with a standard plate-bending vise to attach snugly to the superior surfaces of the pubic rami. The advantages of this simple technique included a short stay in the hospital, rigid fixation, freedom from pain, and restoration of the normal anatomy of both the symphysis pubis and the sacroiliac joints.

More recently, Tile[469] and Mears[289] as well as others[144] have advocated in specific instances the use of internal fixation both anteriorly and posteriorly. The advantages are obvious but the disadvantages are also considerable in that frequently closed fractures are converted to open fractures with an associated increase in bleeding; additionally, the region is one that is not commonly familiar to most orthopaedists (with the exception of the hip and the surgical procedures used in its treatment). Because of the diversity of the types of fractures and dislocations encountered both anteriorly and posteriorly and because of the relative infrequency of the need for open reduction and internal fixation, there is no standard for proceeding in the management of these complicated fractures. These disadvantages are to a great extent overcome by the use of external skeletal fixation devices.

In spite of these advances, contemporary dissatisfaction with problems of both internal and external fixation devices has prompted further attempts to provide ideal methods for pelvic fracture management. Mears[289] has written, ''Attempts to apply internal fixation to these formidable fractures have been associated with catastrophic bleeding and limited success in stabilization of the fractures.'' As confirmed by a recent biomechanical study[171] the simple trapezoid or the quadrilateral external frame with the use of half pins in the iliac crests provides insufficient stability, and residual deformity after correction of Malgaigne type pelvic ring fractures has been widely encountered.[289]

In an attempt to overcome these difficulties, Mears has developed a technique of more rigid external fixation with the use of transfixing pelvic pins. This technique has been employed in a number of complicated pelvic fractures. The method has ''provided rigid stabilization to permit early transfers from bed to chair, partial weight bearing gait and rapid discharge from hospital, usually within a few days of application of the device.''[289] Mears uses a pelvic jig to direct a 6.0 mm threaded pin from a position midway between the anterior superior and anterior inferior iliac inferior spines, exiting at the posterior inferior spines. The pins are usually inserted on each side of the hemipelvis. Then they are connected by standard Vidal frames, both anteriorly and posteriorly.

Considerable study is presently underway, both clinically and in the laboratory, in attempts to define the ideal methods of managing these complex fractures. What follows is a survey of recent contributions to this field.

Gunterberg, Goldie, and Slatis[171] performed ten experiments in which cadaver pelves were experimentally fractured unilaterally, either through the sacroiliac joint and the symphysis pubis, or through the sacrum or ilium and the pubic rami. In seven other experiments there were eight bilateral fractures, both posteriorly and anteriorly. Subsequently, a trapezoidal fixation frame was assembled after three pins had been affixed to the iliac crests bilaterally. The results indicated that ipsilateral fractures could be stabilized by the external compression frame well enough to permit weight bearing in the upright standing position but that bilateral injuries to the pelvic skeleton, whether oblique or vertical, could not. In consequence of these findings with external fixation, the authors suggested (1) that in bilateral injuries, no weight bearing should be permitted for 3 weeks of immobilization; (2) that unilateral sacroiliac dislocations and unilateral vertical fractures of the sacrum or iliac wing may be allowed immediate weight bearing by crutches; and (3) that unilateral injuries involving oblique fractures of the sacrum or iliac wing may achieve early mobilization with full weight bearing. A similar study by Reimer and co-workers[383] performed on cadaver pelves demonstrated that the most unstable configuration, a bilateral sacroiliac dislocation plus disruption of the symphysis pubis, appeared to be better stabilized with the addition of direct pinning of the sacroiliac joints plus the external fixator. With partial disruptions and unilateral lesions the internal pins offered no advantage *in vitro* over the external fixator used alone.

Brown and co-workers[46] have studied rigidity measurements of external fixators used for unstable pelvic ring fractures in cadaver pelves. A series of fixation devices was used including the Slatis frame, the Bonnel frame, a doubled anterior frame that was coupled and uncoupled, as well as combined anterior and posterior fixation with through and through pins, and, finally, a posteriorly mounted internal fixation device through the sacroiliac joint in conjunction with an anterior trapezoidal frame. Brown and associates found that the Bonnel and Slatis frames withstood fairly equal loads, approximating 100 Newtons; the doubled anterior coronal frames, whether coupled or uncoupled, had a failure load of approximately 200 Newtons, whereas the anterior and posterior pins, and the through and through pins had failure loads of about 400 Newtons. The sacroiliac plate and anterior Slatis frame had a failure load of approximately 700 Newtons.

Nelson and co-workers[319] have continued their investigations into the clinical and biomechanical aspects of pelvic fixation and their results indicated that 5 mm half pins provide greatly improved biomechanical stability over 4 mm pins tested in pelvic external fixation devices. It was also found that double anterior frames are biomechanically more stable than the single anterior frames tested. Internal fixation, performed anteriorly and poste-

riorly, or external fixation, performed anteriorly with posterior internal fixation, can provide physiologic stability in an unstable pelvis with complete disruption of the symphysis and one or both sacroiliac joints. An innovative triangular frame configuration was demonstrated to show significant improvement in pelvic stability and allowed early bed to chair transfers and partial weight bearing.

Riska and co-workers[390] reported on the use of the Hoffmann external fixator in 56 unstable pelvic fractures. The device was applied under general anesthesia after the dislocated pelvis had been reduced. In 16 cases residual dislocation of less than 1.5 cm was noted after the reduction and the reduced position was maintained in 48 out of 51 cases, with a minor redislocation occurring in the remaining three patients and five of the patients succumbing to their injuries. Complications were few: a pin tract infection was noted in one patient, an iliac crest fracture in another patient, and a subsequent exostosis of the iliac crest occurred in one young patient. Results showed that 43 of the patients were symptom-free with regard to the pelvis at the time of review, whereas five patients had residual pain.

Burke and co-workers[52] also studied pelvic fracture stabilization with the Hoffmann external fixator in 12 multiply traumatized patients with severe pelvic fractures. Aside from the fact that this apparatus was well tolerated by all patients, it appeared to facilitate the overall management of the severely injured, from both a medical and nursing aspect. Areas of management that were facilitated included nursing procedures, skin care, mobilization, and the treatment of perineal wounds, colostomies, or suprapubic cystostomies. Seven of the 12 patients did show signs of local inflammation around one or more pins, but in no instance was premature pin removal necessary. The Hoffmann fixation device was in place for an average duration of 72 days, with a range from 55 to 99 days. Each pelvic fracture united with no evidence of instability and, at follow-up, at least 6 months after the fracture, nine of the 12 patients were asymptomatic and two patients had mild sacroiliac pain with strenuous activity. The authors claimed a more anatomical reduction and stabilization, greater control of hemorrhage, reduction of pain, ease of nursing care, and the facilitation of secondary operative procedures for the management of associated intra-abdominal, intrapelvic, perineal, and extremity injuries.

At this time there is much confusion over the indications, methods, materials, and results of the use of external fixators in pelvic fractures. Some of the more obvious points of controversy are whether the pins should be half-pins of 4 mm, 5 mm, or 6 mm diameter, or full pins of 6 mm diameter, the latter being intended to traverse the pelvis; whether pins should be inserted blindly or under direct visualization; which external frame is to be used for which type of fracture; what types of fractures should be treated with combined internal and external fixation; what kind of inventory of materials will be needed for specific fixation frames; and what postreduction and fixation mobilization is possible for various fractures and various devices.

The number of combinations and permutations of techniques available are astounding, and because the number of fractures of the pelvis requiring the kind of management described above is not great and because so few fractures are essentially similar, either in regard to their intrinsic characteristics (open versus closed, fracture versus dislocation) or with regard to extrinsic circumstances (associated injuries, age, sex, size of the patient), no large series has been done so far. Even further from consideration has been the idea to do a controlled study of various methods. Despite the technical difficulties in achieving the goal of satisfactory fracture stability to achieve patient mobility, there is little controversy that such a goal is a desirable ideal which must be sought.

AUTHOR'S PREFERRED METHOD OF TREATMENT

With respect to my indications for operative fixation of unstable pelvic fractures, I would note that the indications for surgical intervention are not yet clear-cut. Nevertheless, it would appear, based on my own observations as well as the available observations of others, that a more surgically oriented posture is warranted in those situations in which multiple system trauma and open injuries of the pelvic area demand freedom from the encumbrances associated with skeletal traction and pelvic slings. This leads to the paradox that the patient who is the most traumatized and, generally, the one least ready to tolerate surgery, is the patient who is given general anesthesia and stabilized, either with internal or external fixation devices. On the other hand, the patient who has sustained an unstable pelvic fracture that is essentially a solitary injury is judged better capable of withstanding the rigors of prolonged, conservative, nonsurgical management.

Philosophical differences about which patients should have surgery for pelvic fractures may take a route similar to that of the gradual recognition and acceptance of intramedullary rodding of appropriate femoral shaft fractures. At one time the patient who could tolerate nonsurgical, "conservative" treatment was treated by traction, followed by a spica. Only those patients who had multiple-system injuries were subjected to either open or closed intramedullary roddings. The more "aggressive," surgical treatment has turned out to be the more beneficial treatment for the patient, and now in most instances a solitary femoral shaft fracture in an adult will be treated with internal fixation. I surmise that the same sort of transitional process is occurring in the management of fractures in patients who have unstable pelvic fractures. The day may well come when all unstable pelvic fractures will be treated with fixation, either external or internal. Actually, my own preference would be for internal fixation both anteriorly and posteriorly, but such violations of the retroperitoneal hematoma with consequent loss of tamponade and potential contamination may constitute risks that are not proportionate to the benefits that accrue from early mobilization. Only the additional use of laboratory testing techniques and the accumulation of information from experienced surgeons will provide the ultimate answer to the ideal treatment for patients with unstable pelvic fractures.

Based on patient complaints of pain in the sacroiliac region after dislocation and the effective relief of these symptoms by subsequent sacroiliac fusion, I believe that an unsound traumatic ankylosis of this joint, which amounts to a chronic subluxation, is painful, and that sacroiliac disruptions should be managed vigorously in the early treatment stages by accurate reduction and maintenance of that reduction. The standard treatment for years has consisted of traction and the use of a pelvic sling for approximately 8 weeks. It is important to keep in mind that the pelvic sling should not be used unless an accurate reduction has been achieved previously by means of traction to bring down any of the pelvic fragments connected to the acetabulum and thereby to the hip; nor should a pelvic sling be used for pelvic fractures in which compression from side to side is an obvious etiologic factor. I discourage full weight bearing for patients with complete sacroiliac dislocations for a total of 16 weeks from the time of injury. In specific instances external fixators have been used to allow the patient minimal mobilization and to facilitate surgical and nursing management of associated injuries. For para-articular fractures I advise 6 weeks of traction and an additional 6 weeks of non-weight bearing if traction, bedrest or a pelvic sling is to be used, since it is my opinion that a sacroiliac dislocation heals more slowly than a para-articular fracture.

If an external fixator is to be used, a considerable reduction in the period of bedrest and hospitalization can be achieved but not, perhaps, to the extent that the enthusiastic optimism of some external fixator advocates would suggest.

It should be remembered that disability from sacroiliac disruption is common, but surprisingly good functional recovery may occur in the face of para-articular malunions. The same is true for malunions of the anterior tie arch of the pubis. Dommisse [117] has pointed out that the pubic ligaments heal by strong scar tissue when reduction of the symphyseal diastasis is reasonably accurate and Taylor[466] noted that chronic symphysis pubis pain has been recorded but that he had not seen such complications in his own series.

Most investigators dealing with reduction and fixation of the disrupted human pelvis accept the assumption that compression is a valuable force to be used in achieving stable repair of the dislocated sacroiliac joint(s). Taking advantage of my familiarity with the compression rod system devised by Paul Harrington for use in correction of spinal deformities, I adapted the heavy compression rod with two number 1279-11 hooks as a means of applying compression between the iliac bones across the sacroiliac joints and into the sacrum (Figs. 13-66 and 13-67). This device was first used in conjunction with bilateral sacroiliac arthrodeses after it was recognized that trans-sacroiliac compression screws of the AO cancellous variety did not provide sufficient compression across the sacroiliac joint, even with the use of washers or small buttress plates that distributed the compression of the screw head over a wider area of the ilium. Adaptation of the Harrington compression apparatus to management of the acute fracture was a natural consequence of the stability found in association with its earlier usage in repair of chronic sacroiliac arthritis. Anteriorly, the use of AO compression plates set at right angles on the superior and anterior surfaces of the parasymphyseal pubis has been the fixation device of my choice.

Other instruments that have been found useful in the open reduction and internal fixation of pelvic fractures and pelvic dislocations include the use of the laminar spreader, which facilitates debridement of the sacroiliac joint of bony fragments as well as of ligamentous debris. Another strong and useful device that has been used for bringing widely separated pubic segments together is the double-jawed Jackson clamp (Fig. 13-68). After the obturator foramina have been sufficiently cleared, the jaws of the bone-holding clamp are attached to the most medial portions of the superior pubic rami on both sides. The handles then are distracted, bringing each jaw, which contains the superior pubic ramus, into close approximation. This procedure allows for an easier application of the AO compression plate beneath the jaws with at least one holding screw on each side. Once the reduction and initial fixation have been achieved, the remaining screws in the first plate and the second plate with its screws can then be inserted with much more ease.

Mears,[49,289] has advocated that, if at all possible, patients who have two or more disruptions of the pelvic ring should have rigid fixation of all fractures simultaneously during a single procedure. He argues that if only one fracture is fixed internally a second disruption may become more displaced as a result of treatment of the first disruption. On the basis of my experience, I would concur with this advice fully.

SEVERE MULTIPLE FRACTURES OF THE PELVIS (INCLUDING FRACTURES OF THE SACRUM)

The fractures sustained in a massive crushing injury are severe and multiple. The pelvic ring is thoroughly demolished, and its stability is destroyed (Figs. 13-69 to 13-73). More important, the forces that led to this musculoskeletal damage have usually caused severe visceral and neurovascular damage. Hemorrhage is greater, genitourinary tract injuries more frequent, and associated injuries more common.

Furey's[143] analysis of most pelvic fractures indicates that nearly all of the complete fractures of the pelvic ring were explosive and of the contrecoup type; that is, the result of exceptional stress with strain to the explosive point, which is usually at the weakest part of the pelvic ring. Thus, in the majority of cases the fracture encountered most frequently was one involving the obturator ring, either through the pubic ramus or through a ramus of the pubis and a ramus of the ischium. Double fracture of the obturator foramen is due to the near impossibility of breaking a rigid ring at a single point with an explosive force. This also explains the reasoning behind the idea that a fracture of the pelvic ring anteriorly may be accompanied by a fracture of the ring elsewhere, usually posteriorly. While the pelvic ring is not entirely rigid, the

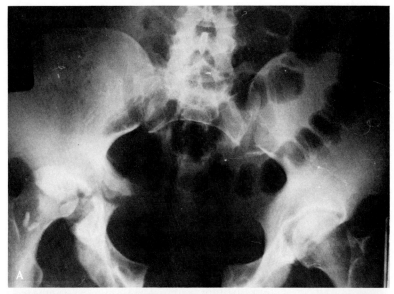

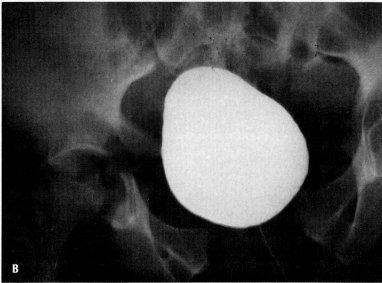

Fig. 13-66. (*A*) Multiple joint disruptions in a 31-year-old, 325-pound policeman who fell 80 feet to a creek bed in a camping accident. A fracture-dislocation of the right hip was present in addition to bilateral sacroiliac disruptions and a wide separation of the symphysis pubis. (*B*) A normal cystogram performed acutely misled treating physicians into believing that the lower tract was intact although a urethrogram taken later dispelled that misconception.

rigidity is sufficient to apply the rule in many cases, thus accounting for a relatively large number of these fractures that do occur.

The diagnosis of severe multiple fractures of the pelvis is more readily achieved than that of isolated fractures. The history and physical examination certainly lead one to suspect disruption of pelvic stability, and x-rays confirm the diagnosis. As will be discussed below, sacral fractures are not easily discovered by routine x-ray studies so that special views may be necessary. In addition, acetabular fractures also can be difficult to detect.

Beyond the principles already elaborated for managment of the double vertical fractures of the pelvis, it is advisable to consider one aspect of multiple severe fractures of the pelvis that is pertinent here; that is the sacral fracture, which is uncommon in isolation but common with multiple fractures.[292,401,522]

The incidence of sacral fractures in association with pelvic fractures is quite variable. Wakeley[491] quoted 4%, Furey[143] quoted 74%, and Noland and Conwell[326] reported a group of 60 pelvic fracture patients of whom 7 had sacral fractures—an inci-

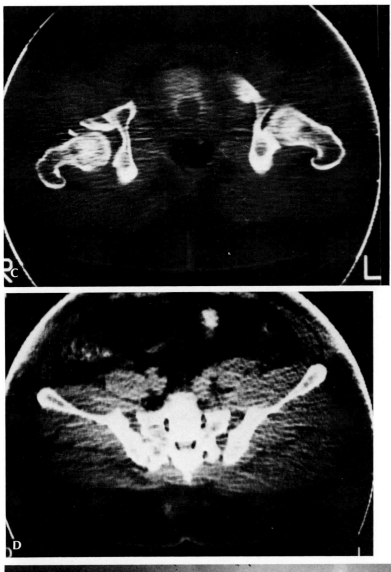

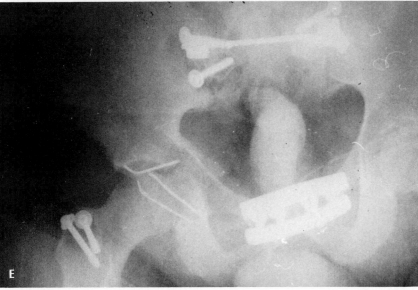

Fig. 13-66 (*Continued*). (*C,D*) CT scans reveal the acetabular fracture and the bilateral sacroiliac disruptions. (*E*) Postoperative film shows two compression plates at the symphysis pubis, two cancellous screws across each sacroiliac joint, and a Harrington compression rod with two Leatherman hooks inserted into the ilia. These wires affix the small posterior rim fracture and two screws affix the osteotomized trochanter.

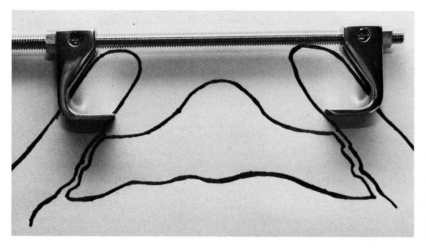

Fig. 13-67. The position of two sharp Leatherman alar hooks in the iliac crests connected by a large (diameter, 3/16 inch [4.8 mm]) Harrington threaded compression rod. This instrumentation was used in the patient depicted in Figure 13-66.

dence of 11.7%. Wakeley[489] found 44 sacral fractures in conjunction with 100 cases of pelvic fractures, and Medelman[292] found 22 cases of sacral fractures in conjunction with 50 consecutive cases of pelvic fractures. Both series yielded a 44% incidence.

Watson-Jones[495] noted that extensive crushing injuries of the pelvis were often accompanied by fractures of the sacrum but that isolated sacral fractures were rare, these being undisplaced linear fractures that recovered rapidly and completely.

Medelman[292] stated that those cases that show several fractures of the anterior half of the pelvis were more likely to show fractures of the sacrum, owing to the fact that such cases undoubtedly were subjected to greater trauma and that, consequently, shearing force exerted on the sacrum was greater.

Bonnin[37] also found that a sacral fracture was usually associated with other pelvic fractures. The sacrum resists compression well, and in the intact pelvis, aside from direct violence, the sacrum can be acted on only by compressive forces. Recognition of the biomechanics of the sacrum and the sacroiliac joint, as well as analysis of the usual types of pelvic fractures, suggests that the sacrum is broken by tension and shear transmitted through the innominate bone. The more common sacral and pelvic injuries are secondary to violence applied to one leg or one side of the body. Thus the sacrum is broken by tension and shear forces, the forces to which all bones offer least resistance. The idea that this violence is transmitted through the innominate bone is in conformity with ideas expressed by Taylor[466] on dislocations of the innominate bone.

Bonnin[37] determined that fractures through the weaker superolateral portion of the sacrum between the first and third sacral foramina can occur in three ways (or four, if pure compression is given its unimportant place): by rotation, by leverage, or by shear.

In injuries caused by rotation there is separation of the pubic symphysis or fractures of the pubic rami. The rotation force hyperextends the affected pelvis around the horizontal axis of the sacroiliac joint so that the pubis is depressed. If the sacroiliac joint does not yield (and Bonnin maintained that the sacroiliac joints offer the greatest resistance to rotation), fracture occurs through the first and second sacral foramina. Uncommonly, the affected innominate bone is rotated in the opposite direction. The direction of the rotation may be noted either by elevation or depression of the affected superior pubic ramus and comparison with the unaffected contralateral side.

In fractures of the sacrum that occur through leverage, the anterior ring is broken, its two halves are widely separated, and once the sacroiliac joint has been maximally opened, the sacrum fractures through the buttresses of the bone between the first and second sacral foramina. Bonnin maintained that the action can be reversed and the pubic symphysis can be made to overlap by compression.

In shearing fractures of the sacrum, the affected half of the pelvis is driven up and back, and the sacrum shears again at its weakest point between the first and third sacral foramina. Bonnin also maintained that the frequency with which sacral fractures are seen depends on the quality of the x-rays and the persistence of the surgeon in looking for sacral fractures.

Because the sacrum is curved and is situated obliquely in relation to the x-ray beam and the x-ray plate, it is visualized only with difficulty on routine anteroposterior views. The problem is com-

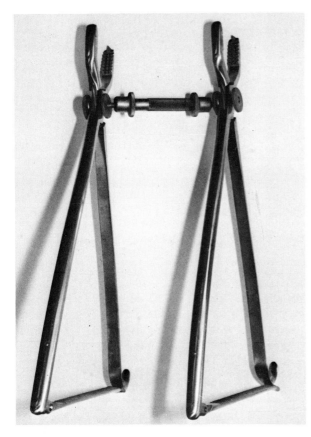

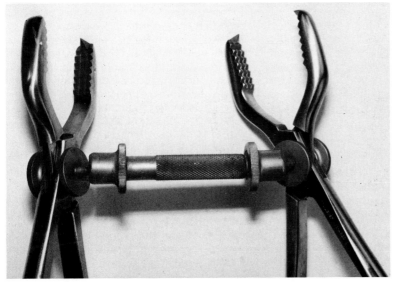

Fig. 13-68. (*Top*) The double Jackson clamp that was used to approximate the pubic bones during reduction and internal fixation, (*Bottom*) Close-up of the connection and jaws of the double Jackson clamp.

plicated by the relative thinness of the compact bone over the anterior and posterior margins of the sacrum. Bonnin maintains that the weakest area of the sacrum runs from the notch between

the articular process for the fifth lumbar vertebra and the lateral mass of the sacrum above and through the first and second foramina to the edge of the sacrum, usually through the third sacral

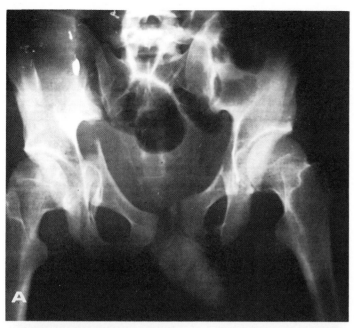

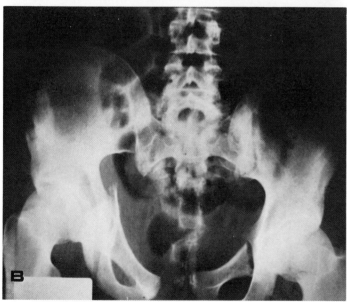

Fig. 13-69. These films demonstrate three eponymic fractures sustained simultaneously by a 20-year-old motorcyclist. The symphyseal dislocation in conjunction with the right sacroiliac disruption together with the cephalad displacement of the intervening fragment represents a Malgaigne fracture. The right ischial and inner acetabular fracture constitutes a Walther's fracture. The fracture of the right iliac wing is a Duverney's fracture. Coincidentally, the patient had fractures of the left superior and inferior rami.

foramen. The upper and lower lateral sacral promontories, which represent the upper and lower borders of the sacroiliac joint, serve as convenient landmarks in true anteroposterior views of the sacrum. The distances from the midline to these promontories can be compared between the affected and unaffected sides in a suspected sacral fracture. Bonnin stressed the value of obstetric views of the pelvis in determining the displacement after pelvic fractures, especially in injuries that cause

forward displacement of the lateral mass of the sacrum on the main mass of the bone. Sacral fractures can be recognized by inspecting the regularity of the superior arches of the anterior sacral foramina and comparing them with the opposite side. The lumbosacral notch should be inspected, and the lateral border of the sacrum should be followed inferiorly into the vicinity of the third sacral foramen. Traction fractures at the attachment of the sacrotuberous ligament are apparent more

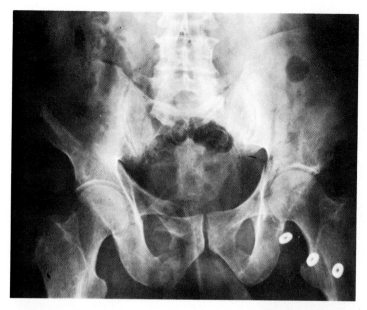

Fig. 13-70. Multiple severe fractures of the pelvis. This 48-year-old male pedestrian sustained multiple fractures of the pelvis including the bilateral superior and inferior pubic ramus fractures (constituting a straddle fracture). The fracture of the left ischium as well as the inner wall of the acetabulum constitutes a Walther's fracture. Additionally, the patient has a fracture through the body of the ilium from the greater sciatic notch to the iliac crest on the left side. The patient also has a vertical fracture of the left sacrum.

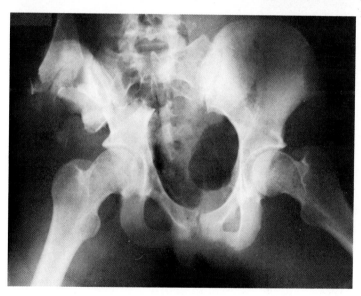

Fig. 13-71. This 19-year-old pedestrian sustained subluxation of the symphysis pubis and a dislocation of the right sacroiliac joint in conjunction with a massively comminuted fracture of the right ilium.

distally along the lateral border of the sacrum above the coccyx. Since the sacrum can be influenced therapeutically only through its ipsilateral pelvis attached to the fractured portion, the usual method for managing sacral fractures is to provide a sling to counterbalance the patient's weight with ipsilateral femoral traction. In undisplaced sacral fractures pelvic reduction is unnecessary. Patients are treated by exercise and physiotherapy.

Although the neurologic complications of pelvic and sacral fractures are dealt with more extensively in a later section of this chapter, it should be noted that sacral fractures with involvement of the first and second sacral nerve roots produce a syndrome characterized by sensory disturbances over the outer side of the foot, weakness of the hamstrings and gluteii, marked weakness of the calf, and diminution or loss of the ankle jerk. Neurologic recovery is slow, and permanent impairment of gait and limitation of activity may ensue.

With respect to the treatment of multiple pelvic fractures, each patient must be studied carefully and frequently by radiography to prevent, if possible, a permanent deformity and physical impair-

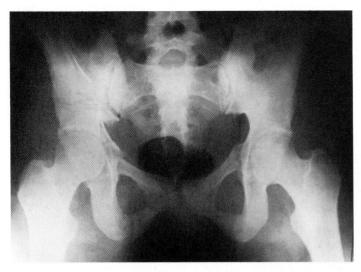

Fig. 13-72. This 33-year-old woman sustained right superior and inferior ramus fractures, a segmental fracture of the left superior ramus, a right acetabular fracture, a transverse fracture of the right ilium, and a subluxation of the right sacroiliac joint. The combination of the right ischial ramus and the inner wall of the acetabulum constitutes Walther's fracture.

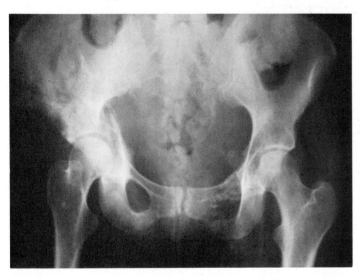

Fig. 13-73. Severe multiple fractures of the pelvis. This 41-year-old woman sustained a series of severe fractures of the pelvis including the left superior and inferior pubic rami, which were comminuted, the right ischial ramus in conjunction with the inner wall of the acetabulum, which constitutes a Walther's fracture, a transverse iliac fracture on the right side just above the acetabular roof, and a fracture of the right iliac wing (Duverney's fracture).

ment. The forces that caused the fractures should, as is generally the case, be counterpoised by therapeutic forces aligned in the opposite directions from the traumatic forces.

TREATMENT

The multitude of methods available for achieving reduction can be appreciated from the fact that Rankin[377] described in his series of 449 cases of pelvic fractures 13 different forms of treatment. Rest in bed with or without sandbags ranked first, and some form of pelvic sling or binder with some extension was second.

Cave[68] emphasized that severe contortions of pelvic contour should not be allowed to persist, especially in women of child-bearing age. He noted that in almost every severe pelvic disruption a large portion of the innominate bone is found to be intact, including a portion of the ilium as well as the superior portion of the acetabulum. "If this fragment is reduced to normal relationship with the sacrum, the other fragments of the hemipelvis both usually assume an acceptable position.[68] Cave felt that traction-suspension of the legs is the treatment of choice, because it does not upset the patient's precarious status and reduces discomfort but does not interfere in the treatment of any other injuries. Simultaneously, it benefits any displace-

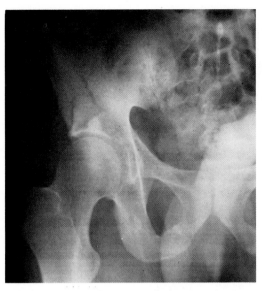

Fig. 13-74. This 22-year-old man sustained a virtually undisplaced fracture into his acetabular weight-bearing surface in an 18-foot fall. Weight bearing was discontinued for 12 weeks.

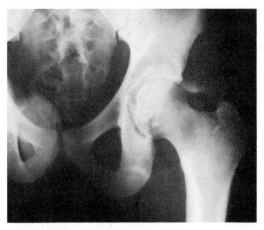

Fig. 13-75. Undisplaced fracture into the acetabulum. This unusual fracture into the left acetabulum involves the non-weight-bearing surface of the acetabular fossa. It is virtually undisplaced and is seen in association with a fracture of the junction of the body of the pubis and the inferior pubic ramus. The fracture was sustained in a fall in a sitting position. The patient's symptoms were treated and weight bearing was begun as soon as the patient felt comfortable.

ments. A pelvic sling assists in reducing or holding a widely opened pelvis, but patients often find the sling uncomfortable and complain of pressure over the trochanters. The sling should not be used when an injured pelvis has collapsed inward or when the femoral head has been driven into or through the acetabulum.

UNDISPLACED FRACTURES INTO THE ACETABULUM (TYPE IV FRACTURES)

While fractures of the acetabulum are in fact fractures of the pelvis, the symptoms and disability of these fractures are those of the hip joint itself and—with the exception of the undisplaced fractures of the acetabulum—are presented in Chapter 14. Since this chapter is limited to undisplaced fractures of the acetabulum (Figs. 13-74 to 13-76), I shall emphasize the necessity of avoiding displacement in a previously undisplaced acetabular fracture, not restoration of fragments.

CLASSIFICATION AND MECHANISM OF INJURY

In general, acetabular fractures are of three types: (1) the rim fracture, commonly called a "dashboard fracture"; (2) central fracture of the acetabulum;

and (3) the ischioacetabular fracture of Walther. While all of these acetabular fractures may be due to common etiologic forces, it should not be presumed that these forces come from only a single direction. This is a matter of some contention. Pearson and Hargadon[347] performed experiments in which a suspended weight was swung against the upper and outer aspect of a cadaver thigh. The momentum of the force was found to determine the extent of the fracture, and, as would be anticipated, the greater the momentum the more likely it was to produce a central dislocation of the femoral head. The pattern of the injuries sustained was fracture of the inferior pubic ramus and fracture of the superior pubic ramus at the point where the superior pubic ramus formed the anterior superior part of the roof and floor of the acetabulum. They concluded from their studies that it did not appear to matter whether the femur was abducted, adducted, or rotated medially or laterally when the fractures were produced.

Knight and Smith[236] stated that the popular concept of the mechanism of central acetabular fracture—the force of a severe blow to the trochanter transmitted up through the femoral neck so that the head of the femur is rammed into the acetabular wall, breaking the continuity of the arcuate line—while not wrong, was incomplete

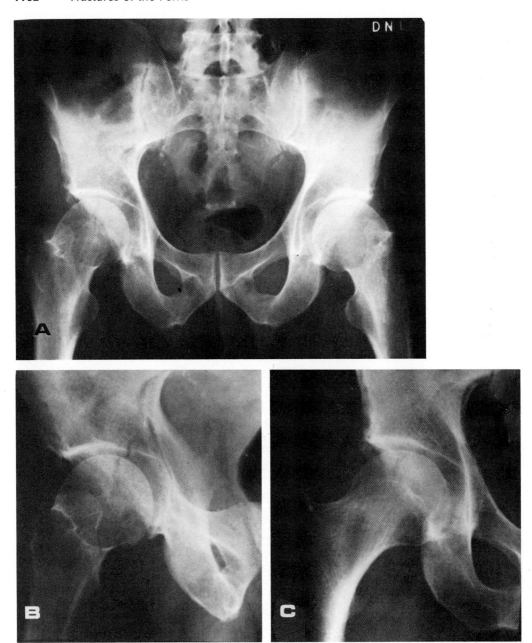

Fig. 13-76. Undisplaced fracture into the acetabulum. (*A*) Anteroposterior view of the pelvis of a 62-year-old man who fell. The presence of an os acetabuli in the same acetabulum (*right*) as an undisplaced fracture complicated the interpretation of this film. External rotation (*B*) and internal rotation (*C*) views of the pelvis and limb defined the existence of the fracture and the os acetabuli more precisely.

both in the anatomy of the fracture and the mechanism of injury. They stated that the classic acetabular fracture was seldom found and that the mechanism of injury, a blow on the trochanter, was probably now a rarity. While head-on impacts are more likely than side impacts in vehicular accidents, it does seem that pedestrians are more likely to suffer lateral forces than head-on forces. Nevertheless, Knight and Smith elucidated the concept that by gradually changing the attitude of the thigh with respect to the pelvis from flexion, adduction, and internal rotation to abduction, extension, and external rotation, the first injury resulting from the knees striking the instrument panel would be a posterior dislocation. The second would be a fracture of the posterior rim with posterior dislocation; the third, a fracture of the posterior rim and posterior vault; the fourth, a central fracture with a major fracture line vertical; the fifth, a central fracture with the major fracture line horizontal; and the sixth, anterior dislocation.

The pathogenetic mechanism described by Knight and Smith[236] also leads to a more detailed type of classification of acetabular fractures as described by Lowell,[263] which he indicates bears many similarities to that described earlier by Judet, Judet, and Letournel[216] in which the acetabulum is divided into anterior and posterior rami that join to form an arc, the apex of which is the acetabular dome. These authors classify their fractures into those involving the anterior or the posterior column, transverse fractures involving both columns, or varying combinations. Lowell[263] classifies fractures of the acetabulum into six categories: (1) linear or undisplaced fractures; (2) inner wall fractures, either with a normal head-dome relationship or with dislocation of the head; (3) posterior fractures and fracture-dislocations, either with a minor or a major single rim fracture, or comminuted with or without a major fragment; (4) fractures of the superior dome, either with or without the normal head-dome relationship; (5) bursting fractures, either with or without the normal head-dome relationship; and (6) anterior fractures, which are either stable or unstable.

RADIOGRAPHIC FINDINGS

Because detection of undisplaced acetabular fractures is difficult, x-ray views in different projections are usually needed to visualize the fracture lines, and the following projections may be obtained, depending on the needs of the particular patient:

1. Standard anteroposterior view.
2. Three fourths internal oblique view (see Fig. 13-12) to show the iliopubic column and the posterior lip of the acetabulum, and three fourths external oblique view (see Fig. 13-13) to show the posterior edge of the iliac bone and the anterior lip of the acetabulum (Fig. 13-77).
3. Thirty-degree lateral view with the thigh at 90° to the pelvis showing the relationship of the femoral head to the acetabulum.

4. Stereoscopic anteroposterior views. Oblique views may be difficult to obtain as they may cause the patient pain as he is turned on the injured side.[236] Also, Pearson and Hargadon warned that in approximately one third of the patients with a fracture of the pelvis after such an injury, the acetabular involvement was not immediately apparent radiographically, but it must be assumed to be present if the x-rays show fractures of the inferior and superior pubic rami. In their experience the fracture of the acetabulum became apparent in later x-rays, usually within 3 months of the injury. The presence of such a concealed fracture of the acetabular floor would, as they noted, appear to be of legal as well as clinical importance.
5. Few studies provide more information than anteroposterior or lateral-medial tomograms if sufficient time is given to visualizing in three-dimensional terms what is extractable from the information on these x-rays. Perhaps more helpful is the information that can be derived from CT scans in delineating the extent and configuration of fractures of the acetabulum. Not only can complex fractures be more readily understood with respect to their pathologic anatomy but otherwise occult fractures may be identified, as well as significant intra-articular loose bodies.[381,393,431]

METHODS OF TREATMENT

Elliott[127] has pointed out that even in acetabular fractures with undetectable displacement both the head of the femur and the acetabulum itself sustain damage. Damage to the femoral head "may have been sustained even though not manifest through damage to the blood vessels of the capsule and the femoral neck itself, particularly the posterior retinacular; through thrombosis of the intramedullary vessels in the head and the neck and intraosseous vessels of the haversian system; or perhaps through an intracellular molecular change from impact to the femoral head," as suggested by Stewart and Milford.[436] Both Elliott and Urist[127,483] pointed out that anatomical integrity of the acetabulum is the critical factor in the end result. While these authors and others[61,528] stressed that disruption of the acetabulum most certainly leads to degenerative changes, one must not assume the converse (i.e., that because x-rays show integrity of the acetabulum following an undisplaced fracture complicating sequelae such as osteonecrosis or osteoarthritis cannot develop). Pearson and Hargadon also stressed

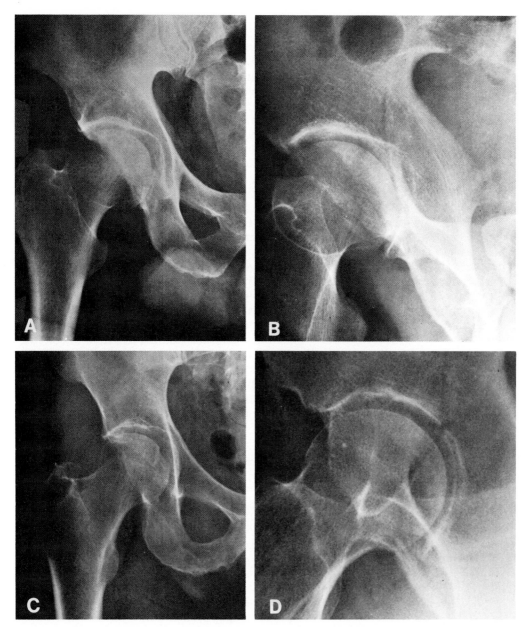

Fig. 13-77. (A) Standard anteroposterior view of a 49-year-old man who fell 5 days earlier sustaining a blow on the greater trochanter. While there is some soft tissue swelling along the inner wall of the iliopubic column, no fracture could be determined in the anteroposterior view. (B) A three fourths external oblique view brings an undisplaced fracture of the iliopubic column into view. (C) An anteroposterior view of a 58-year-old man who sustained a blow against his greater trochanter with a subsequent inability to bear weight. Routine anteroposterior views of the pelvis revealed soft tissue swelling along the inner wall of the iliopubic column and a suggestion of a fracture in the superior portion of the acetabulum. (D) A three fourths external oblique view clearly demonstrated the presence of the undisplaced fracture of the acetabulum.

that osteoarthritic changes might follow acetabular fractures, however mild, and while they admitted that in fractures without central dislocation this was not severe, "its appearance in any particular patient was unpredictable. With central dislocation, osteoarthritis is inevitable, and often severe enough to necessitate operation.[347] It is for this reason that patients with this injury should be treated with bed rest or traction, depending on the extent of the fracture lines and the potential for displacement.

Eichenholtz and Stark[124] analyzed fractures caused by minimum force applied to the greater trochanter with the hip in an abducted position that demonstrated little or no intrapelvic protrusion of the femoral head and no disruption of the lower pelvic cage. They found that such fractures could even be treated by simple bedrest supplemented by light traction for 1 or 2 weeks, if necessary, to relieve pain. They advocated active exercises but stated that weight bearing was contraindicated for a minimum of 4 months. Swimming pool- or Hubbard tank therapy was quite helpful in providing a reduced-gravity environment for active range of motion of the hip. Eichenholtz and Stark emphasized the importance of scrupulous avoidance of early weight bearing in all forms of treatment of fractures involving the inner acetabular wall.

Pearson and Hargadon, analyzing their 110 cases of pelvic fractures in Manchester, found that 80 involved the acetabulum. Twenty-three of them had occult fractures of the acetabulum that were recognized to have a fracture through the inferior pubic ramus and a fracture through the superior pubic ramus at its junction with the ilium. They stressed the necessity of realizing that involvement of the floor of the acetabulum is not usually apparent on the initial anteroposterior x-rays of this group and felt that it was not widely known that such fractures always involve the acetabulum. The remaining 57 patients had obvious involvement of the acetabulum, with 29 of them having had central displacement of the femoral head.

Fourteen of the 23 patients with occult fractures of the acetabulum were reviewed from 1 to 8 years after fracture. These patients had been treated with bed rest from 1 to 6 weeks and had gradually resumed full activity. Eight of the 14 patients had no symptoms; six of the 14 had no abnormal physical findings; and nine of the 14 had no x-ray evidence of arthritic changes. Even the remaining patients had, at most, only mild symptoms, mild limitation of hip motion, and only slight radiographic changes.

Rowe and Lowell,[400] studying 93 acetabular frac-

tures treated initially at the Massachusetts General Hospital, categorized 21 of them as having linear undisplaced fractures that usually (60%) had a single fracture line but sometimes (40%) showed multiple fracture lines. While the fracture line was usually demonstrated clearly on anteroposterior views of the pelvis, oblique views in some instances demonstrated the size and depth of the fracture line more satisfactorily. All of these patients were treated conservatively, and pain disappeared—usually by 3 to 6 weeks. Twenty percent of the patients were out of bed by the end of 1 week, and 90% were out of bed by the eighth week. Half of the patients used crutches for 8 weeks. In this series of undisplaced linear fractures, there is no instance of late traumatic arthritis or avascular necrosis of the femoral head. The clinical result was excellent in 19 and good in two. The anatomical result was excellent in 20 and good in one, demonstrating a very close correlation between clinical and anatomical results. Rowe and Lowell also noted that the length of time that the patient was maintained on no weight bearing and on partial or protected weight bearing may have some relation to the outcome in that the patients who remained in bed longer and did not give up their crutches too early seemed to have a higher incidence of excellent results.

Judet, Judet, and Letournel[216] treated undisplaced fractures of the acetabulum with complete bed rest and gentle passive range of motion exercises and massage for the first 45 days. (They too alerted readers to the possibility of secondary displacement of these fractures.) Crutch walking without weight bearing on the involved limb is allowed for the next 45 days, and then gradual weight bearing is permitted.

Four of eight patients with fractures of the acetabulum in Urist's[483] series had no displacement. Treatment consisted essentially of bed rest or traction for periods up to 8 weeks. No complications were recognized in these four patients, and in the three available to follow-up, the hip joints were rated as normal in one and slightly painful in the other two. These findings reinforce the concept that arthritic symptoms may occur in the absence of displacement of central fractures of the acetabulum and that care and caution must be exercised to avoid early weight bearing. The patient with the normal joint bore no weight for 6 months, while the other two patients available to follow-up were allowed to bear weight after 3 months. The management of traumatic arthritis of the hip after dislocation or acetabular fracture would be dictated largely by the usual considerations given to age, sex, occupation, and so forth—those factors considered in deciding which mode of treatment is warranted in relief of degenerative arthritis of the hip. As is true elsewhere, the use of mold arthroplasties[176] has given way to the use of total hip arthroplasties in these situations.[96]

AUTHOR'S PREFERRED METHOD OF TREATMENT

Elliott advised that treatment of central fractures of the acetabulum without displacement should be handled by the conventional method of combined longitudinal and lateral traction and indicated that a good result usually can be anticipated. I agree that these fractures need to be maintained without displacement, for the prognosis, overall, is much more pessimistic if displacement is allowed to occur following initial examination. For this reason, I believe the lower extremities should be placed in longitudinal traction with lateral traction on the hip accomplished with a sling or band around the thigh in well-muscled or fleshy people. In slender patients I prefer to apply the lateral traction by means of a heavy anteroposterior Steinmann pin through the greater trochanter, or by means of a screw hook or eye hook inserted into the trochanter.[61,231,255,496] Traction should be continued for 6 weeks, followed by no weight bearing for an additional 6 weeks.

WALTHER'S FRACTURE

Milch[301] referred to the ischioacetabular fracture as Walther's fracture (Figs. 13-78 and 13-79). The fracture line passes through the pubic ramus and terminates in the region of the sacroiliac joint. The entire medial wall of the acetabulum is displaced inward—without, however, any protrusion of the femoral head into the acetabulum. Healed, this fracture presents the appearance of a unilateral Otto pelvis. In 1891, Walther[490] produced an ischioacetabular fracture as a result of trying to reproduce central fractures of the acetabulum in cadavers. In the fracture that now bears his name, the ischium as a whole is pushed and tilted inward as a result of a fracture line that passes through the ischiopubic junction, the acetabular cavity, and the ischial spine. Milch noted that the fracture occurs more often than is suspected and has been erroneously included in statistical studies of central fractures of the acetabulum. Milch has also reviewed the literature and noted that Gioia[156] and Leinati[250] had previously recognized the characteristics of the

ischioacetabular fractures. Milch stated that treatment, even early, was difficult. Neither lateral skeletal traction nor a direct reduction through a retroperitoneal incision assured success. I prefer closed attempts and accept a less than perfect reduction rather than risk converting a closed fracture to an open, infected fracture.

COMPLICATIONS OF PELVIC FRACTURES

In the beginning of this chapter, it was noted that fractures of the pelvis are secondary only to those of the skull in terms of interest, mortality, and other complications.[87] Much of this material is detailed more specifically in Chapter 4, but it is essential to enumerate and touch briefly on some complications commonly seen with and specifically related to fractures of the pelvis.

LOSS OF REDUCTION

Loss of reduction is occasionally caused by overeagerness and overconfidence of both the patient and his physician. Within days after the injury, provided serious soft tissue and visceral problems are not persisting, the patient's attitude changes from that of a patient to that of a prisoner. He finds himself trussed up and confined to bed while he feels well in general. As the days go by, he becomes more and more agitated and eager to be out of traction, out of bed, and out of the hospital. If he is sufficiently abrasive, his physician begins to agree with him prematurely, and the patient is allowed freedom earlier than is wise. A loss of correction may ensue. In general, pelvic fractures will heal, but because of the extraordinary weight-bearing stresses and muscle tension crossing the fractures, sufficient time must be allowed for secure union to occur, so that earlier reduction is not lost. I advise patience, courage, and endurance for both the patient and the physician. Removal from traction or cast immobilization and graduated weight bearing is determined by callus formation seen on x-rays and by the patient's reaction to motion, the palpation of subcutaneous sites of earlier disruption, and, finally to weight bearing.[324]

SEPSIS

While a retroperitoneal abscess may develop in conjunction with a closed fracture of the pelvis, as reported by O'Keefe,[326] the problems of sepsis are much more commonly associated with open pelvic

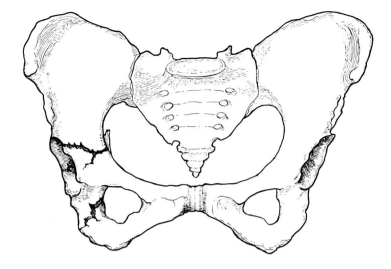

Fig. 13-78. Ischioacetabular fracture of Walther. This illustration shows the fracture passing through the ramus of the ischium terminating in the ilium. The inner wall of the acetabulum is displaced inward.

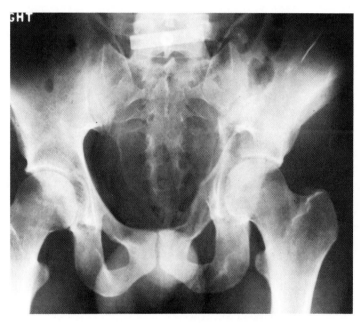

Fig. 13-79. Ischioacetabular fracture of Walther. This male pedestrian sustained a fracture of the left ischium and the inner wall of the acetabulum, extending into the region of the inferior left sacroiliac joint. Note the asymmetry in transverse diameter between the ascending ramus of the ischium on the left side as compared with the right side, indicating a rotation of the fragment on the fracture side.

fractures. In the former instance a retroperitoneal abscess began 25 days after injury and the definitive diagnosis was not made for an additional 56 days. In another patient signs of sepsis did not manifest themselves until 95 days after the trauma and the definitive diagnosis was not made for an additional 17 days. Both patients succumbed to the septic complications of their injuries. Cooke and his co-workers[91] remind us in their case report and review of the literature that septic arthritis of the hip may develop in the absence of osteomyelitis as a sequela of pelvic fracture in patients who also sustained rupture of the bladder or urethra. Six such patients

have been reported in the English literature. The likelihood of contamination of extravasated blood or urine by urologic procedures is overwhelming, and the physician must be alert to the possibility of early diagnosis of a hip infection in conjunction with a pelvic fracture. In addition, every attempt should be made to maintain sterility during catheterization and cystourethrography.

The lethality of open pelvic fractures is dramatically recorded in the works of Maull, Sachatello, and Ernst[288] and Rothenberger and associates.[399] Maull and his co-workers[287] reviewed 12 patients with deep perineal lacerations, of whom seven died. Early deaths were caused by uncontrolled hemorrhage, while late deaths were related to infection in the pelvis. It is their recommendation that a prompt, totally diverting colostomy with irrigation and disimpaction of the defunctionalized rectum be performed, as well as primary repair of urethral injuries. They also attempt to achieve pelvic stability whenever practical by reapproximation of the exposed, widely separated symphysis pubis by means of wire sutures; this is especially advantageous in repairing and protecting a torn urethra.

Rothenberger and his associates[398] reported a series of 604 patients with pelvic fractures of whom 22 (4%) had open fractures. Open pelvic fractures are ten times more likely to occur if the victim is a pedestrian or a motorcyclist. Virtually all patients with open pelvic fractures had sustained multiple injuries, and the mortality rate for an open pelvic fracture was 50%, in contrast to the 10.5% for closed pelvic fractures. Of even greater significance is the fact that the pelvic fracture was the primary cause of death in 73% of those dying with an open pelvic fracture and in only 30% of those dying with closed pelvic fracture. This higher mortality rate was due to increased infection and to increased massive hemorrhage as a result of an associated major vessel injury. Therapeutic goals in the management of patients with open pelvic fractures should be directed at restoration of blood volume, identification and repair of major vessel injuries, and diminution of diffuse retroperitoneal hemorrhage. They advocate that if drainage is necessary, it should be accomplished with a closed system; that an immediate diverting colostomy should be performed; and that antibiotics should be instituted promptly.

Perry[355] extended the same series an additional 2 years, studying overall a group of 738 patients with pelvic fracture. Of the 13 patients with open pelvic fracture who died, hemorrhage, sepsis, or acute renal failure was the primary cause of death in ten patients; hemorrhage was the secondary cause of death in one patient, and two other patients died of associated injuries.

Of considerable interest is the fact that if the mortality figures for the period 1977 to 1978 are found by subtracting the figures from the first article from those in the second article, there are reductions in the mortality rate for both patients with closed pelvic fractures, as well as those with open pelvic fractures, at least in the experience of the reporting physicians. During the years 1970 to 1976, 61 out of 582 patients with closed pelvic fracture died (10.5%); during the period 1970 to 1978, 73 out of 707 patients died (10.3%); and for the period 1977 to 1978, 12 out of 125 patients died (9.6%).

In the open pelvic fracture group the figures are even more dramatic, indicating that once the recognition of the lethal nature of the injury was recognized by the authors, they were much more effective in managing such patients. For example, during the period 1970 to 1976 the mortality rate was 50% (11 of 22 patients died). In the overall period from 1970 to 1978, the mortality rate was 42% (13 of 31 patients died). During the period 1977 to 1978 the mortality rate for open pelvic fractures was only 2 out of 9 (22%). Similar improvements in effective care of patients with open pelvic fractures should be sought by all physicians dealing with this dangerous injury (Table 13-1).

Raffa and Christensen[375] also performed an extensive study on 16 patients with open pelvic fractures. Four were victims of blunt trauma and arrived in the emergency room in hypovolemic shock. Of the 14 patients who were involved in pedestrian-vehicle or motorcycle accidents, there were eight deaths, a mortality rate of 57%. Overall, the mortality rate was 50%. These 16 patients had 81 nonfatal complications, and eight patients had an episode of systemic sepsis during their hospital course.

THROMBOPHLEBITIS

If the problems associated with hemorrhage are successfully combated, then within a few days' time attention must be directed to the prevention of

Table 13-1. Comparison of Mortality Rates for Patients with Open and Closed Fractures of the Pelvis During Different Periods

Years	Open Fracture (Mortality Rate)	Closed Fracture (Mortality Rate)
1970–76*	11/22 (50%)	61/582 (10.5%)
1977–78	2/9 (22%)	12/125 (9.6%)
1970–78†	13/31 (42%)	73/707 (10.3%)

* Rothenberger, D.; Velasco, R.; Strate, R.; Fisher, R. P.; and Perry, J. F., Jr.: Open Pelvic Fracture: A Lethal Injury. J. Trauma, 18:184–187, 1978.
† Perry, J. F.: Pelvic Open Fractures. Clin. Orthop., 151:41–45, 1980.

deep venous thrombosis following pelvic fractures. Although the morbidity and mortality lists of the large series of pelvic fractures rarely mention this diagnosis or pulmonary embolus,[121,324] I believe thrombophlebitis is a frequently unrecognized complication of pelvic fractures due to the combination of disrupted, traumatized vessels, long-term immobilization, and constricting external binders. For this reason I advise antiembolic stockings, the early introduction of active, and, if necessary, passive range of motion exercises of the lower extremities in conjunction with a regimen of anticoagulant therapy.[173] If, as in many cases of pelvic fracture, hemorrhage has been an acute problem, I would advise a delay of 7 to 10 days before initiating an anticoagulant program.

DELAYED UNION AND NONUNION

Delayed union is a term rarely heard in conjunction with pelvic fractures, presumably because of the inability to gather enough fractures that are sufficiently alike that a rigid norm for the chronology of the healing can be made. Likewise, nonunions of pelvic fractures are reported only sporadically,[191] and they seem to be usually of small concern over the long run. But Hundley in 1966[204] reported a series of 20 symptomatic nonunions that developed in a series of 141 pelvic fractures after a variety of treatment regimens, all of which included an "adequate" period of bedrest, and "adequate" reduction of fracture fragments. The nonunions occurred only in severely displaced fractures, and they were attributed to instability of reduction; symptoms were ascribed to movement at the fracture site. Eighteen of the 20 symptomatic nonunions were Malgaigne fractures. Half the nonunions were treated by grafting of the sacroiliac, lumbosacral, or pubic symphysis regions, combined (as necessary) with closed reduction and immobilization in a cast for an average of 3 months or until there was x-ray evidence of union. The ten patients so treated returned to their previous occupation, but the other ten did not.

Elton[128] reported on a fracture of the posterior inferior iliac spine associated with a fracture-dislocation of the pelvis that went on to nonunion. He believes it failed to unite because of its possible attachment to the piriformis, which would have caused traction with every step. Removal of the loose fragments from the greater sciatic notch and stripping of the scar tissue around these fragments led to immediate freedom from symptoms.

MALUNION

Fracture malunion affecting function is uncommon, unless a sacroiliac disruption is present. As Huckstep[434] has noted, little can be done in late cases to correct the already united and consolidated pelvic malunions. The hips, however, can be realigned, arthrodesed, or made mobile to compensate for pelvic obliquity and displacement. He feels that this is a much better method of dealing with severe deformities than trying to perform a massive reconstructive operation on the highly vascular pelvis itself, especially in the older child and adult. In women of child-bearing age alterations in the shape of the pelvic straits may require cesarean section. In mild degrees of displacement there is no indication for operative replacement.

POST-TRAUMATIC ARTHRITIS

Parasacral back pain is a common complication, usually associated with sacroiliac injuries in conjunction with sprains and opened-out pelves. Smith-Peterson and Rogers[444] stated that the diagnosis of sacroiliac joint arthritis depends on a careful history and examination and that x-rays may be corroborative. Knowledge of the etiology—traumatic or nontraumatic—is important, and whether the pain is local or radiating. Insofar as examination goes, the presence of a list and muscle spasm on inspection is important, as well as areas of tenderness determined by palpation, the patient's range of motion when standing, sitting, and lying, the straight leg raising test, compression of iliac crests, and passive lumbar flexion. On x-ray study these authors look for increased density along the margins of the joint, irregularity of the joint line, proliferative changes at the inferior margin of the joint, and malalignment of the symphysis pubis.

Using a posterior approach through the medial portion of the ilium below the posterior superior iliac spine and removing a major bone block, the authors obtained sacroiliac fusion in 21 of 23 cases. They examined microscopically the cartilage and bone removed at surgery and found post-traumatic erosion of the joint cartilage and replacement fibrosis, especially at the junction of the cartilage with the underlying bone but also in the medullary spaces. In some cases replacement fibrosis was so extensive that not a vestige of cartilage was found, and the joint surfaces consisted entirely of fibrous scar tissue. In some cases localized areas of hemorrhage with old blood pigment were seen within the region of fibrosis. The authors reported that

96% of the patients (25 of 26) returned to their previous occupation and that in 89% of the cases (23 of 26) there has been no pain since operation.

MISSILE WOUNDS OF THE PELVIS

Lucas[264] reported a series of 20 patients with missile wounds involving the bony pelvis. While most of the injuries were incurred in combat in the Vietnam war, civilian injuries were also encountered. In addition to bone damage and soft tissue damage inflicted by missiles travelling into or through the bony pelvis, hypovolemic shock and later sepsis are potentially lethal concomitants. The tissue damage sustained in a missile injury is due to the kinetic energy and the fact that tissue fragments are flung from the track of the missile at a velocity only slightly less than that of the missile itself, and such tissue fragments often act as secondary missiles. Simultaneously, cavitation about the missile tract, which is determined by the velocity of the missile, also disrupts tissue. Further destruction may be affected by the tumbling effects of irregular missiles. Lucas stressed that a missile wound of the pelvis is likely to cause injury to the gastrointestinal tract, genitourinary tract, and large vessels, and an exploratory laparotomy is mandatory in nearly all cases.

The type of fracture that a missile produces does not allow classification by any of the standard classification schemes for pelvic fractures, but Lucas was able to note that the most serious fracture, in terms of permanent disability, involved the acetabulum. Much less morbidity was seen with sacroiliac joint involvement. The most common type of fractures in the series were those of the iliac wings. Chronic sepsis occurred in 11 of the 20 patients, four with acetabular involvement, three with sacroiliac involvement, one with iliac wing involvement, and one with ischiopubic involvement. The bacterial flora was usually mixed and almost invariably included one or more gram-negative organisms. Only three of the 20 patients returned to full duty with the Navy or the Marine Corps. Four patients did return to limited duty. Lucas noted that early treatment includes vigorous resuscitative measures—massive blood replacement, supplementary fluids—and early operation including laparotomy and diversion of the fecal or urinary stream. Drainage of the deep pelvis was usually indicated and could be accomplished by coccygectomy.[519]

Intermediate therapy included secondary wound closure 7 to 10 days after injury, in addition to antibiotics, fluids, and other supportive measures. If wound conditions are not favorable for secondary closure, the wound management should continue on an open basis. Later, it may be necessary to perform debridements and the instillation of appropriate antibiotic solution through irrigation-outflow tubes. Intermediate therapy may also involve colostomy closure and reestablishment of the urinary stream. Late surgery may include further attempts at eradication of chronic sepsis, such as a sacrococcygeal excision, a hip fusion, or other procedures to restore function.

ASSOCIATED INJURIES

Concomitant soft tissue injuries and complications, such as visceral rupture and hemorrhagic shock, are common with pelvic fractures. When they are present they are more important than the pelvic skeletal injuries and are largely responsible for the mortalities associated with pelvic fractures (which range from 5% to 20% in the recent literature).[87,141,181,194,254,350] It is therefore essential to be aware of guidelines for their diagnosis and management. (Some of these traumatic problems have been discussed elsewhere in association with fractures in general, but with pelvic fractures there is sufficient need to emphasize some of the special characteristics of these combined injuries.)

The incidence of associated injuries directly attributable to pelvic fractures is quite variable but can run as high as 54%,[125] and the variation is explained by differences in the cause of the trauma. The higher percentages are attributed to crushing injuries seen in industrial accidents and pedestrian involvement in motor vehicle accidents as well as motorcycle rider injuries; the lower percentages are seen in conjunction with series made up largely of occupants of vehicles in motor vehicle accidents. In one series[317] of 703 patients with pelvic fractures, due in large part to mining accidents (41%), 63% of the patients had accompanying intrapelvic or extrapelvic injuries. The associated intra-abdominal injuries that occurred in 40 cases (5.7%) included 23 lacerations of the serosamesentery or peritoneum, 16 perforations or lacerations of the small or large intestine, seven ruptures of the diaphragm, and four injuries to large vessels.

The relation of associated injuries with the severity of the pelvic fracture is one that is naturally anticipated, and such expectation is borne out in practice. Chapman,[71] using the classification of Trunkey and colleagues,[478] showed a dramatic

Table 13-2. Relation of Type of Pelvic Fracture to Mortality and Morbidity

	Number	Mortality	Morbidity	Respiratory Distress Syndrome
Crush	23	5 (21.7%)	16 (69.5%)	8 (34.7%)
Unstable	61	7 (11.4%)	28 (45.9%)	13 (19.4%)
Stable	89	4 (4.5%)	27 (30.3%)	7 (7.8%)

(Chapman, M.: Management of Pelvic Fractures. West. J. Med., **120**:421–424, 1974)

Table 13-3. Relation of Blood Loss to Type of Pelvic Fracture

Type of Fracture	A Number of Patients	B Number of Patients Transfused	C Per Cent of Patients Transfused	D Total Number of Units Whole Blood	D/A Units of Whole Blood per Patient	D/B Units of Whole Blood per Transfused Patient
I	54	15	28	75	1.4	5.0
II	80	24	30	87	1.1	3.5
III	45	30	67	335	7.4	11.2
IV	17	4	24	16	0.9	4.0

Type I: Fractures without a break in the pelvic ring. These include fractures of the wing of the ilium, a single pubic or ischial ramus, fracture of the anterior superior iliac spine, the ischial tuberosity, sacrum, or coccyx.
Type II: Fractures with a single break in the pelvic ring. These include fractures of both rami of one side, separation of the pubic symphysis, or separation of the sacroiliac joint.
Type III: Fractures with a double break in the pelvic ring. Included here are double vertical fractures and severe multiple fractures.
Type IV: Fractures of the acetabulum.

(Hauser, C. W., and Perry, J. F., Jr.: Massive Hemorrhage from Pelvic Fractures. Minnesota Med., **49**:285–290, 1966.)

correlation between the severity of the fracture and mortality, morbidity, and respiratory distress syndrome (Table 13-2).

HEMORRHAGE

Pelvic fractures inevitably produce bleeding and hematoma formation; it is the source and size of the hematoma that is important. Depending on whether the patient is bleeding from marrow vessels or from torn pelvic and lumbar arteries and veins, the amount of blood in the extraperitoneal or retroperitoneal spaces is greater or less, and it is in the management of the bleeding that considerable discussion of alternative treatments results.

The incidence of significant hemorrhage has apparently increased in proportion to the doggedness of surgeons and, later, of pathologists in searching for sites of blood loss. One study[181] of 196 patients with fractures of the pelvis showed that 77 of the patients received, or should have received, transfusions. In 63 of these patients the blood loss was judged to be primarily from the pelvic fracture rather than from concurrent injuries. Nineteen of the 63 died, a mortality of 30%, and of 24 patients who received more than 5 units of blood, 13 died, a mortality of 54%. This contrasted with a mortality rate of only 8% among patients who did not require transfusion. Overall, approximately 40% of all pelvic fracture patients require a transfusion. This study showed also that fractures with a double break in the pelvic ring (type III injury) required transfusions 2½ times more often than types I, II, or IV injuries. Patients with type III injuries needed, on the average, 2½ times more blood than patients with type I, II, or IV fractures who received transfusions (Table 13-3).

Braunstein and co-workers,[43] after reviewing 200 consecutive cases of fatally injured pedestrians, were impressed that pelvic fractures were a cause of severe and often unrecognized retroperitoneal bleeding, and that, in the face of "more dramatic and more symptomatic injuries, the amount of concealed retroperitoneal hemorrhage may not be appreciated in assessing the need for vigorous supportive therapy." Post-traumatic anemia, direct visualization of retroperitoneal collections of blood at the time of laparotomy for concurrent intra-abdominal injuries, and postmortem examinations led to what had been overlooked episodes of pelvic fracture and hemorrhage. In autopsy studies of the 200 fatally injured pedestrians, 90 were found to have pelvic fractures. Of the 90, 69 had significant injuries in other body areas. But 21 had only important pelvic injuries in association with significant retroperitoneal bleeding, which either was the direct cause of death or contributed substantially to the fatal outcome. In another study[43] of 500 pedestrians struck by automobiles whose injuries were not fatal, only 20 (4%) had pelvic fractures—many fewer than the 90 out of 200 (45%) in the fatal pedestrian series—indicating that pelvic fractures occur more often with severe trauma or are more often a contributing factor to death.

Peltier[350] stated categorically that in his series of 186 patients hemorrhage was the most serious complication. Six of the 17 fatalities (35%) in his series were directly attributable to hemorrhage or shock. In Weil's[500] series, 13.7% died, and 17 of the 35 deaths were due to shock and hemorrhage.

Hauser and Perry,[181] in their series of 196 patients with pelvic fracture, found an overall mortality of 19.4% and a mortality of 7.7% due primarily to pelvic fracture. Of these 15 mortalities, nine were ascribed to hemorrhage alone. Three were type II, and six were type III, substantiating the logical hypothesis that the more severe the pelvic fracture, the greater the risk of hemorrhage and death from hemorrhage. Eight of the nine were pedestrians.

Conolly and Hedberg,[87] in their study of 200 pelvic fracture patients, determined that the major cause of death was hemorrhagic shock or renal failure secondary to shock producing 21 of the 28 fatalities (75%).

DIAGNOSIS

The diagnosis of significant hemorrhage from pelvic fractures is frequently delayed or overlooked, and the signs and symptoms are often confusing.[42] It may be that either the signs are minimal or they are ascribed to concomitant injuries that turn the surgeon's eye away from the undramatic closed fracture of the pelvis. In other instances there is little doubt about the diagnosis due to the absence of concomitant injuries and the presence of unmistakable signs of traumatic shock due to hemorrhagic hypovolemia. The patient is in pain and is developing rigidity of the abdomen. He is pale, sweaty, and restless and his extremities are cool. He has a thready, rapid pulse, hypotension, and a diminished urinary output due to serious blood volume deficit. A pulse over 100 per minute suggests a 20% blood volume deficit; a systolic pressure of less than 100 mm. Hg suggests a 30% blood volume deficit.[77,166,525] On physical examination bruises may be seen with expanding ecchymoses extending over the anterior abdominal wall. There may be boggy fullness in the flank regions, as well as the gluteal regions and the proximal thighs. The hematoma may become superficial above the inguinal ligament or in the scrotum (Milch called this Destot's sign[300]).

Plain x-ray studies define the extent of the fractures and reveal the blunting of the psoas margins. Cystourethrograms and excretory urograms for characterization of possible genitourinary tract injuries may also, in fact—through displacement of ureters, bladder, and urethra—signal the presence of significant retroperitoneal hemorrhage.

Continued monitoring of the central venous pressure in conjunction with arterial pressure and urinary output provide the best survey of peripheral perfusion, especially if trends in these determinations can be followed.

While hemoglobin and hematocrit determinations are used to follow blood losses and replacement, they are of little benefit in measuring the acute changes that occur in the severely injured patient with hemorrhage from pelvic fractures.

In practice I have gained little clinical benefit from the use of blood volume estimators, for measurement of either plasma volume or red cell mass. This approach is limited by the technical inaccuracies of the method when volumes are changing rapidly from continued hemorrhage or blood replacement and when shock states have altered the usual vascular capacities. Additionally, repetition of this type of study is limited by practical as well as methodologic handicaps, so that isolated readings, if obtained, are of limited value.

The retroperitoneal hematoma is responsible for other complications aside from shock. Intrapelvic bleeding envelops the bladder and rectum, tracks up the paraspinal gutters, moves into the renal regions, the subhepatic area, and the posterior portion of the diaphragm, and spreads into the leaves of the mesentery of the intestine. This leads to signs that simulate intraperitoneal visceral injury—abdominal muscle spasm, guarding, rigidity, tenderness, and hypoactive bowel sounds and the distention of ileus.

Intra-abdominal injuries are reported in 8.2% to 19% of pelvic fracture patients,[254] and most of these injuries are hepatic and splenic lacerations.[254,262,350,478,511] It is important to realize that retroperitoneal hematomas can rupture into the peritoneal cavity, so this possibility should not be dismissed.[20] Frequent clinical examination of the abdomen as well as review of the patient's overall status are essential, and often the question can be answered only by a diagnostic peritoneal tap, with or without the use of sterile lavage, or by a laparotomy. Peritoneal lavage, suggested by Root and coworkers in 1965,[395] is the natural evolution of Salomon's[408] idea in 1906 of peritoneal puncture for diagnostic purposes. Diagnostic peritoneal lavage (DPL) is performed by the introduction of a peritoneal dialysis tube into the abdominal midline under local anesthesia. Gumbert and colleagues[170] advised a lower abdominal site, but Hawkins and colleagues[182] noted that an extraperitoneal hematoma can lift the peritoneal floor to the umbilicus and suggested an upper abdominal site. If gross blood is not aspirated, 1000 ml of Ringer's lactate solution is injected (in adults). The infusion bottle is placed lower than the abdomen to create a siphon. The test is considered positive when a salmon-pink fluid is obtained. Gumbert and coworkers recorded a 97% accuracy, with only one false-positive, out of 53 patients studied. Since 31 of their 53 patients had associated head or chest injuries, which complicate the diagnosis of intraperitoneal injury, they considered peritoneal lavage lifesaving, especially in the unconscious patient in whom general anesthesia and a laparotomy could be critical. One prospective study of 315 patients with blunt abdominal trauma showed that in conscious patients with obvious physical findings who were operated on without diagnostic peritoneal lavage (DPL), a diagnostic accuracy of 96% was achieved. In patients with altered states of consciousness, DPL was performed for equivocal physical findings, and an overall accuracy of 97% was achieved with a concomitant 50% reduction in the rate of normal findings at laparotomy.

The advantages of open paracentesis lavage for the diagnosis of abdominal trauma over the percutaneous method has been studied in a randomized prospective fashion by Pachter and Hofstetter,[336] who divided 210 consecutive patients into two groups of 105 each. They reported no false-negative diagnoses in either group. Their accuracy rate for the open method was 98.1% and 91.4% for the percutaneous method. In addition, there were six major complications with the percutaneous method, whereas there were no major complications with the open method. They concluded that the open method is superior to the percutaneous method.

Some have advocated laparoscopy in the diagnosis and management of intra-abdominal trauma[142]

but others[453] believe that peritoneal lavage is superior in that it allows continuous monitoring of the patient's intraperitoneal status. Those advocating the use of emergency laparoscopy believe that its advantages are that it can be quickly performed and rapidly gives detailed information concerning the location and type of injury, as well as the amount of intra-abdominal bleeding.

Klaue,[235] in his review of 71 patients with blunt abdominal trauma and pelvic fracture, found peritoneal lavage positive in 28 patients in whom laparotomy was performed; a ruptured retroperitoneal hematoma not requiring surgery was the final diagnosis in eight patients, whereas 16 patients had significant intra-abdominal lesions, most commonly splenic rupture. Two patients were known to have had false-positive results because of the direct puncture of a large retroperitoneal hematoma. Out of 12 patients with a weakly positive lavage, only one case with a ruptured diaphragm needed operation. In 31 patients with negative lavage there was also one false-negative result because of a diaphragmatic rupture in conjunction with a torn spleen which had herniated into the left thorax. Klaue concluded that any patient with a pelvic fracture suspected of having intra-abdominal injury should have a diagnostic tap and lavage, and that to avoid the puncture of a large retroperitoneal hematoma leading to false-positive results the tap should be performed in the upper abdomen. In addition, any patient with a pelvic fracture and a positive tap should be explored since intra-abdominal lesions requiring surgery will be found in more than 50% of cases. Weak positive or negative results can be considered reliable, justifying further conservative treatment with close observation for the next 24 hours.

Other authors[112] have found evidence for false-positive peritoneal lavage due to retroperitoneal hematoma. Similar diagnostic errors with peritoneal lavage in patients with pelvic fractures were reported by Hubbard and his co-workers,[197] who found that 61 of 222 patients with pelvic fractures underwent diagnostic peritoneal lavage as a part of their initial evaluation. Twenty-six of the 61 had negative lavage results; it was later determined that there were no false-negative results in this group. Of the 35 patients with a positive lavage result, ten (29%) were found to have false-positive lavage results with no intraperitoneal source of the bleeding. It was their opinion that four of the eight deaths in the group were due to uncontrollable bleeding that resulted from exploration of the retroperitoneal hematoma. These data suggest that a negative lavage result is highly reliable but that positive lavage results should be interpreted with caution.

In summary, the likelihood of a false-positive DPL depends on the amount of retroperitoneal bleeding and on the length of time between the injury and the diagnostic peritoneal lavage; this is due to the fact that red blood cells can enter the peritoneal cavity by diapedesis. False positives can be further reduced by going into the abdomen in the supraumbilical region, thereby avoiding the extraperitoneal hematoma seen with the pelvic fracture. An ambiguously positive DPL might be followed by an open paracentesis lavage, or by laparoscopy, in an effort to avoid what might otherwise be an unnecessary laparotomy.

Additional information can be obtained by performance of emergency abdominal CT scans, which has been recognized as a highly sensitive and specific imaging method for a wide variety of intraperitoneal and retroperitoneal traumatic lesions. In the study of Federle and co-workers[133] of more than 200 cases of acute blunt abdominal trauma, there were no false-positive or false-negative CT interpretations except for a single case in which residual peritoneal lavage fluid was mistaken for intraperitoneal blood. The authors believe that CT scans have major advantages over other radiologic techniques, including angiography, and may obviate peritoneal lavage and exploratory laparotomy in some instances.[133]

INDICATIONS FOR LAPAROTOMY

Laparotomy should not be denied to a patient with multiple injuries who shows obvious signs of intraperitoneal visceral rupture, but on the other hand, it should not be undertaken lightly. Laparotomy increases the possibility of ventilatory insufficiency through diaphragmatic splinting and disturbance of the ventilation of basal pulmonary segments.[184] There are, however, good indications for laparotomy, including clear-cut evidence of intraperitoneal bleeding or visceral perforation obtained by means of radiography, urography, angiography, or paracentesis. Less widely accepted findings that indicate laparotomy include the presence of an expanding, palpable suprapubic hematoma, x-ray evidence of bone fragments driven into the pelvis, and continuing blood loss that cannot be ascribed to associated injuries. If the suspected intraperitoneal bleeding or perforation is found, it can be managed in the standard fashion via hemostasis, splenectomy, colostomy, hepatic suture, or bladder repair. It is when only extraperitoneal bleeding is found that no satisfactory answer exists.

Hawkins and associates[182] emphasized that the surgeon is faced, basically, with two questions: (1) whether to do a laparotomy and (2) how to control pelvic bleeding if it is found at operation. They stressed that these two questions are essentially unrelated in that apprehension over controlling pelvic bleeding should not affect the decision to perform laparotomy after pelvic fracture. Virtually all surgeons concede that the small nonenlarging retroperitoneal hematoma should not be disturbed, lest the mechanical tamponade effect be destroyed and bacterial contamination be introduced. The recommendation of Ravitch,[380] that surgery for the direct control of pelvic bleeding "should not be considered unless the patient shows signs of continuing severe hemorrhage after administration of more than 20 pints of blood," represents an opinion popular among trauma surgeons, but it is not universally accepted. Quinby,[372] recognizing the importance of speedy action, advised that if a full blood volume replacement given in the first hour after arrival at the hospital does not produce sustained circulatory response, a major arterial injury requiring prompt direct attention must be considered. He also recommended major vein repair over ligature, which can cause shunting of the lower extremity venous return into an uncontrollable swamp of injured pelvic venous plexuses.

In dealing with the situation in which uncontrolled massive arterial hemorrhage is suspected and in which continued blood transfusions are no longer sustaining the patient, Miller advocated surgical exploration and direct control of the source of bleeding. Also stressing the time factor in the preoperative decision-making period, he emphasized the need for awareness of the possibility of massive arterial hemorrhage in the pelvis, frequent blood pressure determinations with charting in relation to fluid therapy, as well as reduction of unnecessary sources of induced hypotension, such as movement of the patient and extensive x-ray examinations. On the basis of the anatomy of the hypogastric (internal iliac) artery's major branches and their position in relation to the bony pelvis, as well as on the basis of actual case experiences, Miller suggested that ligation is a reasonable and effective maneuver in massive hemorrhage. This procedure has been used safely and effectively by gynecologists for uncontrollable bleeding of the female genital tract without evidence of ischemic necrosis.[30,382] While others[136,180,194,418] have subsequently reported on its effectiveness in stemming massive arterial bleeding in pelvic fractures, hypogastric artery ligation has not gained wide acceptance[313,341] because the rich collateral blood flow of the hypogastric arteries prevents ischemic necrosis, and so makes it a safe procedure, but can also render it futile. In addition, experimental work has shown that ligation of the internal iliac artery and its branches has no effect on internal iliac venous pressure.[150]

Riska and associates,[391] in dealing with 42 patients who had an average of 39 units of blood transfused, came to the conclusion that operative control of the hemorrhage was warranted and found the midline approach most useful, although other surgical incisions were sometimes used singly or in combination. Although aware of arteriography, they believed it was seldom indicated because "of its limited value in the detection of bleeding arteries, and because the examination took too much time." In their series only three of the 12 deaths could be attributed to pelvic bleeding, although it is not stated whether the surgery contributed to two deaths from later sepsis.

The unusual maneuver of dividing the pubic symphysis has been reported to enable surgeons to expose, identify, and ligate arterial bleeders in the retropubic area without unfortunate sequelae.[451]

ANGIOGRAPHY

Athanasoulis and his co-workers[12] and Margolies and colleagues[285] introduced the use of emergency pelvic angiography to assess vascular damage and to localize hemorrhage. Although it is generally accepted that the major source of bleeding is venous, venography has not enjoyed the same measure of success in demonstrating the site of hemorrhage as arteriography.[526] In their series of bilateral femoral venograms in 25 patients, Reynolds and colleagues[385] could demonstrate only one venous bleeding point and concluded that identification of bleeding from the venous plexus or lesser veins is not feasible by transfemoral venography. On the other hand, transfemoral aortography, followed by selective localized angiography, can demonstrate sites of active bleeding. After the identification of such bleeding points, hemorrhage can be controlled by selective arterial catheterization for subsequent infusion either of vasopressors, autologous clotted blood, gelatin foam sponge, detachable silicone balloons or a number of other foreign materials of varying composition.[13,513] Occlusion of the torn vessel may also be accomplished by means of inflated intra-arterial balloon catheters, which may be used temporarily, pending stabilization of the patient's condition and use of permanent occlusion devices.[12,282,339,428] While I advised in the first edition of this textbook that this regimen does require

a degree of multi-specialty expertise and cooperation that is not available in every hospital, during the ensuing years that expertise has become more and more widely available, to the point where virtually every major trauma center may be expected to have such facilities.

Arteriographic evaluation is ordinarily performed through the femoral artery opposite the side most seriously traumatized. In pelvic fracture patients it is advised that a midstream aortogram with "a catheter tip above the aortic bifurcation" is advisable in order to demonstrate bilateral bleeding sites in the pelvis that would not be demonstrated if a more distal position were chosen.[13,460] Since most bleeding in pelvic trauma has been demonstrated to be within the branches of the hypogastric arteries, selective hypogastric arteriograms are also performed. As bleeding sites are identified, the catheter is moved as closely as possible to the point of extravasation. Following injection of the contrast fluid, repeat films are required over the next 20 seconds to demonstrate accumulation of the extravasated dye. Control of the hemorrhage is obtained by embolization of one of the occlusive materials as previously indicated. Arteriography is repeated after the embolization to verify the effectiveness of the occlusion.

In a series of 324 patients with pelvic fractures admitted over a 5-year period, the Massachusetts General Hospital team evaluated 30 patients by means of angiography for massive bleeding.[283,460] Two patients were eliminated because of inadequate follow-up, and in 20 of the remaining 28 there was at least one arterial bleeding site noted. Embolization of the bleeding vessels was performed in 18 patients. Of the two patients who did not undergo embolization, one required surgical intervention for other injuries and the other had a tight proximal stenosis of the bleeding vessel precluding embolization. In eight patients no bleeding site was demonstrated; these patients eventually stabilized hemodynamically. Subsequent to arterial embolization, there was a dramatic decrease in blood requirements, although mortality remained high due to associated injuries. One complication was the distal embolization of a pledget of surgical gelatin foam into the femoral artery, requiring surgical embolectomy. Most authors reporting on the use of transcatheter arterial embolization hesitate to make a definite statement about when the procedure should be performed, but because of its low risk they suggest prompt examination of patients in whom the pelvic injury predisposes to massive bleeding.

If after arterial embolization has been performed

and no further arterial bleeding source is identified, and there is still continuing blood loss in the patient, consideration should be given to performing a venous examination. Venous disruptions cannot be managed through the angiographic catheter in the same manner as arterial bleeding since the flow of blood is directed from the site of injury towards the heart. A balloon catheter, however, may be inflated intravascularly as a potential means of locally tamponading an iliac venous laceration, but in general a surgical repair is necessary.[339,389]

Arteriography has several advantages in the management of patients with pelvic fractures. First, accurate definition of the site of arterial bleeding can usually be ascertained. If injury to a major trunk is identified, early exploration should ensue. More commonly, the bleeding site is identified in a distal branch of the hypogastric system, and the arterial hemorrhage may be controlled effectively by embolization techniques, thereby avoiding operation. Advocates of angiography note that embolization via the transcatheter method specifically localizes its effect to the bleeding vessels, so that the tamponade of the retroperitoneum is not violated, and it is reported that "hemostasis is more effective because the emboli are discharged peripherally where there is less chance of collateral flow supplying the bleeding site."[460]

However, the arteriographic approach to the primary management of the pelvic fracture also has some pitfalls. Extra motion is required to move the patient from the stretcher to the x-ray table, and this can cause renewed bleeding and progression of shock. More important, placing the bleeding, critically injured trauma victim in the x-ray suite, where a less than ideal resuscitation capability usually exists, is risky. It is essential that the angiography suite should be equipped not only with the appropriate radiographic equipment but also with monitoring and life-support facilities to allow for the continuing intensive care of the patient during the performance of the study. One must weigh these risks against the possible therapeutic benefits of embolization. Most pelvic fractures are accompanied by predominantly venous bleeding, and experimental evidence shows that control of hypogastric arterial inflow will not slow the associated venous hemorrhage. It must also be borne in mind that *this regimen does require a degree of multi-specialty expertise and cooperation that is not available in every hospital.* Quinby[371,372] was skeptical that a local infusion of vasopressors can control large vessel hemorrhage.

Most other clinicians have also abandoned va-sopressors for pelvic trauma hemorrhage. Quinby cautioned, too, that angiography deserves a trial if the patient's condition is stable enough for him to go through the necessary manipulation. Quinby's scheme is reminiscent of *"Catch-22"*: the patient can have angiography only if his condition is "stable," but if his condition is "stable" he doesn't need angiography, and so angiography is not done. If the patient is "unstable" he cannot tolerate angiography, even though he needs it, and so angiography is not done. In either instance, angiography is not done. The frustration of attending to a patient who is exsanguinating internally, with the likely sequelae of shock, renal failure, or respiratory distress with hypoxia, led in one instance to the induction of controlled hypotension using a ganglionic blocking agent, trimethaphan camphor sulfonate (Arfonad), after bilateral internal iliac artery ligation had failed to alter a clinical picture of shock.[193] This was an extraordinary example of the possible alternatives that exist in the extreme situation. Other approaches, including the use of external compression, are under study and appear promising.

THE G-SUIT

Gardner and Storer[146] accidentally discovered the capacity of the antigravity or G-suit to control intra-abdominal bleeding (using the principle of circumferential pneumatic compression first described by Crile in 1903)[98] when a postpartum patient, after receiving 55 units of blood, was placed in a G-suit to maintain blood pressure. Paradoxically, bleeding stopped. After it was later used for postoperative bleeding in aneurysmectomies and in a case of uncontrollable rectal bleeding complicated by portal hypertension, the method was subjected to laboratory investigation. It was concluded that circumferential pneumatic compression applied to the body below the diaphragm causes compression of the vascular bed and redistribution of blood to the structures above the level of compression. In addition to increasing blood volume to the vital structures, the G-suit raises blood pressure and diminishes bleeding by means of the circumferential compression, or loop stress, which it applies to the vascular tree. This force overcomes the tangential tension in the vessel wall, which is largely responsible for the bleeding. According to Gardner and Storer, the law of LaPlace* would indicate that this

---

* Tension in a vessel wall (dynes/cm) equals the excess pressure inside the vessel over that outside (dynes/cm²) times the radius (in cm) of the vessel.

mechanism is more effective if the bleeding is from either smaller arteries or veins.

Wangensteen and his co-workers,[491,492,493] in laboratory investigations, found that the transmural pressure was identical when hemorrhage ceased in both test and control dogs and that local counterpressure raised the final blood pressure by an amount equal to the counterpressure exerted. In both intact and hemorrhaged animals they found that the use of external counterpressure caused an increase in arterial blood pressure, cardiac output, stroke volume, and peripheral vascular resistance, but arterial pH and blood gas value patterns developed that were representative of a severe metabolic acidosis. This derangement, while benefited by mechanical ventilation, was believed to have diminished the survival time of the test animals as compared to animals that were subjected to hemorrhagic shock without the subsequent use of the modified G-suit.

Despite the seemingly inconclusive evidence as to the effectiveness of the G-suit in the experimental situation, there have been some promising preliminary clinical studies that suggest that the salvage rate in those catastrophic hemorrhages from pelvic fractures can be improved. Kaplan[222] has used the redistribution-of-blood-volume aspect of the technique to counteract the pooling of venous blood in shock and to create "an emergency autotransfusion" by means of pneumatic trousers, which also have been used by rescue squads at accident scenes.

Batalden and co-workers[23] have demonstrated the usefulness of the G-suit and reported on their experience with ten patients with severe pelvic trauma. A G-suit is available in their trauma unit and is used for each patient with recognized intraabdominal or intrapelvic trauma from the time such a diagnosis is made until the laparotomy is begun or until bleeding ceases. In addition to providing an autotransfusion of 1000 ml of autologous blood within 1 to 2 minutes of application, blood loss is diminished, and subsequent transfusions are fewer. The device is also used in patients with no evidence of intraperitoneal bleeding or visceral disruption whose pelvic fractures and continued shock indicate intrapelvic extraperitoneal bleeding. At present, G-suits are available that have three separate chambers (torso and the lower limbs) that can be individually pressurized and depressurized to allow evaluation, treatment, and gradual discontinuation of the external counterpressure. The suit is applied at a pressure of 20 to 25 mm Hg and periodically (at least every 6 hours) the suit is deflated, the skin

is inspected, and the clinical evidence for or against recurrence of the hemorrhage is reviewed. While suspicious abdomens may require much more frequent observations in the early postadmission hours, the use of the G-suit helps to immobilize the pelvic fractures themselves and does not seriously complicate lower extremity fracture care.

Flint and colleagues[137] use a pressure of 40 mm Hg in the abdominal compartment and 50 mm Hg in the extremity compartments. Because the G-suit compromises diaphragmatic excursion, mechanical respiratory assistance using endotracheal intubation is advised when the suit is to be used for extended periods. This precaution is not necessary if the G-suit is used for the rapid transport of a trauma victim to a nearby hospital. Kaplan and co-workers[222] advise, however, that its application may result in an undesirable sensation of difficulty in breathing, as well as triggering urination, defecation, or emesis. They also state that the device is contraindicated in cases of pulmonary edema or congestive heart failure. Pelligra and Sandberg,[348] in their review of the development and experiences of many with the G-suit, state that the presence of renal disease and cerebral edema are also probable contraindications to its use.

MAJOR ARTERIAL INJURY

The rarity of gangrene of the lower extremity as a complication of a pelvic fracture may be assessed from the fact that Mock and Tannehill,[304] in a review of the literature covering 65 years and 3108 cases, found only 13 cases in which injuries to the external iliac or femoral vessels were described. Ferguson and colleagues[134] confirmed the rarity of this finding. Lawson and Wainwright[247] believed, though, that the closed variety of arterial trauma with intimal tears and arterial thrombosis have been more common in their experience than the lacerated arterial injury in pelvic fractures. Limb ischemia and hypotension were the typical presenting features of these cases. Two of their 38 patients with pelvic fracture had this complication. In a report of lower limb ischemia complicating a fracture of the pelvis Wilson[517] noted that the occluded femoral artery was in immediate relation to a fragment of the superior pubic ramus, which impinged against the artery and which was more obvious on moving the pelvis. Moore[307] found 13 vascular injuries in 1307 cases, an incidence of 1%. In addition to transection and intimal tears, other forms of arterial injury include contusion with subsequent thrombosis, laceration, arteriovenous fistula and false aneurysm.

As described earlier, the internal iliac or hypogastric artery is much more vulnerable than the external iliac or the femoral, which has a more direct course across the pelvis and a better muscular buffer between itself and the bony pelvis.[467] Smith and co-workers,[442] however, stress that the superior gluteal artery is also at significant risk in pelvic fractures. Nonetheless, the gravity of the consequences impels a brief outline of the diagnosis and treatment of these vascular injuries.

The frequent examination and notation of findings of both lower extremities for color, pulsations, temperature—and, where possible, for sensory and motor function—is a first-order requirement. Commonly, hypovolemic shock will cause modifications in these physical findings, but if they persist, then one of two unpleasant conclusions must be drawn: either the leg is not being perfused or the patient is not being perfused. Neither bodes well. If, after shock has been successfully offset, there are still signs of diminished flow to one leg or the other, the next step is to avoid ascribing the hypoperfusion to "vascular spasm," an error that has often delayed the proper recognition and treatment of major vascular injuries. Specifically motivated to reduce the delay in the treatment of patients with major vascular injuries related to pelvic fractures, Rothenberger and colleagues[397] attempted to define more clearly the clinical features of such patients and reviewed their experience with 604 pelvic fracture patients. Only eight patients (1.3%) had major vascular injuries, but if the group was more rigidly defined as "pedestrians in shock at admission," of the 25, seven (28%) had a vascular injury; of 13 "pedestrians with open pelvic fractures," six (46.2%) had a vascular injury; and of eight "pedestrians in shock at admission and with open pelvic fractures," five (62.5%) had a major vascular injury. In consequence of this last finding, it is advised that "prompt operative exploration of all pedestrians admitted in hemorrhagic shock with open pelvic fractures characterized by a double break in the pelvic ring, should reduce the 83% mortality currently associated with this combination of injuries."

ANGIOGRAPHY

Whether the vessel is completely transected, leading usually to occlusion of the lumen by constriction and retraction, or partially severed, leading to recurrent bleeding and the later complications of a false aneurysm or an arteriovenous fistula,[63] or is subjected to an intimal tear with occlusion of the lumen by thrombosis, the best next step is angiography. Saletta and Freeark[407] advised arteriography whenever (1) pulses distal to the fracture site diminish or disappear following reduction of the fracture, (2) a bruit is auscultated, (3) extremely large or pulsating hematomas are noted, or (4) there is severe or recurrent hemorrhage through an open wound. Angiography is extremely useful in localizing the site of injury, and later in assessing the results of the repair as well as the patency of the distal arterial tree. Sensitivity to the iodide in the dye is the single serious contraindication to this study. An arterial injury can be diagnosed on free extravasation or extravasation into a false aneurysm, premature venous filling indicating an arteriovenous fistula, irregularity of the lumen contour, or complete block of the contrast column.

OPERATIVE TREATMENT

While the presence of pelvic fracture and possibly other injuries may complicate the surgical repair, the operative treatment of a vascular injury follows standard precepts, including the prepping of a sufficiently large area of the patient to give access to the vessels proximal to the injury and access to a vein graft if necessary, and to obtain proximal and distal control of the injured vessel. The decision to resect and reanastomose or to graft depends on the local circumstances of the injury. Extraction of a clot by a Fogarty catheter and irrigation of the distal arterial tree with heparinized saline (5000 u/ 50 ml saline) are performed before anastomosis.

The need for early reduction and immobilization of pelvic fractures as an important factor in the successful management of intrapelvic hemorrhage has been stressed by Orr,[334] Peltier,[350] and others. Reapproximating fracture surfaces exerts a pressure on marrow vessels, and limiting unnecessary motion facilitates the benefits of a tamponade effect. To reduce the number of moves to which the trauma patient is subjected during his transportation from the accident scene to the formulation of a definitive plan of therapy, Root and VanTyn[396] have devised a safe, effective, comfortable, light, radiolucent, durable, economical litter, which can be adapted to the use of simple traction devices (Fig. 13-80).

Management plans for the control of retroperitoneal hemorrhage from pelvic fractures have been suggested by a number of authors.[137,267,287,523,526] There has been considerable variation in their approaches to this problem. One author[524] stated, "Retroperitoneal hematomas should be routinely

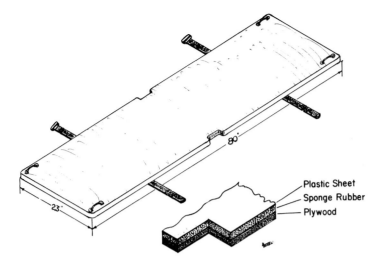

Plastic Sheet
Sponge Rubber
Plywood

Fig. 13-80. This litter, devised by Root and VanTyn, is safe, effective, comfortable, light, radiolucent, and durable. (Root, H. D., and VanTyn, R. A.: A Device and Method for the Atraumatic Transportation of the Injured Patient. Surgery, **58**:32, 1965.)

explored; intraperitoneal pelvic hematomas should *not*, except if there is uncontrollable blood loss."

This opinion is so out of step with most surgical thinking that a follow-up conversation with the author corroborated my impression that it was an unintended transposition of the words "retroperitoneal" and "intraperitoneal" during the publishing process.* Another author[287] writes, "Intraoperative hemostasis probably has little to offer over tamponade by the intact retroperitoneum."

McAvoy and Cook[267] pose three questions that summarize the problems presented by a pelvic fracture patient: "(1) Does the patient have associated intra-abdominal visceral injuries that necessitate prompt exploratory laparotomy? (2) Does the patient have bleeding from the region of the fractures as his sole cause of shock? (3) If hypovolemia is due to retroperitoneal extravasation alone, when should transfusional therapy be abandoned for an attempt at direct control?" To answer the first question they advocate a diagnostic peritoneal lavage, urethrogram, cystogram, and intravenous pyelogram. If these studies reveal a surgically repairable lesion, then a laparotomy is performed; if not, then angiography is used to ascertain the bleeding point or visceral injury. Transcatheter embolization with absorbable gelatin sponge rather than autologous clot is the treatment of choice; if unsuccessful, open retroperitoneal control of hemorrhage may be considered.

Flint and colleagues[137] recognized that postmortem studies of patients with fatal pelvic fractures showed multiple lacerations of small- and medium-sized arteries and veins more commonly than single vessel injuries, and understanding that occlusion of a single inflow-trunk would have little effect on the richly collateralized circulation of the pelvis, depended on the external counterpressure suit to immobilize the fracture and control retroperitoneal hemorrhage. For high-risk pelvic fracture patients (those with unstable type III or multiple crushing fractures) resuscitation is begun in the operating room, where a urethrogram and cystogram are performed, as well as a diagnostic peritoneal lavage. Once the pelvic fracture has been identified as the primary source of hemorrhage and other injuries have been appropriately treated, the patient is transferred to the intensive care unit.

If bleeding continues at a rate that would require transfusion of more than 2000 ml of blood in an 8-hour period after initial resuscitation, the G-suit is used. Arterial pressure, central venous pressure, arterial gas tensions, urine output, and transfusion requirements are monitored closely. If no blood is required after 8 hours the suit is deflated but left in place; if no blood is required in the ensuing 12 hours, the suit is removed. If hemorrhage control is not achieved within 2 hours after application of the G-suit, pelvic angiography is performed and embolization attempted. In the patient group treated by this protocol, only two of 22 patients were subjected to hypogastric artery ligation, and this was because of external bleeding from an open pelvic fracture; otherwise, the authors deemed this procedure "rarely successful," and attempts to open retroperitoneal hematomas were unsuccessful due to "torrential hemorrhage." This program led to statistically significant reductions in overall mortality and in shock-related deaths (Table 13-4) among two groups of patients treated at the same institution, one before the use of the G-suit and

* Wotkyns, R. S.: Personal communication.

Table 13-4. Pelvic Fracture—Mortality

Group	Number of Patients	Deaths	Patients Admitted in Shock	Death from Hemorrhage
I	18	12 (67%)	14	9
II	22	6 (27%)*	17	2†

Group I: Before use of G-suit and treatment algorithm.
Group II: After use of G-suit and treatment algorithm.

* p < 0.05.
† p < 0.01.
(Flint, L.M.; Brown, A.; Richardson, J.D.; and Polk, H. C.: Definitive Control of Bleeding from Severe Pelvic Fractures. Ann. Surg., **189**:709–716, 1979.)

the other after its introduction and the formulation of the treatment algorithm.

Maull[526] and Sachatello[287] and McMurtry and colleagues[277] created treatment algorithms that are very similar to that of Yap.[526] I have modified those algorithms according to my evaluation of appropriate management protocols (Fig. 13-81). After initial assessment and resuscitation, a urethrogram and cystogram are performed; if positive, appropriate treatment (*vide infra*) is instituted. A DPL is performed; if positive, laparotomy is performed. If the DPL is negative and the patient is still unstable according to Flint's[137] criteria (*vide supra*) then a G-suit is applied. If the patient still does not achieve hemodynamic stability, an arteriogram is performed followed by arterial embolization, balloon occlusion, or, in the last instance, by direct surgical repair or ligation. If at laparotomy a stable retroperitoneal hematoma is found, and the patient is unstable the G-suit is used, but if the patient is stable, then expectant, supportive care is provided. If a rapidly expanding hematoma is found retroperitoneally, an operative arteriogram is performed and, if positive, the same three therapeutic modalities are considered.

In summary, the problem of hemorrhage associated with pelvic fractures is one that demands: (1) awareness of its potential, especially when other injuries may be expected to distract the surgeon, (2) persistence in managing hemorrhage with generous amounts of whole blood, and (3) in the face of continuing failure in the unusual situation, courage to use innovative therapy as a means of saving life.

INJURIES OF THE LOWER URINARY TRACT

It is anticipated that in most situations the orthopaedic or trauma surgeon will be able to enlist the aid of a urologist in the managment of these injuries. However, in some instances such consultation may not be available, and the orthopaedist or traumatologist may be forced to independently manage at least the early stages of some of these injuries. For this reason the sections on treatment concern themselves with the acute management of urinary tract injuries in greater detail than ordinarily would be necessary.

Pelvic fractures are attended by an extravasation of hemorrhage and a regional accumulation of extracellular fluid. In fractures of the anterior pubis the bladder is lifted cephalad and displaced away from the side of the injury, and the ensuing inflammatory response may produce spasm of the bladder sphincter. This combination of bladder displacement, urethral stretch, and sphincter spasm more often than not produces temporary acute urinary retention. Hematuria is another common finding associated with pelvic fractures, but, as will be seen, little or no pathognomonic significance can be attached to its presence or absence. This is so despite the fact that it has been stated that if, in the presence of minor pelvic fractures, clear urine is voided spontaneously, it can be concluded that the lower urinary tract is intact.[275]

Hematuria secondary to pelvic trauma, whether blunt or penetrating, requires immediate radiologic investigation. Three x-ray studies will, in general, visualize the entire urinary tract: (1) retrograde urethrogram, (2) cystogram, and (3) intravenous pyelogram.[25] The timing and selection of a particular study is determined by previously obtained information regarding the patient. If a urethral injury is suspected in men on the basis of blood at the urethral meatus, evidence of trauma to the penis and scrotum from a "straddle" injury, a "high-riding" prostate on rectal examination, a wide diastasis of the symphysis or a type III fracture etc., then a urethrogram should be performed before urethral catheterization. Some[25] advocate a

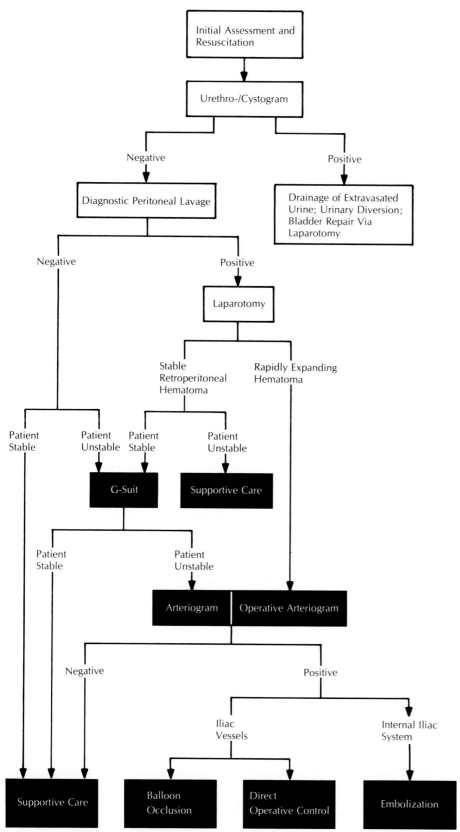

Fig. 13-81. Outline of early management of intraperitoneal and retroperitoneal soft tissue injuries associated with pelvic fractures.

urethrogram for any pelvic fracture in men, while others[241] advise that "conventional radiographic studies such as intravenous urogram and, especially, a retrograde cystogram must be done in all patients with pelvic fractures, even in the absence of urinary symptomatology and pertinent laboratory findings." I would not embark on such a diagnostic work-up solely on the basis that a pelvic fracture is present as it is almost unheard of to have a lower urinary tract injury, for example, as the result of a type I pelvic fracture. For all type III fractures and for type II fractures with hematuria, the admonition should be heeded, however. If the urethrogram is normal, a urethral catheterization is performed, followed by a cystogram and post-evacuation washout film. If the cystogram is normal or if the urethrogram or cystogram is abnormal, an intravenous pyelogram should be performed to rule out the presence of upper genitourinary tract injury before treatment of the urethral or bladder injury. Colapinto[82] especially advocates a dynamic retrograde urethrogram, which involves exposure of the films as the contrast medium is being injected, and categorizes urethral injuries as to whether the urethra is stretched (type I), torn above the urogenital diaphragm (type II), or torn below the diaphragm (type III).

A Suggested Routine for Evaluation of Urologic Trauma in Association with Pelvic Fracture*

1. Transfer of patient to a proper stretcher
2. Rapid history, including previous urologic status
3. Thorough physical examination, including rectal and vaginal examinations and a possible diagnostic peritoneal lavage
4. Initial x-ray examination of the pelvis
5. Urethral catheterization or urethrogram (see text for priority)
6. Cystogram and postevacuation film of bladder when indicated
7. Intravenous excretory urography when indicated
8. Cystoscopy and retrograde pyelography when indicated

---

* After Orkin,[330] Scott,[416] Cass and Ireland,[64] and Benson and Brewer[25]

INCIDENCE OF GENITOURINARY INJURIES

The major lower urinary tract injuries associated with pelvic fractures are rupture of the urethra and rupture of the urinary bladder. A combination of these two injuries may also be seen. The incidence of these urinary tract injuries in association with pelvic fractures is reported, variously, from less than 1% to over 21%. In an analysis of approximately 4750 cases of pelvic fracture from the literature, I compute that the average rate of major lower urinary tract complication is 13%. Urethral injuries tend to occur twice as commonly as bladder injuries, although this varies considerably from series to series. Older series, made up of mining accidents and industrial trauma, usually give evidence of higher percentages of major urinary tract injuries than the more modern series, in which the injuries are largely the result of vehicular trauma. Trafford[474] determined in a study of 28,000 emergency surgical admissions that 412 patients were admitted with pelvic fracture, and 19 had an associated posturethral rupture (an incidence of about 5%).

Levine and Crampton[254] analyzed the records of 425 patients with fractures of the pelvic girdle seen in a 10-year span at a suburban hospital near a number of busy parkways and highways. They found an overall incidence of 3.5% for major trauma to the lower portion of the urinary tract. While this is considerably less than in earlier reported series, the urinary tract was the most frequent site of associated major injuries, and of the 15 patients who sustained major associated urinary tract injuries, four died, a mortality of 26%.

While past attempts to correlate the type of pelvic fracture with the type of urinary trauma and to use this information predictably have not been generally successful, it has been noted that patients with symphyseal separations and fractures of the pubic rami have a higher incidence of urinary tract involvement than do those without pubic ramus involvement. Patients with fractures of both pubic rami have an even higher urinary tract injury rate than those with single ramus fractures.[135,474] However, this correlation is quite rough, and the first film of a patient with a fractured pelvis should not lead to an unfounded surmise as to whether or not the patient has also sustained vesical or urethral damage.

At the outset, all pelvic fracture patients must be assumed to have urinary tract injuries until proved otherwise. As further information is obtained regarding the type of trauma sustained, the classification of the pelvic fracture from the initial x-ray examination, and the findings of the physical examination, the physician can assign an appropriate priority rating to the urologic work-up. It must be stressed at the outset of a discussion on urinary tract injuries in association with pelvic trauma that little or no significance can be ascribed to any single symptom or physical sign, with, perhaps, the exception of a rectal examination that reveals upward and posterior displacement of the prostate. The presence or absence of bleeding from the urethra or of slight or marked hematuria cannot be used as dependable signs of the status of the injury. Hematuria is most commonly seen as a result of contusion of the urethral or vesical bladder mucosa, but such statistical probability does not provide diagnostic reliability. Similarly, while the inability to void may signify rupture of either the posterior urethra or the bladder, it may also be present in a patient with no injuries of the lower urinary tract who voided just prior to the accident or in whom the pain of the pelvic fracture has caused a loss of ability to micturate voluntarily. Blood at the tip of the urethra is frequently reported as diagnostic of lower urinary tract rupture, but it may, in fact, be associated with contusion of the kidneys without associated lower tract damage. Also, the presence or relative absence of pain in conjunction with pelvic fractures is not a useful guide to the presence of other associated injuries in the pelvic region, nor should the passage of a catheter into the bladder and the drainage of urine guarantee that the bladder is intact, since such catheters have drained urine occasionally directly from the peritoneal space. A sense of complacency should not be tolerated, even if the patient has voided grossly clear urine voluntarily. In the presence of either gross or microscopic hematuria (10 red blood cells per high-power field), a cystogram, and in the male, a urethrogram, should always be performed to rule out more definitely the possibility of urinary tract injuries.

RUPTURES OF THE ANTERIOR URETHRA

Ruptures of the anterior urethra in association with pelvic fractures are uncommon, although they may be seen in the so-called straddle injuries in which the victim is struck in the perineal region, pinching the anterior urethra in two under the arch of the pubis while sustaining simultaneous injury to the pelvic skeleton.

DIAGNOSIS

The diagnosis is facilitated by a history of the mechanism of injury, which should immediately arouse the suspicion of such an injury to the urethra, as well as by a physical examination, which frequently reveals hematoma or ecchymosis of the perineal region and genitalia. The skin of the perineum may not be broken, and gross blood may be present at the urethral meatus. The patient

should be encouraged not to void until the diagnosis is established, for additional urinary extravasation only complicates therapy. The urethrogram, in my opinion, should be done before the cystogram, if there is strong evidence on physical examination of urethral injury, rather than performing the cystogram first, as is usually done. This will inform the physician whether passage of a catheter into the bladder is likely to be successful before attempts to do so are initiated.

In addition, the passage of a catheter may turn an incomplete urethral tear into a complete one. It would be preferable to delay the catheterization until the urethrogram has been performed, but in many instances the trauma patient is catheterized immediately on entering the emergency room; in such a situation when the patient is already catheterized and urethral injury is suspected, a peri-catheter urethrogram can be performed to evaluate the presence of an injury (see Fig. 13-66B).[274]

Conclusive diagnostic evidence can be obtained only on a urethrogram taken as the dye (20 ml Renografin—30%) is injected into the urethra with a syringe and a Brodny clamp.[65] Penetration of Buck's fascia permits extravasation behind Scarpa's fascia in the abdominal wall into the scrotum and into the perineum, where it is limited by Colles' fascia. Since Scarpa's fascia is attached to the fascia lata of the thigh at Poupart's ligament, there is usually no extravasation into the thighs (Figs. 13-82 and 13-83).

TREATMENT

The extravasation of dye through an anterior urethral rupture is diagnostic and allows for early treatment. If the urethrogram reveals an incomplete tear and if Buck's fascia has not been ruptured, urine extravasation will be limited to the penis. The possibility of passing a catheter then exists, and it should be attempted gently. The first attempt should be with a 5-ml Foley catheter, No. 16 to 22 French, depending on meatal size, but of as large a caliber as possible. If it is passed successfully it should not be removed, as the next attempt may not be so productive. If unsuccessful, the second should be with a soft rubber, Coudé-tipped straight catheter or a filiform. There should be no third attempt. If it does not pass or if the rupture is complete, then no other trials of catheterization are advisable until definitive surgical repair is under way. If catheterization is successful and the urethral rupture is incomplete, an indwelling urethral catheter should be left in place for several days. This,

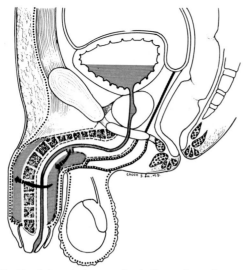

Fig. 13-82. Partial anterior urethral disruption allows extravasation of urine into the penis. The extravasation is limited by Buck's fascia, which is intact.

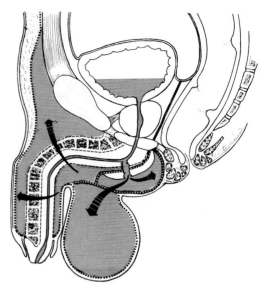

Fig. 13-83. Total disruption of the anterior urethra with penetration of Buck's fascia permits extravasation behind Scarpa's fascia in the abdominal wall and into the scrotum and the perineum, where it is limited by Colles' fascia, which is an extension of Scarpa's fascia. Since Scarpa's fascia is attached to the fascia lata of the thigh at Poupart's ligament, there is usually no extravasation of urine into the thighs.

plus the early application of cold compresses and the institution of antibiotic therapy usually suffices for urethral contusions or incomplete ruptures without widespread extravasation. When catheterization cannot be performed or if there is extensive extravasation of urine, it is obviously a much more significant injury and requires operative management.

The principles underlying the treatment of extensive anterior urethral injuries are (1) drainage of extravasated urine and blood, (2) urinary diversion, and (3) restoration of the continuity of the injured urethra. In occasional instances a soft urethral catheter can pass the complete rupture, but it should not be considered as the sole method of achieving these three goals, since its very presence tends to increase the likelihood of infection developing in the extravasated urine and hematoma, leading to abscess formation, necrosis of the urethral segment, and the eventual development of either urethral strictures or a urethral fistula. Accordingly, cystostomy should be done in virtually all instances when urinary extravasation is present. It is also advisable to perform immediate suture of the severed urethral ends via a perineal approach, to employ a small inlying urethral splinting catheter, and to maintain cystostomy drainage for at least 2 weeks. The perineum and all extravasated areas should be drained "high, wide, and unhandsome[411] with rubber drains if there has been urine extravasation.

If the patient's general status or local factors preclude primary anterior urethral repair, a suprapubic cystotomy is performed, the extravasated fluids are drained, and a secondary reconstructive operation is planned.

RUPTURE OF THE POSTERIOR URETHRA

Rupture of the urethra at or above the urogenital diaphragm is the most common major injury of the lower urinary tract seen in association with pelvic fractures; conversely, pelvic fractures are the most common reason for a posterior urethral rupture.[172] The incidence of a urethral disruption among patients with a fractured pelvis varies from 25% in Vermooten's report[486] to 5% by Holdsworth.[188] Wilkinson[516] reports an incidence of 11% in 1400 cases and Mitchell[303] reports a rate of 4.7%. The membranous urethra is ruptured more often than the prostatic portion, and this is understandable in view of the fact that basically the walls of the prostatic urethra are the substance of the prostate itself. In children the incidence of proximal posterior urethral damage appears to be higher, and the higher incidence may be related to the immaturity of the prostate. Membranous urethral ruptures are classified by Colapinto and Mac-Cullum[83] as type I injuries in which the prostate or urogenital diaphragm is dislocated but the membranous urethra is merely stretched and not severed; in type II injuries the membranous urethra is ruptured above the urogenital diaphragm at the apex of the prostate; and in type III injuries the membranous urethra is ruptured above and below the urogenital diaphragm. The authors advocate the use of dynamic retrograde urethrography in patients with a suspected posterior urethral rupture.

Trafford,[474] in his series of 37 posterior urethral ruptures, found that each was in conjunction with a pelvic fracture and that in general these ruptures are associated with severe fractures, especially those with major separation or displacement of the symphysis pubis and fractures of the pubic rami.

Anatomically, the membranous urethra is fixed by virtue of its attachment to the urogenital diaphragm. The urogenital diaphragm, as described previously, is anchored anteriorly to the pubis and posteriorly to the ischial ramus and tuberosity and to the lower edge of the sacrotuberous ligament. As the membranous urethra passes through the urogenital diaphragm, it is bound firmly to it and has little mobility. On the other hand, the apex of the prostate is not bound as rigidly to the urogenital diaphragm, triangular ligament, or by any strong fibrous structure.

It should be noted that the rupture of the urethra associated with fracture of the pelvis is virtually limited to the male. The shortness and relative mobility of the female urethra, and the absence of structures and attachments like those that render the male urethra immobile make this difference quite understandable. A major urinary tract injury in a female with a fractured pelvis is almost of necessity a bladder rupture.

Because a transverse crushing injury of the pelvis is the commonest cause of rupture of the posterior urethra, it is postulated that the transverse diameter of the pelvis is shortened and the anteroposterior diameter is lengthened, causing a sudden and severe stretching of the soft parts in the sagittal plane.[481] The membranous urethra is stretched and drawn out, and it ruptures at the most vulnerable, weakest point—the apex of the prostate. The puboprostatic ligaments are also ruptured by the same action. The loss of the puboprostatic ligaments and the pressure of the extravasated blood and urine in the space of Retzius cause the neck of the bladder, together with the prostate, to be pushed upward and backward, causing the posterior dislocation of

the prostate, which can be palpated on rectal examination. The proximal and distal segments of the torn urethra are, as a rule, displaced laterally in proportion to the amount of bone displacement.

On rare occasions bony spicules may penetrate the urethra or bladder, and there is a theoretical possibility that a urethral rupture may occur without any associated fractures, as when the momentum of the person with a full bladder is suddenly arrested and the momentum of that full bladder tears the apex of the prostate from the triangular ligament. Violent movement of the triangular ligament in any direction causes snapping off or shearing of the urethra at the prostatomembranous region.

The dangers related to these complications are twofold. First, the extravasation of the urine may result in very severe infection or necrosis, and second, urethral injuries may result in strictures, fistulae, urinary incontinence, or impotence.

The major factor leading to severe and difficult urethral strictures is reported to be the uncorrected displacement of the pelvic bones,[157] so that reduction of pelvic disruptions may be required for urinary tract repairs.

Urinary extravasation from the posterior urethra is intrapelvic and may be either prevesical or perivesical with extension into the paraspinal gutters. Neglected extravasation is frequently followed by virulent, spreading cellulitis with widespread abscess formation and necrosis of the urethra and surrounding tissues. Manifestations of toxemia follow, as well as the possibility of gas-forming bacteria. It is for this reason that prompt effective diagnosis and treatment are necessary.

DIAGNOSIS

The possibility of a urethral injury must be borne in mind with any patient with fractures of the pelvis, especially if the pubic rami are involved. Pain in the lower part of the abdomen is an inconstant finding, and it must be remembered that the pain associated with a fractured pelvis masks any other pain due to the severed urethra. Inability to micturate combined with a desire to do so is a common complaint. With partial rupture, micturition is often normal, but the urine is usually blood-stained. Patients in whom urethral damage is suspected must be warned not to attempt to urinate, lest unnecessary extravasation is caused. Blood at the external meatus is a useful sign of possible urethral injury, but it is not pathognomonic.

Physical signs of extravasation behind the urogenital diaphragm occur late and cannot be relied on as significant assists in the diagnosis of this injury. A distended bladder that is palpable or percussible implies that the bladder is intact and if lower urinary tract trauma has occurred, it is at the prostatomembranous urethra. Usually, however, because of pain and spasm, it is difficult to palpate the lower portion of the abdomen. Consequent to such a rupture, blood from the periprostatic veins and urine from the bladder escape into the perivesical tissues and retropubic space and form a large extravasation. This extravasation is usually held in the pelvis above the urogenital diaphragm but in severe comminution of the pelvis, the soft tissues may also be torn, so that the perineum and scrotum are bruised and swollen.

Diagnosis of a complete rupture of the posterior urethra is facilitated if the patient is unable to urinate, if the bleeding is observed from the external urethral meatus, if the physician cannot pass a catheter, and—most reliably—if rectal examination, reveals the prostate to be retracted upward and backward out of its normal position and a boggy, fluctuant mass is palpable in its place (Fig. 13-84). If such a finding is made on rectal examination, most urologists deplore even gentle attempts at the passage of a catheter and suggest that if a doubt exists, direct urethrography by the injection of 20 ml of dilute, water-soluble pyelographic medium such as Endographin, Renografin, Urographin, or Hypaque should be performed. In the male, the nozzle of an Asepto syringe is inserted into the urethral meatus with the syringe held so as to prevent the contrast material from leaking out of the urethra, or a Brodny clamp can be used.[65] During the injection, an anteroposterior x-ray is taken. Then, after positioning the patient in the oblique position, the urethra is again injected, and an oblique x-ray is obtained of the urethra and bladder. This technique demonstrates any break in the continuity of the anterior, membranous, or prostatic urethra. The extravasated contrast agent may be indistinguishable from that caused by extraperitoneal rupture of the bladder. If no break in the continuity of the anterior urethra or posterior urethra is seen, the bladder can then be filled by further injection through a urethral catheter, after which anteroposterior and oblique films of the bladder are obtained. This should be performed in all patients who have evidence of microscopic or gross hematuria following pelvic trauma. Others maintain that a urethrocystogram should be performed on all patients with a disrupting pelvic fracture, regardless of what the clinical findings

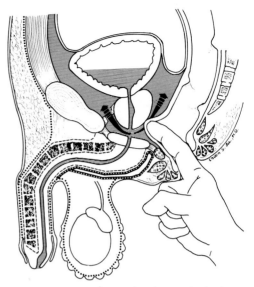

Fig. 13-84. Rectal examination reveals the prostate to be retracted upward and backward out of its normal position. This is pathognomonic of posterior disruption of the urethra. The mobility of the prostate is due to the fact that the puboprostatic ligaments have been disrupted. Extravasation of urine occurs into the extraperitoneal perivesical space.

have been or what the urinalysis shows. I would agree with that dictum for type III fractures.

Because the female urethra is short, mobile, and free of rigid attachments, it is rarely injured in association with pelvic fractures. Seven incomplete tears in females were reported by Simpson-Smith in his series of 381 traumatic urethral ruptures,[436] and one complete rupture has been recorded by Casselman and Schillinger.[66]

TREATMENT

As with anterior urethral ruptures,[403] establishment of adequate urinary diversion by the use of a suprapubic cystostomy, reestablishment of normal alignment and contour of the injured urethra by the use of a urethral splint, and drainage of extravasated urine and blood from the perivesical space are the chief measures in the management of ruptures of the prostatomembranous urethra. Rutherford's article of 1904[403] was the classic. A quarter century later a number of authors[17,29,527] advised reconstitution of urethral continuity by the direct repair of the divided urethra via a perineal approach, and in 1934, Ormond and Cathran[332] introduced the idea of traction on a urethral catheter to assist in achieving urethral continuity. The use of delayed urethroplasty after initial management is advocated by others.[29,303,309] Initial management consists of avoiding urethral catheterization and performing a retrograde urethrogram. A cystogram is done if no urethral injury is detected and then an excretory urogram (IVP) is obtained. If posterior urethral injury is suspected by extravasation on retrograde urethrography, simple cystostomy is advocated as the only immediate surgical therapy.

Late genitourinary tract complications can be expected frequently. They are independent of the mode of therapy initially used, and these complications appear to be most directly related to the severity of the initial injury. It bears repeating that the three commonest late genitourinary tract complications seen in association with pelvic fractures include urethral strictures, urinary incontinence, and impotency.[116]

With the advent and widespread use of antibiotics, there has been a tendency to disregard the principle of urinary diversion, but there can be little justification for such a policy, in view of the considerable hazard and difficulty if there is no adequate and efficient safety valve for the evacuation of urine from the lower tract.

The management of the patient with a torn prostatomembranous urethra is best achieved by bringing the resuscitated patient to the operating theater, placing him supine in moderate Trendelenburg position, and making a low midline abdominal incision. This approach gives direct access to the peritoneal cavity, which should be opened and explored through a small incision to exclude intraperitoneal injuries and to inspect the back of the bladder. After the peritoneal incision has been closed without drains, the retropubic space is dissected, the blood clot and urine are cleared out, and a cystostomy is then performed allowing for further inspection of the inner wall of the bladder.

One surgical method for the reestablishment of urethral alignment is the two-catheter technique described by Reynolds[386] involving the retrograde passage of one catheter through the distal urethra and the downward passage of a second catheter from the bladder into the prostatic portion of the urethra. The tip of each catheter is grasped and brought up out of the prevesical space, and the catheter tips are then sutured together. The distal catheter should be a No. 18 to 22 Foley catheter with a 30-ml bag.

A second method of obtaining urethral continuity is to use metal bougies, which can be put into contact using the metallic sound as they touch for assistance. The deep portion of the penile bougie is led blindly into the bladder, where it is a simple matter to attach one end of a straight catheter over the tip of the bougie, to withdraw the bougie, and then to secure the end of the straight catheter via suture to the bladder end of a Foley balloon catheter, which can then be drawn into the bladder and inflated. The majority of authors do not attempt direct suture of the urethra at the urethrovesical junction, because it is impractical, time-consuming, and extremely difficult.

By 1 pound of traction on the Foley catheter the urethra is realigned, and undue elongation of the posterior urethra and separation of the severed urethral ends are minimized. In addition, several anchoring stitches should be taken in the prostatic capsule using heavy silk, and they should be led via long, straight needles through the perineum, where the suture ends can be tied over buttons. If too much traction is applied on just the Foley catheter, there is a risk of causing ischemic necrosis to the external sphincter of the bladder, which may subsequently lead to incontinence. It should also be recalled that traction on the penile catheter should be directed at an angle of 45° to horizontal, in order to avoid necrosis of the urethral mucosa opposite the suspensory ligament of the penis. Traction can be applied either through an overhead frame with pulleys and weights, or by attaching the Foley catheter to a rubber band that is in turn taped to the distal thigh. The rubber band serves to minimize tension created by abduction and adduction of the hip. The 1 pound traction may be discontinued at the end of 1 week.

A heavy silk suture through the vesical end of the splinting catheter is led out through the cystostomy wound to the abdominal wall, or the splinting catheter may be sutured to the vesical end of the cystostomy catheter. In either fashion, this acts as insurance against the unplanned loss of the splinting Foley catheter, which without the retention suture would require a second operation for reinstallation. It is also advisable to drain the space of Retzius for 48 hours with a rubber drain.

It should not be felt, however, that the traction catheter method detailed above is not without its disadvantages. Weems[499] has noted with justification that it entails a considerable amount of surgery for a traumatized patient and that anatomic orientation is quite difficult due to frequently uncontrollable bleeding. As has already been stated, operation to manage bleeding in pelvic fractures is frequently a discouraging undertaking, and, of necessity, a suprapubic cystostomy enters the extraperitoneal space, which in turn causes a loss of the tamponade effect that is relied on for spontaneous cessation of hemorrhage. Because of a recent contention that a significant number of these posterior urethral injuries are actually incomplete at the time of the initial examination, there is always the risk of converting the incomplete injury into a complete one, either by surgical manipulation or by necrosis of the urethra pursuant to infection and trauma from the traction catheter. A fourth problem with the standard management is that it converts a closed sterile hematoma into an open, and therefore contaminated, hematoma. In addition, Weems has maintained that approximately three fourths of the patients managed in the standard fashion get a stricture, and while they may respond to nonoperative treatment, many develop severe strictures that require operation to avoid serious disabilities due to obstructive uropathy and infection. He also claims that manipulation of the urethra might increase the likelihood of impotence, which represents a significant complication in these individuals.

The alternative approach, which has been introduced in Europe, is to do as little as possible during the early period after the injury, even to the point of recommending that no urethrogram be done. If the patient cannot void or if he has a bloody discharge from his urethral meatus, a suprapubic tube is simply put into the bladder, and nothing else is done until several weeks later when the urethrogram is made. If severe damage to the urethra has occurred and if secondary operations will be necessary, the patient convalesces for an additional 2 to 3 months until pelvic scars have softened and the traumatic reaction has subsided. Obviously, if the urethra is intact and the patient can void, the suprapubic catheter is simply removed. Proponents of this method have argued that the extravasation of sterile urine is not a serious problem, and Weems supports this contention, believing that if the urine escapes into the retroperitoneum or into the peritoneum and is uninfected, it will be absorbed without significant reaction. He has admitted that if the urine is contaminated or becomes infected, it carries a different prognosis. Because of his faith in the competency of the bladder neck, even in the face of complete transection of the urethra at the prostatic apex, he believes that the cystostomy drainage provides perfectly adequate urinary diversion. A strong argument in favor of this form of management is that it avoids contamination in the hematoma, since it is undisturbed and unopened. In a great majority of cases, it does not become infected and there is spontaneous resorption of this hematoma with remarkably little fibrosis in the pelvis. In two series consisting of 37 patients, the results were deemed extremely encouraging compared with the standard method of management. Theoretically, as soon as the cystostomy is performed, the urine within the bladder is contaminated, and I have less faith in the competency of the sphincter mechanism, especially in anesthetized patients and in patients receiving goodly amounts of medication for sedation and analgesia.

While urethral rupture secondary to pelvic fracture in the female must be considered extremely rare according to the literature reviews, it must be recognized that the general features and principles of management would be the same as for the male. A suprapubic cystostomy should be performed unless a catheter can be passed easily into the bladder. Because it is located along the anterior vaginal wall, it may be possible to repair it under direct vision. Stricture and incontinence are likely complications of such an injury. Details of the subsequent management of posterior urethral injury may be obtained from a urology text.

In cases in which the diagnosis of the posterior urethral rupture has been made quite a while after the injury, the only alternative may be to open up the space of Retzius, remove the infected clot and urine, and perform a cystostomy. Once the acute problems have subsided an attempt to restore continuity of the urethral segments can be performed. If such a repair is not possible, a more permanent form of diversion such as a permanent suprapubic cystostomy, an ileal conduit, or bilateral ureterostomies may have to be performed.

COMPLICATIONS

Complications of posterior urethral rupture include stricture formation, stone formation (especially if associated injuries demand prolonged recumbency), fistulae, impotence, and incontinence.

Recumbency calculi can be minimized. They are due to a combination of urinary stasis, a raised level of urinary calcium, and infection. Urinary stasis can be prevented by assuring an adequate intake of fluid and by avoiding a permanent dorsal decubitus position. Decalcification of bone can be prevented by exercise and massage of the uninjured limbs. Routinely, antibiotics are given and the patient is encouraged to drink freely. Urinary acidification lessens the chance of urinary infection and also prevents the deposition of the soft triple phosphate calculi.

Chambers and Balfour[70] reported the incidence of impotence following rupture of the urethra in association with pelvic fractures ranging from 42% in their series to over 50% in Young's series.[527]

Froman and Stein[141] note that about one half of their 29 patients with posterior urethral disruptions complained of impotence. Ward-McQuaid[494] reported similarly pessimistic results in urethral ruptures with pelvic fractures. He found that four of six patients with ruptured urethra and pelvic fracture failed to retain normal sexual function. While a neuromuscular mechanism with disruption of the greater and lesser cavernous nerves that supply the corpus cavernosa[2] is believed responsible, a vascular cause is not altogether ruled out,[473,527] and it is apparent that the incidence of impotence varies with the severity of the injury to the lower urinary tract.

Others also suggest that impotence is primarily related to the severity of the fracture and the soft tissue injuries rather than to the specific surgical technique used in the repair of urethral disruptions. Of 36 patients with urethral injuries and pelvic fractures in whom data were available, 13 (36%) were impotent.[157] Impotence (failure of erection, failure to achieve orgasm, failure to ejaculate, or retrograde ejaculation) was found by King[233] in 13 of 31 (42%) men under 60 who had had a urethral injury with a pelvic fracture, whereas 3 of 59 (5%) had this complication after a pelvic fracture without an injury to the urethra. In Gibson's[154] series of 44 patients, 14 (32%) were impotent, and in an earlier report he lists a 50% impotence rate in a series of 126 patients recorded in the literature.[153]

PARTIAL RUPTURES OF THE POSTERIOR URETHRA

It should be noted that when difficulty is encountered in passing a urethral catheter in the situation of a partial rupture of the posterior urethra, the urethrogram demonstrates extravasation of the medium in the area superior to the urogenital diaphragm. Therefore, the injury cannot be differentiated from an extraperitoneal rupture of the bladder, and this distinction can be made only at the time of operation. If, on the other hand, no difficulty is encountered in passing the catheter into the bladder and a cystogram is basically normal, a sense of complacency may lead to failure to perform a urethrogram in conjunction with the cystogram. Because partial rupture of the posterior urethra cannot be differentiated from extraperitoneal rupture of the bladder on the basis of contrast radiography, operative intervention is indicated, including a suprapubic cystostomy, prevesical drainage, and a urethral splinting catheter.

Levine and Crampton[254] have reported that up to one-third of the patients who sustain pelvic fractures have hematuria without demonstrable renal, vesical, or urethral injury. Therefore, the diagnosis of vesical or urethral contusion can be made—but only by exclusion after appropriate x-ray studies of both the upper and lower urinary tracts have been performed. This problem is usually self-limiting and clears up spontaneously.

BLADDER INJURIES

Because bladder contusions are self-limiting and respond to conservative treatment, it is difficult to assess their incidence. On the other hand, rupture of the bladder occurs in approximately 4% of the reported cases of pelvic fracture. Earlier series gave a higher incidence than most recent series owing to the severe crushing injuries previously reported in industrial and mining accidents. Watson-Jones[496] noted that bladder rupture is not associated with isolated fractures of the sacrum, coccyx, iliac wing, ischium, or acetabulum. The mechanism of injury leading to rupture of the bladder can be due either to perforation by pelvic bone fragments or to the tearing of the dome of the bladder due to sudden compression of the distended viscus.[273] Entrapment of the bladder within the pelvic fracture has been recorded.[241] Whether the bladder injury is penetrating or nonpenetrating, it is quite obvious that the distended bladder is more liable to rupture than the empty one.

The empty bladder cannot be injured by a nonpenetrating force unless the pelvic circle is broken. The distended bladder, however, can be ruptured intraperitoneally by a sudden force of the lower abdominal region, with or without fracture of the pelvis. Kaiser and Farrow,[220] in their excellent review, noted that 11 of their 12 patients with bladder rupture had sustained a disruption of the pelvic ring. One patient, who sustained a fracture of the superior pubic ramus on one side and the inferior ramus on the opposite side, had no discernible disruption of the pelvic ring. It was surmised that this patient had had a distended bladder at the time of the injury and, therefore, had sustained an intraperitoneal rupture of the bladder. The ease with which a toy rubber balloon can be broken is proportional to the tension with which it has been inflated, and the same is true for the bladder. If the bladder is empty when a stable pubic fracture is incurred, there is little or no risk of rupture. But, if it is full and tense, it may rupture with the mere transmitted impact of a fall, whether or not a pubic fracture is also incurred.[275]

As previously noted, bladder ruptures in the past have been more common in men who have been engaged in manual labor occupations, but as wider use of the motor vehicle has occurred, there has been an increase in the number of women who have sustained lower urinary tract injuries in conjunction with pelvic fractures. Cass and Ireland[64] reported a 4:3 preponderance of men to women in the period 1960 to 1971 in reporting 68 patients with blunt external trauma.

Bladder ruptures can be intraperitoneal, extraperitoneal, or combined, and may occur with urethral injuries as well. The fully distended bladder usually ruptures at its dome into the intraperitoneal space, while partially distended bladders can also rupture anteriorly, posteriorly, or extraperitoneally into the space of Retzius. Intraperitoneal rupture of the bladder in asssociation with pelvic fractures occurs approximately one-fourth as often as extraperitoneal rupture.[369] The fully distended bladder is weakest at its dome, where it has a peritoneal reflection off the anterior abdominal wall, and a sudden blow to the region can cause the bladder to burst; in the male, the rupture may also occur at the posterior bladder surface. The sudden entrance of a large volume of even sterile urine causes a serious peritonitis, and previously contaminated urine or extravasated urine that becomes contaminated as a result of instrumentation or surgery will undoubtedly cause bacterial peritonitis.

Extraperitoneal rupture leads to extravasation of urine in the perivesical tissues, and in conjunction with the hemorrhage associated with the pelvic fracture a very severe cellulitis and phlegmon usually develops if the extravasation goes undiagnosed or untreated. Eighty percent of the ruptures of the bladder occurring with fractured pelves have usually been reported to be extraperitoneal,[15,220,369] but one recent series[65] showed an equal incidence of intra- and extraperitoneal ruptures in conjunction with pelvic fractures. Extraperitoneal ruptures are much more commonly associated with fractures of the pelvis that involve disruption of the anterior ring, including bilateral fractures of both the superior and inferior rami (butterfly fracture) as well as serious disruptions including Malgaigne fractures and diastasis of the symphysis pubis. The mechanism of this injury is believed to be one in which the trauma causes anterior crushing of the pelvis, which in turn leads either to perforation of the extraperitoneal portion of the bladder with a bony spicule or to disruption of the bladder wall by tearing and ripping of the pubovesical ligaments or pelvic fascia. Extraperitoneal injuries commonly occur along the anterolateral bladder wall close to the vesical neck, leading to urinary extravasation into the space of Retzius, which may then dissect retroperitoneally up into the paracolic gutters, through the sciatic notch into the buttocks, or via the inguinal canal into the scrotum. Combined intraperitoneal and extraperitoneal ruptures of the bladder due to pelvic fractures are uncommon but have been reported.

DIAGNOSIS

While signs and symptoms may be delayed in appearing, and are "disastrously misleading,[101] the earliest common findings in bladder rupture are shock in association with lower abdominal pain, inability to void, and bleeding from the urethra (although bleeding is not as common or as brisk as it is in urethral ruptures). It may be impossible to differentiate the shock from the hemorrhage that commonly is associated with pelvic fractures to at least some extent. In other instances shock is not an invariable finding. The signs of peritoneal irritation are minimal soon after injury, but later the classical signs of peritonitis may be expected. During the earlier phase, there is no generalized abdominal spasm or rebound, and peristalsis is active. Later, signs of peritoneal irritation with distention as well as generalized tenderness and rigidity develop.

Extraperitoneal rupture of the bladder also gives evidence of lower abdominal tenderness, and percussion of the region in the suprapubic area reveals dullness due to extravasation of urine and blood. A vague mass may be felt on vaginal or rectal examination. As urinary extravasation continues, the tissues so undermined give a doughy, indurated, edematous feeling, which on occasion might lead to the development of collections of hemorrhagic urine, which gives the signs of free fluid in the subcutaneous spaces. After 24 hours the patient with an extraperitoneal extravasation begins to show signs of toxemia, as undrained extravasated urine causes tissue necrosis and cellulitis. When contaminated, this process is much more devastating and lethal.

The rather late appearance of signs of intraperitoneal irritation seen in association with extravasation of urine may be useful in distinguishing a bladder rupture from the rupture of other abdominal organs, which would be more likely to give earlier signs of peritoneal irritation. The diagnostic usefulness of a peritoneal tap needs no emphasis at this point. The presence of ileus is of little assistance as it may be present even without associated bladder injury in the presence of pelvic fractures. After 24 hours the patient with an intraperitoneal rupture also gives evidence of toxemia with distention, nausea and vomiting, fever, and leukocytosis.

Despite the fact that the patient states that he has not voided just prior to the injury, he is unable to void spontaneously. Usually, a survey flat-plate of the abdomen reveals the pelvic fractures and should raise the suspicion of major urinary tract injury. As described in the section on urethral injuries, under sterile conditions, a Foley catheter should be introduced gently into the bladder. If this is unsuccessful, a second equally gentle attempt should be made with a Coudé-tipped straight catheter. If no urine is obtained as the catheter enters the ruptured bladder, this is highly suggestive of a rupture, if there is a history of the patient not having voided recently. Occasionally, clear urine may be obtained, but this does not exclude rupture, because the urine may be withdrawn from the abdominal cavity through a rent in the bladder. While catheterization and cystography do carry the risk of contaminating the extravasated fluids, the information gained should lead to a prompt diagnosis and more than balances such a risk. The retrograde cystogram is the most significant single procedure for diagnosing a ruptured bladder (Fig. 13-85).[126,369] A cystogram should be performed by instilling, by gravity flow or gentle injection, 250 ml of a 30% solution of the medium used for excretory urography. If the anteroposterior view shows no extravasation, an additional 150 ml is instilled, and another film is taken. The second dose tends to overcome the tamponade effect of the perivesical hemorrhage and hematoma. The bladder is emptied, given a saline wash-out, and another film is taken to detect extravasations obliterated by a bladder full of dye (Fig. 13-86).[65]

The use of air cystograms is not widely advocated at the present time for patients with pelvic fractures, because it can be extremely harmful and painful to get the patient into the upright position in order to demonstrate free air under the diaphragmatic leaves. Similarly, the method of measuring the amount of returned fluid after a quantity of known volume has been injected into the bladder is quite useless and has led to a number of false-positive and false-negative interpretations. Cystoscopy is not recommended routinely because of a number of factors: the positioning of the patient may aggravate hemorrhaging, large ruptures preclude the distention of the bladder, and the presence of blood or a blood clot makes visualization difficult.

Through all these maneuvers, the overriding principle must be to gain as much information as possible in order that a positive diagnosis can be made with as little strain to the patient as is possible in view of his multiple injuries.

At the conclusion of the cystogram, during which anterior and oblique films of the bladder region have been obtained, a urethrogram should be performed in all male patients, using 20 ml of a 30% urographic medium. Again, anterior, posterior, and oblique views are made. During the urethrogram, it is essential to remember that x-ray examination should be done during the continued injection of the medium.

In male patients, the cystogram is done before

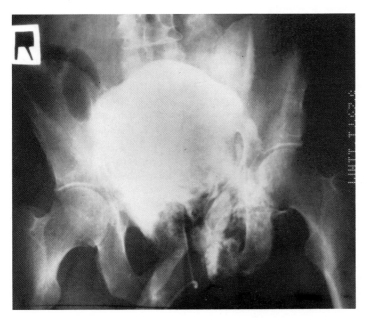

Fig. 13-85. Radiopaque contrast material entered the ruptured bladder and exited into the extraperitoneal perivesical space following cystogram.

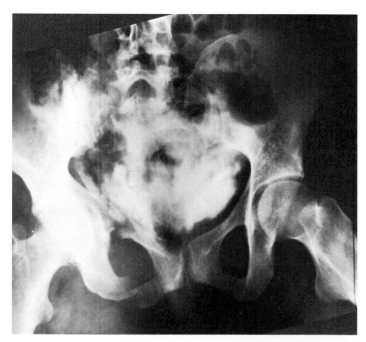

Fig. 13-86. This postvoiding cystogram demonstrates the continued presence of extraperitoneal perivesical contrast material following voiding and saline wash-out. The rupture was at the inferior portion of the bladder.

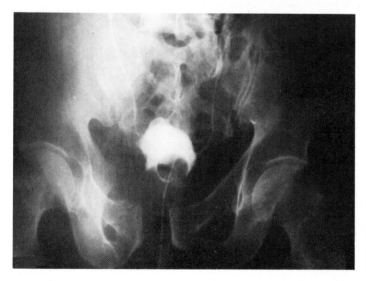

Fig. 13-87. This intravenous pyelogram was performed after a normal cystourethrogram was obtained in this patient, who has a Malgaigne fracture. The film shows bladder filling 20 minutes after injection of the intravenous contrast agent.

the urethrogram, except in two situations: (1) when there is a high index of suspicion of anterior urethral injury (*e.g.*, a straddle fracture), and (2) when it is impossible to pass a catheter into the bladder.

If hematuria has been detected and the cystogram and urethrogram are both negative, it is, in my opinion, advisable to perform an intravenous pyelogram, provided the patient can tolerate the procedure and provided his systolic blood pressure is over 100 mm Hg (Fig. 13-87). This information

can provide evidence of renal trauma or trauma to the ureters as a result of nonpenetrating external forces.

With intraperitoneal rupture of the bladder, the contrast medium accumulates in the dependent portions of the peritoneal cavity, especially in the paracolic recesses. There may also be scalloped filling defects in the contrast medium produced by loops of intestine. Large ruptures give a spectacular sunburst appearance to the abdominal x-ray.

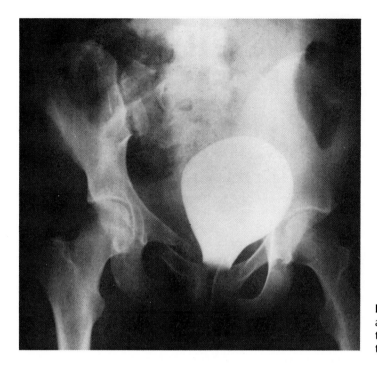

Fig. 13-88. The perivesical hematoma lifts and compresses the bladder neck causing the upside down teardrop pattern seen on the cystogram.

Extraperitoneal ruptures lead to the accumulation of the contrast agent in the perivesical spaces, although if the extravasation has been extensive this contrast agent may, in fact, diffuse through the extravasated urine to distant locations. But oblique films should facilitate differentiating this extravasation from a purely intraperitoneal extravasation.

In some instances the cystogram is typical—with an hourglass configuration to the opaque medium. The lower half represents the partially filled bladder, and the contrast material in the pelvic peritoneal cavity represents the upper half of the hourglass. An upside-down "tear-drop" pattern indicates only perivesical hematoma lifting and compressing the bladder neck (Fig. 13-88).

The unequivocal diagnosis of extraperitoneal bladder rupture is impossible by clinical examination alone. Proper cystographic results require the injection of 400 ml of a 30% solution of the contrast media used for intravenous pyelography in sterile saline. The appearance of extravasated contrast medium usually shows a well-filled bladder with extravasation in the neck area. If the rent is large, however, the bladder may not be identifiable, since all of the contrast solution escapes. These x-ray examinations should be performed with the patient on a Bradford frame or a special litter that reduces the need for manipulation of the patient and his fractured pelvis.

TREATMENT

The treatment of bladder ruptures in association with pelvic fractures is direct surgial intervention, as quickly as is feasible. The principles underlying the treatment of bladder rupture include diversion of the urinary flow by means of a suprapubic cystostomy, the drainage of extravasated urine and blood from the space of Retzius operatively and postoperatively, and the identification and repair of bladder wall lacerations. In extraperitoneal ruptures the rent is sutured directly. The space of Retzius is drained, and the bladder is decompressed by a urethral catheter as well as with a suprapubic tube. The suprapubic drainage should be provided with a large Pezzer type catheter of at least 30 Fr caliber. The space of Retzius should be irrigated with saline, and Penrose drains should be brought out through separate stab wounds. In the presence of known extraperitoneal extravasation, the decision to perform an intraperitoneal exploration as well depends on factors determined during the surgical procedure.

With respect to intraperitoneal ruptures, a laparotomy should be performed to permit the aspiration of urine and blood from the abdomen as well as exploration of its contents. The tear in the bladder should be repaired with chromic catgut sutures, and the peritoneum should be closed without drainage. The anterior extraperitoneal portion of the bladder should then be opened and drained with a large Pezzer catheter. Penrose drains should be laid into the space of Retzius bilaterally and brought out through separate stab wounds. The closure is accomplished with the cystostomy tube exiting from the superior portion of the skin incision.

In cases where rectal ruptures have communicated wtih bladder ruptures, a suprapubic cystostomy, closure of the bladder wall, drainage of the perivesical spaces with Penrose drains, and a diverting colostomy provide the best opportunity for avoiding a rectovesical fistula.

COMPLICATIONS

The complications of bladder ruptures—provided the patient does not succumb acutely to shock, hemorrhage, and distant injuries—are largely those of sepsis. Cellulitis and abscess formation in the peritoneal as well as the extraperitoneal spaces of the pelvis leading to osteomyelitis of the pelvis and pyarthrosis are not uncommon.[168,228,284,296,322,433] Bladder neck fibrosis (if this area has been traumatized) and bladder stone formation are also frequent complications.

Without treatment, bladder ruptures have a 100% mortality. Since the early 1900s, when the principles of urinary diversion began to gain foothold in surgical practice and as more patients had the benefit of the repair of their bladder perforations, mortality rates of bladder rupture in association with pelvic fractures have been reduced to less than a half of their previous high. Recent death rates of 30% to 45% have been recorded in patients with bladder trauma, pelvic fractures, and associated multiple injuries.[15,64,329,369] Cass and Ireland[64] report a mortality rate of 16% in such patients with bladder contusions, 22% with intraperitoneal rupture, and 53% with extraperitoneal rupture, but they ascribe the mortality to the associated injuries. They also correlated increasing death rates with advancing age of the patient (16% in the 0- to 29-year age group, 24% in the 30- to 59-year age group, and 67% in the 60- to 80+ age group, although the degree of associated injuries was similar in each age group).

No discussion on bladder injuries should fail to stress the necessity of prompt diagnosis by clinical signs with the aid of x-ray, by cystourethrography, and the extreme importance of prompt suprapubic cystostomy with good drainage of extravasated urine.

URETERAL INJURIES

The association of ureteral disruptions with pelvic fractures is rare, but they may occcasionally be seen in crush injuries, or in situations in which tension is imposed by extreme hyperextension of the lumbar spine and by sudden acceleration.[7] Shepherd[430] notes that the peritoneum is not usually torn, and what occurs most commonly is a slow urinary extravasation into the retroperitoneal space, usually at the brim of the pelvis. The condition can be recognized by the absence of ureteral visualization on intravenous pyelography followed by the subsequent extravasation of the contrast material.[19] Additional diagnostic evidence of the ureteral injury consists of demonstrating an opaque ureteral catheter outside of the normal course of the ureter. Confirmatory diagnostic studies include a retrograde ureterogram.[65]

Lateral deflection of the ureters on excretory urography may be caused by pelvic hematoma without signifying injury of the ureters themselves. The same is true for retrograde opaque catheters being deflected by the pelvic and retroperitoneal hematoma. Clinical findings in a patient with an unrecognized rupture of the ureter are the onset of toxic symptoms with palpation of a fluid mass in the flank. Failure to recognize the ureteral injury may result in a hydronephrosis due to stricture. Stickel and Howse[457] reported on 85 cases of ureteral trauma found in the English literature, and only four of the cases were associated with fracture of the bony pelvis. Interestingly, all four resulted from motor vehicle accidents that involved children. The diagnosis frequently is delayed until a urinary fistula may develop. Hematuria is either microscopic or not present at all. It may be necessary to perform a reanastomosis with fine chromic catgut sutures over a stent. Other important principles in the treatment of ureteral injuries include splinting, extraperitoneal drainage from the site of repair, and urinary diversion, which can usually be accomplished by transureteral catheter drainage or by nephrostomy or ureterostomy.[65,228]

GYNECOLOGIC INJURY

Injuries to other perineal organs are rarely associated with pelvic fractures. With respect to vaginal injuries, Siegel[433] proposed a routine that includes a history to establish whether the patient is pregnant or menstruating, an adequate pelvic examination (under anesthesia if necessary), and immediate closure of the vaginal laceration. Antibiotic coverage is essential. Peltier[350] reported two patients with vaginal lacerations. Both died—one of intrapelvic hemorrhage, and the other of amyloidosis secondary to recurrent pelvic abscesses due to septic contamination of the retroperitoneal hematoma. Levine and Crampton[254] reported the survival of a patient with a 10-cm separation of the symphysis pubis, a severe anterior vaginal wall laceration, and prolapse of the bladder into the defect. Ikpeme and Morison[205] recorded the successful repair of a vaginal avulsion, which they believed to have been caused by violent compression within the pelvis that led to bilateral fractures of the superior and inferior pubic rami. Froman and Stein[141] also reported on two patients with vaginal laceration. In one, a pubic bone fragment was found free in the vagina, but healing was prompt. In the other patient, the pubic fragment created a vesicovaginal fistula and posteriorly there was a third-degree laceration of the vagina extending into the rectum. Immediate surgical repair prevented the development of a urinary fistula. The same authors reported four instances of pelvic fractures in patients in the last trimester of pregnancy, all four babies were stillborn, and two mothers succumbed (one to a placental detachment that led to exsanguination). In the latter instance the authors hypothesize that a cesarean section at the time of laparotomy for the intraperitoneal rupture of the bladder might have been more judicious. Peltier[350] reported two cases, one in the last trimester and one in the second trimester, that proceeded to normal delivery. Speer and Peltier[449] reviewed the obstetrical outcomes of six patients who were pregnant at the time of the pelvic fracture and five patients who subsequently became pregnant after the pelvic fracture had been sustained. In the first group there was a fetal loss of 33% (2 of 6 patients), and in the latter group there was no fetal loss although one of the five patients had to undergo a cesarean section. They also accumulated 51 additional cases from published sources and found that nine of 26 (34.6%) pregnant at the time of the fracture had lost their fetuses. Three of 25 (12%) who became pregnant subsequent to the pelvic fracture also sustained fetal loss, and ten required cesarean section. Osmond-Clark and Gissane[335] recorded the intrauterine fracture of the fetal skull.

TESTICULAR INJURY

Because the normal testis is mobile, it is not readily injured, but if contused or avulsed, it can usually be retained due to its good local blood supply. Conolly and Hedberg[87] mentioned having had two testicular avulsions in their series.

BOWEL AND RECTAL INJURY

While bowel injury is rarely associated with pelvic fractures[10,47,109,265,306] the diagnosis is difficult and frequently lethal. Prolonged ileus should prompt consideration of this unusual associated injury.

Since World War II, the accepted management of major rectal wounds has been fecal diversion via colostomy, drainage of the retrorectal space, closure of the rectal wound when possible, and the use of systemic antibiotics. The largest series of rectal injuries associated with pelvic fracture, to my knowledge, is the dozen patients of Froman and Stein. They describe four types: (1) a linear laceration from the anal verge to midrectum; (2) extraperitoneal laceration anteriorly, usually associated with disruption of the posterior urethra; (3) intraperitoneal rupture; and (4) anorectal avulsion with either the rectum drawn up into the sacral hollow or prolapse. Nine of the 12 patients had major urinary tract injuries, and despite diversional colostomy in nine patients, two developed fecal fistulas of the anterior abdominal wall. Mathieson and Mann[285] also recorded a rare anal avulsion secondary to violent compression of the pelvic floor causing distortion of the pelvis and urogenital diaphragm and destroying the anchorages of the anal canal.

ABDOMINAL WALL INJURY

Ryan[405] reported on a small series of hernias related to pelvic fractures. Two patients sustained rupture of the rectus abdominis muscle at its attachment to the pubis on the side opposite to maximum bone displacement. These hernias were due to anteroposterior compression forces that divided the attachment from the upper edge of the pubic crest. Two other patients developed direct hernias through the posterior wall of the inguinal canal with the tear in the canal being in line with a fracture of the superior ramus of the pubis or body of the pubis. These hernias were related to lateral or vertical forces that fractured not only the superior pubic ramus but also the posterior wall of the inguinal canal. Levine and Crampton reported on four cases from their own series with diaphragmatic ruptures and noted four others in the literature.[234,341] Peltier[350] observed that the major abdominal injury overlooked in his series was diaphragmatic hernia (four in a series of 186 patients); the diagnosis was not made early in any of the cases, and three patients were late in convalescence before symptoms attracted attention.

NEUROLOGIC INJURY

The incidence of neurologic deficits in conjunction with pelvic fractures is quite variable, and the availability of reliable studies is limited. Patterson and Morton[341] reported a 1.2% incidence in 809 patients with pelvic fracture. A later series by the same authors reviews 1500 pelvic fractures and 34 associated neurologic deficits (an incidence of 2.3%).[342] Lam[242] recorded an incidence of 0.75% in 1889 cases culled from the literature, but in his personal series, he had nine patients with nerve injury in a group of 100 pelvic fractures. G. C. Davis is cited by Scudder[417] as having found a 2% incidence. Junge[218] quoted an incidence between 0.41 and 0.75%, based on a literature survey. Huittinen and Slatis[202] surveyed 85 patients with double vertical pelvic fractures and found an incidence of 46%; they extrapolated that since these fractures comprise 25% of all pelvic fractures, nerve lesions are expected in 10% to 12% of an unselected series of pelvic fractures. This figure certainly is much higher than the figure quoted by other authors, which runs between 0.5% and 2%. Huittinen and Slatis found lesions of variable severity, with the greatest predominance occurring at L5 and S1 roots. In most instances several roots from L4 to S5 were affected. All patients had an associated sacroiliac injury that was in close approximation of the lumbosacral trunk. Bonnin[37] stated that in his series of cases, radiographically obvious fractures of the sacrum were present in 45% of the patients with pelvic ring fractures, and he found that the sacral fractures are localized around the first and second anterior and posterior foramina. Bonnin noted that injuries to the nerve tissue from pelvic fractures may be due to stretching, small fragments of bone, surrounding hemorrhage, fibrous tissue and callus contraction, and bone pressure when the displacement is considerable. Frequently, symptom onset is delayed, and few signs may be elicited at the time of the first examination, while more marked features may appear later.

Wakeley[489] in his review of 100 cases of fractures of the pelvis noted no case of injury to the sacral nerves at the time of accident and only one at a later date, due to compression from excessive callus

formation. He did not find this surprising insofar as the sacral foramina are roughly double the size of the nerves they transmit, and therefore there is ample room for some callus formation without encroaching upon the nerves.

Bonnin described sacral root stretching in five patients and differentiated these nerve lesions from intrathecal compression of the roots at higher levels by the absence of local pain. He also held that the sacral fracture was responsible for the cauda equina injury, noting that the sacral injuries are frequently overlooked. Bonnin felt that the most characteristic feature of the syndrome is the distribution of the muscle paresis caused by pressure or division of the first or second sacral nerves. The peroneal and anterior tibial compartments are slightly affected, and mostly there is marked weakness of plantar flexion at the ankle with loss of the ankle jerk and loss of power in the hamstrings and gluteii. The loss of these three posterior groups of muscles of the lower extremity (calf, hamstrings, and buttock) characterizes the lesion; the calf muscles are more markedly paralyzed than the other groups. The ankle jerk will be lost if there is serious damage to the first sacral root. Sensory changes associated with injuries of the first and second sacral nerves lead to alterations in sensation, paresthesia, and referred pain on the outside of the calf and the lateral half of the foot. Pain is not a prominent feature of the syndromes in which the first and second sacral roots are stretched, because once the nerve has been either completely or partially divided, it is rendered painless unless the remaining fibers are stretched or stimulated by some other method. Because nerves of the bladder and bowel issue below the second sacral nerve root and because sacral fractures are usually unilateral, bowel and bladder disturbances are not usually anticipated.

Bonnin strongly advocated early exercises against graduated resistance to offset disuse atrophy. He felt that the prognosis is good for these cauda equina injuries, especially from a functional standpoint, although there may be some persistent weakness and muscle wasting. In the severe cases, however, the prognosis is not good, and a permanent partial disability due to calf weakness as well as gluteal weakness will persist.

Goodell's[163] careful study of three patients with nerve injury complicating pelvic fractures (including surgical exploration) has provided some additional understanding of the problem. He believes that sacral fractures can cause root tearing by forceful shearing at the fracture lines, and that in others movement of the part of the fracture or dislocated pelvic ring could result in traction on the nearby peripheral nerves. One patient with a transverse comminuted fracture of the sacrum and no associated pelvic fractures sustained disruption of sacral roots as they passed through the fracture site. In this instance the sacral trauma was direct. Most sacral fractures, however, are indirect and are associated with at least one other pelvic fracture. In these instances the most commonly reported neurologic deficit is weakness in the gluteii, hamstrings, and plantar flexors, with cutaneous sensory defects of the buttocks and posterior aspect of the lower limb and lateral aspect of the foot. In his second patient with traumatic disruption of the pelvic ring including symphyseal and sacroiliac separations, Goodell believed that the unilateral sensory and motor deficits corresponding to the L5-S1 segments were due to avulsion forces beyond the sacral foramina and that forceful displacement of the hemipelvis at the moment of fracture caused excessive traction on the affected nerves. Goodell's third patient, who also sustained a severe sacroiliac dislocation, displayed a total sensory and motor loss in the ipsilateral leg. Clinical evidence indicated an injury to all roots contributing to the lumbosacral plexus proximal to the origin of the posterior and primary rami. So Goodell postulated (on the basis of additional information obtained by myelography and by surgical exploration) that the tearing of the L5 and the sacral nerve roots could have occurred because of sciatic nerve traction, and that the hyperextension of the hip and backward displacement of the hemipelvis could have placed traction directly on the nerves arising from the lumbar plexus.

Goodell believed that avulsion of lumbosacral nerve roots occurred at, or just beyond, the vertebral foramina, but he admitted that the data are insufficient to draw a firm conclusion. He also noted that in each of his three cases, although multiple nerves had been torn, myelographic diverticula were present at only one or two levels. He found, too, that the significance of myelographically demonstrable arachnoidal diverticula is different at cervical and lumbosacral levels. Whereas intraspinal root avulsion in the cervical region is usually associated with irregular outpouching at the foramen, diverticula have not been reported following extraspinal tearing of the proximal components of the brachial plexus. In contrast, in the lumbosacral region, diverticula were not related to avulsion of the root from the cord but to avulsions at, or distal to, the foramina.

Patterson and Morton[341] characterized the trauma associated with their series of ten cases as severe and crushing, with pelvic ring continuity broken anteriorly and posteriorly in 12 of their cases. It was recognized that a disproportionately high number of patients sustained neurologic damage when sacral fracture or sacroiliac disruption was a component of their pelvic fractures. An inadequate record of neurologic findings is the outstanding characteristic of the charts in these cases, according to the authors, and accounts for the difficulty in detailing the actual onset of the palsy, its recovery, if any, and the true nature of the defect that generally is loosely referred to as sciatic nerve palsy.

In their subsequent series, Patterson and Morton[342] again stress that neurologic complications are frequently missed due to poor evaluations and reporting. Since most lesions were peripheral rather than root avulsions, they had the potential for recovery. The authors recommend early electrodiagnostic testing and myelography.

Barnett and Connolly[22] reviewed the literature regarding lumbosacral nerve root avulsion intradurally and accumulated a total of 14 cases. Their work and that of Huittinen[199] on postmortem dissections demonstrates that surgical exploration is not advisable. Patients with flaccid paralysis, sensory loss, and the persistence of causalgic or sciatic pain should suggest a possible root avulsion that can be confirmed by myelography.

Harris and co-workers[176] reported four cases of lumbar nerve root avulsion associated with dislocation of, or fracture adjacent to, the sacroiliac joint. Myelographic evidence of diverticula at the roots did not signify complete avulsion of the nerve roots as in the cervical root avulsion, and recovery could occur. The level of the neurologic deficit did not always correspond to the location of the diverticula.

While the sciatic nerve is the peripheral nerve most often affected, Carruthers and Logue[63] reported in a series of 72 pelvic fracture patients three cases of obturator paralysis, all of which recovered spontaneously.

In Bonnin's article on sacral fractures and associated injuries of the cauda equina, he stresses the necessity of comparing both lower extremities to determine the degree of disuse atrophy. Confirmation, by means of a tape measure, that one limb has more extensive muscle loss than the opposite limb with paresis of specific muscle groups should indeed point to the presence of a previously unnoticed nerve lesion.

I sincerely acknowledge a debt of gratitude to the orthopaedic surgery and radiology staffs of Northwestern Memorial Hospital, Chicago, Illinois, St. Francis Hospital, Evanston, Illinois and Hennepin County Hospital, Minneapolis, Minnesota. Particular thanks are due to Drs. Lee F. Rogers, Ramon B. Gustilo, and the late Dr. John J. Fahey. I am also indebted to the late Dr. Choon-Shick Lee for his art work and to Muriel Hughes and Karen Ferry for their secretarial assistance.

REFERENCES

1. Abbate, C.: Avulsion Fracture of the Ischial Tuberosity. A Case Report. J. Bone Joint Surg., 27:716–717, 1945.
2. Abbott, A. C.: Rupture of the Urethra. Canad. Med. Ass. J., 20:634–637, 1929.
3. Adams, J. C.: Fractures of the Pelvis. *In* Adams, J. C. (ed.): Outline of Fractures. Edinburgh, E. & S. Livingstone, 1960.
4. Adams, J. D.: Report of a Case of Fracture into the Acetabulum with Separation at the Sacroiliac Synchondrosis without Clinical Symptoms. Boston Med. Surg. J., 158:432–433, 1907.
5. Adrey, J.: Hoffmann's External Anchorage Coupled in Arrangement. Paris, Gead, 1971.
6. Ahmad, W., and Polk, H. C., Jr.: Blunt Abdominal Trauma. Arch. Surg., 111:489–492, 1976.
7. Ainsworth, T.; Weems, W. L.; and Merrell, W. H.: Bilateral Ureteral Injury due to Non-penetrating External Trauma. J. Urol., 96:439–442, 1966.
8. Almond, G., and Vernon, E.: Iliac Skeletal Cross Traction. J. Bone Joint Surg., 41B:779–781, 1959.
9. Apley, A. G.: A System of Orthopaedics and Fractures. London, Butterworth, 1963.
10. Arnold, G. J.: A Case of Fracture of the Pelvis with Nipping of Small Intestine Between the Fragments. Lancet, 1:1157, 1907.
11. Ashhurst, A. P. C.: Fractures of the Pelvis. Ann. Surg., 49:433–440, 1909.
12. Athanasoulis, C. A.: Angiography to Assess Pelvic Vascular Injury. New Engl. J. Med., 284:1329, 1971.
13. Athanasoulis, C. A.: Therapeutic Applications of Angiography. New Engl. J. Med., 302:1117–1124, 1174–1179, 1980.
14. Ayella, R. J.; DePriest, R. W., Jr.; Khaneja, S. C.; Maekawa, K.; Soderstrom, C. A.; Rodriguez, A.; and Cowley, R. A.: Transcatheter Embolization of Autologous Clot in the Management of Bleeding Associated with Fractures of the Pelvis. Surg. Gynecol. Obstet., 147:849–852, 1978.
15. Bacon, S. K.: Rupture of the Urinary Bladder: Clinical Analysis of 147 Cases in the Past Ten Years. J. Urol., 49:432–435, 1943.
16. Baijal, E.: Multiple Fractures of the Pelvis with an Unusually Wide Disruption of the Symphysis Pubis Sustained in an Accident Shortly after Childbirth: A Case Report. Injury, 6:57–59, 1974.
17. Bailey, H.: Rupture of the Urethra. Br. J. Surg., 15:370–384, 1928.
18. Baker, W. J., and Graf, E. C.: The Management of the Urinary Tract in Fractures of the Bony Pelvis. A.A.O.S. Instructional Course Lectures, 11:245–260, 1954.
19. Baker, W. J., and Graf, E. C.: Management of Urinary Tract Injuries in Fracture of the Bony Pelvis. Surg. Clin. North Am., 55:295–304, 1955.
20. Banks, H.: Ruptured Urethra: A New Method of Treatment. Br. J. Surg., 15:262–263, 1927.
21. Barlow, B.; Rottenberg, R. W.; and Santulli, T. V.: Angiographic Diagnosis and Treatment of Bleeding by Selective Embolization Following Pelvic Fracture in Children. J. Pediatr. Surg., 10:939–941, 1975.
22. Barnett, H. G., and Connolly, E. S.: Lumbosacral Nerve Root Avulsion: Report of a Case and Review of the Literature. J. Trauma, 15:532–535, 1975.
23. Batalden, D. J.; Wickstrom, P. H.; Ruiz, E.; and Gustilo, R. B.: Value of the G Suit in Patients with Severe Pelvic Fracture. Arch. Surg., 109:326–328, 1974.
24. Baylis, S. M.; Lansing, E. H.; and Glas, W. W.: Traumatic Retroperitoneal Hematoma. Am. J. Surg., 103:477–480, 1962.
25. Benson, G. S., and Brewer, E. D.: Hematuria: Algorithms for Diagnosis: Hematuria in the Adult and Hematuria Secondary to Trauma. J.A.M.A., 246:993–995, 1981.
26. Berg, P. M.: Acute Pelvic Disruption, The Bucking Horse Injury. Orthop. Trans., 3:271, 1979.
27. Berry, F. B.: Trauma and the Urinary Bladder. [Editorial] Arch. Surg., 66:582–584, 1953.
28. Berry, J. M.: Fracture of the Tuberosity of the Ischium due to Muscular Action. J.A.M.A., 59:1450, 1912.
29. Berry, N. E.: Traumatic Rupture of the Bladder and Urethra. Can. Med. Ass. J., 22:475–483, 1930.
30. Binder, S. S., and Mitchell, G. A.: The Control of Intractable Pelvic Hemorrhage by Ligation of the Hypogastric Artery. South. Med. J., 53:837–843, 1960.
31. Blount, W. P.: Fractures in Children. Baltimore, Williams & Wilkins, 1955.
32. Bogart, L.: Rupture of the Urinary Bladder. Urol. Cutan. Rev., 43:310–313, 1939.
33. Bohler, J., and Ender, H. G.: Acetabular Fractures: Morphology and Management. *In* The Hip Society: The Hip, Proceedings of The Hip Society. pp. 197–209. St. Louis, C. V. Mosby, 1975.
34. Böhler, L.: The Treatment of Fractures. New York, Grune & Stratton, 1956.
35. Bonnel, F.: Problemes therapeutiques des fracas du cotyle (Apport du fixateur externe). Montpellier Chir., 19, 6:160–163, 1973.
36. Bonnel, F.: Codification du Fixateur Externe Dans Les Traumatismes du Bassin. Ann. Chir., 30:131–134, 1976.
37. Bonnin, J. G.: Sacral Fractures and Injuries to the Cauda Equina. J. Bone Joint Surg., 27:113–127, 1945.
38. Boobbyer, G. N.: External Fixation with the Coat Hanger Method in Treatment of Unstable Fractures of the Pelvis. Injury, 11:254–256, 1979.
39. Boorstein, S. W.: Central Fracture of the Acetabulum. J.A.M.A., 86:617–619, 1926.
40. Boorstein, S. W.: Fractures of the True Pelvic Ring. Am. J. Surg., 7:633–643, 1929.
41. Borkowski, W.: Avulsion Fracture of the Anterior Superior Spine of the Ilium. Chir. Narz. Ruchu., 5:473–481, 1932.

42. Braunstein, P. W., and Draper, J. W.: Fracture of the Pelvis and Complicating Injuries. *In* Wade, P. A. (ed.): Surgical Treatment of Trauma. New York, Grune & Stratton, 1960.

43. Braunstein, P. W.; Skudder, P. A.; McCarroll, J. R.; Musolino, A.; and Wade, P. A.: Concealed Hemorrhage Due to Pelvic Fracture. J. Trauma, **4**:832–838, 1964.

44. Brooke, R.: The Sacro-iliac Joint. J. Anat., **58**:299–305, 1924.

45. Broomhead, R.: Sacro-iliac Dislocation Reduced by Hoke's Traction. Proc. Soc. Med., **27**:576–579, 1933.

46. Brown, T. D.; Stone, J. P.; Schuster, J. H.; and Mears, D. C.: Rigidity Measurements of External Fixators Used for Unstable Pelvic Ring Fractures, 27th Annual ORS. Las Vegas, Nevada, 1981.

47. Buchanan, J. R.: Bowel Entrapment by Pelvic Fracture Fragments: A Case Report and Review of the Literature. Clin. Orthop., **147**:164–166, 1980.

48. Bucholz, R. W.: The Pathological Anatomy of Malgaigne Fracture-Dislocations of the Pelvis. J. Bone Joint Surg., **63A**:400–404, 1981.

49. Bucholz, R. W., and Mears, D. C.: An Unstable Fracture of the Pelvis. *In* A. B. Ferguson, Jr., (ed): Orthop. Consultation, **3**:1–10, 1982.

50. Bucknill, T. M., and Blackburne, J. S.: Fracture-Dislocations of the Sacrum: Report of Three Cases. J. Bone Joint Surg., **58B**:467–470, 1976.

51. Burgi, S.: Luxations of the Os Innominatum. J. Chir. (Paris), **49**:536–561, 1937.

52. Burke, D. L.; Miller, A.; and Kerner, M.: Pelvic Fracture Stabilization with Hoffman External Fixation. Orthop. Trans., **4**:336–337, 1980.

53. Burnham, A. C.: Fractures of the Pelvis. Ann. Surg., **61**:703–715, 1915.

54. Butt, A. J., and Perry, J. Q.: Ureteral Injury Complicating Fracture of the Bony Pelvis. South Surg., **16**:1139–1142, 1950.

55. Byrnes, D. P.; Russo, G. L.; Ducker, T. B.; and Cowley, R. A.: Sacrum Fractures and Neurological Damage. J. Neurosurg., **47**:459–462, 1977.

56. Bystrom, J.; Dencker, H.; Joderling, J.; and Meurling, S.: Ligation of the Internal Iliac Artery to Arrest Massive Hemorrhage following Pelvic Fracture. Acta Chir. Scand., **134**:199–202, 1968.

57. Cahill, G. F.: Rupture of the Bladder and Urethra. Am. J. Surg., **36**:653–662, 1937.

58. Caldwell, C. E.: Fractures of the Pelvis and their Complications. Ohio Med. J., **15**:798–800, 1919.

59. Callahan, J. J.: Fractures of the Pelvis. Indust. Med., **6**:651–654, 1937.

60. Campbell, M. F.: Rupture of the Bladder. Surg. Gynecol. Obstet. **49**:540–560, 1929.

61. Campbell's Operative Orthopaedics. Crenshaw, A. H. (ed.). St. Louis, C. V. Mosby, 1971.

62. Carabalona, P.; Rabischong, P.; Bonnel, F.; Perruchon, E.; and Peguret, F.: Apports du fixateurs externes dans les disjonctions du pubis et de lárticulation sacro-iliaque. (Etude biomecanique et resultats cliniques). Montpellier Chir., **19**:61–70, 1973.

63. Carruthers, F. W., and Logue, R. M.: Treatment of Fractures of the Pelvis and their Complications. A.A.O.S. Instructional Course Lectures, **10**:50–56, 1953.

64. Cass, A. S., and Ireland, G. W.: Bladder Trauma Associated with Pelvic Fractures in Severely Injured Patients. J. Trauma, **13**:205–212, 1973.

65. Cass, A. S., and Ireland, G. W.: Urinary Tract Trauma. Minnesota Med., **57**:15–18, 1974.

66. Casselman, R. C., and Schillinger, J. F.: Fractured Pelvis with Avulsion of the Female Urethra. J. Urol., **117**:385–386, 1977.

67. Castle, M. E., and Orinion, E. A.: Prophylactic Anticoagulation in Fractures. J. Bone Joint Surg., **52A**:521–528, 1970.

68. Cave, E. F.: Fracture of the Acetabulum. *In* Wilson, P. D. (ed.): Management of Fractures and Dislocations. Philadelphia, J. B. Lippincott, 1938.

69. Cave, E. F.: (ed.): Fractures and Other Injuries. Chap. 24. Chicago Year Book Publishers, 1958.

70. Chambers, H. L., and Balfour, J.: The Incidence of Impotence following Pelvic Fracture with Associated Urinary Tract Injury. J. Urol., **89**:702–703, 1963.

71. Chapman, M.: Management of Pelvic Fractures. West. J. Med., **120**:421–424, 1974.

72. Chavez, C. J.: Urethral Injuries Associated with Pelvic Fractures. South. Med. J., **64**:565–573, 1971.

73. Chenoweth, D. R.; Cruickshank, B.; Gertzbein, S. D.; Goldfarb, P.; and Janosick, J.: A Clinical and Experimental Investigation of Occult Injuries of the Pelvic Ring. Injury, **12**:59–65, 1981.

74. Christopher, F.: Fracture of the Anterior Superior Spine of the Ilium. J.A.M.A., **100**:113–114, 1933.

75. Chunn, C. F.: Wounds of the Rectum. Surg. Clin. North Am., **38**:1649–1659, 1958.

76. Clark, S. S., and Prudencio, R. F.: Lower Urinary Tract Injuries Associated with Pelvic Fractures: Diagnosis and Management. Surg. Clin. North Am., **52**:183–201, 1972.

77. Clarke, R., and Fisher, M. R.: Assessment of Blood Loss following Injury. Br. J. Clin. Pract., **10**:746–769, 1956.

78. Cleaves, E. N.: Fracture or Avulsion of the Anterior Superior Spine of the Ilium. J. Bone Joint Surg., **20**:490–491, 1938.

79. Coffield, K. S., and Weems, W. L.: Experience with Management of Posterior Urethral Injury Associated with Pelvic Fracture. J. Urol., **117**:722–724, 1977.

80. Cohen, H. H.: Avulsion Fracture of the Ischial Tuberosity. J. Bone Joint Surg., **19**:1138–1140, 1937.

81. Colachis, S. C. Jr.; Worden, R. E.; Bechtol, C. O.; and Strohm, B. R.: Movement of the Sacroiliac Joint in the Adult Male; A Preliminary Report. Arch. Phys. Med. Rehab., 490–498, 1963.

82. Colapinto, V.: Trauma to the Pelvis: Urethral Injury. Clin. Orthop., **151**:46–55, 1980.

83. Colapinto, V., and McCallum, R. W.: Injury to the Male Posterior Urethra in Fractured Pelvis: A New Classification. J. Urol., **118**:575–580, 1977.

84. Coley, B. L.: Central Fracture of the Acetabulum. J. Bone Joint Surg., **23**:458–464, 1925.

85. Colp R., and Findlay, R. T.: Fractures of the Pelvis. Surg. Gynecol. Obstet., **49**:847–853, 1929.

86. Connes, H.: In Hoffman's Double Frame External. Paris, Gead, Anchorage, 1973.

87. Conolly, W. B., and Hedberg, E. A.: Observations on Fractures of the Pelvis. J. Trauma, **9:**104–111, **1969.**

88. Constantin, H. M., and Felton, L. M.: Separation of the Urethra from the Bladder due to Fracture of the Pelvis. J. Urol., **68:**823–830, 1952.

89. Conway, F. M.: Fractures of the Pelvis. A Clinical Study of 56 Cases. Am. J. Surg., **30:**69–82, 1935.

90. Conwell, H. E.: The Treatment of Certain Complicated Fractures of the Pelvis. Am. Surgeon, **18:**297–306, 1952.

91. Cooke, C. P., III; Levinsohn, E. M.; and Baker, B. E.: Septic Hip in Pelvic Fractures with Urologic Injury: A Case Report, Review of the Literature, and Discussion of Pathophysiology. Clin. Orthop., **147:**253–257, 1980.

92. Cooper, A.: A Treatise on Fractures and Dislocations of the Joints. London, Churchill, 1842.

93. Corlette, C. E.: Fracture of the Anterior Inferior Spine of the Ilium. Med. J. Aust., **14:**682–683, 1927.

94. Cottalorda, J.: Experimental Studies in Fracture of the Acetabulum. Lyon Chir., **20:**32–42, 1923.

95. Cotton, F. J.: Dislocations and Joint Fractures. Philadelphia, W. B. Saunders, 1924.

96. Coventry, M. B.: The Treatment of Fracture-Dislocation of the Hip by Total Hip Arthroplasty. J. Bone Joint Surg., **56A:**1128–1134, 1974.

97. Crane, J. J.: Rupture of the Urinary Bladder. Urol. Cutan. Rev., **36:**614–619, 1932.

98. Crile, G. W.: Blood Pressure in Surgery. Philadelphia, J. B. Lippincott, 1903.

99. Crosbie, A. H.: Rupture of the Urinary Bladder. J. Urol., **12:**431–437, 1924.

100. Cubbins, W. R.; Conley, A. H.; and Callahan, J. J.: Fractures of the Acetabulum. Surg. Gynecol. Obstet., **51:**387–393, 1930.

101. Culp, Ormond S.: Treatment of Ruptured Bladder and Urethra: Analysis of 86 Cases of Urinary Extravasation. J. Urol., **48:**266–286, 1942.

102. Culver, H., and Baker, W. J.: Rupture of the Urinary Bladder. J. Urol., **43:**511–531, 1940.

103. Cunningham's Textbook of Anatomy. Brash, J. C. (ed.) London, Oxford Press, 1951.

104. Curry, G. J.: Fractures of the Pelvis J. Bone Joint Surg., **21:**384–386, 1939.

105. Curry, G. J., and Lyttle, S. N.: Treatment of Multiple Severe Complex Injuries. Am. J. Surg., **83:**703–710, 1952.

106. d'Aubigne, M. R.: Management of Acetabular Fractures in Multiple Trauma. J. Trauma, **8:**333–340, 1968.

107. Day, L.: Open Book Pelvis: Symphysis Pubis Diastasis. Orthop. Trans., **2:**226–227, 1978.

108. Delort, P.: Quelques considerations sur le mecanisme, la symptomatologie et le traitement des fractures du le bassin en general. Paris Thesis, Vol. 15, 1898–99.

109. Derian, P. S., and Purser, T.: Intra-articular Small Bowel Herniation Complicating Central Fracture-Dislocation of the Hip. J. Bone Joint Surg., **48A:**1614–1621, 1966.

110. Derry, D. E.: The Influence of Sex on the Position and Composition of the Human Sacrum. J. Anat. Physiol., **46:**184–192, 1912.

111. Desault, P. J.: A Treatise on Fractures, Luxations, and Other Affections of the Bones. Ed. by Bichat, Fry and Kammerer, pp. 280–324, 1805.

112. deVries, J. E., and van der Slikke, W.: False Positive Peritoneal Lavage Due to Retroperitoneal Haematoma. Injury, **12:**191–193, 1980.

113. DeWeerd, J. H.: Case of the Severely Injured Patient—Urologic Aspects. J.A.M.A. **165:**1916–1921, 1957.

114. DeWeerd, J. H.: Management of Injuries to the Bladder, Urethra, and Genitalia. Surg. Clin. North Am., **39:**973–987, 1959.

115. DeWitt, R. F.: Method of Treatment of Fractures of the Acetabulum. J. Bone Joint Surg., **24:**690–691, 1942.

116. Diokno, A. C.: Late Genitourinary Tract Complications Associated with Severe Pelvic Injury. Surg. Gynecol. Obstet., **150:**150–154, 1980.

117. Dommisse, G. F.: Diametric Fractures of the Pelvis. J. Bone Joint Surg., **42B:**432–443, 1960.

118. Dommisse, G. F.: Function and Anatomy of the Pelvic Joints. J. Bone Joint Surg., **43B:**400, 1961.

119. Dorsey, J. S.: Inguinal Aneurism Cured by Tying the External Iliac Artery in the Pelvis. Philadelphia, 1811.

120. Dudgeon, H.: Pelvic Fractures and Dislocations Reduced by Turnbuckles. J. Bone Joint Surg., **24:**354–358, 1942.

121. Dunn, W., and Morris, H. D.: Fractures and Dislocations of the Pelvis. J. Bone Joint Surg., **50A:**1639–1648, 1968.

122. Duverney, J. G.: Traite des Maladies des Os. Vol. 1. Paris, De Bure l'Aíné, 1751.

123. Dwyer, B. E.: Assessment of Blood Loss after Trauma. *In* Nash, T. (ed.): The Medical and Surgical Management of Road Injuries. Sydney, Australia, E. J. Dwyer Pty. Ltd., 1969.

124. Eichenholtz, S. N., and Stark, R. N.: Central Acetabular Fractures. J. Bone Joint Surg., **46A:**695–714, 1964.

125. Eid, A. M.: Non-urogenital Abdominal Complications Associated with Fractures of the Pelvis. Arch. Orthop. Traumat. Surg., **98:**35–40, 1981.

126. Eliason, E. L., and Johnson, J.: Fractures of the Pelvis. Surg. Clin. North Am., **17:**1571–1584, 1937.

127. Elliott, R. B.: Central Fractures of the Acetabulum. Clin. Orthop., **7:**189–201, 1956.

128. Elton, R. C.: Fracture-Dislocation of the Pelvis followed by Non-union of the Posterior Inferior Iliac Spine. J. Bone Joint Surg., **54A:**648–649, 1972.

129. Emmett, J. L., and Witten, D. M.: Clinical Urography. Philadelphia, W. B. Saunders, 1971.

130. Engel, G. C., and Suigmaster, L.: Ligation of Internal Iliac Arteritis to Facilitate Abdominoperineal Resection for Malignancy of the Rectum. Surgery, **52:**867–870, 1962.

131. Farrington, J. D.: Severe Pelvic Fractures Treated by Fixed Skeletal Traction. J. Bone Joint Surg., **28:**150–152, 1946.

132. Faruzzi, E.: Le fratture isolate del sacro. G. Med. Milit., **106:**739–743, 1956.

133. Federle, M. P.; Crass, R. A.; Jeffrey, R. B.; and Trunkey, D. D.: Computed Tomography in Blunt Abdominal Trauma. Arch Surg., **117:**645–650, 1982.

134. Ferguson, I. A., Sr.; Byrd, W. M.; and McAfee, D. K.: Experiences in the Management of Arterial Injuries. Ann. Surg., **153:**980–986, 1961.

135. Flaherty, J. J.; Kelley, R.; Burnett, B.; Bucy, J.; Surian, M.; Schildkraut, D.; and Clarke, B. G.: Relationship of Pelvic Bone Fracture Patterns of Injuries of Urethra and Bladder. J. Urol., **99:**297–300, 1968.

136. Fleming, W. H., and Bowen, J. C. III: Control of Hemorrhage in Pelvic Crush Injuries. J. Trauma, **13**:567–570, 1973.

137. Flint, L. M.; Brown, A.; Richardson J. D.; and Polk, H. C.: Definitive Control of Bleeding from Severe Pelvic Fractures. Ann Surg., **189**:709–716, 1979.

138. Forsee, G. G.: Clinical Observations on Pelvic Fractures. Am. J. Surg., **38**:145–149, 1924.

139. Fountain, S. S.; Hamilton, R. D.; and Jameson, R. M.: Transverse Fractures at the Sacrum. J. Bone Joint Surg., **59A**:486–489, 1977.

140. Francis, C. C.: The Human Pelvis. St. Louis, C. V. Mosby, 1952.

141. Froman, C., and Stein, A.: Complicated Crushing Injuries of the Pelvis. J. Bone Joint Surg., **49B**:24–32, 1967.

142. Fuchs, E.; Bechtler, H.; Merkel, R.; Franke, D.; Hennig, K.; and Scheffler, W.: Die Notfall-Laparoscopie in der Unfallchirurgie. Unfallheilkunde, **81**:601–603, 1978.

143. Furey, W. W.: Fractures of the Pelvis with Special Reference to Associated Fractures of the Sacrum. Am. J. Roentgenol., **47**:89–96, 1942.

144. Gamble, J. G.; Simmons, S. C.; and Freedman, M. T.: The Symphysis Pubis: Anatomy and Pathology of a Commonly Neglected Joint. Read at A.A.O.S., New Orleans, Jan. 21, 1982.

145. Garcia, A., Jr.: Fractures of the Pelvis. In Bick, E. M. (ed.): Trauma in the Aged. New York, McGraw-Hill, 1960.

146. Gardner, W. J., and Storer, J.: The Use of the G-suit in Control of Intraabdominal Bleeding. Surg. Gynecol. Obstet., **123**:792–798, 1966.

147. Gardner, W. J.; Taylor, H. P.; and Dohn, D. F.: Acute Blood Loss Requiring Fifty-eight Transfusions; Use of Antigravity Suit as Aid in Postpartum Intra-abdominal Hemorrhage. J.A.M.A., **167**:985–986, 1958.

148. Gay, C. C. F.: Fracture of the Floor of the Acetabulum. N.Y. Med. J., **40**:699–701, 1884.

149. Geckeler, E. O.: Fractures and Dislocations. Baltimore, Williams & Wilkins, 1943.

150. Ger, R.; Condrea, H.; and Steichen, F. M.: Traumatic Intrapelvic Retroperitoneal Hemorrhage: An Experimental Study. J. Surg. Res., **9**:31–34, 1969.

151. Gerlock, A. J., Jr.: Hemorrhage Following Pelvic Fracture Controlled by Embolization: Case Report. J. Trauma, **15**:740–742, 1975.

152. Gertzbein, S. D., and Chenoweth, D. R.: Occult Injuries of the Pelvic Ring. Clin. Orthop., **128**:202–207, 1977.

153. Gibson, G. R.: Impotence Following Fractured Pelvis and Ruptured Urethra. Br. J. Urol., **42**:86–88, 1970.

154. Gibson, G. R.: Urological Management and Complications of Fractured Pelvis and Ruptured Urethra. J. Urol., **111**:353–355, 1974.

155. Gilmour, W. R.: Acute Fractures of the Pelvis. Ann. Surg., **95**:161–166, 1932.

156. Gioia, T.: Exceptional Variedad di Fractura isquio-acetobular. (Fractura de Walther por Causa indirecta.) La Semina Medica di Buenos Aires, **36**:725, 1929.

157. Glass, R. E.; Flynn, J. T.; King, J. B.; and Blandy, J. P.: Urethral Injury and Fractured Pelvis. Br. J. Urol., **50**:578–582, 1978.

158. Glynn, M. K., and Dunlop, J. B.: Eight Lateral Compression Injuries of the Pelvis Treated by the Hoop Apparatus of Lardennois. Injury, **12**:305–309, 1981.

159. Godfrey, J. D.: Major and Extensive Soft Tissue Injuries Complicating Skeletal Fractures. J. Bone Joint Surg., **44A**:753–766, 1962.

160. Godfrey, J. D.: Trauma in Children. [Avulsion Fracture Anterior Inferior Iliac Spine] J. Bone Joint Surg., **46A**:442–443, 1964.

161. Godshall, R. W., and Hansen, C. A.: Incomplete Avulsion of a Portion of the Iliac Epiphysis. J. Bone Joint Surg., **55A**:1301–1302, 1973.

162. Goldthwait, J. E., and Osgood, R. B.: A Consideration of the Pelvic Articulations from an Anatomical, Pathological, and Clinical Standpoint. Boston Med. Surg. J., **152**:595–601, 1905.

163. Goodell, C. L.: Neurological Deficits Associated with Pelvic Fractures. J. Neurosurg., **24**:837–842, 1966.

164. Goodwin, M. A.: Myositis Ossificans in the Region of the Hip Joint. Br. J. Surg. **46**:547–549, 1959.

165. Gordon-Taylor, G.: Complicated Injuries of the Urinary Tract. Br. J. Urol., **12**:1–28, 1940.

166. Grant, R. T., and Reeve, E. B.: Observations on the General Effect of Injury in Man with Special Reference to Wound Shock. Medical Research Council Special Report, Series No. 277. London, H. M. Stationery Office, 1951.

167. Greene, J. J., and Smith, D. H.: Fractures of the Pelvis; Analysis of 79 Cases. Arch. Surg., **38**:830–852, 1939.

168. Grieco, M. H.: Pseudomonas, Arthritis, and Osteomyelitis. J. Bone Joint Surg., **54A**:1693–1704, 1972.

169. Gross, A.: Stabilization of Pelvic Fractures with Hoffman External Fixation: The French Experience. In Brooker, A. F., Edwards, C. C. (eds.): External Fixation—The Current State of the Art, pp. 123–132. Baltimore, Williams & Wilkins, 1979.

170. Gumbert, J. L.; Froderman, S. E.; and Mercho, J. P.: Diagnostic Peritoneal Lavage in Blunt Abdominal Trauma. Ann. Surg., **165**:70–72, 1967.

171. Gunterberg, B.; Goldie, I.; and Slatis, P.: Fixation of Pelvic Fractures and Dislocations. Acta Orthop. Scand., **49**:278–286, 1978.

172. Hand, J. R.: Surgery of the Penis and Urethra. In Campbell, M. F., and Harrison, J. H. (eds.): Urology. Philadelphia, W. B. Saunders, 1963.

173. Hansen, E. H.; Jessing, P.; Lindewald, H.; Ostergaard, P.; Olesen, T.; and Malver, E. I.: Hydroxychloroquine Sulphate in Prevention of Deep Venous Thrombosis following Fractures of the Hip, Pelvis, or Thoracolumbar Spine. J. Bone Joint Surg., **58A**:1089–1093, 1976.

174. Harding, M. C.: Fractures of the Pelvis. Calif. West. Med., **31**:320–322, 1929.

175. Harris, W. H.: Traumatic Arthritis of the Hip after Dislocation and Acetabular Fractures: Treatment by Mold Arthroplasty. J. Bone Joint Surg., **51A**:737–755, 1969.

176. Harris, W. R.; Rathbun, J. B.; Wortzman, G.; and Humphrey, J. G.: Avulsion of Lumbar Roots Complicating Fracture of the Pelvis. J. Bone Joint Surg., **55A**:1436–1442, 1973.

177. Harrison, J. H.: The Treatment of Rupture of the Urethra, Especially when Accompanying Fractures of the Pelvic Bones. Surg. Gynecol. Obstet., **72**:622–631, 1941.

178. Hartmann, K.: Blasen- und Harnrohrenverletzungen bei Beckenbrüchen. Arch. Klin. Chir., **282:**943–948, 1955.

179. Hauser, C. W.: Initial Treatment of Pelvic Fractures. Lancet, **86:**285–286, 1966.

180. Hauser, C. W., and Perry. J. F., Jr.: Control of Massive Hemorrhage from Pelvic Fractures by Hypogastric Artery Ligation. Surg. Gynecol. Obstet., **121:**313–315, 1965.

181. Hauser, C. W., and Perry, J. F., Jr.: Massive Hemorrhage from Pelvic Fractures. Minnesota Med., **49:**285–290, 1966.

182. Hawkins, L.; Pomerantz, M.; and Eiseman, B.: Laparotomy at the Time of Pelvic Fracture. J. Trauma. **10:**619–623, 1970.

183. Haymaker, W., and Woodhall, B.: Injuries of the Peripheral Nerves Derived from the Lumbar Plexus. *In* Haymaker, W., and Woodhall, B. (eds.): Peripheral Nerve Injuries. Philadelphia, W. B. Saunders, 1945.

184. Haymaker, W., and Woodhall, B.: Injuries of the Sacral Plexus and its Constituent Nerves. *In* Haymaker, W., and Woodhall, B. (eds.): Peripheral Nerve Injuries. Philadelphia, W. B. Saunders, 1945.

185. Heller, J.: Catch-22. New York, Simon & Schuster, 1961.

186. Hirsch, L.: Fractures of the Pelvis. Beitr. Klin. Chir., **132:**441, 1924.

187. Holdsworth, F. W.: Dislocation and Fracture-Dislocations of the Pelvis. J. Bone Joint Surg., **30B:**461–466, 1948.

188. Holdsworth, F. W.: Injury to the Genito-urinary Tract Associated with Fractures of the Pelvis. Proc. R. Soc. Med., **56:**1044–1046, 1963.

189. Hollinshead, W. H.: Anatomy for Surgeons: The Thorax, Abdomen and Pelvis, Vol. 2. New York, Paul B. Hoeber, 1956.

190. Hollinshead, W. H.: Anatomy for Surgeons: The Back and Limbs, Vol. 3. New York, Paul B. Hoeber, 1958.

191. Holm, C. L.: Treatment of Pelvic Fractures and Dislocations. Clin. Orthop., **97:**97–107, 1973.

192. Holm, O. F.: Diagnosis of Rupture of Urinary Bladder. Acta. Radiol., **24:**198–205, 1943.

193. Hopkins, R. W.; Fratianne, R.; Penn, J.; Sabga, G.; and Simeone, F. R.: Controlled Hypotension in the Management of Severe Hemorrhage. Ann. Surg., **160:**669–680, 1964.

194. Horton, R. E., and Hamilton, S. G. I.: Ligature of the Internal Iliac Artery for Massive Hemorrhage Complicating Fracture of the Pelvis. J. Bone Joint Surg., **50B:**376–379, 1968.

195. Howard, F. M., and Meany, R. P.: Stress Fracture of the Pelvis during Pregnancy. J. Bone Joint Surg., **43A:**538–540, 1961.

196. Howell, J. B.: Pelvic Fractures. Mississippi Doctor, **21:**273–276, 1944.

197. Hubbard, S. G.; Bivins, B. A.; Sachatello, C. R.; and Griffen, W. O. Jr.: Diagnostic Errors with Peritoneal Lavage in Patients with Pelvic Fractures. Arch. Surg., **114:**844–846, 1979.

198. Hughes, C. W.: Vascular Injuries in the Orthopaedic Patient. J. Bone Joint Surg., **40A:**1271–1280, 1958.

199. Huittinen, V. M.: Lumbosacral Nerve Injury in Fracture of the Pelvis. A Postmortem Radiographic and Pathoanatomical Study. Acta. Chir. Scand., (Suppl) **429:**3–43, 1972.

200. Huittinen, V. M., and Slatis, P.: Fractures of the Pelvis. Trauma Mechanism, Types of Injury and Principles of Treatment. Acta. Chir. Scand., **137:**576–580, 1971.

201. Huittinen, V. M., and Slatis, P.: Fractures of the Pelvis. Trauma Mechanism, Types of Injury and Principles of Treatment. Acta. Chir. Scand., **138:**563–569, 1972.

202. Huittinen, V. M., and Slatis, P.: Nerve Injury in Double Vertical Pelvic Fractures. Acta. Chir. Scand., **138:**571–575, 1972.

203. Huittinen, V. M., and Slatis, P.: Postmortem Angiography and Dissection of the Hypogastric Artery in Pelvic Fractures. Surgery, **73:**454–462, 1973.

204. Hundley, J. M.: Ununited Unstable Fractures of the Pelvis. J. Bone Joint Surg., **48A:**1025, 1966.

205. Ikpeme, J. O., and Morison, C. R.: Vaginal Avulsion Complicating Pelvic Fracture. Br. J. Surg., **57:**317–318, 1970.

206. Innes, B.: Management and Results of Bladder and Urethral Injuries Complicating Fractures of the Pelvis. J. Bone Joint Surg., **47B:**600, 1965.

207. Irving, M. H.: Exostosis Formation after Traumatic Avulsion of the Anterior Inferior Iliac Spine. Report of Two Cases. J. Bone Joint Surg., **46B:**720–722, 1964.

208. Jahss, S. A.: Injuries Involving the Ilium. A New Treatment. J. Bone Joint Surg., **17:**338–346, 1935.

209. Jahss, S. A.: Injuries Involving the Pelvis. Am. J. Surg., **43:**394–403, 1939.

210. Jenkins, D. H. R., and Young, M. H.: The Operative Treatment of Sacro-Iliac Subluxation and Disruption of the Symphysis Pubis. Injury, **10:**139–141, 1978.

211. Jewett, E. L.: A Method for Treating Displaced Fractures of the Pelvis. J. Bone Joint Surg., **21:**177–181, 1939.

212. Johnson, H. F.: Derangements of the Coccyx. Nebraska State Med. J., **21:**451–457, 1936.

213. Johnson, R.: Stabilization of Pelvic Fractures with Hoffman External Fixation: The Colorado Experience. *In* Brooker, A. F., and Edwards, C. C. (eds.): External Fixation—The Current State of the Art, pp. 133–150. Baltimore, Williams & Wilkins, 1979.

214. Johnston, R. M., and Jones, W. W.: External Skeletal Pin Fixation (Hoffman) for Unstable Pelvis Fractures. Orthop. Trans., **3:**17–18, 1979.

215. Jones, D. B.: March Fracture of the Inferior Pubic Ramus. Radiology, **41:**586–588, 1943.

216. Judet, R.; Judet, J.; and Letournel, E.: Fractures of the Acetabulum: Classification and Surgical Approaches for Open Reduction. J. Bone Joint Surg., **46A:**1615–1646, 1964.

217. Judet, R.; Judet, J.; Lord, G.; and Orlandini, J.: Etude critique du traitement chirurgical de 20 observations de "disjonction traumatique de la symphyse pubienne." Presse Med., **73:**1787–1792, 1965.

218. Junge, H.: Neurological Complications of Fractures of the Pelvis. Mschr. Unfallh., **55:**1–6, 1952.

219. Kadish, L. J.; Stein, J. M.; Kotler, S.; Meng, C. H.; and Barlow, B.: Angiographic Diagnosis and Treatment of Bleeding Due to Pelvic Trauma. J. Trauma, **13:**1083–1085, 1973.

220. Kaiser, T. F., and Farrow, F. C.: Injury of the Bladder and Prostatomembranous Urethra Associated with Fracture of

the Bony Pelvis. Surg. Gynecol. Obstet., **120**:99–112, 1965.

221. Kapandji, I. A.: The Physiology of the Joints. Vol. 3, 2nd ed, pp. 52–71. Edinburgh, Churchill-Livingstone, 1974.

222. Kaplan, B. C.; Civetta, J. M.; Nagel, E. L.; Nussenfeld, S. R.; and Hirschman, J. C.: The Military Anti-Shock Trouser in Civilian Pre-Hospital Emergency Care. J. Trauma, **13**:843–848, 1973.

223. Kaplan, B. H.: Pneumatic Trousers Save Accident Victims' Lives. J.A.M.A., **225**:686, 1973.

224. Karaharju, E. O., and Slatis, P.: External Fixation of Double Vertical Pelvic Fractures with a Trapezoid Compression Frame. Injury, **10**:142–145, 1978.

225. Katzen, B. T.; Rossi, P.; Passariello, R.; and Simonetti, F.: Transcatheter Therapeutic Arterial Embolization. Diagn. Radiol., **120**:523–531, 1976.

226. Kaufman, J. J.: Cutaneo-osteovesical Fistula. Report of a Case Following Fracture of the Pelvis, Rupture of the Bladder, and Hip Fusion. J. Bone Joint Surg., **33A**:1017–1020, 1951.

227. Kaufman, J. J.: Bladder and Urethral Trauma. Trauma, **3**:77–128, 1963.

228. Kaufman, J. J.: Injuries to the Genitourinary System. *In* Nahum, M. (ed.): Early Management of Acute Trauma. St. Louis, C. V. Mosby, 1966.

229. Kelley, J.: Ischial Epiphysitis. J. Bone Joint Surg., **45A**:435, 1963.

230. Kerr, W. S., Jr.; Margolies, M. N.; Ring, E. J.; Waltman, A. C.; and Baum, S. N.: Arteriography in Pelvic Fractures with Massive Hemorrhage. J. Urol., **109**:479–482, 1973.

231. Key, J. A., and Conwell, H. E.: Management of Fractures, Dislocations and Sprains. St. Louis, C. V. Mosby, 1951.

232. Kicklighter, J. E.: Traumatic Rupture of Urinary Bladder. South. Med. J., **47**:837–841, 1954.

233. King, J.: Impotence after Fractures of the Pelvis. J. Bone Joint Surg., **57A**:1107–1109, 1975.

234. Kisner, C. D.: Injuries of the Urethra with Special Reference to those Occurring in Fractures of the Pelvis. South African Med. J., **32**:1105, 1958.

235. Klaue, P.: Indikationen zur Laparotomie nach stumpfem Korpertrauma mit Beckenfraktur Die Rolle der Peritoneallavage. Unfallheilkunde, **82**:327–330, 1978.

236. Knight, R. A., and Smith, H.: Central Fractures of the Acetabulum. J. Bone Joint Surg., **40A**:1–16, 1958.

237. Köhler, A.: Borderlands of the Normal and Early Pathologic in Skeletal Roentgenology, 10th ed. Case, J. T. (trans.). New York, Grune & Stratton, 1956.

238. Koster, H., and Kasman, L.: Treatment of Fractures of the Pelvis. J. Bone Joint Surg., **19**:1130–1133, 1937.

239. Koven, B.: Fracture of the Rim of the Acetabulum. Am. J. Surg., **2**:267–268, 1927.

240. Kreuscher, P. H.: Fractures of the Pelvis. Indust. Med., **5**:185–186, 1936.

241. Kumar, R.; Schaff, D. C.; and Ostrowski, E.S.: Entrapped Urinary Bladder: Complication of Pelvis Trauma. Urology, **16**:82–83, 1980.

242. Lam, C. R.: Nerve Injury in Fracture of the Pelvis. Ann. Surg., **104**:945–951, 1936.

243. Langan, A. J.: The Use of the Jones Splint in the Treatment of Fracture of the Pelvis and of the Neck of the Femur. J. Bone Joint Surg., **17**:435–442, 1935.

244. Langloh, N.D.; Johnson, E. W., Jr.; and Jackson, C.B.: Traumatic Sacroiliac Disruptions. J. Trauma, **12**:931–935, 1972.

245. Lardennois, R.: Huit cas d'enforcement due cotyle traites par l'appareil a areau. Ann. Chir., **13**:769–773, 1959.

246. Lavenson, G. S., and Cohen, A.: Management of Rectal Injuries. Am. J. Surg., **120**:522–526, 1971.

247. Lawson, L. J., and Wainwright, D.: Massive Hemorrhage Following Pelvic Fracture. Report of a Case. J. Bone Joint Surg., **50B**:380–382, 1968.

248. Leadbetter, G. W.: Fractures of the Pelvis. South. Med. J., **25**:742–745, 1932.

249. Leimbacher, E.: Injuries of the Pelvis. J. Bone Joint Surg., **25**:828–833, 1943.

250. Leinati, F.: Sopra un nuova case di frattura ischio-acetabuloare (frattura di Walther). Chir. Org. Movimento, **20**:416–420, 1936.

251. Letournel, E.: L'osteosynthese des fractures du bassin. *In* Actualities Orthopediques de l'Hospital Raymond Poincare, Vol. 8. Masson Edit., 1970.

252. Letournel, E.: Annotation to Karaharju, E. O. and Slatis, P. Injury, **10**:145–148, 1978.

253. Letournel, E.: Acetabulum Fractures: Classification and Management. Clin. Orthop. **151**:81–106, 1980.

254. Levine, J. I., and Crampton, R. S.: Major Abdominal Injuries Associated with Pelvic Fractures. Surg. Gynecol. Obstet, **116**:223–226, 1963.

255. Levine, M. A.: A Treatment of Central Fractures of the Acetabulum. J. Bone Joint Surg., **25**:902–906, 1943.

256. Lewin, P.: The Coccyx—its Derangements and their Treatment. Surg. Gynecol. Obstet., **45**:705–706, 1927.

257. Lewis, M. M., and Arnold, W. D.: Complete Anterior Dislocation of the Sacro-iliac Joint. J. Bone Joint Surg., **58A**:136–138, 1976.

258. Leydig, S. M., and Key, J. A.: Treatment of Fractures of the Pelvis. Surg. Gynecol Obstet., **69**:508–514, 1939.

259. Lich, R., Jr., and Howerton, L. W.: Anatomy and Surgical Approach to Male Urogenital Tract. *In* Campbell, M. F., and Harrison, J. H. (eds.): Urology, Philadelphia, W. B. Saunders, 1963.

260. Lichtblau, S.: Dislocation of the Sacroiliac Joint. J. Bone Joint Surg., **44A**:193–198, 1962.

261. Lombardo, L. J.: Heyman, A. M.; and Barnes, R. W.: Injuries of the Urinary Tract due to External Violence. J.A.M.A., **172**:1618–1622, 1960.

262. Looser, K. G., and Crombie, H. D., Jr.: Pelvic Fractures: An Anatomic Guide to Severity of Injury. Am. J. Surg., **132**:638–642, 1976.

263. Lowell, J. D.: Fractures of the Acetabulum. *In* Kane, W. J. (ed): Current Orthopaedic Management. New York, Churchill-Livingstone, 1981.

264. Lucas, G. L.: Missile Wounds of the Bony Pelvis. J. Trauma, **10**:624–633, 1970.

265. Lunt, H. R. W.: Entrapment of Bowel within Fractures of the Pelvis. Injury, **2**:121–126, 1970.

266. Lynch, K. M., Jr.: Traumatic Urinary Injuries: Pitfalls in their Diagnosis and Treatment. J. Urol., **77**:90–95, 1957.

267. McAvoy, J. M., and Cook, J. H.: A Treatment Plan for

Rapid Assessment of the Patient with Massive Blood Loss and Pelvic Fractures. Arch. Surg., **113:**986–990, 1978.

268. McCague, E. J., and Semans, J. H.: The Management of Traumatic Rupture of the Urethra and Bladder Complicating Fracture of the Pelvis. J. Urol., **52:**36–41, 1944.

269. McCarroll, J. R.; Braunstein, P. W.; Cooper, W.; Helpern, M.; Seremetis, M.; Wade, P. A.; and Weinberg, S.: Fatal Pedestrian Automotive Accidents. J.A.M.A., **180:**127–133, 1962.

270. McCarroll, J. R.; Braunstein, P. W.; Musolino, A.; Skudder, P. A.; and Wade, P. A.: The Pathology of Pedestrian Automotive Accident Victims. J. Trauma, **5:**421–426, 1965.

271. MacGuire, C. J.: Fracture of the Acetabulum. Ann. Surg., **83:**718–719, 1926.

272. McKay, H. W.; Baird, H. H.; and Justis, H. R.: The Management of Ureteral Injuries. J.A.M.A., **154:**202–205, 1954.

273. MacKinnon, K. J., and Susset, J. H.: Urinary Complications of Fractures of the Pelvis. *In* Moseley, H. F. (ed.): Accident Surgery, Vol. 2. New York, Appleton-Century-Crofts, 1964.

274. McLaughlin, A. P. III, and Pfister, R. C.: Double Catheter Technique for Evaluation of Urethral Injury and Differentiating Urethral from Bladder Rupture. Radiology, **110:**716–719, 1974.

275. McLaughlin, H. L.: Fractures of the Hips. *In* Moseley, H. F. (ed.): Accident Surgery, Vol. 2. New York, Appleton-Century-Crofts, 1964.

276. MacLean, L. D.; Duff, J. H.; Scott, H. M.; and Peretz, D. I.: Treatment of Shock in Man Based on Hemodynamic Diagnosis. Surg. Gynecol. Obstet., **120:**1–16, 1965.

277. McMurtry, R.; Walton, D.; Dickinson, D.; Kellam, J.; and Tile, M.: Pelvic Disruption in the Polytraumatized Patient. Clin. Orthop., **151:**22–30, 1980.

278. McNealy, R. W., and Willems, J. D.: Fractures of the Pelvis. Am. J. Surg., **8:**573–580, 1930.

279. Magnus, G.: Uber Beckenbruche, Behandlung und Resultate. Arch. Klin. Chir., **167:**667–670, 1931.

280. Malgaigne, J. F.: Treatise on Fractures. Philadelphia, J. B. Lippincott, 1859.

281. Marberger, M.; Wilbert, D.; and Ahlers, J.: Beckenfrakturen ohne Klinisch Manifeste Harntraktverletzung-Urologische Spatmorbiditat. Helv. Chir. Acta, **44:**339–343, 1977.

282. Margolies, M. N.; Ring, E. J.; Waltman, A. C.; Kerr, W. S., Jr.; and Braum, S.: Arteriography in the Management of Hemorrhage from Pelvic Fractures. New Engl. J. Med., **287:**317–321, 1972.

283. Matalon, T. S. A.; Athanasoulis, C. A.; Margolies, M. N.; Waltman, A. C.; Novelline, R. A.; Greenfield, A. J.; and Miller, S. E.: Hemorrhage with Pelvic Fractures: Efficacy of Transcatheter Embolization. Am. J. Radiol., **133:**859–863, 1979.

284. Mathe, C. P.: Management of Intractable Cystitis Associated with Vesical Fistula and Osteomyelitis of Pelvic Girdle. Report of Three Cases Following Traumatic Rupture of the Bladder and Fractured Pelvis. J. Urol., **43:**543–560, 1940.

285. Mathieson, A. J., and Mann, T. S.: Rupture of the Posterior Urethra and Avulsion of the Rectum and Anus as a Complication of Fracture of the Pelvis. Br. J. Surg., **52:**309–311, 1965.

286. Matthews, D. N.: Recent Advances in the Surgery of Trauma. London, J. & A. Churchill, 1963.

287. Maull, K. I., and Sachatello, C. R.: Current Management of Pelvic Fractures: A Combined Surgical-Angiographic Approach to Hemorrhage. South Med. J., **69:**1285–1289, 1976.

288. Maull, K. I.; Sachatello, C. R.; and Ernst, C. B.: The Deep Perineal Laceration—An Injury Frequently Associated with Open Pelvic Fractures: A Need for Aggressive Surgical Management. J. Trauma, **17:**685–696, 1977.

289. Mears, D. C.: The Management of Complex Pelvic Fractures. *In* Brooker, A. F., Edwards, C. C.: External Fixation: The Current State of the Art, pp. 151–177. Baltimore, Williams & Wilkins, 1979.

290. Mears, D. C., and Fu, F.: External Fixation in Pelvic Fractures. Orthop. Clin. North Am., **11:**465–479, 1980.

291. Mears, D. C., and Fu, F. H.: Modern Concepts of External Skeletal Fixation of the Pelvis. Clin. Orthop., **151:**65–72, 1980.

292. Medelman, J. P.: Incidence of Associated Fractures of the Sacrum. Am. J. Roentgenol., **42:**100–103, 1939.

293. Medical News: Injected Blood Clots can Stop Bleeding. J.A.M.A., **230:**952–954, 1974.

294. Metzmaker, J. N., and Pappas, A. M.: Avulsion Fractures of the Pelvis. Orthop. Trans., **4:**52, 1980.

295. Meyer, T. L., and Wiltberger, B.: Displaced Sacral Fractures. Am. J. Orthop., **4:**187, 1962.

296. Meyer, W. C., and Fahey, J. J.: Fracture of the Pelvis and Rupture of the Bladder Complicated by Pyogenic Arthrosis. J. Urol., **68:**297–301, 1952.

297. Michels, L. M.: Wounds of the Urinary Bladder: An Analysis of 155 Cases. Ann. Surg., **123:**999–1002, 1946.

298. Milam, D. F., and Miyakawa, G.: Urinary Tract Complications of Pelvic Fractures. Am. Surg., **29:**424–428, 1963.

299. Milch, H.: Avulsion Fracture of the Tuberosity of the Ischium. J. Bone Joint Surg., **8:**832–838, 1926.

300. Milch, H.: Ischio-acetabular (Walther's) Fracture. Bull. Hosp. Joint Dis., **16:**7–13, 1955.

301. Milch, H., and Milch, R. A.: Fractures of the Pelvic Girdle. *In* Milch, H., and Milch, R. A.: Fracture Surgery. New York, Paul B. Hoeber, 1959.

302. Miller, W. E.: Massive Hemorrhage in Fractures of the Pelvis. South. Med. J., **56:**933–938, 1963.

303. Mitchell, J. P.: Injuries to the Urethra. Br. J. Urol., **40:**649–670, 1968.

304. Mock, H. E., and Tannehill, E. H.: Fractured Pelvis Complicated by Gangrene of Extremity—Amputation under Refrigeration Anesthesia. Surg. Gynecol. Obstet., **78:**429–433, 1944.

305. Monohan, P. R. W., and Taylor, R. G.: Dislocation and Fracture–Dislocation of the Pelvis. Injury, **6:**325–333, 1975.

306. Moore, J. R.: Pelvic Fractures: Associated Intestinal and Mesenteric Lesions, Can. J. Surg., **9:**253–261, 1966.

307. Moore, J. R.: Intra-abdominal Visceral Injuries Associated with Pelvic Fracture. [Unpublished data]

308. Moore, J. R.: Genito-urinary Tract Injuries Associated with Pelvic Fracture. [Unpublished data]

309. Morehouse, D. D.; Belitsky, P.; and MacKinnon, K.: Rupture of the Posterior Urethra. J. Urol., **107**:255–258, 1972.

310. Morson, C.: Discussion on Rupture of the Urethra and its Treatment. Proc. R. Soc. Med., **35**:287–289, 1942.

311. Motamed, H. A.: Fractures of the Acetabulum. Int. Surg., **59**:20–24, 1974.

312. Motsay, G. J.; Alho, A.; Butler, B.; Perry, J.; and Lillehei, R.: Iliac Vein Trauma with Pelvic Fracture. Postgrad. Med., **51**:133–136, 1972.

313. Motsay, G. J.; Manlove, C.; and Perry, J. F., Jr.: Major Venous Injury with Pelvic Fracture. J. Trauma, **9**:343–346, 1969.

314. Moyson, F. R.; Duprez, A.; Bremer, G.; and DeGraef, J.: Evaluation et traitment du shock traumatique dans les fractures du leassin. Acta Chir. Belg., **56**:406–421, 1957.

315. Müller, J.; Bachmann, B.; and Berg, H.: Malgaigne Fracture of the Pelvis: Treatment with Percutaneous Pin Fixation. J. Bone Joint Surg., **60A**:992–993, 1978.

316. Muller, K. H., und Muller-Farber, J.: Die Osteosynthese mit dem Fixateur externe am Becken. Arch. Orthop. Trauma. Surg., **92**:273–283, 1978.

317. Müller-Farber, J., and Decker, S.: Das stumpfe Bauchtrauma als Komplikation der Beckenfrakturen. Unfallheilkunde, **82**:89–100, 1979.

318. Müller-Farber, J., and Müller K. H.: Stabile und Instabile Beckenringfrakturen. Arch. Orthop. Trauma. Surg., **93**:29–41, 1978.

319. Nelson, D. D.; Rubash, H. E.; and Mears, D. C.: Clinical and Biomechanical Aspects of Pelvic Fixation. Presented at Am. Acad. Orthop. Surg., Jan. 21, 1982, New Orleans.

320. Neuhof, H., and Cohen, J.: Abdominal Puncture in the Diagnosis of Acute Intraperitoneal Disease. Ann. Surg., **83**:454–462, 1926.

321. Newland, D. E.: Genitourinary Complications of Pelvic Fractures. J.A.M.A., **152**:1515–1520, 1953.

322. Nicholson, J. T.; Sherk, H. H.; Christides, S.; and Wilder, H.: Hip Sepsis Complicating Pelvic Fractures and Urologic Trauma. Clin. Orthop., **76**:21–26, 1971.

323. Noland, L.: Fractures of the Pelvis. Am. J. Surg., **38**:608–611, 1937.

324. Noland, L., and Conwell, H. E.: Acute Fractures of the Pelvis. J.A.M.A., **94**:174–178, 1930.

325. Noland, L., and Conwell, H. E.: Fracture of the Pelvis. Surg. Gynecol. Obstet., **56**:522–525, 1933.

326. O'Keefe, T. J.: Retroperitoneal Abscess. A Potentially Fatal Complication of Closed Fracture of the Pelvis. J. Bone Joint Surg., **60A**:1117–1121, 1978.

327. Okelberry, A. M.: Fractures of the Floor of the Acetabulum. J. Bone Joint Surg., **38A**:441–442, 1956.

328. Orator, V.: The End-Results in Fractures of the Pelvis. Arch. Klin. Chir., **74**:387, 1928.

329. Orkin, L. A.: Bedside Urological X-ray Examination of the Severely Injured Patient. Surg. Gynecol. Obstet., **94**:693–702, 1952.

330. Orkin, L. A.: The Diagnosis of Urological Trauma in the Presence of Other Injuries. Surg. Clin. North Am., **33**:1473–1495, 1953.

331. Orkin, L. A.: Traumatic Avulsion of the Bladder Neck and Prostate Complicating Fractures of the Pelvis. Am. J. Surg., **89**:840–853, 1955.

332. Ormond, J. K., and Cathran, R. M.: Simple Method of Treating Complete Severance of Urethra Complicating Fracture of the Pelvis. J.A.M.A., **102**:2180–2181, 1934.

333. Ormond, J. K., and Fairey, P. N.: Urethral Rupture at Apex of Prostate. J.A.M.A., **149**:15–18, 1952.

334. Orr, H. W.: Osteomyelitis and Compound Fractures of the Pelvis. Surg. Gynecol. Obstet., **54**:673–679, 1932.

335. Osmond-Clark, H., and Gissane, W.: The Abdomen and Pelvis, *In* London, P. S. (ed.): A Practical Guide to the Care of the Injured. Edinburgh, E. & S. Livingstone, 1967.

336. Pachter, H. L., and Hofstetter, S. R.: Open and Percutaneous Paracentesis and Lavage for Abdominal Trauma. Arch. Surg., **116**:318–319, 1981.

337. Papavoine, L. N.: Observation—d'un accouchement mortel: par suite de fracture et de deformation consecutive du bassin. J. Progres, **12**:234–244, 1828.

338. Parker, O. W.: Fractures of the Pelvis. Minnesota Med., **14**:29–41, 1931.

339. Paster, S. B.; Van Houten, F. X.; and Adams, D. F.: Percutaneous Balloon Catheterization. J.A.M.A., **230**:573–575, 1974.

340. Paton, D. F.: The Pathogenesis of Anterior Tibial Syndrome. J. Bone Joint Surg., **50B**:383–385, 1968.

341. Patterson, F. P., and Morton, K. S.: Neurologic Complications of Fractures and Dislocations of the Pelvis. Surg. Gynecol. Obstet., **112**:702–706, 1961.

342. Patterson, F. P., and Morton, K. S.: Neurological Complications of Fractures and Dislocations of the Pelvis. J. Trauma, **12**:1013–1023, 1973.

343. Patterson, F. P., and Morton, K. S.: The Cause of Death in Fractures of the Pelvis. J. Trauma, **13**:849–856, 1973.

344. Payne, R. F., and Thomson, J. L.: Myelography in Lumbosacral Plexus Injury. Br. J. Radiol., **42**:840–845, 1969.

345. Peabody, C. W.: Disruption of Pelvis with Luxation of the Innominate Bone. Arch. Surg., **21**:971–994, 1930.

346. Peacock, A. H., and Hain, R. F.: Injuries of Urethra and Bladder. J. Urol., **15**:563–582, 1926.

347. Pearson, J. R., and Hargadon, E. J.: Fractures of the Pelvis Involving the Floor of the Acetabulum. J. Bone Joint Surg., **44B**:550–561, 1962.

348. Pelligra, R., and Sandberg, E. C.: Control of Intractable Abdominal Bleeding by External Counterpressure. J.A.M.A., **241**:708–713, 1979.

349. Peltier, L. F.: Joseph Francois Malgaigne and Malgaine's Fracture. Surgery, **44**:777–784, 1958.

350. Peltier, L. F.: Complications Associated with Fractures of the Pelvis. J. Bone Joint Surg., **47A**:1060–1069, 1965.

351. Peltier, L. F.: Complications of Pelvic Fractures. Hosp. Med., **2**:88–93, 1967.

352. Peltier, L. F.: Historical Note: Joseph Francois Malgaigne and Malgaine's Fracture. Clin. Orthop., **151**:4–7, 1980.

353. Pennal, G. F., and Massiah, K.: Non-union Fractures of the Pelvis. J. Bone Joint Surg., **57A**:1022, 1975.

354. Pennal, G. F.; Tile, M.; Waddell, J. P.; and Garside, H.: Pelvic Disruption: Assessment and Classification. Clin. Orthop., **151**:12–21, 1980.

355. Perry, J. F.: Pelvic Open Fractures. Clin. Orthop., **151**:41–45, 1980.

356. Perry, J. F., Jr., and McClellan, R. J.: Autopsy Findings in 127 Patients Following Fatal Traffic Accidents. Surg. Gynecol. Obstet., **119:**586–590, 1964.

357. Petkovic, S. A.: A Clinical Study of Urethral Injuries. J. Urol., **75:**81–94, 1956.

358. Pick, M. P.: A Classification of Fractures of the Pelvis. Proc. R. Soc. Med., **48:**96–98, 1955.

359. Pierce, J. M., Jr.: Genitourinary Injuries in the Multiply Injured Patient. Orthop. Clin. North Am., **1:**75–91, 1970.

360. Poigenfurst, J.: Beckenringbruche und ihre Behandlung. Unfallheilkunde, **82:**309–319, 1979.

361. Poirier, P., and Charpy, A.: Traite d'Anatomie Humaine, Vol. 3, 2nd ed. Paris, Masson et Cie, 1904.

362. Pokorny, M.; Pontes, J. E.; and Pierce, J. M., Jr.: Urological Injuries Associated with Pelvic Trauma. J. Urol., **121:**455–457, 1979.

363. Poole-Wilson, D. S.: The Treatment of Injuries of the Urethra and Bladder. *In* Carling, E. R., and Ross, J. P. (eds.): British Surgical Practice. London, Butterworth, 1954.

364. Prather, G. C.: War Injuries of the Urinary Tract. J. Urol., **55:**94–118, 1946.

365. Prather, G. C.: Bladder Injuries: Treatment, Past and Present. N.Y. J. Med., **53:**318–323, 1953.

366. Prather, G. C.: Injuries of the Bladder. J.A.M.A., **154:**205–207, 1954.

367. Prather, G. C.: Injuries of the Bladder. *In* Campbell, M. C., and Harrison, J. H. (eds.): Urology, Vol. 1, 2nd ed. Philadelphia, W. B. Saunders, 1963.

368. Prather, G. C.: Injuries of the Bladder. *In* Campbell, M. C., and Harrison, J. H. (eds.): Urology, Vol. 1, 3rd ed. Philadelphia, W. B. Saunders, 1970.

369. Prather, G. C., and Kaiser, T. C.: Bladder in Fracture of Bony Pelvis: Significance of "Tear Drop Bladder" as shown by Cystogram. J. Urol., **63:**1019–1030, 1950.

370. Quain, E. P.: Rupture of the Bladder Associated with Fracture of the Pelvis. Surg. Gynecol. Obstet., **23:**55–62, 1916.

371. Quinby, W. C., Jr.: Fractures of the Pelvis and Associated Injuries in Children. J. Pediat. Surg., **1:**353–364, 1966.

372. Quinby, W. C., Jr.: Pelvic Fractures with Hemorrhage. New Engl. J. Med., **284:**668–669, 1971.

373. Radley, T. J.; Liebig, C. A.; and Brown, J. R.: Resection of the Body of Pubic Bone, the Superior and Inferior Pubic Rami, the Inferior Ischial Ramus and the Ischial Tuberosity. A Surgical Approach. J. Bone Joint Surg., **36A:**855–858, 1954.

374. Raf, L.: Double Vertical Fractures of the Pelvis. Acta Chir. Scand., **131:**298–305, 1966.

375. Raffa, J., and Christensen, N. M.: Compound Fractures of the Pelvis. Am. J. Surg., **132:**282–286, 1976.

376. Ralston, E. L.: Handbook of Fractures. St. Louis, C. V. Mosby, 1967.

377. Rankin, L. M.: Fractures of the Pelvis. Ann. Surg., **106:**266–277, 1937.

378. Ratliff, R. K., and Isaacson, A. S.: Intraperitoneal Rupture of Urinary Bladder Complicating Fracture of the Pelvis; Technics of Repair. Arch. Surg., **57:**681–685, 1948.

379. Ravdin, I. S., and Ellison, E. H.: Hypogastric Artery Ligation in Acute Pelvic Trauma. Surgery, **56:**601–602, 1964.

380. Ravitch, M. M.: Hypogastric Artery Ligation in Acute Pelvic Trauma. Surgery, **56:**601–602, 1964.

381. Redman, H. C.: Computed Tomography of the Pelvis. Radiol. Clin. North Am., **15:**441–448, 1977.

382. Reich, W. J., and Nechtrow, M. J.: Ligation of Internal Iliac (Hypogastric) Arteries: a Life-saving Procedure for Uncontrolled Gynecologic and Obstetric Hemorrhage. J. Int. Coll. Surg., **36:**157–168, 1961.

383. Reimer, B.; Gustilo, R. B.; Johnson, W.; and Simon, F.: Unpublished Data.

384. Reynolds, B. M., and Balsano, N. A.: Venography in Pelvic Fractures. A Clinical Evaluation. Ann. Surg., **173:**104–106, 1971.

385. Reynolds, B. M.; Balsano, N. A.; and Reynolds, F. X.: Pelvic Fractures. J. Trauma, **13:**1011–1014, 1973.

386. Reynolds, C. J.: Diagnosis and New Treatment of Traumatic Rupture of Posterior Urethra. South. Med. J., **35:**825–828, 1942.

387. Rieser, C., and Nicholas, E.: Diagnosis of Bladder Rupture: Unusual Features. J. Urol., **90:**53–57, 1963.

388. Ring, E. J.; Athanasoulis, C.; Waltman, A. C.; Margolies, M. N.; and Baum, S.: Arteriographic Management of Hemorrhage Following Pelvic Fracture. Diagn. Radiol., **109:**65–70, 1973.

389. Ring, E. J.; Waltman, A. C.; Athanasoulis, C.; Smith, J. C. Jr.; and Baum, S.: Angiography in Pelvic Trauma. Surg. Gynecol. Obstet., **139:**375–380, 1974.

390. Riska, H. B.; von Bonsdorf, H.; Hakkinen, S.; Jaroma, H.; Kiviluoto, O.; and Paavilainen, T.: External Fixation of Unstable Pelvic Fractures. Int. Orthop., **3:**183–188, 1979.

391. Riska, E. B.; von Bonsdorf, H.; Hakkinen, S.; Jaroma, H.; Kiviluoto, O.; and Paavilainen, T.: Operative Control of Massive Haemorrhage in Comminuted Pelvic Fractures. Int. Orthop., **3:**141–144, 1979.

392. Robertson, R. C.: Fracture of the Anterior-superior Spine of the Ilium. J. Bone Joint Surg., **17:**1045–1048, 1935.

393. Rogers, L. F.; Novy, S. B.; and Harris, N. F.: Occult Central Fractures of the Acetabulum. Amer. J. Roentgenol., **124:**96–101, 1975.

394. Rogge, E. A., and Romano, R. L.: Avulsion of the Ischial Apophysis. J. Bone Joint Surg., **38A:**442, 1956.

395. Root, H. D.; Hauser, C. W.; McKinley, C. R.; LaFave, J. W.; and Mendiola, R. P., Jr.: Diagnostic Peritoneal Lavage. Surgery, **57:**633–637, 1965.

396. Root, H. D., and VanTyn, R. A.: A Device and Method for the Atraumatic Transportation of the Injured Patient. Surgery, **58:**327–329, 1965.

397. Rothenberger, D. A.; Fischer, R. P.; and Perry, J. F., Jr.: Major Vascular Injuries Secondary to Pelvic Fractures: An Unsolved Clinical Problem. Am. J. Surg., **136:**660–662, 1978.

398. Rothenberger, D. A.; Fisher, R. P.; Strate, R. G.; Velasco, R.; and Perry, J. F., Jr.: The Mortality Associated with Pelvic Fractures. Surgery, **84:**356–361, 1978.

399. Rothenberger, D.; Velasco, R.; Strate, R.; Fisher, R. P.; and Perry, J. F., Jr.: Open Pelvic Fracture: A Lethal Injury. J. Trauma, **18:**184–187, 1978.

400. Rowe, C. R., and Lowell, J. D.: Prognosis of Fractures of the Acetabulum. J. Bone Joint Surg., **43A:**30–59, 1961.

401. Rowell, C. E.: Fracture of Sacrum with Hemisaddle Anes-

thesia and Cerebrospinal Fluid Leak. Med. J. Aust., **1:**16, 1965.

402. Rush, L. V., and Rush, H. L.: Avulsion of the Anterior Superior Spine of the Ilium. J. Bone Joint Surg., **21:**206–207, 1939.

403. Rutherford, H.: On Ruptured Urethra: Its Treatment by Combined Drainage. Lancet, **2:**751–753, 1904.

404. Ryan, E. A.: Hernias Related to Pelvic Fractures. Surg. Gynecol. Obstet., **133:**440–446, 1971.

405. Ryan, W. J.: Fractures of the Pelvis. Ann. Surg., **71:**347–359, 1920.

406. Sahlstrand, T.: Disruption of the Pelvic Ring Treated by External Skeletal Fixation. J. Bone Joint Surg., **61A:**433–434, 1979.

407. Saletta, J. D., and Freeark, R. J.: Vascular Injuries Associated with Fractures. Orthop. Clin. North Am., **1:**93–102, 1970.

408. Salomon, H.: The Diagnostic Puncture of the Abdomen. Berl. Klin. Wchnschr., **43:**45–46, 1906.

409. Salzberg, A. M.; Fuller, W. A.; and Hoge, R. H.: The Surgical Management of Profuse Hemorrhage from Uterine Carcinoma. Surg. Gynecol. Obstet., **97:**773–775, 1953.

410. Santaella, R. A.: Trauma to Pelvic Girdle and Urethra and its Treatment. Br. J. Urol., **18:**135–137, 1946.

411. Sargent, M. F.: Injuries of the Genital Tract. In Campbell, M., and Harrison, J. H. (eds.): Urology, Vol. 2. Philadelphia, W. B. Saunders, 1954.

412. Sashin, D.: A Critical Analysis of the Anatomy and the Pathologic Changes of the Sacro-iliac Joints. J. Bone Joint Surg., **12:**891–910, 1930.

413. Schmiedt, E.: Frakturen und Luxationen im Beckenbereich. Unfallheilkunde, **82:**331–339, 1979.

414. Schroeder, K. E., and Pryor, M.: Bilateral Sacroiliac Dislocations in an Adolescent: A Case Report. Clin. Orthop., **143:**191–193, 1979.

415. Schunke, G. B.: The Anatomy and Development of the Sacro-iliac Joint in Man. Anat. Rec., **72:**313–331, 1938.

416. Scott, W. W.: Trauma of the Genitourinary System. In Ballinger, W. F., II; Rutherford, R. B.; and Zuidema, G. D. (eds.): The Management of Trauma. Philadelphia, W. B. Saunders, 1968.

417. Scudder, C. L.: The Treatment of Fractures, 9th ed. Philadelphia, W. B. Saunders, 1923.

418. Seavers, R.; Lynch, J.; Ballard, R.; Jernigan, S.; and Johnson, J.: Hypogastric Artery Ligation for Uncontrollable Hemorrhage in Acute Pelvic Trauma. Surgery, **55:**516–519, 1964.

419. Seitzman, D. M.: Repair of Severed Membranous Urethra by Combined Approach. J. Urol., **89:**433–438, 1963.

420. Selakovich, W., and Love, L.: Stress Fractures of the Pubic Ramus. J. Bone Joint Surg., **36A:**573–576, 1954.

421. Semans, J. H.: Neurogenic Disease of the Bladder. The Surgical Management of its Complications. J. Urol., **6:**820–832, 1949.

422. Semba, R. T.; Yasukawa, K.; Gustilo, R. B.; and Kuslich, S. D.: Critical Analysis of Results of Malgaigne Fractures of the Pelvis. Presented at Am. Acad. Orthop. Surg., Jan. 21, 1982, New Orleans.

423. Seright, W.: Traumatic Closed Rupture of the Upper Ureter. Br. J. Surg., **46:**511–514, 1959.

424. Sever, J. W.: Obstetrical Paralysis. Surg. Gynecol. Obstet., **44:**547–549, 1927.

425. Sever, J. W.: Fractures of the Pelvis. New Engl. J. Med., **199:**16–30, 1928.

426. Sever, J. W.: Traumatic Separation of the Symphysis Pubis. New Engl. J. Med., **204:**355–357, 1931.

427. Sharp, I. K.: Plate Fixation of Disrupted Symphysis Pubis. J. Bone Joint Surg., **55:**618–620, 1973.

428. Sheldon, G. F., and Winestock, D. P.: Hemorrhage from Open Pelvic Controlled Intraoperatively with Balloon Catheter. J. Trauma, **18:**68–70, 1978.

429. Shepherd, J. A.: Intraperitoneal and Retroperitoneal Hemorrhage. In Shepherd, J. A.: Surgery of the Acute Abdomen, 2nd ed. Baltimore, Williams & Wilkins, 1968.

430. Shepherd, J. A.: Ureter: Genito-urinary System. In Shepherd, J. A.: Surgery of the Acute Abdomen, 2nd ed. Baltimore, Williams & Wilkins, 1968.

431. Shirkhoda, A.; Brashear, H. R.; and Staab, E. V.: Computer Tomography of Acetabular Fractures. Radiology, **135:**683–688, 1980.

432. Siegel, P., and Mengert, W. F.: Internal Iliac Artery Ligation in Obstetrics and Gynecology, J.A.M.A., **178:**1059–1062, 1961.

433. Siegel, R. S.: Vesico-vaginal Fistula and Osteomyelitis. J. Bone Joint Surg., **53A:**583–586, 1971.

434. Silva, J. F.: Management of Neglected Trauma. Springfield, Charles C Thomas, 1972.

435. Silver, C. M., and Rusbridge, H.: A Treatment for Displaced Fractures of the Pelvis. J. Bone Joint Surg., **27:**154–156, 1945.

436. Simpson-Smith, A.: Traumatic Rupture of the Urethra; 8 Personal Cases with a Review of 381 Recorded Ruptures. Br. J. Surg., **24:**309–332, 1936–1937.

437. Skillern, P. G., and Pancoast, H. K.: Fracture of the Floor of the Acetabulum. Ann. Surg., **60:**92–97, 1912.

438. Slatis, P.: Injuries in Fatal Traffic Accidents. Acta Chir. Scand., (Suppl) **297:**1–40, 1962.

439. Slatis, P., and Huittinen, V. M.: Double Vertical Fractures of the Pelvis. Acta Chir. Scand., **138:**799–807, 1972.

440. Slatis, P., and Karaharju, E. O.: External Fixation of the Pelvic Girdle with a Trapezoid Compression Frame. Injury, **7:**53–56, 1975.

441. Slatis, P., and Karaharju, E. O.: External Fixation of Unstable Pelvic Fractures: Experiences in 22 Patients Treated with a Trapezoid Compression Frame. Clin. Orthop., **151:**73–80, 1980.

442. Smith, K.; Ben-Menachem, Y.; Duke, J. H., Jr.; and Hill, G. L.: The Superior Gluteal: An Artery at Risk in Blunt Pelvic Trauma. J. Trauma, **16:**273–279, 1976.

443. Smith, M. J. V.; Nanson, E. M.; and Campbell, J. M.: An Unusual Case of Closed Rupture of the Ureter. J. Urol., **83:**277–278, 1960.

444. Smith-Peterson, M. N.; Rogers, W. A.: End-Result Study for Arthrodesis of the Sacro-iliac Joint for Arthritis—Traumatic and Non-traumatic. J. Bone Joint Surg., **8:**118–136, 1926.

445. Solonen, K. A.: The Sacroiliac Joint in the Light of Anatomical, Roentgenological, and Clinical Studies. Acta. Orthop. Scand., **27**(Suppl):12–127, 1957.

446. Sommer, G.: Traumatic Rupture of Symphysis. Beitr. Klin. Chir., **165**:607–618, 1937.

447. Sparrow, J. D.: Traumatic Separation of the Symphysis Pubis. J.A.M.A., **94**:27–28, 1930.

448. Speed, K.: Text-Book of Fractures and Dislocations. Philadelphia, Lea & Febiger, 1935.

449. Speer, D. P., and Peltier, L. F.: Pelvic Fractures and Pregnancy. J. Trauma, **12**:474–479, 1972.

450. Spence, H. M., and Boone, T. B.: Injuries of the Ureter due to External Violence. Am. Surg., **24**:423–430, 1958.

451. Spencer, F. C., and Robinson, R. A.: Division of the Pubis for Massive Hemorrhage from Fractures of the Pelvis. Clin. Orthop., **7**:189–201, 1956.

452. Spencer, F. C., and Robinson, R. A.: Division of the Pubis for Massive Hemorrhage from Fractures of the Pelvis. Arch. Surg., **78**:535–537, 1959.

453. Steenblock, U., and Durig, M.: Die Diagnostik des stumpfen Bauchtraumas—Peritoneallavage oder Notfall-Laparoskopie? Unfallheilkunde, **82**:530–532, 1979.

454. Stern, W. G.: Fracture-Dislocation of Sacro-iliac Joint Reduced by Well Leg Traction Method. Am. J. Surg., **32**:179–185, 1936.

455. Stevens, A. R., and Delzell, W. R.: Traumatic Injuries of the Bladder. J. Urol., **38**:475–485, 1937.

456. Stewart, M. J., and Milford, L. H.: Fracture-Dislocation of the Hip. J. Bone Joint Surg., **36A**:315–342, 1954.

457. Stickel, D. L., and Howse, R. R.: Injuries of the Ureter due to External Violence. Ann. Surg., **154**:137–141, 1961.

458. Stimson, L. A.: Fractures and Dislocations. Philadelphia, Lea & Febiger, 1917.

459. Stirling, W. C., and Belt, N.: Traumatic Rupture of the Bladder with Perivesical Extravasation. J.A.M.A., **92**:2006–2008, 1929.

460. Stock, J. R., and Harris, W. H.: The Role of Diagnostic and Therapeutic Angiography in Trauma to the Pelvis. Clin. Orthop., **151**:31–40, 1980.

461. Stone, H. H.; Rutledge. B. A.; and Martin, J. D., Jr.: Massive Crushing Pelvic Injuries. Am. Surg., **34**:869–878, 1968.

462. Sullivan, C. R.: Fractures of the Pelvis. A.A.O.S. Instructional Course Lectures, **18**:92–101, 1961.

463. Sutro, C. J.: The Pubic Bones and their Symphysis. Arch. Surg., **32**:823–841, 1936.

464. Swinney, J.: Traumatic Lesions of the Urethra. *In* Matthews, D. N. (ed.): Recent Advances in the Surgery of Trauma. London, J. & A. Churchill, 1963.

465. Tachdjian, M. O.: Fractures of the Pelvis. *In* Tachdjian, M. O.: Pediatric Orthopaedics. Philadelphia, W. B. Saunders, 1973.

466. Taylor, R. G.: Pelvic Dislocations. Br. J. Surg., **30**:126–132, 1942.

467. Thomford, N. R.; Curtiss, P. H.; and Marable, S. A.: Injuries of the Iliac and Femoral Arteries Associated with Blunt Skeletal Trauma. J. Trauma, **9**:126–134, 1969.

468. Thompson, K.: Fractures of the Pelvis Requiring Surgical Treatment. J. Bone Joint Surg., **45A**:437, 1963.

469. Tile, M.: Pelvic Fractures: Operative Versus Nonoperative Treatment. Orthop. Clin North Am., **11**:423–464, 1980.

470. Tile, M., and Pennal, G. F.: Pelvic Disruption: Principles of Management. Clin. Orthop., **151**:56–64, 1980.

471. Tool, C.: Intraperitoneal Rupture of the Urinary Bladder. J. Urol., **58**:431–434, 1947.

472. Torok, G.: Bilateral Sacroiliac Joint Dislocation with Intrapelvic Intrusion of the Intact Lumbosacral Spine and Sacrum. J. Trauma, **16**:930–934, 1976.

473. Trafford, H. S.: Traumatic Rupture of the Posterior Urethra. Br. J. Urol., **27**:165–171, 1955.

474. Trafford, H. S.: Types of Fractures of the Pelvis with Associated Urethral Ruptures and Relative Frequency. Postgrad. Med. J., **34**:656–657, 1958.

475. Trafford, H. S.: The Management of Urethral Injuries Associated with Pelvic Fractures. J. Bone Joint Surg., **47B**:376, 1965.

476. Treasure, R.: Spontaneous Fractures of the Pelvis in Middle-Aged Women. J. Bone Joint Surg., **45B**:223, 1963.

477. Trunkey, D.; Hays, R. J.; and Shires, G. T.: Management of Rectal Trauma, J. Trauma, **13**:411–415, 1973.

478. Trunkey, D. D.; Chapman, M. W.; Lim, R. C., Jr.; and Dunphy, J. E.: Management of Pelvic Fractures in Blunt Trauma Injury. J. Trauma, **14**:912–923, 1974.

479. Turner-Warwick, R.: A Personal View of Immediate Management of Pelvic Fracture Urethral Injuries. Urol. Clin. North Am., **4**:81–93, 1977.

480. Turner-Warwick, R.: Complex Traumatic Posterior Urethral Strictures. J. Urol., **118**:564–574, 1977.

481. Uhle, C. A. W., and Erb, H. R.: Reconstruction of the Membranous Urethra. Case Reports. J. Urol., **52**:42–60, 1944.

482. Urist, M. R.: Injuries to the Hip Joint. Am. J. Surg., **74**:586–597, 1947.

483. Urist, M. R.: Fractures of the Acetabulum. Ann. Surg., **127**:1150–1164, 1948.

484. Urist, M. R.: Fracture-Dislocation of the Hip Joint. J. Bone Joint Surg., **30A**:699–727, 1948.

485. Van Urk, H.; Perlberger, R. R.; and Muller, H.: Selective Arterial Embolization for Control of Traumatic Pelvic Hemorrhage. Surgery, **83**:133–137, 1978.

486. Vermooten, V.: Rupture of the Urethra—A New Diagnostic Sign. J. Urol., **56**:228–236, 1946.

487. Vidal, M. J.: Diagnosis and Management of Urethral Injuries. Med. Arts Sci., **9**:1–10, 1955.

488. Vidal, M. J.: Notre experience du fixateur extern de'Hoffmann. A propos de 46 observations. Les indications de son emploi. Montpellier Chir., **14, 4**:451–460, 1968.

489. Wakeley, C. P. G.: Fractures of the Pelvis: An Analysis of 100 Cases. Br. J. Surg., **17**:22–29, 1930.

490. Walther, C.: Recherches experimentelles sur certains fracturas de la cavietecotyloide. Bull. Soc. Anat. Paris, **5**:561, 1891.

491. Wangensteen, S. L.; deHoll, J. D.; Ludewig, R. M.; and Madden J. J., Jr.: The Detrimental Effect of the G-Suit in Hemorrhagic Shock. Ann. Surg., **170**:187–192, 1969.

492. Wangensteen, S. L.; Eddy, D. M.; and Ludewig, R. M.: The Hydrodynamics of Arterial Hemorrhage. Surgery, **64**:912–921, 1968.

493. Wangensteen, S. L.; Ludewig, R. M.; Cox, J. M.; Lynk, J. N.: The Effect of External Counter-Pressure on Arterial Bleeding. Surgery, **64**:922–927, 1968.

494. Ward-McQuaid, J. N.: Abdominal and Urological Injuries. J. Bone Joint Surg., **45B**:801, 1963.

495. Watson-Jones, R.: Dislocations and Fracture-Dislocations of the Pelvis. Br. J. Surg., **25**:773–781, 1938.

496. Watson-Jones, R.: Fractures and Joint Injuries. Baltimore, Williams & Wilkins, 1957.

497. Watts, W. B.: An Analysis of 48 Cases of Pelvic Fracture. Southwest Med., **9**:293–297, 1925.

498. Weems, W. L.: Management of Genitourinary Injuries in Patients with Pelvic Fractures. Ann. Surg., **189**:717–723, 1979.

499. Weems, H. S.; Newman, J. H.; and Florence, T. J.: Trauma of the Lower Urinary Tract. New Engl. J. Med., **234**:357–364, 1946.

500. Weil, G. C.; Price, E. M.; and Rusbridge, H. W.: The Diagnosis and Treatment of Fractures of the Pelvis and their Complications. Am. J. Surg., **44**:108–116, 1939.

501. Weil, M. H.; Shubin, H.; and Rosoff, L.: Fluid Repletion in Circulatory Shock. J.A.M.A., **192**:668–674, 1965.

502. Weisl, H.: The Ligaments of the Sacro-Iliac Joint Examined with Particular Reference to Their Function. Acta Anat., **20**:201–213, 1954.

503. Weisl, H.: The Movements of the Sacro-Iliac Joint. Acta Anat., **23**:80–91, 1955.

504. Weitzner, I.: Fracture of the Anterior Superior Spine of the Ilium in One Case and Anterior Inferior in Another Case. Am. J. Roentgenol., **33**:39–40, 1935.

505. Welch, C. S., and Powers, S. R., Jr.: The Essence of Surgery. Philadelphia, W. B. Saunders, 1958.

506. Wesson, M. B.: Fasciae of the Urogenital Triangle. J.A.M.A., **81**:2024–2030, 1923.

507. Westerborn, A.: Fractures and Dislocations of the Pelvis. Acta Chir. Scand., **63**[Suppl.]:7–375, 1928.

508. Westerborn, A.: Breitrage zur Kenntnis der Beckenbrucke und Becken-Luxationer. Acta Chir. Scand., **8**(Suppl):7–375, 1928.

509. Weyrauch, H. M., Jr., and Peterfy, R. A.: Tests for Leakage in Early Diagnosis of Rupture of the Bladder. J. Urol., **44**:264–273, 1940.

510. Wheeler, W.: Fractures of the Pelvis and Lower Extremity. Lancet, **11**:313–316, 1925.

511. Whiston, G.: Internal Fixation for Fractures and Dislocations of the Pelvis. J. Bone Joint Surg., **35A**:701–706, 1953.

512. White, R. I.: Selected Techniques in Interventional Radiology. J.A.M.A., **245**:741–744, 1981.

513. White, R. I. Jr.; Kaufman, S. L.; Barth, K. H.; DeCaprio, V.; and Strandberg, J. D.: Therapeutic Embolization with Detachable Silicone Balloons, J.A.M.A., **241**:1257–1260, 1979.

514. Wiesel, S. W.; Zeide, M. S.; and Terry, R. L.: Longitudinal Fractures of the Sacrum: Case Report. J. Trauma, **19**:70–71, 1979.

515. Wilenius, R.: Uber Beckenbruche. Acta Chir. Scand., **79**(Suppl):1–134, 1943.

516. Wilkinson, F. O. W.: Rupture of the Posterior Urethra. Lancet, **1**:1125–1129, 1961.

517. Wilson, J. N.: Fracture of the Pelvis Complicated by Ischaemia of the Lower Limb. J. Bone Joint Surg., **34B**:68–69, 1952.

518. Wilson, J. N.: The Management of Acute Circulatory Failure. Surg. Clin. North Am., **43**:469–495, 1963.

519. Winegarner, F. G.: Coccygectomy for Drainage of Pelvic Abscesses after Pelvic Wounds. Am. J. Surg., **121**:249–250, 1971.

520. Winter, J. E., and Marsh, H. O.: Traumatic Separation of the Symphysis Pubis. Orthop. Trans., **2**:221, 1978.

521. Wishner, J. G., and Mayer, L.: Separation of the Symphysis Pubis. Surg. Gynecol. Obstet., **49**:380–386, 1929.

522. Woodward, A. H., and Kelly, P. J.: An Unusual Fracture of the Sacrum. Minnesota Med., **57**:465–466, 1974.

523. Worland, R. L., and Keim, H. A.: Displaced Fractures of the Major Pelvis. Clin. Orthop., **112**:215–217, 1975.

524. Wotkyns, R. S.: Pelvic Fractures. *In* Eiseman, B., and Wotkyns, R. S. (eds.): Surgical Decision Making. Philadelphia, W. B. Saunders, 1978.

525. Wylie, W. D., and Churchill-Davidson, H.: A Practice of Anaesthesia. London, Lloyd-Luke, 1966.

526. Yap, S. N. L.: The Management of Traumatic Pelvic Retroperitoneal Hemorrhage. Surg. Rounds, 34–44, March, 1980.

527. Young, H. H.: Treatment of Complete Rupture of the Posterior Urethra Recent or Ancient by Anastomosis. J. Urol., **21**:417–449, 1929.

528. Young, H. H.: Lesions of the Hip Joint: Primary Acetabular Pathologic Changes and Primary Synovial Changes. Proc. Staff Meet. Mayo Clin., **29**:41–43, 1954.

14

Fractures and Dislocations of the Hip*   *Jesse C. DeLee*

FRACTURES OF THE NECK OF THE FEMUR

The quotation "We come into the world under the brim of the pelvis and go out through the neck of the femur" reflects the defeatist attitude that has long been held by medical and lay personnel toward femoral neck fractures.[90] The history of the development of treatment rationale for femoral neck fractures parallels the historical development of orthopaedic surgery itself. Specific milestones have included the principle of reduction by dynamic traction,[276,329] the importance of anatomical reduction and its maintenance in plaster,[434,435,436] the development of stable internal fixation devices,[111,198,199,358,359,376,377,422] and finally the development of implant arthroplasty[301] that led to the era of total joint replacement. In spite of these advances in the management of femoral neck fractures, in certain situations we must still refer to this entity as "The Unsolved Fracture."[386]

HISTORICAL REVIEW

Ambrose Paré, the famous French surgeon, recognized the existence of hip fractures over 400 years ago.[320] Sir Astley Cooper, however, appears to have been the first to attempt to delineate clearly between fractures of the femoral neck, or intracapsular fractures, and other fractures and dislocations about the hip.[96] He believed that nonunion of

intracapsular fractures was related to the loss of blood supply to the proximal fragment, that most femoral neck fractures would eventually heal but with a fibrous union, and that such patients would suffer "permanent lameness." He stated, however, that it was possible that the neck of the femur might be broken without tearing the periosteum or "reflected ligament" on the neck. In such cases, ossific union was possible without deformity.

Phillips, in 1867, introduced a technique for longitudinal and lateral traction to be used in the treatment of femoral neck fractures to eliminate "shortening or other deformity."[329] Maxwell, in 1876, reported the successful use of this technique.[276] Ruth, in 1921, advocated closed reduction and maintenance of the reduction in a "Phillips splint" for 8 weeks and non-weight bearing for 6 to 12 months post-traction.[345] He recognized the use of the capsular ligament as a "splint" to maintain the reduction.

Senn, in 1883, was able to obtain a higher rate of union of femoral neck fractures in dogs by using internal fixation.[358,359] As a result of this research, Senn made the following statement: "The only cause for nonunion in the case of an intracapsular fracture is to be found in our inability to maintain coaptation and immobilization of the fragments during the time required for bone union to take place." Nearly 100 years later, the successful treatment of femoral neck fractures is still dependent on these principles.

With the advent of x-ray, in 1902 Whitman advocated careful reduction and holding reduced fractures in a spica cast.[434,435,436] His results were never published,[88] but a series from St. Luke's Hospital noted a 30% union rate.[139] Watson-Jones subsequently estimated a union rate of approximately 40% from this method.[428] Cotton, 9 years later, recommended artificial impaction of fracture fragments by blows from a heavy mallet applied to the padded trochanter before cast application.[98] Wilkie,[439] in 1927, modified the Whitman method by using bilateral short leg casts connected by a transverse bar instead of a spica cast for fracture immobilization.

The first to have nailed a hip fracture appears to have been von Langenbeck, in 1850.[422] Konig, in 1875,[244] and Nicolaysen, in 1897,[313] advocated the use of nails in serious cases. In 1908, Davis reported the use of ordinary wood screws for the fixation of femoral neck fractures.[111] Similar screws for internal fixation were used by DaCosta in 1907,[109] Delbet in 1919,[113] and Martin and King in 1920.[271] A quadriflanged nail, designed to obtain better fixation, was developed by Hey-Groves in 1916, but it was made of unsatisfactory material.[198,199] Smith-Peterson, in 1931, using a triflanged nail, reported a series of open nailings in which he advocated reduction, impaction, and internal fixation.[377] The development and standardization of biocompatible metals by Venable and Stuck was an essential step in the success of this technique.[415,416,417,418,419] Smith-Petersen's technique was simplified by the introduction of the cannulated nail by Johansson in 1932[223,224] and Westcott in 1934.[433] This advancement allowed the surgeon to reduce the fracture closed and then fix the fracture blindly using the cannulated nail over a guide pin. While the triflanged nail was a major advancement in the treatment of this difficult fracture, it proved to be no panacea, and since then many surgeons have evaluated other forms of internal fixation.

A side plate was added to the triflanged nail by Thornton[403] in 1937. This ultimately led to the development of a solid nail plate by Jewett in 1941.[222] Telescoping nails or screws, which allow gradual impaction at the fracture site, were introduced by Schumpelick and Jantzen,[357] Pugh,[334] Massie,[273,274] Badgley,[21] and Clawson.[85] A screw that provided dynamic compression at the fracture site was introduced by Virgin and MacAusland in 1945.[421]

Moore, in 1934,[295] Gaenslen,[159] Telson and Ransohoff,[400] and Knowles,[241] in 1936, independently advocated the use of multiple pins for the internal stabilization of femoral neck fractures. Harmon, in 1944,[188] added a side plate to incorporate these pins. Deyerle perfected a side plate that also acted as a template for pin insertion and allowed the sliding of multiple pins in 1958.[119]

The use of bone grafts, alone or in combination with other methods of internal fixation, has been recommended by many authors[3,232,238,323] in an effort to decrease the incidence of nonunion and aseptic necrosis following femoral neck fracture.

Following the introduction of a stainless steel prosthesis by Moore and Böhlman in 1940,[301] other prosthetic designs were introduced by Judet,[229] Thompson,[401,402] and Moore.[298] Surgeons frustrated with the problems of management of femoral neck fractures subsequently turned to primary prosthetic replacement.[172,202,266] Improving results with total hip replacement have led some to recommend its use in certain femoral neck fractures.[367,368] The number of prostheses, both of the hemiarthroplasty and total joint arthroplasty type, currently available indicates that none are totally satisfactory. The search, therefore, continues for a more rational approach to the treatment of this complex fracture. A complete treatise on this subject is not possible, but the following section is an attempt to place treatment of the complex femoral neck fracture on a rational, physiologic basis.

ANATOMY

VASCULAR ANATOMY

Femoral neck fractures have all the problems associated with healing of intracapsular fractures elsewhere in the body. The hip joint capsule is a strong fibrous structure that encloses the femoral head and most of its neck. The capsule is attached anteriorly at the intertrochanteric line; however, posteriorly the lateral half of the femoral neck is extracapsular.[319] That portion of the neck that is intracapsular has essentially no cambium layer in its fibrous covering to participate in peripheral callus formation in the healing process.[150,319,326,356,364] Therefore, healing in the femoral neck area is dependent on endosteal union alone.[150,319,325,327,328,356] Unless the fracture fragments are carefully impacted, synovial fluid can lyse blood clot formation and thereby destroy another mode of secondary healing by the prevention of the formation of cells and scaffolding that would allow for vascular invasion of the femoral head. In addition, it is significant that for all practical purposes the femoral head is rendered largely avascular by a displaced fracture.[360] Union of the fracture can occur in spite of an avascular fragment,[73] although the incidence of nonunion is increased.[27,210,319,327,328,364] Even with optimum treatment, signs of aseptic necrosis and later segmental collapse occur.

The arterial supply to the proximal end of the femur has been studied extensively.[14,15,60,83,97,106,107,123,193,206,230,308,309,310,409,410,411,432,440] The description by Crock seems the most appropriate because it is based on three-plane analysis and provides a standardization of anatomical nomenclature.[106,107] Crock describes the arteries of the proximal end of the femur in three groups: (1) an extracapsular arterial ring located at the base of the femoral neck; (2) ascending cervical branches of the extracapsular arterial ring on the surface of the femoral neck; (3) the arteries of the round ligament.

The extracapsular arterial ring is formed poste-

riorly by a large branch of the medial femoral circumflex artery (Fig. 14-1 *bottom*) and anteriorly by branches of the lateral femoral circumflex artery (Fig. 14-1 *top*). The superior and inferior gluteal arteries also have minor contributions to this ring.

The ascending cervical branches arise from the extracapsular arterial ring.[319] Anteriorly, they penetrate the capsule of the hip joint at the intertrochanteric line; and posteriorly, they pass beneath the orbicular fibers of the capsule.[97] The ascending cervical branches pass upward under synovial reflections and fibrous prolongations of the capsule toward the articular cartilage that demarcates the femoral head from its neck. These arteries are known as retinacular arteries, described initially by Weitbrecht[193,424,430] (Fig. 14-1). This close prox-

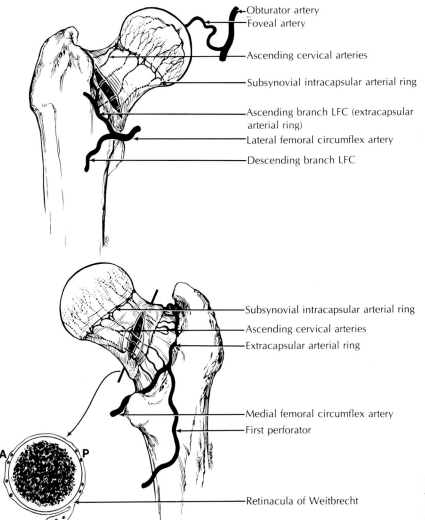

- Obturator artery
- Foveal artery
- Ascending cervical arteries
- Subsynovial intracapsular arterial ring
- Ascending branch LFC (extracapsular arterial ring)
- Lateral femoral circumflex artery
- Descending branch LFC

- Subsynovial intracapsular arterial ring
- Ascending cervical arteries
- Extracapsular arterial ring

- Medial femoral circumflex artery
- First perforator

A   P

- Retinacula of Weitbrecht

Fig. 14-1. Vascular anatomy of the femoral head and neck. (*Top*) Anterior aspect. (*Bottom*) Posterior aspect.

imity of the retinacular arteries to bone puts them at risk of injury in any fracture of the femoral neck.[319]

As the ascending cervical arteries traverse the superficial surface of the neck of the femur, they send many small branches into the metaphysis of the femoral neck.[97,206] Additional blood supply to the metaphyses arises from the extracapsular arterial ring and may include anastomoses with intramedullary branches of the superior nutrient artery system, branches of the ascending cervical arteries, and the subsynovial intra-articular ring. In the adult, there is communication through the epiphyseal scar between the metaphyseal and epiphyseal vessels when the femoral neck is intact.[106,410] This excellent vascular supply to the metaphysis explains the absence of avascular changes in the femoral neck as opposed to the head.

The ascending cervical arteries can be divided into four groups (anterior, medial, posterior, and lateral) based on their relationship to the femoral neck. Of these four, the lateral provides most of the blood supply to the femoral head and neck.[34,97,85,106,107,319] At the margin of the articular cartilage on the surface of the neck of the femur these vessels form a second ring that Chung has termed the *subsynovial intra-articular arterial ring*.[83] This ring was initially termed the circulus articuli vasculosis by William Hunter in 1743. Trueta and Harrison mentioned an incomplete subsynovial ring in 1953.[410] The ring can be complete or incomplete depending on anatomical variation, with complete rings being more common in male specimens.[83]

At the subsynovial intra-articular ring, epiphyseal arterial branches arise that enter the head of the femur. Disruption of this arterial ring has significance in high intracapsular fractures. Indeed, Claffey[84] demonstrated that in all femoral neck fractures that communicate with the point of entry of the lateral epiphyseal vessels, aseptic necrosis occurred (Fig. 14-2).

Once the arteries from the subsynovial intra-articular ring penetrate the femoral head, they are termed the *epiphyseal arteries*. Two distinct groups of vessels within the femoral head were described by Trueta as the lateral epiphyseal and inferior metaphyseal arteries.[409] However, Crock believes that these two groups of arteries actually arise from the same arterial ring and hence are both epiphyseal arteries.[106,107]

The artery of the ligamentum teres is a branch of the obturator or the medial femoral circumflex artery[97,206] (see Fig. 14-1 *top*). The *functional* presence of this artery has been variably reported in

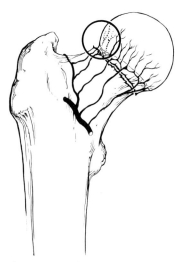

Fig. 14-2. A fracture line in the femoral neck may communicate with the point of entry of the lateral epiphyseal vessels into the bone of the femoral head-neck junction. Claffey[84] demonstrated that when this fracture pattern was present, all cases developed aseptic necrosis of the femoral head. When the fracture of the neck occurred distal to the entry of these vessels, the superior retinaculum that contained the lateral epiphyseal vessels was stripped of bone, allowing considerable displacement without damage to or tension on these vessels.

the literature.[14,15,78,84,206,326,410,432] Howe and associates[206] found that, although the vessels of the ligamentum teres did supply vascularity to the femoral head, they were often inadequate to assume the major nourishment of the femoral head following a displaced fracture. Claffey also reported that simple patency of the vessels of the ligamentum teres does not make them capable of keeping the head alive if all other sources of blood supply are interrupted.[84] Wertheimer and Lopes[432] found that only one-third of patients studied had a large artery of the ligamentum teres that supplied a substantial portion of the femoral head blood supply.

Trueta[410] believed that the femoral epiphyseal blood supply in the adult arose largely from the lateral epiphyseal arteries that enter the head posterosuperiorly and secondarily from the medial epiphyseal artery entering through the ligamentum teres. Sevitt also demonstrated that the superior retinacular and lateral epiphyseal vessels were responsible for the majority of femoral head circulation.[361] The vessels in the ligamentum teres (medial epiphyseal) were unimportant in most femoral heads, being responsible only for a small area of subsynovial circulation.[410] Anastomoses between the artery of the ligamentum teres and other arteries of the head and neck are variable.

Clinical Significance of Vascular Anatomy

Femoral head circulation arises, therefore, from three sources: intraosseous cervical vessels that cross the marrow spaces from below, the artery of the ligamentum teres (medial epiphyseal vessels), and chiefly by the retinacular vessels, branches of the extra-capsular arterial ring, which run along the femoral neck beneath the synovium. When a femoral neck fracture occurs, the intraosseous cervical vessels are disrupted; femoral head nutrition is then dependent on remaining retinacular vessels and those functioning vessels in the ligamentum teres.[360] The amount the femoral head supplied by the medial epiphyseal vessels varies from a very small area just beneath the fovea to the entire head.[361,432] The injection studies of Trueta and Harrison[410] and Judet and colleagues[230] demonstrate anastomoses between the various groups of vessels within the femoral head. In practice, however, such anastomoses may frequently be insufficient to nourish the whole head. Sevitt and Thompson believed that anastomoses between the subfoveal vessels and other vessels in the femoral head may be insufficient to support viability.[361]

The femoral head has for some time been recognized to be avascular, either partially or totally, in the majority of cases following displaced femoral neck fractures.[14,15,54,55,73,74,325,326,327,360] Phemister, Catto, and others have demonstrated that revascularization occurs through the remaining blood supply by the process of creeping substitution.[73,74,93,360] Bonfiglio* emphasized that although such revascularization through the marrow spaces may occur rapidly, actual *repair* of the necrotic bone is a much slower process, thereby setting the stage for late segmental collapse.

This revascularization after the vascular insult arises from three sources[326,327,360]: first, from areas of the femoral head that remain viable, especially the subfoveal area supplied by the medial epiphyseal vessels.[73,74] The importance of this source of revascularization is dependent on intraosseous vascular anastomoses between the medial and lateral epiphyseal vessels. Every attempt should be made, therefore, to protect the remaining vascular supply to the femoral head following fracture. The possibility that increased pressure within the hip joint will damage the already tenuous circulation has been mentioned by several authors, including De-

* Bonfiglio, M.: Personal communication, 1982.

yerle, who recommends aspiration of the hip if surgery is delayed more than a few hours and a decompressive capsulotomy in all cases at the time of internal fixation.[121,384,385]

The second source of revascularization is from vascular ingrowth across the fracture site. This is known to be slower than from the subfoveal area.[73,74] If the fracture site is first stabilized by fibrous tissue, this tissue may prevent vascular ingrowth into the head. In addition, the ingrowing vascular buds can be repeatedly torn by motion at a poorly stabilized fracture site.[73] Increased stability that protects these vascular buds may be the explanation for the reported decreased incidence of aseptic necrosis after open reduction and posterior bone grafting in femoral neck fractures.[289] Although revascularization across the fracture can be slow and incomplete,[73,74] studies by Ray in 1964 demonstrate that a bone graft can be revascularized within hours and suggest lumen-to-lumen connection of existing blood vessels.[338,339] Bonfiglio has demonstrated revascularization of the subchondral zone within 2 weeks of a grafting procedure.[50] These facts favor the prompt reduction and stable fracture fixation in the treatment of femoral neck fractures with the hope that the metaphyseal vessels may promptly reestablish and restore circulation before late segmental collapse occurs.

Third, revascularization occurs from vascular tissue growing in from that part of the femoral head not covered by articular cartilage.[360]

When discussing aseptic necrosis, it is important to differentiate aseptic necrosis and late segmental collapse.[264] Aseptic necrosis describes the infarct that occurs *early* following a femoral neck fracture, either secondary to the fracture, the reduction,[196,372] or the pinning.[60,61] In contrast, late segmental collapse is a term used to identify the collapse noted in the femoral head that occurs *late* in the course of the vascular insult.[73,74] The incidence of late segmental collapse is considerably less than that of aseptic necrosis.[264]

The x-ray appearance of aseptic necrosis is that of increased density. This density may be secondary to new bone being laid down on necrotic spicules, which produces an absolute increase in density,[325] to a relative increase in density owing to the osteoporosis of disuse present in surrounding vascular bone,[73] or to calcification that may be present in the necrotic marrow.[45] The x-ray appearance of late segmental collapse is that of flattening and fracture in the subchondral bone and articular cartilage overlying the infarct. This produces joint incongruity and arthritis.[264]

The position achieved at reduction is a significant factor in the development of an avascular episode and subsequent late segmental collapse. Valgus and rotatory malposition are known to affect the foveal blood supply,[196,372] and a higher incidence of aseptic necrosis has been recorded by Garden in all malreductions, whether they are in the extremes of valgus, varus, retroversion, or anteversion.[164,166]

Linton also suggested that a large nail may increase the incidence of aseptic necrosis.[259,260] The position of the nail in the femoral head can interfere with blood supply. Brodetti[60,61] and Claffey[84] both demonstrated that nails in the superior aspect of the femoral head can inadvertently interrupt the lateral epiphyseal vessels that supply a majority of the blood to the femoral head. Also, inadvertent perforation of the fovea in a patient whose head is dependent on the medial epiphyseal vessels for revascularization could change a partial necrosis to a total head necrosis.[73,74]

Finally, the use of screw fixation can result in rotation of the femoral head on its axis, leading to further compromise of the vessels of the ligamentum teres.[136,264]

Attempts to determine the viability and vascularization of the femoral head at the time of surgery have not been rewarding. Oxygen tension measurements,[444] venography,[209] isotopes,[10,55,224] intraosseous pressure,[14,15] and isotope clearance[205] all indicate a significant degree of disturbance in the vascular supply to the femoral head following fracture. Even using these time-consuming tests, the correlation between vascular findings and the clinical end result has never been more than about 80% accurate, and for this reason these techniques must still be considered research tools of little practical value in the management of the acute femoral neck fracture. Improved accuracy has been reported with Technetium-99m-sulfur colloid bone marrow scanning.[33,239,291] Although this method of determining femoral head vascularity is readily available, many patients with bone scan evidence of altered vascularity do not develop late segmental collapse or significant symptoms. The surgeon is, therefore, unable to determine from the scan which patients require initial treatment of the vascular insult to prevent long-term adverse sequelae.

In summary, there are two sources of viability of the femoral head after a displaced femoral neck fracture. First, the residual uninjured vascular supply may be sufficient to sustain the femoral head. Second, revascularization from the neck of the femur or surrounding soft tissue may occur *before* late segmental collapse. The aim of treatment,

therefore, is early anatomical reduction, impaction, and rigid internal fixation to protect existing circulation and to allow revascularization to occur *before* segmental collapse takes place.

SKELETAL ANATOMY

The femoral head is not a perfect sphere, and the joint is only congruous in the weight-bearing position.[72,425] This fact alone tends to cast doubt on the statement of those authors who suggest that reduction and fixation in any but the anatomical position are acceptable.

In 1838 the internal trabecular system of the femoral head was first described by Ward,[427] the orientation being along lines of stress with thicker lines coming from the calcar and rising superiorly into the weight-bearing dome of the femoral head. Forces acting in this arcade are largely compressive. Lesser trabecular patterns extend from the inferior region of the foveal area across the head and superior portion of the femoral neck into the trochanter, and hence to the lateral cortex. The presence of osteoporosis is important, especially in patients being considered for internal fixation, as the ability of osteoporotic bone to hold an internal-fixation device is minimal and hence such bone may affect treatment alternatives.[183] Singh (see p. 1258) used the trabecular pattern seen on x-rays of the upper end of the femur as an index for the diagnosis and grading of osteoporosis.[370] This system is based on the presence or absence of the five normal groups of trabeculae in the proximal femur as described by Ward[427] (Fig. 14-3). Although Khairi and associates found difficulty in interpreting the Singh index,[237] we use it as a *general* indication of the degree of osteoporosis present in the proximal femoral fragments as noted on the initial x-rays.

According to Harty[194] and Griffin,[177] the calcar femorale is a dense vertical plate of bone extending from the posterior medial portion of the femoral shaft under the lesser trochanter and radiating laterally to the greater trochanter, serving to reinforce the femoral neck posteroinferiorly (Fig. 14-4).[194] The calcar femorale is thickest medially and gradually thins as it passes laterally.[177]

The external and internal geometry of the femur and its effect on experimental fracture production has been well described.[20,155,156,347,348] Rydell, using a femoral prosthesis with a strain gauge, has made considerable contributions regarding the forces acting on the femoral head.[347,348] He showed that standing on one leg generated a force 2.5 times body weight in that hip. In one-leg support, with a cane in the *opposite* hand, the force across the hip

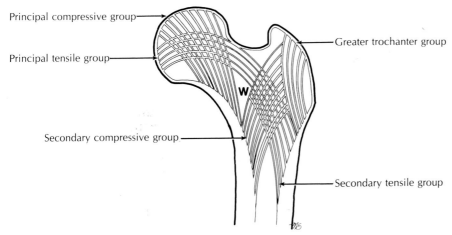

Fig. 14-3. Anatomy of the bony trabeculae in the proximal end of the femur. In a nonosteoporotic femur, all five groups of bony trabeculae are readily evident on x-ray. Ward's triangle (W) is a small area in the neck of the femur that contains thin and loosely arranged trabeculae only.

is reduced to body weight. At rest with two-leg support, there was a force of approximately half body weight across each hip joint, while standing with the hip and knee flexed 90° increased the force to near body weight across the flexed hip. Running was noted to increase these forces to five times body weight.[335] Rydell also found that lifting the leg from a supine position with the knee straight produces a force of 1.5 times body weight across the hip joint.[347,348]

ETIOLOGIC FACTORS

QUALITY OF BONE

Femoral neck fractures are uncommon in young patients with normal bone[17,333] and in older patients in races in which osteoporosis is uncommon such as the American Negro[136,137,139,140,180,294] and the South African Bantu.[380] The average age of patients with femoral neck fractures is 3 years younger than those with trochanteric fractures, both occurring most commonly in the eighth decade.[5]

Studies suggest that femoral neck fractures should be considered fractures through pathological bone secondary to either osteomalacia[394] or osteoporosis.[396] An association between osteomalacia and femoral neck fractures has been suggested by Alffram,[5] Chalmers and associates,[76] and Jenkins and associates.[219] Anderson and associates[6] reported osteomalacia in 4% of unselected elderly females, and Chalmers and associates[76] revealed that 12% of patients with osteomalacia initially present with femoral neck fractures.[76] Hodkinson was unable to

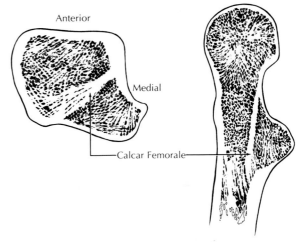

Fig. 14-4. (*Left*) The calcar femorale is a vertical plate of bone that originates in the posteromedial portion of the femoral shaft under the lesser trochanter, and radiates laterally toward the posterior aspect of the greater trochanter. (*Right*) The calcar femorale fuses with the posterior aspect of the femoral neck superiorly and extends distally anterior to the lesser trochanter and fuses with the posteromedial aspect of the femoral diaphysis.

demonstrate an increased incidence of osteomalacia in patients with femoral neck fractures. However, he did show a high incidence of low calcium and phosphorus products in their blood analysis.[204]

Although osteomalacia may be an underlying cause in some patients, the more commonly held concept is that femoral neck fractures are preceded by the development of osteoporosis.[246,257,423] Hip fracture patients have bone that is more osteoporotic than age and sex match controls, as has been documented by iliac biopsy photomicrographs,[394] x-ray analysis of femoral neck films,[394] lumbar spine films,[257,263,315,394] and metacarpal cortical thickness evaluation.[315,394]

The history of minor trauma associated with most femoral neck fractures further suggests that these fractures are secondary to primary skeletal pathology.[396] In addition, femoral neck fractures are much more common in elderly women. Frangakis believed that this was secondary to the senile osteoporosis seen in women in advanced age.[149] Barnes and co-workers demonstrated an increasing degree of osteoporosis in advancing age, especially in women.[28] Bonfiglio believed that women suffer from fractures of the neck of the femur because of "osteoporosis secondary to inactivity and aggravated by disease."[50]

Not only does osteoporosis play a role in the etiology of femoral neck fractures, it also plays an important role in their treatment.[183,252] Osteoporotic bone leads to more marked comminution of the posterior cortex[37,259,353,354] and to decreased quality of internal fixation secondary to the inability of the bone to hold internal fixation devices.[183,414] Arnold demonstrated a relationship between the failure rate of internal fixation and nonunion and the presence of osteoporotic bone.[12]

MECHANISM OF INJURY

The majority of patients suffering femoral neck fractures have experienced trivial or minor injuries. Indeed, only a few involve major trauma.[24] Kocher suggested two mechanisms of injury in femoral neck fractures.[242] The first is that of a fall producing a direct blow over the greater trochanter.[242] This mechanism was confirmed by Linton.[259] The second mechanism is that of lateral rotation of the extremity.[242] In this mechanism the head is firmly fixed by the anterior capsule and iliofemoral ligaments while the neck rotates posteriorly. The posterior cortex impinges on the acetabulum, and the neck buckles. This mechanism is compatible with the marked posterior comminution of the neck emphasized by Scheck[353,354,355] and is favored by Backman,[20] Banks,[24] Klenerman,[240] and Lowell.[262,263,264] A third recently suggested mechanism is cyclical loading, which produces micro- and macro- fractures.[412] It has been shown that forces within physiologic limits can produce fractures in osteoporotic bone.[157,178,404] It is suggested that a stress

fracture of this type becomes complete following a minor torsional injury that precedes the fall the patient identifies with the fracture. It has been shown that muscles produce an axial load along the longitudinal axis of the femoral neck and, coupled with external pressure, help to detemine the fracture pattern.[21,203,286]

In the case of young patients with femoral neck fractures, the resultant trauma is major, usually resulting in a direct force along the shaft of the femur with or without a rotational component.[333] The increased magnitude of trauma involved leads to more marked soft tissue stripping and comminution, which give rise to the increased incidence of failure in treatment of these fractures in young adults.[333]

CLASSIFICATION

CLASSIFICATION BASED ON *PATIENT* CHARACTERISTICS

1. Femoral neck fracture in the elderly patient
   a. Impacted fractures
   b. Displaced fractures
2. Fractures of the femoral neck diagnosed late
3. Femoral neck fracture in the young adult below 40 years of age
4. Stress fracture of the femoral neck
5. Ipsilateral fracture of the femoral neck and femoral shaft
6. Femoral neck fractures in patients with Paget's disease
7. Femoral neck fractures in patients with Parkinson's disease
8. Fractures of the femoral neck in patients with spastic hemiplegia
9. Postradiation fracture of the femoral neck
10. Pathologic femoral neck fractures secondary to metastatic disease of bone

CLASSIFICATION BASED ON *FRACTURE* CHARACTERISTICS

The three common classifications of femoral neck fractures are those based on (1) anatomical location of the fracture[428] (2) the direction of the fracture angle[324] and (3) displacement of the fracture fragments.[164]

Anatomical Location

Some authors classify intracapsular fractures of the neck of the femur anatomically into subcapital and transcervical types.[10,18,34,136,236,428] The so-called base of the neck fracture is extracapsular and therefore is not included in this discussion. The term *subcapital* is used to describe fractures that occur immediately beneath the articular surface of the femoral head along the old epiphyseal plate.[240] A transcervical fracture refers to a fracture passing across the femoral neck between the femoral head and the greater trochanter.[240] Klenerman and Marcuson[240] and Garden[167] suggest that the exact location of the fracture in the femoral neck cannot be determined distinctly by x-rays. Bayliss and colleagues[34] believed that there is no functional difference in subcapital and transcervical fractures. Askin and Bryan[17] agree that subcapital and transcervical fractures are essentially the same and that any identified difference is artifactual secondary to x-ray parallax. In addition, Klenerman and associates were unable to find a true transverse cervical femoral neck fracture in their series, the fractures being all of the subcapital type.[240] Banks, on the other hand, divided his patients anatomically into four types: classical subcapital fracture, wedge subcapital fracture, inferior beak fracture, and mid-neck fracture.[24] In essence, his first three types are all of the subcapital variety. He, too, found the transcervical type to be extremely rare. Owing to the relative infrequency of true transcervical fractures and the difficulty of describing the fractures by x-ray as noted in the above series, we have not used this classification.

Fracture Angle (Pauwels' Classification)

Pauwels divided femoral neck fractures into three types based on the direction of the fracture line across the femoral neck.[324] Type I is a fracture 30° from the horizontal; type II, 50° from the horizontal; and type III, 70° from the horizontal (Fig. 14-5). Type I fractures are therefore much more horizontal than type III, which are almost vertical. Pauwels

attributed nonunions in type III to the increased shearing force of this vertical fracture.[324] However, Boyd and Salvatore were unable to demonstrate a direct relationship between the angle of the fracture and the incidence of aseptic necrosis or nonunion.[57] Type II fractures had a 12% nonunion and 33% aseptic necrosis rate as compared to type III fractures with only 8% nonunion and 30% aseptic necrosis rate.[57] Also, Cassebaum and Nugent[69] and Ohman and colleagues[316] could find no relation between end results and Pauwels' fracture types.

Pauwels' classification is based on the x-ray shadow of the fracture line. Garden stated that,[167] because the femoral neck is spiral in shape, it is the *x-ray projection of the fracture line* and not the fracture line itself that varies in obliquity with rotation of the distal fragment. Garden found the fracture line to be remarkably constant at 50° from the horizontal on the frontal x-ray.[165] He believed that any change in obliquity is the result of a misinterpretation of the x-ray examination. He believed, therefore, that Pauwels' classification was a better measure of reduction than an indication of the angle at which the femoral neck was broken.[167] Linton[259] stressed that the direction of the fracture line on the x-ray could be altered by changing the direction of the beam *or* position of the limb. To be accurate, the x-ray must be made with the femoral neck parallel to the film. This is difficult and is rarely obtained because of pain. Linton also found that the inclination of the fracture surface did not vary greatly, with over 85% being between 45° and 60°. He proposed that the various types of femoral neck fractures represented different stages of the same displacing movement.[259] Owing to the findings of Garden[165] and Linton[259] and the fact that Boyd and Salvatore[57] found little difference in the nonunion and aseptic necrosis rates of type II and III fractures, we have elected not to use Pauwels' classification system.

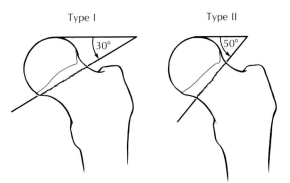

Type I   Type II

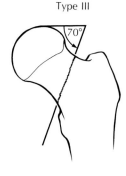

Type III

Fig. 14-5. Pauwels' classification of femoral neck fractures is based on the angle the fracture forms with the horizontal plane. As a fracture progresses from type I to type III, the obliquity of the fracture line increases and, theoretically, the shear forces at the fracture site also increase.

Fracture Displacement (Garden Classification)

Garden proposed a classification system based on the degree of displacement of the fracture noted on *pre*reduction x-rays[162,163,164,165,166,167] (Fig. 14-6). Garden agreed with Linton, who suggested that the various types of subcapital fractures were actually different degrees of displacement of a single fracture type.[259]

The Garden I fracture is an incomplete or impacted fracture. In these fractures, the trabeculae of the inferior neck are still intact. This group includes the "abducted impaction fracture." A Garden II fracture is a complete fracture without displacement. The x-ray demonstrates that the weight-bearing trabeculae are interrupted by a fracture line across the entire neck of the femur. A Garden III fracture is a complete fracture with partial displacement. In this fracture, there are frequently shortening and external rotation of the distal fragment. The retinaculum of Weitbrecht[430] remains attached to, and maintains continuity between, the proximal and distal fragments. In the Garden III fracture the trabecular pattern of the femoral head does not line up with that of the acetabulum, demonstrating incomplete displacement between the femoral fracture fragments. A Garden IV fracture is a complete fracture with total displacement of the fracture fragments. In this fracture all continuity between the proximal distal fragments is disrupted. The femoral head assumes a normal relationship in the acetabulum. Therefore, the trabecular pattern of the femoral head lines up with the trabecular pattern of the acetabulum.

Garden believes that in the Garden I and II fractures the challenge of the femoral neck fracture has been solved. Garden III and IV fractures are those that still have a significant degree of failure associated with their management.[167]

DIAGNOSIS

STRESS FRACTURES AND IMPACTED FRACTURES

Patients with stress fractures and those with impacted fractures may complain of only slight pain in the groin or referred along the medial side of the knee. They may be able to walk with an antalgic limp and therefore delay seeking treatment, thinking that they are suffering only from a muscle problem.[264]

Physical examination reveals no obvious clinical deformity. Only minor discomfort is produced by active or passive range of motion of the hip, but usually some muscle spasm is associated with the extremes of motion. Percussion over the greater trochanter is particularly painful. Failure to recognize nondisplaced stress fractures or impacted fractures may result in fracture displacement on weight bearing. This complication can be avoided if all patients complaining of hip or thigh pain after an injury, or those exposed to stress (*e.g.* military recruits, joggers), are *assumed* to have a fractured hip.[136] If the initial x-rays are negative, but pain persists, the patient should still be suspected of having a femoral neck fracture. He should be placed on crutches and additional x-rays obtained in 10 to 14 days. By this time the osteolysis associated with early fracture union should demonstrate the fracture line. In some cases, x-ray tomograms or bone scans may be required in the diagnosis of these fractures.[332] A correct diagnosis is the reward for a high index of suspicion in these patients.

DISPLACED FRACTURES

In patients with *displaced* intracapsular fractures, there is pain in the entire hip region. The patient lies with the leg in external rotation, abduction, and slight shortening. These patients do not present with the extreme deformity present in dislocations of the hip or that seen in intertrochanteric fractures because of the partially intact capsule.[264] Efforts to move the leg to elicit crepitus are condemnable. The limb should be splinted when the diagnosis is suspected. Buck's traction is applied to prevent further soft-tissue injury and to protect the remaining vascular supply to the femoral head.[264,384,385]

The diagnosis in displaced fractures is easily confirmed by routine x-ray. X-ray evaluation of the fracture type, the degree of posterior comminution, and the presence or absence of osteoporosis are essential *prior* to selection of the treatment regimen. The routine x-ray evaluation of a patient with a hip fracture should include a true anteroposterior view with the maximum degree of internal rotation possible, and a lateral x-ray.[225] If these views cannot be obtained on arrival, they should be taken under anesthesia just prior to selecting the desired treatment approach.

TREATMENT

IMPACTED AND NONDISPLACED FRACTURES (GARDEN I AND GARDEN II)

The impacted or "abduction" fracture of the femoral neck is distinctly different from an undisplaced fracture. Impacted fractures constitute 15% to 20% of femoral neck fractures[89,104,143] and are usually classified as Garden I fractures. The undisplaced

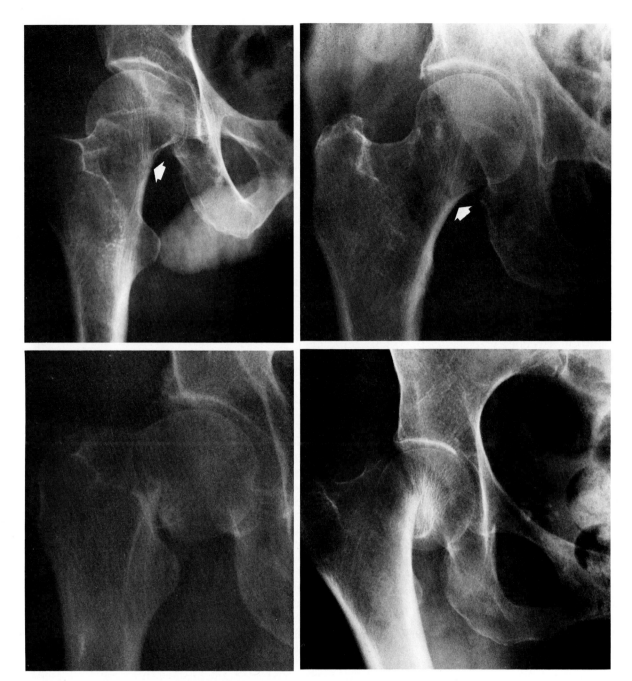

Fig. 14-6. Garden's classification of femoral neck fractures.[167] (*Top left*) Stage I fractures are incomplete or impacted. The trabeculae of the inferior neck may remain intact. The femoral head is tilted in a posterolateral direction. (*Top right*) Stage II fractures are complete fractures of the femoral neck without displacement. The x-ray demonstrates that the weight-bearing trabeculae are interrupted by a fracture line across the entire neck of the femur, but their alignment is undisturbed. (*Bottom left*) Stage III fractures are complete with partial displacement. The trabecular pattern of the femoral head does not line up with the trabecular pattern of the acetabulum, demonstrating incomplete displacement between the femoral neck fracture fragments. (*Bottom right*) Stage IV fractures are complete with total displacement of the fracture fragments. All continuity between the proximal and distal fragments is disrupted, therefore the trabecular pattern of the femoral head lines up with the trabecular pattern of the acetabulum.

fracture, on the other hand, has no bone impaction and hence no inherent stability; these correspond to Garden II fractures. Displacement is likely in undisplaced fractures unless they are internally fixed.[319]

Smith,[375] in 1845, stated, "osseous union of intracapsular fractures is most likely to occur when the fracture is impacted." In the impacted fracture, the femoral neck cortex is driven into the cancellous femoral head, which assumes a valgus or abducted position.[24,139] Although varus impacted fractures have been mentioned, Lowell found *all* such fractures displaced after conservative treatment, indicating no inherent stability.[264] He believed, therefore, that all fractures showing any degree of varus *or* exhibiting retroversion greater than 30° at initial examination were unstable and required internal fixation.[264]

Bony impaction lends a certain degree of inherent stability to the fracture.[131,316,319] Owing to this stability, the patient may have minimal pain even on weight bearing and does not demonstrate the shortening or external rotation deformity seen in displaced fractures.[64,185,264] Because of this inherent stability at the fracture site, two approaches to treatment have arisen: operative[64,149,319] and nonoperative.[7,131,201]

MacAusland and colleagues[269] advised that impacted fractures should be treated the same as other femoral neck fractures to prevent displacement and nonunion. This philosophy is shared by Fielding,[136] Frangakis,[149] Moore,[299] and Pankovich.[319]

Christopher[82] recommended immediate application of a short spica cast and the use of a 2-inch heel lift on the uninvolved leg for impacted fractures. Hilleboe and co-workers[201] recommended conservative treatment of impacted fractures, as did Crawford.[104,105] According to Crawford, the advantages of conservative treatment include avoiding an operation as well as the expense and unnecessary use of hospital beds. He believed that the main disadvantage of conservative treatment was the risk of disimpacting the fracture. Crawford's criteria for inclusion as an impacted fracture are: no shortening or external rotation of the limb, little discomfort on active or passive motion to the hip, the ability to perform active internal rotation of the limb, and impaction on both anteroposterior *and* lateral x-rays. He manages the patients in bed, avoiding external rotation. As soon as the patient is comfortable, she is taught to walk without bearing weight on the extremity. The patient walks this way for at least 4 months or until the fracture is healed. It is apparent that very cooperative patients

who are agile and alert enough to resist weight bearing are a *prerequisite* of this form of treatment. In spite of specific selection of patients and strict adherence to the treatment regimen, the incidence of loss of reduction of these fractures varies from 8%[104,141,143,185] to 20%.[13,141,185,201,263] Bentley,[36,37] on the other hand, showed that in his series 100% of impacted fractures treated by internal fixation healed.

In addition, impacted fractures treated conservatively are reported to develop aseptic necrosis in 13%[57] to 44% of patients.[105,131,143] Bentley[36] reported aseptic necrosis in 14% of patients treated conservatively and in only 18% of those treated operatively at 3 years. This helps substantiate Brodetti's contention[60] that internal fixation devices do not increase the incidence of aseptic necrosis.

The cause of aseptic necrosis in impacted or valgus fractures is thought to be kinking of the lateral epiphyseal vessels and tethering of the medial epiphyseal vessels in the ligamentum teres as the head assumes an extreme valgus position.[131,141] Garden strongly supported the concept of malreduction leading to aseptic necrosis, but he believed that impacted valgus fractures should not be disimpacted, as this would "exchange" the natural healing properties of the stable fracture for the known hazards of the unstable fracture.[166] On the other hand, Moore believed that fractures impacted in valgus should be reduced and nailed.[298] However, in spite of the risk of aseptic necrosis in valgus impacted fractures, disimpaction to decrease valgus is not recommended because not all patients with aseptic necrosis develop symptoms.[36]

Author's Preferred Method of Treatment

Impacted Fractures. Because of the need for absolute patient cooperation in closed (nonoperative) treatment, the risk of disimpaction with closed treatment (which may require secondary surgery), and the fact that aseptic necrosis does not seem to be increased with internal fixation, I favor internal fixation with multiple pins such as Hagie, Knowles, or Moore's pins. Larger implants, such as compression hip screws or other nail-plate devices, may increase the risk of disimpaction at surgery and are therefore avoided.[136]

Conservative treatment is considered only if the patient has an *impacted* fracture that is several weeks old and is walking without pain, or if the patient is medically unfit for surgery. Even in the second group of patients I prefer percutaneous pinning under local anesthesia, because, if disimpaction occurs, these patients are not candidates for the more extensive salvage procedures that may be required.

Nondisplaced Fractures.   Garden II, or undisplaced fractures, on the other hand, do not have the inherent bony stability seen in impacted fractures. These fractures, therefore, are likely to displace in almost every case when treated by conservative means. For this reason, I routinely treat these fractures by closed reduction and internal fixation. I prefer a sliding compression hip screw with a single Knowles pin above the sliding screw to prevent rotation in these fractures. Multiple pins are an alternative form of internal fixation, but they do not allow as safe postoperative weight bearing as the compression hip screw.

DISPLACED FRACTURES (GARDEN III AND IV)

Nonoperative Treatment

Historically, femoral neck fractures were treated with longitudinal and lateral traction for up to 8 weeks, followed by non-weight bearing for up to 6 months.[276,329,345] Whitman introduced closed reduction in abduction and spica cast immobilization to improve treatment results.[434,435,436] However, both traction and closed reduction followed by casting resulted in unacceptable rates of deformity and nonunion.[88,139,428] More important, the immobilization they require often leads to fatal pulmonary complications. It is because of these problems that nonoperative treatment of displaced femoral neck fractures is *rarely*, if ever, indicated.[363] Even in patients with severe medical complications in whom general or spinal anesthesia is deemed too great a risk, percutaneous pin fixation under local anesthesia can provide improved anesthetic safety and fracture stability.[2,12,241,243]

However, severe associated medical conditions or mental deterioration (particularly in a *non*ambulatory patient) may influence the physician to select a totally nonoperative approach. In this *limited* number of patients the fracture can be managed by "skillful neglect." This is done by ignoring the fracture while mobilizing the patient commensurate with pain tolerance. Early mobilization will avoid the dreaded systemic complications associated with other forms of nonoperative treatment. It is important to remember that, unlike intertrochanteric fractures, femoral neck fractures treated in this manner may result in *both* deformity *and* nonunion, which may later be symptomatic.

Although well-leg traction, introduced by Anderson for conservative treatment of hip fractures, might maintain fracture alignment and reduce the incidence of nonunion,[8,9,330] the immobilization that results from the bilateral long leg casts required for its application may defeat the purpose of nonoperative treatment.

Operative Treatment

In displaced fractures of the femoral neck (Garden III and IV fractures) the goal is anatomical reduction, impaction, and stable internal fixation.[28,122,166,378] Those fractures with significant posterior femoral neck comminution present special problems that are discussed later.[353,354,355]

In view of the bony and vascular anatomy of the femoral neck, it would appear that displaced fractures should be handled as an emergency with treatment being instituted as quickly as possible *without* additional risk to the patient.[122,253] Most patients, when first seen, are in the optimum medical condition to undergo operative treatment. Further unnecessary delays may cause a deterioration in the general medical status.[122,253,319,363]

According to Massie, when surgery is performed within 12 hours of injury, there is a 25% incidence of aseptic necrosis. The incidence rises to 30% with a delay of 13 to 24 hours; to 40%, between 24 to 48 hours; and to 100% after 1 week.[275] This direct relationship between the time from injury to internal fixation and the complications of aseptic necrosis and nonunion have also been reported by Brown and Abrami,[62] and Soto-Hall and colleagues.[385] Graham,[174] however, was unable to relate these two factors. Finally, Barnes and colleagues[28] found that a delay of operation of up to 1 week did not affect union or the incidence of late segmental collapse.

Müssbichler's[309] arteriographic studies demonstrated better arterial flow in the remaining vessels to the femoral head with the limb in neutral or slight internal rotation. These studies suggest that the fractured femoral neck should be immobilized in traction in an effort to reduce the external rotation deformity at the fracture site.[122] Cleveland and associates[88] also stressed the need for correcting rotational displacement to improve arterial blood flow. In addition, Deyerle recommends traction to prevent additional soft-tissue damage and aspiration of the hip joint to reduce intra-articular pressure from hemorrhage as initial steps in the management of patients with femoral neck fractures.[121,122]

Reduction Techniques.   An acceptable reduction is the *key* factor in decreasing the risk of aseptic necrosis and nonunion. Moore demonstrated that when the fragments are not anatomically reduced, actual bony contact at the fracture site is only half as much as appears on x-ray.[299] This decreased area of contact reduces the area for blood vessels to grow from the base of the neck into the femoral head. Moore believed that this was a significant factor in the incidence of aseptic necrosis and delayed union[299] (Fig. 14-7). Cleveland and associates[88] stressed the need for correction of *rotational* displacement of the proximal fragment to improve bony apposition and union.

The methods recommended to achieve reduction must be well understood because the fracture reduction is one of the few determining factors under the surgeon's control. Although the fracture can be reduced by closed or open means, closed reduction, *if* acceptable, is preferable to an open reduction, which is done *only* if the closed reduction fails.[264]

Closed Reduction. Many surgeons favor closed reduction on the fracture table, which then allows for the insertion of internal fixation devices under two-plane x-ray control or image intensification. Although multiple methods of closed reduction have been described,[144,256,276,329,345,377,434] none have been documented to be superior.

Smith[374] has emphasized the importance of the retinaculum of Weitbrecht in obtaining fracture reduction. He compared this retinaculum to the binding of a book; external rotation opens the book and internal rotation closes it, thereby reducing the fracture. The different techniques used for closed reduction of femoral neck fractures can be divided into those performed with the hip in extension and those performed with the hip in flexion.

CLOSED REDUCTION WITH THE HIP IN EXTENSION. Whitman described a reduction method that involved traction on the limb in *extension* followed by internal rotation and abduction.[434] Massie[275] added the concept of *forceful* internal rotation, which, if unsuccessful, was to be repeated with increased internal rotation strength. Green,[175] however, recommended reduction in near full extension by *gentle* longitudinal traction combined with internal rotation. Garden agreed that a *gentle* reduction is more desirable and successful than techniques using vigorous manipulation.[167] Additionally, a strenuous or careless reduction may complete damage to the remaining intact blood vessels and therefore increase the rate of nonunion and aseptic necrosis.[149,167]

McElvenny[280] believed that an anatomical position could *not* be maintained in a fracture through the femoral neck. He compared this to an attempt to appose the ends of two fingernails for stability purposes. He recommended a reduction in which the medial portion of the femoral neck was *medial* and *beneath* the corresponding medial cortex of the femoral head. This produced a slight medial shift of the femoral neck and resulted in marked bone stability, owing to the elimination of shear and angulation forces at the fracture site (Fig. 14-8). McElvenny was quick to emphasize that, although much had been written about a "valgus reduction," the valgus position did not in itself lend bony stability. He believed that stability was the result of the medial portion of the neck fragment being medial and underneath the head fragment.[279] In addition, he felt that a true subcapital fracture (through the old epiphyseal scar) could not be

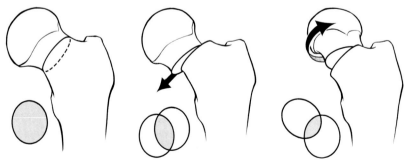

Fig. 14-7. As one progresses from an anatomical reduction (*left*), to increasing degrees of displacement at the fracture site (*center* and *right*), the area of bony contact between the fracture surfaces of the proximal and distal fragments is decreased. This decreased area of surface contact reduces the cross-sectional area through which blood vessels can grow from the base of the neck into the femoral head. Moore[299] believed that this decreased contact area is a factor in the development of aseptic necrosis and delayed union or nonunion.

Anatomical   Underreduced   Overreduced

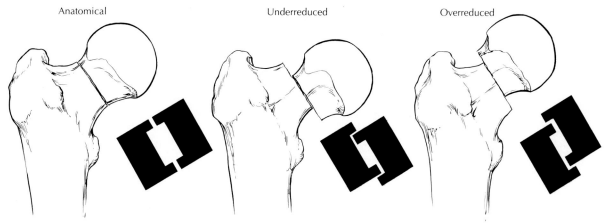

Fig. 14-8. McElvenny's concept[279] of reduction is that either anatomical (*left*) or underreduced (*center*) femoral neck fractures are inherently unstable. He therefore strived to achieve an overreduced position (*right*) in which the medial cortex of the distal fragment lies medial to the medial cortex of the femoral head and neck fragment.

rendered stable by *any* form of reduction and that a concomitant osteotomy was necessary to ensure its stability and union.[282] McElvenny[280] described a reduction technique in which both feet are bound to the fracture table with the hips in extension. Traction is applied to both lower extremities. The affected limb is then externally rotated and heavier traction applied. Next, the assistant rotates the foot internally at the same time as the operator rotates the limb internally at the knee. Full internal rotation occurs with little effort. When full internal rotation is obtained, the operator places his hands on the greater trochanter and pushes firmly posteriorly and medially. With traction maintained, the limb is adducted to the neutral position. At this point the reduction is checked by x-rays.[280] If more valgus is required, traction is reapplied to the affected leg, and an adduction force is applied at the knee while simultaneously pushing inward over the trochanter.

Deyerle[119,120,121,122] places the patient on a fracture table with a pelvic anchor attachment to lift the opposite limb well out of the way for good lateral x-rays. The involved limb is bound to the foot plate of the fracture table. Strong traction is applied with the leg parallel to the body and the foot slightly rotated externally. After the fracture is overreduced with respect to length, the foot is internally rotated until it is at an angle of approximately 40° with the floor. (An assistant rotates the knee as the foot is rotated to take stress off the ligaments of the knee.) At this point, two hands are placed *anterior* to the greater trochanter and a

force is applied directly posteriorly while the pelvis is held firmly on the opposite side to prevent rotation. This maneuver reduces the fracture in the lateral plane. Next, an overreduced position of the head is achieved by traction on the involved leg (parallel to the body) and direct pressure is applied laterally over the greater trochanter, pushing toward the center post of the fracture table.[122]

CLOSED REDUCTION WITH HIP FLEXION. Leadbetter[255,256] championed reduction of femoral neck fractures in full hip flexion. In his technique, the affected leg is flexed at the hip to 90° and traction (with slight adduction of the femoral shaft) is applied along the axis of the femur. In this position the thigh is internally rotated. The leg is then circumducted into abduction (maintaining internal rotation) and brought down to table level in extension. Leadbetter evaluated the reduction with the so-called "heel/palm test" in which the heel is placed in the palm of an outstretched hand. If reduction is complete, the leg will not spontaneously rotate externally. Although this reduction frequently produces satisfactory alignment on x-ray, the head may be rotated on the femoral neck, resulting in a nonanatomical configuration.

Smith-Petersen and colleagues recommended reduction by gentle traction in *slight* hip flexion while counterpressure is maintained on the pelvis. This is followed by internal rotation, abduction, and extension. The limb is then supported on a stool at the side of the table with the knee flexed.[134,269,377]

Owing to a lack of satisfaction with previous reduction methods, Flynn[144] introduced a manipulation technique based on anatomical detail. The fracture is disimpacted by gentle flexion of the hip in slight abduction with traction in the axis of the femoral neck. While this traction is maintained, the hip is extended and medially rotated to a degree comparable with the range of these motions in the opposite hip. Although Flynn[144] reported acceptable reductions in *all* patients using this method, Compton was unable to demonstrate any improvement in the accuracy of reduction with this method.[95]

Following fracture reduction, impaction of the fracture, particularly in cases with severe comminution, has been recommended.[94,98,122,319] This concept is based on the idea that impacted fractures are known to be stable and to heal readily. Impaction is obtained by the use of several blows to the lateral aspect of the greater trochanter following reduction.[98,99] The danger of overreduction into a valgus position with its known complications must be considered when using this technique.[166,319,372]

The influence of the technique of closed reduction on end results has *not* been clearly defined in the literature. In addition, the number of closed reduction attempts that should be made in an effort to obtain an acceptable reduction is not known. The surgeon should keep in mind the theoretical risks of repeated manipulation versus those of an open reduction.

Evaluation of Reduction. *Radiographic Evaluation.* Following closed reduction, high-quality x-rays are essential to evaluate the acceptability of the reduction. Cotton emphasized the need for *both* anteroposterior and lateral x-rays to evaluate the quality of reduction.[98] McElvenny emphasized that the accuracy of reduction of the inferior aspect of the head-neck fragment must be confirmed on a true lateral x-ray of the hip made with the limb fully rotated internally.[281,282] However, Simon and Wyman, using multiple views of the hip in different degrees of flexion and internal rotation, demonstrated that most reductions thought to be "acceptable" after two-plane x-ray were indeed far from anatomical.[369] Lowell[264] demonstrated experimentally that all x-ray images of an *anatomical* femoral head-neck junction reveal the convex outline of the femoral head meeting the concave outline of the femoral neck *regardless* of the x-ray projection. This outline produces the image of an "S"-shaped curve. In *no* instance does the concave outline of the femoral neck appear *tangent* to the femoral head to form an unbroken "C"-shaped curve (Fig. 14-9). Therefore, if the x-ray image reveals an unbroken "C"-shaped curve, the fracture is *not* reduced.

There is some disagreement among authors as to what constitutes an *acceptable* reduction. A varus reduction is known to result in an increased incidence of nonunion of the fracture.[81,264] Barnes and colleagues[28] reported that the rate of nonunion approaches 55% in those fractures with 20° residual varus displacement after reduction. A valgus reduction is favored by some authors because of increased bony stability at the fracture, especially in patients with extensive posterior comminution.[12,37,280,353,355] Banks believes that fracture fragments are adequately reduced if they are in an anatomical slight valgus position with 2 mm to 3 mm separation of the fracture site at the medial calcar.[24] However, Garden,[166] Frangakis,[149] and others[81,84,264] have demonstrated that excessive valgus (*i.e.,* a Garden angle of greater than 185°; see below) results in a markedly increased incidence of aseptic necrosis. In addition, anteversion or retroversion at the fracture site of greater than 20° has been shown to increase the incidence of nonunion.[28,353,420] Finally, rotational displacement about the axis of the femoral neck has been shown to compromise the remaining blood supply.[372] This rotational displacement may be impossible to detect by x-ray.[149]

Due to the problems associated with such malreductions, most authors favor as near anatomical reduction of femoral neck fractures as is possible.[62,144,164,166] Authors stressing anatomical reduction believe that it allows maximum opportunity for the reestablishment of the vascular supply.[121] Anatomical reduction also prevents the stretching of vessels in the ligamentum teres and the introduction of abnormal forces along the internal architecture of the femoral head.[372] Finally, an anatomical reduction prevents the joint incongruity present in a valgus reduction caused by the fact that the femoral head is not perfectly spherical.[74,166,245]

Christophe and associates compared the results of varus, valgus, and anatomical position of the femoral head following reduction and nailing. They found no cases of aseptic necrosis or nonunion in patients in which the head was in an anatomical position.[81]

Garden has extensively investigated the effect of the quality of reduction on both early and late results in femoral neck fractures.[164,165,166,167] He found that an "acceptable reduction" decreased the incidence of aseptic necrosis, nonunion, and degenerative joint disease. In an effort to standardize the term "acceptable reduction," he developed an *alignment index* by which the surgeon can objectively evaluate the reduction.[166] The alignment

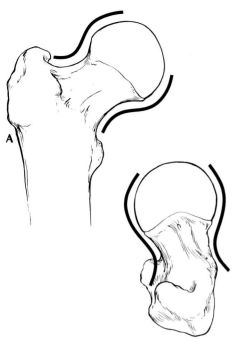

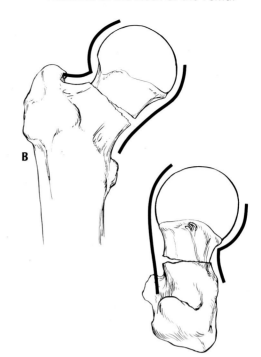

Fig. 14-9. (*A*) According to Lowell,[264] the x-ray appearance of an anatomical femoral head and neck junction shows the convex outline of the femoral head meeting the concave outline of the femoral neck *regardless* of the projection on x-ray. This outline produces the image of an S or reversed S curve. Therefore, the outline of the femoral neck is never tangent to the outline of the femoral head in a reduced femoral neck fracture. (*B*) An incompletely reduced fracture.

index is measured on the anteroposterior and lateral x-rays taken following reduction. These x-rays *must* be of excellent quality to allow identification of the bony trabeculae accurately. In the frontal anteroposterior view, the angle formed by the central axis of the medial trabecular system in the capital fragment and the medial cortex of the femoral shaft is measured. In the normal femoral head and neck, this angle measures approximately 160°. On the lateral x-ray, the central axis of the head and the central axis of the neck normally lie in a straight line (180°) (Fig. 14-10).[167] Garden believes that an alignment index *postreduction* within the range of 155° to 180° on *both* the frontal and lateral views is an acceptable reduction, resulting in a high percentage of union and a low rate of late segmental collapse.[166] Indeed, when the alignment index was less than 155° or greater than 180° on either view, the incidence of aseptic necrosis rose from 7.3% to 53.8% in his series.[167] Although Edholm and colleagues[128] were unable to substantiate this relationship, Frangakis[149] confirmed that a valgus reduction of greater than 20° had a catastrophic result on the head, resulting in ischemia in 80% of

cases. Barnes and colleagues[28] and Smyth and colleagues[378] have also confirmed the relationship of the alignment index to the later development of aseptic necrosis and nonunion.

Stability of Reduction. The evaluation of the lateral x-ray *post*reduction to identify posterior comminution of the femoral neck is critical in selecting treatment alternatives. The effect on stability of posterior comminution at the fracture site has been emphasized by Scheck.[353,354,355] Posterior comminution leads to the loss of a buttressing effect posteriorly with subsequent loss of reduction and nonunion. Garden reported that only type III and IV fractures develop nonunion[164] and that this is because of an *unstable* reduction secondary to comminution posteriorly and inferiorly at the fracture site.[164] Banks also recognized that posterior comminution was an important factor in nonunion, demonstrating that over 60% of patients with nonunion had posterior comminution at the time of initial treatment.[25]

The presence of posterior comminution has led to treatment modifications in Garden III and IV fractures in an effort to restore posterior stability.

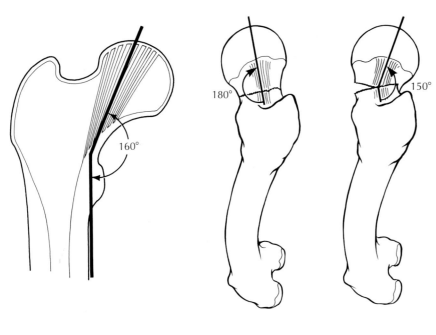

Fig. 14-10. Garden's alignment index.[167] (*Left*) In the frontal view, the angle formed by the central axis of the medial trabecular system in the capital fragment and the medial cortex of the femoral shaft is measured. In the normal femoral head and neck this measures 160°. (*Center*) In the lateral view, the central axis of the head and the central axis of the neck lie in a straight line at 180°. According to Garden, an acceptable reduction can be expressed as an alignment index (following reduction) within the range of 160° to 180° on both the frontal and lateral views. (*Right*) An unacceptable reduction in the lateral view.

Garden's low-angle fixation nailing,[163] the posterior muscle pedicle bone graft,[287,289,290] double screw osteosynthesis,[272] and the triangle fixation described by Smyth[378] have all been suggested. The posterior muscle pedicle bone graft attempts to *augment* the cortical defect by primary bone grafting, while low-angle nailing and triangle fixation attempt to restore stability by means of an internal fixation device. Although the union rate in these series is the same, approaching 90%, the posterior muscle pedicle graft has a lower incidence of aseptic necrosis.[287,289,290] In addition, Scheck[353,354] and Frangakis[149] demonstrated that, even with correct placement, internal fixation devices may not alter the effect of the posterior comminution.

Open Reduction. If the fracture is not acceptably reduced after two attempts at closed reduction, consideration must be given to open reduction.[235,253,264,278] However, open reduction can be a difficult and hazardous procedure. McElvenny believed that open reduction of a femoral neck fracture was the most difficult surgical procedure about the hip,[278] and Cleveland reported that up to 50% of fractures treated by open reduction actually displaced during the process of nailing.[86] Cave[75] and Scheck[353] also expressed hesitancy in performing an open reduction for fear of damage to the remaining blood supply and difficulty in controlling the ''spinning femoral head.'' In addition, Green[175,176] expressed reservations about open reduction because of the limited space available for manipulation of the fracture even under direct visualization.

In spite of these reservations, Banks[24] demonstrated that open reduction was associated with a decreased incidence of both nonunion and aseptic necrosis when compared to a group of patients in whom an inadequate closed reduction was accepted. Therefore, should closed reduction fail, open reduction and internal fixation under direct vision must be considered *if* the patient is not a candidate for prosthetic hemiarthroplasty.

Usually, open reduction is performed through an anterior or anterolateral approach (Watson-Jones) in an effort to avoid further damage to the remaining blood supply and to provide room for fracture manipulation.[235,264] However, if x-rays reveal an inadequate closed reduction *and* the presence of marked posterior comminution, a posterior approach with muscle pedicle bone grafting as described by Meyers and associates may be considered.[287,288,289] This approach has the advantages of providing a vascularized bone graft plus additional cancellous bone directly to the area of the posterior bony defect. This method has been shown to result in a high rate of union and a low incidence of aseptic necrosis.[287,288,289] Although it has not proved to be a problem to the original authors,[290] the risk to the remaining posterior blood supply by this posterior approach *must* be considered.[235] Bonfiglio* has expressed concern that the posterior approach can easily result in damage to the posterior blood supply to the femoral head, thereby putting the femoral head at risk for aseptic necrosis and

* Bonfiglio, M.: Personal communication, 1982.

late segmental collapse. He also emphasized that, although the posterior muscle pedicle graft does provide excellent posterior *bony* stability, it does not provide *structural* support to the anterior-superior portion of the femoral head where necrosis can give rise to late segmental collapse.

Operative Techniques (Methods of Internal Fixation). In a textbook of this nature, it is not possible to give a detailed account of all the types of internal fixation available for fracture treatment or the indications proposed by each advocate. It must be emphasized that whatever technique is selected, the reduction must be done gently and accurately, as no device will overcome a poor reduction.[215] Rigid fixation must be achieved by impaction at the fracture site as well as by proper placement of the internal fixation device. No currently available internal fixation device will indefinitely withstand the cyclic loads that are applied to the hip in normal daily activities unless there is a sharing of these loads by external protection, adjacent bone, or both.[264] The surgeon should be thoroughly familiar with the technical problems associated with the particular device under consideration.

Multiple Pins. Multiple pin fixation with Knowles,[12,22,241] Moore,[2,295,296,297,299,302] or other pins[159,243,283,400] has been advocated as the simplest method of internal fixation of femoral neck fractures. This method can be done percutaneously, often under local anesthesia, thereby reducing the risk of operative morbidity, blood loss, and infection in the elderly patient.[2,12,241,243] One must remember, however, that these poor risk patients may be quite osteoporotic, with bone not strong enough to support this means of fixation. On the other hand, such pins are ideal in impacted fractures of the femoral neck, as they can be inserted without fear of fracture displacement.[215]

Moore[295,296,299] recommended the use of four pins widely separated but parallel in placement. He found an increased incidence of nonunion if the pins were allowed to converge. Such parallelism of the pins has been found essential by most authors.[2,12,22,241,243,295,296] Peripheral (not central) placement of the pins, whether in the shape of a parallelogram,[295,296,299] a box,[12,264] or a triangle,[12] is deemed necessary for increased stability of fixation and for the prevention of rotation of the proximal fragment. Arnold recommends placing the pins into the subchondral bone of the femoral head to ensure maximal proximal fixation.[12]

Arnold and associates[12] and Kofoed and associates[243] report excellent results in using this method, even in displaced fractures. Most of their failures were secondary to osteoporotic bone,[12] comminution at the fracture site,[12] or a poor reduction.[243] Following fixation with multiple pins, most authors allow patients to be up in a chair, with weight bearing on crutches *only* to the extent of the weight of the limb until fracture union is present.[241,295,296,299]

Deyerle, using the basic principle of multiple pins, recommended an increased number of pins to improve proximal fracture fixation.[119,120,121,122] Because the lateral cortex of the femur is often thin and frequently inadequate to provide good fixation, he developed a metal template to hold the pins more securely while simultaneously permitting them to slide.[119,120,121,122] This implant therefore allows for impaction at the time of surgery *and* with subsequent weight bearing. The side plate provides better fixation to the femoral shaft, a design modification felt by Haboush to be essential in femoral neck fractures.[181,182] The holding power of 8 to 12 of these pins placed parallel in the neck and head of the femur is significantly greater than that which can be achieved by any single-type screw or nail. In addition, each pin constitutes 1% of the cross-sectional diameter of the neck, while a Smith-Petersen triflanged nail occupies only about 6% of the cross-sectional diameter.[122] This adds to the strength of the implant compared to a nail device.[120]

The Deyerle technique, however, is very demanding, and shortcuts lead only to disaster. An anatomical or slightly valgus reduction, as described by Deyerle,[119,120,122] is essential in order to insert the maximum number of pins into the femoral head. If any pin is accidentally advanced through the subchondral plate, the pin tract must be left empty or the pin will continue to advance into the joint rather than to slide with impaction. Deyerle reported 1.8% nonunion and only 9% aseptic necrosis[122] in a series of femoral neck fractures treated in this manner. Although the series of Metz and associates[286] approached these results, Chapman and associates[79] and Ryan and associates[346] reported a significantly higher incidence of both nonunion and aseptic necrosis following the use of the Deyerle apparatus.

Asnis* has recently introduced a system of cannulated screws that provide improved pullout, and bending and torque strengths as compared with Knowles-type pins. An adjustable guide is available to ensure parallel insertion. This improved proximal fixation may prove valuable in treating femoral neck fractures.

---

* Asnis, S.: Personal communication, February 26, 1981.

Fixed-Angle Nail. The original technique of femoral neck fixation with the triphalangeal nail of Smith-Petersen[223,375,377] is now outdated.[319] Dickson[125] and Haboush[181,182] demonstrated improved fixation of femoral neck fractures by implants with a side plate attached to the lateral femoral shaft. A Smith-Petersen nail to which a side plate is attached at varying angles[403] or the one-piece Jewett nail was designed to give such improved fixation.[222] These two devices are relatively easy to use, but their simplicity is outweighed by two major disadvantages:[222] (1) the reduced head may be knocked off during insertion of the nail secondary to the force required; (2) in order to ensure maximum nail fixation in the head, the nail must be within 1 cm of the subchondral bone, and if the fracture impacts further, a nail in this position may penetrate the head into the acetabulum. Riska and associates[342] demonstrated good results when two modified Smith-Petersen nails were used in conjunction with an adequate reduction. Barnes and associates,[28] however, demonstrated that the failure rate was consistently 20% higher following Smith-Petersen-type nailing, and Frandsen and associates[147] demonstrated a 10% increase in nonunion with Smith-Petersen nails compared to a sliding nail plate. The Smith-Petersen nail and the fixed nail plate were important steps in the history of the treatment of this fracture, but, in my opinion, both have now been superceded by a variety of techniques that incorporate the sliding principle.

Sliding or Telescoping Nails. The principle of a sliding or telescoping nail is said to have been introduced in the 1940s by Dr. Henry Briggs.[138] The advantages of a sliding nail-plate device include improved fixation in the femoral head, firm fixation to the femoral shaft, and collapsibility which ensures continuous impaction at the fracture site while lessening the chance of nail penetration through or cutting out of the femoral head.[21,29,41,63,137,138,147,148,215,225,273] Several designs of these implants are available. Pugh and Ken developed a 135° sliding nail in the 1950s,[334,407] and both inventors marketed identical nails under their individual names.[407] These devices were designed to be placed low in the femoral head on the anteroposterior and centrally on the lateral x-ray. Massie[273] introduced a 150° sliding nail in an effort to place the nail in the weight-bearing axis of the femoral neck.[20] He recommended placement of the nail on the calcar so that downward displacement is resisted by a shortened lever arm extending proximally from the point of nail-calcar contact.[273]

He reported an increased healing rate and a decreased incidence of nonunion and early aseptic necrosis.[274,275] However, Brown and Court-Brown[63] were able to find no significant difference in results between the 135° and 150° devices. When using these devices, the barrel must not cross the fracture site and there must be sufficient potential slide remaining in the nail after insertion.[175,215,334] Regardless of the particular type of device used, it is essential to obtain maximal holding capacity in the head. This usually necessitates the use of a 135° device for most individuals when an anatomical reduction is obtained. It is important to remember that 150° devices of any type often come to rest in the rather weak bone of the anterior-superior quadrant of the femoral head unless a valgus reduction and low nail placement are obtained.

Jacobs and associates[215] reported that the only advantage of these sliding implants is a decreased incidence of joint penetration. Jacobs and associates and Rau and associates[337] emphasize that a sliding device will *not* compensate for a poor reduction. Fielding[138] reported a 90% union rate with the Pugh nail and found all failures related to poor reduction or faulty nailing technique. In an analysis of failures of the sliding nail, Brown and Court-Brown[63] also found poor reduction, poor implant placement, and inadequate nail depth to be responsible factors. It must be emphasized again, therefore, that although sliding nail-plate devices have produced improved results in femoral neck fractures, a stable and acceptable reduction is still a *prerequisite* for their use.

Screw and Sliding Screw Fixation. Frankel has demonstrated that the cancellous bone in the femoral head is the limiting factor in the strength of an internal fixation system.[152,153,154] Subsequently, biomechanical testing has shown that a large threaded screw provides better internal fixation than a triphalanged nail.[61,189] The flat surfaces of a screw provide a larger area per unit force, and therefore there is less tendency for a screw to cut through the bone. These studies suggest that a screw will provide better fixation in the femoral head than will a nail.

Charnley devised a compression screw that provided dynamic continuous compression, but there were frequent problems with loss of compression and the need for a secondary operation.[80,187] An implant consisting of a screw (for improved fixation) fitted to a sliding barrel (to allow controlled impaction) was introduced by Schumpelick and Jantzen in 1955[357] and popularized in a modified form by Clawson[85] as the sliding compression hip screw. In addition to a shaft plate and a sliding mechanism, the compression hip screw has a blunt nose to decrease the incidence of joint penetration. Compression at the fracture site can be obtained at surgery by a special screw in the sliding mechanism.[85] Jamming, or failure of the compression hip screw to slide, has been related by Kyle and associates[248] to three *independent* factors: (1) engagement of the screw in the barrel (deep engagement of the screw in the barrel permits sliding); (2) high-angle screw plates (150°), which have better sliding characteristics than low-angle (130°) plates; (3) 316L stainless steel implants, which develop galling in the barrel and will jam, especially when using 130° plates. Clawson reported 87% union in patients treated with this device. He recommended its use in younger patients and emphasized the need for anatomical reduction. Cassebaum and Parkes[70] reported union in 82% of displaced femoral neck fractures. The majority of fractures were secondary to inadequate reduction and postoperative infection. Rau and associates[337] reported a high incidence of unsatisfactory results with this device when there was inadequate reduction, alignment, or depth of screw insertion. They emphasized the necessity of a good reduction and the need for technical accuracy when using this implant. A theoretical disadvantage of this implant is that the screw has the potential to rotate the femoral head during its insertion,[136,264,272] a factor that may increase the incidence of aseptic necrosis.[372] Placing an accessory pin in the femoral head above the screw or in an extraosseous location to stabilize the fracture before screw insertion will prevent this problem.[227] A recent modification of the sliding hip screw was introduced by Calandruccio, who added two threaded pins above the screw to improve fixation and control rotation of the head fragment.[371] The AO group has also introduced a sliding compression hip screw for the treatment of femoral neck fractures because of the advantages mentioned above.

Nail Placement. The ideal location for nail placement in the femoral head has been subject to much controversy.[28,50,61,63,87,136,211,278,334] Bonfiglio[50] suggests central placement on the anteroposterior and lateral x-rays to provide favorable conditions for settling of the fracture. He believed that eccentrically placed nails would tilt the head into a poor position for proper settling. Cleveland and Bailey[87] and McElvenny[278] agree with central placement. However, Fielding,[136] Pugh,[334] and Hunter[211] recommend placement of the nail inferiorly on the anteroposterior x-ray and slightly posteriorly on the

lateral x-ray to allow impaction and to prevent the nail from cutting out of the head in external rotation and adduction. Barnes and associates[28] found the central position most satisfactory, resulting in a higher rate of union than in those fractures with low and posterior placement. A particular problem of low nail placement is the fact that the inferior aspect of the femoral head is dome shaped and does not allow as deep insertion of the nail. Although the controversy over central versus inferior and posterior nail placement is unsettled, there is a consensus that the superior and anterior portion of the head should be avoided.[63,87,264,334]

The depth of nail placement is also critical in obtaining proximal fixation. Brown and Abrami[62] warn against inadvertent penetration of the femoral head articular cortex, as this shell of bone provides the downward pressure needed for collapse in sliding implants. Brown and Court-Brown[63] showed a definite increase in failure rate if the tip of the nail is *more* than 12 mm from the femoral head subchondral articular surface. Additionally, a stress riser effect is present at the tip of the nail, and if it is not inserted deeply enough, fractures of the neck at the tip of the nail have been reported.[23,214,343] The current recommendations are that for best fixation the nail should be advanced to within 0.5 cm of the articular surface of the femoral head.[62,138]

Posterior Muscle Pedicle Bone Grafting. Recognizing that accurate reduction, impaction, and rigid internal fixation are essential in treating femoral neck fractures has led some investigators to advocate the use of a bone graft based on a muscle pedicle, in addition to routine internal fixation.[200,231,232,287,288,289,397] Not only will this *theoretically* provide an additional source of vascular supply for the femoral head, which may have been rendered ischemic by the fracture, but it also allows reduction and impaction of the fracture under direct vision.[287,288,289]

Stuck and Hinchey[397], in 1944, used a pedicle bone graft based on the vastus lateralis and keyed into the *anterior* femoral neck. They demonstrated increased vascularity in the femoral head. Frankel and Derian[151] repeated the experiment and found that subcapital femoral circulation could indeed be introduced by such a graft. Hewson[200] suggested the use of a pedicle graft from the gluteus maximus applied to the femoral neck fracture to increase both vascularity *and* fracture stability.

Judet and colleagues[231,232] introduced a pedicle graft taken from the *posterior* intertrochanteric crest with preservation of muscle attachments and blood supply. They demonstrated acceleration of union and prevention of pseudarthrosis using this graft and internal fixation. Meyers and colleagues,[287,288,289] expanding the work of Judet and colleagues, recommend a bone graft taken with the insertion of the quadratus femoris muscle posteriorly. This pedicled graft is applied to the femoral neck fracture *posteriorly* after open reduction and internal fixation with Hagie pins (Fig. 14-11). They emphasized two advantages of this method. First, since 70% of patients[289,353,354,355] have significant posterior bony comminution, fracture stability is enhanced by the buttressing effect of the posterior bone graft. Second, the graft will serve as an additional source of blood supply to the femoral head. These authors recommended this method in displaced fractures of the femoral neck except in patients who are nonambulatory; those with a life expectancy of less than 2 years; and those patients unable to cooperate with the postoperative program because of senility, psychosis, mental retardation, Parkinsonism, or cerebral vascular accident with residual hemiplegia or spasticity. They reported union in 90% of *displaced* femoral neck fractures, with late segmental collapse in only 8% of patients followed at least 18 months.[288,289] Although criticism of the technique has arisen because of possible damage to the remaining posterior vascular supply to the femoral head,* the authors stress that their approach avoids the *superior* aspect of the head and neck wherein lies the all-important lateral epiphyseal vessels.[287] Meyers reports no problem with this surgical approach, noting only 5% late segmental collapse in his hands.†

Postoperative Management After Nailing

Since the introduction of internal fixation for femoral neck fractures, there has been controversy over when unguarded weight bearing can be instituted following surgery.[174] A long period without weight bearing after internal fixation was generally a part of the treatment regimen in classical nailing.[222,314,334] This was considered necessary because of instability of the fracture and because early compression was thought to increase the possibility of necrosis of the femoral head.[314] Indeed, King[238] reported an increased incidence of poor results when weight bearing was allowed before fracture union. However, as early as 1937, Moore[297] noted no increase in complications following early weight bearing postoperatively. More recently Abrami and Stevens,[1] Garden,[163] Graham,[174] and Nieminen[314]

report that early weight bearing results in *no* increase in postoperative complications. Additionally, attempting to maintain a patient non-weight bearing is frequently frustrating for the surgeon, the therapist, the patient, and his family. Furthermore, the use of a bedpan and the practice of straight leg raising of the unoperated limb while in bed have been shown to produce considerable stress across the femoral neck.[335,347,348] Those advocating non-weight bearing to protect the fracture also *must* remember that approximately half the body weight is transferred across the hip even in so-called "non-weight bearing."[347] If the knee and hip are fully flexed, these forces approximate body weight.[347] After consideration of these factors, it is my opinion that, *provided* a stable internal fixation is achieved, the advantages of early partial weight bearing far outweigh the risks in a cooperative patient.

Author's Preferred Method of Treatment

Displaced femoral neck fractures are treated on a fracture table to aid in reduction and in obtaining good quality x-rays. In displaced (Garden III and IV) fractures I prefer a gentle closed reduction with the patient on a fracture table, using a maneuver similar to that described by Green[175] and Smith-Petersen.[264] The hip is *slightly* flexed, and traction is applied in abduction and external rotation. The limb is then internally rotated and brought in to full extension. If this reduction is unacceptable and posterior comminution of a significant degree is *not* noted on the lateral x-ray, a McElvenny-type reduction is performed. Although my goal is an *anatomical* reduction of all femoral neck fractures, for practical purposes I use the alignment index of Garden as a guideline to an acceptable reduction. I have found that the limiting factor in the use of Garden's alignment index is the need for excellent quality x-rays to determine the angles. Such quality x-rays may not be possible in an operating room setting.

I do not strive for a valgus reduction because it may place stress on the remaining vessels in the ligamentum teres[372] and the lateral epiphyseal vessels[68,166] and may also alter the relationship of the femoral head and acetabulum, thereby predisposing to degenerative change.[166] However, if the reduction maneuver produces a valgus position, consideration of both the patient and fracture characteristics may lead me to accept valgus alignment with its inherent difficulties rather than to risk losing the stability it affords by attempting another reduction.

It must be emphasized that in some cases a

---

* Bonfiglio, M.: Personal communication, 1982.

† Meyers, M. H.: Personal communication, November 5, 1981.

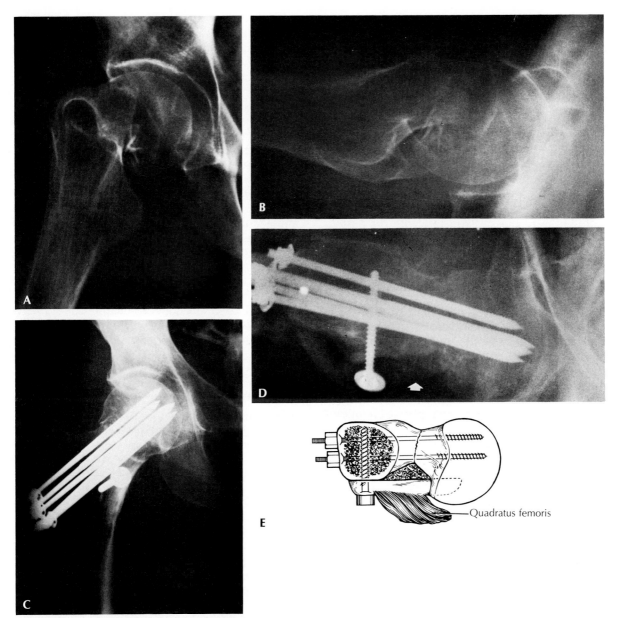

Fig. 14-11. (*A*) Anteroposterior and (*B*) lateral x-rays of a displaced femoral neck fracture in a 40-year-old man. (*B*) Note the posterior comminution. (*C*) Postoperative anteroposterior and (*D*) lateral x-rays demonstrating reduction and internal fixation of the fracture with Haggie pins, and application of a posterior muscle pedicle graft (*arrow*) based on the quadratus femoris muscle. (*E*) The posterior muscle pedicle graft supports the femoral head and neck fragment posteriorly where comminution is most severe. Extra cancellous bone from the posterosuperior iliac spine can be added if the muscle pedicle graft does not completely fill the posterior defect.

reduction within Garden's acceptable alignment index cannot be obtained by closed means. It is then the surgeon's decision as to whether or not an open reduction, hemiarthroplasty, or acceptance of the reduction and nailing *in situ* is indicated. In patients in whom an acceptable reduction is not obtained after two closed manipulations, I do not hesitate to proceed to an open reduction through an anterolateral Watson-Jones approach.[235] If marked posterior comminution of the femoral neck is noted on the postreduction x-ray (and prosthetic hemiarthroplasty is *not* considered an alternative) I prefer open reduction and muscle-pedicle bone grafting as described by Meyers and colleagues.[287,*,288,289,290] I prefer this technique because of the ability to obtain an anatomical reduction under direct vision and because of the buttressing and revascularization effect of the pedicled graft.[151,200,285,397] As this procedure is more demanding and requires longer operating time, the patient's general condition is an *extremely* important factor in deciding on this technique. In addition, the patient must be mentally and physically able to cooperate with the postoperative treatment plan. For these reasons, I usually reserve posterior muscle pedicle bone grafting for the younger patients in this group. Internal fixation in these patients is supplied by Knowles pins or occasionally by the sliding compression hip screw, depending on the size of the femoral neck. It is important to emphasize the use of cancellous bone grafting *in addition* to the muscle pedicle graft to fill in all fracture defects posteriorly.

After I obtain an acceptable reduction (by closed or open means), internal fixation with the sliding compression hip screw augmented by a single Knowles pin superiorly to help prevent rotational displacement is my treatment of choice. I recommend inserting two guide pins (one for the screw and one superiorly) *before* insertion of the screw to prevent rotation of the femoral head during reaming.[70] The gluteus maximus femoral insertion is used as a guide for the satisfactory placement of the implant.[216] In those cases in which the x-rays suggest that the femoral head does not have adequate bone present for firm screw fixation (*i.e.*, very high subcapital fractures), I prefer to use four Knowles pins placed in a boxlike arrangement for fixation. Although the technique results in adequate fixation, early weight bearing is not possible in such cases.

In patients with severe associated medical problems that make a general anesthetic a great risk, I prefer closed reduction and percutaneous pin fixation under local anesthesia, using four Knowles pins. I have found this to be a very acceptable means of treatment in patients with such medical problems.

If internal fixation is stable, patients are allowed partial weight bearing on a walker postoperatively and weight bearing is progressed as they gain control of the limb. I prefer to keep the patients

* Meyers, M. H.: Personal communication, November 5, 1981.

partial weight bearing (with toe touching only) for 6 to 8 weeks prior to the initiation of full weight bearing. The patients are then progressed from a walker to a cane as tolerated. This progression of weight bearing is obviously dependent on the patient's ability to follow postoperative rehabilitation instructions. If the patient's ability to comprehend and cooperate with such a rehabilitation program is questionable, consideration should be given to primary hemiarthroplasty.

If fracture stability is poor, or if the patient is unable to cooperate because of confusion or spasticity, careful transfer to the sitting position and exercises for the upper extremity are instituted immediately. Weight bearing is then instituted when there is x-ray evidence of fracture healing.

In those younger patients who are not candidates for hemi- or total joint arthroplasty, repeat x-rays and medullary bone scans are obtained for the early detection of aseptic necrosis. If this diagnosis is made prior to subchondral collapse, bone grafting or osteotomy can be considered in an effort to salvage the femoral head.

PROSTHETIC REPLACEMENT IN ACUTE FEMORAL NECK FRACTURES

Hemiarthroplasty

Moore and Böhlman, in 1940[301] introduced the first metallic replacement prosthesis in a patient following removal of a giant cell tumor of the proximal femur. This prosthesis was the prototype of the Austin Moore endoprosthesis.[298,300] The Judet brothers, in 1950,[229] introduced a short-stemmed artifical femoral head made of acrylic for arthroplasty of the hip joint. These short-stemmed acrylic prostheses were noted to deteriorate shortly after insertion, and their use was abandoned.[129,202,395] Thompson, in 1954, introduced an intramedullary prosthesis designed mainly for use as salvage prosthesis, especially in patients with nonunion of the femoral neck in whom a shortened femoral neck had resulted from bony resorption.[401,402] Following the lead of Moore and Thompson, multiple other prostheses were introduced for use in the proximal femur. The successful use of these prostheses in salvage situations such as nonunion and aseptic necrosis (which were thought to occur in 40 to 50% of cases) led quickly to their application in the acute treatment of displaced femoral neck fractures.[7] The advantages initially given for primary prosthetic replacement include:

1. Primary prosthetic replacement provides for immediate mobilization with weight bearing. This permits the elderly patient to return to activity

and to avoid the complications of immobilization.[7,28,68,101,202,208,300,381] Owing to the development of improved internal fixation devices that permit early weight bearing in femoral neck fractures, this advantage is becoming less important. However, it remains the primary indication for prosthetic hemiarthroplasty.

2. Primary prosthetic hemiarthroplasty eliminates the complications of aseptic necrosis, nonunion, and fixation failure that occur when this fracture is treated by primary internal fixation. At best this is a theoretical advantage. Boyd and Salvatore pointed out in 1964[57] that 56% of displaced femoral neck fractures progress to union without complications. In addition, they found that only 18% of femoral neck fractures treated by internal fixation required secondary surgery. Primary prosthetic replacement is not indicated solely to prevent this 18% reoperation rate. Also, it is important to remember that all primary hemiarthroplasties are not asymptomatic and that reoperation may be necessary in some of these patients.[57]

The disadvantages of resorting to primary hemiarthroplasty in acute femoral neck fractures include:

1. Function following hemiarthroplasty, although good, is never equal to that of the patient's own femoral head.[57]
2. The surgical procedure required for insertion of a prosthesis is considered by some authors to be more extensive than that required for an uncomplicated internal fixation.[7,57,101,336,349] However, the mortality and morbidity rates reported by several authors are not significantly different in patients treated by primary prosthetic replacement and those treated by internal fixation.[173,331,341,365,382]

Owing to these relative disadvantages of the primary use of prosthetic hemiarthroplasty, definite indications must be present before this method of treatment is selected over primary internal fixation.

Indications for Hemiarthroplasty

Hinchey and Day,[202] in considering the indications for and long-term follow-up of, Austin Moore prosthetic hemiarthroplasty, presented five indications for its use in acute femoral neck fractures:

1. Poor general health that would prevent a secondary operation.
2. Parkinson's disease, hemiplegia, or other neurologic disease.[267,306]
3. Pathologic fracture of the femoral neck.

4. The need for rapid mobilization of the patient (*i.e.,* as in blind patients in whom rapid mobilization is necessary in order to maintain familiarity with their environment.)
5. Patients who are *physiologically* 70 years of age (not *chronological* age).

Thompson[129,401,402] listed the "three P's" as indications for prosthetic hemiarthroplasty: Parkinson's disease, Paget's disease, and porosis. Included in the "porosis" group were patients with spastic hemiplegia, the aged and blind, and those who had undergone electroshock therapy. He emphasized, however, that prosthetic replacement should be undertaken in only about 10% of all femoral neck fractures.[129,401,402]

Other authors have added, as indications, displaced high subcapital fractures,[170] extremely vertical Pauwels type III fractures,[101,371] irreducible fractures,[68,94,101,102,170] severe osteopenia,[170,280] and implant failure following open reduction and internal fixation.[94,101,102,280] Many of these indications are considered to be relative, with the primary consideration being the condition of the patient with respect to his life expectancy, his associated medical problems, and his ability to undergo rehabilitation.

Contraindications to the insertion of an endoprosthesis include preexisting sepsis, an active young patient, and preexisting disease of the acetabular articular cartilage secondary to osteoarthritis or rheumatoid arthritis.[94,133,170,280,371]

The use of an endoprosthesis as primary treatment of displaced femoral neck fractures is on the decline in the past decade, with more emphasis on primary stable internal fixation and preservation of the femoral head.[213] Currently, primary hemiarthroplasty is considered in the treatment of femoral neck fractures *only* when stable internal fixation or the cooperation and rehabilitation after such internal fixation are not possible secondary to fracture characteristics or patient considerations.

Choice of a Prosthesis

Although multiple prostheses have been developed, the most common types in use today are the Austin Moore and Thompson prostheses. These prostheses differ in the amount of the femoral head and neck they are designed to replace. Ideally, both prostheses should be inserted so that the distance between the superior aspect of the lesser trochanter and the acetabulum is anatomically restored.[129] This will restore the length of the abductor mechanism and thereby help to prevent a postoperative limp. The Austin Moore prosthesis is designed for those patients in whom there is ½ to ¾ inch of remaining femoral neck *above* the lesser trochanter.[7,129,298,300] On the other hand, Thompson designed his prosthesis for patients in whom there was limited femoral neck. Therefore, he recommended excision of the femoral neck at the base.[7,129,402] In addition, the collar of the Moore prosthesis is more transverse than that of the Thompson prosthesis, a fact that increases the ability of the neck to receive the compression stresses inserted on it.[129] The more vertical angle of the collar on the Thompson prosthesis tends to allow sinking of the prosthesis into the medullary cavity.[129]

Accurate sizing of the femoral head prosthesis to the acetabulum is *critical* in achieving a good long-term result.[7,202,335,349] If the femoral head is too large, equatorial contact occurs, resulting in a tight joint with decreased motion and pain.[349] If the head is too small, polar contact occurs with increased stress over a reduced area. This leads to erosion, superomedial prosthetic migration, and pain.[349] Neck length is also critical in that, if the neck is left excessively long, reduction may be difficult and pressure on the acetabular cartilage is increased.[349]

Fixation of the Prosthesis

The classical means of fixation of the femoral endoprosthesis is a so-called interference fit.[94,129,133,280] This fit is obtained by careful reaming followed by driving the prosthesis into the shaft of the femur. Moore initially designed his prosthesis with fenestrations in the stem in an effort to induce "self-locking."[133,298,300] This was based on the concept that the fenestrations would allow bone to grow into them, thereby producing rigidity of fixation of the prosthesis. Although the fenestrations lead to some rotatory stability,[129,158,202,220] Eftekhar pointed out that because the prosthesis and bone have different moduli of elasticity, the prosthesis can never be rigidly fixed in bone.[129] In addition to a tight interference fit, the femoral collar of these prostheses is designed to rest on the cut end of the femoral neck in the calcar area to aid in support.[94,129,130,349] Loosening and distal migration of the prosthesis occur when the interference fit fails.[4,195,202,349]

Follacci and Charnley[145] introduced the use of methyl methacrylate for immediate stabilization of a prosthetic hemiarthroplasty in the femoral medullary canal. Methyl methacrylate provides immediate stabilization and therefore decreases the dependence on an interference fit. The principal advantage of methyl methacrylate is excellent fixation of the prosthesis (even in osteoporotic bone),

which allows immediate mobilization and weight bearing.[35,381] Follacci and Charnley believed that the load-bearing capacity of a cemented endoprosthesis was markedly improved over that of a noncemented prosthesis. This is because the load applied to a cemented prosthesis is distributed over a much larger surface area through the cement interface with the bony interstices.[145] They compared a group of cemented versus noncemented Thompson prostheses and found the cemented group to increased acetabular erosion and incidence of in however, that boring of the prosthesis into the acetabulum was more likely in the cemented group, owing to the lack of motion at the prosthesis-bone interface. This problem was particularly prominent in patients with diseased acetabular cartilage. Wrighton and Woodyard[445] reported improved results with cemented Thompson prostheses when compared to interference-fit Moore prostheses in the treatment of fresh femoral neck fractures. Mears and Cruess,[284] and Welch and co-workers[431] noted similar results using cemented endoprostheses. On the contrary, Tressler and Johnson[406] found that penetration of the acetabulum was common and painful, as a result of which only 20 of 44 patients had an excellent result following cemented endoprosthetic replacement. Recently, Beckenbaugh and colleagues[35] demonstrated good results in patients with cemented endoprostheses; however, their patients were carefully selected and were only minimally ambulatory. These authors also noted an increased risk of sepsis and acetabular erosion with the use of methyl methacrylate. In addition to increased acetabular erosion and incidence of infection, the use of methyl methacrylate with an endoprosthesis increases difficulty at reoperation should this be necessary.[170] Finally, a femoral shaft fracture *below* the prosthetic stem of a cemented endoprosthesis may be difficult to heal and especially difficult to revise.[170]

Owing to the complications of increased acetabular erosion, infection, and difficulty in revision, the use of methyl methacrylate with an endoprosthesis can be recommended only in patients in whom there is failure of the interference fit at surgery.[68] Such failure occurs secondary to poor reaming technique,[68] severe osteoporosis of the proximal femur in which the cancellous bone is too weak to give an interference fit,[170] and pathologic fractures.

Surgical Approach

Moore initially recommended the use of a posterior surgical approach for the insertion of his endoprosthesis.[298,300] Although Coventry,[101] using the

Gibson[168] approach for prosthetic hemiarthroplasty, noted no cases of postoperative dislocation, the posterior approach has been related to an increased incidence of posterior dislocation in the postoperative period.[7,110,443] Anderson and co-workers,[7] using the posterior approach, reported that postoperative dislocation occurred in those patients with flexion-adduction contracture of the hip *prior* to fracture. In these patients, they suggested a different approach, probably anterior, in an effort to preserve the intact posterior capsule and prevent posterior dislocation. Wood[443] compared the anterior and posterior surgical approaches for prosthesis insertion and found a higher incidence of sepsis and dislocation when the posterior approach was used. The closeness of the incision to the anus and the resection of the posterior capsule needed for exposure were believed to be important causative factors in these two unrelated complications.

Because of these problems noted with the posterior approach, the anterior approach has been recommended by several authors.[77,110,202,365,443] D'Arcy and Devas[110] found a decreased incidence of dislocation following an anterolateral approach and Sikorski and Barrington[365] noted decreased mortality and morbidity with an anterolateral approach. Wood[443] noted that, although the anterior approach reduced the dislocation rate, it was associated with a higher incidence of femoral shaft fracture and poor prosthesis positioning. Finally, Barr and colleagues[31] were unable to document a definite superiority of either surgical approach.

The Burwell-Scott modification of the Watson-Jones incision,[65,202] which uses a high posterior skin incision combined with an anterior capsular incision into the hip joint, combines the advantages of both the anterior and posterior surgical approaches. The high posterior skin incision is further away from the anus and allows for posterior displacement of the femoral shaft for exposure, while the anterior capsular incision preserves the posterior capsule, resulting in improved stability. Using this approach, Hinchey and Day[202] reported only a 2% combined incidence of sepsis and dislocation.

Position of the Prosthesis

The endoprosthesis should be inserted into the medullary canal in a neutral or slight valgus position, avoiding varus, anteversion, or retroversion.[202,331,349] Although Polyzoides[331] found that a varus tilt of the prosthesis did not affect results, a neutral or slight valgus position is preferred.[202] Excessive retroversion can lead to an external rotation deformity and an increased risk of dislocation with internal rotation. Anteversion can lead

to intoeing and dislocation in external rotation. In patients with osteoporotic bone, or those with a previously inserted nail, penetration of the lateral femoral cortex is possible, and must be avoided.[349]

Complications Following Hemiarthroplasty

Complications following endoprosthetic replacement can be divided into early and late.

Early Complications. *Mortality.* The reported mortality rate following hemiarthroplasty varies from 10%[202] to 41%.[212] Difficulty in comparing mortality statistics in the literature arises from the fact that some authors report in-hospital mortality;[12,158,173,350] others, mortality at 6 months;[202,212] and still others, mortality at 1 year.[395] Recent series have demonstrated a small difference in the mortality rates between patients treated by primary internal fixation versus those undergoing prosthetic replacement.[173,220,226,331,341,365,382] However, Johnson and Crothers,[226] and Salvati and co-workers,[349] emphasized that if correct indications are used, patients undergoing hemiarthroplasty should be older and more debilitated than those undergoing primary internal fixation. Therefore, they should have a higher mortality rate. It is important to remember that mortality following a primary femoral head prosthesis for acute fracture is substantially higher than femoral head replacement as an elective reconstructive procedure.[350,395]

Fracture of the Femur. Anderson and colleagues noted a fracture of the femur in 4.5% of all patients at the time of endoprosthetic replacement.[7] Almost all fractures occur when the surgeon attempts to reduce the prosthesis.[7,202] Most of these fractures are nondisplaced and involve either the greater trochanter or the neck of the femur.[202,212,395] They can often be treated simply with delayed weight bearing on a cane, with or without cerclage wiring.[7,202] Fractures that occur in the shaft of the femur can be treated by primary internal fixation or in traction.[7] With the advent of methyl methacrylate, stability of both the prosthesis and the fracture of the calcar or proximal shaft can be obtained at the time of surgery. Often, methyl methacrylate combined with a long-stem prosthesis (which extends more distally than the tip of a standard prosthesis) will give good stability to femoral shaft fractures.

Fractures that occur *following* surgery are more difficult to manage than those seen at the time of operation.[322,438] Femoral shaft fractures following prosthetic hemiarthroplasty occur in approximately 3% of all patients.[180] Whittaker and colleagues[438] classified these fractures into three types: type I, fractures involving the trochanter; type II, fractures occurring in that part of the femoral shaft protected by the intramedullary prosthesis; and type III, fractures distal to the tip of the prosthesis. Types I and II are stable fractures and can be treated by bed rest and delayed weight bearing.[438] Type III fractures are unstable and can be treated by traction, internal fixation, or the use of a long-stem prosthesis with methyl methacrylate cement.[438] The use of a long-stem prosthesis with methyl methacrylate cement allows the most rapid mobilization of the patient.

Dislocation. The incidence of dislocation following endoprosthetic replacement varies in reported series. Anderson and associates[7] and Hinchey and Day[202] reported a dislocation rate of 1% or less, while Lunt[268] reported a 10% dislocation rate. Factors associated with dislocation include too much anteversion or retroversion of the prosthesis,[349] posterior capsulectomy,[202] and excessive postoperative flexion or rotation with the hip adducted.[349] It is also important to remember that infection is a frequent cause of dislocation, being present in up to one third of dislocated femoral head prostheses.[350] Therefore, in the absence of a definite mechanical etiology, infection *must* be ruled out.

With prompt recognition and reduction, dislocation is not likely to jeopardize the end result.[349,350] Once a dislocation is noted, reduction under general anesthesia is indicated. If several attempts at closed reduction fail, open reduction is indicated. Following reduction, immobilization in abduction and extension until soft-tissue healing occurs is recommended.[349]

Sepsis. The incidence of postoperative sepsis varies from 2%[7,68,77,202] to 20%.[437] As mentioned previously, the incidence seems to be increased in patients in whom a posterior surgical approach is used.[77,212,443] Sepsis may be evident immediately postoperatively or may be diagnosed following discharge from the hospital.[170] Early infections may be either superficial or deep.[349] In the immediate postoperative period, incisional pain, inflammation with drainage, and temperature elevation are noted in superficial infections. Early deep infections vary in their presentation from an acute, potentially fatal clinical course with septic shock to a mild low-grade infection with pain in the upper groin or thigh.[349]

Late deep infections are more difficult to detect.[103] Unusual pain, dislocation, persistent thigh swelling, an elevated sedimentation rate, and finally x-ray evidence of bone erosion suggest the diagnosis.

Aspiration of the hip with culture and sensitivity of the aspirant may confirm the suggested diagnosis.[103] If this is negative, synovial biopsy for culture may be required.[103]

In those patients in whom the infection is diagnosed in the immediate postoperative period, incision and debridement, followed by closed suction-irrigation and intravenous antibiotics, may salvage the prosthesis.[170,267,349] Infections that are diagnosed later usually cannot be salvaged without removal of the prosthesis.[94,103,170] Infection following an endoprosthetic replacement has been reported to result in an extremely high mortality rate.[302,437,443]

Late Complications. *Pain.* The principal late complication of endoprosthetic replacement is pain.[91,437] Although Hinchey and Day[202] reported good long-term results in 84% of patients, and Sharma and Sankaran[362] in over 90% of patients, other authors report good long-term results in only 50% to 60% of patients because of pain.[68,91,437] It is important that both Moore and colleagues[303] and Hinchey and Day[202] found functional limitations after surgery were more dependent on *preexisting* medical conditions than on failure of the prosthesis itself.

Hip pain may be present without x-ray change or may be associated with prosthetic loosening or with distal or proximal prosthetic migration.[103,170,437] Loosening and migration are evidenced initially by a sudden onset of pain in the hip, thigh, groin, or knee, which is increased by rotational stress or weight bearing. Later, inability to perform straight leg raising and deterioration of the abductor muscle power secondary to pain are present.

Loosening is detected on x-ray by the presence of a radiolucent zone around the prosthesis.[103,170,349] In questionable cases, push-pull or rotation films may be helpful.[103,349] Distal migration or settling of the prosthesis is best assessed by comparing recent and earlier x-rays. Calcar resorption,[170] or a change in distance from the collar of the prosthesis to the lesser trochanter, is suggestive.[349] Proximal migration of the prosthesis is noted on x-ray as protrusion of the femoral head into the acetabulum, usually with a concomitant loss of joint space.[103,133,170,349] If clinical signs and symptoms are significant and loosening or migration is present, revision to total hip arthroplasty may be indicated.[94,133]

It is important to recognize that some endoprostheses remain painful without *signs* of sepsis, migration, or loosening.[133] In these patients, it is possible that articular cartilage wear and the involvement of the underlying bone are the cause for pain.[145,170] The surgeon must remember that pain, either idiopathic or associated with signs of loosening or migration, is frequently associated with sepsis.[110] Before revision, therefore, sepsis *must* be carefully excluded.

Heterotopic Ossification. Periarticular ossification after endoprosthetic replacement has been reported to occur in 25%[349] to 40%[317] of patients. However, this ossification significantly interfered with hip function in only 6% of Ornsholt and Esperen's patients.[317] Salvati and colleagues also reported that in most cases the ossification is minimal and does not interfere with hip function.[349] In the unusual instance in which hip motion is markedly restricted, surgical excision of the ossification may be considered.[349]

Author's Preferred Method of Treatment

Patient Selection. I consider the ideal treatment for displaced femoral neck fractures to be anatomical reduction and stable internal fixation because this results in better hip function than that noted in patients following prosthetic replacement. However, endoprosthetic replacement is used as a primary means of treatment if the patient meets certain criteria. *Relative* indications for primary prosthetic replacement in acute displaced femoral neck fractures include:

1. Displaced femoral neck fractures in patients whose *physiological* age is over 70. This means that the patient's life expectancy is *less* than 5 years.
2. Patients whose medical condition is so tenuous that a second salvage procedure is not feasible.
3. Femoral neck fractures through neoplastic, pathologic lesions of the femoral neck.
4. Displaced femoral neck fractures in patients who need to become fully ambulatory quickly because of other illnesses (*i.e.,* blindness).
5. Those patients with associated uncontrolled conditions such as Parkinson's disease, spastic hemiplegia, or mental deterioration in whom internal fixation is not likely to withstand the rigors of their associated medical condition.
6. Fracture of the femoral neck with dislocation of the femoral head. In this instance, the characteristics of the fracture and the patient's age are extremely important considerations. Prosthetic hemiarthroplasty in the younger patient (below age 40) should be undertaken *only* in extreme circumstances.
7. Failure of internal fixation in a recently operated

femoral neck fracture. Evaluation of the acetabulum is critical to make certain that acetabular injury does not dictate total hip arthroplasty.
8. Patients with psychosis or severe mental deterioration who are unable to cooperate with the postoperative regimen required following reduction and internal fixation of the fracture.

It must be emphasized that, no matter what the indication for endoprosthetic replacement (in reference to fracture type, degree of displacement, and so forth), the surgeon must consider the *age* of the patient. In any patient with a life expectancy of more than 5 years and a high level of activity, consideration should be given to a procedure designed to salvage the femoral head.

The author considers as absolute contraindications to prosthetic hemiarthroplasty the following: previous sepsis, severe disease in the acetabular articular cartilage, and a young patient in whom alternative procedures for salvaging the femoral head are feasible.

Operative Technique. The operation is performed under antibiotic coverage. Antibiotics are given immediately preoperatively and for 48 hours postoperatively. Aspirin for thromboembolic prophylaxis is used unless more complete anticoagulation is necessary (see p. 1252).

I prefer the use of the Burwell-Scott modification of the Watson-Jones approach.[65] This incision is away from the anal area, thereby decreasing the chance of contamination. It also allows for an anterior entrance into the hip joint, thereby preserving the stability of the posterior capsular structures. Complete muscle relaxation with general or spinal anesthesia is essential when using this approach.

I prefer an interference-type fit in most endoprosthetic replacements. Methyl methacrylate is used only in pathologic fractures and in those cases in which the interference fit is not stable at surgery. Owing to increased acetabular erosion, infection rate, and difficulty with revision, I try not to use methyl methacrylate in those patients in whom total hip arthroplasty may be indicated in the future. Additionally, if an active urinary tract infection is present, I prefer not to use methyl methacrylate because of the risk of infection about the prosthesis by organisms from the urinary tract if postoperative catheterization is required.

I prefer a solid-stem Austin Moore prosthesis if adequate femoral neck stock (½ to ¾ inch) remains. In those cases in which less than ½ inch of femoral neck remains, a Thompson prosthesis is selected. Owing to the size and shape of the stem of the Thompson prosthesis, I find that an acceptable interference fit is often not possible. Therefore, this prosthesis requires stabilization with methyl methacrylate more frequently than the Austin Moore prosthesis. It is for this reason that I try not to use the Thompson prosthesis unless femoral neck length is at an absolute minimum.

Postoperatively, an abduction pillow splint is kept between the patient's legs during hospitalization. Patients are allowed to dangle their extremities from the bed the first postoperative day and stand by the bed on the second postoperative day. Ambulation with progressive weight bearing as tolerated is then allowed. Physical therapy to restore strength in the hip abductors, flexors, and extensors is encouraged.

TOTAL HIP ARTHROPLASTY IN ACUTE FEMORAL NECK FRACTURES

Total hip arthroplasty is now widely performed to salvage such complications of femoral neck fractures as nonunion and aseptic necrosis.[92,129,130,367] It is also used extensively to manage failed endoprostheses inserted primarily for femoral neck fractures. The short-term results of total hip arthroplasty for nonunion, aseptic necrosis, and failure of internal fixation of femoral neck fractures have been uniformly good.[92,258] There remain, however, no guidelines for the use of total hip arthroplasty in the management of *acute* femoral neck fractures. Sim and Stauffer[367,368] recommend total hip arthroplasty in patients with:

1. Femoral neck fractures who have associated hip disease.
2. Those with contralateral hip disease.
3. Elderly patients with femoral neck fractures in whom internal fixation historically has a high potential for failure.[367,368]

These authors prefer total hip arthroplasty to cemented hemiarthroplasty in the elderly patient because of improved functional capacity and a greater predictability of outcome.

Although considered an indication for primary total hip arthroplasty, preexisting hip disease associated with femoral neck fracture is not common.[318,391,413] Östrup reports that osteoarthritis of the hip, although associated with femoral neck fractures, is more commonly seen in association with intertrochanteric fractures.[318] Both Stephen[391] and Vahvanen[413] noted that subcapital fractures of the femur in patients with rheumatoid arthritis

have a very poor union rate and that loss of fixation occurred in a high percentage of their patients. Because of these problems, Eftekhar recommends primary total hip replacement in patients with coexisting osteoarthritis, rheumatoid arthritis, severe osteoporosis, and pathologic conditions with acetabular involvement such as Paget's disease.[129]

Coates and Armour[92] suggested total hip arthroplasty in elderly patients with Garden III and IV femoral neck fractures. His goal was to avoid the high incidence of complications following internal fixation of these subcapital fractures,[28,92] and the acetabular erosion and migration seen following hemiarthroplasty.[92] Although the mortality and postoperative infection rate were comparable to those found following hemiarthroplasty, the dislocation rate was much higher.[92] Importantly, both the infection and dislocation rates were higher than those noted following elective total hip arthroplasty. Additionally, Sim and Stauffer[367] reported medical complications in 21% and surgical complications in 22% of patients undergoing primary total hip replacement for femoral neck fracture.

Bipolar Prostheses

There is recent interest in prostheses having in common the interposition of an inner prosthetic bearing within the implant.[39,127,258,261,398,405] These implants consist of a femoral component (stabilized by interference fit or methyl methacrylate into the medullary canal) that articulates by snap fit into the high-density polyethylene liner of a metallic cup that moves freely within the patient's acetabulum (Fig. 14-12). These prostheses allow motion *both* at the prosthetic inner bearing and at the prosthetic bearing-acetabular surface. The design is aimed at reducing the friction and impact forces at the prosthesis-acetabular cartilage interface[39,251,258,261,405] (noted in conventional femoral hemiarthroplasty) by allowing additional motion at the femoral head-polyethylene bearing interface. The difference in frictional torque between the prosthetic femoral head-polyethylene bearing and the metallic cup-articular cartilage interface are designed to concentrate motion at the prosthetic femoral head-polyethylene interface. Theoretically, by decreasing motion at the acetabular surface, the articular cartilage wear that results in acetabular wandering and pain[127,251,258] is reduced. In addition, these implants are easily converted to a total hip arthroplasty.[39,258]

The two designs most commonly used in this country are the Bateman[127,258,261] (Fig. 14-12) and Giliberty prostheses.[39,251,405] Drinker and Murray[127] reported a series of Bateman prostheses that were compared to cemented Thompson prostheses. They noted no significant differences in hip ratings between these two groups. They also found in the Bateman prostheses that, although inner bearing motion did occur, the degree was not predictable, and it decreased over a period of time. It was their conclusion that the ultimate relationship between the presence of inner bearing motion and the development of pain and protrusio in the acetabulum is not yet known.

Long and Knight[261] concluded that the Bateman prosthesis offers no advantage over the conventional Moore prosthesis in elderly patients, especially if they are debilitated, confused, or minimally ambulatory. Postoperative dislocations, although not common, were difficult to manage and required a second operative procedure in all cases.[127,251,258] Langan[251] reported good short-term results using the Giliberty bipolar prosthesis. However, at 1 year postoperatively movement of the cup was noted to be absent in 86% of patients. This may lead later to acetabular erosion and migration. Bhuller[39] reported a high rate of disassembly, dislocation, mortality, and prolonged hospitalization following the use of the Giliberty prosthesis. He found no advantage to this prosthesis in the treatment of femoral neck fractures in the elderly.

Although the use of these prostheses has not proved more advantageous than conventional methods in treating patients with fresh fractures, their use in patients with late segmental collapse and those with tumors of the femoral head and neck is promising. Perhaps with improvements in design, their application in the treatment of fresh fractures can be expanded.

Author's Preferred Method of Treatment

I reserve primary total hip arthroplasty for three groups of patients. First, patients suffering a femoral neck fracture who have preexisting symptomatic diseased acetabular cartilage in the *ipsilateral* hip. Although unusual, this is seen in patients with rheumatoid arthritis, preexisting osteoarthritis, Paget's disease, and occasionally with aseptic necrosis. The patient's physiologic age is critical in considering whether or not, even in this small group of patients, total hip replacement is indicated. Those patients under the age of 60 with a normal life expectancy and activity are not good candidates for total hip replacement, in my opinion.

Second, total hip replacement is considered in patients who are candidates for hemiarthroplasty (under the criteria listed on p. 1235) and who have

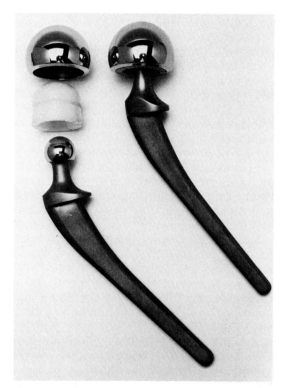

Fig. 14-12. Bateman's universal proximal femoral prosthesis. (*Left*) Disassembled prosthesis consisting of the femoral component, a polyethylene liner, and the metallic cup. (*Right*) The assembled prosthetic components. Motion occurs between the femoral head and polyethylene liner, and also between the metallic cup and the acetabular articular cartilage.

preexisting disease in the *contralateral* hip. The patient with an endoprosthesis in one hip who suffers a fracture of the *contralateral* hip is a particularly good candidate for total hip arthroplasty. This is because of the rather poor functional quality noted in patients with bilateral endoprosthetic replacement.[124,357]

Third, total hip replacement is used in those femoral neck fractures associated with metastatic disease in the ipsilateral acetabulum. In these patients hemiarthroplasty may lead to rapid migration or, worse, may not provide pain relief. Total hip replacement is a more certain solution for this problem.

I have been reticent to extend my criteria beyond these, owing to the complication rate of total hip arthroplasty. Currently, my experience with the Bateman and Giliberty type prostheses is too limited to give definite indications for their use in acute femoral neck fracture management.

FRACTURES OF THE NECK OF THE FEMUR DIAGNOSED LATE

Fractures of the femoral neck diagnosed late present unique problems in management.[3,197,238,290,371] The old or untreated femoral neck fracture will obviously in time blend with those fractures that are termed "delayed" or "nonunions." King[238] termed an untreated fracture of the femoral neck 3 weeks old an "ununited fracture." Reich[340] termed fractures of the neck of the femur "ununited" if they had been untreated 6 weeks from the time of injury. It is beyond the scope of this chapter to discuss the treatment of truly ununited fractures of the neck of the femur. However, the treatment of those fractures that have gone unrecognized for a period of up to 3 months following injury will be considered.

Coventry[101,102] and Eftekhar[130] both concluded that open reduction and internal fixation of femoral neck fractures after 10 days was not useful and recommended prosthetic hemiarthroplasty in those patients. Sisk[371] recommends prosthetic hemiarthroplasty in those cases left unreduced and untreated for more than 3 weeks after fracture. Meyers and colleagues[290] reported a series of 32 patients undergoing posterior muscle pedicle bone grafting and internal fixation 30 to 90 days after fracture of the femoral neck. They reported a 72% union rate, but follow-up was not adequate to give meaningful information regarding aseptic necrosis. Meyers and colleagues recommended this procedure only if adequate femoral neck remained. Henderson[197] recommended that bone grafts *not* be used in ununited fractures of the neck of the femur if the femoral head were avascular. However, Phemister[327] stressed the difficulty in determining the viability of the femoral head clinically or by x-ray in patients with previous femoral neck fractures. Meyers and colleagues believe that avascularity of the femoral head is not a contraindication to bone grafting in undiagnosed femoral neck fractures.

Author's Preferred Method of Treatment

I consider patients in whom a femoral neck fracture has been unreduced and untreated for several weeks after injury to be in two groups.

In the first group are patients who are *not* candidates for prosthetic hemiarthroplasty by the parameters of physiologic age, life expectancy, associated disease, and other factors. I strongly recommend attempting to salvage the femoral head in these patients even in the presence of aseptic necrosis of the femoral head. I have been satisfied with the posterior muscle pedicle bone graft described by Meyers and colleagues.[290] The use of supplemental iliac crest bone graft in addition to the posterior muscle pedicle graft at the time of internal fixation has been required in every case. If aseptic necrosis of the femoral head is present, bone grafting may not prevent late segmental collapse even though the femoral neck fracture heals. Consideration is then given to osteotomy, arthrodesis, or arthroplasty.

In the second group are those patients who are candidates for prosthetic arthroplasty. Treatment in these patients consists of hemiarthroplasty or total hip replacement, depending on the presence or absence of acetabular articular cartilage involvement.

TRAUMATIC FEMORAL NECK FRACTURES IN YOUNG ADULTS

Femoral neck fractures in young adults are considered as a separate group, owing to the fact that these fractures occur in normal bone and are distinctly uncommon.[19,235,247] As stressed by McDougall,[277] this bone is very hard and considerable violence is required for it to fracture. In addition to the relative rarity of the injury, the high incidence of aseptic necrosis and nonunion reported in the management of these fractures is distinctly different from that seen in the elderly age group.[233,247,274,333,448]

The age group of 20 to 40 years is selected because this age reflects the adult vascular pattern and also the period of greatest skeletal mineral density.[17] Protzman and Burkhalter[333] described 21 cases of femoral neck fractures in patients between the ages of 20 and 40 years that resulted in a 62% nonunion rate and 90% aseptic necrosis rate. Massie[274] reported ten patients between the ages of 20 and 40 with femoral neck fractures. Of these, six developed aseptic necrosis and five developed a delayed union or nonunion. Kuslich and Gustilo[247] reported 20 femoral neck fractures in young adults in whom the nonunion rate was 25% and the aseptic necrosis rate was 45%, again reinforcing the poor results associated with this fracture. These tragic results were also reflected by Badgley[21] and Cave.[75] On the other hand, Askin and Bryan[17] reported that in 17 patients between the ages of 20 and 40 with femoral neck fractures, the aseptic necrosis rate was only 18.7% with none of the fractures developing nonunion. However, only *six* of these seventeen patients had clinically normal hip joints subsequent to the fracture. It is believed that technical difficulties in obtaining adequate reduction and stable internal fixation in the dense bone in this age group help to explain such poor results.

Protzman and Burkhalter[333] emphasized three basic differences between these femoral neck fractures and those in the elderly patient. First, they are distinctly uncommon, as they could locate only 43 reported cases in the literature in patients younger than 40 years of age. Second, the results of treatment as reported are notably poorer than those in the more elderly patients. Third, there is a significant difference in the severity of trauma causing this fracture in the young adult. High kinetic energy is required to cause a nonpathologic femoral neck fracture in the young adult, often resulting in associated skeletal or visceral injuries. Protzman and Burkhalter believed that this fracture should be included with femoral neck fractures in the pediatric age group and with displaced stress fractures of the femoral neck, both of which have rather dismal results.[333] They related the nonunion and aseptic necrosis rates directly to the high-energy trauma responsible for the fractures. No resulting recommendations of treatment were given based on their patients. It is important to note that theirs was a retrospective review and that they were unable to make any statement regarding the type or quality of reduction or the stability of fixation present in the cases reported.

Cave[75] encouraged anatomical reduction in all femoral neck fractures but stated that in this younger age group it is particularly important. He recommended, therefore, that if one closed reduction fails, the surgeon should proceed directly to an open reduction through an anterior approach. Badgley[21] also performed open reduction in the majority of patients in his series. However, a series comparing open reduction versus closed reduction in femoral neck fractures in young patients is not available for analysis.

Meyers[287] reported the use of a posterior muscle pedicle graft in 23 patients under the age of 40 with femoral neck fractures. He had no cases of late segmental collapse and only one nonunion. Neither the quality of reduction nor a detailed analysis of these patients was presented.

Author's Preferred Method of Treatment

If concomitant injuries allow, the fracture is treated as an emergency in an effort to preserve what blood supply remains to the proximal (head) fragment. I believe that open reduction and internal fixation of displaced femoral neck fractures in young adults is essential if an *anatomical* reduction is not obtained by simple closed manipulation. If the fracture is undisplaced or if anatomical reduction is obtained by a simple manipulation and there is *minimal* posterior comminution, the fracture is internally fixed with multiple AO cancellous screws, a compression hip screw and anterotation pin, or multiple Knowles pins, depending on the level of the fracture.

In all these cases, consideration is given to bone grafting, especially in displaced fractures. I have been pleased with Meyers'[287] modification of the posterior muscle pedicle bone graft in managing displaced fractures, with posterior comminution. Several steps in this technique must be emphasized. First, experience is necessary to know how to place the patient prone on the fracture table. Second, it is *essential* that an anatomical reduction be obtained prior to internal fixation and bone grafting. Third, the posterior bony defect resulting from comminution must be filled with cancellous bone from the posterior iliac crest, over which is applied the quadratus femoris muscle pedicle bone graft (see Fig. 14-11). The cancellous bone and the muscle pedicle graft restore stability in the fracture area and are essential to prevent loss of fixation, malunion or delayed union, and aseptic necrosis.

All patients postoperatively are managed non-weight bearing for 6 weeks. Although spica cast fixation is not a part of Meyers'[287] postoperative recommendations, I have found that following repair of a femoral neck fracture, young patients are sometimes difficult to manage on a partial weight-bearing basis. Therefore, consideration is given in each patient to the use of a hip spica with a hinged knee during these first 6 weeks. If comminution present at the fracture site results in internal fixation that is less stable than desired, I believe that spica cast protection is essential.

Protected weight bearing is begun 6 weeks after surgery. Unprotected weight bearing is allowed when x-rays, either routine or tomographic, demonstrate fracture union. A technetium-99m-sulfur colloid bone scan is obtained initially and 6 weeks after fracture to determine the vascularity of the femoral head.[239,291]

STRESS FRACTURES

Blecher first reported a stress fracture of the neck of the femur in 1905.[43] Subsequently, in 1944, Branch reported two cases of displaced femoral neck fractures, neither of which healed.[59] Since then, stress fractures of the femoral neck have been described by many authors.[44,117,118,132,169,207,218,293,304,311,332,426,442]

The occurrence of a stress fracture is dependent

on two factors: the degree of force applied and the strength of the bone involved.[311] Stress fractures can occur in normal bone undergoing repeated submaximal stresses or in diseased bone undergoing repeated minimal stresses.[311] Stress fractures of the femoral neck are seen, therefore, in two groups of patients: (1) young persons with normal bone experiencing strenuous activity to which they are not accustomed[44,117,169] (*e.g.,* military recruits); and (2) older persons with minimal stress to osteopenic bone.[117,293] Stress fractures have been found to be distinctly unusual in the black population in both the younger *and* older age groups.[207] Preexisting alignment abnormalities such as coxa vara may increase the risk of femoral neck stress fracture (Fig. 14-13).

The subtlety of symptoms associated with impending stress fractures is often responsible for the diagnosis' being missed. A patient in one of the two groups above who demonstrates pain in the hip or knee with exertion, limitation of hip motion, or localized anterior tenderness, in spite of negative x-rays, *has* a femoral neck stress fracture until proven otherwise. All lab values are usually normal.[304] Tenderness is often minimal, owing to the soft tissue overlying the femoral neck.

Although x-rays may be negative initially, they often reveal endosteal or subperiosteal callus 10 to 14 days later.[304] A bone scan is often positive before an x-ray diagnosis is made[332] (Fig. 14-14). An intensive search should be aimed at the opposite hip to rule out bilateral fractures as mentioned by Devas.[117]

Ernst first reported the high incidence of complications of displaced femoral neck stress fractures.[132] He believed that the time required for healing was longer in stress fractures than in other fractures. Blickenstaff and Morris[44,304] confirmed these findings, reporting nine displaced fractures, four of which never united and three of which required two operations to achieve union. Owing to the poor results following displacement of a stress fracture, Walsh treated two cases of displaced stress fractures with bone grafting, one primarily and one secondarily.[426] Both fractures healed without untoward sequelae.

Devas has described two types of femoral neck stress fractures recognized by x-ray.[117,118] One, a "distraction" or *transverse* fracture, is perpendicular to the axis of the femoral neck. Almost all stress fractures in patients over the age of 60 are of this type. The second type, a "compression" fracture,

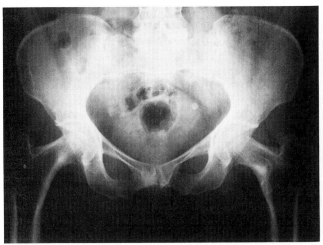
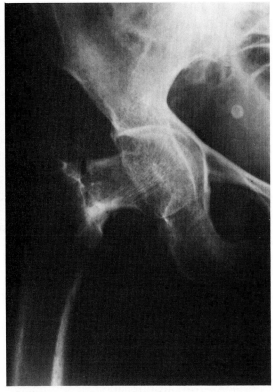

Fig. 14-13. (*Left*) Preexisting coxa vara in a 52-year-old woman with osteomalacia who presented with pain in her right hip. (*Right*) Displacement of a stress fracture secondary to a twisting injury.

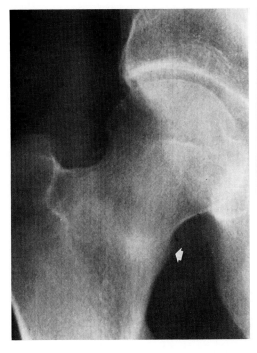

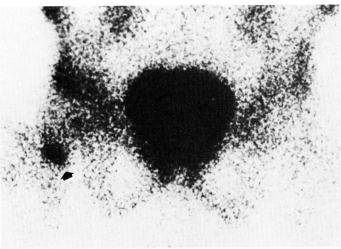

Fig. 14-14. (*Left*) A compression-type femoral neck stress fracture (*arrow*). (*Right*) This bone scan confirms a stress fracture by increased uptake in the right femoral neck (*arrow*).

begins as a "haze" of internal callus in the inferior part of the femoral neck (Fig. 14-15). This type accounts for one half of the stress fractures under the age of 60.[117,118] Devas believed that treatment of the "distraction" fracture was a surgical emergency because of its propensity to displace. Although symptoms may be severe, the likelihood of displacement of the compression type is thought to be less.[117,118] Devas recommended surgical treatment of both types of stress fractures in the older patient. Compression type fractures in young people must also be considered for surgical treatment unless "good grounds" for conservative treatment are present.[117,118] Indeed, Pankovich[319] recommends internal fixation of all stress fractures, transverse and compression, as a means of increasing the reliability of treatment.

Blickenstaff and Morris[44,304] reported extensive experience with femoral neck stress fractures in young military recruits. They divided these fractures into three types:

Type I: Patients with endosteal or periosteal callus without a definite fracture line.
Type II: Patients in whom a fracture line is present without displacement.
Type III: Displaced stress fractures.

They recommended bed rest followed by progressive weight bearing in type I, conservative treatment (including a plaster spica)[44] or internal fixation[304] in type II, and reduction and internal fixation in type III fractures. In type III fractures, complications including malunion, nonunion, and aseptic necrosis were common. In fact, only two of nine displaced fractures healed without complication. They concluded that the osteoporosis that develops early at the fracture site is a factor that interferes with union.

Author's Preferred Method of Treatment

Owing to the great disability resulting from *displaced* femoral neck fractures in young patients, early diagnosis and treatment *before* displacement are essential.[26,304] A high index of suspicion, mandatory bed rest, and bone scans or repeated x-rays until the diagnosis is made are indicated in high-risk patients. The same tenacity in diagnosis is pursued in the older patient with hip pain, whether or not it is precipitated by trauma.

For stress fractures in young patients, I follow a treatment regimen modified from Blickenstaff and Morris.[44,304] Type I fractures are treated in the hospital with bed rest until the pain subsides and the hip has a full range of motion. Then partial weight bearing is begun. In young patients whose reliability is questionable, a spica cast is considered, as recommended by Howland.[207] If the endosteal or periosteal callus is located on the lateral (tension)

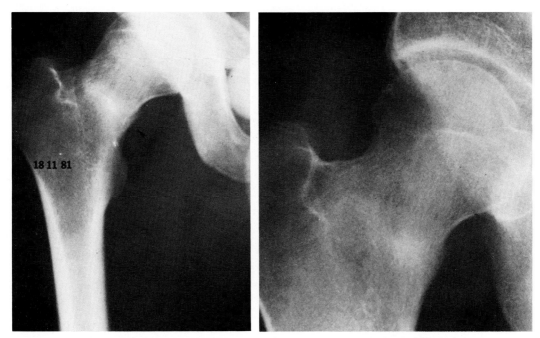

Fig. 14-15. (*Left*) A transverse or distraction-type femoral neck stress fracture as described by Devas.[117,118] The fracture line is perpendicular to the axis of the femoral neck (*arrows*). (*Right*) A compression-type stress fracture of the femoral neck. (Note the haze of internal callus on the inferior part of the femoral neck.) The compression-type fracture is *not* perpendicular to the axis of the femoral neck.

side of the femoral neck, consideration is given to prophylactic pinning, particularly in the unreliable patient. Type II (complete but nondisplaced) fractures are treated by internal fixation with multiple Knowles pins or AO cancellous screws. I believe that the use of a large nail can result in rotation, tilting, or displacement of the femoral head in these cases. Type III fractures are treated by internal fixation after anatomical reduction (closed if possible) with a compression hip screw supplemented by a bone graft applied either posteriorly as a muscle pedicle graft or laterally through the femoral neck. Osteotomy of the femur is added if preexisting coxa vara is felt to be contributing to the stress fracture. Postoperative immobilization in a plaster spica for 6 weeks is used in all young patients with type III fractures and in those patients with type I and II fractures that appear to be unreliable.

In the older patient, treatable metabolic bone disease is ruled out (*i.e.*, osteomalacia) once the stress fracture is diagnosed. In a patient with a normal life expectancy whose stress fracture is in osteopenic bone, I attempt to achieve union and salvage the femoral head as described for the younger patient *if* the bone will hold an internal

fixation device. Salvage procedures for failure of treatment of type III fractures (*i.e.*, hemiarthroplasty or total hip arthroplasty) are much more appropriate in this group than in younger patients. In patients whose physiologic age or physical condition warrants prosthetic femoral head replacement, this procedure is performed primarily in displaced stress fractures.

IPSILATERAL FRACTURE OF THE FEMORAL NECK AND SHAFT

The occurrence of fractures of the femoral neck and shaft in the *same* limb poses a difficult problem in management.[16,38,112,115,270,351] Since the original description by Delaney and Street,[112] only a few cases have been reported.[16,38,115,270,351]

Knowledge of this combination of injuries is important because in almost one half of the cases reported in the literature the femoral neck fracture was initially missed.[38] Only in the series of Dencker[115] and Bernstein[38] was the femoral neck fracture diagnosed initially in all cases. The reason for the missed diagnosis is that the usual external rotation deformity of the hip fracture is masked by the deformity of the femoral shaft fracture.[270] Careful clinical and x-ray evaluation of the joint above and below a femoral shaft fracture (to detect associated femoral neck or patellar fracture) will prevent such missed diagnoses.[38,115,270]

This combination of injuries most commonly occurs in cases of severe trauma such as automobile or motorcycle accidents.[38,112,115] Schatzker and Barrington[351] and MacKenzie[270] believe the mechanism of injury to be longitudinal compression along the axis of the femur with the hip in a position of abduction. With the hip abducted, the femoral head is stable in the acetabulum and cannot dislocate posteriorly. If all the energy is not dissipated at the femoral fracture, a fracture-dislocation of the hip or a femoral neck fracture will result.[38,115]

The resulting femoral neck fracture is frequently of the Pauwels' III type according to Schatzker and Barrington.[351] Also, Bernstein[38] and Delaney and Street[112] noted a high incidence of patellar fracture associated with this combination of injuries, a fact that tends to support this mechanism.[351]

The end result of this injury complex is *most* dependent on when the correct diagnosis is made.[270] MacKenzie[270] stressed not only the importance of obtaining x-rays of the hip and knee in patients with femoral shaft fractures but also the necessity for *careful* evaluation of these x-rays in an effort to detect a nondisplaced femoral neck fracture that might later displace.

Treatment alternatives are based on the patient's age, the location of femoral shaft fracture, and the degree of displacement of the femoral neck fracture.[38,270] Treatment alternatives include:

1. Traction for *both* fractures.[270] This method is very likely to result in nonunion or varus of the femoral neck fracture[38] and should be considered only when the associated hip fracture is nondisplaced and extracapsular.[270]
2. Intramedullary nailing of the femoral shaft fracture and accessory internal fixation of the femoral neck fracture.[112] Delaney and Street utilized Knowles pins placed around a Küntscher rod, while Dencker[115] used a Nystrom nail for the femoral neck fracture and an intramedullary nail for the shaft fracture in this combination of fractures.[112]
3. Internal fixation of the femoral neck fracture combined with plating of the femoral shaft fracture.[38,351] A nail-plate device with a long side plate can be used to stabilize *both* fractures if the femoral shaft fracture is proximal.[38,351]
4. Internal fixation of the fracture of the femoral neck fracture followed by treating the femoral

shaft fracture in traction.[38,270] The presence of an associated patella fracture limits the use of this approach.[38]
5. Treatment of both the femoral neck and shaft fractures with a single intramedullary device.[16,351]

The prognoses in these injuries is dependent on an early diagnosis of the femoral neck fracture. Bernstein reported that if the hip is treated in traction (either because it is initially missed or because of the surgeon's preference) the result is nonunion or varus.[38] For this reason most authors propose internal fixation of the femoral neck.[16,38,112,115,270,351] The femoral shaft fracture will usually heal whether it is treated by compression plating, intramedullary nailing, or traction.[270] MacKenzie[270] reports a high incidence of second operations *even* when the diagnosis is correct initially. He believes that reduction and internal fixation of the femoral neck fracture and traction for the shaft fracture or intramedullary nailing of the femur and *stable* pinning of the femoral neck are the most reliable procedures in these injuries. Schatzker and co-workers[351] suggest internal fixation of *both* fractures for the best results.

Author's Preferred Method of Treatment

I also emphasize the necessity of diagnosing the femoral neck fracture *initially*. Careful evaluation of good quality hip x-rays is *mandatory* in all patients with femoral shaft fractures if the femoral neck fracture is to be detected.

The specific treatment modality chosen for the femoral neck and femoral shaft fracture is dependent on the characteristics of each particular fracture.

Stable internal fixation of the femoral neck fracture with Knowles pins or a sliding compression hip screw and antirotation Knowles pin is the *key* to the management of these complex fractures. The femoral shaft fracture can be managed in traction followed by a cast brace, compression plating, or intramedullary nailing, the choice being dependent on the characteristics of the femur fracture and the patient's associated injuries. In cases in which the femoral shaft fracture is in the proximal femur, I prefer a compression hip screw with long side plate to stabilize both fractures. In patients with associated patella fractures, stabilization of both the femoral neck and shaft is essential to allow the early range of motion necessary following patellar repair or excision. If the femur fracture is in the mid-shaft, I prefer intramedullary nailing or plate fixation, depending on the fracture characteristics. The femoral neck fracture is treated with Knowles pins or sliding compression hip screw, depending on the method selected for the shaft fracture.

FRACTURE OF THE NECK OF THE FEMUR IN PATIENTS WITH PAGET'S DISEASE

Nicholas and Killoran[312] believed that the incidence of Paget's disease is much more common than is reflected in the literature and actually depends on the extent of the x-ray survey performed on each patient. According to Barry, femoral neck fractures are less common than either intertrochanteric or subtrochanteric fractures in patients with Paget's disease.[32] Lake[249] found fractures in patients with Paget's disease to be more common in the earlier vascular phase than in the later sclerotic phase of the disease.

Pathologic fracture of the neck of the femur through bone involved with Paget's disease presents a formidable problem. In pathologic femoral neck fractures resulting from malignant disease, compromise in standard treatment plans can often be accepted because of limited life expectancy. However, in patients with Paget's disease this is not possible due to the fact that life expectancy is not likely to be shortened.[312]

Fractures through a femoral neck involved with Paget's disease often will not heal.[292,312,390,428] Nicholas and Killoran[312] believed that nonunion in these fractures was usually secondary to a poor reduction, distraction, and failure of internal fixation. These technical problems are more apt to occur in Paget's disease, owing to both the deformity of bone and the inherent characteristics of pagetoid bone. In addition, Lake concluded that in the vascular phase fractures unite rapidly, whereas union is difficult to achieve when the disease is in the sclerotic phase.[249]

For these reasons, the displaced fracture of the femoral neck in Paget's disease still represents an unsolved problem. Grundy[179] reported nonunion in all his patients with displaced femoral neck fractures whether they were treated by open or closed means. Barry,[32] impressed by such poor results, recommended treating nondisplaced fractures with bed rest and gave no firm recommendation for the management of displaced fractures. Dove[126] noted a 75% nonunion rate in fractures treated conservatively or by reduction and internal fixation. Patients treated by primary prosthetic replacement fared much better, with 78% resuming their preoperative ambulatory status. Milgram also suggested replacement arthroplasty over internal

fixation, because of the poor rate of union following displaced fractures through pagetoid femoral neck.[292] He did point out that such patients may be prone to develop fractures below the stem of the prosthesis if this area is involved in the pagetoid process.[292] Contrary to Milgram's findings, both Barry[32] and Nicholas and Killoran[312] reported that the results of prosthetic replacement of the femoral head in patients with Paget's disease are unsatisfactory, presumably because of acetabular involvement with Paget's disease. Stauffer and Sim[390] suggest that total hip arthroplasty would seem to offer the best chance of salvage following failure of internal fixation of these fractures.

Author's Preferred Method of Treatment

The possibility of excessive bleeding in the vascular phase of Paget's disease and the dense bone present in the sclerotic phase (which makes internal fixation quite difficult) are problems that *must* be considered prior to treatment selection.

In patients with a nondisplaced (but not stress) fracture of the femoral neck through pagetoid bone, internal fixation with either Knowles pins or a sliding compression hip screw is preferred. I have found such nondisplaced (not stress) fractures to be unusual in patients with Paget's disease.

In patients with displaced fractures of the femoral neck *through* pagetoid bone, two treatment alternatives are available. If the acetabulum does not appear to be involved in the pagetoid process, primary endoprosthetic replacement is the treatment of choice. If, however, there is concomitant involvement of the acetabulum, and especially if there were prefracture symptoms of hip pain, stiffness, and so forth, total hip arthroplasty is the recommended treatment. Before either of these operations is undertaken, the surgeon *must* have a complete x-ray evaluation of the proximal shaft of the femur to determine whether or not excessive bowing will make prosthetic insertion difficult or impossible. The surgeon must also be prepared to manage excessive bleeding at surgery that may occur following fracture through pagetoid bone, especially if the disease is in the vascular phase.

I have found total hip arthroplasty to be an excellent salvage technique for patients with Paget's disease whose femoral neck fractures have failed to heal following internal fixation.

FEMORAL NECK FRACTURES IN PATIENTS WITH PARKINSON'S DISEASE

Parkinson's disease, a disorder of late life caused by a lesion in the brain stem, is characterized by signs ranging from a mild tremor to complete incapacitation secondary to rigidity and tremor.[100] Patients with Parkinson's disease who suffer fractures of the proximal femur are known to have higher morbidity and mortality than patients in the normal population.[100] Osteoporosis and contractures may make surgical exposure, rigid nail fixation, and secure prosthetic insertion difficult. In addition, the associated tremor and impaired balance often preclude good functional recovery.[344] The poor results noted in displaced femoral neck fractures have led to the recommendation for primary endoprosthetic replacement in patients with Parkinson's disease.[202,371]

Soto-Hall[383] stressed that the rhythmic tremor associated with parkinsonism becomes aggravated with bed rest. He believed that in mild cases of parkinsonism, if a valgus or "over reduction" could be obtained, nail fixation would hold. However, in severe cases he believed that nail osteosynthesis would break down secondary to the powerful rhythmic tremor. Therefore, he recommended the use of a prosthesis in such cases. Soto-Hall pointed out that this treatment regimen was necessary because no medications were available at the time that would control the severe parkinsonism tremor.[383]

Coughlin, and Templeton[100] noted a 6-month mortality rate of 60% in patients with Parkinson's disease who suffer femoral neck fractures. They noted that patients undergoing endoprosthetic replacement suffered a 37% dislocation rate and a 75% mortality rate. However, the surgical approach they used for the arthroplasty was not mentioned, and patients were not allowed to begin ambulation until 5 to 7 days after surgery. These two factors may have been responsible for the high dislocation and mortality rates. Because of poor results with endoprosthesis, Coughlin and Templeton[100] recommended closed reduction and pinning of femoral neck fractures in these patients.

Rothermel and Garcia[344] reported excellent restoration of function when primary endoprosthetic replacement was used in patients with displaced femoral neck fractures. These authors concluded that in patients whose disease was well controlled medically with Levodopa, the indications for replacement prosthesis were the same as in the general population.

Author's Preferred Method of Treatment

Patients with uncontrolled Parkinson's disease who suffer displaced femoral neck fractures are usually treated by primary prosthetic replacement. In the younger patient with minimal rigidity who is well controlled on medications, consideration is given to reduction and internal fixation with a sliding compression hip screw supplemented by a Knowles pin above the screw to prevent rotation. The choice between these two approaches is based on patient age *and* severity of the associated Parkinson's disease. Impacted or nondisplaced fractures are treated by internal fixation using multiple Knowles pins or a sliding compression hip screw and supplementary Knowles pin.

FEMORAL NECK FRACTURES IN PATIENTS WITH SPASTIC HEMIPLEGIA

Femoral neck fracture in patients with hemiplegia is a relatively common complication, having been reported to occur in up to 10% of hemiplegics.[383] In spite of this frequency, there is little literature dealing with this subject.

These fractures may occur at the time of the cerebral vascular accident or, more commonly, later when the physical weakness and limb deformity that follow the cerebral vascular accident precipitate a patient's fall. In such patients, the fracture usually occurs on the hemiplegic side,[371,383] and the patient presents with varying degrees of flexion and adduction contracture associated with hypertonicity of the muscles.[383] Because of the hypertonicity, muscle forces about the hip make reduction of femoral neck fractures difficult. In addition, the associated soft-tissue contractures make the surgical approach more difficult.[383] Tronzo[408] reports that such patients do poorly if the femoral neck fracture is nailed, and he therefore recommends primary endoprosthetic replacement. Similarly, Hinchey and Day,[202] Gingras and colleagues,[170] and Sisk[371] consider spastic hemiplegia an indication for prosthetic hemiarthroplasty.

Soto-Hall[383] believed that if reduction and internal fixation of a femoral neck fracture are to be considered in a patient with spastic hemiplegia, the flexion and adduction deformity *must* be reduced by tenotomy *prior* to reduction. He emphasized the need for the release of the contracted muscles inserting into the anterior-superior iliac spine in order to regain full hip extension, which is necessary prior to reduction. Soto-Hall did not outline specific indications for internal fixation versus hemiarthroplasty in these femoral neck fractures. He did, however, emphasize that, if prosthetic replacement is considered, correction of muscle imbalance is as important as it is following reduction and internal fixation, because flexion-adduction deformity, if not treated, can lead to subluxation or dislocation postoperatively.[383]

Author's Preferred Method of Treatment

In selecting the choice between reduction and internal fixation, or primary hemiarthroplasty, the degree of spasticity resulting from the cerebrovascular accident is critical. In patients with minimal spasticity and minimal flexion-adduction deformity who have been ambulatory prior to the injury, consideration is given to reduction and internal fixation with a compression hip screw and an "anterotation" Knowles pin.

In those patients with marked spastic hemiplegia following cerebral vascular accident, primary hemiarthroplasty is performed. In these patients, consideration is given to an anterior surgical approach that will allow muscle release and will preserve the posterior structures intact, thereby decreasing the likelihood of dislocation. Of course, in severely debilitated patients, skilled neglect may be indicated in the management of these fractures.

POSTIRRADIATION FRACTURES OF THE FEMORAL NECK

Following irradiation of the pelvis for malignancy, fractures have been noted to occur in the femoral neck and less often in the acetabulum.[40,171,240,254,266,373,389,392,399] The most frequently involved malignancies are carcinoma of the cervix, uterus, and ovary.[254] Such fractures occur in approximately 1.5% of all patients receiving pelvic radiation.[254,392,399] Because pelvic radiation is a factor in etiology, there is a high rate of bilateral involvement, varying from 20%[1] to 40%.[254] The interval between the initial exposure to radiation therapy and the appearance of the pathologic fracture varies significantly, ranging from 5 months to 12 years.[40]

Clinical Course

The presenting complaint is usually the spontaneous onset of pain in the hip, groin, or medial thigh. The pain may be referred to the knee and occasionally takes the form of sciatica.[392] It is characteristic of these fractures that pain antedates the proven fracture for a considerable period of time, averaging 1.7 months in Smith's series.[373] Initially, the pain is rarely incapacitating and is noticed only with prolonged walking and standing. There is a gradual increase in the severity of pain accompanying increased weight-bearing activity.

Physical examination initially may be negative or reveal nothing more than a restriction of rotation of the affected hip, especially internal rotation. Later, pain is noted at the extremes of all rotational movements. When fracture displacement occurs, signs of coxa vara become more evident.[392] Generally, a history of trauma is *not* obtained from these patients.

On x-ray, the earliest sign is an irregular transverse line of increased density in the femoral neck.[389] On the anteroposterior x-ray, when the fracture line is incomplete it is noted as a separation in the lateral margin of the femoral neck with concomitant minimal varus deformity.[373] As weight bearing continues, the head goes into more varus as this fissure enlarges. A complete fracture, although evident, is not as definable as that in a traumatic fracture. One of the characteristics of the fracture is this coxa vara deformity on the anteroposterior x-ray with minimal, if any, displacement in the lateral view. Angulation on the lateral x-ray is seen normally with femoral neck fractures associated with trauma.[373] One should recognize that acetabular changes occur in patients following irradiation, and such changes should not be considered to be definite signs of metastatic disease.[254]

The differential diagnosis includes a pathologic fracture through a metastatic malignant lesion. However, metastatic lesions to the neck of the femur from primary cervical and uterine carcinomas have been noted to be distinctly rare.[40,399] Therefore, Bonfiglio* stresses avoiding the use of additional radiation to the hip in these patients under the mistaken assumption that this might represent metastatic disease. The differential diagnosis would also include a fracture secondary to major trauma through irradiated bone. The characteristic lack of lateral displacement on the x-ray and a definite history of trauma should differentiate these two entities.

Pathology

Stephenson and Cohen[392] noted a loss of trabecular bulk in association with a loss of cellular elements in the marrow prior to fracture. They did not note a decrease in blood supply to the area as being responsible for such changes. In fact, they mentioned an increase in blood supply postirradiation.

Bonfiglio[48] reported that the dose of irradiation received by the hip joint is below that which will produce complete devitalization. This may explain the lack of interference with the healing and repair response he noted microscopically.[48] Both Bonfiglio[48] and Leabhart and Bonfiglio[254] report osteoporosis with little evidence of necrosis microscopically. Goodman and Sherman[171] noted extensive marrow fibrosis and edema but were not always able to

---

* Bonfiglio, M.: Personal communication, 1982.

demonstrate osteoporosis. Both Leabhart and Bonfiglio[254] and Goodman and Sherman[171] believed that postirradiation fractures occur in a manner similar to stress fractures. That is, bone metabolism is affected by the radiation resulting in weakened trabecular bone that cannot withstand the normal shearing stresses of daily activity.[48]

Treatment Considerations

One must remember that all series have demonstrated the tendency of these fractures to heal when displacement has not been complete.[40,254,373] Therefore, early diagnosis before displacement occurs is critical.

Bickel recommended simple internal fixation with pins or a nail, possibly supplemented with a bone graft, for these fractures. He also noted aseptic necrosis to be quite rare after these fractures.[40]

Leabhart and Bonfiglio classify these fractures into four types.[254] Type I is a fracture with slight varus deformity, while type IV is a fracture with complete displacement. Types II and III represent gradations of severity of varus displacement of the femoral neck fracture. Their recommendation for the treatment of type I fractures is pinning in situ. In type II and possibly type III fractures, manipulation may be required before pinning. They suggested the addition of a bone graft with internal fixation to aid healing in those fractures that have been manipulated. In fractures with complete displacement (type IV), reconstructive procedures such as prosthetic arthroplasty is suggested. A close follow-up for symptoms in the opposite hip is mandatory, owing to the high incidence of bilaterality of these fractures.

If the patient's life expectancy is limited because of the primary malignancy, the surgeon should strive to restore painless function and ambulation as simply as possible. In these cases, a cemented prosthetic hemiarthroplasty may be indicated.

Author's Preferred Method of Treatment

If the patient's life expectancy is not seriously shortened by the malignancy and the fracture has minimal to moderate displacement (type I or II), I would recommend pinning in situ without manipulative disruption of the fracture. Displaced fractures (types III and IV) are treated by manipulation, pinning, and supplementary bone grafting through the femoral neck if life expectancy is not compromised. In those cases in which life expectancy is limited, a prosthetic hemiarthroplasty or total hip replacement is preferred.

FEMORAL NECK FRACTURES THROUGH METASTATIC DISEASE TO BONE

Pathologic fractures occurring through metastatic lesions about the hip are common, comprising 30% to 50% of pathologic fractures reported in some series.[42,190,221,307,321] Pathologic fractures through the femoral neck result in considerable morbidity secondary to pain and loss of function and require treatment to restore mobility and ensure quality of life.

Francis and colleagues[146] initially recommended resection of the femoral head and neck for metastatic lesions with extensive bone destruction. This technique is effective in relieving pain but results in an unstable hip. Irradiation of the fracture alone, without fracture stabilization, is known to prevent callus formation and hence result in nonunion.[42] Therefore, Parrish and Murray[321] introduced prosthetic replacement for femoral head and neck fractures secondary to neoplastic disease as an effective means of achieving rapid mobilization and pain relief. In those cases in which bone stock was not ideal, they recommended a long-stem prosthesis with therapeutic irradiation postoperatively. They recommended a delay in weight bearing until an osteoblastic response had occurred. This approach is patterned after that of Bonarigo and Rubin[47] which includes a combination of internal fixation and irradiation as a means of limiting the expansion of metastatic bone disease.

The introduction of methyl methacrylate facilitated immediate stabilization by prosthetic hemiarthroplasty.[190,221,250,307,352,366] This enabled earlier mobilization of the patient without the pain often present at an unstable fracture site.[250,366] Murray and Parrish[307] believed that a solid-stem (Austin Moore or Thompson) prosthesis, secured with methyl methacrylate, is the procedure of choice in pathologic fracture of the femoral neck. In a large series of pathologic fractures, Lane and associates[250] reported total hip arthroplasty in patients with femoral neck fractures who also have acetabular involvement. Harrington and associates[190] also recommend total hip arthroplasty in those cases in which both the femoral neck and acetabulum are involved with the disease.

In impending fractures of the femoral neck, with neoplastic lesions occupying greater than 50% of the femoral neck, Cameron and colleagues[67] recommended prophylactic pinning. Lane and colleagues[250] established criteria for endoprosthetic replacement in impending fractures of the hip that include: (1) a painful intramedullary lytic lesion equal to or greater than 50% of the cross-sectional diameter of the bone; (2) a painful lytic lesion involving a length of cortex equal to or more than the cross-sectional diameter of the bone, or more than 2.5 cm in axial length; and (3) a lesion of bone in which pain is unrelieved after radiation therapy.

The general preoperative considerations in these patients include those outlined by Parrish and Murray[321]: (1) the patient's condition must be sufficiently good and life expectancy long enough to justify the surgical procedure; (2) the surgeon must be convinced that the operation is more beneficial than closed treatment; (3) the quality of bone, both proximal and distal to the fracture, should be adequate for stable fixation. (In view of the advantages of methyl methacrylate, this is less important, although it should be considered); (4) the procedure *must* expedite the mobilization of the patient and the reduction of pain, or facilitate general care.

Author's Preferred Method of Treatment

My major indication for operating on pathologic femoral neck fractures is pain. Secondarily, I aim for patient mobilization. Careful evaluation of the patient is essential so that the goals of pain relief, mobilization, and maintained function are attained *without* excess risk to the patient. I prefer a solid-stem Austin Moore prosthetic hemiarthroplasty stabilized with methyl methacrylate for metastatic lesions resulting in fractures of the femoral neck. A careful x-ray evaluation is performed to make certain that the acetabulum and distal femoral shaft are not involved. If acetabular involvement is noted, total joint arthroplasty is recommended. If a lesion is noted farther down the femoral shaft, a long-stem prosthesis is used with methyl methacrylate to stabilize the involved femoral shaft area.

Those patients with an implending fracture of the femoral neck due to neoplastic lesions and who fit Lane's criteria are treated by a cemented primary hemiarthroplasty. I believe that the stresses across the hip joint in the area of the femoral neck are too great to warrant simple prophylactic pinning in these patients.

COMPLICATIONS OF FEMORAL NECK FRACTURES

THROMBOEMBOLIC PHENOMENA

Venous thromboembolic disease is reported to be the leading cause of death in patients suffering orthopaedic trauma who survive a minimum of 7 days after injury.[142] Although the incidence of *documented* venous thromboembolic disease in patients with fractures of the upper end of the femur is known to be at least 40%,[71,108,305,379,393] less than one fourth of these patients have *clinical* symptoms of either venous thrombosis or pulmonary embolism.[108,184,191,305] Owing to this high incidence of thromboembolic disease in patients suffering fractures of the proximal femur, some form of prophylaxis is recommended by most authors.[71,184,191,305,379]

Although physical methods aimed at prophylaxis, including antiembolic stockings,[379] limb elevation,[192] exercises,[192,379] and early mobilization,[379] are important *adjuncts* in prevention, they are only partially successful. Coumadin and other anticoagulants are known to be effective prophylactic agents,[71,184,191] but the frequency of bleeding complications and difficulty with dose regulation make their routine use difficult. Low-dose Heparin anticoagulation has not been found effective in patients undergoing hip surgery.[191] Dextran, although an effective anticoagulant, presents associated problems, including anaphylaxis, renal shutdown, and bleeding complications.[191]

Because of the complications associated with the above anticoagulants, there is increasing interest in the use of aspirin as a prophylactic agent.[114,191,379,446] The basis for this use of aspirin lies in its antiplatelet activity.[114,191,446] Aspirin also has other advantages: economy; no need for laboratory tests before administration; and few side-effects. Zechert[446] reported a significant reduction in thromboembolism in patients with hip fractures who received aspirin compared to those receiving a placebo. However, Harris and colleagues[191] reported that the protective effect of low-dose aspirin (1.2 grams per day) is limited to male patients undergoing total hip replacement. Recently, Snook and colleagues[379] demonstrated significant protection in *both* male and female patients with hip fractures who receive 600 mg b.i.d. This controversy surrounding the efficacy of aspirin in women has not been settled conclusively. It is important to remember that patients with a *documented* previous history of thromboembolic disease require more definitive anticoagulation therapy than aspirin.[114,191] In such patients, Warfarin, low molecular weight Dextran, or Heparin is used instead of aspirin. In addition, patients on aspirin prophylaxis who develop thromboembolic phenomena must be anticoagulated with one of the above agents in an effort to prevent pulmonary embolism.

Author's Preferred Method of Treatment

Because of the decrease in the incidence of pulmonary emboli in all patients, the rarity of fatal pulmonary emboli, and the low incidence of bleeding complications noted with aspirin, I use aspirin, 600 mg b.i.d., in patients with hip fractures who have no previous history of thromboembolic disease.[114,191,379] Patients are maintained on this dosage for 3 weeks postfracture. Classical anticoagulation methods such as Warfarin, Dextran, or Heparin are used in patients with previous thromboembolic disease and in those who develop such problems while on aspirin prophylaxis. Careful clinical examination on a daily basis is essential to diagnose venous thromboembolic phenomena *early* so that more complete anticoagulation can be instituted prior to pulmonary embolization.

INFECTION

Postoperative infection with concomitant osteomyelitis, septic arthritis, and possibly septic dislocation is catastrophic.[30] Barr demonstrated that infected femoral neck fractures are much more likely to have joint involvement than infected intertrochanteric fractures.[29,30] Femoral neck fractures are intracapsular and, therefore, deep sepsis of these fractures is likely to involve the hip joint.[30]

When infection with joint involvement occurs, healing of the femoral neck fracture will *not* occur, and a prompt salvage or reconstructive procedure such as a shaft arthroplasty is recommended.[30] Salvage of the femoral head and neck is usually not possible if the hip joint is involved in the infection.[30] A complete discussion of the diagnosis, treatment, management, and results of such infections is found under the section on complications of intertrochanteric fractures on page 1274.

Perioperative antibiotics have been shown to significantly reduce the incidence of postoperative hip infections significantly. Therefore, I recommend their use on a routine basis in patients undergoing surgical treatment of femoral neck fractures. A more detailed discussion of the use of perioperative antibiotics is found under the section on intertrochanteric fractures (see p. 1271).

NONUNION

In the past, nonunion following femoral neck fractures was noted in a large percentage of patients. Indeed, Catto[74] found that *one third* of all femoral neck fractures failed to heal following internal fixation. With recent improvements in internal fixation devices and with an improved understanding of the importance of a stable reduction and internal fixation, some authors now report nonunion below 5%.[29,122] However, recently Barnes and co-workers[28] found a union rate of only 74% in a large number of femoral neck fractures treated by different surgeons. At present, most series reflect a union rate of 85% to 95% following reduction and internal fixation of displaced femoral neck fractures.[12,79,140,226,286,288]

The temporal criteria used to diagnose a nonunion of the femoral neck are not certain, but most authors agree that there should be evidence of healing between 6 and 12 months postfracture.[25,56,160] Many factors such as operative technique, vascularity, and comminution have been incriminated as causes of nonunion following femoral neck fractures.[25,27,69,87,140,210,327,329] Either inadequate reduction or poor internal fixation technique was present in all cases of nonunion in the series reported by Fielding and associates.[140] Cleveland and Bailey[87] also noted the direct correlation between a poor reduction and internal fixation and the incidence of nonunion. Barnes and colleagues[28] also reported that the quality of reduction directly affects union. Indeed, Cassebaum and Nugent[69] reported that with accurate reduction and stable internal fixation they could predict union in 93% of their patients. DePalma[116] noted that open reduction of the fracture and shearing stresses present in fractures with a vertical inclination increased the risk of nonunion. In these patients he recommended a primary osteotomy to change the vertical shear force to a compression force at the fracture site.

Phemister[327] emphasized that the lack of a cambium layer of the periosteum of the femoral neck makes this fracture at high risk for nonunion owing to a resultant decrease in healing potential. Hulth[210] reported that avascularity of the head of the femur contributes to nonunion because in such a situation healing callus can come only from the neck-shaft side of the fracture. Barnes and colleagues,[28] Boyd,[54] and Phemister[327] have also noted a marked increase in nonunion in patients with aseptic necrosis of the femoral head following fracture.

Comminution at the fracture site, especially posteriorly, was noted by Banks to be present in over 60% of patients who later developed nonunion.[25] Scheck also noted the relationship of posterior comminution and nonunion.[353,354,355] Barnes and colleagues[28] also reported that both the rate and percentage of union decrease as the patient's age and degree of osteoporosis increase.

Treatment

A complete treatise on the treatment of nonunion of the femoral neck is beyond the scope of this book, but a brief review is pertinent for better understanding of the treatment of this difficult fracture.

Phemister[327] emphasized that even in nonunions of a long-standing nature, the femoral head may retain its normal contour and the cartilage space and articular cortex may remain intact. If this situation is present, healing of the nonunion will result in a functional hip joint.

In evaluating the patient with a nonunion of the femoral neck, the surgeon must determine if the head is viable, the degree of femoral neck resorption that has occurred, and the degree of osteoporosis present. After these three factors are analyzed, the surgeon has two choice: (1) to salvage the patient's own femoral head, or (2) to discard the femoral head in favor of an endoprosthesis or total hip replacement.[94]

If the femoral head is viable and there is adequate femoral neck remaining, the nonunion can be treated by osteotomy,[124,217] cortical bone grafting,[3,50,51,52,53,161,429] cancellous bone grafting,[122,124,125] or a combination of osteotomy and bone grafting.[124,125,160] Bone grafting alone is reserved for recent cases of nonunion with minimal resorp-

tion of the femoral neck, a normal neck shaft angle, and preferably a viable femoral head.[124,125,429] Some authors recommend osteotomy alone in such cases to promote union.[124,125,160] The Dickson geometric osteotomy with bone grafting is indicated in the femoral neck nonunion with a viable femoral head and varus displacement due to a loss of fracture reduction. The advantages of this osteotomy include its ease of performance, the immediate stability it provides, and the fact that it converts the shear forces of a vertical fracture to the compressive forces of a transverse fracture (Fig. 14-16). If inadequate femoral neck remains because of excessive resorption, a reconstruction such as the Brackett or Colonna procedures may be indicated.[217]

Since the majority of patients with nonunion of the femoral neck have associated aseptic necrosis[327,429] in which there may be significant disruption of the articular cartilage of the femoral head or acetabulum, prosthetic arthroplasty may be indicated. To be a candidate for prosthetic arthroplasty, the patient must meet the criteria outlined in the section on prosthetic arthroplasty (see p. 1235). In such patients, prosthetic hemiarthroplasty is indicated if the articular cartilage of the acetabulum is normal. If the acetabular cartilage is deteriorated, total hip replacement is the procedure of choice.[429] The age and activity level of the patient *must* be considered

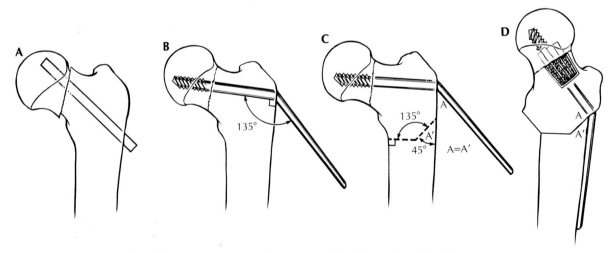

Fig. 14-16. Dixon's geometric osteotomy. (*A*) Nonunion of the femoral neck with a nail device in place. (*B*) Insertion of a sliding compression hip screw. Note that the hip screw is inserted at an angle of 90° *to the lateral femoral cortex*. (*C*) An osteotomy is performed near the level of the lesser trochanter so that the angle of the osteotomy is 135° and the distance A equals the distance A'. (*D*) The osteotomy is completed and rotated into position. At this point bone grafting of the anterior aspect of the femoral neck can be performed if indicated through a cortical window.

before prosthetic arthroplasty of any type is selected (see p. 1234 under treatment of femoral neck fractures).

ASEPTIC NECROSIS

Aseptic necrosis of the femoral head following femoral neck fracture is one of the two major long-term complications of this injury (nonunion being the other). Catto[73,74] has emphasized the importance of distinguishing between aseptic necrosis and late segmental collapse. Aseptic necrosis, the actual death of bone secondary to ischemia, is an *early* phenomenon following fracture of the femoral neck and can be considered a microscopic event.[12,33,73,74] Late segmental collapse is the collapse of the subchondral bone and articular cartilage that overlies the infarcted bone. This collapse results in joint incongruity, pain, and eventually degenerative joint disease.[326] This collapse occurs *late* in the sequence of the ischemic event and is recognized as a *clinical* entity. Not all patients with aseptic necrosis will develop late segmental collapse,[73,74] as those femoral heads with partial necrosis may revascularize and repair before routine stresses on the hip result in collapse of the infarcted area.

The reported incidence of aseptic necrosis following femoral neck fractures is extremely variable. Sevitt[360] reports that 84% of patients suffering femoral neck fractures have partial or total aseptic necrosis of the femoral head. Catto[73] found evidence of partial or total aseptic necrosis in 66% of patients suffering displaced femoral neck fractures. Fielding and colleagues[140] believe that no method of treatment of femoral neck fractures will result in less than 11% aseptic necrosis, as this is the incidence noted in nondisplaced fractures.

The incidence of late segmental collapse following femoral neck fracture varies from 7% to 27%.[12,28,140,164,274,286,288,334] Recently, Barnes and colleagues[28] noted late segmental collapse in 27% of patients suffering Garden type III and IV displaced femoral neck fractures. They also report that the frequency of late segmental collapse is higher in women than men. The incidence of late segmental collapse rises substantially in patients who undergo reoperation after failure of reduction and fixation on the first attempt.[447]

Vascularity of the femoral head following femoral neck fracture is dependent on preservation of the remaining vascular supply and on revascularization and repair of the necrotic areas *before* collapse of the necrotic segment can occur. All the vessels within the femoral neck and most of the retinacular vessels are disrupted in widely displaced fractures.[360] If such displacement occurs, femoral head survival is dependent on the vessels of the ligamentum teres and the subfoveal arterial anastomosis between these vessels and those of the lateral epiphyseal vessels.[360] The terminal branches of the lateral epiphyseal vessels and the vessels of the ligamentum teres anastomose in the subfoveal area.[230,410,441] There are two reasons why this communication does not always provide adequate nutrition for femoral head survival when all the retinacular vessels have been completely disrupted. First, the quality of the vessels of the ligamentum teres is variable.[97,206] In some patients, the vessel is very small and does not actually reach the femoral head.[432,440,441] Second, the degree of anastomosis between the vessels of the ligamentum teres (the medial epiphyseal vessels) and the remaining vessels in the femoral head (the lateral epiphyseal vessels) is variable and incomplete.[361]

If the femoral head is rendered avascular following a fracture, revascularization occurs as vessels grow into the necrotic areas from three sources.[360] First, in cases of partial necrosis, ingrowth can occur from the remaining viable portions of the head, such as the subfoveal area.[326,360] Second, vascular ingrowth can occur across the uniting fracture line from the femoral neck fragment.[360] This is a slower process than ingrowth from the subfoveal area.[326,327,360] It is important to remember that these tender vascular buds can be repeatedly torn if there is persistent motion at the fracture site owing to poor fracture stabilization.[360] Finally, some vascular ingrowth can occur from tissue over that part of the femoral head not covered by articular cartilage.[360] Anatomical reduction and stable internal fixation are the major factors that help preserve the remaining blood supply and provide the stability necessary for these revascularization buds to grow into the area of necrosis.[41,73,74,326,360] Revascularization is known to be more rapid and complete under these conditions.[13,41,196,299] In addition, Moore demonstrated that in a poor reduction the surface area for blood vessels to grow up the remaining neck is decreased, so that the incidence of aseptic necrosis and late segmental collapse is increased when the fracture is poorly reduced[299] (see Fig. 14-7).

Although Phemister[326] believed that the fate of the head of the femur (with regard to viability) is sealed at the time of the fracture, there exists a time between the injury and final fixation of the fracture in which protection by splinting of the extremity may protect the remaining vascular supply to the femoral head.[264] In addition, other authors have demonstrated that vascular injury can also occur at the time of reduction or internal fixation.[73,74,136,264,372]

Smith[372] demonstrated that excessive rotation about the longitudinal axis, or excessive valgus at the time of reduction, may obstruct the remaining blood supply in the ligamentum teres. Fielding[136] and Lowell[264] mention that insertion of a screw for fixation may rotate the femoral head fragment, thereby obstructing the remaining blood supply in the capsule and ligamentum teres.[88] In addition to the rotational displacements with screw insertion, some investigators have demonstrated that a nail placed superiorly and laterally in the femoral head may disrupt the lateral epiphyseal vessels and therefore increase the risk of aseptic necrosis.[60,66,84]

Boyd and Salvatore[57] reported that only 18% of patients suffering femoral neck fractures required a second operation for any complication, and Barnes and colleagues[28] reported that only 30% of patients suffering late segmental collapse required further surgery. One must remember that late segmental collapse *may not* result in a symptomatic hip, although Boyd and George[56] concluded that all patients with late segmental collapse will develop arthritic changes if they bear weight long enough.

Radiographic Diagnosis

The x-ray appearance of aseptic necrosis is that of increased bone density. This increased density may be secondary to: new bone being laid down on necrotic spicules, producing an absolute increase in bony density[46,325]; a relative increase in density owing to the osteoporosis of disuse present in the surrounding vascular bone[73,325]; and finally because of calcification that may be present in the necrotic marrow.[45] X-ray evidence of aseptic necrosis, however, may not be present for up to 6 months following the injury.

Early diagnosis of aseptic necrosis may allow treatment intervention to prevent the late segmental collapse that results in arthritic symptoms. Many different methods of diagnosing aseptic necrosis of the femoral head *prior* to this collapse have been suggested in the past.[11,33,54,55,58,68,205,209,224,291,444] Most of these techniques have proved to be inaccurate and to require such specialized equipment as to be impractical. However, the recent introduction of medullary and cortical bone scanning suggests that this method may be both accurate and practical in the early diagnosis of aseptic necrosis.[33,239,265,291] It is important to remember, however, as emphasized by Bauer and co-workers[33] that even those femoral heads determined to be avascular by scanning may

function well and *not* undergo late segmental collapse. Therefore, a positive scan does not in itself necessarily dictate surgical treatment.[33]

Treatment

A detailed discussion of treatment of aseptic necrosis following femoral neck fracture is beyond the scope of a book such as this. According to Calandruccio and Anderson, the treatment alternatives include symptomatic treatment, osteotomy of the femur, bone grafting, endoprosthetic replacement, and total hip arthroplasty.[66]

When avascular changes are identified by x-ray or by bone scanning, the patient should be treated with protective weight bearing and managed according to symptomatology. Bonfiglio and colleagues report 78% satisfactory results following bone grafting in aseptic necrosis.[49,51,52,53] Weinstein[429] reported similar results in patients with healed femoral neck fractures and aseptic necrosis when treated by tibial bone grafting. These authors, however, emphasize that the procedure is demanding and that poor technique *guarantees* a poor clinical result.[51] The best results in these series have occurred when treatment is instituted *before* collapse of the femoral head occurs.[49,51,52,53,387,429] If late segmental collapse is present in the younger patient, osteotomy is indicated in an effort to salvage the femoral head.[66]

In many older patients, the condition is seldom severe enough to warrant any further surgery.[264] In older patients with collapse of the femoral head and increasing pain, prosthetic replacement is the treatment of choice if the acetabular cartilage is intact.[349,350,429] If the cartilage is not intact, total hip replacement must be considered.

INTERTROCHANTERIC FRACTURES

Classically, an intertrochanteric fracture occurs along a line between the greater and lesser trochanters[534] (Fig. 14-17). Theoretically, this fracture is totally extracapsular; however, the distinction between an intertrochanteric and a basilar femoral neck fracture is not always clear. In intertrochanteric fractures the internal rotators of the hip remain attached to the distal fragment, while usually some of the short external rotators are still attached to the proximal head and neck fragment.[535] This fact is important in reducing the fracture because, in order to align the distal fragment with the proximal one, the leg must usually be held in some degree of external rotation.[534]

Early authors placed most emphasis on intracapsular femoral neck fractures and paid relatively little attention to the extracapsular intertrochanteric fracture because of the fact that these fractures usually healed regardless of the mode of treatment.[517,575] Extracapsular intertrochanteric fractures occur through cancellous bone, which has an excellent blood supply.[577] If there is no interference with the healing process, the fracture will unite promptly. Even if left untreated, the fracture usually stabilizes within 8 weeks and allows weight bearing within 12 weeks. However, marked varus of the head and neck with an associated external rotation deformity usually results in a short leg gait limp.

Morris[539] found extracapsular fractures to be four times as common as femoral neck fractures and to occur primarily in the elderly. Cleveland,[470,471] Evans,[488] Morris,[539] Norton,[548] and Riska[559] reported patients with intertrochanteric fractures to be 10 to 12 years older than patients with intracapsular femoral neck fractures. The average age reported in these patients is 66 to 76 years of age.[449,459,472,477,542] The ratio of females to males ranges from 2 to 1[569] to 8 to 1.[470,477] Cleveland[470] and Weiss and colleagues[589] believed that intertrochanteric fractures occur more commonly in women because of metabolic bone changes.

MECHANISM OF INJURY

Intertrochanteric fractures almost invariably occur as a result of a fall, involving both direct and indirect forces.[470,491] Mulley and Espley[543] demonstrated that the hemiplegic patient was much along the axis of the femur or directly over the side secondary to impaired locomotor function and disuse osteoporosis on that side. Direct forces act along the axis of the femur or directly over the greater trochanter to result in an intertrochanteric fracture.[528,533] Indirect forces, including pull of the iliopsoas muscle on the lesser trochanter and the abductors on the greater trochanter, have also been incriminated as a cause of the fracture.[491]

CLINICAL DIAGNOSIS

The limb is usually markedly shortened with as much as 90° of external rotation deformity.[528] The external rotation deformity is usually greater than that seen in patients with intracapsular fractures. There may be swelling in the hip region and, if seen later, there is usually ecchymosis over the greater trochanter.[528] Intertrochanteric fractures are rarely open fractures, but if such injury occurs,

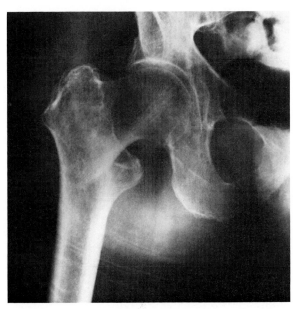

Fig. 14-17. A stable intertrochanteric fracture.

wound management outlined in Chapter 3 is indicated. Stabilization by internal fixation should not be attempted until there is primary wound healing with no evidence of infection.

Attempts to move the fractured limb are painful and should be avoided. Immediate immobilization of the fractured limb with Buck's skin traction or sandbags is necessary to prevent further soft-tissue damage and additional bony comminution.[486,527]

RADIOGRAPHIC FINDINGS

After the limb is immobilized, a true anteroposterior x-ray in *internal* rotation and a lateral x-ray are taken to confirm the diagnosis and, more importantly, to delineate the fracture pattern. The anteroposterior x-ray taken in *internal* rotation is useful in determining fracture obliquity *and* the quality of bone present. If this film is taken in external rotation, the greater trochanter rotates posteriorly and overlies part of the fracture line, obscuring radiographic detail. The lateral x-ray is extremely important to determine the size, location, and comminution of posterior fracture fragments and, hence, to help determine the presence or absence of fracture stability.[525,527,528] If traction has been applied using a Thomas splint for transportation, this splint must be removed *before* x-rays are made or it will interfere with proper assessment of the fracture.

QUALITY OF BONE

Intertrochanteric fractures frequently occur through osteoporotic or[491,515,524,589] osteomalacic bone,[497,515] and occasionally through pagetoid bone.[484] The presence of osteoporosis in intertrochanteric fractures is important because fixation of the proximal fragment depends *entirely* on the quality of cancellous bone present.[524,592] Although medial cortical abutment will restore fracture stability, good quality bone in the head and neck is essential for fixation of the proximal fragment.[491]

Because of its importance in determining fracture stability, some means of measuring the degree of osteoporosis is essential. Singh[576] introduced a method of determining the degree of osteoporosis by the x-ray evaluation of trabecular patterns of the proximal femur (Fig. 14-18). He graded the degree of osteoporosis from 1 to 6, with grade 1 being severely osteoporotic and grade 6 being normal bone. Laros and Moore,[524] using this grading system, found those patients with Singh grade 3 or lower (osteoporotic) had an increased incidence of complications of fixation. The incidence

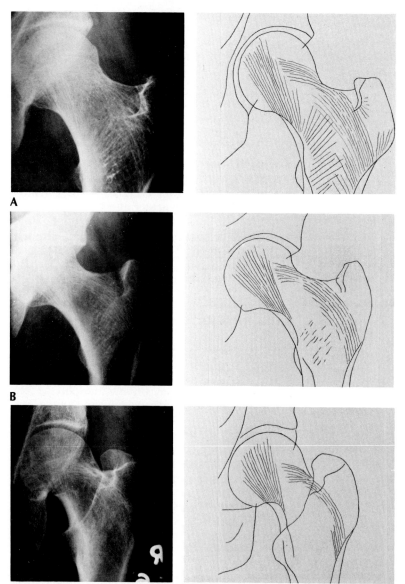

Fig. 14-18. Singh's index of osteoporosis. (*A*) Grade VI: All the normal trabecular groups are visible and the upper end of the femur seems to be completely occupied by cancellous bone. (*B*) Grade V: The structure of principal tensile and principal compressive trabeculae is accentuated. Ward's triangle appears prominent. (*C*) Grade IV: Principal tensile trabeculae are markedly reduced but can still be traced from the lateral cortex to the upper part of the femoral neck.

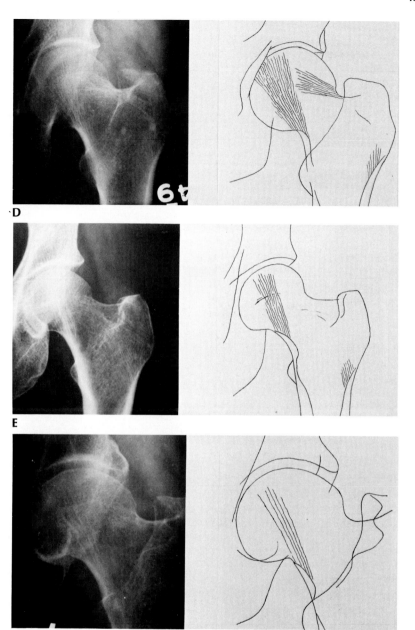

Fig. 14-18 (*Continued*). (*D*) Grade III: There is a break in the continuity of the principal tensile trabeculae opposite the greater trochanter. This grade indicates definite osteoporosis. (*E*) Grade II: Only the principal compressive trabeculae stand out prominently; the others have been more or less completely resorbed. (*F*) Grade I: Even the principal compressive trabeculae are markedly reduced in number and are no longer prominent. (From Singh, M.; Nagrath, A.R.; and Maini, P.S.: Changes in the Trabecular Pattern of the Upper End of the Femur as an Index to Osteoporosis. J. Bone Joint Surg., **52A:**457–467, 1970.)

of complications of fixation in osteoporotic patients (grades 1 to 3) with two-part *stable* fractures was found to be the same as in comminuted *unstable* fractures occurring in normal bone (grades 4 to 6). Not surprisingly, therefore, they found that most complications occurred in severely osteoporotic (grade 3 or less), four-part, unstable fractures.

Although there is question as to the accuracy of measuring the degree of osteoporosis by the Singh method, it is an important tool to provide an *estimate* of the degree of osteoporosis present.[237] If the bone is osteoporotic, Laros and Moore[523,524] found that, by placing the nail of a nail-plate device *low* in the femoral head, the incidence of cutting out could be decreased. Harrington[493] and Muhr and co-workers[541] recommended the use of methyl methacrylate to reinforce and improve proximal fixation in such osteoporotic patients with intertrochanteric fractures. Neither author found an increase in infection, nonunion, or aseptic necrosis. One must remember that this technique does increase the complexity of the procedure and that nonunion may result if the methyl methacrylate gets between bony fragments.

FRACTURE GEOMETRY AND STABILITY

When there is cortical instability on one side of a fracture due to cortical overlap or destruction, a fracture tends to collapse in the direction of such instability.[487] A truly stable intertrochanteric fracture, therefore, is one that, when reduced, has cortical contact *without* a gap medially *and* posteriorly.[567,592] This contact will prevent fracture displacement into varus or retroversion when forces are applied to the proximal femur.[487,567] It is important prior to treatment to distinguish by x-ray stable and unstable intertrochanteric fractures based on fracture geometry and the ability to restore cortical contact medially and posteriorly by reduction.

In a stable fracture (see Fig. 14-17), the medial cortices of the proximal and distal fragments are not comminuted and there is no displaced fracture of the lesser trochanter. Conversely, unstable intertrochanteric fractures are seen in two situations.[476] First, fractures with *reversed* obliquity in which there is a marked tendency toward medial displacement of the shaft secondary to adductor muscle pull are unstable[458,476,487,591,593] (Fig. 14-19). Comminution of the greater trochanter and adjacent posterolateral shaft of the femur will also predispose to such medial shaft migration.[544] This medial shaft migration may result in penetration of the internal fixation device into the joint.[544] Second, intertrochanteric fractures in which there is no contact between the proximal and distal fragments owing to comminution *or* displacement of fracture fragments medially and posteriorly are unstable. The classic example of the unstable intertrochanteric fracture is the so-called four-part fracture of Dimon and Hughston[480,481] (Fig. 14-20). The importance of the lesser trochanter as a key to evaluating instability of intertrochanteric fractures has been pointed out by several authors.[468,480,481,482,483,514] However, the mere presence of a lesser trochanteric fragment does not constitute instability.[520] The size *and* displacement of the fragment are the critical factors in this evaluation. Owing to the posteromedial location of the lesser trochanter, when this structure is fractured *and* displaced, a defect results at the posterior and medial aspects of the fracture surfaces. The medial

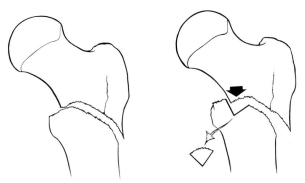

Fig. 14-19. (*Left*) An intertrochanteric fracture with reversed obliquity. These fractures are unstable because of a marked tendency toward medial shaft migration. (*Right*) By notching the distal fragment, the proximal fragment can be impacted into the notch, therefore stabilizing the fracture.

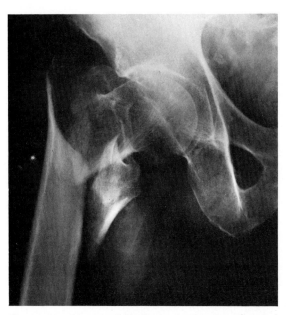

Fig. 14-20. An unstable, four-part intertrochanteric femoral fracture with severe comminution. Note the large posteromedial fragment.

defect results in a tendency for varus displacement and the posterior defect in a tendency to displacement in retroversion, either of which can result in bending, breaking, or cutting out of the implant.[480,546] Up to 60% of intertrochanteric fractures are unstable and hence at risk for these complications.[481,487,508,540]

Efforts to prevent the complications of unstable fractures have taken two approaches: (1) the design of stronger implants in an effort to prevent breakage and displacment;[499,513,590] and (2) methods to restore bony contact medially and posteriorly by anatomical reduction *or* displacement osteotomy.[480,569,592] Frankel[489] pointed out that up to 75% of the load in weight bearing can be taken up by the bone fragments in contact at the fracture site with the rest of the stability being provided by the nail. It is important, therefore, to recognize that the ultimate stability of an intertrochanteric fracture treated surgically is dependent on *both* the stability of the fracture fragments and the strength of the implant.[513,515] No device will alone withstand the cyclical loads present after unstable fixation of an intertrochanteric fracture.[556,592]

The complications of varus displacement, cutting out, breaking, bending, and penetration of the device could *theoretically* be prevented by treatment selection based on the accurate determination of fracture stability. Ganz and colleagues[491] found that the primary cause of failure in treatment of intertrochanteric fractures has been poor evaluation of fracture stability *preoperatively*. Laskin and colleagues[525] have rightly suggested that the *final* determination of stability is best obtained at operation with the fracture fragments exposed. The difficulty in accurately determining fracture stability is emphasized by the fact that so-called stable fractures, even when reduced anatomically and internally fixed, will occasionally displace.[468,542]

CLASSIFICATION OF INTERTROCHANTERIC FRACTURES

As emphasized by Jensen,[507,508] a classification system of fractures must serve two functions. First, it must relate the possibility of obtaining a primary stable and anatomical fracture reduction. Second, it must allow the surgeon to predict the risk of secondary loss of this fracture reduction following internal fixation.

Several classification systems of intertrochanteric fractures have been proposed. Boyd and Griffin[459] presented a classification system based on the ease of obtaining and maintaining fracture reduction. They divided intertrochanteric fractures into four types (Fig. 14-21). Tronzo[586] modified this classification by dividing their type III fractures into two separate groups, thereby resulting in five fracture types. Evans[487] presented a simpler classification based on dividing fractures into *stable* and *unstable* groups. He further divided the unstable fractures into those in which stability could be restored by anatomical or near anatomical reduction and those

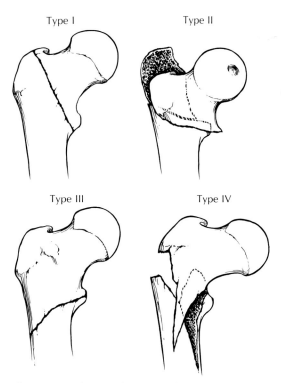

Fig. 14-21. The Boyd and Griffin classification of trochanteric fractures (Redrawn from Boyd, H. B., and Griffin, L. L.: Classification and Treatment of Trochanteric Fractures. Arch. Surg., **58:**853–866, 1949.)

in which anatomical reduction would not create stability (Fig. 14-22). Jensen found this classification to be the most accurate system in predicting the possibility of anatomical reduction and also the possibility of secondary fracture displacement after nailing.[507] From the standpoint of simplicity and accuracy, I have found Evans' concept of classification into stable or unstable fractures to be the most satisfactory.

TREATMENT

Early reports of intertrochanteric fractures favored closed treatment in traction.[457,577] However, an increase in mortality and morbidity associated with such closed treatment led to recommendations for internal fixation of these fractures.[471,488,516,521,526]

It is difficult to compare accurately mortality figures for intertrochanteric fractures treated operatively with those treated conservatively. In most series, those patients treated conservatively have been older, have had more associated medical

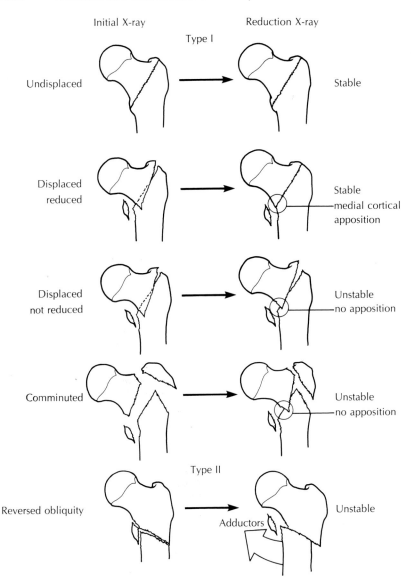

Fig. 14-22. Evans's classification of intertrochanteric fractures are divided into two main types depending on the direction of the fracture. In type I the fracture line extends upward and outward from the lesser trochanter. In type II the fracture line is one of reversed obliquity. Stability in type I fractures is obtained by anatomical medial cortical reduction. Type II fractures have a tendency toward medial displacement of the femoral shaft and, hence, retain a degree of instability.

problems, and were, therefore, higher risk surgical candidates. Several recent reports[498,501,573] have noted that open reduction and internal fixation may increase patient comfort, facilitate nursing care, and decrease hospitalization stay but may not effect a difference in mortality. Because intertrochanteric fractures will usually unite (often in acceptable position) when treated closed,[490] the keys in choosing operative versus nonoperative treatment are the patient's prior ambulatory status and medical condition.[573]

The goal of treatment of an intertrochanteric fracture must be restoration of the patient to his preoperative status at the earliest possible time. If

the patient was confined to bed and chair prior to injury, the goal of treatment is pain relief. If prior to injury the patient was active and vigorous, the treatment should return him to this preoperative status.[563] Both of these goals can best be achieved through reduction and internal fixation in a stable fashion that allows early mobilization of the patient.[491,570,579]

It is my belief that the overwhelming majority of intertrochanteric fractures should be treated operatively for ease of nursing care, rapid mobilization, decreased mortality, and restoration of function.[570] However, conservative treatment may be considered in certain situations.

NONOPERATIVE TREATMENT

The indication for nonoperative treatment of intertrochanteric fractures is unclear. Murray and Frew[544] reported a 10% mortality in patients treated conservatively; however, these patients were younger than the normal for intertrochanteric fractures and hence could tolerate traction better. In general, operative treatment should be undertaken in patients in whom the risk of anesthesia and surgery do not outweigh the benefits of open reduction.[570] Friedenberg and colleagues[490] suggested that the terminal patient, a patient with an old fracture, and a nonambulatory patient who was comfortable with the fracture were all indications for conservative treatment. Rowe[563] recommended conservative treatment if the fracture could not be stabilized adequately by open reduction.

Conservative treatment regimens include simple support with pillows or splinting to the opposite limb,[471] Buck's traction,[471] well-leg traction or external fixation,[450,451] plaster spica immobilization,[471,577] Russell's balanced traction[471,575] and skeletal traction through the distal femur.[453,468,550] Nonoperative treatment of intertrochanteric fractures may follow one of two fundamentally different approaches. The first, as suggested by Shaftan and colleagues,[573] is early mobilization. These patients are mobilized immediately, just as if they had been treated operatively. They are *not* treated in traction but are given analgesics and placed in a chair daily. If, after chair mobilization, the physical condition improves, they are begun on non-weight-bearing crutch walking. Shaftan reported that fracture pain after a few days is rarely more severe than wound pain following open reduction.[573] He also stressed that nonoperative treatment by his technique did not prevent fracture healing or weight bearing. The mortality of patients with conservatively and operatively treated fractures were the same in his series. This fact was particularly impressive since the closed treatment patients generally had more associated illnesses. However, in selecting this approach, one immediately accepts a deformity of varus, external rotation, and shortening because the fracture itself is essentially ignored.

The second approach is traction to maintain alignment of the fracture so that varus, shortening, and external rotation do not ensue. Aufranc and associates[453] recommended skeletal traction in balanced suspension for 10 to 12 weeks. The leg is kept in slight abduction, which allows easier reduction and maintenance of the normal head-neck angle. The patient is then mobilized and allowed partial weight bearing until fracture healing is solid.

Aufranc noted that partial weight bearing may be required for 6 months before good fracture stability is obtained, and that varus displacement could occur as late as 3 to 4 months post fracture. Clawson[468] also used longitudinal skeletal traction in certain unstable fractures. He stressed the need to adjust rotation of the limb, to use serial x-rays to evaluate fracture reduction, and to encourage a daily program of exercises. He noted early callus by the third week, and patients became ambulatory in 10 to 12 weeks.

Well-leg traction as described by Anderson and colleagues[451] and Childress[466] is an alternative to open reduction or neglect of the fracture with its resultant deformity. This technique allows the patient to be moved from bed to chair and eliminates the cumbersome apparatus required by skeletal traction. However, using the normal limb for countertraction can lead to skin problems and ulceration, especially in this elderly group.

If conservative treatment is elected, especially those methods requiring prolonged traction, great care must be taken to avoid the secondary complications of pneumonia, urinary tract infection, pressure sores over the sacrum and heels, equinus contractures of the foot, and thromboembolic disease.

OPERATIVE TREATMENT

If operative treatment is selected, it is important to consider this an urgent, and *not* an emergency, procedure.[488,579] Ring[558] warned against delaying surgery to improve the medical condition because he believed that such problems would not substantially improve with long-term medical treatment. McNeill[536] noted a tenfold increase in mortality when the operation was delayed (for *non*medical reasons) over 48 hours following admission. These facts support the need for urgent internal fixation of an intertrochanteric fracture and for avoiding any unnecessary delays.

The goal of surgical treatment is to fix a stably reduced fracture internally. I agree with Kaufer and associates[515,516] that the strength of the fracture fragment-implant assembly is determined by five variables: (1) bone quality; (2) fragment geometry; (3) reduction; (4) implant design; and (5) implant placement. Of these five, bone quality and fracture geometry, which were discussed above, are beyond the control of the surgeon. The surgeon therefore has within his control the quality of reduction and the choice and placement of the implant to achieve a stably reduced internal fixation of an intertrochanteric fracture.

Reduction

A stable reduction of an intertrochanteric fracture requires providing medial and posterior cortical contact between the major proximal and distal fragments in order to resist varus and posterior displacing forces.[515] Such restoration of normal anatomy is the ideal goal, but unfortunately anatomical reduction of a comminuted intertrochanteric fracture is difficult, if not impossible, to achieve. Therefore, a nonanatomical but *stable* reduction is indicated in those fractures in which an anatomical stable reduction cannot be obtained.

Intertrochanteric fractures can be reduced by open or closed means. Initially, the displaced fracture should undergo a closed reduction that is evaluated to see if it meets the criteria of fracture stability. Closed reduction under anesthesia is obtained by direct traction, slight abduction, and usually slight external rotation.[535] May and Chacha[535] found that intertrochanteric fractures with only slight involvement of the greater trochanter reduced better in neutral rotation, while slight external rotation was required for more extensive and comminuted fractures. Longitudinal traction is applied to restore the normal neck-shaft angle. Such traction uses remaining soft-tissue attachments to the bone fragments as an aid to restoring fracture alignment.[533] Massie believed that this was the most important step in reducing an intertrochanteric fracture.[534] He also emphasized reduction in slight (15° to 20°) external rotation to close the defect that occurs in most comminuted intertrochanteric fractures posterolaterally. He recommended evaluating a lateral x-ray postreduction, and, if fracture separation was present posteriorly, limb rotation was used to correct this separation. In noncomminuted linear fractures *without* displacement, the limb is simply fixed to the table in neutral or slight internal rotation before surgery is commenced.[488,535] Satisfactory results can be expected with most internal fixation devices used in such stable intertrochanteric fractures.[472,481,499,569] In my opinion, the degree of rotation required for reduction is variable, depending on the degree of comminution.[492] This can be determined at the time of surgery by palpation anteriorly and posteriorly as the limb is rotated.

After the manipulation is performed, the reduction is evaluated for stability. If the surgeon feels that stability of the fracture has not been restored, open anatomical reduction is indicated.[580] Occasionally, there is some residual posterior displacement at the fracture site that requires the femur to be lifted anteriorly to secure an anatomical reduc-

tion at the time of surgery. Greider and Horowitz found that approximately 10% of fractures were not stably reduced by manipulation and required open reduction.[492]

Certain fracture patterns should suggest the need for open reduction. Tronzo[586] noted difficulty in closed reduction of specific intertrochanteric fractures in which the lesser trochanter remained intact *and* there was a large spike on the proximal fragment (Fig. 14-23). In these fractures, the iliopsoas tendon remains attached to the lesser trochanter, and the long spike on the head-neck fragment often gets caught between the iliopsoas and the lesser trochanter. Even with strong traction, this fracture tends to remain in varus. However, simple surgical release of the ilipsoas tendon off the lesser trochanter will allow reduction. Also, the intertrochanteric fracture with reversed obliquity requires special surgical treatment.[458,586] For stability, these fractures require open reduction and notching of the distal shaft so that the neck fragment will be impacted into the notch in the shaft to prevent medial migration of the shaft[586] (see Fig. 14-19).

If after closed and then open reduction, the surgeon still believes that the fracture is unstable,

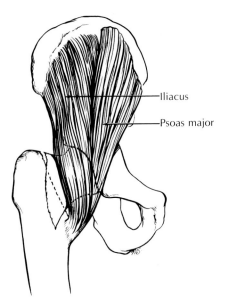

Fig. 14-23. An irreducible intertrochanteric fracture secondary to iliopsoas muscle obstruction. The long spike on the head-neck fragment is caught between the iliopsoas and the lesser trochanter. The varus position remains, even with the application of strong traction. Release of the iliopsoas insertion from the lesser trochanter will allow reduction.

he must resort to some nonanatomical means to restore fracture stability.

Unstable Intertrochanteric Fractures

The unstable intertrochanteric fracture is a serious and difficult problem. Inadequate treatment often results in significant complications. These include failure of the fixation device, delayed union or nonunion, penetration of the device through the femoral head or neck with destruction of the hip joint, multiple operations with increased incidence of infection, and a high morbidity and mortality unless the patient can be mobilized safely. Therefore, some degree of bony stability must be obtained in these fractures. The following are techniques that are used to obtain a stable reduction of unstable intertrochanteric fractures:

Anatomical Stable Reduction

Open Anatomical Reduction and Internal Fixation. Open anatomical reduction and internal fixation of unstable intertrochanteric fractures has been mentioned by Laskin and associates[525] and Riska.[559] Reduction and fixation of a displaced lesser trochanteric fragment to the femoral shaft in an effort to provide a stable buttress for reduction to the proximal fragment have also been suggested.[514,590] Wardle[587] mentions that this method is difficult, time consuming, and often not successful. These techniques are of limited value, especially in cases in which there is comminution of the lesser trochanteric fragment, or in which extensive surgical exposure is required to attain an anatomical reduction. However, young patients in whom the anatomical restoration of the hip joint *biomechanics* is important may be candidates for this extensive procedure.

Nonanatomical Stable Reduction

Internal Fixation of the Fracture in the Varus Position. Cram[476] and Evans[488] mention internal fixation of unstable intertrochanteric fractures in their *displaced* varus position. Fracture stability exists in the displaced position because of medial contact between the two major fragments. However, this technique is the least satisfactory type of nonanatomical reduction because of the limp and shortening that result from union in the displaced (varus) position.

The Use of a Sliding Screw or Nail-Plate Device (without first obtaining bony stability). The use of a sliding device theoretically allows an unstable fracture to impact and thereby seek its

own stability. Jacobs and colleagues[505] demonstrated that, as the sliding device shortens with settling of the unstable fracture, the lever arm acting on the nail-plate junction shortens, thereby reducing the force on the implant. Clawson[469] and Ecker and colleagues[486] noted that unstable fractures treated with a sliding device underwent shortening and medial displacement, but the fracture went on to prompt union. Although shortening of up to 1 cm occurred, the head did not fall into varus, nor did the fixation device cut through the head and damage the acetabulum.

The surgeon must remember that, if he elects to treat *unstable* intertrochanteric fractures with a sliding screw or nail-plate device *without* obtaining bony stability, success rests on the ability of the device to slide. If the device impinges, it will act as a solid-angle nail plate and result in either cutting out or penetration of the head as these unstable fractures settle into a position of stability. Indeed, Wolfgang and co-workers[592] noted that unstable intertrochanteric fractures treated with a sliding screw *without* obtaining bony stability had a 21% rate of mechanical failure. This rate was reduced to 10% when bony stability was obtained prior to use of the sliding hip screw.

I too believe that sliding screw or nail-plate devices are the most satisfactory for treating unstable intertrochanteric fractures *after* a stable reduction is obtained. If a stable reduction is inadvertently not obtained at the time of operation, the sliding apparatus is "forgiving"; it allows for subsequent displacement to achieve stability.

Wayne County or Valgus Reduction. In this reduction, the shaft of the femur is displaced *lateral* to the medial cortex of the femoral neck, thereby creating a buttressing force to resist varus displacement[516] (Fig. 14-24). This is referred to as the medial cortical overlap technique by Stover and colleagues.[580] This technique is helpful in unstable fractures with only *slight* medial and posterior cortical instability.[580] If more cortical instability is present, one must resort to an osteotomy.[580]

Elective Osteotomy of the Femoral Shaft to Achieve Stability. Elective medial displacement of the femoral shaft to achieve medial cortical stability followed by solid-angle nail-plate fixation has been described by many authors.[453,458,480,481,500,528] Dimon and Hughston reported that four-part fractures (see Fig. 14-20) with a posterior or medial gap after reduction (an unstable reduction) collapsed into varus.[481] This collapse resulted in the

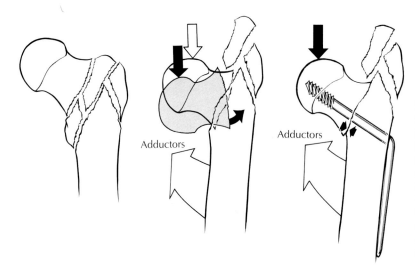

Fig. 14-24. The Wayne County reduction. (*Left*) An unstable intertrochanteric fracture. (*Center*) Reduction without medial cortical apposition or overlap is unstable and will result in femoral neck shortening and varus displacement. (*Right*) The Wayne County reduction. The proximal fragment is medially displaced to create medial cortical overlap that resists femoral neck shortening and varus displacement.

Adductors

Adductors

nail's penetrating the acetabulum; bending, breaking, or cutting through the head, or in the nail plate's pulling off the side of the shaft of the femur in 51% of conventionally nailed unstable fractures. In their hands, the addition of the medial displacement osteotomy (Fig. 14-25) reduced the incidence of these complications to 8%. Naiman and associates[546] believe that, in addition to four-part intertrochanteric fractures, oblique intertrochanteric fractures with a thin greater trochanteric component, and intertrochanteric fractures in which the greater trochanter is fractured during nail insertion are indications for medial displacement osteotomy.

Failure of fixation following medial displacement osteotomy varies from 10%[473,481] to 30%.[498,524] Harrington and Johnston[494] added the use of the sliding compression hip screw for fixation *after* medial displacement osteotomy and found the results to be improved over those obtained when using a fixed nail-plate device.

Roberts and colleagues[560] reported that patients undergoing medial displacement osteotomy have a poor functional result compared to patients with anatomically nailed intertrochanteric fractures. This is secondary to a decreased range of hip and knee motion and shortening of the limb. Shortening after medial displacement osteotomy has ranged from 1 to 2.5 cm.[486,494,525,546] This shortening does not seem to be related to early weight bearing. Although the functional differences after medial displacement may reflect in part the greater magnitude of the original injury in unstable fractures, the surgeon must be willing to accept the shortening and possibly a limp when choosing osteotomy to stabilize an intertrochanteric fracture.

Sarmiento introduced a valgus osteotomy for the unstable intertrochanteric fracture in an effort to gain medial cortical stability[566] (Fig. 14-26). This technique changes the fracture plane from vertical to near horizontal and creates contact between the medial and posterior cortex of the proximal and distal fragments. The advantage of this valgus osteotomy is that valgus realignment of the proximal fragment makes up for the loss of length at the osteotomy site so that limb lengths remain equal.[566]

Sarmiento warns of two possible errors in the technique of this valgus osteotomy. First, if the osteotomy is made too transverse, it places the head in an exaggerated valgus position. This may result in the leg's being too long or in the hip's being unstable. To avoid this, Sarmiento recommends that the medial end of the osteotomy exit 1 cm below the fracture surface medially to compensate for the increased length caused by the valgus osteotomy. Kaufer also warns against an excessive valgus reduction because it results in increased demands on abductor power to stabilize the pelvis in single stance phase. This increased abductor force increases the joint reaction force, which can lead to a limp and arthritic changes.[515] In addition, an excessive valgus reduction results in an incongruous hip joint, which may also lead to arthritic changes.

The second potential error is creation of an external rotation deformity after nailing. This can be prevented by attaching the shaft to the proximal fragment in slight internal rotation. Sarmiento also mentions that in some fractures medial comminution is so extensive that osteotomy will not create enough bony contact to ensure stability.[568]

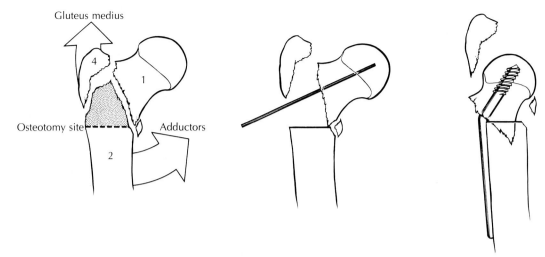

Fig. 14-25. Dimon and Hughston's technique of medial displacement osteotomy to stabilize an unstable four-part intertrochanteric fracture (see text). *(Left)* In a four-part fracture the adductor muscle pull tends to displace the fracture into varus secondary to a lack of medial cortical apposition. The *dotted line* indicates a transverse osteotomy at the level of the lesser trochanter. *(Center)* A guide wire inserted centrally into the head and neck fragment (position confirmed on x-ray). *(Right)* The femoral shaft is displaced medially and the spike on the head and neck is impacted into the femoral shaft.

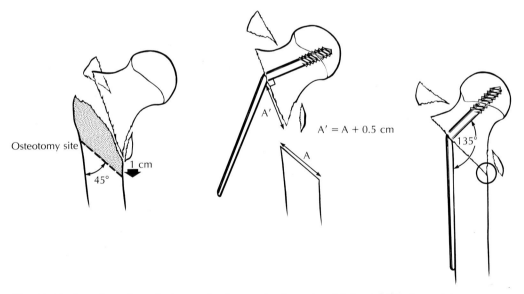

Fig. 14-26. Sarmiento's technique of valgus osteotomy to obtain stability in an unstable intertrochanteric fracture. *(Left)* An oblique osteotomy (approximately 45°) of the distal fragment begins slightly below the flare of the greater trochanter and exits 1 cm distal to the apex of the fracture. *(Center)* The guide wire and then the implant are inserted at 90° to the plane of the fracture. The distance of the point of entry of the guide wire from the medial cortex (A') is 0.5 cm (half the width of the implant) greater than the width of the osteotomized surface of the distal fragment (A). *(Right)* The fracture is reduced and impacted. Medial cortical apposition and, hence, stability, is restored.

Augmentation with Methyl Methacrylate.
Recently the use of methyl methacrylate to augment medial stability has been recommended in comminuted intertrochanteric fractures.[493] Although no complications were reported with its use, the addition of methyl methacrylate increases the magnitude of the operation and may introduce complications of nonunion and delayed union.

Choice of an Implant

Once a stable reduction has been obtained, either anatomically or by one of the nonanatomical means discussed above, an implant must be chosen to provide fixation of the fracture fragments. Jensen and colleagues demonstrated that in stable intertrochanteric fractures the choice of implant did not affect results,[511] but in unstable fractures the sliding hip screw was the most suitable implant.[510]

There are basically four types of implants available: (1) fixed nail-plate devices; (2) sliding nail-plate devices; (3) intramedullary devices; and (4) replacement prostheses. Both fixed nail and sliding nail-plate devices are available in varying angles, of which 150° and 135° are the most commonly used. Stephens[579] recommended the use of a 150° nail to approximate the angle of the resultant force of the body weight and pull of the abductors. Inman demonstrated this angle to be approximately 155° from the vertical.[502] Massie also recommended using a 150° nail, which would allow insertion of the implant along the weight-bearing axis, thereby ensuring that force transmission occurred across bone and not as torque across the implant.[533] He stressed that if a 150° angle nail were used, the fracture must be overreduced in a valgus position to prevent the insertion of the implant into the superior and anterior aspect of the head. Petersen and co-workers[552] stressed the importance of the 150° nail because of the resultant *decrease* in the varus moment arm on the implant.

In spite of the biomechanical advantage of the 150° nail, most authors recommend the use of a 135° nail.[541,586] Wolfgang and colleagues[592] found that the use of a 150° side plate often resulted in unacceptably high placement of the lag screw in sliding screw-plate fixation. Mulholland and Gunn[542] reported two problems with the 150° nail. First, it resides in the relatively weak bone in the anterior/superior part of the femoral head. Second, because it necessarily enters the shaft below the fracture in thick cortical bone, the angle of entry has to be exact, as the bone at the entry hole is too thick to permit crushing to correct minor errors of angle insertion. In addition, they found no difference in fracture impaction between 135° and 150° plates. For these reasons they recommended the 135° nail in most fractures.

Fixed-Angle Devices.
The fixed-angle nail-plate devices of Holt,[499] Jewett,[512] and others[583,584,591] have been the most commonly used in the past. Owing to the fact that they do not allow controlled collapse and impaction at the fracture site without penetration of the femoral head, a stable reduction (anatomical or nonanatomical) prior to nail insertion is *essential* to prevent these complications. Jacobs and co-workers[503,504,505] have demonstrated an increased incidence of joint penetration with fixed nail-plate devices. Therefore, although fixed-angle nail plates are satisfactory in the hands of those experienced with their use, the sliding devices give the surgeon a slight advantage, especially with fractures in which the stability has been misjudged.

Sliding Nail-Plate Devices.
Sliding nail-plate devices were introduced independently by Schumpelick and Jantzen,[572] Pugh,[554] and Massie[533] in the 1950s. Deyerle's plate with multiple pins also provides for sliding of the pins with fracture impaction.[479]

There is a definite recent trend toward the use of these devices.[501,515,584] Their advantages include the fact that they permit deeper insertion of the nail or screw without fear of lateral penetration of the joint. They also allow controlled collapse of the fracture site without penetration of the femoral head.[503] This controlled collapse improves the weight-bearing capacity of the implant by a reduction of the moment arm.[508] Therefore, the telescoping nails maximize bony contact and hence fracture stability, thereby decreasing implant failure.[492]

These sliding nail-plate and screw devices have either sharp ends to aid in insertion (Massie and Pugh nails) or blunt ends to resist penetration (compression hip screw). The sliding compression hip screw introduced by Schumpelick and Jantzen[572] and reported by Clawson[469] combines a blunt end to resist penetration and screw threads to increase fixation in the proximal fragment.[503,529] This is a definite advantage over the sharp ends present on sliding nail-plate devices.[533] However, these sliding hip-screw devices demand more accuracy in insertion to prevent complications.[592] Clawson[469] pointed out that to ensure impaction, the barrel of the hip-screw device must not cross the fracture site. There must also be enough room for the implant to collapse before the screw impinges on the barrel because, when such impingement occurs, the device acts as a fixed-angle plate.[542] Jamming, or failure of the hip screw to slide, also results in the implant's functioning as a fixed-angle plate. According to Kyle and colleagues,[522] the potential for jamming is *decreased* by maximum engagement (more than 2.5 cm) of the screw in the barrel and by using a 150° screw plate instead of a 30° implant. Wolfgang and colleagues[592] emphasize that failure of the lag screw to telescope can also occur as the result of impingement of the sleeve of the side plate on the base of proximal fragment. These authors also reported metal failure by side-plate or lag-screw fracture in patients in whom the fracture reduction was felt to be unsatisfactory. Because the screw occupies a larger part of the head of the femur (up to 10%) than a nail-plate device, if a second insertion is needed, Doherty and Lyden[482] suggested that consideration should be given to a fixed-angle device low in the head to ensure proximal fixation.[482] Finally, owing to recent reports of disengagement of the sliding screw from the barrel, some authors[463,485] now recommend leaving the compression screw in the sliding device to prevent disengagement.

Although the sliding device is more technically demanding, Laros and Moore found fewer complications of fracture and nonunion with them than with fixed-angle devices.[524] Jacobs and co-workers[504,505] noted a decreased incidence of joint penetration using a sliding compression screw as compared to fixed-nail devices. The low incidence of complications found after *anatomical* nailing of *unstable* fractures by Friedenberg and colleagues,[490] Sahlstrand,[565] and Mulholland and Gunn[542] emphasize the value of the sliding compression hip screw in the treatment of intertrochanteric fractures.

Intramedullary Devices. The complications of nail-plate fixation, including postoperative mortality, delayed union and nonunion, and wound infection, led to the development of intramedullary devices for the fixation of intertrochanteric fractures.[481,496,518,557,558,564] Owing to the fact that these nails are inserted into the medullary canal along the lines of force, the bending moment on them is considerably less than on a standard nail-plate device (Fig. 14-27).[452,518,532,555] Martinek and associates[532] demonstrated that, even if medial cortical support is lacking, flexible intramedullary nails and a valgus reduction can provide a stable osteosynthesis. This should lead to a decrease in implant failure.

Two types of intramedullary devices have gained

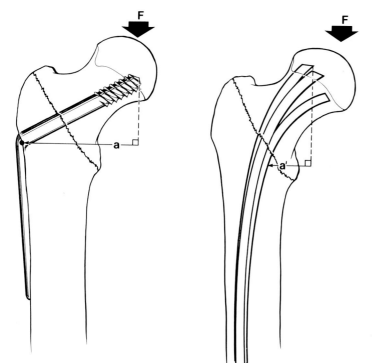

Fig. 14-27. The bending moment acting on the proximal fragment is reduced by the ratio of a to a' when intramedullary fixation is used.

popularity. First, Ender, in 1970, reported the use of multiple flexible condylocephalic nails that were to be introduced through the distal femur for the stabilization of intertrochanteric fractures without opening the fracture site. Advantages were said to include a decrease in operative mortality,[564] minimal surgical trauma secondary to not opening the fracture site,[519,551] decreased blood loss,[519,564] and decreased operation time.[452,519] Although initial reports were encouraging, subsequent investigations demonstrate significant complications.[549] Chapman and associates[465] reported as complications: the nails' backing out of the medullary canal, perforation of the nails through the femoral head, and rotational deformity at the fracture site. Raugstad and colleagues[555] found that 70% of patients, and Kuderna and colleagues[519] reported that 50% of patients, had a rotational deformity after fixation with Enders nails. Olerud suggested that the malrotation in unstable fractures can be prevented if the nails are bent into 25° of anteversion before insertion.[549] Richmond and colleagues[557] recommended wide abduction and internal rotation of the distal fragment to prevent malrotation and to improve fracture stability.

In addition to malrotation, knee pain, stiffness, and supracondylar fractures have been reported as significant complications.[555] Owing to the fact that secondary displacement occurred in 64% of unstable intertrochanteric fractures treated with Ender's nails and that 46% required reoperation, Jensen[509] concluded that Ender's nails were inadequate fixation for unstable intertrochanteric fractures.

The second type of intramedullary device is the single nail described first by Küntscher and subsequently by Harris.[496] Harris designed this single nail to prevent the external rotation deformity and distal nail migration noted with the Ender's type nails.[519]

I have found the single Harris-type nail useful in stable fractures in patients in whom minimal operative trauma is desired as a means of rapidly mobilizing the patient. However, a Wilkie boot is often necessary postoperatively in unstable fractures to prevent malrotation at the fracture site.

One must remember that these intramedullary methods of treatment of intertrochanteric fracture require extensive operative experience with the technique and expensive operating equipment, including image intensification.

Prosthetic Hemiarthroplasty. Although prosthetic replacement is popular in femoral neck fractures, its use for intertrochanteric fractures has not gained widespread support.[561,578] Rosenfeld and colleagues[561] reported the use of prosthetic replacement for intertrochanteric fractures of the femur in debilitated patients. Pinder and associates[553] reported the use of a Leinbach-type femoral head-neck prosthesis in 225 complex intertrochanteric fractures with excellent clinical results and a prompt return to preoperative status. Stern and Goldstein[578] report successful use of the Leinbach prosthesis in a select group of intertrochanteric fractures. Their indications for use of the Leinbach prosthesis include failed internal fixation of an intertrochanteric fracture and a severely comminuted, unstable intertrochanteric fracture in an elderly, debilitated patient. The prosthesis permitted ambulation in 86% of these patients within 1 week of surgery without the complications of thrombophlebitis, pneumonia, decubiti, malunion, and nonunion noted following internal fixation of intertrochanteric fractures in this high-risk group of patients. Therefore, in patients with severe osteoporosis and in whom proximal fixation with any type of device is questionable, the use of prosthetic replacement of the Leinbach type may be considered.

Nail Placement in the Femoral Head

The ideal location for placement of a nail in the femoral head has been the subject of controversy.[489,529,542,591] Mulholland and Gunn,[542] in a retrospective study, found that central placement of the nail on the anteroposterior and lateral x-rays with deep penetration of the head was optimum. They did not, however, evaluate nail placement in the inferior and posterior quadrants. Wilson and associates[591] agree that the center of the head on the anteroposterior and lateral x-ray is the ideal position. Evans[488] suggested placing the nail in the center of the femoral head on the lateral but low on the calcar on the anteroposterior x-ray. Wolfgang and colleagues[592] recommend placement of the pin in the central position on both the anteroposterior and lateral, believing that low posterior placement results in less rotational stability, inviting motion of the proximal fragment on the eccentrically placed device. Finally, Kaufer[515] recommended placing the nail-plate device in the posterior/inferior quadrant of the head on the lateral and low on the calcar on the anteroposterior so that the nail would have to "plow through" a maximum amount of bone before cutting out of the femoral head.

Despite the controversy over whether central nail placement on the anteroposterior and lateral x-ray, or low placement on the anteroposterior and posterior/inferior placement on the lateral x-ray is the most ideal for nail-plate devices, there is uniformity of agreement that the anterior and superior aspects of the femoral head should be avoided, owing to the increased risk of the device's cutting out.[566]

The depth of nail insertion is also important. In the elderly osteoporotic patient, the femoral neck itself is little more than a hollow tube. Therefore, in order to gain proximal purchase, it is essential to insert the nail or screw well into the femoral head.[516,523] Kaufer recommends placing the internal fixation device within 2 cm of the subchondral bone for maximum purchase.[515,516] In addition to poor proximal fixation, failure to place the screw deep enough into the femoral head can produce a stress riser effect in the femoral neck. A stress fracture of the femoral neck at the tip of the nail secondary to this mechanism has been reported by Baker,[454] Cameron and colleagues,[464] and Tronzo.[586]

Special Considerations

Prophylactic Antibiotics. The use of perioperative (pre- and postoperative) antibiotics in the treatment of intertrochanteric fractures of the hip is strongly recommended by most authors.[462,492,525,582] Boyd and associates,[460] Burnett and associates,[462] and Tengve and associates[582] all reported a significant decrease in postoperative wound infection in those patients receiving antibiotics immediately preoperatively and for a period of 72 hours postoperatively. As Burnett and associates[462] stressed, these fractures frequently occur in patients with serious underlying disease. It is this particular subgroup of patients that is most at risk for operative infection. Prophylactic antibiotics in these patients help to decrease operative infection from contamination from other body cavity sites, airborne infection in the operating room, and breaks in surgical technique.

Fracture Table. The use of a fracture table in these fractures is controversial.[483,492,525,528] Doppelt[483] considered a fracture table optional, while Greider and Horowitz[492] recommends the fracture table in all patients. Wolfgang and colleagues[592] recommend the use of the fracture table because of the good x-ray control it allows. Both Doppelt[483] and Lowell[528] recommend a *regular* operating table with the entire leg draped free in comminuted fractures. This technique enables the *surgeon* to manipulate the leg in order to obtain reduction. On the other hand, Lowell recommended the use of a fracture table only for stable fractures requiring little manipulation.[528]

Patient Positioning. Most authors recommend positioning the patient supine on the table for internal fixation.[483,492,525,592] A straight lateral incision is used.[483] Should the reduction be difficult or unacceptable, this can be extended anteriorly into a Watson-Jones incision for open reduction of the fracture site. However, Davis and Frymoyer[478] and Harrington and colleagues[495] suggested placing the patient in a lateral position with a straight lateral approach to the intertrochanteric area. The advantages of this approach are improved visualization of the fracture site, decreased need for retraction, decreased dependency on x-ray control (owing to exposure anteriorly and posteriorly of the fracture fragments), and decreased hydrostatic pressure of venous blood.

The Lesser Trochanter as a Guide. Schultz[571] recommends using the lesser trochanter as an exact reference point for insertion of a nail-plate device. He noted that a point on the lateral cortex of the femur directly opposite the lesser trochanter will allow consistently accurate insertion of a 135° angle nail. For a 150° angle nail, a site is selected 2 cm *distal* to the lower edge of the lesser trochanter on the lateral cortex for insertion of the nail. Tronzo[585] also recommends using the lesser trochanter as a guide for nail insertion. In addition, he recommends the use of an extramedullary guide pin carefully placed on the anterior neck of the femur to use as an anteversion guide in directing the surgeon's insertion of the nail. This technique is very helpful in positioning the intramedullary guide pin (Fig. 14-28).

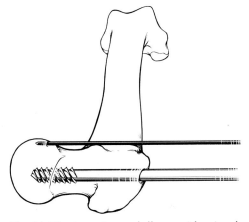

Fig. 14-28. An extramedullary guide pin placed beneath the vastus intermedius, along the anterior neck of the femur, and into the flare of the femoral head is an excellent anteversion guide for final guide wire insertion.

In addition, Clawson,[468,469] Massie,[533] and others[542,552,592] recommend the insertion of a guide wire into the femoral head and neck *prior* to insertion of the implant. X-ray confirmation of guide-wire position assures accurate placement in the proximal fragment.

Special Patient Considerations

Intertrochanteric Fractures in Patients with Paget's Disease. Intertrochanteric fractures are seen occasionally in patients with Paget's disease.[484] Conservative treatment resulted in 72% mortality in Dove's series. Open reduction and internal fixation with a two-piece nail-plate device resulted in union in 86% of cases.[484]

Intertrochanteric Fractures in Patients with Parkinson's Disease. Patients with Parkinson's disease who suffer a hip fracture have a higher mortality and morbidity than the normal population.[475,562] Coughlin and Templeton[475] report an overall 6 month mortality of 47% in patients with Parkinson's disease and hip fractures. The mortality in subcapital fractures was 60% while that in intertrochanteric fractures was only 27%. The authors believe this difference partially results from the fact that their patients with intertrochanteric fractures were considerably younger than the corresponding patients with femoral neck fractures.

The tremor and impaired balance plus the osteoporosis in Parkinson's patients results in prolonged rehabilitation and a higher complication rate after treatment of a hip fracture.[475,562] Rothermel and Garcia found that, by adequately managing patients on Levodopa in an effort to minimize neurological disease, a significant improvement in both survival and ambulatory status was obtained.[562] Coughlin and Templeton[475] found a higher mortality and morbidity in patients on drug therapy; however, this may be secondary to the fact that the patients on medication were more severely involved with the disease. Both authors recommended open reduction and internal fixation of intertrochanteric fractures in patients with Parkinson's disease.

Postoperative Management

There are three approaches to the postoperative management of patients with intertrochanteric fractures. First, the hip is protected with bed rest and supplementary traction until soft-tissue healing is present. Crutch walking is then initiated, but no weight is borne until there is x-ray evidence of healing.[472] Second, the patient is allowed up in a chair immediately after operation and begins a crutch-walking program with partial weight bearing, as tolerated.[592] Third, some authors believe that, if the fracture is stable at the time of operative treatment and is securely internally fixed, early weight bearing is advantageous in obtaining union and is important in patient rehabilitation.[499,540,568,590,592]

The decision on postoperative weight bearing must be determined on an *individual* basis.[592] Those patients with mental confusion and poor control of balance may not be able to cooperate with an early weight-bearing program (either partial or total weight bearing). In addition, the surgeon must consider the bony stability of the internal fixation, the quality of bone, and the type of implant used.[592] Wolfgang and colleagues[592] recommend only bed to chair activity postoperatively until x-rays demonstrate healing in patients with an unstable reduction, osteoporosis, poor implant placement, or an inability to cooperate with a non- or partial weight-bearing program. If the surgeon's goal of rehabilitation is to return patients to their prefracture status at the earliest possible time, early weight bearing is advantageous in those patients who were ambulatory preoperatively, provided no untoward results are foreseen. At the very least, the patient should be mobilized from the bed to a sitting position the day after surgery, to decrease the incidence of pulmonary, thromboembolic, and urinary tract complication.

Author's Preferred Method of Treatment

On arrival of the patient, five pounds of Buck's traction is applied to the involved limb. Good quality anteroposterior and lateral x-rays are obtained. Following thorough medical evaluation, the decision as to whether the patient will be treated operatively or nonoperatively is made . If surgery is selected, this is treated as an urgent (not emergency) operative procedure. I prefer to perform the internal fixation within 48 hours after admission. Antibiotics are given immediately preoperatively and for 72 hours after surgery.

The x-rays are carefully studied to determine whether the fracture is stable or unstable. Stable intertrochanteric fractures are treated by closed reduction on a fracture table and internal fixation using a sliding compression hip screw. To fulfill the criteria of stability, a reduction must have anatomical medial cortical apposition *or* slight overcorrection in the valgus position (a Wayne County-type reduction). I favor the use of the sliding compression hip screw for two reasons. First, if the estimation of fracture stability made by x-ray and at operation is incorrect, implant sliding allows secondary impaction and stabilization of the fracture site. This may prevent nail penetration or cutting out. Second, the screw provides better fixation in the proximal fragment than other nail-plate devices.

Those fractures that are unstable by radiographic evaluation are treated on a standard operating table with the entire leg draped free. I believe that it is essential to obtain bony stability in all such cases. Those fractures with minimal medial and posterior cortical comminution are managed with a Wayne County-type valgus reduction. In severely comminuted unstable fractures in elderly patients, either medial displacement or valgus osteotomy is performed.

I prefer valgus intertrochanteric osteotomy because it does not result in the shortening noted with a medial displacement osteotomy. However, both methods are used, depending on individual fracture geometry.

I am hesitant to perform a medial displacement or valgus osteotomy in a young patient (below the age of 40) because of the alterations in hip biomechanics induced by these procedures. In this age group I prefer open anatomical reduction and internal fixation of unstable fractures. The sliding compression hip screw is used in all cases and an iliac crest bone graft is applied medially, especially if the medial cortex is not *anatomically* restored. These patients are treated in a spica cast postoperatively if fixation or stability is in question.

The postoperative management is individualized. Patients who were nonambulatory before surgery are treated by dangling their feet off the bed the day after surgery with rapid progression to sitting in a wheelchair. Ambulatory patients dangle their feet the first day postoperatively and are transferred to a bed-to-chair situation the second postoperative day. The decision on weight bearing is dependent on bony stability, fixation of the implant, quality of the bone, and most importantly on the patient's ability to cooperate with the rehabilitation program. Those patients who were ambulatory preoperatively, in whom stable internal fixation is obtained, and who can cooperate with a rehabilitation program are begun on partial weight bearing as soon as possible. However, if there is any question of fracture stability, bone quality, or ability to cooperate, I prefer to delay weight bearing for 6 to 12 weeks to allow early fracture consolidation.

If the nonoperative approach to the fracture is chosen, I prefer one of two methods. If the patient was nonambulatory before the fracture, the fracture is simply ignored. Pain medications are given as needed and the patient is mobilized to the sitting position in the first 2 or 3 days. Buck's traction used intermittently may be helpful in the first few days to decrease pain in these patients. Once the pain is minimized, the patient is returned to his or her prefracture environment.

If the patient was ambulatory before the fracture, and I do not wish to accept shortening, varus, and external rotation, skeletal traction through the distal femur is instituted. Care is taken to ensure adequate reduction and to prevent rotational deformity. Patients are kept in traction 8 to 12 weeks until the fracture is nontender and callus is noted on x-ray. Full weight bearing is delayed 4 to 6 months. This method is used *only* in young patients in whom open reduction is not elected and in whom deformity is not acceptable. Its use in most elderly patients is to be condemned because of the morbidity associated with immobilizing these patients by skeletal traction.

PROGNOSIS AND COMPLICATIONS

MORTALITY

Weeden and associates[588] reported that intertrochanteric fractures carry a higher mortality than femoral neck fractures because the patients are older. If these age differences are corrected, however, Alffram[449] found no difference in mortality between intertrochanteric fractures and femoral neck fractures. Indeed, Dahl[477] and Meyn and associates[537] found no difference in mortality by type of hip fracture.

When considering mortality figures, one must be careful that the groups of patients are comparable and that the postoperative time in which mortality figures are calculated is similar. Dahl[477] found that in the first month after fracture the expected mortality was 15 times that for the same age patient; in the second month there was a sevenfold increase in mortality over the unoperated same aged patient; and after the second month, the mortality was the same as for other patients of the same age without a fractured hip. Ganz and colleagues,[491] Jensen,[508] and Moore[538] report a 10% in-hospital mortality rate associated with intertrochanteric fractures. The postoperative mortality in institutionalized patients has been reported by Sherk and co-workers[574] to be higher than that for noninstitutionalized patients. In Sherk's series the mortality was 52% in those treated with open reduction and internal fixation and 55% in those treated closed.

Neimann and Mankin[547] also found that surgical

treatment of hip fractures in institutionalized patients did not always decrease the mortality rate as reported in other patient groups. However, Laskin and associates[525] and Meyn and associates[537] did not find any difference in the postoperative mortality of organic brain syndrome or institutionalized patients as compared to their other patients after operative treatment of intertrochanteric fractures.

WOUND INFECTION

The incidence of postoperative wound infection after operative treatment of intertrochanteric fractures varies from 1.7%[470,472] to 16.9%.[582] Barr,[456] in an excellent discussion of postoperative hip infection, listed the following as significant factors in the development of postoperative infection; (1) a patient population including patients in the seventh, eighth, and ninth decades with decubitus ulcers, bladder infections, and cardiovascular disease; (2) the prolonged operating time that may occur in unstable fractures, thus increasing the risk of infection; (3) a disoriented patient, who may remove his bandage and contaminate the wound; and (4) the proximity of the wound to the perineum. He found infection after intertrochanteric fractures to be twice as common as after femoral neck fractures and divided postoperative infections into four groups.[456] The first group includes early *superficial* sepsis with fever, wound swelling, erythema, and spontaneous drainage. His recommended treatment for these patients was removal of skin sutures, debridement of subcutaneous tissues, and the administration of parenteral antibiotics while allowing the wound to heal secondarily. The second group consisted of those with early *deep* sepsis. In this group of patients the mortality rate was quite high. He recommended extensive early debridement and parenteral antibiotics. Late sepsis patients included those diagnosed from 6 to 24 months after fracture. These patients were divided into those with (group III) and without (group IV) joint involvement. In patients without joint involvement, treatment included removal of the metallic internal fixation device. If the joint was involved in a late deep infection, it was difficult to diagnose and often required an extensive reconstructive procedure for pain relief.

Barr stressed the difficulty in diagnosing postoperative hip infection and found that in most cases a delayed diagnosis was made. Those clues that suggest postoperative infection include spiking fever, aching in the hip region postoperatively, muscle spasm and decreased range of motion, and a sedimentation rate of 30 millimeters or greater. Barr did demonstrate that an infected intertrochanteric fracture was less likely to have joint involvement than an infected femoral neck fracture. Therefore, an attempt at local wound management is worthwhile in hopes of saving the femoral head.

MECHANICAL AND TECHNICAL FAILURES

Varus Displacement. Varus displacement is associated with failure of nail fixation in the proximal fragment and failure to obtain a stable reduction and internal fixation.[592] It is usually accompanied by implant bending, breaking, cutting out of the head, or pulling off the femoral shaft.[480,481,592] Evans[488] found that the incidence of varus displacement after treatment of intertrochanteric fractures by either open or closed methods approximated the percentage of unstable fractures in the series.

Although varus displacement is a relatively common complication following open reduction and internal fixation of hip fractures, Taylor found it to be symptomatic with pain, weakness of the hip, and a short extremity only if the varus were less than 120°.[581] If varus displacement develops postoperatively, the surgeon has three options: (1) accept the varus deformity; (2) attempt to correct the varus with skeletal traction until union occurs; or (3) reoperate. The choice is dependent on patient *and* the fracture characteristics.

Nail Penetration. Nail penetration into the hip joint following fixation of intertrochanteric fractures may account for one third of the treatment failures.[581] Taylor and colleagues[581] found that, even if a nail penetrates the head of the femur into the acetabulum, it may not lead to degenerative joint disease. They concluded that penetration was secondary to too long a nail or to a reversed intertrochanteric fracture with medial shaft migration. They recommended leaving the nail in the penetrated position until union was certain. Wilson and colleagues[591] also noted that nail penetration did not necessarily prejudice the result, finding that only 1.3% required nail removal.

Rotational Deformity. Rotational deformity following internal fixation of intertrochanteric fractures is a well-known problem, especially in unstable fractures. Massie[533,534] stressed avoidance of internal rotation in reducing intertrochanteric fractures to prevent rotational deformity postoperatively. Dimon and Hughston[481] also stressed the need for correct interpretation of rotational alignment at the time of nailing to prevent postoperative deformity.

Nonunion. Owing to the fact that intertrochanteric fractures occur in cancellous bone with good blood supply, nonunion has been found to be uncommon.[455,566] Mulholland and Gunn[542] and Wilson and associates[591] reported the incidence of nonunion to be less than 2%. Laskin and associates[525] noted that union was usually present within 3 months of fracture and that nonunion was secondary to poor bony apposition at the time of surgery. Baker[455] recommended open reduction, renailing, and bone grafting to obtain union in these patients.

Aseptic Necrosis. Intertrochanteric fractures, being mainly extracapsular injuries, have a low incidence of aseptic necrosis.[467,472,522,530,545,566,581] Kyle and associates[521] report an incidence of 0.8%, a figure agreed on by Cleveland and associates,[472] Mann,[530] and Taylor.[581] Importantly, Mann[530] and Claffey[467] were unable to find a significant relationship between nail placement in the superior lateral portion of the femoral head and the incidence of aseptic necrosis.

Stress Fractures of the Femoral Neck. Tronzo[586] reported that, if an intertrochanteric fracture was internally fixed with a nail that did not enter the head, the nail could cut out of the proximal fragment as the patient flexed the hip and rotated the limb, or the nail could act as a stress riser in the femoral neck and result in a subcapital stress fracture. He reported having seen two such cases. Cameron[464] and Laskin[525] also reported this complication. Accurate replacement of the nail *deep* into the head will avoid this problem.

Miscellaneous Complications. Evans[488] reported one patient with peritonitis secondary to a guide pin's violating the pelvis during hip nailing, and one patient with gangrene secondary to a dissecting aneurysm not noted preoperatively. Both of these complications, although rarely reported in the literature, should be considered when treating intertrochanteric fractures.

PATHOLOGIC INTERTROCHANTERIC FRACTURES

Marcove and Yang[531] found that 40% of patients with pathologic fractures secondary to metastatic carcinoma survived 6 months, and that after this first fracture, 30% survived 1 year or more. Because of this, aggressive treatment of fractures or impending fractures secondary to metastatic disease is indicated. The goal in treating these patients is to improve the quality of life by decreasing pain and maintaining mobility.[474] Coran and associates[474] reported that while local irradiation may relieve pain, fracture healing is inhibited by radiation therapy alone. Such treatment would result in severely limiting patient function if the fracture did not heal. Therefore, it is the combination of internal fixation and irradiation that results in the abolition of pain, maintenance of function, and the limitation of tumor expansion.

Those patients with an intertrochanteric fracture (or an impending intertrochanteric fracture) secondary to metastatic disease and a life expectancy of at least a few months are considered candidates for surgical treatment.[495] Open reduction and internal fixation with a standard nail-plate device[461,471] or with a nail-plate device supplemented with methyl methacrylate have given excellent results.[495] However, in those patients with extensive metastatic disease, use of a hemiprosthesis fixed with methyl methacrylate should be considered.[474] In those patients in whom prosthetic hemiarthroplasty is considered, careful evaluation of the acetabulum for metastatic disease is indicated. The presence of metastatic disease in the acetabulum can result in medial migration of the hemiprosthesis *or* in the persistence of hip pain after hemiarthroplasty. Persistent pain defeats the purpose of operative treatment. Therefore, total hip arthroplasty may be indicated in patients with both intertrochanteric and acetabular involvement.

GREATER TROCHANTERIC FRACTURES

Isolated avulsion or comminuted fractures of the greater trochanter are unusual injuries.[594,599,604] These fractures are seen as two distinctly different types occurring in different age groups. First and most common are epiphyseal separations in young children and adolescents between 7 and 17 years of age.[594] In this type the entire trochanteric apophysis is avulsed and can be displaced up to 6 cm.[594,600,603,604] The second type is a comminuted fracture of the greater trochanter seen in adults (Fig. 14-29). Merlino and Nixon[599] and Milch[600] both demonstrated that this fracture is usually comminuted and only a part of the trochanter is generally involved. The part usually involved is that portion of the trochanter that projects upward and backward from its line of junction with the femoral neck.[600] The fragment is usually displaced superiorly and posteriorly.[600]

The mechanism of injury is specific for each of these two types of fractures. In the child or adolescent the mechanism of injury is a muscle contraction that results in avulsion of the apophysis.[599] The comminuted fracture in the adult is usually secondary to a direct blow to the greater trochanter.[599,600]

CLINICAL DIAGNOSIS

Physical findings include tenderness over the area of the avulsion, a flexion deformity of the hip secondary to pain and spasm,[599] and occasionally a limp.[594,599] Ecchymosis directly over the trochanter is unusual.[600]

Most authors report displacement in the epiphyseal avulsions to be greater than that seen in isolated trochanteric fractures in the adult. Both Merlino and Nixon[599] and Milch[600] believed that the displacement of the trochanteric fracture in an adult was secondary to the short external rotators and not the abductors.

TREATMENT

Treatment of trochanteric avulsions has been controversial. As healing always occurs,[600] treatment should be aimed at improving function after healing. In the adult fracture in which only part of the trochanter is fractured, remaining intact fibers of the gluteus medius usually prevent wide separation of the fracture fragment.

Three types of treatment have been proposed.[599] The first employs wide abduction of the limb to oppose the displaced fragment with its bed. These patients are kept in skin traction and then immobilized either with adhesive strapping from thigh to buttock, hip, groin, and abdomen applied in a fan-shaped fashion[603] or with a spica cast for 6 weeks.[594] An alternative method prescribes bed rest without traction until the symptoms are absent, at which time active motion and partial weight bearing of the limb are permitted. Full weight bearing is delayed for 4 to 6 weeks. Finally, Armstrong[594] and Watson-Jones[606] mention open reduction and internal fixation of the displaced fragment through a straight lateral incision over the greater trochanter. Fixation is obtained with screws, pegs, or

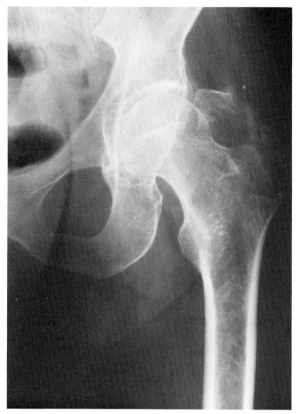

Fig. 14-29. Isolated fracture of the greater trochanter secondary to a direct blow.

suture.[594,606] Merlino and Nixon[599] reserved open reduction for those infrequent cases in which there is marked separation or soft-tissue interposition.

The prognosis in these injuries is uniformly good. If the displacement is slight, conservative treatment results in bony union, while in wider separations fibrous union results.[594,599,600] Function following healing is reported to be excellent.[594,599,600]

I believe generally that, if separation of a large trochanteric fragment is greater than 1 cm and the fragment is not comminuted, consideration should be given to open reduction and internal fixation. Otherwise, these fractures are treated as soft-tissue injuries with protected weight bearing until the patient is asymptomatic. This usually requires several days of bed rest followed by crutches for 3 to 4 weeks.

In the elderly patient, even with separation greater than 1 cm, operative treatment with internal fixation is rarely indicated. In the younger person with displacement of the apophysis greater than 1 cm, it is advisable to repair the fracture fragment internally either with two cancellous screws or a wire loop to secure the fragments. This results in restoration of the abductor mechanism. Postoperatively, the extremity is protected with partial weight bearing on crutches until soft tissue healing is complete. The patient is then allowed to ambulate without weight bearing (toe-touch only) for an additional 3 to 4 weeks, followed by partial weight bearing for another 3 to 4 weeks until limp-free walking is achieved.

ISOLATED AVULSION FRACTURE OF THE LESSER TROCHANTER

This injury is seen most often in children and young adults, with 85% of cases occurring under the age of 20.[595,598] The peak age of incidence is between 12 and 16 years, when the injury is noted to be an apophyseal avulsion.[602] This injury is usually secondary to a forceful contracture of the iliopsoas muscle that avulses the lesser trochanteric apophysis.[595,597,598,601,602]

The injury is also infrequently seen in elderly patients with osteoporosis.[598] Poston[602] believed that this occurred in elderly patients because of rarefaction of the trabecular structure of the lesser trochanter, which resulted in a loss of resistance to iliopsoas contraction.

CLINICAL DIAGNOSIS

Physical examination in these patients reveals tenderness in the femoral triangle.[596,602] Pain can often be reproduced by hip flexion against resistance.[595,596] Ludloff's sign of iliopsoas insufficiency is usually positive.[602] This sign is elicited by having the patient in a seated position and demonstrating that he is unable to lift the leg from the ground. If the trochanteric separation is incomplete and the trochanter retains a partial periosteal attachment, or displacement is inhibited by fibers of insertion of the iliacus muscle (which are often prolonged 1 inch downward and in front of the lesser trochanter to be inserted in the shaft of the femur), a varying range of active flexion is possible.[595,602]

TREATMENT

The treatment of this injury is usually bed rest, *without* plaster, followed by mobilization.[598,605] Sweetman found that patients had active hip flexion without pain 3 weeks after injury following this regimen.[605] Open reduction and internal fixation have been mentioned in cases with wide separation, although a definition of the amount of separation requiring open reduction and internal fixation has not been given.[601,602] Poston[602] concluded that open reduction is unnecessary treatment in view of the excellent results obtained by less dramatic procedures.

I believe that, unless displacement is greater than 2 cm, operative fixation is not indicated and one can expect an excellent result. If displacement is greater than 2 cm in a young athletic patient, replacement of the avulsed fragment with cancellous or cortical screws should be considered. This can be accomplished through a medial approach. The excellent functional results obtained by essentially ignoring the fracture suggest that open reduction is not indicated in the sedentary adult.[598,605]

SUBTROCHANTERIC FRACTURES

Subtrochanteric fractures are those fractures in which a part of the fracture occurs between the lesser trochanter and a point 5 cm distally.[635,668,672] Such fractures are seen as independent entities[617] or as extensions of intertrochanteric fractures. The mechanism of injury is usually direct trauma. These fractures are seen in two groups of patients: older patients suffering a minor fall in which the subtrochanteric fracture occurs through weakened bone; and younger patients with normal bone who are involved in high-energy trauma.[629,668]

The two main problems noted in treating subtrochanteric fractures have been malunion and delayed union or nonunion. Allis, in 1891, recognized the complications of shortening, angular deformity, and rotational malalignment that often result following this fracture.[607] He used muscular force analysis to explain the etiology of these deformities.[607]

Two factors are responsible for a slower rate of union and a higher rate of malunion in subtrochanteric fractures.[609,610,620,660] First, the subtrochanteric area of the femur is composed mainly of cortical bone, which is often comminuted in these fractures.[619,620,629,633,660,666] The cortical bone vascularity and fracture surfaces available for healing are less than in the cancellous bone surfaces in intertrochanteric fractures.[665,670] Second, the large biomechanical stresses present in the subtrochanteric area may result in failure of internal fixation devices *before* bony union occurs.[634,640]

CLASSIFICATION

Several classifications of subtrochanteric fractures have been suggested. Boyd and Griffin[617] divided *all trochanteric* fractures into four types (I–IV). Type III were subtrochanteric fractures and type IV were subtrochanteric fractures with intertrochanteric extensions (see Fig. 14-21). One third of all their trochanteric fractures fell into these two groups. Although they found the highest percentage of complications in type III and type IV fractures, an analysis of specific subtrochanteric fracture patterns was not done.

Fielding and Magliato[635] developed a classification specifically for subtrochanteric fractures that included three types based on the *location* of the primary fracture line in relation to the lesser trochanter. Type I are fractures at the level of the lesser trochanter, type II are within 1 inch below the lesser trochanter, and type III are from 1 to 2 inches below the lesser trochanter (Fig. 14-30). They recognized an increasing incidence of complications following treatment as the fractures became more distal. Unfortunately, this classification does not address the problem of comminution, which is critical in assessing fracture stability.

Seinsheimer[660] proposed a classification based on the number of major fragments and the *location* and *shape* of fracture lines (see below and Fig.

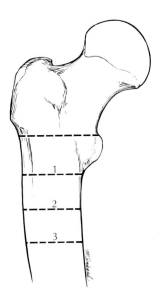

Fig. 14-30. Fielding's classification of subtrochanteric fractures (Redrawn from Fielding. J.W., and Magliato, H.J.: Subtrochanteric Fractures. Surg. Gynecol. Obstet., **122**:555–560, 1966.)

14-31). Although the classification is more cumbersome than other systems, Seinsheimer noted that all implant failures and nonunions occurred in type IIIA and IV fractures. The common denominator in these types is medial cortical comminution that may result in a lack of stability following internal fixation.

Seinsheimer's Classification of Subtrochanteric Fractures[660]

Type I: Nondisplaced fractures; any fracture with less than 2 mm of displacement of the fracture fragments.

Type II: Two-part fractures:
   Type IIA: A two-part transverse femoral fracture.
   Type IIB: A two-part spiral fracture with the lesser trochanter attached to the proximal fragment.
   Type IIC: A two-part spiral fracture with the lesser trochanter attached to the distal fragment.

Type III: Three-part fractures:
   Type IIIA: A three-part spiral fracture in which the lesser trochanter is part of the third fragment, which has an inferior spike of cortex of varying length.
   Type IIIB: A three-part spiral fracture of the proximal one third of the femur, with the third part a butterfly fragment.

Type IV: Comminuted fractures with four or more fragments.

Type V: Subtrochanteric-intertrochanteric fractures; this group includes any subtrochanteric fracture with extension through the greater trochanter.

FRACTURE STABILITY

In considering subtrochanteric fractures, I prefer to use the concept of stable and unstable fractures in place of a specific classification system. It is important to emphasize that the farther down the shaft of the femur the primary fracture line is located, the greater the incidence of delayed union and implant failure.

Stable subtrochanteric fractures are those in which it is possible to reestablish bone-to-bone contact of the medial and posterior femoral cortex anatomically. When this is possible, an internal fixation device will act as a tension band on the lateral femoral cortex, and impaction and weight bearing can occur directly through the medial cor-

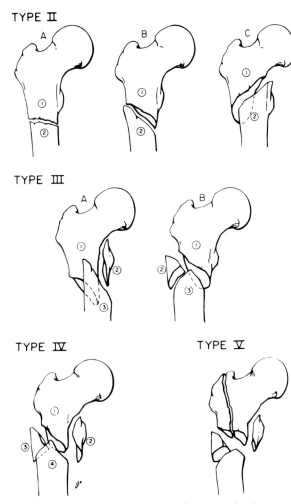

TYPE II

TYPE III

TYPE IV   TYPE V

Fig. 14-31. Seinsheimer's classification of subtrochanteric fractures[660] (see text for description). (From Seinsheimer, F.: Subtrochanteric Fractures of the Femur. J. Bone Joint Surg., **60A**:300–306, 1978.)

tex.[637,651,660] In unstable fractures, medial cortical apposition is not attainable secondary to comminution *or* fracture obliquity.[660] In this situation, there is inadequate medial cortical support. Any lateral plate (or intramedullary device) will be subjected mainly to bending stress and the loads will concentrate in one area of the implant. This will result in implant failure or loss of fixation.[660,670,671] This concept of stability is particularly important in treating those fractures distal to the lesser trochanter, because in more proximal fractures stability can often be restored by osteotomy or medial displacement as recommended for intertrochanteric fractures.[623,631,656]

CLINICAL DIAGNOSIS

Depending on the extent of the fracture, the clinical picture resembles that in a patient with an intertrochanteric or femoral shaft fracture. Open fractures, although uncommon, do occur and signify severe soft-tissue and bone injury.[629] Because the forces required to produce this fracture are substantial, associated injuries, both of the same extremity and especially elsewhere in the body, should be suspected.[629,630,641,667] Hemorrhage in the thigh may be significant, and the patient should be monitored for hypovolemic shock.[629] Emergency splinting with a Thomas splint will prevent further soft-tissue damage and hemorrhage. Associated vascular and neurologic injury is not common in subtrochanteric fractures.

RADIOGRAPHIC DIAGNOSIS

Anteroposterior and true lateral x-rays are necessary to assess the extent of the fracture clearly. As in all patients with femoral fractures, an x-ray of the pelvis is essential to rule out associated dislocation of the hip or pelvic fracture. The x-ray of the hip and pelvis is viewed to determine the presence or degree of osteoporosis in elderly patients *before* a decision regarding open versus closed treatment is made.[652,662]

TREATMENT

Recommendations concerning the most successful method of treating subtrochanteric fractures are confusing for two reasons. First, reports on the treatment of subtrochanteric fractures have included other hip fractures, especially intertrochanteric fractures, making analysis difficult.[617,639,650,653] Second, subtrochanteric fractures have usually been considered as a homogeneous group, whether they occur from minor trauma in older patients with osteopenia or from high-energy trauma in younger patients with normal bone.[609,612,614,632,638,640,641,653,660,661,666,668,672] Watson and associates[668] separated young patients with the high-energy, comminuted, subtrochanteric fractures from the older patients whose fractures were inflicted by minor trauma. He was able to demonstrate a difference in prognosis between the two groups. Consideration of these two groups *separately* is essential when planning the treatment of subtrochanteric fractures and in predicting their outcome.[629,668]

NONOPERATIVE TREATMENT

The treatment of choice in severely comminuted subtrochanteric fractures, especially in young patients in which *stable* internal fixation cannot be obtained, and in open subtrochanteric fractures, is nonoperative.[629,660,661,670] In the past the nonoperative treatment of these fractures resulted in high rates of morbidity and mortality.[625,650,662] Beaver and Bach,[614] Cech and Sosna,[620] and Watson and associates[668] reported that closed treatment of these fractures often resulted in varus angulation and rotational deformity. The problem of nonunion and the morbidity associated with the spica cast were minimized with the development of cast bracing, which reduced the time required for union of femoral shaft fractures and allowed patients mobility during treatment.[626,627,644,649,655] However, Mooney[649] and Sarmiento[656] reported angulation and shortening as significant complications in patients with subtrochanteric fractures treated in a cast brace. The use of a modified cast brace with pelvic band applied with the hip in 20° abduction and a contralateral shoe lift, designed to prevent this varus angulation in subtrochanteric fractures, has been reported.[629] Significant shortening, angulation, and rotational deformity were avoided in a series of comminuted and open subtrochanteric fractures treated in this fashion.[629]

OPERATIVE TREATMENT

Open reduction and internal fixation to restore anatomy and allow early mobilization is the treatment of choice in subtrochanteric fractures *provided* a stable osteosynthesis can be obtained at the time of operation.[612,620,629] However, because subtrochanteric fractures are often comminuted, stable internal fixation may be difficult to achieve.[619,661,665,670,671] These fractures extend into diaphyseal bone, which has decreased vascularity and therefore poorer healing potential. This increases the need for stable internal fixation to reduce implant failure.

Forces exceeding 1200 pounds per square inch were demonstrated in the subtrochanteric area by Koch[645] and by Frankel and Burstein.[637] Forces of a similar magnitude secondary to muscular pull *alone* have been reported.[637,671] Such *in vivo* bending forces load the medial femoral cortex in the compression mode and the lateral cortex in tension. Schatzker and Waddell[658] have shown that the compression strains are considerably greater than the tension strains.[658] These large stresses on the medial cortex in the subtrochanteric area make cortical restoration at the time of open reduction and internal

fixation mandatory to prevent cyclical loading and failure of any device used on the tension side of the femur. Velasco and Comfort[666] reported that as little as 2 mm separation of the medial cortex will lead to medial collapse and lateral plate bending. In most reports of subtrochanteric fractures, those patients with severe medial cortical comminution have consistently had an increase in failure rate secondary to these biomechanical and anatomical considerations.[617,620,634,658,660]

Choice of Implants

Many internal fixation devices have been recommended for use in subtrochanteric fractures because of the incidence of complications reported after surgical treatment.[609,620,640,641,658,672] Each of these devices has advantages in certain types of subtrochanteric fractures,[619] and their selection should be based on the individual fracture anatomy.

Fixed-Angle Nail Plates. The use of fixed-angle nail plates of the Jewett type in subtrochanteric fractures has met with mixed results.[638,640,647,663,667] Froimson[638] reported that the heavy-duty Jewett nail, supplemented by circumferential wire and screws when indicated, was reliable in the management of the unstable comminuted subtrochanteric fracture. Postoperatively, however, his patients did not begin partial weight bearing for 2 months. Hanson and Tullos[640] demonstrated an 88% union rate after a single operation using a nail-plate device. They recognized that implant failure was secondary to the nonunion and not the reverse. Fielding[633,634,635] noted an increasing incidence of nonunion and implant failure with fixed-angle nail plates as the fracture site moved distally (57% of his type III fractures failed to unite). However, he believed that internal fixation with a strong Jewett nail, possibly supplemented by an anterior plate and bone grafting, was the best method then available.[635] Fielding and Magliato[635] recommended a valgus reduction and nail-plate fixation in type I fractures wherein the lateral cortex of the proximal fragment is placed inside the lateral cortex of the distal fragment to increase bony stability and prevent medial migration of the distal fragment.[631,656] They recognized that this technique was not possible in more distal type II and III fractures.[633,635] Zickel[673] also noted that neither medial displacement nor osteotomy was useful if the fracture line extended into the femoral shaft.[672–674]

More recently, a high incidence of varus deformity, acetabular penetration, and implant failure associated with the Jewett nail led Teitge[663] to discontinue the use of this type implant for routine use in subtrochanteric fractures. Waddell[667] also reported a high incidence of nonunion and implant failure associated with the use of fixed-angle plates of the Jewett or McLaughlin type, especially in comminuted fractures in the subtrochanteric area.

AO Blade Plate. Both Schatzker and Waddell[658,667] recommend the use of the AO blade plate in selected subtrochanteric fractures. They believe that it is best suited for those fractures that are slightly more distal in the subtrochanteric region so that an accessory cancellous screw can be inserted beneath the blade into the calcar to increase proximal fixation.

Asher and associates[612] and Cech and Sosna[620] also recommended the use of the AO blade plate and stressed the importance of restoring medial cortical stability by the use of interfragmentary compression of medial cortical fragments. Velasco and Comfort[666] supported the use of the blade plate, especially in fractures that were transverse or with multiple large fractures that could be anatomically reduced to restore medial stability. Waddell[667] reported failure with the AO blade in 20% of fractures. He related failure to poor reduction of fracture fragments and hence loss of medial cortical support and to the initiation of weight bearing too early in the postoperative course.

Sliding Compression Hip Screw. Waddell reported satisfactory results in 21 of 24 subtrochanteric fractures using the sliding compression hip screw.[667] Although the side plate has increased strength, this does not nullify the importance of medial buttress reconstitution, as even the most massive plate will undergo fatigue failure.[658] Berman and co-workers[615] reported 38 consecutive subtrochanteric fractures using the compression hip nail. They stressed interfragmentary screw fixation to secure comminuted fractures to the main fragments, the use of the Hirschorn device (used to produce compression beneath the plate) for compression of short oblique and transverse fractures, and bone grafting in all cases with comminution. Using these methods, they had no nonunions, implant failures, or varus dislacement.

The large proximal screw in the compression hip screw system obtains better purchase in the proximal fragment than do nail-plate devices.[667] The large sliding screw has a blunt nose, which results in less penetration of the femoral head and acetabulum in those fractures that self-impact after nailing.[658,667] The ability of the screw shaft to slide in the collar of the plate allows for impaction at the fracture surfaces, a fact of considerable importance in Fielding type I fractures. The sliding will also permit slight medial displacement of the shaft in relationship to the head and neck fragment. This tends to reduce the bending moment and resulting forces that lead to collapse of the medial buttress and varus displacement.[658] For this sliding to occur, the plate must not be fixed with screws into the proximal fragment. Therefore, the implant is most useful in the most proximal of subtrochanteric fractures.[658] Schatzker and Waddell[658] recommend the use of the sliding compression hip screw in *high* subtrochanteric fractures in which medialization of the shaft and impaction of the fracture are possible. They suggested that low fractures do better with AO slide-plate fixation if the medial cortex can be reconstituted.

Intramedullary Devices. *Intramedullary Nails.* Theoretically, in subtrochanteric fractures intramedullary fixation decreases the stress on the implant as compared to nail-plate devices (Fig. 14-32). The use of an intramedullary rod does, however, present some difficulties.[658,660,667] First, in fractures involving the subtrochanteric area of the proximal femur, the medullary canal and the trochanteric area do not provide good stable purchase on the proximal fragment.[658,667] This results in varus angulation of the proximal fragment and, frequently, rotational instability of the distal fragment. This is particularly true in high subtrochanteric fractures. Schatzker and Waddell[658] reserve intramedullary nailing for the occasional young patient with a low transverse or short oblique fracture in the isthmus area of the femur. Winter and Clawson[670] recommend intramedullary nailing only if there is an intact ring of cortical bone on the proximal fragment *2 cm* below the lesser trochanter. Clawson and colleagues[624] recommended closed intramedullary nailing in those subtrochanteric fractures located in such a position that adequate stabilization could be obtained by intramedullary rod fixation.

The introduction of special intramedullary nails such as the Grosse-Kempf nail, which allow the insertion of proximal and distal transfixing or locking screws have extended the indications for *closed* intramedullary nailing in subtrochanteric fractures. The presence of a proximal locking screw provides rotational stability to the fracture, and prevents shortening and varus angulation. These devices are useful only in subtrochanteric fractures below the level of the lesser trochanter and without involve-

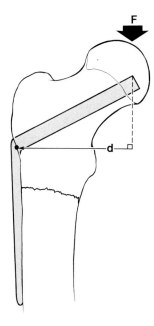 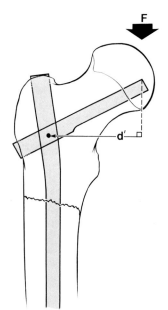

Fig. 14-32. The moment arm (d) on a nail-plate device is greater than the moment arm (d') on an intramedullary device (Zickel nail). Since the force (F) remains the same, the torque (torque = F × d) on the nail-plate is greater than the torque on the Zickel nail.

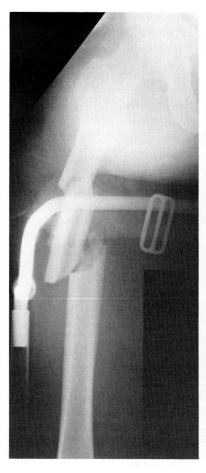 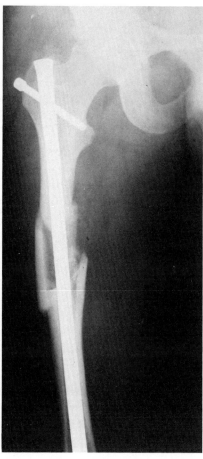

Fig. 14-33 (*Left*) Comminuted, segmental fracture in the subtrochanteric area of the right femur, extending into the diaphysis. (*Right*) The fracture 3 months after closed intramedullary nailing with a Grosse-Kempf locking nail.

ment of the greater trochanter (Fig. 14-33). The ability to insert these devices without opening the fracture site and further devascularizing fracture fragments should improve union in these fractures. The exact indications for use of locking nails in the management of subtrochanteric fractures awaits further clinical investigation.

Aronoff and colleagues[609,610] reported intramedullary fixation to be safer than nail-plate fixation. However, supplementary internal fixation was required in two thirds of their patients and external plaster support in 20% of their patients postoperatively. These authors stressed the use of this technique in the patient who has had a failed nail-plate device.

To improve fixation of the proximal fragment, the Sampson rod, a stepped, fluted intramedullary rod with extreme bending strength and excellent torsional control, was developed. Heiple and colleagues[641] reported no failure of the implant and union in all patients in their series. Zickel,[674] however, has expressed concern over reaming the large

hole (up to 18 mm) at the base of the femoral neck that is required for introduction of the Sampson-type rod.

Zickel Nail. Cuthbert and Howat[628] reported the use of a Küntscher "Y" nail for improved proximal fixation in subtrochanteric fractures. Zickel designed and introduced a similar intramedullary device that provides supplementary internal fixation by means of a nail into the head and neck fragment.[672,674,675] This device consists of three parts: (1) a specially designed intramedullary rod; (2) a modified Smith-Petersen nail that penetrates the rod as does Küntscher's "Y" nail;[628] (3) a set screw used to assemble the intramedullary rod and the nail (Fig. 14-34).

The advantages of these implants are: (1) improved proximal fragment fixation due to the Smith-Petersen nail,[672] and (2) resistance to medial migration of the shaft secondary to the enlarged proximal portion of the intramedullary nail.[664,672] The impaction and early patient mobilization are thought to restore the medial cortical bony buttress

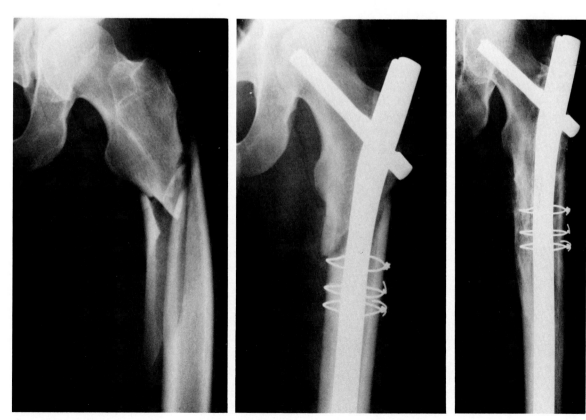

Fig. 14-34. (*Left*) A comminuted subtrochanteric fracture. (*Center*) Internal fixation obtained with a Zickel nail supplemented with cerclage wire. (*Right*) The fracture 12 months later demonstrating solid union.

even in comminuted fractures.[672] In 84 subtrochanteric fractures in which the Zickel nail was used by its inventor, the problems of varus displacement and protrusion of the device into the hip joint were not encountered and only one mechanical failure was reported.[672] It is important to remember that 26 of these 84 patients required accessory fixation because of comminution,[672] and that even Zickel considers using a nail plate in comminuted intertrochanteric fractures in which the subtrochanteric component is small.[674] Beaver and Bach,[614] DiStefano and associates,[632] and Templeton and Saunders[664] have similarly demonstrated excellent union rates with the Zickel device.

Technical complications, including intraoperative trochanteric comminution, rotational malalignment of the femoral shaft, and perforation of the head or neck of the femur have been reported with the Zickel nail.[648,672] Winter and colleagues[671] reported significant mechanical or technical intraoperative problems in 21% of patients. Comminution of the greater trochanter[640,672] and structural abnormalities of the hip or femur are particularly important causes of such problems. However, Winter and colleagues concluded that, if properly performed, the procedure will result in early ambulation and fracture union.

Schatzker and Waddell[658] and Asher and coworkers[612] expressed dissatisfaction with the device, owing to a lack of control of rotational stability of the distal fragment. One additional problem with the use of the Zickel nail is the consideration of whether or not the nail needs to be removed following fracture healing, especially in a young patient. If the nail in the neck of the femur is not inserted deep enough, stress fractures can occur at the tip of the nail through the femoral neck. Such faulty insertion is an indication for removal. Also, the tip of the intramedullary rod can *theoretically* act as a stress riser and result in distal femoral fracture. Although Zickel[673] recommends nail removal only if the patient is symptomatic, I have reservations about leaving such a device in a young patient indefinitely.

Ender's Nail. Ender's condylocephalic nail has been recommended for use in intertrochanteric and subtrochaneric fractures.[646,652,654,658] Russin and Sonni[654] recommended Ender's nails in subtrochanteric fractures because of the reduced surgical trauma required for their insertion, decreased blood loss, uniform distribution of stress, and superior healing potential. However, Schatzker and Waddell[658] report that subtrochanteric fractures are often difficult to reduce closed for Ender's nailing and,

therefore, open reduction is often needed. Opening the fracture essentially nullifies the theoretical advantage of a lesser surgical procedure for the patient. These authors did suggest that the nails were useful in the elderly and in fractures too comminuted to reconstruct surgically. Pankovich and Tarabishy[652] found the complications of proximal or distal nail migration and loss of fixation to be highest in subtrochanteric fractures as compared to intertrochanteric fractures treated with Ender's nails. All patients with osteoporotic bone (Singh's grade 1, 2, or 3) had major complications following Ender's nailing in their series.[652] Kuderna and associates[646] also reported that additional stabilization is often needed in subtrochanteric fractures treated with Ender's nails.

The Use of a Supplementary Bone Graft

The use of a supplementary bone graft, especially along the medial cortex in cases with severe comminution, has been recommended by several authors.[667,670,672] Velasco and Comfort[666] recommend bone grafting any time there is a gap medially after fracture fixation. Schatzker and Waddell[658] also recommend filling any remaining gap in the medial cortex with cancellous bone at the time of the initial operation. Early incorporation of the bone graft helps protect the fixation device from the varus deforming forces that are present owing to lack of the medial cortical bone support.[667]

Postoperative Management

Postoperative mangement must be individualized based on the patient, the fracture characteristics, and the stability of the internal fixation obtained. Initiation of weight bearing too soon postoperatively was found by Waddell to be one of the major causes of fracture healing complications.[667] After internal fixation of fractures in which there is significant medial comminution and loss of medial support, most authors recommend delaying weight bearing for up to 8 weeks.[620,638,658,667] Postoperative use of a modified spica or cast brace should be considered if fracture stability or patient cooperation is questionable.

AUTHOR'S PREFERRED METHOD OF TREATMENT

In the initial x-ray evaluation of the patient, I attempt to determine whether or not a *stable* internal fixation is possible. In those patients in whom internal fixation is indicated for their overall management, and whose fractures are amenable to stable internal fixation, operative treatment is chosen.

I do not recommend any one type of internal fixation device, but attempt to choose the particular device I believe will best provide fracture stability.[619]

In low transverse or short oblique subtrochanteric fractures with a ring of 1 inch of intact bone below the lesser trochanter, I prefer closed intramedullary nailing using a standard or a locking nail.[624] In fractures above this level without trochanteric extension, I consider a locking nail or the Zickel nail with accessory fixation of the medial buttress.

In higher subtrochanteric fractures (Fielding zone 1) and especially those with trochanteric extension, I prefer the sliding compression hip screw. Medial bony stability is obtained by interfragmental compression of bony fragments or by medial displacement or valgus reduction when comminution is severe. I do not recommend use of a fixed-angle nail plate for the reasons given above.

I prefer to augment most cases of internal fixation with an autogenous cancellous bone graft from the ipsilateral iliac crest. Absolute indications for bone grafting include those fractures that cannot be anatomically reduced and in which a medial gap remains, and those fractures in which extensive dissection medially has been required for anatomical internal fixation.

I do not hesitate to use a modified cast brace with pelvic band and knee hinges postoperatively to allow early knee motion in patients who are not likely to comply with our postoperative regimen or in whom fixation is not stable. Postoperatively, partial weight bearing only is allowed for 6 to 8 weeks when the compression hip screw is used. Full weight bearing is permitted when there is

x-ray evidence of healing. In patients treated with an intramedullary or Zickel nail, partial weight bearing on crutches is allowed when muscular control of the limb is present. Progression to full weight bearing is allowed within the limits of pain.

In those patients in whom the preoperative x-ray evaluation suggests that comminution is too severe to allow stable internal fixation, and in open fractures, I choose nonoperative treatment.[629] Open fractures are treated by wound debridement, fracture reduction, and traction. Wounds are left open and undergo delayed secondary closure.

The principle of closed treatment is to align the distal fragment with the proximal fragment as described initially by Hibbs.[642] Skeletal traction with a pin at the level of the tibial tubercle or distal femur is instituted. If the lesser trochanter is still attached to the proximal fragment, the iliopsoas becomes a deforming force causing flexion and external rotation of the proximal fragment.[609,610] The 90°-90° position is used in this situation to align the distal fragment (Fig. 14-35).

In some instances marked abduction of the distal fragment is necessary to compensate for the hip abductor force on the proximal fragment. The 90°-90° position with hip abduction is held for 3 weeks. In the fourth week, hip flexion is slowly decreased until the limb is flat on the bed. Serial x-rays are taken as hip flexion is decreased to ensure that angulation does not occur at the fracture site. When the limb is flat on the bed, a quadrilateral cast brace with a pelvic band holding the limb in 15°-20° of abduction is applied.

If the lesser trochanter is avulsed as part of the fracture, it is no longer a deforming force and the 90°-90° position is not necessary. These patients

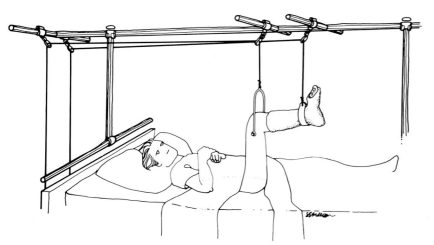

Fig. 14-35. 90-90 traction used in the nonoperative treatment of subtrochanteric fractures. Skeletal traction can be applied with a femoral or tibial pin. This technique is excellent for wound care in open fractures. (DeLee, J.C.; Clanton, T.O.; and Rockwood, C.A.: Closed Reduction of Subtrochanteric Fractures of the Femur in a Modified Cast-Brace. J. Bone Joint Surg., **63A:**773, 1981.)

can be treated in routine balanced suspension before cast brace application. Anatomical restoration of the neck-shaft angle obtained in traction is maintained in the cast. The opposite limb is elevated with a 1½- to 2-inch shoe lift in an effort to shift the center of gravity over the fractured limb, thereby removing the varus stress present during weight bearing (Fig. 14-36). The patient ambulates in this cast with hinges at the knee until union is present.

When using any closed method of treatment I emphasize that the patient's fracture *must* be reduced in traction.[620,629] A closed reduction performed at the time of instituting skeletal traction is helpful in obtaining acceptable alignment.

COMPLICATIONS

The most common complications following subtrochanteric fractures are nonunion, malunion, and implant failure.[609,610,613,618] Both Baker[613] and Boyd and Lipinski[618] noted that the majority of trochanteric fracture nonunions occurred in fractures with subtrochanteric components. The incidence of nonunion and implant failure can be minimized by strict adherence to the principles of stable internal fixation, especially restoring the medial cortical buttress.[657] In established nonunion, excision of the scar tissue and internal fixation with a nail plate[618] or intramedullary device[609,610,611] supplemented by bone grafting have yielded good results.

PATHOLOGIC SUBTROCHANTERIC FRACTURES

Fracture through pathologic bone in the subtrochanteric area is seen with considerable frequency.[621,622,643] This results mainly from the high stresses noted in the subtrochanteric area.[634,637,645] Normal bone in the subtrochanteric area is adapted to withstand these tremendous forces. However, in those conditions in which bone strength is altered, pathologic fracture is likely to occur. Pathologic fractures are seen in systemic disorders such as osteomalacia, renal dystrophy, osteopetrosis, Paget's disease, and osteogenesis imperfecta.[621,661] Indeed, Chalmers and associates[622] reported subtrochanteric fractures as the *presenting* symptom in 3 of 37 patients with osteomalacia.

In addition to metabolic bone disease, the subtrochanteric area is a common location for pathologic fractures secondary to neoplastic metastatic disease.[648,657,659,675] In patients with metastatic tumors, the loss of bone substance prior to fracture adds to the difficulty in management. Excellent

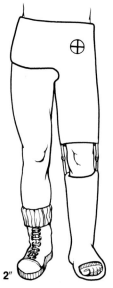

Fig. 14-36. Modified cast-brace with a pelvic band and shoe lift on the contralateral limb for the closed treatment of comminuted or open subtrochanteric fractures. The 2-inch shoe-lift shifts the center of gravity (⊕) over the fractured hip and therefore decreases the tendency for varus malalignment at the fracture site.

results using the Zickel nail in pathologic fractures have been reported by Zickel and Mouradian[675] and by Mickelson and Bonfiglio.[648]

In considering patients with pathologic subtrochanteric fractures, the remainder of the shaft of the femur must be evaluated to make certain that the metabolic process (*i.e.*, Paget's disease) has not altered the bony architecture (increased anterior bowing, and so forth) that could severely limit the choice of type of internal fixation device. In patients with neoplastic metastatic disease, lesions distal to the fracture should be considered when stabilization is undertaken, as they will act as stress risers if not protected by the internal fixation device.

AUTHOR'S PREFERRED METHOD OF TREATMENT

In pathologic fractures or impending pathologic fractures in the subtrochanteric area, I have been pleased with the use of the Zickel nail. The advantages of the Zickel nail are that it will stabilize the proximal fragment and *also* protect the distal femur from further metastatic lesions producing pathologic fractures. One must remember, in considering pathologic fractures secondary to metabolic disease, that the distal shaft may have a curvature in it that does not allow intramedullary rod fixation. Stability can sometimes be improved by the addition of methyl methacrylate to the intramedullary Zickel nail in metastatic lesions.[657] Rotational stability may be a problem postoperatively, but splinting with a Wilkie boot and early quadriceps muscle contraction and leg control exercises tend to limit this instability and allow early mobilization.

DISLOCATIONS AND FRACTURE-DISLOCATIONS OF THE HIP

Dislocation of the hip, with or without an associated acetabular or femoral head fracture, was once thought to be an infrequent injury.[680,846] However, over the past decade these injuries have become more common.[730] They should be considered major injuries because the forces necessary to cause them are considerable. In addition to the obvious disruption of the femoral head-acetabular relationship noted on x-ray, there is often significant associated local soft-tissue injury.[856] Small osseous or cartilaginous fragments often remain in the joint space as the result of the primary injury and may prevent a congruous reduction. This can lead to severe degenerative arthritis.[725,726,728,729,730] As such dislocations frequently result from automobile or automobile-pedestrian accidents, significant injury elsewhere in the body is often present and must

be considered.[716,728,730,737,777,780,812] Up to 50% of these patients suffer fractures elsewhere at the time of dislocation.[842]

Because of the frequency with which injuries about the pelvis are missed in severely traumatized patients, a routine x-ray of the pelvis is indicated in all patients involved in major trauma.[730,839] Fracture or fracture-dislocation of the hip can be easily missed when there is an associated ipsilateral extremity fracture that obscures the clinical deformity of the hip dislocation[712,714,723,733,750,753,757,775, 82,858,867] (see Fig. 14-60). This fact emphasizes the rule of *always* visualizing on x-ray the joint above and below any diaphyseal fracture.[710,869]

Dislocations and fracture-dislocations of the hip are orthopaedic emergencies. A careful physical examination and detailed x-ray assessment of the extent of bony injury for thorough evaluation of the joint, possibly including polytomography or computed tomography, are essential.[758,772,827,833,837]

SURGICAL ANATOMY

The anatomy of the hip, especially the precarious blood supply to the femoral head[683,719,810,814,844] (see Fig. 14-1) and the close proximity of the sciatic nerve,[677,681,715,730,741,746,754,766,788] (Fig. 14-37) are important considerations in the treatment and complications of all dislocations and fracture-disloca-

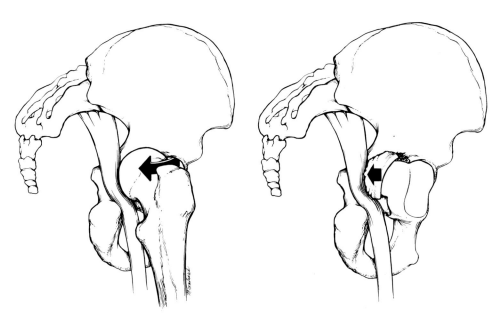

Fig. 14-37. (*Left*) Sciatic nerve impingement by the posteriorly dislocated femoral head. (*Right*) Sciatic nerve impingement by a posterior acetabular fracture fragment in a posterior fracture-dislocation of the hip.

tions about the hip. Special anatomical considerations of the various types of dislocations of the hip are presented separately with the discussion of the mechanism of injury and individualized treatment regimens for each type of dislocation.

CLASSIFICATION

Numerous classifications of hip dislocations are recorded in the literature. In this presentation dislocations will be grouped according to the relationship of the femoral head to the acetabulum: anterior, posterior, and central.[679,680,685,686,691,699,760,767,823,843,849] Each of these three are classified by the

system we have found most useful in delineating the pathology, directing treatment approach, and projecting a prognosis.

ANTERIOR DISLOCATION

In anterior dislocations of the hip, the femoral head rests *anterior* to the coronal plane of the acetabulum. They are classified after a modification of the method of Epstein[728] (Fig. 14-38):

Type I: Superior dislocations (include pubic[686,717,836] and subspinous[686] dislocations).

Type IA: No associated fracture (simple dislocation).

Type IB: Associated fracture of the head of the femur (transchondral or indentation type).

Type IC: Associated fracture of the acetabulum.

Type II: Inferior (includes obturator,[679,860] thyroid,[686,840] and perineal[698,738,846] dislocations).

Type IIA: No associated fracture (simple dislocation).

Type IIB: Associated fracture of the head of the femur (transchondral or indentation type).

Type IIC: Associated fracture of the acetabulum.

Type IA

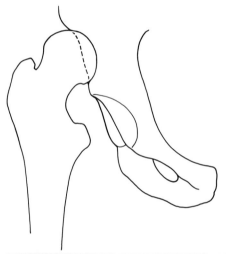

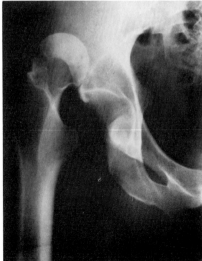
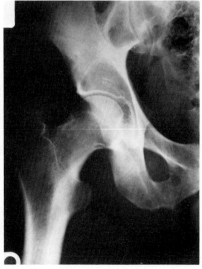

Fig. 14-38. Anterior dislocation of the hip Type I: Superior dislocations (pubic and subspinous). Type IA, simple dislocation (no associated fracture).

Prereduction   Postreduction

POSTERIOR DISLOCATION

In posterior dislocations of the hip the femoral head rests *posterior* to the coronal plane of the acetabulum. Posterior dislocations are classified after the method of Thompson and Epstein.[849] This classification excludes all central protrusion-type fractures that do *not* have an associated posterior dislocation of the hip (Fig. 14-39):

Type I: With or without minor fracture.
Type II: With a large single fracture of the posterior acetabular rim.
Type III: With comminution of the rim of the acetabulum with or without a major fragment.
Type IV: With fracture of the acetabular floor.

Type V: With fracture of the femoral head.

Thompson and Epstein's[849] type V fracture-dislocation has been subclassified into four types according to Pipkin[811] (Fig. 14-40):

Type I: Posterior dislocation of the hip with fracture of the femoral head *caudad* to the fovea centralis.
Type II: Posterior dislocation of the hip with fracture of the femoral head *cephalad* to the fovea centralis.
Type III: Type I or type II with associated fracture of the femoral neck.
Type IV: Type I, II, or III with associated fracture of the acetabulum. (*Text continues on p. 1295.*)

Type IB

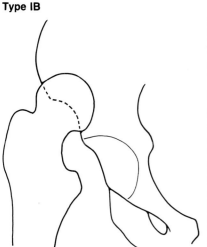

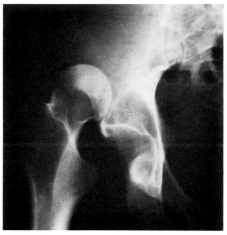

Prereduction

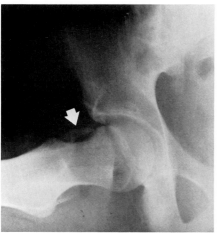

Postreduction

Fig. 14-38 (*Continued*). Type IB, associated femoral head fracture (*arrow* shows transchondral fracture of the femoral head). (*Continues on p. 1290.*)

Type IC

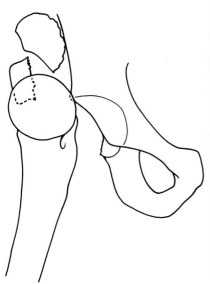

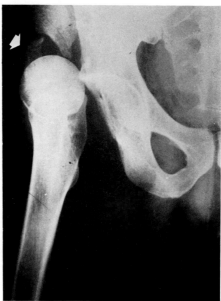

Prereduction

Fig. 14-38 (*Continued*). Type IC, associated acetabular fracture (*arrows*). (Courtesy of Herman Epstein, M.D.)

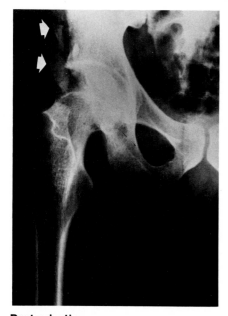

Postreduction

Type IIA

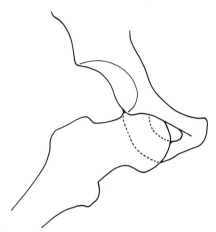

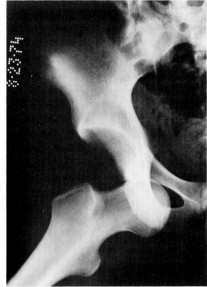

Prereduction

Fig. 14-38 (*Continued*). Type II: Inferior dislocations (obturator, thyroid, or perineal). Type IIA, simple dislocation (no associated fracture). (*Continues on p. 1292.*)

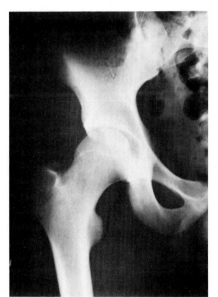

Postreduction

Type IIB

Type IIC

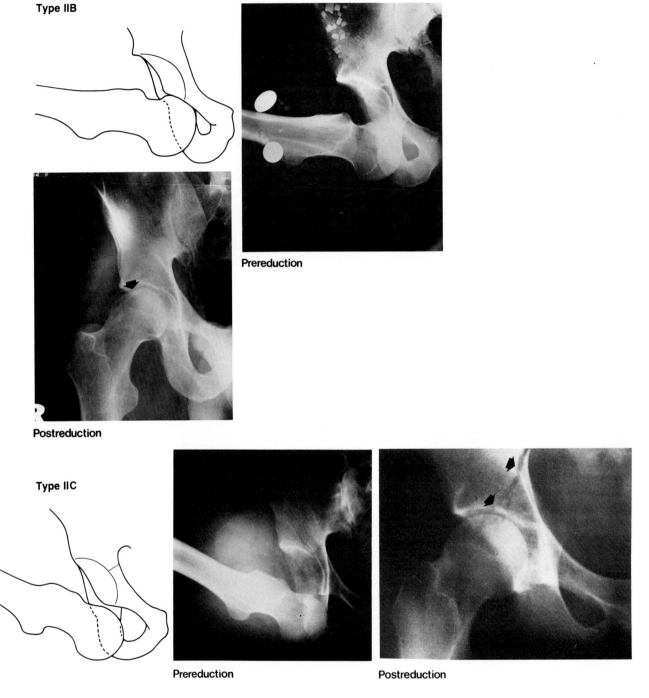

Prereduction

Postreduction

Prereduction

Postreduction

Fig. 14-38 (*Continued*). Type IIB, associated femoral head fracture (*arrow* shows indentation fracture of the femoral head). Type IIC, associated acetabular fracture (*arrows*).

Type I

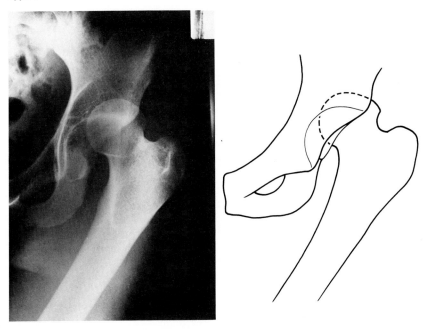

Type II

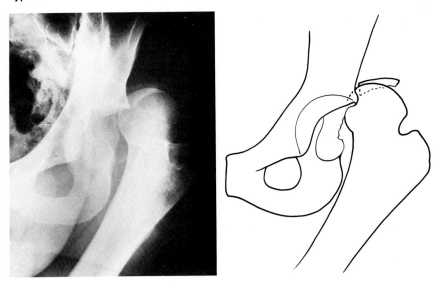

Fig. 14-39. Posterior dislocations of the hip.[796] Type I: With or without minor fracture. Type II: With a large single fracture of the posterior acetabular rim. (*Continues on p. 1294.*)

Type III

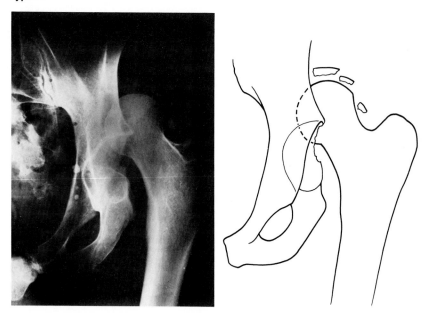

Type IV

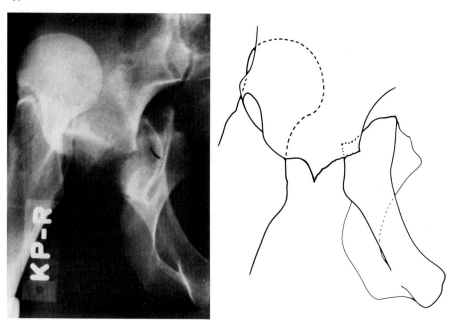

Fig. 14-39 (*Continued*). Type III: With comminution of the rim of the acetabulum with or without a major fragment. Type IV: With a fracture of the acetabular floor.

CENTRAL ACETABULAR FRACTURE-DISLOCATION

In central acetabular fracture and fracture-dislocations, a fracture involving the medial acetabular wall or the superior weight-bearing dome of the acetabulum is present with or without associated central displacement of the femoral head. Several classification systems have been presented.[701,710,722,724,740,779,807,809,823,834,843,850] However, none of these classifications is complete in its ability to suggest fracture anatomy, treatment alternatives, surgical approaches, and prognosis. Therefore, central fracture-dislocations of the hip are classified after a modification of the method of Rowe and Lowell,[823] which we have found useful in suggesting treatment principles and in determining prognosis.[779] This classification basically divides acetabular fractures by the epiphyseal divisions of the developing acetabulum. However, one must be familiar with the anatomical classification of Judet and associates[760] because of its value in selecting the correct surgical approach required in these complex fractures should open reduction be required (Fig. 14-41).

1. Undisplaced fractures (either single line or stellate types).
2. Inner wall fractures.
   A. Femoral head concentrically reduced beneath the dome on initial films.
   B. Femoral head not reduced under the acetabular dome but is centrally dislocated.
3. Superior dome fractures.
   A. The gross outline of the acetabular dome is intact and congruous with the femoral head.
   B. Gross outline of the acetabular dome is not intact and not congruous with the femoral head.
4. Bursting fractures (all elements of the acetabulum are involved).
   A. Fractures in which congruity remains between the femoral head and acetabular dome.
   B. Fractures in which there is incongruity between the femoral head and acetabular dome.

(*Text continues on p. 1299.*)

Type V

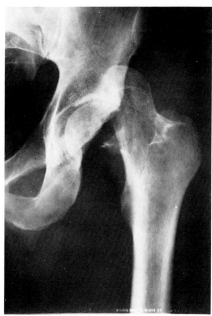
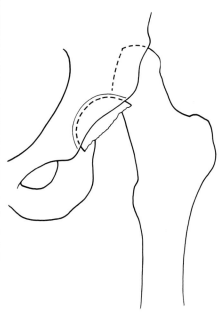

Fig. 14-39 (*Continued*). Type V: With a fracture of the femoral head.

Type I

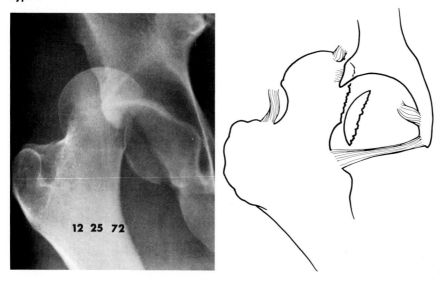

Type II

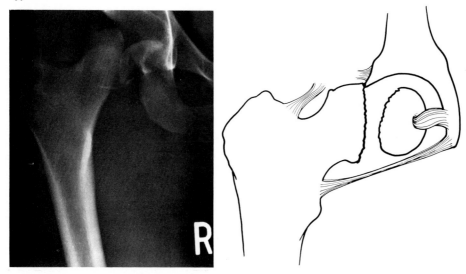

Fig. 14-40. Posterior dislocation of the hip with a femoral head fracture.[762] Type I: Femoral head fracture *caudad* to the fovea centralis. Type II: Femoral head fracture *cephalad* to the fovea centralis.

Type III

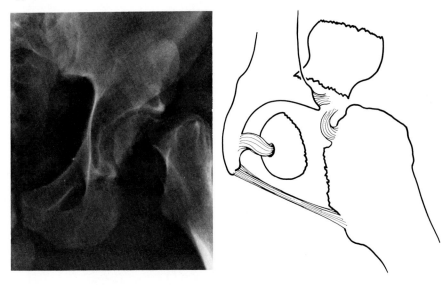

Type IV

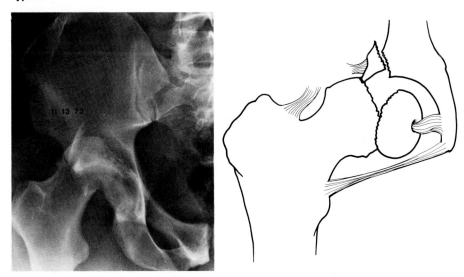

Fig. 14-40 (*Continued*). Type III: Type I or II with associated femoral neck fracture. Type IV: Type I, II, or III with associated acetabular fracture.

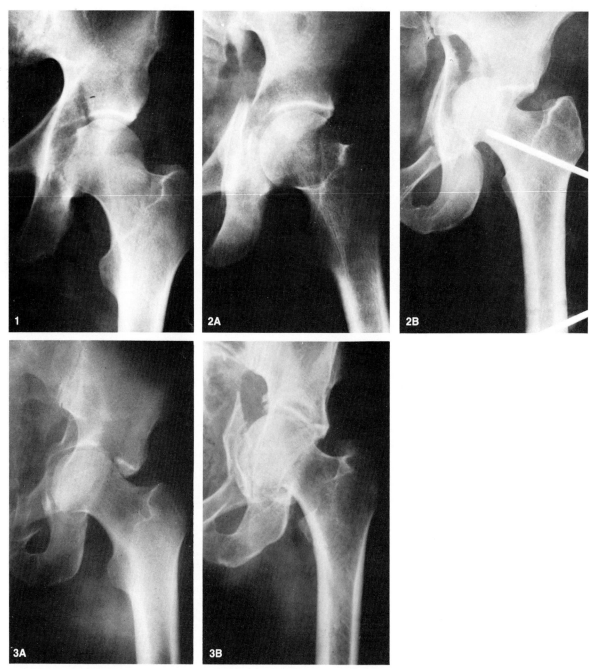

Fig. 14-41. Central acetabular fracture-dislocation.[737] 1. Undisplaced fracture (either single or stellate fracture). 2. Inner wall fractures. 2A. The femoral head is concentrically reduced beneath the acetabular dome on the initial x-rays. 2B. The femoral head is not concentrically reduced beneath the acetabular dome (which is intact), but is centrally dislocated. 3. Superior dome fractures. 3A. The gross outline of the acetabular dome is intact and is congruous with the femoral head. 3B. The gross outline of the acetabular dome is not intact and not congruous with the femoral head. (The fracture through the acetabular dome is so close to the apex that when the head is reduced beneath the dome, it will dislocate unless stabilized by traction or internal fixation.)

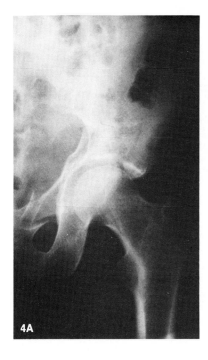
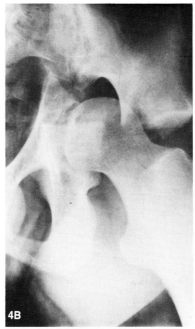

Fig. 14-41 (*Continued*). Bursting Fractures (all elements of the acetabulum involved). 4A. Congruity remains between the femoral head and acetabular dome. Proximal and medial migration of the femoral head is noted. However, the dome is similarly displaced so that a good relationship remains between the femoral head and acetabular dome. 4B. Incongruity exists between the femoral head and acetabular dome. The femoral head is displaced medially and proximally, but the dome is tilted superiorly, resulting in joint incongruity.

ANTERIOR DISLOCATIONS

Anterior dislocations comprise 10% to 15% of traumatic dislocations of the hip.[703,713,730,778,869] They occur in automobile accidents when the knee strikes the dashboard with the thigh abducted, in falls from heights, or secondary to a blow to the back of the patient while in a squatted position.[676,728,730,731,778,785] The neck of the femur or greater trochanter impinges on the rim of the acetabulum and thereby levers the head of the femur out of the acetabulum through a tear in the anterior hip capsule. The degree of hip flexion determines whether a superior or inferior type of anterior dislocation results. Pringle[815] demonstrated that the obturator (inferior) type dislocation was the result of simultaneous hip abduction, external rotation, and flexion. Abduction, external rotation, and hip extension were seen to result in the pubic or iliac (superior) types of anterior dislocation.

These mechanisms of dislocation often result in associated femoral head fractures. A shear fracture of the femoral head may occur as the femoral head passes superiorly over the anterior-inferior rim of the acetabulum,[713,731,826,827] resulting in a transchondral-type fracture (Fig. 14-38 type IB). Generally, such transchondral fractures are easily seen on routine x-rays.[713] In inferior-type (obturator or thyroid) dislocations, the sharp anterolateral margin of the obturator foramen may indent the anterior-superior aspect of the femoral head, resulting in the so-called indentation fracture[676,693,713,720,734] (See Fig. 14-38 type IIB). A high index of suspicion and occasionally polytomography are needed to document the presence of these indentation fractures.[713]

CLINICAL DIAGNOSIS

Owing to the fact that hip dislocations are often secondary to high-energy trauma, careful multi-system evaluation for associated life-threatening injuries is *essential* prior to directing attention solely to the musculoskeletal system. Physical examination of the involved extremity may reveal slight shortening. The position of the limb suggests the diagnosis. In superior dislocations (iliac or pubic type) the hip is extended and externally rotated (Fig. 14-42). In inferior-type dislocations (obturator, thyroid, or perineal type) the hip is abducted, is externally rotated, and is in varying degrees of flexion (Fig. 14-43).

In superior dislocations of the subspinous or iliac type the femoral head is palpable in the vicinity of the anterior superior iliac spine. It is palpable in the groin in pubic types. In inferior-type dislocations a fullness is palpable in the region of obturator foramen.

In all cases of anterior dislocation the circulatory

and neurologic status of the limb must be fully assessed. Trauma to the femoral artery, vein, and nerve have been reported only in the superior-type dislocations or in open anterior dislocations.[690,747,795,799,829]

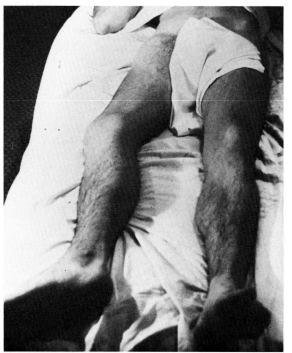

Fig. 14-42. Clinical appearance of a superior-type anterior dislocation of the hip. (Courtesy of Herman Epstein. M.D.)

RADIOGRAPHIC FINDINGS

The diagnosis is readily apparent on routine anteroposterior x-rays of the hip that demonstrate the femoral head to be out of the acetabulum in either a superior or inferior position (see Fig. 14-38). A careful x-ray evaluation of associated bony damage, including fractures of the acetabular rim or floor, femoral head, and femoral neck must be carefully performed to prevent further damage during reduction and to assist the physician in determining the treatment approach and prognosis.[713,813] If questions arise concerning associated femoral head fractures, acetabular fractures, or loose fragments within the joint, polytomography[713,758] or CT scanning is necessary to complete the evaluation.[772,825,833,837]

TREATMENT

Early diagnosis and prompt closed reduction under a general anesthetic is the treatment of choice; however, certain dislocations require open reduction. Multiple attempts at closed reduction are not recommended.[713,730,842,843,856] If the hip cannot be reduced under a general anesthetic with one attempt, an anatomical obstruction to reduction is present and open reduction is recommended.[730] Most authors suggest reduction attempts under general or spinal anesthesia to prevent further articular damage that may result from a forceful closed reduction in the unrelaxed patient.[691,730]

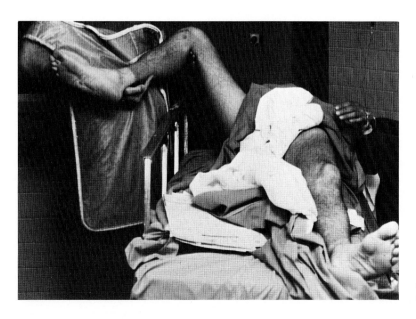

Fig. 14-43. Clinical appearance of an inferior-type anterior dislocation of the hip.

Closed Reduction

Three methods of closed reduction have been reported.

The Gravity Method of Stimson. This maneuver was described primarily for acute posterior dislocations,[845,846] but anterior dislocations can occasionally be reduced by this method.[713] The patient is in the prone position with the lower limbs hanging from the end of the table. An assistant immobilizes the pelvis by applying pressure on the sacrum. The surgeon holds the knee and ankle flexed to 90° and applies gentle downward pressure to the leg just distal to the knee. Gentle rotatory motion of the limb may assist in reduction (Fig. 14-44).

It must be emphasized that superior dislocations of the pubic type in which the hip presents in extension are not amenable to a Stimson maneuver[717] because of the need for further extension to achieve reduction.

The Allis Maneuver. In the Allis[677] maneuver, the patient is placed in the supine position. The knee is flexed to relax the hamstrings. An assistant stabilizes the pelvis and applies a lateral traction force to the inside of the thigh. Longitudinal traction is applied in line with the axis of the femur and the hip is slightly flexed. The surgeon gently adducts and internally rotates the femur to achieve reduc-tion (Fig. 14-45). This is a safe and successful method of reduction.

The Reverse Bigelow Maneuver.[685,686,687,846,859] The position of the hip in the reverse Bigelow maneuver is partial flexion and abduction. Bigelow suggests two methods of reduction. First, the lifting method, in which a firm "jerk" is applied to the flexed thigh. This method will often result in reduction except in pubic dislocations.[685]

If this "lifting method" fails, traction is applied in the line of deformity. The hip is then adducted, sharply internally rotated, and extended (Fig. 14-46). One must be careful in using this technique, since the sharp internal rotation can result in fracture of the femoral neck in osteoporotic bone. Polesky[813] reported a displaced fracture of the femoral neck following attempted closed reduction of an anterior dislocation. Careful scrutiny of pre-reduction x-rays for nondisplaced fractures and adherence to the principle of gentle reduction are required to prevent such complications.

Epstein,[728] DeLee and associates[713] and Walker[859] favor a modification of the Allis technique for reduction of inferior dislocations. Continuous traction is applied in the line of the deformity with gentle flexion of the hip joint. A lateral force is applied to the thigh. Slight internal rotation and adduction are then used to reduce the hip. In superior dislocations, traction strong enough to pull

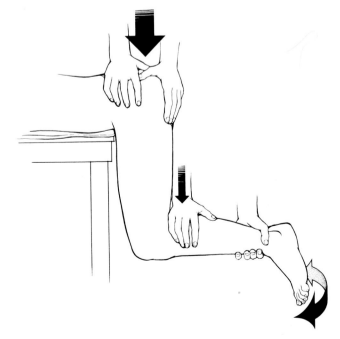

Fig. 14-44. Stimson's gravity method of reduction (see text for description).

the femoral head distal to the acetabulum is applied in the line of the femur. Gentle flexion and internal rotation are then applied. Dingley and Denham[717] reported a case of pubic dislocation of the hip that was irreducible by techniques of reduction involv-

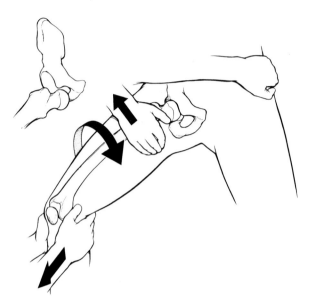

Fig. 14-45. The Allis reduction maneuver for an anterior dislocation of the hip (see text for description).

ing flexion. Reduction was finally accomplished by placing the patient prone and hyperextending the hip. They[717] postulated that hyperextension relaxed the posterior capsule and external rotators, which allowed reduction to be accomplished. It must be emphasized that of the anterior dislocations, the superior type (pubic or subspinous) is distinctly uncommon,[679,713,730] and therefore extensive experience with their management is not available.

Femoral head fracture, either transchondral or indentation type, associated with anterior dislocation of the hip was reported in 8 of 55 cases by Epstein and Harvey[732] and in 17 of 22 cases by DeLee and associates.[713] Urist emphasized that almost all cases have damage to the femoral head, which may be small fractures not visible on x-ray.[856] If pre- or post-reduction films demonstrate an associated transchondral fracture of the femoral head, excision has been recommended.[728,730,731] Indentation fractures, although present in a significant percentage of patients,[713,731,732] do not lend themselves to surgical repair. The importance of recognition of indentation fractures rests in their adverse effect on prognosis.[713,732]

Acetabular fractures associated with anterior dislocations are unusual.[730] Such fractures are treated as individual cases demand, depending on location and displacement of the acetabular fracture.[730,731]

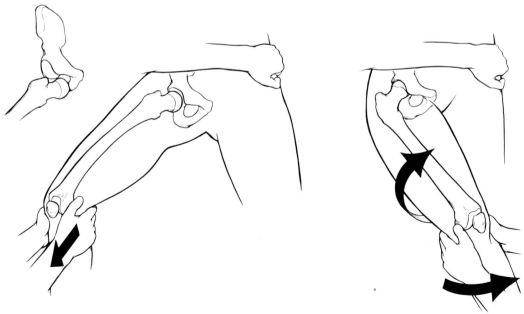

Fig. 14-46. The reverse Bigelow reduction maneuver for an anterior dislocation of the hip (see text for description).

Management After Reduction

Management following closed reduction of an anterior dislocation includes traction.[713,728,731] The recommended period of traction ranges from 8 days[713] to 4 to 6 weeks[679,730] following simple dislocations. Controlled range of motion is instituted during this time to aid articular cartilage nutrition.[713] Care is taken to avoid the extremes of abduction and external rotation of the injured hip to prevent redislocation. A longer period of immobilization may be necessary in dislocations with associated fractures of the acetabulum or femoral head.[730]

Late Diagnosis

The late diagnosis of unreduced anterior hip dislocations is extremely uncommon in the western world.[676,745] Aggarwal and Singh[676] and Hamada[745] suggest osteotomy of the proximal femur as a means of obtaining a functional hip in late, unreduced anterior dislocations. Aggarwal and Singh attempted an open reduction of a chronic dislocation, but this resulted in a painful hip with limited function. The literature does not deal extensively with open reduction of chronic anterior dislocations. However, the surgeon should be fully aware of the possible future need of bone stock for hip arthroplasty as a pain relief procedure in such patients. From this standpoint, although osteotomy may result in good function short term, the long-term results of such procedures are unknown.

COMPLICATIONS AND PROGNOSIS

Early Complications

Neurovascular Compromise. Direct pressure on the femoral artery, vein, or nerve resulting in distal neurovascular compromise has been reported in superior (pubic or subspinous) dislocations[690,747,795,799] and in open dislocations.[829] Inferior-type dislocations do not have a high incidence of associated neurovascular compromise.[713] In cases with neurovascular compromise, immediate reduction of the hip is essential to assure limb viability.

Irreducibility. Anterior hip dislocations may be irreducible by closed means. Obstructions to closed reduction include bony locking in the obturator foramen[826] and interposition of soft tissues, including the rectus femoris,[869] iliopsoas muscle,[730,761] and the anterior hip capsule.[752,759,761,782,783] Therefore, a failed closed reduction under adequate anesthesia dictates open reduction to remove the structure blocking reduction.

Late Complications

Post-traumatic Arthritis. Results following anterior dislocation of the hip initially were thought to be very good in most cases.[843,849] However, recent studies report fair or poor results in one third to one half of cases owing to the development of post-traumatic arthritis.[713,731,732] The factors associated with the development of traumatic arthritis include associated femoral head fractures, acetabular fractures, and aseptic necrosis.[730] Femoral head fractures of the transchondral type[713] and indentation fractures of significant depth[693,713,734] have a high incidence of symptomatic degenerative arthritis. Surgical excision of the transchondral fracture may decrease the incidence of post-traumatic arthritis, but no specific treatment of indentation fractures has been shown to be successful.[713,730,731,732]

Aseptic Necrosis. Aseptic necrosis after uncomplicated anterior dislocation of the hip is less common than in posterior dislocations, having been reported to occur in up to 8% of cases.[691,728,826] Aseptic necrosis may appear from 2 to 5 years after the dislocation.[798,814,843] Delay in reduction or repeated attempts at reduction[730,790,793,844] have been linked to the development of aseptic necrosis. Although early weight bearing may modify the severity of aseptic necrosis, it does not appear to increase the incidence of this complication.[691] The most important factor determining vascularity of the femoral head is the extent of the initial injury.[683,730,844] Epstein and Harvey warn against confusing the x-ray appearance of aseptic necrosis with that of developing traumatic joint disease, especially in patients with indentation fractures.[731]

Recurrent Dislocations. Recurrent anterior dislocation of the hip has been reported by several authors.[708,744,831] Dall and colleagues[708] and Scudese[831] implicate inadequate immobilization during the post reduction period, which fails to allow adequate capsular healing, as the cause of recurrent anterior dislocation.

AUTHOR'S PREFERRED METHOD OF TREATMENT

A thorough x-ray evaluation is essential prior to reduction to identify nondisplaced fractures of the femoral neck that may displace during closed reduction.

Anterior dislocations are managed by closed reduction, usually under general or spinal anesthesia, using a modification of the Allis[677] maneuver. First, countertraction is applied by the use of a sheet in the groin. The pelvis is stabilized by an assistant. In superior dislocations, traction is then applied in the line of the femur and the hip is flexed and gently internally rotated *only* after strong traction pulls the femoral head distal to the acetabulum. In inferior dislocations, flexion of the hip with continuous traction in line of the femur and gentle internal rotation and adduction are used to reduce the hip.

Muscle relaxation obtained with general or spinal anesthesia is preferred, but if there is a significant delay in obtaining anesthesia, I perform the reduction under intravenous analgesia.

Open reduction through an anterior iliofemoral approach[869] is performed (1) in patients in whom closed reduction is not successful; (2) in patients with a transchondral fracture of the femoral head, that is displaced after reduction of the dislocation; or (3) in patients in whom such a fragment prevents closed reduction. These displaced transchondral fracture fragments are usually excised. However, consideration is given to open reduction and internal fixation of such fractures when they involve greater than one third of the weight-bearing surface of the femoral head. Indentation fractures are treated with traction and early hip motion following closed reduction in an effort to restore full range. No surgical treatment for the indentation fracture is presently feasible.

In patients with associated acetabular fractures, treatment is modified in accordance with the type of acetabular fracture and its degree of displacement.

After closed reduction, patients are managed in skin traction in slight flexion and internal rotation until the hip has a painless range of motion, usually in 2 to 3 weeks. Weight bearing is then begun as tolerated. Recurrent dislocation has not been a problem in my experience in spite of this minimal period of immobilization.

POSTERIOR DISLOCATIONS

Posterior dislocations of the hip are becoming more common due to the increasing incidence of high-energy trauma.[730] The mechanism of this injury is usually a force applied to the flexed knee with the hip in varying degrees of flexion.[820,822] If the hip is in the neutral or adducted position at the time of impact, a simple dislocation without acetabular fracture will usually occur. If it is in slight abduction, an associated fracture of the posterior-superior rim of the acetabulum will result.[730,862] The greater the degree of hip flexion the more likely the injury will be a simple dislocation. This mechanism of injury

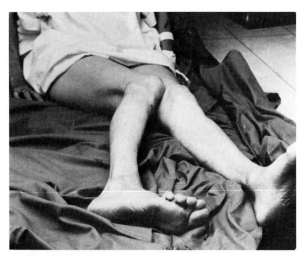

Fig. 14-47. The clinical appearance of a posterior dislocation of the right hip.

most commonly occurs when the knee strikes the dashboard of an automobile during a head-on collision, hence the term "dashboard dislocation" given this injury by Funsten and associates.[734]

CLINICAL DIAGNOSIS

The involved limb is classically shortened, internally rotated, and adducted (Fig. 14-47). Because of the high-energy trauma responsible for posterior dislocations, associated life-threatening injuries are common and their recognition is essential.[730,822] Indeed, Tronzo believes that a patient may be in shock as a result of the hip dislocation alone, and the shock may be corrected by reduction of the hip.[853]

Associated musculoskeletal injuries are also frequent and must be carefully sought. Sciatic nerve injury associated with posterior dislocation is seen in 10% to 14% of cases.[728,756,806,832,843,849] In addition, associated ligamentous injuries to the ipsilateral knee,[737,756] femoral head fractures,[689,696,697,702,704,711,718,762,763,802,811,821,824] and femoral shaft fractures are not uncommon.[712,714,721,733,750,753,757,797,841,858,867] Posterior dislocation of the hip associated with a femoral shaft fracture frequently goes unrecognized because the classical clinical position of the flexed, internally rotated, and adducted limb is not present (see Figs. 14-47 and 14-60).

RADIOGRAPHIC FINDINGS

The diagnosis of posterior fracture or fracture-dislocation of the hip is usually confirmed by a single anteroposterior x-ray (see Fig. 14-39). However, this alone is not satisfactory for evaluation of associated acetabular, femoral head, or femoral neck fractures.[864] These associated fractures must be recognized prior to carrying out any type of reduction. A slightly oblique lateral view of the pelvis is excellent for assessing the acetabulum and is made with the patient lying on the affected side with the body rotated forward at 15° (Fig. 14-48). Urist[856] also recommended a posterior oblique view, in which the injured side is elevated 60° with the patient supine, to demonstrate the posterior acetabular rim in profile. An alternative method of taking oblique x-rays of the acetabulum is that of Judet[760]; the so-called three-quarter internal and external oblique views (see Chapter 13). Finally, a surgical lateral film of the hip is made to show the position of posterior fracture fragments.[864] If positioning the patient for prereduction x-rays is not possible because of pain, these x-rays are taken while under anesthesia *before* reduction.

Three anatomical areas should be carefully scrutinized on the prereduction x-ray: (1) the femoral head for an associated fracture;[762,811,821,864] (2) the

acetabulum to ascertain the presence, size, and location of acetabular fractures;[710,864] and (3) the femoral neck for nondisplaced fractures that might displace when closed reduction is attempted[821] Polytomography[713,758,822,864] and CT scans have recently been used to further delineate fracture fragment size and location[772,825,833,837] (see Fig. 14-51).

Immediately following reduction, repeat x-rays are obtained to ascertain (1) the adequacy of reduction of the dislocation;[700,835] (2) the presence or absence of entrapped fracture fragments in the joint space,[725,759] and (3) the accuracy of reduction of associated femoral head and acetabular fracture fragments to determine the need for open reduction.[762,811,821]

TREATMENT

The treatment of posterior dislocations and fracture-dislocations of the hip is divided between two philosophical groups. Classically, the dislocation or fracture-dislocation is treated by immediate closed reduction, reserving open reduction for those patients in whom (1) closed reduction is not suc-

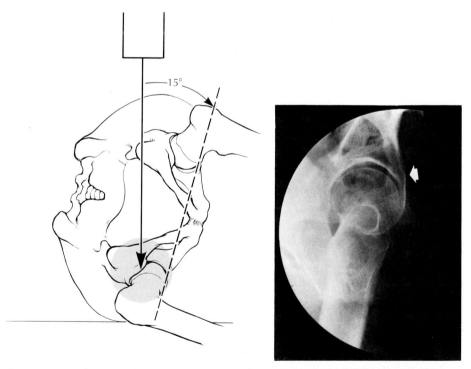

Fig. 14-48. (*Left*) Correct patient positioning for an x-ray to highlight the posterior acetabulum and greater and lesser sciatic notches. The injured side is nearest the film and the patient is tilted 15° from the vertical to prevent superimposition of the normal hip and acetabulum. (*Right*) A 15° oblique lateral view of the pelvis. Note the clarity of posterior acetabulum (*arrow*).

cessful, (2) the reduction is unstable, or (3) fracture fragments are trapped between the joint surfaces following reduction.[677,680,685,686,687,688,699,700,718, 730,748,756,768,770,798,806,835,843,847,864]

More recently, Epstein[725,726,728,729,730,*] has recommended primary open reduction, debridement of the joint, and anatomical internal fixation of fracture fragments of the acetabular rim to increase the incidence of good results. Although he has reported the largest series to date with adequate followup, and demonstrates a significant improvement in results, Epstein's[725,726] concept of primary open reduction is often not possible because associated injuries make general anesthesia and operative open reduction impractical.[822] Whether open or closed reduction is selected, one must remember that most authors are in agreement that early reduction, usually within 12 hours of injury, is essential.[691,730,793,842,843] The treatment of posterior dislocations and fracture-dislocations will be specifically discussed for each type in the Thompson-Epstein classification.[849]

Type I (Posterior Dislocation Without Fracture)

Type I is a simple posterior dislocation without fracture. Both philosophical groups agree that type I posterior dislocations should be reduced by closed means as soon as possible, and certainly within 12 hours.[680,691,725,728,729,730,734,736,756,793,842,843]   Closed reduction by the techniques of Stimson,[845,846] Allis,[677] or Bigelow[685,686,687,688] may be successful. If reduction will be delayed because of associated injuries, one attempt at closed reduction under intravenous analgesics and muscle relaxants in the emergency room is warranted.[729] If reduction by this technique cannot be accomplished with ease, excessive force must not be used. The patient should instead be prepared for reduction under general or spinal anesthesia as soon as possible.

Gravity Method of Stimson.

Although the Stimson maneuver[845,846] (see Fig. 14-44) is believed to be the least traumatic, associated injuries may prevent the prone positioning it requires. The patient is placed in a prone position with the hip flexed over the end of the table. An assistant stabilizes the pelvis by pressure on the sacrum or by extending the opposite limb. The involved hip and knee are flexed 90°. Downward pressure is applied behind the flexed knee. Gentle rotation of the femur may facilitate the reduction.

* Epstein, H.C.: Personal communication, 1981.

The Allis Maneuver. In the Allis maneuver[677] the patient is supine and the pelvis is stabilized by pressure on both anterior spines by an assistant (Fig. 14-49). The essential feature of the Allis maneuver is traction in direct line of the deformity followed by gentle flexion of the hip to 90°. The hip is gently rotated internally and externally with continued longitudinal traction until reduction is achieved.

The Bigelow Maneuver. In the Bigelow maneuver, [685,686,687,688] (Fig. 14-50) the patient lies supine, and an assistant applies countertraction by downward pressure on the anterosuperior iliac spines. The surgeon grasps the affected limb at the ankle with one hand, places the opposite forearm behind the knee, and applies longitudinal traction in the line of the deformity. The adducted and internally rotated thigh is then flexed 90° or more on the abdomen. This relaxes the Y ligament and allows the surgeon to bring the femoral head near the posterior/inferior rim of the acetabulum. While traction is maintained, the femoral head is levered into the acetabulum by abduction, external rotation, and extension of the hip. Since this technique requires more force, it can result in fracture or increased soft-tissue damage to the hip; therefore, it should be used with great care.

Management After Reduction. Following closed reduction, light skin or skeletal traction (5 to 8 pounds) is recommended for comfort and to allow capsular healing. The traction should prevent the hip from being flexed, internally rotated, and adducted (*i.e.,* positions that might result in recurrent dislocation). Traction is maintained until the hip is pain free (several days to 2 weeks) and has a good range of motion.[728] Spica cast immobilization after reduction is condemned because it prevents early range of motion necessary to promote nutrition and healing of the damaged articular cartilage.[728]

The time at which weight bearing is recommended after reduction is a very controversial point.[678,680,688,691,730,768,770,798,806,820,843,847,853] Stuck and Vaughan[847] recommended non-weight bearing for 6 to 12 months after reduction. Brav[691] indicated that overall complications were less frequent when patients were kept from bearing weight for 12 weeks; however, the incidence of aseptic necrosis was unchanged. Epstein recommends resuming weight bearing when pain and spasm disappear.[730] Stewart and associates[842] recommended weight bearing 2 to 4 weeks after reduction. It must be remembered that, although aseptic necrosis may

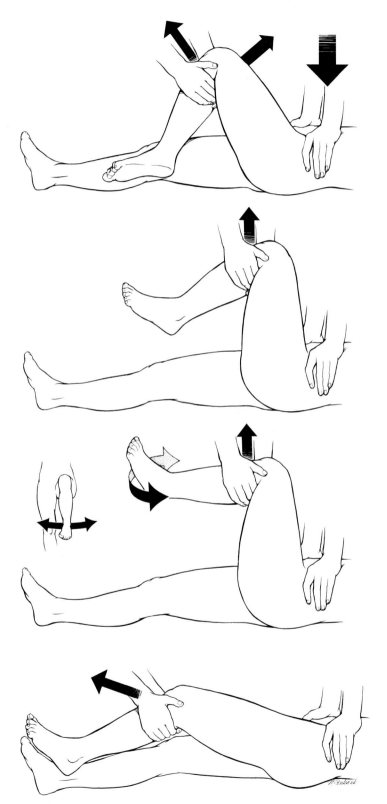

Fig. 14-49. The Allis reduction maneuver for a posterior dislocation of the hip (see text for description).

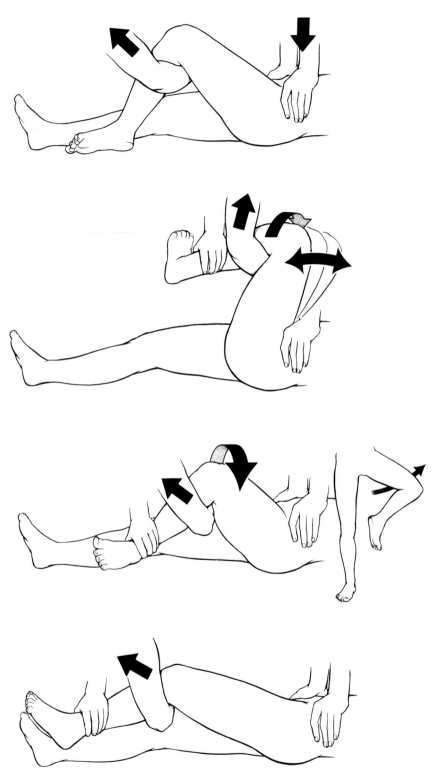

Fig. 14-50. The Bigelow reduction maneuver for a posterior dislocation of the hip (see text for description).

be detected earlier on x-rays if there is generalized disuse osteoporosis of the affected hip secondary to withholding weight bearing, this is an incidental point and not a clinical dictum.

Types II Through IV (Posterior Fracture-Dislocations)

It is in the management of type II through IV posterior fracture-dislocations of the hip that the two philosophies, one recommending primary closed reduction and the other primary open reduction, disagree.

The majority of authors classically recommend that the dislocation with associated acetabular fractures should be reduced by closed means as quickly as possible.[680,691,735,842,843] Stewart and colleagues[842] reported improvement of results with time in patients treated by closed reduction and the reverse in patients treated by open reduction.

Definite indications for open reduction have been given by several authors. Griswold and Herd,[742] in 1929, recommended open reduction to restore stability of displaced posterior acetabular lip fragments that remain displaced after hip reduction. King and Richards[764] recommended closed reduction followed by traction unless (1) there was a large posterior lip fragment that did not reduce (an unstable reduction), (2) a bone fragment was noted in the acetabulum (Fig. 14-51), or (3) a fracture of the femoral head prevented reduction. Armstrong[680] recommended closed reduction except in those cases in which there was a displaced posterior rim fracture associated with a sciatic nerve palsy. Brav[691] and Stewart and Milford[843] recommended open reduction only when attempts at closed reduction failed, when loose fragments were visible within the joint on x-ray, or when the joint was unstable after reduction. Urist[855,856] recommended primary open reduction in dislocations associated with comminuted fractures of the acetabulum. Lipscomb[777] also reserved open reduction for those patients with a displaced large acetabular fragment that results in joint instability, and those in whom a fragment of the acetabulum or femoral head blocks reduction.

Gregory stressed that following successful closed reduction, stability of the joint must be evaluated by carrying the hip through a range of flexion to 90°, with adduction and posterior pressure on the hip.[741] If the hip dislocates again, it is considered to be unstable. The long-term results of nonoperative treatment in such cases are uniformly poor.[699,731,742,764,843] Therefore, operative treatment with internal fixation of the fragment is indicated

to create a stable joint with a congruous articular surface. Primary closed reduction of these injuries may avoid an operative procedure in a significant number of cases where the posterior acetabular fracture is small; however, it is apparent that the secondary dislocation that occurs in the unstable group subjects the articular cartilage to increased trauma.[730]

Epstein reported the largest series of posterior fracture-dislocations in the literature.[730] He has noted bony fragments and debris in the joints of 91% of patients at arthrotomy. He reported significantly better results in type II, III, and IV dislocations after early *primary* open reduction than after closed reduction alone, than when open reduction was performed *after* closed reduction, or than when open reduction was delayed. He also noted better results in patients who underwent open reduction following closed reduction than in those patients treated only by closed reduction.* He therefore recommends *primary* open reduction of all posterior fracture-dislocations of the hip for the following reasons:[726,730]

1. To remove loose fragments of bone and cartilage from the joint space.
2. To restore joint stability and joint congruity by open reduction and internal fixation of large posterior acetabular fragments.
3. To ensure accurate reduction of the dislocation.

Epstein believes that, by accomplishing the above goals, he can delay the onset of osteoarthritis *and* minimize its severity.* I agree that Epstein's concept of *primary* open reduction of fracture-dislocations of the hip is correct *in theory*. However, it is not always possible to have optimum operating conditions for major hip surgery as an emergency procedure. Unless such conditions are met, it is safer to carry out a closed reduction. If, after closed reduction, open reduction is deemed necessary because of instability or retained fragments in the joint, the operative procedure can be carried out in optimum conditions for hip surgery as a semi-emergency procedure. Epstein* has noted an increase in the incidence of poor results when open reduction and joint debridement following closed reduction is performed later than 2 to 3 weeks after the dislocation. However, Rosenthal and Coker[822] reported good results when bony fragments were removed up to 4 weeks after the dislocation.

Regardless of whether one chooses primary open reduction or closed reduction as the treatment of

---

* Epstein, H.C.: Personal communication, 1981.

Prereduction   **Postreduction**

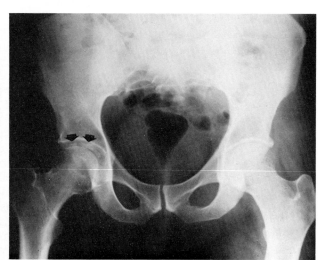

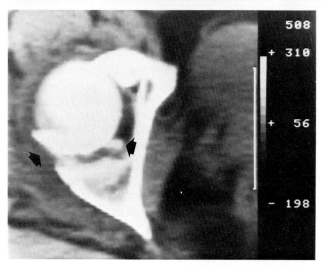

Fig. 14-51. (*Top left*) Posterior fracture-dislocation of the right hip. (*Top right*) A postreduction x-ray shows bone fragments trapped in the acetabulum (*arrows*), resulting in an incongruous reduction. (*Bottom*) Intra-articular fragments confirmed by a CT scan.

choice for posterior fracture-dislocations of the hip, the following are factors considered by most authors to be of prognostic significance in patients with these injuries[680,691,725,727,728,729,730,736,741,756,768,771,777, 793,798,843]:

1. Long-term results are *directly* related to the degree of the initial trauma.[678,691,730,847,855,856,857] This explains the percentage of good results, progressively decreasing from type II to type V injuries.

2. Reduction, either closed or open, should be performed within 12 to 24 hours to ensure the best result.[678,691,730,822,843,849]

3. If closed reduction is selected, it should be attempted only once. If this fails, one should proceed to an open reduction to prevent further damage to the femoral head.[729,798]

Technique of Open Reduction   Open reduction and internal fixation should be carried out through a posterior approach. Epstein[730] and Stewart and Milford[843] report a higher incidence of aseptic necrosis when an anterior approach is used. The technique described by King and Richards[764] is a safe and simple approach involving a muscle-splitting incision through the gluteus maximus that is extended distally as necessary. Other posterior approaches to the hip may be acceptable, provided that exposure allows adequate visualization of the sciatic nerve and sciatic notch.

Once the joint is exposed, it is carefully irrigated to ensure removal of all fragments of bone and cartilage.[730] If the hip has not been reduced previously, it can then be reduced without traumatizing the articular cartilage.[730] Care should be taken not to detach any soft tissues about the head or neck that may further compromise the blood supply. The fracture fragments should then be repositioned to provide an anatomical reduction of the acetabular fracture. This is most easily accomplished when there is a single large fragment, as in a type II injury. Fixation is obtained by cancellous screws, care being taken not to penetrate the acetabular floor (Fig. 14-52).

When several fragments are present, as in a type III injury, reconstruction should be carried out as accurately as possible, using the major fragments to provide a bony buttress. Either multiple pin fixation or fixation with a small malleable plate to ensure stability is satisfactory.[730]

The fractures of the acetabular floor in type IV injuries are treated based on their location and displacement. Epstein[730] found that those patients with displaced fractures of the acetabular dome have uniformly poor results regardless of treatment.

Postoperative Treatment. Skeletal traction of 10 to 15 pounds is used with the hip in extension and slight abduction. Gentle active and passive exercises in traction can be initiated as soon as the patient is comfortable, usually within 3 to 5 days. The hip should not be immobilized in a spica cast unless it is essential to the treatment of other injuries.[730] Immobilization of the joint following an intra-articular fracture has an adverse effect on articular cartilage nutrition, as well as predisposing to the capsular adhesions and muscular atrophy that delay rehabilitation.[728]

As in the case of a simple dislocation, there is no consensus as to how long a patient should be maintained in traction or protected from weight bearing.[691,770,806] Epstein recommends traction for

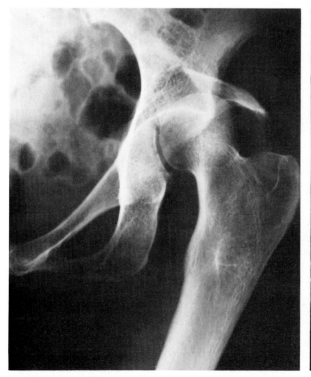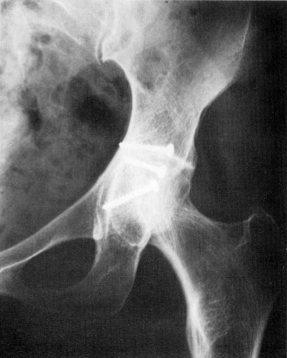

Fig. 14-52. (*Left*) Thompson-Epstein type II posterior fracture-dislocation of the hip. (*Right*) Primary open reduction and internal fixation using cancellous bone screws.

6 to 8 weeks to allow time for the acetabular fractures to heal. This is followed by progressive weight bearing with crutches as tolerated.[728] If internal fixation is not rigid, traction should be maintained for a minimum of 8 weeks, followed by a similar period of protected weight bearing.[730,843] Some authors advocate non-weight bearing for a prolonged period of time to protect the cartilage until a firm fibrocartilaginous surface is established, and to prevent collapse of the avascular hip by reducing the trauma and microfractures during the revascularization phase.[810,847]

Thompson-Epstein Type V Posterior Fracture-Dislocations

In type V posterior fracture-dislocations, there is an associated fracture of the femoral head. This injury was first reported by Birkett in 1869.[689] Christopher found only 15 cases reported up to 1926.[704] With the increasing incidence of motor vehicle accidents, type V fracture-dislocations are becoming more frequent.[702,864] The mechanism of injury, according to Davis,[711] is a force transmitted along the axis of the femur. If the hip is flexed 90° or greater when the force is applied, the head of the femur is forced out over the posterior acetabular rim. This results in a posterior dislocation with or without a fracture of the acetabular rim. If the hip is flexed 60° or less and is in the neutral position (with reference to abduction), the femoral head is driven against the firm posterior/superior acetabular rim, resulting in a combined dislocation and fracture of the femoral head.[711]

The Thompson-Epstein type V posterior fracture-

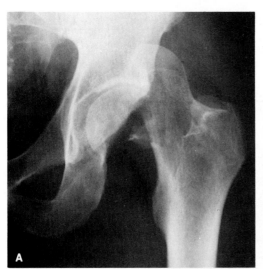
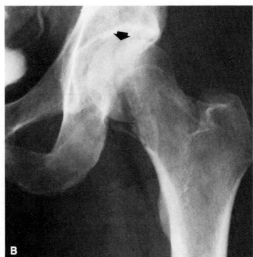
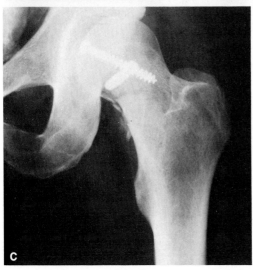

Fig. 14-53. A Pipkin type II fracture of the femoral head associated with posterior dislocation of the hip. (*A*) Initial injury film. (*B*) Post-closed reduction film. The femoral head fracture is not anatomically reduced (*arrow*). (*C*) X-rays taken after open reduction by detaching the ligamentum teres from the femoral head fragment and internal fixation of the femoral head fracture.

dislocations were further divided by Pipkin[811] (see Fig. 14-40). Pipkin type I injuries have a fracture of the femoral head caudad, and type II cephalad to the fovea centralis. In type I fractures, Chakraborti and Miller,[702] Roeder and DeLee,[821] and Stewart[841] recommend closed reduction of the dislocation and x-ray evaluation of the reduction of the femoral head fracture. If the fracture reduces, 6 weeks of traction followed by protective weight bearing is recommended.[739,841] Surgical excision of the fragments is reserved for cases in which closed reduction of the dislocation is unsuccessful (often because the femoral head fragment obstructs reduction)[866] or when there is incongruous reduction of the femoral head fracture.

Stewart[841] believes that internal fixation of the femoral head fracture in type I injuries is unnecessary, since excision of the fragment produces a functional hip. Primary excision of the femoral head fragment and open reduction of the hip have been recommended by Epstein.[730] Gordon and Freiberg[739] recommended excision of the fragment following closed reduction. After excision of this small fragment, the cephalad half of the femoral head usually retains congruity with the acetabulum.[841] However, Kelly and Yarbrough[762] found that those fractures treated by excision did not fare as well as those treated by simple closed reduction.

Type II injuries have been treated in several ways. Pipkin[811] and Kelly and Yarbrough[762] found

that those patients with type II injuries who satisfied criteria for closed treatment had a higher incidence of good results. Butler also recommends primary closed reduction.[697] If this results in a congruous hip joint *and* femoral head fracture reduction, the patient is managed in traction. If the femoral head fracture reduction is not anatomical, he recommends open reduction and internal fixation of the fracture (Fig. 14-53). However, Dowd and Johnson[718] report the successful closed treatment of a type II fracture in spite of an incongruous fracture reduction (Fig. 14-54). Internal fixation of the fracture is also recommended by Sarmiento and Laird.[824] Epstein[730] recommends excision of the fragment if it is no larger than one third of the articular surface.

In type III fractures, there is an associated fracture of the femoral neck. This injury too often occurs at the time of manipulative reduction of type I or II injuries.[821,841] Two alternatives of treatment exist in these patients. The first is open reduction and internal fixation of the femoral neck fracture, followed by treatment of the femoral head fracture as in types I and II.[811] Alternatively, these can be treated by the primary insertion of an endoprosthesis[696,821] or other type arthroplasty.[748]

In type IV fractures, there is a femoral head fracture as in type I, II, or III, associated with an acetabular fracture.[811] The degree of acetabular damage in these patients is the determining factor in planning treatment and in prognosis.[821,841] A

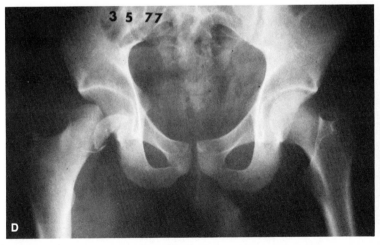

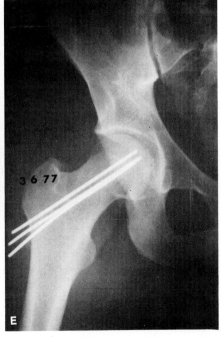

Fig. 14-53 (*Continued*). (*D*) Another case of the Pipkin type II fracture of the femoral head associated with posterior dislocation of the hip. (*E*) Open reduction *without* detaching the ligamentum teres from the femoral head fragment and internal fixation using Kirschner wires inserted through the lateral femoral shaft. This technique is used to preserve the blood supply in the ligamentum teres for the fragment.

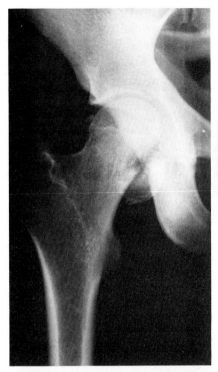

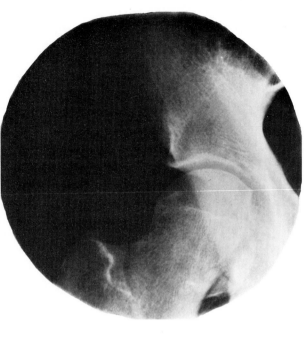

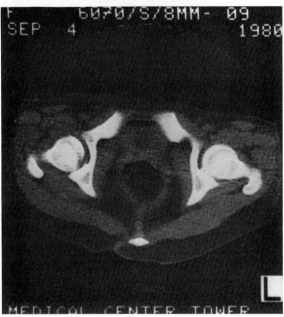

Fig. 14-54. (*Top left*) A Pipkin type I fracture of the femoral head associated with posterior dislocation of the hip. The patient was not a surgical candidate so the *displaced* femoral head fragment was left *in situ*. Polytomography (*top right*) and a CT scan (*bottom*) revealed a congruous reduction of the hip joint. There was full range of motion without crepitus. The fragment healed to the femoral neck, resulting in excellent hip motion and function.

small posterior acetabular fragment may contribute nothing more than a loose body requiring debridement, while a large displaced fracture of the acetabular dome predisposes to a poor result.[730,811,821,856] After selecting treatment for the acetabular fracture, the femoral head fracture is treated as in types I and II.[811,821,828,841]

AUTHOR'S PREFERRED METHOD OF TREATMENT TYPES I–V (THOMPSON AND EPSTEIN[835])

Our routine x-ray hip trauma series includes a single anteroposterior film of the pelvis, a slightly oblique lateral view, and the internal and external oblique views of Judet.[760] Good quality x-rays are essential prior to the initiation of treatment to recognize a nondisplaced femoral neck fracture or a femoral head fracture. These may not be seen on poor quality films. CT scans are used routinely prior to open reduction and in cases where intra-articular fragments are suspected in the joint following closed reduction.

Type I

In type I posterior dislocations I prefer closed reduction under general or spinal anesthesia. However, if evaluation of other injuries will significantly delay the closed reduction, manipulation is performed under intravenous analgesia in the emergency room.

I prefer the Stimson[845,846] maneuver if the patient does not have other injuries that preclude the use of the prone position for closed reduction. My second choice is the Allis[677] maneuver, which is useful in those patients who cannot assume the

prone position. The circumduction maneuver of Bigelow is used only rarely, and with great care owing to the stress it places on the proximal femur, particularly the femoral neck.

After reduction, light skin traction is applied for comfort, and early range of motion is instituted (Fig. 14-55). I agree with Stewart and colleagues[842] that muscle rehabilitation is essential following dislocation. Traction is maintained until the patient has a full active range of motion in the hip. This period of time has varied from 5 days to 2 weeks. The use of the skateboard is beneficial in obtaining full motion, especially abduction (Fig. 14-56). Weight bearing is resumed when comfortable. Prolonged protection from weight bearing, as has been recommended by some authors, is recommended only in those patients at high risk for aseptic necrosis. This group includes those patients in whom reduction is delayed beyond 12 hours after dislocation.

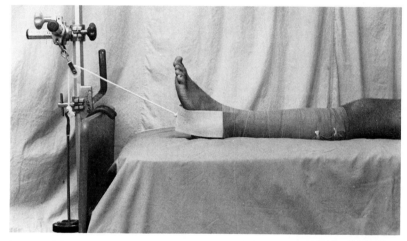

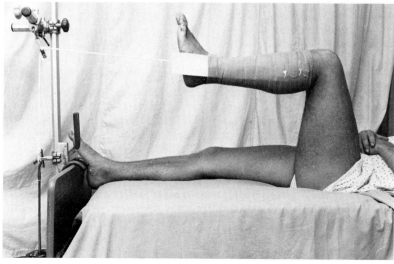

Fig. 14-55. Modified Apley's traction. This type of traction can be applied as skin or skeletal traction depending on hip stability. (*Top*) The thigh rests flat on the bed. (*Bottom*) Distal traction allows active hip and knee flexion.

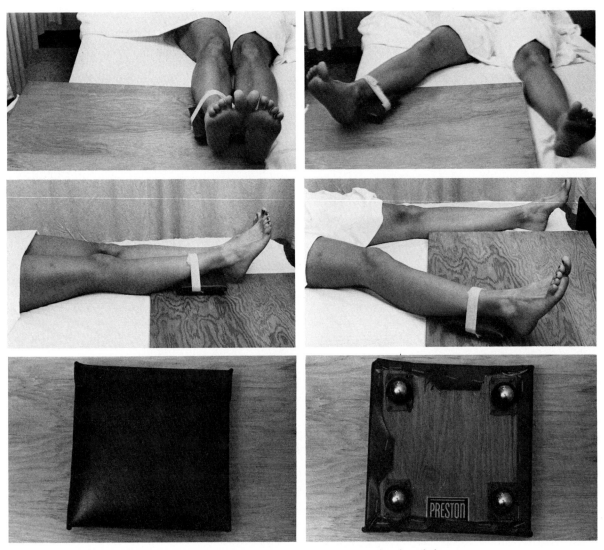

Fig. 14-56. A pad with rollers (skateboard) is applied to the patient's heel and then placed on a piece of plyboard on the patient's bed. This allows active abduction and adduction exercises of the hip. (*Top*) Abduction and adduction viewed from the front. (*Center*) Abduction and adduction viewed from the side. (*Bottom*) Superior and inferior view of the padded roller.

Delayed weight bearing in this group may prevent collapse of the avascular segment before treatment can be instituted.

Type II

In type II posterior fracture-dislocations in which there is a large posterior acetabular fragment significantly displaced, I prefer primary open reduction. The goal of primary open reduction is to restore joint congruity *and* stability just as one attempts in all other intra-articular fractures. Al-

though closed reduction has been reported to effect reduction of these fragments, my experiences have shown that a significant number of the posterior lip fragments remain displaced after the hip is relocated. It is for this reason that I do not do a primary closed reduction but proceed directly to an open reduction to prevent additional articular cartilage damage owing to repeated reduction and dislocation. Following open reduction, patients are managed in traction to encourage range of motion.

If the patient is not an operative candidate

because of other injuries, a closed reduction is performed and the patient is placed in skin traction until open reduction can be performed. If delayed open reduction cannot be performed in the first 2 weeks, the patient is treated in skeletal traction.* After closed reduction, the range of motion of the hip should be complete and without crepitus (which suggests trapped intra-articular fragments). If there is a question regarding the congruency of reduction or the presence of retained intra-articular fragments, a CT scan is obtained. Those patients with hips that are unstable at 70% to 90% of flexion and those with trapped intra-articular fragments warrant open reduction.

In all patients placed in traction, after either primary open reduction and internal fixation or closed reduction, the goal is to obtain a good range of motion of the hip and to restore muscle control. Initially, I use balanced suspension and convert this to Apley's (see Fig. 14-55) type traction after the first 3 to 5 days to maintain knee motion and restore hip extension. The skateboard is used to restore hip abduction and adduction (see Fig. 14-56). In those patients who have undergone *stable* internal fixation, skin traction is maintained until there is a full range of painless hip motion (usually 3 weeks). If internal fixation is not stable, or if the dislocation is treated closed, I maintain skeletal traction for 6 to 8 weeks, depending on the individual situation. Weight bearing is begun as tolerated after traction is discontinued, but not sooner than 6 weeks postreduction.

Type III

In type III posterior fracture-dislocations, the pre-reduction x-rays and CT scan are carefully scrutinized to determine whether or not the posterior rim fragments are large enough to permit stable internal fixation.

In those cases in which stable internal fixation is possible, I proceed to a primary open reduction. If the patient is not a good surgical risk or the posterior acetabular rim appears to be too comminuted, a simple closed reduction is performed. Following closed reduction, new x-rays of the hip are obtained to determine the presence or absence of retained bony fragments in the joint space. Open reduction is performed if closed reduction is unsuccessful, if the reduction is unstable, or if an incongruent reduction results.

After *stable* open reduction and internal fixation of type III injuries, the limb is placed in skeletal

traction until a full range of painless motion is obtained (usually 3 weeks). Weight bearing is progressed within the patient's tolerance, but, again, no sooner than 6 weeks postreduction to allow bony healing.

In patients treated nonoperatively or those in whom stable internal fixation is not obtained, traction is maintained for 6 to 8 weeks to allow adequate acetabular healing. If the reduction is unstable because of posterior comminution, a short leg cast with a posterior bar (Wilkie boot) to hold the limb in external rotation is used in conjunction with traction. Progressive weight bearing is begun after traction.

Type IV

In type IV fractures, primary closed reduction is performed, followed by careful x-ray evaluation of the associated acetabular fracture. The decision for open reduction of the acetabular fracture is based on the same principles delineated in the section on central fracture-dislocations of the acetabulum (see p. 1328). One *must* remember that fractures that communicate with the greater sciatic notch have the potential of damaging the superior gluteal artery. Life-threatening blood loss can occur once the tamponade effect of the fracture is removed at fracture reduction. If the artery retracts into the pelvis, an abdominal approach may be necessary to control the hemorrhage. Consideration of this potential complication must be given during draping of the patient (Fig. 14-57). After reduction, the limb is placed in skeletal traction for 6 to 12 weeks (depending on the acetabular fracture) with early range of motion.

Type V

My preferred treatment of Thompson-Epstein type V posterior fracture-dislocations of the hip will be discussed under each of the four subclassifications (I to IV) presented by Pipkin.[811]

Pipkin Type I. I prefer to perform a primary closed reduction. If the hip joint reduction is congruous and a full range of motion without crepitus is obtained, the limb is placed in skeletal traction for 6 weeks and managed as above. If the fragment blocks hip joint reduction or is in an unacceptable position after reduction, an arthrotomy is performed and the fragment is excised. Skin traction is used after arthrotomy until a full range of motion is obtained. I have found, however, that *anatomical* reduction of the femoral head fracture is not essential. If the head fragment does *not* interfere with

* Epstein, H.C.: Personal Communication, 1981.

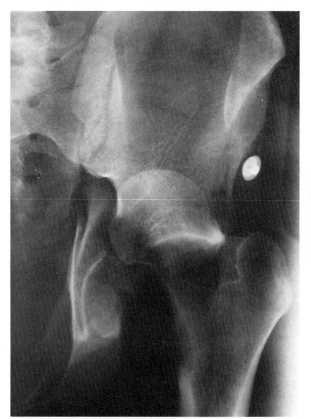

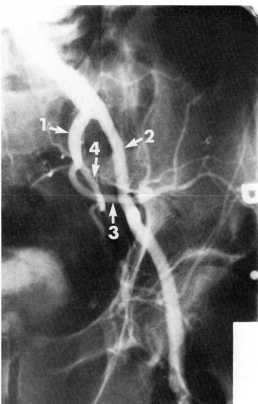

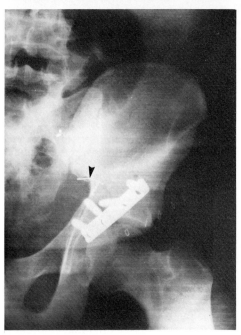

Fig. 14-57. (*Top left*) A transverse fracture of the acetabulum with posterior dislocation of the hip. Note that the fracture communicates with the greater sciatic notch, therefore placing the superior gluteal artery at risk to laceration. (*Top right*) An arteriogram of a normal pelvis demonstrating the proximity of the superior gluteal artery to the sciatic notch. (1, Hypogastric or internal iliac artery; 2, external iliac artery; 3, superior gluteal artery; 4, inferior gluteal artery) (*Bottom*) This x-ray was taken following open reduction and internal fixation in which a plate had been used to stabilize the transverse fracture. The superior gluteal artery was lacerated by the fracture fragment. Reduction of the fracture removed the tamponade effect of the displaced fragment, which resulted in profuse hemorrhage. The superior gluteal artery retracted into the pelvis and required an abdominal approach for control of the hemorrhage. Note the vascular clips used to control hemorrhage.

hip motion, good results can be obtained by leaving it in situ and instituting early motion[822] (see Fig. 14-54). I do not recommend this as a primary treatment modality but find it useful in the patient who is not a surgical candidate.

Pipkin Type II. A primary closed reduction is performed. Careful scrutiny of postreduction x-rays is made to determine the quality of reduction of both the joint *and* the femoral head fracture. If both reductions are adequate, the limb is placed in skeletal traction for 6 weeks.

If the femoral head fracture is not adequately reduced—that is, if there is articular surface incongruity (this may require polytomography or CT scanning for delineation)—an open reduction is performed. It must be emphasized that this can be a difficult surgical procedure often requiring two experienced hip surgeons. At surgery, the hip is redislocated, the joint is irrigated, and all loose fragments are removed. Initially, the large femoral head fragment is left attached to the ligamentum teres and gentle reduction of the hip is performed. The surgeon attempts to reduce the femoral head fracture as the hip is reduced. The reduction of the femoral head fracture is evaluated visually and by intraoperative x-ray. If the reduction is anatomical, the fracture is stabilized using Kirschner wires passed through the lateral femoral cortex (see Fig. 14-53 E). If the fracture reduction is not anatomical, the large fragment is detached from the ligamentum teres and is reattached to the femoral head, using countersunk screws as described by Sarmiento and Laird[824] (see Fig. 14-53). Maintaining the femoral head fragment attachment to the ligamentum teres may supply circulation for fracture healing.

Following open or closed reduction, the limb is placed in skeletal traction and begun on early range of motion for 3 to 6 weeks. Weight bearing as tolerated is instituted 6 weeks after reduction.

Pipkin Type III. I base my decision on the treatment of type III fractures primarily on the age of the patient. In elderly patients who are candidates for endoprosthetic replacement, endoprosthetic hemiarthroplasty is preferred. If the acetabular articular cartilage is damaged, total hip arthroplasty is considered in these elderly patients.

In the younger patient, due consideration is given to open reduction and internal fixation of the femoral neck fracture. The femoral head fracture is then treated by excision or internal fixation de-

pending on size. The addition of a posterior muscle pedicle graft may improve results, although I have little experience with it in these injuries. This approach will restore bone stock for later fusion if nonunion, aseptic necrosis, or arthritic changes of the femoral head occur. Alternatively, hemiarthroplasty or primary arthrodesis is considered.

Pipkin Type IV. I believe that the acetabular fracture dictates the treatment protocol in these patients. The acetabular fracture can vary from an insignificant fracture of the posterior acetabular lip requiring no treatment to displacement of the weight-bearing dome requiring operative reduction. After treatment of the acetabular component (in selected patients), the femoral head fracture is managed as mentioned under types I and II. In elderly patients, primary total hip arthroplasty is considered.

I must emphasize that in the management of posterior fracture-dislocations of the hip, conservative treatment should be used if (1) the patient is not a good surgical candidate, or (2) the surgeon is not certain of his ability to perform a *stable* internal fixation. Skeletal traction until soft-tissue and bone union occur coupled with early range of motion can produce acceptable results.

In my opinion, the only *absolute* indications for open reduction in these injuries are: (1) Irreducibility by closed methods; and (2) incongruity of the reduction due to retained bony fragments within the joint.

Relative indications for open reduction include: (1) sciatic nerve paralysis (persisting after closed reduction) with a displaced posterior acetabular fragment; and (2) joint instability following reduction (these can occasionally be managed in traction).

Following reduction of all posterior dislocations and fracture-dislocations of the hip, patients undergo x-ray examination and bone scans (cortical and medullary)[765,789] every 3 to 6 months for 2 years in an effort to diagnose aseptic necrosis so that treatment may be instituted before collapse occurs.

COMPLICATIONS

Early Complications

Sciatic Nerve Paresis. *Prereduction Paresis.* The sciatic nerve, most commonly the peroneal component,[842] is frequently injured in dislocations or fracture-dislocations about the hip.[728,754,756,806,843,849] Epstein[730] and Stewart and colleagues[842] note this complication in 8% to 19% of patients, being more common in fracture-dislocations (Thompson and Epstein types II to V). The injury is usually one of direct contusion, although partial laceration may occur.[723,788]

These nerve injuries must be recognized early. Nerve tissue does not tolerate pressure, and permanent ischemic changes soon occur.[832] For this reason, it is recommended that a posterior dislocation with neurological involvement be reduced as an *acute* surgical emergency. Pressure may be secondary to persistent dislocation of the femoral head or from a posterior acetabular fracture fragment following a posterior or central fracture-dislocation[767,796,816,843,866] (see Fig. 14-37). The nerve may be directly impaled by a small fragment of bone.[680,840] The posterior lip fragment may be displaced superiorly so that it presses against the sciatic nerve as far proximally as the sciatic notch (Fig. 14-58).

In those patients with simple dislocations, reduction of the dislocation removes all pressure on the nerve and recovery should then begin. These injuries usually represent a neurapraxia or axon-

otmesis, and surgical treatment of the nerve *per se* is not indicated.[832] However, those patients with a persistently displaced posterior lip fracture after reduction of the femoral head are a special group (Fig. 14-58). Open reduction and internal fixation of the displaced acetabular fragment are recommended in an effort to decompress the sciatic nerve.[749,767,788,796,816,857,866]

Postreduction Paresis. Occasionally, a patient with no initial neurologic involvement develops a deficit during the course of treatment. If this occurs immediately following closed reduction, surgical exploration is indicated to make certain that the nerve has not been trapped in the joint.

A postreduction paresis also can occur after unstable dislocations are reduced and subsequently redislocate, in patients with displaced acetabular fragments who are *not* surgical candidates, and in some patients secondary to scar formation during healing.[748] While ideally none of these situations should be allowed to occur, in practice it sometimes happens because concomitant injuries and the patient's general condition prevent surgical treatment. Under such circumstances the following should be

Prereduction   Postreduction

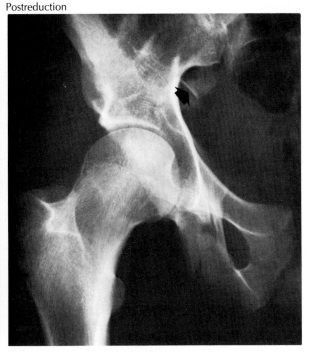

Fig. 14-58. (*Left*) A type IV posterior fracture-dislocation of the hip. The patient had a total sciatic nerve palsy. (*Right*) Following closed reduction, the posterior acetabular lip fragment remained in the sciatic notch, causing direct pressure on the sciatic nerve (*arrow*). Exploration of the nerve and removal of the fragment were performed.

noted: do not use a Thomas splint with the ring posteriorly (the ring acts to draw the sciatic nerve even tighter) and do not extend the knee on a flexed hip (this produces the sciatic stretch test). Most patients under such circumstances complain bitterly of pain and paresthesias in the leg prior to the onset of paralysis. If immediate reduction of the dislocation or fixation of displaced bone fragments is not feasible, the hip should be extended and the knee flexed in order to reduce the sciatic nerve stress.

Late sciatic nerve paralysis has also been reported secondary to ectopic bone formation.[715,749,754,766] Delayed neurolysis at 2 and 4 months[754] after injury has resulted in partial recovery.

In addition to sciatic nerve paralysis, Eisenberg and colleagues[723] reported avulsion of the S1 nerve root and formation of a meningocele after posterior dislocation of the hip. For this reason, a thorough neurological examination is essential to determine whether a sciatic nerve or nerve root lesion is present.

Rehabilitation After Sciatic Nerve Injury. A *well-padded* short leg plaster cast incorporating a tibial pin for traction maintains the foot in the best position and prevents pressure ulcers. Once pressure on the nerve has been relieved by open or closed methods, a treatment program is designed to avoid fixed deformity and ulceration. Passive dorsiflexion assists for the foot and ankle can be used on any traction apparatus. The toes and ankles should be moved passively through a full range of motion several times a day. Unusually severe pain associated with the nerve injury should suggest the possibility of causalgia, and treatment should be instituted quickly to prevent the disability that such problems produce.

As soon as the patient is allowed to be ambulatory, he should be fitted with a light toe-raising appliance and well-padded shoe, and encouraged to walk. Most of the unsatisfactory functional results following sciatic nerve injury are accompanied by fixed deformity and ulceration. Therefore, the best rehabilitation is one aimed at maintaining joint motion and restoring the patient to full ambulatory status as quickly as possible.

The use of electrical muscle stimulation has not proved to be of sufficient value to warrant the expense of the time and money associated with its routine use. The patient should be followed with periodic EMGs and physical examinations after the third week, and standard indications for nerve exploration based on the normal progression of nerve regeneration used. Most series report sub-

sequent functional recovery of the nerve in 60% to 70% of cases.[730,756,832,843,849]

In the case of permanent sciatic paralysis, a light toe-raising appliance can be sufficient for good function. In cases with common peroneal nerve paralysis only, transfer of the tibialis posterior tendon through the interosseous membrane without a triple arthrodesis (if foot and ankle motion are normal) can produce excellent function results. Care must be taken to balance the foot with regard to inversion and eversion.

Irreducible Posterior Dislocations. Three percent to sixteen percent of simple posterior dislocations of the hip require open reduction because of irreducibility.[691,756,807,816,835,849] Canale and Manugian[700] described two groups of irreducible traumatic dislocations of the hip. The first consisted of those dislocations that required open reduction because the hip could not be reduced by closed means. The cause was buttonholing of the femoral head through the hip capsule or interposition of the piriformis muscle between the femoral head and acetabulum, preventing reduction. Hunter also described a patient with the femoral head buttonholed through the posterior capsule,[756] and Slatis and Latvala[835] reported a case in which the piriformis muscle was obstructing the reduction. The second group consisted of patients in whom a reduction was obtained but the reduction was not concentric.[700] Patients with such nonconcentric reductions were more common than those with total obstruction to closed reduction. The obstructions to concentric reduction included presence of an inverted limbus or osteocartilaginous fragments in the joint. Dameron[709] and Paterson[804] both described a torn acetabular labrum that obstructed closed reduction. Even though the initial x-rays may not reveal any osteocartilaginous fragments, oftentimes these can be visualized by tomography, CT scans, or contrast arthrography.[700] The incidence of irreducibility is higher in fracture-dislocations compared to simple dislocations of the hip[835] owing to the presence of these obstructing osseous fragments.[705,730,835,838] Careful scrutiny for these occult osteocartilaginous fragments causing nonconcentric reductions accounted for the higher rate of irreducible dislocations in Canale and Manugian's series[700] (16%) as compared to most other series of simple dislocations, which are in the neighborhood of 3%.[691,756,816,849]

Most authors agree that, if closed reduction fails after at most two attempts under general anesthesia, the surgeon should proceed to an open reduction with the idea of removing the offending obstruction. If the closed reduction is incongruent, a second closed reduction under general anesthesia may be attempted. If the second reduction is incongruent, an open reduction in order to obtain congruency is indicated.[700]

Missed Knee Ligament Injuries. Owing to the fact that most posterior fracture-dislocations occur secondary to a blow on the anterior aspect of the knee, associated knee ligament injuries are common.[730,737,756] Gillespie found that 35 of 135 patients with posterior dislocations had significant associated knee injuries.[737] These injuries are seen in two groups of patients. One group has fractures involving the knee (patella, tibial or femoral condyles) or traumatic chondromalacia. The second group suffers injury to the collateral or cruciate ligaments secondary to varus/valgus or rotation forces being applied to the limb. In my experience, posterior cruciate ligament and posterolateral rotatory instabilities are more commonly associated with posterior hip dislocations. Evidence of a direct blow to the anterior aspect of the tibia should make one suspicious of such an injury. Early recognition and repair should minimize later disability.[730,737]

Recurrent Dislocation in Traction. Even those posterior dislocations or fracture-dislocations that are thought to be stable following reduction have been known to subluxate while being treated in traction.[741] Frequent x-rays demonstrating the relationship of the femoral head to the acetabulum (this may require a true lateral view) are necessary to be certain of the maintenance of reduction. This is particularly important in those patients who are in coma or who have associated injuries that do not allow adequate clinical evaluation of the hip joint.

Late Complications

Recurrent Posterior Dislocations. Recurrent posterior dislocation of the hip unassociated with paralysis, fracture, congenital acetabular dysplasia, or sepsis is very uncommon.[691,781,848] Liebenberg and Dommisse[776] demonstrated a defect and pouch in the posterior hip capsule in two locations following posterior dislocation. A capsular pouch was found between the piriformis and gemellus superior in one instance, and between the gemellus inferior and quadratus femoris in the other. Two theories regarding the etiology of recurrent dislocation have been presented. Liebenberg and Dommisse[776] postulated that a buildup of hydrostatic pressure in the joint cavity owing to a one-way valve in a posterior capsular defect forced the femoral head across the posterior rim and into a pseudocavity. The second theory is that a combination of factors is involved: repeated injury and a chronically intoxicated state,[848] a shallow acetabulum or deficient posterior rim,[852] and massive soft-tissue injury.[781]

Some authors suggest that inadequate immobilization is the etiology of recurrent dislocation.[691] Lutter[781] and Townsend,[852] however, believed that, although recurrent dislocation occurred in only 0.3% to 1.2% of cases, it was likely that greater than 1.2% of all dislocated hips could be classified as having been inadequately mobilized.[781] They believed, therefore, that recurrent dislocation was secondary to a number of factors.[781,848,852]

Treatment recommendations fall into two groups. The first group recommends capsular plication with or without muscle plication.[776,794,852] The second group recommends resection of the pseudocavity and insertion of a bone block at the posterior margin of the acetabular rim to act as a buttress.[848,852] The second alternative is most useful in cases with a deficient posterior acetabular rim.

Author's Preferred Method of Treatment. I have not found recurrent dislocation to be a common problem. Owing to the fact that I immobilize my patients only with traction and for very short periods of time, I do not believe that inadequate immobilization plays a major role in the etiology of recurrent dislocation.

My usual treatment of recurrent posterior dislocation is capsular and muscle plication, unless a posterior acetabular deficit is present that adds to the instability. If such a bony defect is present, a bone block is added. Postoperatively, a spica cast is used for 4 to 6 weeks to allow healing of the soft-tissue plication. Weight bearing is begun when leg control and hip motion have returned. If a bone graft is used, weight bearing is delayed until the bone graft shows evidence of incorporation.

Myositis Ossificans. The incidence of myositis ossificans is reported by Epstein[728,730] to be in the neighborhood of 2%. The occurrence is related to initial muscle damage and hematoma formation and seems to have no relation to when range of motion or weight bearing is begun following reduction.[730,847,188a,864,866] Epstein,[730] Rosenthal and Coker,[822] and Stewart and Milford[843] report an increased incidence of myositis ossificans following open reduction and internal fixation, especially if this is delayed. Gregory[741] and Proctor[816] also reported increased capsular calcification or ossification following surgically treated hip dislocations. This may be secondary to the second traumatic episode (the open reduction) following closed reduction.

Although restriction of motion is not common, cases have been reported in which there was extreme limitation of motion secondary to the myositis.[741] Gregory[741] was unable to find any method of accurately anticipating or preventing myositis ossificans. Therefore, if the initial trauma is severe (as noted by marked swelling, bruising), he recommended disturbing the fracture-dislocation surgically only if absolutely indicated.

Aseptic Necrosis. Aseptic necrosis of the femoral head following posterior dislocation of the hip is a well-recognized complication.[683,691,692,810,843,856] The incidence varies from 6%[678,854] to over 40%.[843] Stewart and Milford[843] noted a marked difference in the incidence of aseptic necrosis in those patients treated by closed (15.5%) and those treated by open reduction (40%). On the other hand, Epstein* has noted a decrease of aseptic necrosis in those patients treated by primary open reduction. It is possible that Stewart and Milford's patients had a higher incidence of aseptic necrosis because the operations were performed through an anterior approach.[843]

The etiology of aseptic necrosis is believed by most authors to be secondary to ischemia caused by damage to the vessels of the ligamentum teres and retinaculum of Weitbrecht.*[807,847,855,856] In addition, Stewart and Milford[843] suggested that the force and counterforce of initial trauma may produce a molecular change that may "precipitate intracellular crystallization sufficient to lead to avascular death of the bone." Epstein agrees with this concept and believes that both of these etiologies are likely contributors to aseptic necrosis.* Brav[691] and Proctor[816] both related the evidence of aseptic necrosis to the degree of initial trauma.

The incidence of aseptic necrosis has been directly related to the time the hip remains dislocated. Brav[691] noticed an increased incidence of aseptic necrosis when primary reduction was delayed longer than 12 hours after injury. A delay in reduction or repeated reductions were also found to be associated with an increased incidence of aseptic necrosis by Funsten,[734] Morton,[793] Nicoll,[798] and Stewart and Milford.[843] Only Paus[806] was unable to discover an increased incidence of aseptic necrosis in those

patients in whom reduction of the dislocation was delayed.

The effect of the time of initiation of weight bearing following reduction of a dislocation is controversial. Brav[691] found no relation between the incidence of aseptic necrosis and the time of initiation of weight bearing; however, he did note that the severity of avascular changes was decreased if weight bearing was delayed for 3 months. Ghormley and Sullivan[736] also recommended a 3-month delay. Stuck and Vaughan[847] believed that weight bearing delayed for 6 months was essential to allow restoration of blood supply and to decrease the risk of further vascular change. Banks[683] and Phemister[810] recommended delayed weight bearing to prevent collapse and to allow for surrounding bone atrophy to make the diagnosis of aseptic necrosis roentgenographically. The general consensus seems to be that delayed weight bearing has no real effect on the incidence of aseptic necrosis, although it may decrease the severity and degree of late collapse if aseptic necrosis does develop.

The time following dislocation when the diagnosis of aseptic necrosis is made is variable. Aseptic necrosis has been reported to occur 2 to 5 years after posterior dislocation of the hip.[812,840] Banks[683] noted that 3 to 4 months after dislocation were required before sufficient atrophy was present in surrounding bone to contrast living and dead bone on x-ray for the purpose of diagnosis. Patients should, therefore, be followed very carefully for a minimum of 2 years and probably longer with repeat x-rays and physical examinations to enhance early diagnosis. Recently, Meyers and associates[789] and Kirchner and Simon[765] reported the use of Technetium 99M-Sulfur colloid bone scanning to determine the vascularity of the femoral head. If accurate, this will allow much earlier diagnosis and treatment before collapse occurs.[789] Although the treatment of aseptic necrosis following dislocation varies from protected weight bearing[683] to bone grafting or other reconstructive procedures,[691,730,777] most authors agree that early diagnosis is essential for successful treatment. Discussion of the diagnosis and treatment alternatives of aseptic necrosis is found under the section on femoral neck fractures (see p. 1255).

Post-Traumatic Arthritis. The incidence of post-traumatic arthritis following posterior dislocation and fracture-dislocation of the hip is variable.[730,793,843,852,854,855,856] Epstein[730] emphasized difficulty in distinguishing aseptic necrosis and degenerative joint disease, especially when a single

---

* Epstein, H.C.: Personal communication, 1981.

x-ray is reviewed after injury. Stewart and Milford[843] reported a 48% incidence of degenerative joint disease after closed reduction and 71% after open reduction. These are the same figures they reported for aseptic necrosis and, indeed, they stated that the incidence of degenerative joint disease and aseptic necrosis are the same. Most authors, however, do not agree with this concept.[691,730,793,854]

The severity of the initial trauma is the major factor in determining the later development of post-traumatic arthritis.[691,776,793,844,849,854] Morton[793] noticed an increased incidence of post-traumatic arthritis following fracture-dislocations as compared to patients with simple dislocations. Epstein found that post-traumatic arthritis, not aseptic necrosis, was the major cause of fair or poor results.[730] He noted a 30% incidence of arthritis in fracture-dislocations (type II to V). Upadhyay and Moulton[854] recognized the direct relationship between the incidence of osteoarthritis and grade of initial trauma. The incidence of post-traumatic arthritis is increased in those patients with associated fractures of the acetabulum (type IV) and femoral head (type V), both of which are secondary to greater initial injury.[730,731] Epstein[730] recommends primary open reduction of posterior fracture-dislocations to reduce the incidence of post-traumatic arthritis by removing bony fragments, restoring stability of the joint, and ensuring accurate reduction. He noted that the incidence of post-traumatic arthritis dropped to 17% in patients who underwent primary open reduction. The treatment of established arthritis is beyond the scope of this chapter.

PROGNOSIS

Urist[855,856] was the first to determine that the overall prognosis following fracture-dislocation or simple dislocation of the hip was directly related to the initial trauma. Most authors since that time have agreed that the severity of initial trauma is the single most important factor in determing long-term prognosis.[690,730,842,849,854] Other factors known to be significant include delay between dislocation and reduction,[822] repeated unsuccessful attempts at reduction,[842] and associated injuries.[842]

UNREDUCED POSTERIOR FRACTURE-DISLOCATIONS OF THE HIP—LATE DIAGNOSIS

Several factors can be responsible for failure to diagnose a posterior dislocation or fracture-dislocation of the hip: (1) failure to examine the hip clinically and radiographically at the time of initial injury;[710,735] (2) a fracture-dislocation, present at the moment of injury, which was unknowingly reduced by ambulance attendants and later resubluxates while the patient is being treated for other injuries,[830,864] and finally (3) a fracture of the ipsilateral femur or a dislocation or fracture of the opposite hip that diverts attention from the presence of the hip dislocation.[691,712,714,750,755]

Any delay in diagnosis and reduction increases the risk of aseptic necrosis and degenerative arthritis and often leads to ankylosis.[694,712,729,751,843] Closed reduction has been advocated as the treatment of choice during the first 3 weeks after dislocation,[735] and indeed Huckstep[755] reported a successful closed reduction 16 months after injury. Garrett and co-workers,[735] however, found no good results in hips reduced 3 days to 3 months after dislocation because of the development of aseptic necrosis. Reduction by heavy traction followed by hip abduction was found to be successful in reducing these old dislocations by Gupta and Shravat[743] without evidence of aseptic necrosis. Although closed reduction may be successful up to 3 months, fibrous tissue begins to fill the acetabulum as early as 3½ weeks following dislocation.[694,735]

Buchanan,[694] in 1920, reported a case in which the hip was reduced surgically 6 months after injury with a good result. He also reviewed the 45 cases that had been reported prior to 1920 in which 80% reported good results. Nixon[800] also reported good results in three cases treated by open reduction 4 weeks or longer after dislocation. Garrett and co-workers[735] recommended that young patients with Thompson-Epstein type I, type II, or type III hip dislocations undergo an attempted closed reduction, even though there is a high risk of aseptic necrosis. Additionally, a young patient with a type II or II fracture-dislocation of less than 3 months' duration should undergo an open reduction, removal of bone fragments, and internal fixation of the acetabular lip fracture.[735] These authors report uniformly poor results in type IV or type V fracture-dislocations and in dislocations greater than 3 months old. Primary reconstruction is recommended in these patients.

Letournel[773] reported that two thirds of the patients who underwent a delayed open reduction and internal fixation of a posterior fracture-dislocation of the hip (over 3 weeks old) developed aseptic necrosis and all patients after 160 days after fracture-dislocation developed this complication.

In addition to reduction, either open or closed, subtrochanteric osteotomy,[755] Girdlestone procedure,[755] arthrodesis,[735] endoprosthetic replacement,[735] cup arthroplasty,[791] and total hip replacement have been recommended in these patients.[735]

Author's Preferred Method of Treatment

Treatment of patients presenting with the missed diagnosis of a posterior fracture-dislocation of the hip must be individualized. Up to 3 weeks, post-injury, closed reduction is attempted. If this fails, open reduction is performed.

In dislocations more than 3 weeks old, young patients with type II and type III dislocations (if the acetabular rim can be stabilized) are treated by open reduction of the hip and internal fixation of the acetabular rim. Patients with type IV and V dislocations and young patients with type II and III dislocations over 3 months old are treated by primary reconstructive procedures, depending on the patient's age, activity, and so forth. In some patients open reduction of the acetabular rim may be a prerequisite to giving adequate bony stock for later total hip replacement.

DISLOCATIONS AND FRACTURE-DISLOCATIONS OF
THE HIP ASSOCIATED WITH FRACTURES OF THE
FEMORAL SHAFT

Fractures of the shaft of the femur associated with anterior (Fig. 14–59),[714,828] posterior (Fig. 14-60),[849] and central fracture-dislocations (Fig. 14-61) of the hip are being reported with increasing frequency.[712,721,750,753,756,782,787,828,861,864] This combination of injuries was first reported in 1823 by Sir Astley Cooper, who recommended reduction of the hip after the femoral shaft fracture had healed.[706] Helal and Skevis[750] speculated that this injury is the result of two forces: the hip joint is dislocated by axial impaction and the femoral shaft fracture occurs after a direct blow to the thigh.

The key to fractures of the femur associated with hip dislocations and fracture-dislocations is recognition of the dislocation. Because of the femur fracture, the clinical deformity of the lower extremity usually associated with dislocations of the hip is absent.[828] Helal and Skevis[750] emphasized the incidence of unrecognized hip fracture-dislocations in patients with femoral shaft fractures, noting that in more than 50% of reported cases the hip dislocation was initially missed. A delay in diagnosis will decrease the chances of a successful closed reduction and increase the risk of aseptic necrosis.[712,721,828] This is the major reason pelvic x-rays are *mandatory* in all patients with major trauma.[710,828] A dislocation of the hip should be suspected if the x-ray of the femoral fracture reveals the proximal femoral fragment in a fixed abducted (anterior hip dislocation) (see Fig. 14-59) or adducted (posterior hip dislocation) position[864] (see Fig. 14-60).

Once the diagnosis is made, preference in treatment should be given to immediate reduction of the hip in an effort to decrease the incidence of

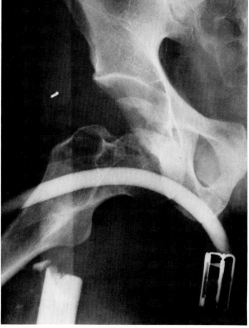

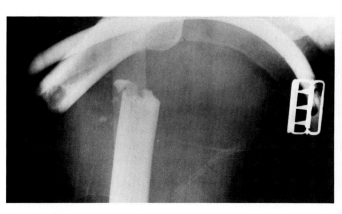

Fig. 14-59. Anterior dislocation of the hip with an associated fractured femoral shaft. (*Left*) The abducted proximal femoral fragment suggests an anterior dislocation of the hip. (*Right*) An x-ray of the hip confirms the anterior dislocation. (Note the fracture of the femoral head.)

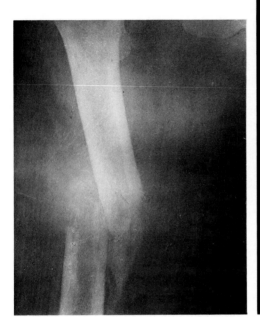
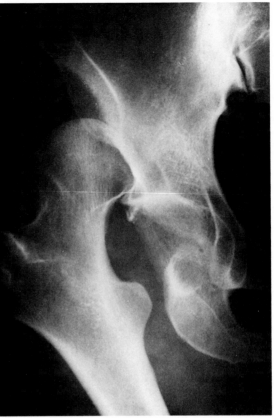

Fig. 14-60. Posterior dislocation of the hip with an associated fractured femoral shaft. (*Left*) The adducted proximal fragment in this healing femoral shaft fracture suggests a posterior dislocation of the hip. (*Right*) An x-ray of the hip confirms the posterior dislocation, which was initially missed.

aseptic necrosis, which is known to be increased with delay in reduction.[712,721,787] Also, Schoenecker and associates[828] believe that the shorter the interval between the dislocation and time of reduction, the greater the chances of a successful closed reduction of the hip dislocation in these cases.

Difficulty in closed reduction of the hip is secondary to the fact that the long lever arm generally used for closed reduction (the femur) is shortened by the fracture. Therefore, one has little control over the proximal fragment for manipulation. Manipulation may, therefore, cause angulation and distraction of the soft parts at the site of the fracture of the femur leading to increased soft-tissue damage. In spite of this, Watson-Jones[862] believed that a gentle Stimson type of closed reduction could be attempted without significant damage at the fracture site. Schoenecher and associates[828] reported successful closed reduction of the hip by gentle

manual traction on the proximal thigh with the hip and knee flexed 90° and countertraction of the pelvis.

Several techniques have been introduced in which a pointed awl,[684] screws,[782] or Steinmann pins[757,867] are used as a means of gaining control of the proximal fragment. After this is done, the proximal fragment can be manipulated and the hip reduced. Following hip reduction, the femoral fracture can be treated by delayed intramedullary nailing[769] or by traction followed by casting.

If the hip is irreducible by closed means, or if, once reduced, it is unstable because of a displaced acetabular or femoral head fragment, open reduction of the dislocation of the hip and internal fixation of the associated fractures are recommended.[712,828] Following this, the fracture of the shaft of the femur can be treated by traction or internal fixation.[828] Primary open reduction of the

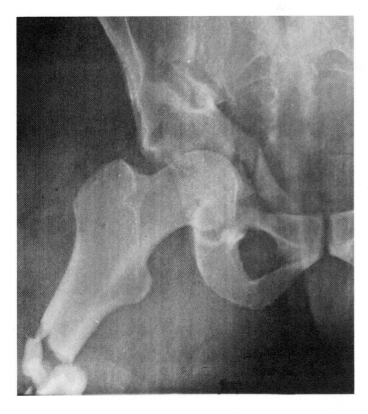

Fig. 14-61. A central fracture-dislocation of the hip with an associated femoral shaft fracture.

dislocated hip and internal fixation of the femoral shaft was recommended by Ehtisham.[721]

Author's Preferred Method of Treatment

Many of these patients have suffered multisystem injury and a major primary orthopaedic procedure is often not possible. In these instances, I first attempt a gentle closed reduction by the Stimson maneuver without rotation of the thigh. If this is unsuccessful, a Steinmann pin is inserted into the proximal femur for manipulation.

If the dislocation is irreducible or unstable, and the patient is a candidate for surgery, open reduction with internal fixation of the acetabular fragments is performed. Treatment of the femoral shaft fracture is dependent on its location and comminution and the patient's condition. If stable internal fixation is possible and the patient is a good surgical candidate, simultaneous intramedullary nailing is performed.

CENTRAL ACETABULAR FRACTURES AND FRACTURE-DISLOCATIONS

Central fracture-dislocations of the acetabulum are occurring with increasing frequency secondary to an increased number of motor vehicle acci-

dents.[760,796] Although Elliott[724] found fracture-dislocations more common in young and middle-aged patients while older patients suffered femoral neck fractures, central acetabular fractures occur in all adult age groups.[722,767,823]

Central fracture-dislocations of the hip are usually the result of a blow to the lateral aspect of the trochanter with the femoral head transmitting the force into the acetabulum.[701,722,779,823,857] Judet[760] mentioned that rarely the femoral head acts as an anvil on which the acetabulum is broken by a violent blow from behind. These fractures can also occur secondary to a force acting along the longitudinal axis of the femur with the hip in abduction. The head of the femur is not a perfect sphere, nor is the acetabulum its perfect match, except in the weight-bearing position. Therefore, forces acting through the femur are concentrated instead of being dispersed equally about the femoral head. The direction, magnitude, and point of application of such force determines the exact pattern of fracture.[760]

In addition to such violent traumatic etiologies, central fracture-dislocation of the hip has been reported secondary to epileptic seizure and electroconvulsive therapy.[792,807]

Associated skeletal[807] and life-threatening

visceral[695,701,710,779,796,807] injuries are common in patients with central fracture-dislocations of the hip because of the severity of the initial trauma (see Fig. 14-61). These injuries may direct attention away from the central fracture-dislocation of the hip and result in its being missed.

CLINICAL DIAGNOSIS

There is usually slight shortening of the involved limb, and severe pain and muscle spasm with attempted motion of the hip.[807] There may be a bruise over the greater trochanter.[807] It is difficult to determine clinically whether or not the femoral head is centrally dislocated into the pelvis or whether a nondisplaced central fracture of the acetabulum is present.[807] Neurologic examination of the involved limb for possible sciatic nerve injury is a requisite. Careful evaluation for other injuries involving the musculoskeletal system, head, chest, and abdomen is essential because of their frequent association.[796,807]

The acetabulum consists largely of cancellous bone, and hemorrhage into these fracture sites may be severe, requiring large quantities of blood to maintain adequate systemic blood volume. The use of 6 to 12 units is not uncommon for a fracture that involves a considerable portion of the pelvis. The extent of hemorrhage and soft-tissue damage can usually be assessed by soft-tissue films of the pelvis. Occasionally, an intravenous pyelogram is helpful because, in patients with considerable hemorrhage, the bladder will be displaced by the hematoma superiorly and toward the opposite side of the pelvis.[796]

RADIOGRAPHIC DIAGNOSIS

Adequate x-ray evaluation of the fracture site is essential. An anteroposterior x-ray of the pelvis will often demonstrate the gross disruption of the femoral head-acetabular relationship. However, internal and external oblique views (see Chapter 13) are essential in delineating fracture lines and displacement. Pearson and Hargadon[807] and Rowe and Lowell[823] noted that up to one third of patients with fractures of the pelvis have acetabular involvement that is not readily apparent from x-ray. Such acetabular involvement is assumed to be present if there are fractures of the superior and inferior pubic rami.[807] Additionally, polytomography,[758] stereo views,[767] and CT scans[833] may be required to delineate fracture lines and displacement for the purpose of treatment.

Although routine x-rays do not demonstrate femoral head injury,[724] there may be cartilaginous damage to the head, or the impact may result in an intracellular molecular change as suggested by Stewart and Milford.[843] Since associated femoral head injury has been related to a poor result,[724] efforts to delineate this damage should be pursued for purposes of prognosis.

TREATMENT

The treatment dilemma facing the orthopaedist dealing with central fracture-dislocations of the acetabulum is that of surgical or nonsurgical treatment. This dilemma is made difficult by the fact that the clinical examination and functional result often do not parallel the radiographic appearance.[740,796,823,843]

The goals of treatment of central fracture-dislocations of the acetabulum are to[684,796,851,868] (1) restore the femoral head-acetabular relationship by reduction of the femoral head; (2) restore stability to the joint; (3) reestablish the joint surfaces; (4) institute early range of motion so as to "round off the fracture fragments."

While attempting to attain these goals, the fracture surgeon must constantly be reminded that even though x-ray appearance may be poor, the patient may demonstrate good hip function with few limitations.[823]

Acute Central Fracture Dislocations of the Acetabulum

Acute central fracture dislocations of the acetabulum can be treated by one of three methods:

1. Traction with or without closed reduction of the femoral head.
2. Open reduction and internal fixation.
3. Primary arthroplasty or arthrodesis.

Traction With or Without Closed Reduction. The nonsurgical treatment of acetabular fractures has many proponents.[682,684,710,722,740,786,796,819,851] Although Levine[774] and Maynard[786] recognized the importance of ligamentous and capsular attachments in manipulative closed reduction or traction to improve fracture alignment, Elliott pointed out that, because of a lack of these specific capsular attachments to the inner wall fragment, open reduction may be necessary to effect reduction of that fragment.[724]

Nonsurgical treatment includes reduction of the femoral head-acetabular relationship followed by traction to maintain this reduction and enable early range of motion.[684,796,868] Reduction of the femoral head under the acetabular dome can be accomplished in two ways. The first is by gentle manipulation under general anesthesia. If such reduction is to be attempted, it should be done in the first 48 to 72 hours before internal hemorrhage begins to clot and the possibility of obtaining reduction decreases. Whitman proposed reduction by longitudinal traction and hip abduction to restore the femoral head beneath the acetabulum.[865] Rowe and Lowell[823] presented two maneuvers for reduction. One is for the patient with a central dislocation of the femoral head, a displaced inner wall fracture, and an *intact* acetabular dome. Longitudinal traction is applied to the limb, followed by hip adduction over a bolster located between the thighs.[779] The second maneuver described by Rowe and Lowell is for bursting-type fractures of the acetabulum.[823] Traction is applied to the injured limb with a Kirschner wire inserted in the proximal tibia. Lateral traction is applied through a swath in the groin held by an assistant. The maneuver begins with the leg in full extension and internal rotation. This is followed by flexion, abduction, and finally circumduction of the leg around to a neutral position while strong lateral traction is maintained. This maneuver places tension sequentially on the anterior, medial, posterior, and finally lateral portions of the hip capsule. The tension on these capsular attachments to the acetabulum results in reduction. Attempted manipulative reduction by the finger inserted in the rectum is mentioned only to be condemned.[724,857]

The second means of obtaining reduction is that of longitudinal or lateral traction.[722,817,818,850,851,857] When longitudinal skeletal traction is to be used for reduction, pins may be placed in distal femur or the tibia, depending on associated injuries.[722,857] Initial weight of 20% of the body is used and is increased in small increments with serial x-rays every 2 hours until reduction is achieved. If reduction is not obtained within the first 24 hours, this method is usually unsuccessful and is not pursued further.

Lipscomb,[777] MacGuire,[784] and Watson[861] advocated the use of crossed wires or screws in the femoral neck and head in addition to longitudinal traction to achieve reduction by providing a *direct* lateral pull (Fig. 14-62). In these techniques the crossed wires and screws should not be left in place longer than absolutely necessary because motion and fat necrosis may lead to pin tract sepsis.

Once the femoral head is reduced beneath a congruous acetabular dome, the position must be maintained by longitudinal traction of 5% to 10% of body weight. Concomitant lateral traction is used if necessary to maintain reduction.[817] Early range

of motion is instituted while in traction.[843] The use of spica cast immobilization following closed reduction, which was introduced by early investigators, is to be condemned.[808,834,865] Most authors agree with Rowe and Lowell[823] that the prognosis depends on the condition of the acetabulum.[740,807,868] Irregularities in the inner wall can frequently be ignored and have little effect on the outcome.[779,823,868] However, traction must be maintained until there is an opportunity for the space on the inner aspect of the acetabulum to fill with mature tissue and fibrocartilage. This requires a minimum of 8 to 12 weeks in traction, followed by protected weight bearing for an additional 3 to 6 months.[771,842,850,851]

Open Reduction and Internal Fixation. Levine reported successful open reduction and internal fixation of a central fracture of the acetabulum in 1943.[774] Okelberry[801] and Pennal[809] reported good short-term results in selected cases of central acetabular fractures. Knight and Smith[767] recommended limited open reduction and internal fixation for certain acetabular fractures, based on the theory that the more perfect reconstruction of the acetabular femoral relationship, the better the results. Their main goal was to restore the weight-bearing dome. They recommended primary closed reduction with a delay of open reduction and internal fixation for 4 to 5 days to allow the patient to stabilize. Their most important contribution was stressing the need for three-dimensional thinking in evaluating these fractures prior to surgical treatment.

Carnesale and associates[701] offered specific indications for open reduction and internal fixation of central fracture-dislocations of the acetabulum: (1) intra-articular fragments that remain displaced; and (2) inability to reduce the acetabular-femoral head relationship. Eichenholtz and Stark[722] added to this list of indications cases in which impingement of the femoral head against the sharp corner of the acetabulum persists despite attempts at reduction by closed means or traction.

D'Aubigne,[710] Judet and associates[760] and Letournel[773] have recommended open reduction and internal fixation of all *displaced* acetabular fractures, based on the theory that the poor results of nonoperative treatment were not secondary to the inability to reduce the femoral head but rather to the inability to reduce the acetabular fracture components. Judet and associates[760] divided acetabular fractures into four elementary fracture patterns and introduced the use of the ¾ internal and ¾ external

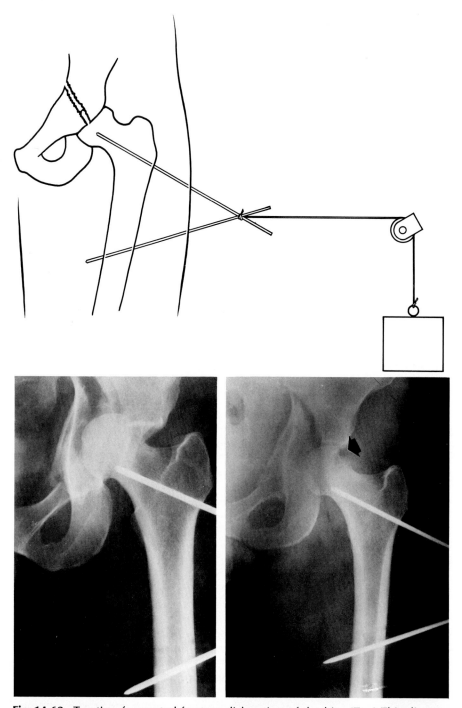

Fig. 14-62. Traction for central fracture-dislocation of the hip. (*Top*) This diagram demonstrates the position of the two Steinmann pins, and the connection to a lateral weight for traction. (*Bottom left*) Steinmann pins were inserted with no lateral traction. (*Bottom right*) Lateral traction applied. Note that the femoral head is now reduced beneath the acetabular dome. The *arrow* denotes an indentation fracture of the femoral head.

oblique x-rays to evaluate various fracture components (see Figs. 13-12 and 13-13). Although the concept of open reduction of all displaced acetabular fractures is not supported by most authors, the method of evaluation and classification of fracture patterns outlined by Judet and associates[760] is essential in planning open reduction and internal fixation of these fractures.

While open reduction and internal fixation of displaced acetabular fractures is *theoretically* sound and should produce the best results, the operative risks and complications are substantial.[760,796] In considering open reduction and internal fixation, four criteria must be met:

1. The patient's condition will permit the extensive surgical procedure required for open reduction and internal fixation of acetabular fractures.
2. The patient's age *and* activity level warrant open reduction of the acetabular fracture and its inherent risks.
3. The fracture fragments that remain displaced must be large enough to ensure a stable internal fixation.
4. The surgeon *must* be experienced in the operative treatment of these fractures.

Primary Arthroplasty   The dismal results from closed treatment of certain central fracture-dislocations of the acetabulum have led some authors to recommended primary arthroplasty[863] or arthrodesis[680] in these injuries. In most series, the number of patients undergoing primary arthroplasty or arthrodesis is too small to formulate definite indications for the use of these procedures.[680,722,740,771,779,863] According to Lowell, inability to restore joint stability or the femoral-head-acetabular relationship are indications for primary arthroplasty.[779] Larson[771] believed that primary reconstruction was *never* a substitute for reduction of the fracture-dislocation and was indicated only when closed reduction failed and open reduction revealed severe articular damage.

COMPLICATIONS

Early Complications

Sciatic Nerve Paresis.   Patterson and Morton[805] emphasized that these neurologic complications are frequently missed and poorly recorded. The injuries are more common when the central acetabular fracture or fracture-dislocation is associated with fractures of the pubic rami anteriorly or the sacrum or ilium posteriorly.[805]

The incidence of associated sciatic nerve palsy is variable and is more common in burst-type fractures as opposed to inner-wall fractures.[779] Although sciatic palsy usually occurs at the time of injury, it has been reported to occur late, either after closed reduction or after the institution of traction.[779] Treatment recommendations include early reduction of the fracture fragments (by closed or open means) to prevent pressure necrosis of the nerve.[796] Where no fracture fragments are impinging on the nerve, careful observation is indicated.[805] Specific treatment recommendations are given in the section on posterior fracture-dislocations with sciatic palsy.

Superior Gluteal Artery Injury.   Anatomically, the main trunk of the superior gluteal artery or one of its major branches may be trapped in fractures communicating with the greater sciatic notch (see Fig. 14-57). Therefore, great care must be exercised in the open treatment of these fractures to prevent iatrogenic injury to this major arterial trunk. Inadvertent laceration and retraction of this artery into the pelvis may necessitate an abdominal approach to control hemorrhage.

Bowel Obstruction.   The symptoms of bowel obstruction after central fracture-dislocation of the acetabulum are most often due to ileus.[695] However, true mechanical obstruction secondary to entrapment in the acetabular fracture fragments has been reported by Derian and Purser,[716] Lunt,[780] and Poilly and Hamilton.[812] These obstructions can occur both acutely and after the institution of traction for treatment.

Thrombobophlebitis.   Patients with acetabular fractures are at a high risk of phebitis.[779] Most surgeons now use an anticoagulation program usually initiated when fracture bleeding has been controlled after 48 to 72 hours.[779] The exact therapeutic regimen is open to question, each author having his own preference.[793,823]

Infection.   Infection of the fracture site after open reduction and internal fixation was reported by Carnesale and associates to occur in 36% of cases done prior to 1970.[701] However, D'Aubigne[710] and Rowe and Lowell[823] report infection rates in the neighborhood of 6%. One must remember that such an infection may prohibit later total joint arthroplasty.

Pin Tract Infection. Pin tract infections, especially those associated with lateral pin sites, have been reported with increasing frequency.[851] A pin tract infection in the greater trochanteric area may lead to osteomyelitis, which could prevent later reconstructive procedures. For this reason, lateral traction should be used for as short a perioid as possible in an effort to decrease the risk of infection.

Recurrent Central Dislocation. Recurrent displacement of the femoral head into the acetabulum because of too short a period of traction has been reported by Judet and associates[760] and Tipton and associates.[851] Judet[760] warns that even nondisplaced fractures may displace if weight bearing is instituted too early. For this reason, he recommends non-weight bearing on crutches for 6 weeks in nondisplaced fractures (Fig. 14-63).

Recommendations for the duration of time in traction are variable in *displaced* fracture dislocations. Tipton and associates[850,851] recommended 12 weeks of traction to allow a new acetabulum ("pseudoacetabulum") to form. They believed that traction must be maintained until there is cancellous bone healing and time for acetabular defects to fill with mature granulation tissue and fibrocartilage so as to prevent later redislocation. This period of traction is followed by protection from weight bearing from 3 to 6 months after fracture.

Myositis Ossificans. MyosItis ossificans is reported to occur in 5% of patients undergoing closed treatment[779,823,843] and in up to 34% of those treated with open reduction.[710,760,823] The significance of myositis ossificans as it relates to function, has been questioned by several authors.[710,760] Delayed open reduction has been associated with an increased incidence of myositis.[741]

Late Complications

Post-traumatic Arthritis and Aseptic Necrosis. Difficulty in accurately separating post-traumatic arthritis and aseptic necrosis has led some authors to consider them together as causes of poor results.[796,818,857] Rowe and Lowell[823] reported these conditions in 26% of their patients, half with primarily post-traumatic arthritis and half with aseptic necrosis. Stewart and Milford[843] and Elliott[724] contend that aseptic necrosis is related to the degree of initial trauma, which causes damage to the capsular vessels, thrombosis of the intramedullary vessels, and intracellular molecular change.

Most series also document a direct relationship between the incidence of post-traumatic arthritis and the severity of the initial damage.[682,722,724,807]

Post-traumatic arthritis is the major cause of poor results. Undisplaced and inner-wall fractures in which the femoral head-acetabular relationship has been restored produce good results in 75% to 80% of cases.[682,722,740,796,823,857] On the other hand, fractures involving the dome of the acetabulum and those in which the anatomical relationship between the femoral head and acetabulum were not restored have produced good results in only 25% to 40% of patients.[682,684,722,779,796] Both Stewart and Milford[843] and Rowe and Lowell[823] demonstrated the uniformly poor results in patients with associated femoral head damage.

Nonunion. Nonunion of central fracture dislocations of the acetabulum is usually seen in untreated fractures or those in whom reduction was not obtained.[707,773] Nonunion may be a cause of pain and should be treated to improve acetabular bone stock before total hip arthroplasty.[707]

DELAYED DIAGNOSIS OF CENTRAL FRACTURE-DISLOCATIONS OF THE ACETABULUM

Central fracture-dislocations of the acetabulum that are diagnosed late present great difficulty in management. Letournel[773] found that after 3 weeks, treatment was difficult secondary to the callus already present about the fracture fragments. His indication for open reduction and internal fixation of delayed diagnosed injuries was an incongruent femoral head and acetabulum. The three prerequisites for delayed open reduction and internal fixation of these injuries are: (1) a normal femoral head; (2) no arthritis present in the hip; and (3) an x-ray demonstrating fracture lines and fragments that can be easily recognized. The goals of delayed open reduction are to restore bone stock to facilitate subsequent total hip replacement, as well as to defer this type of reconstruction in those patients who obtain good clinical results following open reduction. If the displaced acetabular fragments remain in contact with the subluxated femoral head, forming a "neo-congruence," conservative treatment is indicated.

Coventry[707] recommended open reduction and internal fixation of subacute and chronic displaced acetabular fractures as a prerequisite for restoring bony stock for total hip replacement. He also recommended open reduction and internal fixation in *acute* fracture-dislocations in whom the predictable outcome is pain and disability so that total hip

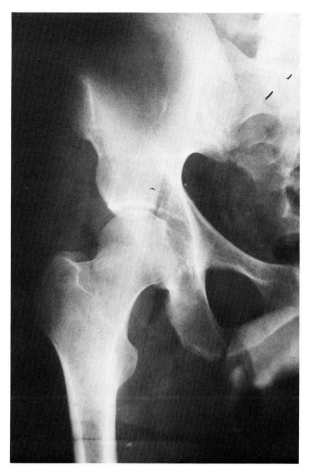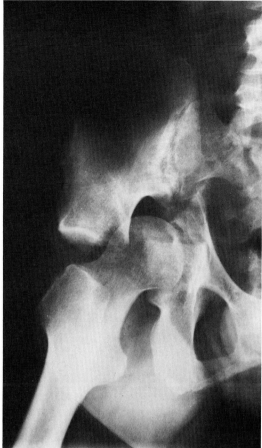

Fig. 14-63. (*Left*) Initial x-ray of a central fracture of the acetabulum. Due to lack of displacement the patient was allowed to bear full weight 2 weeks postinjury. (*Right*) Central displacement of the femoral head 3 weeks postinjury when the patient was full weight bearing on the limb.

arthroplasty will be simpler. Great care and surgical expertise are needed to attempt open reduction in these patients with delayed diagnosis.[773] Although the rationale of restoring anatomy for future reconstruction is sound, one must recall the possibility of postoperative sepsis, which may itself prevent future reconstruction.[701]

AUTHOR'S PREFERRED METHOD OF TREATMENT

I agree in principle with the concept of anatomical restoration of joint surfaces to prevent long-term disability from intra-articular fractures. However, the surgical treatment of central fracture dislocations of the hip is technically demanding and the potential complications substantial.

Although the recommendation of Carnesale and associates[701] to use the "simplest method" that produces the best result seems simplistic, I strive to follow this dictum in the management of central fracture-dislocations of the acetabulum.

Complete clinical evaluation of the patient *and* characteristics of the fracture by routine x-rays, internal and external oblique views, and CT scans are used before a treatment regimen is instituted. In these particular injuries, the ability to define those fractures that require open reduction for good long-term results requires excellent judgment.[722] Associated injuries of the head, chest, abdomen, or other musculoskeletal injuries may limit or compromise the treatment of the acetabular fracture.[710] Although the surgeon should try to avoid such a compromise in treatment, he must remember that a functional hip is oftentimes obtained even though the x-ray reduction is not perfect.

The discussion of treatment of central acetabular fracture and fracture-dislocation will follow the classification of these injuries first introduced by Rowe and Lowell[823] and modified by Lowell.[779]

Undisplaced Fractures

Patients with nondisplaced fractures are treated at bed rest until a satisfactory range of motion in the hip is restored. Following this, non-weight bearing on crutches is continued for a period of 6 to 8 weeks.[823] Weight bearing too soon can result in displacement of fractures that were initially believed to be undisplaced (see Fig. 14-63)

Inner-Wall Fractures

In the management of inner-wall fractures, it is important to remember that, because the superior and posterior acetabular components are intact, there is no need to reduce the medial fragment.[710,722,823,857]

Those fractures in which the femoral head is concentrically reduced beneath the acetabular dome initially are managed with bed rest, skin or skeletal traction, and early range of motion. Although Lowell[779] reported that in none of these patients did the femoral head dislocate medially during treatment, Judet and associates[760] mention this complication in patients who bear weight early. I keep these patients in traction 4 to 6 weeks and prevent full weight bearing for 3 months.

Those fractures in which the femoral head is not initially located beneath the acetabular dome but is centrally dislocated are treated by reduction of the femoral head. If the patient's condition permits, a closed reduction after the method of Lowell[779] is attempted. The use of image intensification during reduction has been helpful. If the patient's condition does not permit, a closed reduction by traction is attempted. Once the femoral head-acetabular relationship has been restored, these patients are maintained in longitudinal skeletal traction for 10 to 12 weeks. Lateral traction, either skeletal or by the use of a sling in the groin, is required to maintain the reduction for 10 to 12 weeks. Range of motion exercises are instituted immediately.[684] Patients are mobilized on crutches and remain non-weight bearing until evidence of fracture healing is seen on x-ray. I agree with Tipton and colleagues[850,851] that in severely displaced fractures, 12 weeks of traction is needed to allow sufficient cancellous healing to let the patient become weight bearing without fear of redislocation.

If the femoral head cannot be reduced under the acetabular dome by closed manipulation or by traction, open reduction is necessary in the younger patient.[796] In the elderly patient one must consider the risks of this major operative procedure. The fact that x-ray appearance often does not parallel clinical function must be remembered.

Superior Dome Fractures

Superior dome fractures, in which the outline of the acetabular dome is intact and there is a congruous relationship between the femoral head and acetabulum, are treated in longitudinal skeletal traction and early range of motion for 8 weeks. The patients are then treated with crutches non-weight bearing until there is x-ray evidence of healing on x-ray before full weight bearing is allowed.

In those superior dome fractures in which the outline of the acetabulum is not intact or congruous with the femoral head, consideration is given to open reduction and internal fixation. If the fracture fragments appear to be large enough to permit internal fixation, and the patient's physical condition permits, open reduction and internal fixation are performed. This is not a procedure to be attempted by surgeons without prior experience in operating on the acetabulum and pelvis. We must stress that thorough understanding of the fracture patterns, anatomy, and surgical approaches described by Judet and associates[760] are essential before open reduction and internal fixation are attempted. After internal fixation, these patients are managed in skeletal traction for 4 to 6 weeks with intensive range of motion exercises. The patients are then progressed to crutch walking, avoiding full weight bearing until there is x-ray evidence of healing.

If fracture fragments are too small, or the patient is not a good surgical risk, I institute skeletal traction with 10% of body weight and early range of motion in an effort to get the "neocongruence" described by Letournel[773] and others.[722,777,866,868] Traction is maintained for 8 to 10 weeks. The patient is then allowed to begin crutch walking partial weight bearing until there is fracture consolidation. The end results are often so poor that early reconstruction may be required.

Bursting Fractures

Bursting fractures in which there is a good relationship between the acetabulum and femoral head are managed in skeletal traction, usually both longitudinal and lateral, for a period of 8 to 12 weeks.[842] Crutch walking non-weight bearing is then instituted, with weight bearing allowed at 3 to 6 months.

In those fractures in which there is a poor relationship between the acetabulum and the femoral head, I attempt a closed reduction under general anesthesia after the technique described by Lowell.[779] If the reduction is successful—that is, if it restores an acceptable acetabular-femoral head relationship, the patient is managed in longitudinal and lateral traction for 12 weeks. He is then allowed to be up on crutches with a 3- to 6-month delay in full weight bearing.

If closed reduction is not acceptable, the surgeon is faced with the decision of accepting an inadequate reduction versus the risks of open reduction and internal fixation. The same considerations mentioned in displaced superior dome fractures are taken to account in making this decision. The author emphasizes that the end results of this fracture treated by traction and early range of motion are surpisingly good in spite of the x-ray appearance.

I have found that the eventual outcome in these injuries depends greatly on the type of fracture-dislocation, which is a reflection of the severity of the injury itself. The condition and congruity of the acetabular dome and femoral head, the adequacy of reduction, and the stability of the hip joint after treatment are the important factors in determining the prognosis.

Because of the incidence of pin tract infections noted in patients with lateral traction, I prefer to avoid lateral traction if possible. I have often been able to use a swathe in the groin in the place of lateral skeletal traction to maintain the femoral head relationship beneath the acetabulum. However, if this is not successful, I do not hesitate to use lateral pin traction after the method of Tipton and colleagues (see Fig. 14-62).[850,851]

Because of the possibility of redislocation of the femoral head centrally, x-rays are taken on a routine basis in patients in traction. If the femoral head was displaced centrally initially, traction for 12 weeks is usually required to prevent redislocation. Full weight bearing is not permitted until 4 to 6 months after fracture, the time at which healing appears on x-ray.

In severely displaced fractures, restoration of bony anatomy by open reduction to prepare for possible future total joint replacement is a theoretical consideration. However, I have been reticent to use this as an absolute indication for open reduction, owing to the potential complications, especially sepsis that might prevent later reconstruction.

Traction in the Treatment of Fractures and Dislocations About the Hip

My regimen for those patients in traction consists of balanced suspension with immediate institution of hip and knee motion. If the situation permits, I prefer a distal femoral pin, especially if a larger longitudinal force is required to maintain reduction. After a short time in this traction, longitudinal traction is applied with the thigh flat on the bed, using a method similar to that which Apley has described for tibial plateau fractures (see Fig. 14-55). This allows the hip to flex and extend fully. A skateboard on the patient's bed is used to institute abduction and adduction and rotation exercises in an effort to maintain these motions of the hip (see Fig. 14-56). Although these patients all eventually lose some hip motion, early attention to range of motion exercise can keep this to a minimum.

The author expresses his appreciation to John J. Hinchey, M.D. of San Antonio, Texas, for his stimulation and guidance, for the standards he sets as a physician and surgeon, and for his encouragement and assistance in completing this chapter.

REFERENCES

Fractures of the Neck of the Femur

1. Abrami, G., and Stevens, J.: Early Weightbearing after Internal Fixation of Transcervical Fracture of the Femur. J. Bone Joint Surg., **46B:**204–205, 1964.
2. Ackroyd, C. E.: Treatment of Subcapital Femoral Fractures Fixed with Moore's Pins: A Study of 34 Cases Followed-Up For Up to 3 Years. Injury, **5:**100–108, 1973–1974.
3. Albee, F. H.: The Bone Graft Peg in Treatment of Fractures of Neck of the Femur. Ann. Surg., **62:**85–91, 1915.
4. Albright, J. P., and Weinstein, S. L.: Treatment for Fixation Complications. Arch. Surg., **110:**30–36, 1975.
5. Alffram, P. A.: An Epidemiologic Study of Cervical and Trochanteric Fractures of the Femur in an Urban Population. Acta Orthop. Scand. (Suppl), **65:**1–109, 1964.
6. Anderson, L.; Campbell, A. E. R.; Dunn, A.; and Runciman, J.: Osteomalacia in Elderly Women. Scottish Med. J., **11:**429, 1966.
7. Anderson, L. D.; Hamsa, W. R.; and Waring, T. L.: Femoral-Head Prostheses. J. Bone Joint Surg., **46:**1049–1065, 1964.
8. Anderson, R.: New Method for Treating Fractures Utilizing the Well Leg for Countertraction. Surg., Gynecol. Obstet., **54:**207–219, 1932.

9. Anderson, R.: The Well-Leg Countertraction Method. Am. J. Surg., **18**:36–50, 1932.

10. Apley, A. G.: A System of Orthopaedics and Fractures. 3rd ed. London, Butterworths, 1968.

11. Arden, G. P., and Veall, N.: The Use of Radioactive Phosphorus in Early Detection of Avascular Necrosis in the Femoral Head in Fractured Neck of Femur. Proc. Roy. Soc. Med., **46**:344–346, 1952–53.

12. Arnold, W. D.; Lyden, J. P.; and Minkoff, J.: Treatment of Intracapsular Fractures of the Femoral Neck. J. Bone Joint Surg., **56A**:254–262, 1974.

13. Arnoldi, C. C., and Lemperg, R. K.: Fracture of the Femoral Neck. Clin. Orthop., **129**:217–222, 1977.

14. Arnoldi, C. C., and Linderholm, H.: Intraosseous Pressures in Patients with Fracture of the Femoral Neck. Acta Chir. Scand., **135**:407–411, 1969.

15. Arnoldi, C. C., and Linderholm, H.: Fracture of the Femoral Neck. Clin. Orthop., **84**:116–127, 1972.

16. Ashby, M. E., and Anderson, J. C.: Treatment of Fractures of the Hip and Ipsilateral Femur with the Zickel Device. Clin. Orthop., **127**:156–160, 1977.

17. Askin, S. R., and Bryan, R. S.: Femoral Neck Fractures in Young Adults. Clin. Orthop., **114**:259–264, 1976.

18. Aston, J. N.: A Short Textbook of Orthopaedics and Traumatology. London, The English Universities Press, 1961.

19. Atkinson, R. E.; Kinnett, J. G.; and Arnold, W. D.: Simultaneous Fractures of Both Femoral Necks: Review of the Literature and Report of Two Cases. Clin. Orthop., **152**:284–287, 1980.

20. Backman, S.: The Proximal End of the Femur. Acta. Radiol. (Suppl.), **146**:1–166, 1957.

21. Badgley, C. E.: Fractures of the Hip Joint; Some Causes for Failure and Suggestions for Success. A.A.O.S. Instructional Course Lectures, **17**:106–116, 1960.

22. Bagby, G. W., and Wallace, G. T.: Femoral Neck Fractures in the Elderly Treated by Multiple Pins (Knowles). Northwest Med., **70**:696–698, 1971.

23. Baker, D. M.: Fractures of the Femoral Neck After Healed Intertrochanteric Fractures: A Complication of Too Short a Nail Plate Fixation. Report of Three Cases. J. Trauma, **15**:73–81, 1975.

24. Banks, H. H.: Factors Influencing the Result in Fractures of the Femoral Neck. J. Bone Joint Surg., **44A**:931–964, 1962.

25. Banks, H. H.: Nonunion in Fractures of the Femoral Neck. Orthop. Clin. North Am., **5**:865–885, October, 1974.

26. Bargren, J. H.; Tilson, D. H.; and Bridgeford, O. E.: Prevention of Displaced Fatigue Fractures of the Femur. J. Bone Joint Surg., **53A**:1115–1117, 1971.

27. Barnes, R.: The Diagnosis of Ischemia of the Capital Fragment in Femoral Neck Fractures. J. Bone Joint Surg., **44B**:760–761, 1962.

28. Barnes, R.; Brown, J. T.; Garden, R. S.; and Nicoll, E. A.: Subcapital Fractures of the Femur. J. Bone Joint Surg., **58B**:2–24, 1976.

29. Barr, J. S.: Experiences with a Sliding Nail in Femoral Neck Fractures. Clin. Orthop., **92**:63–68, 1973.

30. Barr, J. S.: Diagnosis and Treatment of Infections Follow-ing Internal Fixation of Hip Fractures. Orthop. Clin. North Am., **5(4)**:847–864, 1974.

31. Barr, J. S.; Donovan, J. F.; and Florence, D. W.: Arthroplasty of the Hip. J. Bone Joint Surg., **46A**:249–266, 1964.

32. Barry, H. C.: Fractures of the Femur in Paget's Disease of Bone in Australia. J. Bone Joint Surg., **49A**:1359–1370, 1967.

33. Bauer, G.; Weber, D. A.; Ceder, L.; Darte, L.; Egund, N.; Hansson, L. I.; and Stromqvist, B.: Dynamics of Technetium-99m Methylenediphosphonate Imaging of the Femoral Head After Hip Fracture. Clin. Orthop., **152**:85–92, 1980.

34. Bayliss, A. P., and Davidson, J. K.: Traumatic Osteonecrosis of the Femoral Head Following Intracapsular Fracture: Incidence and Earliest Radiological Features. Clin. Radiol., **28**:407–414, 1977.

35. Beckenbaugh, R. D.; Tressler, H. A.; and Johnson, E. W.: Results After Hemiarthroplasty of the Hip Using a Cemented Femoral Prosthesis: A Review of 109 Cases with an Average Follow-up of 36 Months. Mayo Clin. Proc., **52**:349–353, 1977.

36. Bentley, G.: Impacted Fractures of the Neck of the Femur. J. Bone Joint Surg., **50B**:551–561, 1968.

37. Bentley, G.: Treatment of Nondisplaced Fractures of the Femoral Neck. Clin. Orthop., **152**:93–101, 1980.

38. Bernstein, S. M.: Fractures of the Femoral Shaft and Associated Ipsilateral Fractures of the Hip. Orthop. Clin. North Am., **5**:799–818, 1974.

39. Bhuller, G. S.: Use of the Giliberty Bipolar Endoprosthesis in Femoral Neck Fractures. Clin. Orthop., **162**:165–169, 1982.

40. Bickel, W. H.; Childs, D. S.; and Porretta, C. M.: Post Irradiation Fractures of the Femoral Neck. Emphasis on the Results of Treatment. J.A.M.A., **175**:126–134, 1961.

41. Bingold, A. C.: The Science of Pinning the Neck of the Femur. Ann. R. Coll. Surg. Eng., **59**:463–469, 1977.

42. Blake, D. D.: Radiation Treatment of Metastatic Bone Disease. Clin. Orthop., **73**:89–100, 1970.

43. Blecher, A.: Uber den Einfluss des Parade-Marsches auf die Entstehung der Fuss Geschwulst. Med. Klin., **1**:305–306, 1905.

44. Blickenstaff, L. D., and Morris, J. M.: Fatigue Fracture of the Femoral Neck. J. Bone Joint Surg., **48A**:1031–1047, 1966.

45. Bobechko, W. P., and Harris, W. R.: The Radiographic Density of Avascular Bone. J. Bone Joint Surg., **42B**:626–632, 1960.

46. Bohr, H., and Larsen, E. H.: On Necrosis of the Femoral Head After Fracture of the Neck of the Femur. A Microradiographic and Histological Study. J. Bone Joint Surg., **47B**:330–338, 1965.

47. Bonarigo, B. C., and Rubin, P.: Nonunion of Pathologic Fracture After Radiation Therapy. Radiology, **88**:889–898, 1967.

48. Bonfiglio, M.: The Pathology of Fracture of the Femoral Neck Following Irradiation. Am. J. Roent., **70**:449–459, 1953.

49. Bonfiglio, M.: Aseptic Necrosis of the Femoral Head in

Dogs; Effect of Drilling and Bone Grafting. Surg. Gynecol. Obstet., **98:**591–599, 1954.

50. Bonfiglio, M.: Fracture of the Femoral Neck: Early Recognition and Treatment of Complications. J. Iowa Med. Soc., **59:**303–312, 1969.

51. Bonfiglio, M.: Technique of Core Biopsy and Tibial Bone Grafting (Phemister Procedure) For Treatment of Aseptic Necrosis of the Femoral Head. Iowa Orthop. J., **2:**57–62, 1982.

52. Bonfiglio, M., and Bardenstein, M. B.: Treatment by Bone Grafting of Aseptic Necrosis of the Femoral Head and Nonunion of the Femoral Neck (Phemister Technique). J. Bone Joint Surg., **40A:**1329–1346, 1958.

53. Bonfiglio, M., and Voke, E. M.: Aseptic Necrosis of the Femoral Head and Nonunion of the Femoral Neck. J. Bone Joint Surg., **50A:**48–66, 1968.

54. Boyd, H. B.: Avascular Necrosis of the Head of the Femur. A.A.O.S. Instructional Course Lectures, **14:**196–204, 1957.

55. Boyd, H. B., and Calandruccio, R. A.: Further Observations on the Use of Radioactive Phosphorus (P32) to Determine the Viability of the Head of the Femur. J. Bone Joint Surg., **45A:**445–460, 1963.

56. Boyd, H. B., and George, L. L.: Complications of Fractures of the Neck of the Femur. J. Bone Joint Surg., **29:**13–18, 1947.

57. Boyd, H. B., and Salvatore, J. E.: Acute Fracture of the Femoral Neck: Internal Fixation or Prosthesis? J. Bone Joint Surg., **46A:**1066–1068, 1964.

58. Boyd, H. B.; Zilversmit, D. B.; and Calandruccio, R. A.: The Use of Radioactive Phosphorus (P32) to Determine the Viability of the Head of the Femur. J. Bone Joint Surg., **37A:**260–269, 1955.

59. Branch, H. E.: March Fractures of the Femur. J. Bone Joint Surg., **26:**387–391, 1944.

60. Brodetti, A.: The Blood Supply of the Femoral Neck and Head in Relation to the Damaging Effects of Nails and Screws. J. Bone Joint Surg., **42B:**794–801, 1960.

61. Brodetti, A.: An Experimental Study on the Use of Nails and Bolt Screws in the Fixation of Fractures of the Femoral Neck. Acta Orthop. Scand., **31:**247–271, 1961.

62. Brown, J. T., and Abrami, G.: Transcervical Femoral Fracture. J. Bone Joint Surg., **46B:**648–663, 1964.

63. Brown, T. I. S., and Court-Brown, C.: Failure of Sliding Nail-Plate Fixation in Subcapital Fractures of the Femoral Neck. J. Bone Joint Surg., **61B:**342–346, 1979.

64. Bunata, R. E.; Fahey, J. J.; and Drennan, D. B.: Factors Influencing Stability and Necrosis of Impacted Femoral Neck Fractures. J.A.M.A., **223:**41–44, 1973.

65. Burwell, H. N., and Scott, D.: A Lateral Intermuscular Approach to the Hip Joint for Replacement of the Femoral Head by a Prosthesis. J. Bone Joint Surg., **36B:**104–108, 1954.

66. Calandruccio, R. A., and Anderson, W. E.: Post-Fracture Avascular Necrosis of the Femoral Head: Correlation of Experimental and Clinical Studies. Clin. Orthop., **152:**49–84, 1980.

67. Cameron, H. U.; Fornasier, V. L.; and McNab, I.: Pathological Fractures of the Femoral Neck. Can. Med. Assoc. J., **111:**791–792, 1974.

68. Carnesale, P. G., and Anderson, L. D.: Primary Prosthetic Replacement for Femoral Neck Fractures. Arch. Surg., **110:**27–29, 1975.

69. Cassebaum, W. H., and Nugent, G.: The Predictability of Bony Union in Displaced Intracapsular Fractures of the Hip. J. Trauma, **3:**421–424, 1963.

70. Cassebaum, W. H., and Parkes, J. C.: Treatment of Displaced Intracapsular Fractures of the Hip Utilizing the Richards Screw. J. Bone Joint Surg., **55A:**1309, 1973.

71. Castle, M. E., and Orinion, E. A.: Prophylactic Anticoagulation in Fractures. J. Bone Joint Surg., **52A:**521–528, 1970.

72. Cathcart, R. F.: The Shape of the Normal Femoral Head and Results From Clinical Use of More Normally Shaped Nonspherical Hip Replacement Prostheses. J. Bone Joint Surg., **54A:**1559, 1972.

73. Catto, M.: A Histological Study of Avascular Necrosis of the Femoral Head after Transcervical Fracture. J. Bone Joint Surg., **47B:**749–776, 1965.

74. Catto, M.: The Histological Appearances of Late Segmental Collapse of the Femoral Head After Transcervical Fracture. J. Bone Joint Surg., **47B:**777–791, 1965.

75. Cave, E. F.: Fractures of the Femoral Neck. A.A.O.S. Instructional Course Lectures, **17:**79–93, 1960.

76. Chalmers, J.; Barclay, A.; Davison, A. M.; MacCloud, D. A. D.; and Williams, D. A.: Quantitative Measurements of Osteoid in Health and Disease. Clin. Orthop., **63:**196–209, 1969.

77. Chan, R. N.-W., and Hoskinson, J.: Thompson Prosthesis for Fractured Neck of Femur. J. Bone Joint Surg., **57B:**437–443, 1975.

78. Chandler, S. B., and Kreuscher, P. H.: A Study of the Blood Supply of the Ligamentum Teres and its Relation to the Circulation of the Head of the Femur. J. Bone Joint Surg., **14:**834–846, 1932.

79. Chapman, M. W.; Stehr, J. H.; Eberle, C. F.; Bloom, M. H.; and Bovill, E. G.: Treatment of Intracapsular Hip Fractures by the Deyerle Method. J. Bone Joint Surg., **57A:**735–744, 1975.

80. Charnley, J.; Blockey, N. J.; and Purser, D. W.: The Treatment of Displaced Fractures of the Neck of the Femur by Compression. A Preliminary Report. J. Bone Joint Surg., **39B:**45–65, 1957.

81. Christophe, K.; Howard, L. G.; Potter, T. A.; and Driscoll, A. J.: A Study of 104 Consecutive Cases of Fracture of the Hip. J. Bone Joint Surg., **35A:**729–735, 1953.

82. Christopher, F.: Treatment of Impacted Fracture of the Neck of the Femur. J. Bone Joint Surg., **22:**161–167, 1940.

83. Chung, S. M. K.: The Arterial Supply of the Developing Proximal End of the Human Femur. J. Bone Joint Surg., **58A:**961–970, 1976.

84. Claffey, T. J.: Avascular Necrosis of the Femoral Head. J. Bone Joint Surg., **42B:**802–809, 1960.

85. Clawson, D. K.: Intracapsular Fractures of the Femur Treated by the Sliding Screw Plate Fixation Method. J. Trauma, **4:**753–756, 1964.

86. Cleveland, M.: A Critical Survey of Ten Years' Experience

with Fractures of the Neck of the Femur. Surg. Gynecol. Obstet., **74:**529–540, 1942.

87. Cleveland, M., and Bailey, W. L.: An End-Result Study of Intracapsular Fracture of the Neck of the Femur. Surg. Gynecol. Obstet., **90:**393–405, 1950.

88. Cleveland, M., and Bosworth, D. M.: Fractures of the Neck of the Femur: A Critical Analysis of Fifty Consecutive Cases. Surg. Gynecol. Obstet., **66:**646–656, 1938.

89. Cleveland, M., and Fielding, J. W.: A Continuing End-Result Study of Intracapsular Fracture of the Neck of the Femur. J. Bone Joint Surg., **36A:**1020–1030, 1954.

90. Cleveland, M., and Fielding, J. W.: Intracapsular Fracture of the Neck of the Femur. A.A.O.S. Instructional Course Lectures, **12:**35–43, 1955.

91. Coates, R.: A Retrospective Survey of Eighty-one Patients with Hemiarthroplasty for Subcapital Fracture of the Femoral Neck. J. Bone Joint Surg., **57B:**256, 1975.

92. Coates, R. L., and Armour, P.: Treatment of Subcapital Femoral Fractures by Primary Total Hip Replacement. Injury, **11:**132–135, 1979–1980.

93. Coleman, S. S., and Compere, C. L.: Femoral Neck Fractures. Pathogenesis of Avascular Necrosis, Nonunion, and Late Degenerative Changes. J. Bone Joint Surg., **39A:**1419, 1957.

94. Collins, H. R.: Replacement Endoprostheses in the Treatment of the Damaged Hip. Orthop. Clin. North Am., **2:**75–91, 1971.

95. Compton, E. H.: Accuracy of Reduction of Femoral Subcapital Fractures. Injury, **9:**71–73, 1977–1978.

96. Cooper, A. P.: A Treatise on Dislocations and on Fractures of the Joints, 2nd ed. London, Longman, Hurst, 1823. (Reprinted in Clin. Orthop., **92:**3–5, 1973.)

97. Cosentino, R.: Extra Osseous Circulation of the Proximal End of the Femur in the Adult. Congreso Argentino de Cirugia, Actas Fasc. 11, 1964.

98. Cotton, F. J.: Artificial Impaction in Hip Fractures. Am. J. Orthop. Surg., **8:**680–683, 1911.

99. Cotton, F. J., and Morrison, G. M.: Hip Fractures. Valgus Position: Accidental or Engineered. J. Bone Joint Surg., **20:**461–468, 1938.

100. Coughlin, L., and Templeton, J.: Hip Fractures in Patients with Parkinson's Disease. Clin. Orthop., **148:**192–195, 1980.

101. Coventry, M. B.: Fresh Fractures of the Hip Treated with Prosthesis. A.A.O.S. Instructional Course Lectures, **16:**292–298, 1959.

102. Coventry, M. B.: An Evaluation of the Femoral Head Prosthesis After Ten Years of Experience. Surg. Gynecol. Obstet., **109:**243–244, 1959.

103. Coventry, M. B.: Salvage of the Painful Hip Prosthesis. J. Bone Joint Surg., **46A:**200–212, 1964.

104. Crawford, H. B.: Conservative Treatment of Impacted Fractures of the Femoral Neck. J. Bone Joint Surg., **42A:**471–479, 1960.

105. Crawford, H. B.: Experience with the Non-operative Treatment of Impacted Fractures of the Neck of the Femur. J. Bone Joint Surg., **47A:**830–831, 1965.

106. Crock, H. V.: A Revision of the Anatomy of the Arteries Supplying the Upper End of the Human Femur. J. Anat. (London), **99:**77–88, 1965.

107. Crock, H. V.: An Atlas of the Arterial Supply of the Head and Neck of the Femur in Man. Clin. Orthop., **152:**17–27, 1980.

108. Culver, D.; Crawford, J. S.; Gardiner, J. H.; and Wiley, A. M.: Venous Thrombosis After Fractures of the Upper End of the Femur. J. Bone Joint Surg., **52B:**61–69, 1970.

109. DaCosta, J. C.: Nailing of a Fracture of the Femoral Neck. Am. J. Orthop. Surg., **5:**351, 1907–1908.

110. D'Arcy, J., and Devas, M.: Treatment of Fractures of the Femoral Neck by Replacement with the Thompson Prostesis. J. Bone Joint Surg., **58B:**279–286, 1976.

111. Davis, G. G.: The Operative Treatment of Intracapsular Fracture of the Neck of the Femur. Am. J. Orthop. Surg., **6:**481–483, 1908–1909.

112. Delaney, W. M., and Street, D. M.: Fracture of the Femoral Shaft with Fracture of Neck of Same Femur. J. Int. Coll. Surg., **19:**303–312, 1953.

113. Delbet, P.: Resultat eloigne d'un visage pour fracture transcervicale du femur. Bull. Mem. Soc. Chir. Paris, **45:**305–317, 1919.

114. DeLee, J. C., and Rockwood, C. A.: Current Concepts Review: The Use of Aspirin in Thromboembolic Disease. J. Bone Joint Surg., **62A:**149–152, 1980.

115. Dencker, H.: Femoral Shaft Fracture and Fracture of the Neck of the Same Femur. Acta. Chir. Scand., **129:**597–605, 1965.

116. DePalma, A. F.: Wedge Osteotomy for Fresh Intracapsular Fractures of the Neck of the Femur. J. Bone Joint Surg., **32A:**653–662, 1950.

117. Devas, M.: Stress Fractures. New York, Churchill Livingstone, 1975.

118. Devas, M. B.: Stress Fractures of the Femoral Neck. J. Bone Joint Surg., **47B:**728–738, 1965.

119. Deyerle, W. M.: Absolute Fixation with Contact Compression in Hip Fractures. Clin. Orthop., **13:**279–297, 1959.

120. Deyerle, W. M.: Multiple Pin Peripheral Fixation in the Fractures of the Neck of the Femur: Immediate Weight-Bearing. Clin. Orthop., **39:**135–156, 1965.

121. Deyerle, W. M.: Plate and Peripheral Pins in Hip Fractures: Two-Plane Reduction, Total Impaction and Absolute Fixation. Curr. Pract. Orthop. Surg., **3:**173–207, 1966.

122. Deyerle, W. M.: Impacted Fixation Over Resilient Multiple Pins. Clin. Orthop., **152:**102–122, 1980.

123. Dickerson, R. C., and Duthie, R. B.: Diversion of Arterial Blood Flow to Bone: A Preliminary Report. J. Bone Joint Surg., **45A:**356–364, 1963.

124. Dickson, J. A.: The High Geometric Osteotomy with Rotation and Bone Graft for Ununited Fractures of the Neck of the Femur. J. Bone Joint Surg., **29:**1005–1018, 1947.

125. Dickson, J. A.: The "Unsolved" Fracture. J. Bone Joint Surg., **35A:**805–822, 1953.

126. Dove, J.: Complete Fractures of the Femur in Paget's Disease of Bone. J. Bone Joint Surg., **62B:**12–17, 1980.

127. Drinker, H., and Murray, W. R.: The Universal Proximal Femoral Endoprosthesis. A Short Term Comparison with Conventional Hemiarthroplasty. J. Bone Joint Surg., **61A:**1167–1174, 1979.

128. Edholm, P.: Lindblom, K.; and Maurseth, K.: Angulations in Fractures of the Femoral Neck With and Without

Subsequent Necrosis of the Head. Acta. Radiol. (Diag.) (Stockholm), **6:**329–336, 1967.

129. Eftekhar, N. S.: Status of Femoral Head Replacement in Treating Fracture of Femoral Neck. I. Hemiarthroplasty vs. Total Arthroplasty. Orthop. Rev., **2:**15–23, 1973.

130. Eftekhar, N. S.: Status of Femoral Head Replacement in Treating Fracture of the Femoral Neck. II. The Prosthesis and Surgical Procedure. Orthop. Rev., **2:**19–30, 1973.

131. Eklund, J., and Eriksson, F.: Fractures of the Femoral Neck: with Special Regard to the Treatment and Prognosis of Stable Abduction Fractures. Acta Chir. Scand., **127:**315–337, 1964.

132. Ernst, J.: Stress Fracture of the Neck of the Femur. J. Trauma, **4:**71–83, 1964.

133. Evarts, C. M.: Endoprosthesis as the Primary Treatment of Femoral Neck Fractures. Clin. Orthop., **92:**69–76, 1973.

134. Eyre-Brook, A. L., and Pridie, K. H.: Intracapsular Fractures of the Neck of the Femur. Final Results of 75 Consecutive Cases Treated by the Closed Method of Pinning. Br. J. Surg., **29:**115–138, 1941.

135. Fairbank, T. J.; Femoral Neck Fractures. Proc. Roy. Soc. Med., **63:**43–46, 1970.

136. Fielding, J. W.: Displaced Femoral Neck Fractures. Orthop. Rev., **2:**11–17, 1973.

137. Fielding, J. W.: Pugh Nail Fixation of Displaced Femoral Neck Fractures. Clin. Orthop., **106:**107–116, 1975.

138. Fielding, J. W.: The Telescoping Pugh Nail in the Surgical Management of the Displaced Intracapsular Fracture of the Femoral Neck. Clin. Orthop., **152:**123–130, 1980.

139. Fielding, J. W.; Wilson, H. J.; and Zickel, R. E.: A Continuing End-Result Study of Intra-capsular Fracture of the Neck of the Femur. J. Bone Joint Surg., **44A:**965–974, 1962.

140. Fielding, J. W.; Wilson, S. A.; and Ratzan, S.: A Continuing End-Result of Displaced Intracapsular Fractures of the Neck of the Femur Treated with the Pugh Nail. J. Bone Joint Surg., **56A:**1464–1472, 1974.

141. Finney, D. C. W.; Jones, B. B.; and Eaton, G. O.: Fractures of the Hip. Am. Surg., **25:**8–11, 1959.

142. Fitts, W. T.; Lehr, H. B.; Bitner, R. L.; and Spelman, J. W.: An Analysis of 950 Fatal Injuries. Surgery, **56:**663–668, 1964.

143. Flatmark, A. L., and Lone, T.: The Prognosis of Abduction Fracture of the Neck of the Femur. J. Bone Joint Surg., **44B:**324–327, 1962.

144. Flynn, M.: A New Method of Reduction of Fractures of the Neck of the Femur Based on Anatomical Studies of the Hip Joint. Injury, **5:**309–317, 1973–1974.

145. Follacci, F. M., and Charnley, J.: A Comparison of the Results of Femoral Head Prosthesis With and Without Cement. Clin. Orthop., **62:**156–161, 1969.

146. Francis, K. C.; Higinbotham, N. L.; Carroll, R. E.; Jacobs, B.; and Graham, W. D.: The Treatment of Pathological Fractures of the Femoral Neck by Resection. J. Trauma, **2:**465–473, 1962.

147. Frandsen, P. A.: Osteosynthesis of Displaced Fractures of the Femoral Neck. Acta Orthop. Scand., **50:**443–449, 1979.

148. Frandsen, P. A., and Jorgensen, F.: Osteosynthesis of Medial Fractures of the Femoral Neck by Sliding Nail-Plate Fixation. Acta Orthop. Scand., **48:**57–62, 1977.

149. Frangakis, E. K.: Intracapsular Fractures of the Neck of the Femur. J. Bone Joint Surg., **48B:**17–30, 1966.

150. Frangenheim, P.: Studien uber Schenkelhalsfrakturen und die Vorgange bei ihrer Heilung. Deutsche Zeitschr. f. Chir., **83:**401–455, 1906.

151. Frankel, C. J., and Derian, P. S.: The Introduction of Subcapital Femoral Circulation by Means of Autogenous Muscle Pedicle. Surg. Gynecol. Obstet., **115:**473–477, 1962.

152. Frankel, V. H.: Mechanical Factors for Internal Fixation of the Femoral Neck. Acta Orthop. Scand., **29:**21–42, 1959.

153. Frankel, V. H.: Mechanical Principles for Internal Fixation of the Femoral Neck. Acta Chir. Scand., **117:**427–432, 1959.

154. Frankel, V. H.: The Femoral Neck Function: Fracture Mechanism Internal Fixation. Springfield, Charles C. Thomas, 1960.

155. Frankel, V. H., and Burstein, A. H.: Force and Energetics of Femoral Neck Fractures. Proceedings Dixieme Congress International de Chirugie, Orthopaedique et de Traumatologie, Paris, 1966.

156. Fredensborg, N., and Nilsson, B. E.: The Bone Mineral Content and Cortical Thickness in Young Women with Femoral Neck Fracture. Clin. Orthop., **124:**161–164, 1977.

157. Freeman, M. A. R.; Todd, R. C.; and Pirie, C. J.: The Role of Fatigue in the Pathogenesis of Senile Femoral Neck Fractures. J. Bone Joint Surg., **56B:**698–702, 1974.

158. Furey, J. G.; Spencer, G. E.; and Pierce, D. J.: Use of Hip Prosthesis in Femoral Neck Fractures. J.A.M.A., **177:**100–103, 1961.

159. Gaenslen, F. J.: Subcutaneous Spike Fixation of Fresh Fractures of the Neck of the Femur. J. Bone Joint Surg., **17:**739–748, 1935.

160. Gaertner, R. L., and Deyerle, W. M.: Nonunion of the Femoral Neck and Avascular Necrosis of the Femoral Head: Treatment with Bone Grafts. South Med. J., **70:**1039–1044, 1977.

161. Gallie, W. E., and Lewis, F. I.: Ununited Fracture of the Neck of Femur in Aged. J. Bone Joint Surg., **22:**76–80, 1940.

162. Garden, R. S.: The Structure and Function of the Proximal End of the Femur. J. Bone Joint Surg., **43B:**576–589, 1961.

163. Garden, R. S.: Low-Angle Fixation In Fractures of the Femoral Neck. J. Bone Joint Surg., **43B:**647–663, 1961.

164. Garden, R. S.: Stability and Union in Subcapital Fractures of the Femur. J. Bone Joint Surg., **46B:**630–647, 1964.

165. Garden, R. S.: Scientific Thinking and Clinical Research. Pro. Mine Med. Off. Assoc., Johannesburg, **47:**47–52, 1967.

166. Garden, R. S.: Malreduction and Avascular Necrosis in Subcapital Fractures of the Femur. J. Bone Joint Surg., **53B:**183–197, 1971.

167. Garden, R. S.: Reduction and Fixation of Subcapital Fractures of the Femur. Orthop. Clin. North Am., **5:**683–712, 1974.

168. Gibson, J. M. C.: Early Weight-Bearing in Fractures of

the Femoral Neck. J. Roy. Coll. Surg. Edinb., **9**:213–214, 1964.

169. Gilbert, R. S., and Johnson, H. A.: Stress Fractures in Military Recruits: A Review of Twelve Years' Experience. Milit. Med., **131**:716–721, 1966.

170. Gingras, M. B.; Clarke, J.; and Evarts, C. M.: Prosthetic Replacement in Femoral Neck Fractures. Clin. Orthop., **152**:147–157, 1980.

171. Goodman, A. H., and Sherman, M. S.: Postirradiation Fractures of the Femoral Neck. J. Bone Joint Surg., **45A**:723–730, 1963.

172. Goodwin, R. A.: The Austin-Moore Prosthesis in Fresh Femoral Neck Fractures. Am. J. Orthop., **10**:40–41, 1968.

173. Gossling, H. R., and Hardy, J. H.: Fracture of the Femoral Neck: A Comparative Study of Methods of Treatment in 400 Consecutive Cases. J. Trauma, **9**:423–429, 1969.

174. Graham, J.: Early or Delayed Weight-Bearing After Internal Fixation of Transcervical Fracture of the Femur. J. Bone Joint Surg., **50B**:562–569, 1968.

175. Green, J. T.: Management of Fresh Fractures of the Neck of the Femur. A.A.O.S. Instructional Course Lectures, **17**:94–105, 1960.

176. Green, J. T., and Gay, F. H.: High Femoral Neck Fractures Treated by Multiple-Nail Fixation. A Survey of 100 Cases. Clin. Orthop., **11**:177–183, 1958.

177. Griffin, J. B.: The Calcar Femorale Redefined. Clin. Orthop., **164**:211–214, 1982.

178. Griffiths, W. E. G.; Swanson, S. A. V.; and Freeman, M. A. R.: Experimental Fatigue Fracture of the Human Cadaveric Femoral Neck. J. Bone Joint Surg., **53B**:136–143, 1971.

179. Grundy, M.: Fractures of the Femur in Paget's Disease of Bone. J. Bone Joint Surg., **52B**:252–263, 1970.

180. Gyepes, M.; Mellins, H. Z.; and Katz, I.: The Low Incidence of Fracture of Hip in Negro. J.A.M.A., **181**:1073–1074, 1962.

181. Haboush, E. J.: Photoelastic Stress and Strain Analysis in Cervical Fractures of the Femur. Bull. Hosp. Joint Dis., **13**:252–258, 1952.

182. Haboush, E. J.: Biomechanics of Femoral Nail and Nail-Plate Insertions in Fractures of the Neck of the Femur. Bull. Hosp. Joint Dis., **14**:125–137, 1953.

183. Halpin, P. J., and Nelson, C. L.: A System of Classification of Femoral Neck Fractures with Special Reference to Choice of Treatment. Clin. Orthop., **152**:44–48, 1980.

184. Hamilton, H. W.; Crawford, J. S.; Gardiner, J. H.: and Wiley, A. M.: Venous Thrombosis in Patients with Fracture of the Upper End of the Femur. J. Bone Joint Surg., **52B**:268–289, 1970.

185. Hansen, B. A., and Solgaard, S.: Impacted Fractures of the Femoral Neck Treated by Early Mobilization and Weight-Bearing. Acta Orthop. Scand., **49**:180–185, 1978.

186. Hansen, B. R.: Femoral Fractures After Moore Arthroplasty. Acta Orthop. Scand., **44**:509–515, 1973.

187. Hargadon, E. J., and Pearson, J. R.: Treatment of Intracapsular Fractures of the Femoral Neck with the Charnley Compression Screw. J. Bone Joint Surg., **45B**:305–311, 1963.

188. Harmon, P. H.: Teatment of Trochanteric, Subtrochanteric

and Transcervical Fractures of the Upper Femur by Fixation with Plastic Plate and Stainless Steel Screws. Guthrie Clin. Bull., **14**:10–18, 1944.

189. Harrington, I. J., and Tountas, A. A.: Femoral Fractures Associated with Moore's Prosthesis. Injury, **11**:23–32, 1979–1980.

190. Harrington, K. D.; Johnston, J. O.; Turner, R. H.; and Green, D. L.: The use of Methylmethacrylate as an Adjunct in the Internal Fixation of Malignant Neoplastic Fractures. J. Bone Joint Surg., **54A**:1665–1676, 1972.

191. Harris, W. H.; Athanasoulis, C. A.; Waltman, A. C.; and Salzman, E. W.: High and Low-Dose Aspirin Prophylaxis Against Venous Thromboembolic Disease in Total Hip Replacement. J. Bone Joint Surg., **64A**:63–66, 1982.

192. Hartman, J. T.; Altner, P. C.; and Freeark, R. J.: The Effect of Limb Elevation in Preventing Venous Thrombosis. J. Bone Joint Surg., **52A**:1618–1622, 1970.

193. Harty, M.: Blood Supply of the Femoral Head. Br. Med. J., **2**:1236–1237, 1953.

194. Harty, M.: The Calcar Femorale and the Femoral Neck. J. Bone Joint Surg., **39A**:625–630, 1957.

195. Hawkins, L.: Hip Prostheses: Fifteen Years Experience. J. Iowa Med. Soc., **56**:465–471, 1966.

196. Hayes, A. G., and Groth, H. E.: The Influence of Rotational Malpositions on Intracapsular Fracture of the Femoral Neck. Surg. Gynecol. Obstet., **124**:40–48, 1967.

197. Henderson, M. S.: Ununited Fracture of the Neck of the Femur Treated by the Aid of the Bone Graft. J. Bone Joint Surg., **22**:97–106, 1940.

198. Hey-Groves, E. W.: Some Contributions to the Reconstructive Surgery of the Hip. Br. J. Surg., **14**:486–517, 1926–1927.

199. Hey-Groves, E. W.: Treatment of Fractured Neck of the Femur with Special Regard to the Results. J. Bone Joint Surg., **12**:1–14, 1930.

200. Hewson, J. S.: Treatment of Intracapsular Fracture of the Hip with Primary Pedicle Bone Graft From Greater Trochanter. Clin. Orthop., **76**:100–110, 1971.

201. Hilleboe, J. W.; Staple, T. W.; Lansche, E. W.; and Reynolds, F. C.: The Nonoperative Treatment of Impacted Fractures of the Femoral Neck. South. Med. J., **63**:1103–1109, 1970.

202. Hinchey, J. J., and Day, P. L.: Primary Prosthetic Replacement in Fresh Femoral Neck Fractures. J. Bone Joint Surg., **46A**:223–240, 1964.

203. Hirsch, C., and Frankel, V. H.: Analysis of Forces Producing Fractures of the Proximal End of the Femur. J. Bone Joint Surg., **42B**:633–640, 1960.

204. Hodkinson, H. M.: Fracture of the Femoral Neck in the Elderly, Assessment of the Role of Osteomalacia. Geront. Clin., **13**:153–158, 1971.

205. Holmquist, B., and Alffram, P. A.: Prediction of Avascular Necrosis Following Cervical Fracture of the Femur Based on Clearance of Radioactive Iodine From the Head of the Femur. Acta Orthop. Scand., **36**:62–69, 1965.

206. Howe, W. W.; Lacey, T.; and Schwartz, R. P.: A Study of the Gross Anatomy of the Arteries Supplying the Proximal Portion of the Femur and the Acetabulum. J. Bone Joint Surg., **32A**:856–866, 1950.

207. Howland, J.: Stress Fractures of the Femoral Neck. Am. J. Orthop. Surg., **11**(2):46–51, 1969.

208. Hsu, J. D.: Rehabilitation of Patients Suffering from Fracture of the Hip. Md. State Med. J., **18**:85–87, 1969.

209. Hulth, A.: Intra-osseous Venographies of Medial Fractures of the Femoral Neck. Acta Chir. Scand., (Suppl.) **214**:7–112, 1956.

210. Hulth, A.: The Inclination of the Fracture Surfaces and its Relation to the Rate of Healing in Femoral Neck Fractures. Acta Chir. Scand., **121**:309–314, 1961.

211. Hunter, G.: Treatment of Fractures of the Neck of the Femur. Can. Med. Assoc. J., **117**:60–61, 1977.

212. Hunter, G. A.: A Comparison of the Use of Internal Fixation and Prosthetic Replacement for Fresh Fractures of the Neck of the Femur. Br. J. Surg., **56**:229–232, 1969.

213. Hunter, G. A.: Should We Abandon Primary Prosthetic Replacement for Fresh Displaced Fractures of the Neck of the Femur? Clin. Orthop., **152**:158–161, 1980.

214. Hunter, G. A., and Mehta, A.: Subcapital Fracture of the Hip: A Rare Complication of Intertrochanteric Fracture of the Femur. Can. J. Surg., **20**:165–169, 1977.

215. Jacobs, B.; Wade, P. A.; and Match, R.: Intra-capsular Fractures of the Femoral Neck Treated by the Pugh Nail. J. Trauma, **5**:751–760, 1965.

216. Janecki, C. J.: The Gluteus Maximus Femoral Insertion. Clin. Orthop., **123**:16–18, 1977.

217. Janes, J. M.: Some Complications of Hip Fractures. Minn. Med., **52**(2):1787–1799, 1969.

218. Jeffrey, C. C.: Spontaneous Fractures of the Femoral Neck. J. Bone Joint Surg., **44B**:543–549, 1962.

219. Jenkins, D. H. R.; Roberts, J. G.; Webster, D.; and Williams, E. O.: Osteomalacia in Elderly Patients with Fracture of the Femoral Neck. J. Bone Joint Surg., **55B**:575–580, 1973.

220. Jensen, J. S., and Holstein, P.: A Long Term Follow-up of Moore Arthroplasty in Femoral Neck Fractures. Acta Orthop. Scand., **46**:764–774, 1975.

221. Jensen, T. M.; Dillon, W. L.; and Reckling, F. W.: Changing Concepts in the Management of Pathological and Impending Pathological Fractures. J. Trauma, **16**:496–502, 1976.

222. Jewett, E. L.: One Piece Angle Nail For Trochanteric Fractures. J. Bone Joint Surg., **23**:803–810, 1941.

223. Johansson, S.: On the Operative Treatment of Medial Fractures of the Femoral Neck. Acta Orthop. Scand., **3**:362–385, 1932.

224. Johansson, S. H.: Prognostic Assessment in Fractured Neck of the Femur Using I^{131} and Venography. Acta Chir. Scand., **123**:298–306, 1962.

225. Johnson, C. R.: A New Method for Roentgenographic Examination of the Upper End of the Femur. J. Bone Joint. Surg., **14**:859–866, 1932.

226. Johnson, J. T. H., and Crothers, O.: Nailing Versus Prosthesis for Femoral-Neck Fractures. J. Bone Joint Surg., **57A**:686–692, 1975.

227. Jones, K. G.: Extraosseous Placement of Guide Wire for Blind Stabilization of the Proximal Femur. Clin. Orthop., **72**:265–268, 1970.

229. Judet, J., and Judet, R.: The Use of an Artificial Femoral Head for Arthroplasty of the Hip Joint. J. Bone Joint Surg., **32B**:166–173, 1950.

230. Judet, J.; Judet, R.; LaGrange, J.; and Dunoyer, J.: A Study of Arterial Vascularization of the Femoral Neck in the Adult. J. Bone Joint Surg., **37A**:663–680, 1955.

231. Judet, R.: Treatment of Fractures of the Femoral Neck by Pedicled Graft. Acta Orthop. Scand., **32**:421–427, 1962.

232. Judet, R.; Judet, J.; Lord, G.; Roy-Camille, R.; and Letournel, E.: Treatment of Fractures of the Femoral Neck by Pedicled Graft. Presse. Med., **69**:2452–2453, 1961.

233. Kaltas, D. S.: Stress Fractures of the Femoral Neck in Young Adults: A Report of Seven Cases. J. Bone Joint Surg., **63B**:33–37, 1981.

234. Kavlie, H., and Sundal, B.: Primary Arthroplasty in Femoral Neck Fractures. Acta Orthop. Scand., **45**:579–590, 1974.

235. Keller, C. S., and Laros, G. S.: Indications for Open Reduction of Femoral Neck Fractures. Clin. Orthop., **152**:131–137, 1980.

236. Key, J. A., and Conwell, H. E.: The Management of Fractures, Dislocations and Sprains, 7th ed. St. Louis, C. V. Mosby, 1961.

237. Khairi, M. R. A.; Cronin, J. H.; Robb, J. A.; Smith, D. M.; and Johnston, C. C.: Femoral Trabecular-Pattern Index and Bone Mineral Content Measurement by Photon Absorption in Senile Osteoporosis. J. Bone Joint Surg., **58A**:221–226, 1976.

238. King, T.: The Closed Operation for Intracapsular Fracture of the Neck of the Femur. Br. J. Surg., **26**:721–748, 1938–1939.

239. Kirschner, P. T., and Simon, M. A.: Current Concepts Review: Radioisotopic Evaluation of Skeletal Disease. J. Bone Joint Surg., **63A**:673–681, 1981.

240. Klenerman, L., and Marcuson, R. W.: Intracapsular Fractures of the Neck of the Femur. J. Bone Joint Surg., **52B**:514–517, 1970.

241. Knowles, F. L.: Fractures of the Neck of the Femur. Wis. Med. J., **35**:106–109, 1936.

242. Kocher, T.: Beitrage zur Kentruss einiger praktisch wichtiger Fracturformen. Basel and Leipzig, Carl Sallman, 1896.

243. Kofoed, H., and Alberts, A.: Femoral Neck Fractures. Acta Orthop. Scand., **51**:127–136, 1980.

244. Konig, S.: Congress, Irith Sitzeing, 12, 1875.

245. Kotani, P. T.; Oonishi, H.; Shikita, T.; and Hamaguchi, T.: Study on the Surface Shape and Contours of the Femoral Head and Acetabulum of the Human Joint. Bull. Hosp. Bone Joint Dis., **36**:81–108, 1975.

246. Kranendonk, D. H.; Jurist, J. M.; and Lee, H. G.: Femoral Trabecular Patterns and Bone Mineral Content. J. Bone Joint Surg., **54A**:1472–1478, 1972.

247. Kuslich, S. D., and Gustilo, R. B.: Fractures of the Femoral Neck in Young Adults. Proceedings of A.A.O.S., J. Bone Joint Surg., **58A**:724, 1976.

248. Kyle, R. F.; Wright, T. M.; and Burstein, A. H.: Biomechanical Analysis of the Sliding Characteristics of Compression Hip Screws. J. Bone Joint Surg., **62A**:1308–1314, 1980.

249. Lake, M.: Studies of Paget's Disease (Osteitis Deformans). J. Bone Joint Surg., **33B:**323–335, 1951.

250. Lane, J. M.; Sculco, T. P.; and Zolan, S.: Treatment of Pathological Fractures of the Hip by Endoprosthetic Replacement. J. Bone Joint Surg., **62A:**954–959, 1980.

251. Langan, P.: The Giliberty Bipolar Prosthesis: A Clinical and Radiographical Review. Clin. Orthop., **141:**169–175, 1979.

252. Laros, G. S., and Spiegel, P. G.: Rigid Internal Fixation of Fractures. Editorial Comments. Clin. Orthop., **138:**2–3, 1979.

253. Larson, C. B.: Treatment of Acute Fractures of the Neck of the Femur. A.A.O.S. Instructional Course Lecture, **11:**72–80, 1954.

254. Leabhart, J. W., and Bonfiglio, M.: The Treatment of Irradiation Fracture of the Femoral Neck. J. Bone Joint Surg., **43A:**1056–1067, 1961.

255. Leadbetter, G. W.: A Treatment for Fracture of the Neck of the Femur. J. Bone Joint Surg., **15:**931–940, 1933.

256. Leadbetter, G. W.: Closed Reduction of Fractures of the Neck of the Femur. J. Bone Joint Surg., **20:**108–113, 1938.

257. Lender, M.; Makin, M.; Robin, G.; Steinberg, R.; and Menczel, J.: Osteoporosis and Fractures of the Neck of the Femur: Some Epidemiologic Considerations. Isr. J. Med. Sci., **12:**596–600, 1976.

258. Liebowitz, S.: New Concepts in Femoral Head Replacement: Clinical Experiences. Bull. Hosp. Joint Dis., **38:**57–58, 1977.

259. Linton, P.: On Different Types of Intracapsular Fractures of the Femoral Neck. Acta Chir. Scand., (Suppl. 86) **90:**1–122, 1944.

260. Linton, P.: Types of Displacement in Fractures of the Neck of the Femur. J. Bone Joint Surg., **31B:**184–189, 1949.

261. Long, J. W., and Knight, W.: Bateman UPF Prosthesis in Fractures of the Femoral Neck. Clin. Orthop., **152:**198–201, 1980.

262. Lowell, J. D.: Fractures of the Hip. N. Engl. J. Med., **274:**1418–1425, 1966.

263. Lowell, J. D.: Fractures of the Hip (Concluded). N. Engl. J. Med., **274:**1480–1490, 1966.

264. Lowell, J. D.: Results and Complications of Femoral Neck Fractures. Clin. Orthop., **152:**162–172, 1980.

265. Lucie, R. S.; Fuller, S.; Burdick, D. C.; and Johnston, R. M.: Early Prediction of Avascular Necrosis of the Femoral Head Following Femoral Neck Fractures. Clin. Orthop., **161:**207–214, 1981.

266. Lukawska, J. T.: Fractures of the Neck of the Femur and the Pelvis After X-ray Therapy in Cancer of the Uterus. Pol. Med. J., **7:**965–973, 1968.

267. Lunceford, E. M.: Use of the Moore Self-Locking Vitallium Prosthesis in Acute Fractures of the Femoral Neck. J. Bone Joint Surg., **47A:**832–841, 1965.

268. Lunt, H. R. W.: The Role of Prosthetic Replacement of the Head of the Femur as Primary Treatment for Subcapital Fractures. Injury, **3:**107–113, 1971.

269. MacAusland, W. R.; MacAusland, A. R.; and Lee, H. G.: Fractures of the Neck of the Femur. Surg. Gynecol. Obstet., **58:**679–698, 1934.

270. MacKenzie, D. B.: Simultaneous Ipsilateral Fracture of the Femoral Neck and Shaft: Report of 8 Cases. S. A. Med. J., **45:**459–467, 1971.

271. Martin, E. D., and King, A. C.: Preliminary Report on a New Method of Treating Fractures of the Neck of the Femur. New Orleans Med. Surg. J., **75:**710–715, 1923.

272. Martinelli, B., and Paschina, E.: Double Screw Osteosynthesis in the Treatment of Fractures of the Femoral Neck. Bull. Hosp. Bone Joint Dis., **35:**45–60, 1974.

273. Massie, W. K.: Functional Fixation of Femoral Neck Fractures; Telescoping Nail Technic. Clin. Orthop., **12:**230–255, 1958.

274. Massie, W. K.: Fractures of the Hip. J. Bone Joint Surg., **46A:**658–690, 1964.

275. Massie, W. K.: Treatment of Femoral Neck Fractures Emphasizing Long Term Follow-up Observations on Aseptic Necrosis. Clin. Orthop., **92:**16–62, 1973.

276. Maxwell, T. J.: Intra-Capsular Fracture of Neck of the Femur. Chicago Med. J. Examiner, **33:**401–404, 1876.

277. McDougall, A.: Fracture of the Neck of the Femur in Childhood. J. Bone Joint Surg., **43B:**16–28, 1961.

278. McElvenny, R. T.: The Roentgenographic Interpretation of What Constitutes Adequate Reduction of the Femur Neck Fractures. Surg. Gynecol. Obstet., **80:**97–106, 1945.

279. McElvenny, R. T.: Management of Intracapsular Hip Fractures. Surg. Clin. North Am., **29:**31–58, 1949.

280. McElvenny, R. T.: The Immediate Treatment of Intracapsular Hip Fracture. Clin. Orthop., **10:**289–323, 1957.

281. McElvenny, R. T.: Concepts and Principles in the Treatment of Intracapsular Fractures of the Hip. Am. J. Orthop., **2:**161–164, 1960.

282. McElvenny, R. T.: The Importance of the Lateral X-ray Film in Treating Intracapsular Fractures of the Neck of the Femur. Am. J. Orthop., **4:**212–215, 1962.

283. McQuillan, W. M.; Abernethy, P. J.; and Guy, J. G.: Subcapital Fractures of the Neck of the Femur Treated by Double-Divergent Fixation. Br. J. Surg., **60:**859–866, 1973.

284. Mears, T. S., and Cruess, R. L.: Evaluation of the use of Acrylic Cement in Anchoring Medullary Stem Femoral Head Prosthesis in the Hip. Proceedings of the First Open Scientific Meeting of the Hip Society, p. 139. St. Louis, C. V. Mosby, 1973.

285. Medgyesi, S.: Bone Growth in the Femoral Head Following Pedicled Bone Grafting. Acta Orthop. Scand., **42:**82–93, 1971.

286. Metz, C. W.; Sellers, T. D.; Feagin, J. A.; Levine, M. I.; Onkey, R. G.; Dyer, J. W.; and Eberhard, E. J.: The Displaced Intracapsular Fracture of the Neck of the Femur. J. Bone Joint Surg., **52A:**113–127, 1970.

287. Meyers, M. H.: The Role of Posterior Bone Grafts (Muscle-Pedicle) in Femoral Neck Fractures. Clin. Orthop., **152:**143–146, 1980.

288. Meyers, M. H.; Harvey, J. P.; and Moore, T. M.: Treatment of Displaced Subcapital and Transcervical Fractures of the Femoral Neck or Muscle-Pedicle-Bone Graft and Internal Fixation. J. Bone Joint Surg., **55A:**257–274, 1973.

289. Meyers, M. H.; Harvey, J. P.; and Moore, T. M.: The Muscle Pedicle Bone Graft in the Treatment of Displaced

Fractures of the Femoral Neck: Indications, Operative Technique and Results. Orthop. Clin. North Am., **5**:779–792, 1974.

290. Meyers, M. H.; Harvey, J. P.; and Moore, T. M.: Delayed Treatment of Subcapital and Transcervical Fractures of the Neck of the Femur with Internal Fixation and a Muscle Pedicle Bone Graft. Orthop. Clin. North Am., **5**:743–756, 1974.

291. Meyers, M. H.; Telfer, N.; and Moore, T. M.: Determination of the Vascularity of the Femoral Head with Technetium-99m-sulfur-colloid. Diagnostic and Prognostic Significance. J. Bone Joint Surg., **59A**:658–664, 1977.

292. Milgram, J. W.: Orthopaedic Management of Paget's Disease of Bone. Clin. Orthop., **127**:63–69, 1977.

293. Miller, L. F.: Bilateral Stress Fracture of the Neck of the Femur. J. Bone Joint Surg., **32A**:695–697, 1950.

294. Moldawer, M.; Zimmerman, S. J.; and Collins, L. C.: Incidence of Osteoporosis in Elderly Whites and Elderly Negroes. J.A.M.A., **194**:859–862, 1965.

295. Moore, A. T.: Fracture of the Hip Joint (Intracapsular): A New Method of Skeletal Fixation. J. South Carolina Med. Assoc., **30**:199–205, 1934.

296. Moore, A. T.: Fracture of the Hip Joint: A New Method of Treatment. Int. Surg. Digest, **19**:323–330, 1935.

297. Moore, A. T.: Fracture of the Hip Joint: Treatment by Extra-Articular Fixation with Adjustable Nails. Surg. Gynecol. Obstet., **64**:420–436, 1937.

298. Moore, A. T.: Metal Hip Joint: A New Self-Locking Vitallium Prothesis. South Med. J., **45**:1015–1019, 1952.

299. Moore, A. T.: Hip Joint Fracture (A Mechanical Problem) A.A.O.S. Instructional Course Lectures, **10**:35–49; 1953.

300. Moore, A. T.: The Self-Locking Metal Hip Prosthesis. J. Bone Joint Surg., **39A**:811–827, 1957.

301. Moore, A. T., and Böhlman, H. R.: Metal Hip Joint: A Case Report. J. Bone Joint Surg., **25**:688–692, 1943.

302. Moore, A. T., and Green, J. T.: Fractures of the Neck of the Femur Treated by Internal Fixation with Adjustable Nails: End Result Studies. South. Surg., **9**:684–689, 1940.

303. Moore, R. H.; Premer, R. F.; and Gustilo, R. B.: Femoral Neck Fractures. Minn. Med., **56**:358–362, 1973.

304. Morris, J. M., and Blickenstaff, L. P.: Fatigue Fractures. Springfield, Illinois, Charles C. Thomas, 1967.

305. Moskovitz, P. A.; Ellenberg, S. S.; Feffer, H. L.; Kenmore, P. I.; Neviaser, R. J.; Rubin, B. E.; and Varma, V. M.: Low-Dose Heparin for Prevention of Venous Thromboembolism in Total Hip Arthroplasty and Surgical Repair of Hip Fractures. J. Bone Joint Surg., **60A**:1065–1070, 1978.

306. Mulley, G., and Espley, A. J.: Hip Fracture After Hemiplegia. Postgrad. Med. J., **55**:264–265, 1979.

307. Murray, J. A., and Parrish, F. F.: Surgical Management of Secondary Neoplastic Fractures about the Hip. Orthop. Clin. North Am., **5**:887–901, 1974.

308. Müssbichler, H.: Arterial Supply to the Head of the Femur. Acta Radiol. **46**:533–546, 1956.

309. Müssbichler, H.: Arteriographic Findings in Necrosis of the Head of the Femur After Medial Neck Fracture. Acta Orthop. Scand., **41**:77–90, 1970.

310. Müssbichler, H.: Arteriographic Investigation of the Hip In Adult Human Subjects. Acta Orthop. Scand., (Suppl.) **132**:4–39, 1970.

311. Nand, S., and Shukla, R. K.: Fatigue Fracture of the Femoral Neck. Int. Surg., **61**:31–34, 1976.

312. Nicholas, J. A., and Killoran, P.: Fracture of the Femur in Patients with Paget's Disease. J. Bone Joint Surg., **47A**:450–461, 1965.

313. Nicolaysen, J.: Lidt om Diagnosen og Behandlingen af Fractura colli femoris. Nordiskt Med. Arkiv., **8**:1, 1897.

314. Nieminen, S.: Early Weightbearing After Classical Internal Fixation of Medial Fractures of the Femoral Neck. Acta Orthop. Scand., **46**:782–794, 1975.

315. Nilsson, B. E.: Spinal Osteoporosis and Femoral Neck Fracture. Clin. Orthop., **68**:93–95, 1970.

316. Ohman, U.; Björkegren, N.; and Fahlström, G.: Fracture of the Femoral Neck. Acta Chir. Scand., **135**:27–42, 1969.

317. Ornsholt, J., and Espersen, J. O.: Para-Articular Ossifications after Primary Prosthetic Replacement Ad Modum Austin T. Moore. Acta Orthop. Scand., **46**:643–650, 1975.

318. Östrup, L. T.: Fracture of the Femoral Neck in Cases With Coxarthrosis on the Affected Side. Acta Orthop. Scand., **41**:559–564, 1970.

319. Pankovich, A. M.: Primary Internal Fixation of Femoral Neck Fractures. Arch. Surg., **110**:20–26, 1975.

320. Paré, A.: The Work of that Famous Chirurgion, Ambroise Paré. Translated out of Latin and Compared with the French by Tho. Johnson. Book XV, London, T. Cotes and R. Young, 1634.

321. Parrish, F. F., and Murray, J. A.: Surgical Treatment for Secondary Neoplastic Fractures. J. Bone Joint Surg., **52A**:665–686, 1970.

322. Parrish, T. F., and Jones, J. R.: Fracture of the Femur Following Prosthetic Arthroplasty of the Hip. J. Bone Joint Surg., **46A**:241–248, 1964.

323. Patrick, J.: Intracapsular Fractures of the Femur Treated with a Combined Smith-Petersen Nail and Fibular Graft. J. Bone Joint Surg., **31A**:67–80, 1949.

324. Pauwels, F.: Der Schenkenholsbruck, em mechanisches Problem. Grundlagen des Heilungsvorganges. Prognose und kausale Therapie. Stuttgart, Beilageheft zur Zeitschrift fur Orthopaedische Chirurgie, Ferdinand Enke, 1935.

325. Phemister, D. B.: Repair of Bone in the Presence of Aseptic Necrosis Resulting From Fractures, Transplantations, and Vascular Obstruction. J. Bone Joint Surg., **12**:769–787, 1930.

326. Phemister, D. B.: Fractures of the Neck of the Femur, Dislocation of the Hip and Obscure Vascular Disturbances Producing Aseptic Necrosis of the Head of the Femur. Surg. Gynecol. Obstet., **59**:415–440, 1934.

327. Phemister, D. B.: The Pathology of Ununited Fractures of the Neck of the Femur with Special Reference to the Head. J. Bone Joint Surg., **21A**:681–693, 1939.

328. Phemister, D. B.: Treatment of the Necrotic Head of the Femur in Adults. J. Bone Joint Surg., **31A**:55–66, 1949.

329. Phillips, G. W.: Fracture of the Neck of the Femur: Treatment by Means of Extension with Weights, Applied in the Direction of the Axis of Limb, and also Laterally in

Axis of Neck: Recovery without Shortening or Other Deformity. Am. J. Med. Sci., **LVIII:**398–400, 1869.

330. Pierce, R. O., and Powell, S. G.: The Treatment of Fractures of the Hip by Roger Anderson Well-Leg Traction. Clin. Orthop., **151:**165–168, 1980.

331. Polyzoides, A. J.: Prosthetic Replacement after Femoral Neck Fractures (Short and Long-Term Follow-up). Injury, **2:**283–286, 1971.

332. Prather, J. L.; Nusynowitz, M. L.; Snowdy, H. A.; Hughes, A. D.; McCartney, W. H.; and Bagg, R. J.: Scintigraphic Findings in Stress Fractures. J. Bone Joint Surg., **59A:**869–874, 1977.

333. Protzman, R. R., and Burkhalter, W. E.: Femoral-Neck Fractures in Young Adults. J. Bone Joint Surg., **58A:**689–695, 1976.

334. Pugh, W. L.: A Self-Adjusting Nail-Plate for Fractures about the Hip Joint. J. Bone Joint Surg., **37A:**1085–1093, 1955.

335. Radin, E. L.: Biomechanics of the Human Hip. Clin. Orthop., **152:**28–34, 1980.

336. Raine, G. E. T.: A Comparison of Internal Fixation and Prosthetic Replacement for Recent Displaced Subcapital Fractures of the Neck of the Femur. Injury, **5:**25–30, 1973–1974.

337. Rau, F. D.; Manoli, A.; and Morawa, L. G.: Treatment of Femoral Neck Fractures with the Sliding Compression Screw. Clin. Orthop., **163:**137–140, 1982.

338. Ray, R. D.: Viability of Bone. In Proceedings of the Conference on Aseptic Necrosis of the Femoral Head. St. Louis, National Institute of Health, United States Public Health Service, 1964.

339. Ray, R. D., and Sabet, T.: Bone Grafts: Cellular Survival Versus Induction—An Experimental Study in Mice. J. Bone Joint Surg., **45A:**337–344, 1963.

340. Reich, R. S.: Ununited Fracture of the Neck of the Femur Treated by High Oblique Osteotomy. J. Bone Joint Surg., **23:**141–158, 1941.

341. Riley. T. B. H.: Knobs or Screws? A Prospective Trial of Prosthetic Replacement Against Internal Fixation of Subcapital Fractures. J. Bone Joint Surg., **60B:**136, 1978.

342. Riska, E. B.: von Bonsdorff, H.; Hakkinen, S.; Jaroma, H.; Kiviluoto, O.; and Paavilainen, T.: Subcapital Fractures of the Femur Treated with Two Thin Smith-Petersen Nails. Acta Orthop. Scand., **48:**494–498, 1977.

343. Ross, P. M., and Kurtz, N.: Subcapital Fracture Subsequent to Zickel Nail Fixation: A Case Report. Clin. Orthop., **147:**131–133, 1980.

344. Rothermel, J. E., and Garcia, A.: Treatment of Hip Fractures in Patients with Parkinson's Syndrome on Levodopa Therapy. J. Bone Joint Surg., **54A:**1251–1254, 1972.

345. Ruth, C. E.: Fractures of the Femoral Neck and Trochanters. J.A.M.A., **77:**1811–1815, 1921.

346. Ryan, J.R.; Salciccioli, G. C.; and Pederson, H. E.: Deyerle Fixation for Intracapsular Fractures of the Femoral Neck. Clin. Orthop., **144:**178–182, 1979.

347. Rydell, N.: Forces Acting on the Femoral Head-Prosthesis. Acta Orthop. Scand. (Suppl.), **88:**7–132, 1966.

348. Rydell, N.: Biomechanics of the Hip Joint. Clin. Orthop., **92:**6–15, 1973.

349. Salvati, E. A.; Artz, T.; Aglietti, P.; and Asnis, S. E.: Endoprostheses in the Treatment of Femoral Neck Fractures. Orthop. Clin. North Am., **5:**757–777, 1974.

350. Salvati, E. A., and Wilson, P. D.: Long-Term Results of Femoral-Head Replacements. J. Bone Joint Surg., **54A:**1355–1356, 1972.

351. Schatzker, J., and Barrington, T. W.: Fractures of the Femoral Neck Associated with Fractures of the Same Femoral Shaft. Can. J. Surg., **11:**297–305, 1968.

352. Schatzker, J., and Ha'eri, G. B.: Methylmethacrylate as an Adjunct in Internal Fixation of Pathologic Fractures. Canad. J. Surg., **22:**179–182, 1979.

353. Scheck, M.: Intracapsular Fractures of the Femoral Neck. J. Bone Joint Surg., **41A:**1187–1200, 1959.

354. Scheck, M.: Management of Fractures of the Femoral Neck. J. Bone Joint Surg., **47A:**819–829, 1965.

355. Scheck, M.: The Significance of Posterior Comminution in Femoral Neck Fractures. Clin. Orthop., **152:**138–142, 1980.

356. Schmorl, G.: Die pathologische Anatomie der Schenkelhalsfrakturen. Munchen. Med. Wschr., **71:**1381–1385, 1924.

357. Schumpelick, W., and Jantzen, P. M.: A New Principle in the Operative Treatment of Trochanteric Fractures of the Femur. J. Bone Joint Surg., **37A:**693–698, 1955.

358. Senn, N.: Fractures of the Neck of the Femur with Special Reference to Bony Union After Intracapsular Fracture. Trans. Am. Surg., Assoc., **1:**333–441, 1883.

359. Senn, N.: The Treatment of Fractures of the Neck of the Femur by Immediate Reduction and Permanent Fixation. J.A.M.A., **13:**150–159, 1889.

360. Sevitt, S.: Avascular Necrosis and Revascularization of the Femoral Head After Intracapsular Fractures. J. Bone Joint Surg., **46B:**270–296, 1964.

361. Sevitt, S., and Thompson, R. G.: The Distribution and Anastomoses of Arteries Supplying the Head and Neck of the Femur. J. Bone Joint Surg., **47B:**560–573, 1965.

362. Sharma, S., and Sankaran, B.: Primary Replacement Arthroplasty of the Hip in Femoral Neck Fractures: A Study of 145 Cases. Int. Surg., **65:**259–263, 1980.

363. Sherk, H. H.; Snape, W. J.; and Loprete, F. L.: Internal Fixation Versus Nontreatment of Hip Fractures in Senile Patients. Clin. Orthop., **141:**196–198, 1979.

364. Sherman, M. S., and Phemister, D. B.: The Pathology of Ununited Fractures of the Neck of the Femur. J. Bone Joint Surg., **29:**19–40, 1947.

365. Sikorski, J. M., and Barrington, R.: Internal Fixation Versus Hemiarthroplasty for the Displaced Subcapital Fracture of the Femur: A Prospective Randomized Study. J. Bone Joint Surg., **63B:**357–361, 1981.

366. Sim, F. H.: Daugherty, T. W.; and Ivins, J. C.: The Adjunctive Use of Methylmethacrylate in the Fixation of Pathological Fractures. J. Bone Joint Surg., **56A:**40–48, 1974.

367. Sim, F. H., and Stauffer, R. N.: Management of Hip Fractures by Total Hip Arthroplasty. Clin. Orthop., **152:**191–197, 1980.

368. Sim, F. H., and Stauffer, R. N.: Total Hip Arthroplasty in

Acute Femoral Neck Fractures. A.A.O.S. Instructional Course Lectures, **29**:9–16, 1980.

369. Simon, W. H., and Wyman, E. T.: Femoral Neck Fractures: A Study of the Adequacy of Reduction. Clin. Orthop., **70**:152–160, 1970.

370. Singh, M.; Nagrath, A. R.; and Maini, P. S.: Changes in the Trabecular Pattern of the Upper End of the Femur as an Index of Osteoporosis. J. Bone Joint Surg., **52A**:457–467, 1970.

371. Sisk, T. D.: Fractures. *In* Edmonson, A. S., and Crenshaw, A. H. (eds.): Campbell's Operative Orthopaedics. St. Louis, C. V. Mosby, 1980.

372. Smith, F. B.: Effects of Rotary and Valgus Malpositions of Blood Supply to the Femoral Head. J. Bone Joint Surg., **41A**:800–815, 1959.

373. Smith, F. M.: Fracture of the Femoral Neck as a Complication of Pelvic Irradiation. Am. J. Surg., **87**:339–346, 1954.

374. Smith. L. D.: The Role of Muscle Contraction or Intrinsic Forces in the Causation of Fractures of the Femoral Neck. J. Bone Joint Surg., **35A**:367–383, 1953.

375. Smith, R. W.: A Treatise on Fractures in the Vicinity of Joints, p. 111. Dahlin, Hodges and Smith, New York, Samuel S. and William Wood, 1845.

376. Smith-Petersen, M. N.: Treatment of Fractures of the Neck of the Femur by Internal Fixation. Surg. Gynecol. Obstet., **64**:287–295, 1937.

377. Smith-Petersen, M. N.; Cave, E. F.; and Van Gorder, G. W.: Intracapsular Fractures of the Neck of the Femur. Arch. Surg., **23**:715–759, 1931.

378. Smyth, E. H. J., and Shah, V. M.: The Significance of Good Reduction and Fixation in Displaced Subcapital Fractures of the Femur. Injury, **5**:197–209, 1973–1974.

379. Snook, G. A.; Chrisman, O. D.; and Wilson, T. C.: Thromboembolism after Surgical Treatment of Hip Fractures. Clin. Orthop., **155**:21–24, 1981.

380. Solomon, L.: Osteoporosis and Fracture of the Femoral Neck in the South African Bantu. J. Bone Joint Surg., **50B**:2–13, 1968.

381. Soreide, O.; Lerner, A. P.; and Thunold, J.: Primary Prosthetic Replacement in Acute Femoral Neck Fractures. Injury, **6**:286–293, 1974–1975.

382. Soreide, O.; Mölster, A.; and Raugstad, T. S.: Internal Fixation Versus Primary Prosthetic Replacement in Acute Femoral Neck Fractures: A Prospective, Randomized Clinical Study. Br. J. Surg., **66**:56–60, 1979.

383. Soto-Hall, R.: Treatment of Transcervical Fractures Complicated by Certain Common Neurological Conditions. A.A.O.S. Instructional Course Lectures, **17**:117–120, 1960.

384. Soto-Hall, R.; Johnson, L. H.; and Johnson, R.: Alterations in the Intra-Articular Pressure in Transcervical Fractures of the Hip. J. Bone Joint Surg., **45A**:662, 1963.

385. Soto-Hall, R.; Johnson, L. H.; and Johnson, R.: Variations in the Intra-articular Pressure of the Hip Joint in Injury and Disease. J. Bone Joint Surg., **46A**:509–516, 1964.

386. Speed, K.: The Unsolved Fracture. Surg. Gynecol. Obstet., **60**:341–351, 1935.

387. Springfield, D. S., and Enneking, W. J.: Surgery for Aseptic Necrosis of the Femoral Head. Clin. Orthop., **130**:175–185, 1978.

388. St. Clair Strange, F. G.: The Hip. London, William Heinemann Medical Books Limited, 1965.

389. Stampfli, W. P., and Kerr, H. D.: Fractures of the Femoral Neck Following Pelvic Irradiation. Am. J. Roentgenol., **57**:71–83, 1947.

390. Stauffer, R. N., and Sim, F. H.: Total Hip Arthroplasty in Paget's Disease of the Hip. J. Bone Joint Surg., **58A**:476–478, 1976.

391. Stephen, I. B. M.: Subcapital Fractures of the Femur in Rheumatoid Arthritis. Injury, **11**:233–241, 1979–1980.

392. Stephenson, W. H., and Cohen, B.: Post-irradiation Fractures of the Neck of the Femur. J. Bone Joint Surg., **38B**:830–845, 1956.

393. Stevens, J.; Fardin, R.; and Freeark, R. J.: Lower Extremity Thrombophlebitis in Patients with Femoral Neck Fractures: A Venographic Investigation and a Review of the Early and Late Significance of the Findings. J. Trauma, **8**:527–534, 1968.

394. Stevens, J.; Freeman, P. A.; Nordin, B. E. C.; and Barnett, E.: The Incidence of Osteoporosis in Patients with Femoral Neck Fracture. J. Bone Joint Surg., **44B**:520–527, 1962.

395. Stinchfield, F. E.; Cooperman, B.; and Shea, C. E.: Replacement of the Femoral Head by Judet or Austin-Moore Prosthesis. J. Bone Joint Surg., **39A**:1043–1058, 1957.

396. Stott, S.; Gray, D. H.; and Stevenson, W.: The Incidence of Femoral Neck Fractures in New Zealand. N. Zealand Med. J., **91**:6–9, 1980.

397. Stuck, W. G., and Hinchey, J. J.: Experimentally Increased Blood Supply to the Head and Neck of the Femur. Surg. Gynecol. Obstet., **78**:160–163, 1944.

398. Suman, R. K.: Prosthetic Replacement of the Femoral Head for Fractures of the Neck of the Femur: A Comparative Study. Injury, **11**:309–316, 1979–1980.

399. Taton, J., and Lukawska, K.: Fractures of the Neck of the Femur and the Pelvis after X-ray Therapy in Cancer of the Uterus. Pol. Med. J., **12**:965–973, 1968.

400. Telson, D. R., and Ransohoff, N. S.: Treatment of Fractured Neck of the Femur by Axial Fixation with Steel Wires. J. Bone Joint Surg., **17**:727–738, 1935.

401. Thompson, F. R.: Vitallium Intramedullary Hip Prosthesis; Preliminary Report. New York State J. Med., **52**:3011–3020, 1952.

402. Thompson, F. R.: Two and a Half Years' Experience with a Vitallium Intramedullary Hip Prosthesis. J. Bone Joint Surg., **36A**:489–500, 1954.

403. Thornton, L.: The Treatment of Trochanteric Fracture of the Femur: Two New Methods. Piedmont Hosp. Bull., **10**:21–37, 1937.

404. Todd, R. C.; Freeman, M. A. R.; and Pirie, C. J.: Isolated Trabecular Fatigue Fractures of the Femoral Head. J. Bone Joint Surg., **54B**:723–728, 1972.

405. Trenkle, W. A.; Giliberty, R. P.; and Weiss, C. A.: Giliberty Low Friction Multiaxial Endoprosthesis Poster Session, 48th Annual Meeting, Am. Acad. Orthop. Surg., Las Vegas, Nevada, 1981.

406. Tressler, H. A., and Johnson, E. W.: Cited by Sledge, C.

B.: In the Hip, Proceedings of the Fifth Open Scientific Meeting of the Hip Society, p. 124. St. Louis, C. V. Mosby, 1977.

407. Tronzo, R. G.: Hip Nails for All Occasions. Orthop. Clin. North Am., **5**:479–491, 1974.

408. Tronzo, R. G.: Surgery of the Hip Joint. Philadelphia, Lea & Febiger, 1973.

409. Trueta, J.: The Normal Vascular Anatomy of the Human Femoral Head During Growth. J. Bone Joint Surg., **39B**:358–394, 1957.

410. Trueta, J., and Harrison, M. H. M.: The Normal Vascular Anatomy of the Femoral Head in Adult Man. J. Bone Joint Surg., **35B**:442–461, 1953.

411. Tucker, F. R.: Arterial Supply to the Femoral Head and its Clinical Importance. J. Bone Joint Surg., **31B**:82–93, 1949.

412. Urovitz, E. P. M.; Fornasier, V. L.; Risen, M. I.; and NacNab, I.: Etiological Factors in the Pathogenesis of Femoral Trabecular Fatigue Fractures. Clin. Orthop., **127**:275–280, 1977.

413. Vahvanen, V.: Femoral Neck Fracture of the Rheumatoid Hip Joint. Acta Rheum. Scand., **17**:125–136, 1971.

414. Van Audekercke, R.; Martens, M.; Mulier, J. C.; and Stuyck, J.: Experimental Study on Internal Fixation of Femoral Neck Fractures. Clin. Orthop., **141**:203–212, 1979.

415. Venable, C. S., and Stuck, W. G.: A General Consideration of Metals For Buried Appliances in Surgery. Int. Abst. Surg., **76**:297–304, 1943.

416. Venable, C. S., and Stuck, W. G.: Muscle-flap Transplant for Relief of Painful Monarticular Arthritis (Aseptic Necrosis) of Hip. Ann. Surg., **123**:641–655, 1946.

417. Venable, C. S., and Stuck, W. G.: The Internal Fixation of Fractures. Springfield, Illinois, Charles C. Thomas, 1947.

418. Venable, C. S., and Stuck, W. G.: Results of Recent Studies and Experiments Concerning Metals Used In Internal Fixation of Fractures. J. Bone Joint Surg., **30A**:247–250, 1948.

419. Venable, C. S.; Stuck, W. G.; and Beach, A.: The Effects on Bone of the Presence of Metals; Based on Electrolysis. Ann. Surg., **105**:917–938, 1937.

420. Viano, D. C., and Stalnakir, R. L.: Mechanisms of Femoral Fracture. J. Biomech., **13**:701–715, 1980.

421. Virgin, H., and MacAusland, W. R.: A Continuous Traction Screw for Fixation of Fractures of the Hip. Ann. Surg., **122**:59–67, 1945.

422. Von Langenbeck, B.: Verhandl, d. deutsch. p. 92. Gesellsch. f. Chir. 1878.

423. Vose, G. P., and Lockwood, R. M.: Femoral Neck Fracturing: its Relationship to Radiographic Bone Density. J. Gerontol., **20**:300–305, 1965.

424. Walmsley, T.: A Note on the Retinacula of Weitbrecht. J. Anat., **51**:61–64, 1917.

425. Walmsley, T.: The Articular Mechanism of the Diarthroses. J. Bone Joint Surg., **10**:40–45, 1928.

426. Walsh, R. J.: Displaced Stress Fractures of the Neck of the Femur Treated with Bone Grafting. Surg. Gynecol. Obstet., **132**:503–504, 1971.

427. Ward, F. O.: Human Anatomy. London, Renshaw, 1838.

428. Watson-Jones, R.: Fractures and Joint Injuries, 4th ed. Baltimore, Williams & Wilkins, 1955.

429. Weinstein, S. L.: Femoral Neck Fractures: Complications of Internal Fixation. J. Iowa Med. Soc., **65**:17–20, 1975.

430. Weitbrecht, J.: Syndesmologia sive Historia Ligamentorum Corporis Humani guain Seeundum. Observationes Anatomicas Concinnavit et Figuris ad Objecta Reentia Adumbratis Illustravit, pp. 139–141. Petropoli, Typographia Academiae Scientiarum, 1742.

431. Welch, R. B.; Taylor, L. W.; Wynne, G. F.; and White, A. H.: Results with the Cemented Hemiarthroplasty for Displaced Fractures of the Femoral Neck. In the Hip, Proceedings of the Fifth Open Scientific Meeting of the Hip Society, p. 87. St. Louis, C. V. Mosby, 1977.

432. Wertheimer, L. G., and Fernandes Lopes, S. D. L.: Arterial Supply of the Femoral Head. J. Bone Joint Surg., **53A**:545–556, 1971.

433. Westcott, H. H.: A Method for the Internal Fixation of Transcervical Fractures of the Femur. J. Bone Joint Surg., **16**:372–378, 1934.

434. Whitman, R.: A New Method of Treatment for Fractures of the Neck of the Femur, Together with Remarks on Coxa Vara. Ann. Surg., **36**:746–761, 1902.

435. Whitman, R.: The Abduction Method Considered as the Standard Routine in the Treatment of Fractures of the Neck of the Femur. J. Orthop. Surg., **2**:547–553, 1920.

436. Whitman, R.: The Abduction Method Considered as the Exponent of a Treatment for all Forms of Fracture at the Hip in Accord with Surgical Principles. Am. J. Surg., **21**:335–344, 1933.

437. Whittaker, R. P.; Abeshaus, M. M.; Scholl, H. W.; and Chung, S. M. K.: Fifteen Years' Experience With Metallic Endoprosthetic Replacement of the Femoral Head for Femoral Neck Fractures. J. Trauma, **12**:799–806, 1972.

438. Whittaker, R. P.; Sotos, L. N.; and Ralston, E. L.: Fractures of the Femur About Femoral Endoprostheses. J. Trauma., **14**:675–694, 1974.

439. Wilkie, D. P. D.: The Treatment of Fracture of the Neck of the Femur. Surg. Gynecol. Obstet., **44**:529–530, 1927.

440. Wolcott, W. E.: Circulation of the Head and Neck of the Femur. J.A.M.A., **100**:27–34, 1933.

441. Wolcott, W. E.: The Evolution of the Circulation in the Developing Femoral Head and Neck. Surg. Gynecol. Obstet., **77**:61–68, 1943.

442. Wolfgang, G. L.: Stress Fracture of the Femoral Neck in a Patient with Open Capital Femoral Epiphyses. J. Bone Joint Surg., **59A**:680–681, 1977.

443. Wood, M. R.: Femoral Head Replacement Following Fracture: An Analysis of the Surgical Approach. Injury, **11**:317–320, 1979–1980.

444. Woodhouse, C. F.: An Instrument for the Measurement of Oxygen Tension in Bone. J. Bone Joint Surg., **43A**:819–828, 1961.

445. Wrighton, J. D., and Woodyard, J. E.: Prosthetic Replacement for Subcapital Fractures of the Femur: A Comparative Survey. Injury, **2**:287–293, 1971.

446. Zeckert, F.; Khon, P.; and Vormittag, E.: Prophylaxis of Thromboembolic Diseases in Traumatological Patients. A Randomized Double Blind Study with Acetylsalicylic

Acid, p. 281. In Fourth International Congress on Thrombosis and Hemostasis, Vienna, 1973.

447. Zetterberg, C.; Irstam, L.; and Anderson, G. B. J.: Subcapital Fractures of the Femur. Acta Orthop. Scand., 50:451–455, 1979.

448. Zolczer, L.; Kazár, G.; Manninger, J.; and Nagy, E.: Fractures of the Femoral Neck in Adolescence. Injury, 4:41–46, 1972–1973.

Intertrochanteric Fractures

449. Alffram, P. A.: An Epidemiologic Study of Cervical and Trochanteric Fractures of the Femur in the Urban Population. Acta Orthop. Scand. (Suppl.) 65:1–109, 1964.

450. Anderson, R., and McKibbin, W. B.: Intertrochanteric Fractures. J. Bone Joint Surg., 25:153–168, 1943.

451. Anderson, R. A.: A New Method for Treating Fractures, Utilizing the Well Leg for Countertraction. Surg. Gynecol. Obstet., 54:207–219, 1932.

452. Aprin, H., and Kilfoyle, R. M.: Treatment of Trochanteric Fractures with Ender Rods. J. Trauma, 20:32–42, 1980.

453. Aufranc, O. E.; Jones, W. N.; and Turner, R. H.: Severely Comminuted Intertrochanteric Hip Fracture. J.A.M.A., 199:140–143, 1967.

454. Baker, D. M.: Fractures of the Femoral Neck After Healed Intertrochanteric Fractures: A Complication of too Short a Nail Plate Fixation. J. Trauma, 15:73–81, 1975.

455. Baker, H. R.: Ununited Intertrochanteric Fractures of the Femur. Clin Orthop., 18:209–219, 1960.

456. Barr, J. S.: Diagnosis and Treatment of Infections Following Internal Fixation of Hip Fractures. Orthop. Clin. North Am., 5:847–864, 1974.

457. Bartels, W. P.: The Treatment of Intertrochanteric Fractures. J. Bone Joint Surg., 21:773–775, 1939.

458. Boyd, H. B., and Anderson, L. D.: Management of Unstable Trochanteric Fractures. Surg. Gynecol. Obstet., 112:633–638, 1961.

459. Boyd, H. B., and Griffin, L. L.: Classification and Treatment of Trochanteric Fractures. Arch. Surg., 58:853–866, 1949.

460. Boyd, R. J.; Burke; J. F.; and Colton, T.: A Double Blind Clinical Trial of Prophylactic Antibiotics in Hip Fractures. J. Bone Joint Surg., 55A:1251–1258, 1973.

461. Bremner, R. A., and Jelliffe, A. M.: The Management of Pathological Fracture of the Major Long Bones From Metastatic Cancer. J. Bone Joint Surg., 40B:652–659, 1958.

462. Burnett, J. W.; Gustilo, R. B.; Williams, D. N.; and Kind, A. C.: Prophylactic Antibiotics in Hip Fractures. J. Bone Joint Surg., 62A:457–461, 1980.

463. Cameron, H. U., and Graham, J. D.: Retention of the Compression Screw in Sliding Screw Plate Devices. Clin. Orthop., 146:219–221, 1980.

464. Cameron, H. U.; Pilliar, R. M.; Hastings, D. E.; and Fornasier, V. L.: Iatrogenic Subcapital Fracture of the Hip. Clin. Orthop., 112:218–220, 1975.

465. Chapman, M. W.; Bowman, W. E.; Csongradi, J. J.; Day, L. J.; Trafton, P. G.; and Bovill, E. G.: The Use of Ender's Pins in Extracapsular Fractures of the Hip. J. Bone Joint Surg., 63A:14–28, 1981.

466. Childress, H. M: Well Leg Traction: An Efficient But Neglected Procedure. Clin. Orthop., 51:127–136, 1967.

467. Claffey, T. J.: Avascular Necrosis of the Femoral Head. J. Bone Joint Surg., 42B:802–809, 1960.

468. Clawson, D. K.: Intertrochanteric Fracture of the Hip. Am. J. Surg., 93:580–587, 1957.

469. Clawson, D. K.: Trochanteric Fractures Treated by the Sliding Screw Plate Fixation Method. J. Trauma, 4:737–756, 1964.

470. Cleveland, M.; Bosworth, D. M.; and Thompson, F. R.: Intertrochanteric Fractures of the Femur. J. Bone Joint Surg., 29:1049–1067, 1947.

471. Cleveland, M.; Bosworth, D. M.; and Thompson, F. R.: Management of the Trochanteric Fracture of the Femur. J.A.M.A., 137:1186–1190, 1948.

472. Cleveland, M.; Bosworth, D. M.; Thompson, F. R.; Wilson, H. J.; and Ishizuka, T.: A Ten Year Analysis of Intertrochanteric Fractures of the Femur. J. Bone Joint Surg., 41A:1399–1408, 1959.

473. Conrad, J. J.: Medial Displacement Fixation of Unstable Intertrochanteric Fractures of the Hip. Bull. Hosp. Joint Dis., 32:54–62, 1971.

474. Coran, A. G.; Banks, H. H.; Aliapoulios, M. A.; and Wilson, R. E.: The Management of Pathologic Fractures in Patients with Metastatic Carcinoma of the Breast. Surg. Gynecol. Obstet., 127:1225–1230, 1968.

475. Coughlin, L., and Templeton, J.: Hip Fractures in Patients with Parkinson's Disease. Clin. Orthop., 148:192–195, 1980.

476. Cram, R. H.: The Unstable Intertrochanteric Fracture. Surg. Gynecol. Obstet., 101:15–19, 1955.

477. Dahl, E.: Mortality and Life Expectancy After Hip Fractures. Acta Orthop. Scand., 51:163–170, 1980.

478. Davis, P. H., and Frymoyer, J. W.: The Lateral Position in the Surgical Management of Intertrochanteric and Subtrochanteric Fractures of the Femur. J. Bone Joint Surg., 51A:1128–1134, 1969.

479. Deyerle, W. M.:Surgical Impaction over a Plate and Multiple Pins for Intertrochanteric Fractures. Orthop. Clin. North Am., 5:615–628, 1974.

480. Dimon, J. H.: The Unstable Intertrochanteric Fracture. Clin. Orthop., 92:100–107, 1973.

481. Dimon, J. H., and Hughston, J. C.: Unstable Intertrochanteric Fractures of the Hip. J. Bone Joint Surg., 49A:440–450, 1967.

482. Doherty, J. H., and Lyden, J. P.: Intertrochanteric Fractures of the Hip Treated with the Hip Compression Screw. Clin. Orthop., 141:184–187, 1979.

483. Doppelt, S. H.: The Sliding Compression Screw: Today's Best Answer for Stabilization of Intertrochanteric Hip Fractures. Orthop. Clin. North Am., 11:507–523, 1980.

484. Dove, J.: Complete Fractures of the Femur in Paget's Disease of Bone. J. Bone Joint Surg., 62B:12–17, 1980.

485. Dunn, E. J., and Skinner, S. R.: Disengagement of a Sliding Screw Plate. J. Bone Joint Surg., 58A:1027–1028, 1976.

486. Ecker, M. L.; Joyce, J. J.; and Kohl, E. J.: The Treatment of Trochanteric Hip Fractures using a Compression Screw. J. Bone Joint Surg., 57A:23–27, 1975.

487. Evans, E. M.: The Treatment of Trochanteric Fractures of the Femur. J. Bone Joint Surg., **31B:**190–203, 1949.

488. Evans, E. M.: Trochanteric Fractures. J. Bone Joint Surg., **33B:**192–204, 1951.

489. Frankel, V. H.: Mechanical Fixation of Unstable Fractures About the Proximal End of the Femur. Bull. Hosp. Joint Dis., **24:**75–84, 1963.

490. Friedenberg, Z. B.; Gentchos, E.; and Rutt, C.: Fixation in Intertrochanteric Fractures of the Hip. Surg. Gynecol. Obstet., **135:**225–228, 1972.

491. Ganz, R.; Thomas, R. J.; and Hammerle, C. P.: Trochanteric Fractures of the Femur: Treatment and Results. Clin. Orthop., **138:**30–40, 1979.

492. Greider, J. L., and Horowitz, M.: Clinical Evaluation of the Sliding Compression Screw in 121 Hip Fractures. South. Med. J., **73:**1343–1348, 1980.

493. Harrington, K. D.: The use of Methylmethacrylate as an Adjunct in the Internal Fixation of Unstable Comminuted Intertrochanteric Fractures in Osteoporotic Patients. J. Bone Joint Surg., **57A:**744–750, 1975.

494. Harrington, K. D., and Johnston, J. O.: The Management of Comminuted Unstable Intertrochanteric Fractures. J. Bone Joint Surg., **55A:**1367–1376, 1973.

495. Harrington, K. D.; Johnston, J. O.; Turner, R. H.; and Green, D. L.: The use of Methylmethacrylate as an Adjunct in the Internal Fixation of Malignant Neoplastic Fractures. J. Bone Joint Surg., **54A:**1665–1676, 1972.

496. Harris, L. J.: Closed Retrograde Intramedullary Nailing of Peritrochanteric Fractures of the Femur with a New Nail. J. Bone Joint Surg., **62A:**1185–1193, 1980.

497. Hodkinson, H. M.: Fracture of the Femur as a Presentation of Osteomalacia. Geront. Clin., **13:**189–191, 1971.

498. Holland, W. R.; Weiss, A. B.; and Daniel, W. W.: Medial Displacement Osteotomy for Unstable Intertrochanteric Femoral Fractures. South. Med. J., **70:**576–578, 1977.

499. Holt, E. P.: Hip Fractures in the Trochanteric Region: Treatment with a Strong Nail and Early Weight-Bearing. J. Bone Joint Surg., **45A:**687–705, 1963.

500. Hughston, J. C.: Unstable Intertrochanteric Fractures of the Hip. J. Bone Joint Surg., **46A:**1145, 1964.

501. Hunter, G. A.: The Results of Operative Treatment of Trochanteric Fractures of the Femur. Injury, **6:**202–205, 1974–1975.

502. Inman, V. T.: Functional Aspects of the Abductor Muscles of the Hip. J. Bone Joint Surg., **29A:**607–619, 1947.

503. Jacobs, R. R.; Armstrong, H. J.; Whitaker, J. H.; and Pazell, J.: Treatment of Intertrochanteric Hip Fractures with a Compression Hip Screw and a Nail Plate. J. Trauma, **16:**599–603, 1976.

504. Jacobs, R. R., and McClain, O.: *In Vitro* Strain Patterns in "Intertrochanteric Fractures" Internally Fixed With Nail-Plate or Compression Screw-Plate. Surg. Forum, **27:**511–514, 1976.

505. Jacobs, R. R.; McClain, O.; and Armstrong, H. J.: Internal Fixation of Intertrochanteric Hip Fractures: A Clinical and Biomechanical Study. Clin. Orthop., **146:**62–70, 1980.

506. Jensen, J. S.: Mechanical Strength of Sliding Screw-Plate Hip Implants. Acta Orthop. Scand., **51:**625–632, 1980.

507. Jensen, J. S.: Classification of Trochanteric Fractures. Acta Orthop. Scand., **51:**803–810, 1980.

508. Jensen, J. S.: Trochanteric Fractures. Acta Orthop. Scand. (Suppl.), **188:**1–100, 1981.

509. Jensen, J. S., and Sonne-Holm, S.: Critical Analysis of Ender Nailing in the Treatment of Trochanteric Fractures. Acta Orthop. Scand., **51:**817–825, 1980.

510. Jensen, J. S.; Sonne-Holm, S.; and Tondevold, E.: Unstable Trochanteric Fractures: A Comparative Analysis of Four Methods of Internal Fixation. Acta Orthop. Scand., **51:**949–962, 1980.

511. Jensen, J. S.; Tondevold, E.; and Sonne-Holm, S.: Stable Trochanteric Fractures: A Comparative Analysis of Four Methods of Internal Fixation. Acta Orthop. Scand., **51:**811–816, 1980.

512. Jewett, E. L.: One-Piece Angle Nail for Trochanteric Fractures. J. Bone Joint Surg., **23:**803–810, 1941.

513. Johnson, L. L.; Lottes, J. O.; and Arnot, J. P.: The Utilization of the Holt Nail for Proximal Femoral Fractures. J. Bone Joint Surg., **50A:**67–78, 1968.

514. Jones, J. B.: Screw Fixation of the Lesser Trochanteric Fragment. Clin. Orthop., **123:**107, 1977.

515. Kaufer, H.: Mechanics of the Treatment of Hip Injuries. Clin. Orthop., **146:**53–61, 1980.

516. Kaufer, H.; Matthews, L. S.; and Sonstegard, D.: Stable Fixation of Intertrochanteric Fractures. J. Bone Joint Surg., **56A:**899–907, 1974.

517. Key, J. A.: Internal Fixation of Trochanteric Fractures of the Femur. Surgery, **6:**13–23, 1939.

518. Kolind-Sorensen, V.: Comminuted Intertrochanteric Fracture of the Femoral Neck. Acta Orthop. Scand., **46:**651–653, 1975.

519. Kuderna, H.; Böhler, N.; and Collon, D. J.: Treatment of Intertrochanteric and Subtrochanteric Fractures of the Hip by the Ender Method. J. Bone Joint Surg., **58A:**604–611, 1976.

520. Kumar, V.: The Syndrome of the Fracture of the Lesser Trochanter in Adults: A Neglected Aspect of the Trochanteric Fracture. Injury, **4:**327–334, 1972–1973.

521. Kyle, R. F.; Gustilo, R. B.; and Premer, R. F.: Analysis of Six Hundred and Twenty-two Intertrochanteric Hip Fractures. J. Bone Joint Surg., **61A:**216–221, 1979.

522. Kyle, R. F.; Wright, T. M.; and Burstein, A. H.: Biomechanical Analysis of the Sliding Characteristics of Compression Hip Screws. J. Bone Joint Surg., **62A:**1308–1314, 1980.

523. Laros, G. S.: The Role of Osteoporosis in Intertrochanteric Fractures. Orthop. Clin. North Am., **11:**525–537, 1980.

524. Laros, G. S., and Moore, J. F.: Complications of Fixation in Intertrochanteric Fractures. Clin. Orthop., **101:**110–119, 1974.

525. Laskin, R. S.; Gruber, M. A.; and Zimmerman, A. J.: Intertrochanteric Fractures of the Hip in the Elderly: A Retrospective Analysis of 236 Cases. Clin. Orthop., **141:**188–195, 1979.

526. Leydig, S. M., and Brookes, T. P.: Treatment of Pertrochanteric Fracture of the Femur with a Lag Bolt. J. Missouri Med. Assoc., **37:**354–357, 1940.

527. Lowell, J. D.: Fractures of the Hip. N. Engl. J. Med., **274:**1418–1425, 1966.

528. Lowell, J. D.: Fractures of the Hip (Concluded). N. Engl. J. Med., **274:**1480–1490, 1966.

529. Malerich, M. M.; Laros, G. S.; Wade, T.; and Yamada, R.: Four Fragment Intertrochanteric Hip Fractures: A Biomechanical Study. Trans. Orthop. Res. Soc., **2:**242, 1977.

530. Mann, R. J.: Avascular Necrosis of the Femoral Head Following Intertrochanteric Fractures. Clin. Orthop., **92:**108–115, 1973.

531. Marcove, R. C., and Yang, D. J.: Survival Times After Treatment of Pathologic Fractures. Cancer, **20:**2154–2158, 1967.

532. Martinek, H.; Egkher, E.; Wielke, B.; and Spangler, H.: Experimental Tests Concerning the Biomechanical Behaviour of Pertrochanteric Osteosyntheses. Acta Orthop. Scand., **50:**675–679, 1979.

533. Massie, W. K.: Extracapsular Fractures of the Hip Treated by Impaction Using a Sliding Nail-Plate Fixation. Clin. Orthop., **22:**180–202, 1962.

534. Massie, W. K.: Fractures of the Hip. J. Bone Joint Surg., **46A:**658–690, 1964.

535. May, J. M. B., and Chacha, P. B.: Displacements of Trochanteric Fractures and Their Influence on Reduction. J. Bone Joint Surg., **50B:**318–323, 1968.

536. McNeill, D. H.: Hip Fractures: Influence of Delay in Surgery on Mortality. Wis. Med. J., **74:**129–130, 1975.

537. Meyn, M. A.; Hopson, C.; and Jayasankar, S.: Fractures of the Hip in the Institutionalized Psychotic Patient. Clin. Orthop., **122:**128–134, 1977.

538. Moore, M.: Treatment of Trochanteric Femoral Fractures with Special Reference to Complications. Am. J. Surg., **84:**449–452, 1952.

539. Morris, H. D.: Trochanteric Fractures. South. Med. J., **34:**571–578, 1941.

540. Morrison, D.; Mrstik, L. L.; and Weingarden, T. L.: Management of Unstable Intertrochanteric Fractures of the Hip. J. Am. Osteopath. Assoc., **77:**793–802, 1978.

541. Muhr, G.; Tscherne, H.; and Thomas, R.: Comminuted Trochanteric Femoral Fractures in Geriatric Patients: The Results of 231 Cases with Internal Fixation and Acrylic Cement. Clin. Orthop., **138:**41–44, 1979.

542. Mulholland, R. C., and Gunn, D. R.: Sliding Screw Plate Fixation of Intertrochanteric Femoral Fractures. J. Trauma, **12:**581–591, 1972.

543. Mulley, G., and Espley, A. J.: Hip Fracture After Hemiplegia. Postgrad. Med. J., **55:**264–265, 1979.

544. Murray, R. C., and Frew, J. F. M.: Trochanteric Fractures of the Femur. J. Bone Joint Surg., **31B:**204–219, 1949.

545. Müssbichler, H.: Arterial Supply of the Head of the Femur. Acta Radiol. Scand., **46:**533–546, 1956.

546. Naiman, P. T.; Schein, A. J.; and Siffert, R. S.: Medial Displacement Fixation for Severely Comminuted Intertrochanteric Fractures. Clin. Orthop., **62:**151–155, 1969.

547. Neimann, K. M. W., and Mankin, H. J.: Fractures about the Hip in an Institutionalized Patient Population. II. Survival and Ability to Walk Again. J. Bone Joint Surg., **50A:**1327–1340, 1968.

548. Norton, P. L.: Intertrochanteric Fractures. Clin. Orthop., **66:**77–81, 1969.

549. Olerud, S.; Stark, A.; and Gilström, P.: Malrotation Following Ender Nailing. Clin. Orthop., **147:**139–142, 1980.

550. Pandey, S.: A Modified Conservative Treatment of Trochanteric Fractures. Int. Surg., **53:**201–205, 1970.

551. Pankovich, A. M., and Tarabishy, I. E.: Ender Nailing of Intertrochanteric and Subtrochanteric Fractures of the Femur. J. Bone Joint Surg., **62A:**635–645, 1980.

552. Petersen, C. A.; Pasternak, H. S.; and Kraus, H.: Use of 150 Degree Nail Plate Combination in Intertrochanteric Fractures of the Hip. J. Trauma, **14:**236–241, 1974.

553. Pinder, R. C.; Durnin, C. W.; and Cook, D. A.: The Leinbach Prosthesis in the Treatment of Complex Intertrochanteric Fractures. Paper presented at A.A.O.S. Meeting, Las Vegas, March, 1981.

554. Pugh, W. L.: A Self-Adjusting Nail-Plate for Fractures about the Hip Joint. J. Bone Joint Surg., **37A:**1085–1093, 1955.

555. Raugstad, T. S.; Molster, A.; Haukeland, W.; Hestenes, O.; and Olerud, S.: Treatment of Pertrochanteric and Subtrochanteric Fractures of the Femur by the Ender Method. Clin. Orthop., **138:**231–237, 1979.

556. Rennie, W., and Mitchell, N.: Compression Fixation of Peritrochanteric Fractures and Early Weight Bearing. Clin. Orthop., **121:**157–162, 1976.

557. Richmond, J. C.; Kazes, J. A.; and MacAusland, W. R.: An Evaluation of Three Current Techniques of Internal Fixation for Intertrochanteric and Subtrochanteric Fractures of the Hip. Orthopaedics, **4:**895–898, 1981.

558. Ring, P. A.: Treatment of Trochanteric Fractures of the Femur. Br. Med. J., **1:**654–656, 1963.

559. Riska, E. B.: Trochanteric Fractures of the Femur. Acta Orthop. Scand., **42:**268–280, 1971.

560. Roberts, A.; Rooney, T.; Loupe, J.; Roberts, F.; and Wickstrom, J.: A Comparison of the Functional Results of Anatomic and Medial Displacement Valgus Nailing of Intertrochanteric Fractures of the Femur. J. Trauma, **12:**341–346, 1972.

561. Rosenfeld, R. T.; Schwartz, D. R.; and Alter, A. H.: Prosthetic Replacement for Trochanteric Fractures of the Femur. J. Bone Joint Surg., **55A:**420, 1973.

562. Rothermel, J. E., and Garcia, A.: Treatment of Hip Fractures in Patients with Parkinson's Syndrome on Levodopa Therapy. J. Bone Joint Surg., **54A:**1251–1254, 1972.

563. Rowe, C. R.: The Management of Fractures in Elderly Patients is Different. J. Bone Joint Surg., **47A:**1043–1059, 1965.

564. Russin, L. A., and Sonni, A.: Treatment of Intertrochanteric and Subtrochanteric Fractures with Ender's Intramedullary Rods. Clin. Orthop., **148:**203–212, 1980.

565. Sahlstrand, T.: The Richards Compression and Sliding Hip Screw System in the Treatment of Intertrochanteric Fractures. Acta Orthop. Scand., **45:**213–219, 1974.

566. Sarmiento, A.: Intertrochanteric Fractures of the Femur: 150-Degree-Angle Nail-Plate Fixation and Early Rehabilitation: A Preliminary Report of 100 Cases. J. Bone Joint Surg., **45A:**706–722, 1963.

567. Sarmiento, A.: Avoidance of Complications of Internal Fixation of Intertrochanteric Fractures. Clin. Orthop., **53:**47–59, 1967.

568. Sarmiento, A.: Unstable Intertrochanteric Fractures of the Femur. Clin. Orthop., **92:**77–85, 1973.

569. Sarmiento, A., and Williams, E. M.: The Unstable Intertrochanteric Fracture: Treatment with a Valgus Osteotomy

and I-Beam Nail-Plate. J. Bone Joint Surg., **52A**:1309–1318, 1970.

570. Schneider, M.: Hip Fractures in Elderly Patients. J.A.M.A., **239**:106–107, 1978.

571. Schultz, R. J.: The Lesser Trochanter as a Guide for the Operative Fixation of Hip Fractures. Orthop. Clin. North Am., **5**:529–532, 1974.

572. Schumpelick, W., and Jantzen, P. M.: A New Principle in the Operative Treatment of Trochanteric Fractures of the Femur. J. Bone Joint Surg., **37A**:693–698, 1955.

573. Shaftan, G. W.; Herbsman, H.; and Pavlides, C.: Selective Conservatism in Hip Fractures. Surgery, **61**:524–527, 1967.

574. Sherk, H. H.; Crouse, F. R.; and Probst, C.: The Treatment of Hip Fractures in Institutionalized Patients. Orthop. Clin. North Am., **5**:543–550, 1974.

575. Siler, V. E., and Caldwell, J. A.: Treatment of Intertrochanteric Fractures of the Femur by Modification of Russell Balanced Traction. Am. J. Surg., **47**:431–442, 1940.

576. Singh, M.; Nagrath, A. R.; and Maini, P. S.: Changes in Trabecular Pattern of the Upper End of the Femur as an Index of Osteoporosis. J. Bone Joint Surg., **52A**:457–467, 1970.

577. Speed, K.: Treatment of Fracture of the Femur. Arch. Surg., **2**:45–91, 1921.

578. Stern, M. B., and Goldstein, T. B.: The use of the Leinbach Prosthesis in Intertrochanteric Fractures of the Hip. Clin. Orthop., **128**:325–331, 1977.

579. Stevens, D. B.: Method of Operative Treatment for Intertrochanteric Fractures of the Femur. Curr. Pract. Orthop. Surg., **7**:56–77, 1977.

580. Stover, C. N.; Fish, J. B.; and Heap, W. R.: Open Reduction of Trochanteric Fracture. N. Y. State J. Med., **71**:2173–2181, 1971.

581. Taylor, G. M.; Neufeld, A. J.; and Nickel, V. L.: Complications and Failures in the Operative Treatment of Intertrochanteric Fractures of the Femur. J. Bone Joint Surg., **37A**:306–316, 1955.

582. Tengve, B., and Kjellander, J.: Antibiotic Prophylaxis in Operations on Trochanteric Femoral Fractures. J. Bone Joint Surg., **60A**:97–99, 1978.

583. Thornton, L.: The Treatment of Trochanteric Fractures of the Femur: Two New Methods. Piedmont Hosp. Bull., **10**:21, 1937.

584. Tronzo, R. G.: Hip Nails for All Occasions. Orthop. Clin. North Am., **5**:479–491, 1974.

585. Tronzo, R. G.: Use of an Extramedullary Guide Pin for Fractures of the Upper End of the Femur. Orthop. Clin. North Am., **5**:525–527, 1974.

586. Tronzo, R. G.: Special Considerations in Management. Orthop. Clin. North Am., **5**:571–583, 1974.

587. Wardle, E. N.: The Prevention of Deformity in Intertrochanteric Fractures of the Femur. Postgrad. Med. J., **43**:385–399, 1967.

588. Weeden, R.; Rosenthal, H.; and Miller, P.: Mortality Statistics on Fractured Hips (1935–1955). J. Bone Joint Surg., **39A**:1218, 1957.

589. Weiss, N. S.; Ure, C. L.; Ballard, J. H.; Williams, A. R.; and Daling, J. R.: Decreased Risk of Fractures of the Hip and Lower Forearm with Postmenopausal use of Estrogen. N. Engl. J. Med., **303**:1195–1198, 1980.

590. Weissman, S. L., and Salama, R.: Trochanteric Fractures of the Femur. Clin. Orthop., **67**:143–150, 1969.

591. Wilson, H. J.; Rubin, B. D.; Helbig, F. E. J.; Fielding, J. W.; and Unis, G. L.: Treatment of Intertrochanteric Fractures with Jewett Nail: Experience with 1,015 Cases. Clin. Orthop., **148**:186–191, 1980.

592. Wolfgang, G. L.; Bryant, M. H.; and O'Neill, J. P.: Treatment of Intertrochanteric Fracture of the Femur Using Sliding Screw Plate Fixation. Clin. Orthop., **163**:148–158, 1982.

593. Wright, L. T.: Oblique Subcervical (Reverse Intertrochanteric) Fractures of the Femur. J. Bone Joint Surg., **29**:707–710, 1947.

Isolated Trochanteric Fractures

594. Armstrong, G. E.: Isolated Fracture of the Great Trochanter. Ann. Surg., **46**:292–297, 1907.

595. Eikenbary, C. F.: Avulsion or Fracture of the Lesser Trochanter. J. Orthop. Surg., **3**:464–468, 1921.

596. Hamsa, W. R.: Epiphyseal Injuries About the Hip Joint. Clin. Orthop., **10**:119–124, 1957.

597. Howard, F. M., and Piha, R. J.: Fractures of the Apophyses in Adolescent Athletes. J.A.M.A., **192**:150–152, 1965.

598. Kewenter, Y.: A Case of Isolated Fracture of the Lesser Trochanter. Acta Orthop. Scand., **2**:160–165, 1931.

599. Merlino, A. F., and Nixon, J. E.: Isolated Fractures of the Greater Trochanter. Int. Surg., **52**:117–124, 1969.

600. Milch, H.: Avulsion Fracture of the Great Trochanter. Arch. Surg., **38**:334–350, 1939.

601. Milgram, J. E.: Muscle Ruptures and Avulsions with Particular Reference to the Lower Extremities. A.A.O.S. Instructional Course Lectures, **10**:233–243, 1953.

602. Poston, H.: Traction Fracture of the Lesser Trochanter of the Femur. Br. J. Surg., **9**:256–258, 1921–1922.

603. Ratzan, M. C.: Isolated Fracture of the Greater Trochanter of the Femur. J. Int. Coll. Surg., **29**:359–363, 1958.

604. Rigamonti, L.: Four Cases of Isolated Fractues of the Greater Trochanter. Archivio. Di. Ortopedia (Milano), **71**:107–113, 1958.

605. Sweetman, R. J.: Avulsion Fracture of the Lesser Trochanter. Nurs. Times, **68**:122–123, 1972.

606. Watson-Jones, R.: Fractures and Joint Injuries, Vol. 2, 4th ed., pp. 653–654. Edinburgh, E&S Livingstone, 1955.

Subtrochanteric Fractures

607. Allis, O. H.: Fracture of the Upper Third of the Femur Exclusive of the Neck. Med. News, **59**:585–590, 1891.

608. Anderson, R.; McKibbin, W. B.; and Burgess, E.: Intertrochanteric Fractures. J. Bone Joint Surg., **25**:153–168, 1943.

609. Aronoff, P. M.; Davis, P. M.; and Wickstrom, J. K.: Intramedullary Nail Fixation as Treatment of Subtrochanteric Fractures of the Femur. J. Trauma, **11**:637–650, 1971.

610. Aronoff, P. M.; Davis, P. M.; and Wickstrom, J. K.: Subtrochanteric Fractures of the Femur Treated by Intra-

medullary Nail Fixation. South. Med. J., **65**:147–153, 1972.

611. Ashby, M. E., and Anderson, J. C.: The Use of the Zickel Device for a Malunited Subtrochanteric Femur Fracture. J. Nat. Med. Assoc., **69**:623–624, 1977.

612. Asher, M. A.: Tippett, J. W.; Rockwood, C. A.; and Zilber, S.: Compression Fixation of Subtrochanteric Fractures. Clin. Orthop., 117:202–207, 1976.

613. Baker, H. R.: Ununited Intertrochanteric Fractures of the Femur. Clin. Orthop., **18**:209–220, 1960.

614. Beaver, R. H., and Bach, P. J.: Zickel Nail: A Retrospective Study of Subtrochanteric Fractures. South Med. J., **71**:146–149, 1978.

615. Berman, A. T.; Metzger, P. C.; Bosacco, S. J.; Symanowicz, D. B.; and Cesare, J. G.: Treatment of the Subtrochanteric Fracture with the Compression Hip Nail: A Review of Thirty-eight Consecutive Cases. Orthop. Trans., **3**:255–256, 1979.

616. Boyd, H. B., and Anderson, L. D.: Management of Unstable Trochanteric Fractures. Surg. Gynecol. Obstet., **112**:633–638, 1961.

617. Boyd, H. B., and Griffin, L. L.: Classification and Treatment of Trochanteric Fractures. Arch. Surg., **58**:853–866, 1949.

618. Boyd, H. B., and Lipinski, S. W.: Nonunion of Trochanteric and Subtrochanteric Fractures. Surg. Gynecol. Obstet., **104**:463–470, 1957.

619. Campbell, R. D.: The Problem of Subtrochanteric Fractures of the Femur. J. Trauma, **11**:719–720, 1971.

620. Cech, O., and Sosna, A.: Principles of the Surgical Treatment of Subtrochanteric Fractures. Orthop. Clin. North Am., **5**:651–662, 1974.

621. Chalmers, J.: Subtrochanteric Fractures in Osteomalacia. J. Bone Joint Surg., **52B**:509–513, 1970.

622. Chalmers, J.; Conacher, W. D. H.; Gardner, D. L.; and Scott, P. J.: Osteomalacia: A Common Disease in Elderly Women. J. Bone Joint Surg., **49B**:403–423, 1967.

623. Clawson, D. K.: Trochanteric Fractures Treated by the Sliding Screw-Plate Fixation Method. J. Trauma, **4**:737–752, 1964.

624. Clawson, D. K.; Smith, R. F.; and Hansen, S. T.: Closed Intramedullary Nailing of the Femur. J. Bone Joint Surg., **53A**:681–692, 1971.

625. Cleveland, M.; Bosworth, D. M.; and Thompson, F. R.: Intertrochanteric Fractures of the Femur. J. Bone Joint Surg., **29**:1049–1067, 1947.

626. Connolly, J. F.; Dehne, E.; and LaFollette, B.: Closed Reduction and Early Cast-Brace Ambulation in the Treatment of Femoral Fractures. J. Bone Joint Surg., **55A**:1581–1599, 1973.

627. Connolly, J. F.; King, P.; and Dehne, E.: *In Vivo* Measurements of Femoral-Fracture Immobilization with Early Weightbearing. J. Bone Joint Surg., **54A**:1127–1128, 1973.

628. Cuthbert, H., and Howat, T. W.: The use of the Küntscher Y Nail in the Treatment of Intertrochanteric and Subtrochanteric Fractures of the Femur. Injury, **8**:135–142, 1976.

629. DeLee, J. C.; Clanton, T. O.; and Rockwood, C. A.: Closed Treatment of Subtrochanteric Fractures of the Femur in a Modified Cast-Brace. J. Bone Joint Surg., **63A**:773–779, 1981.

630. Dencker, H.: Shaft Fractures of the Femur: A Comparative Study of the Results of Various Methods of Treatment in 1,003 Cases. Acta Chir. Scand., **130**:173–184, 1965.

631. Dimon, J. H., and Hughston, J. C.: Unstable Intertrochanteric Fractures of the Hip. J. Bone Joint Surg., **49A**:440–450, 1967.

632. DiStefano, V. J.; Nixon, J. E.; and Klein, K. S.: Stable Fixation of the Difficult Subtrochanteric Fracture. J. Trauma, **12**:1066–1070, 1972.

633. Fielding, J. W.: Subtrochanteric Fractures. Clin. Orthop., **92**:86–99, 1973.

634. Fielding, J. W.; Cochran, G. V. B.; and Zickel, R. E.: Biomechanical Characteristics and Surgical Management of Subtrochanteric Fractures. Orthop. Clin. North Am., **5**:629–649, 1974.

635. Fielding, J. W., and Magliato, H. J.: Subtrochanteric Fractures. Surg. Gynecol. Obstet., **122**:555–560, 1966.

636. Forster, I. W., and Lindsay, J. A.: Image Intensifier as an Aid to Insertion of the Zickel Nail Apparatus for Proximal Femoral Fractures. Injury, **11**:148–154, 1979–1980.

637. Frankel, V. H., and Burstein, A. H.: Orthopaedic Biomechanics. Philadelphia. Lea & Febiger, 1970.

638. Froimson, A. I.: Treatment of Comminuted Subtrochanteric Fractures of the Femur. Surg. Gynecol. Obstet., **131**:465–472, 1970.

639. Goldenberg, R. R., and Santoro, A. J.: The Conservative Treatment of Trochanteric Fractures of the Femur. Bull. Hosp. Joint Dis., **12**:27–40, 1951.

640. Hanson, G. W., and Tullos, H. S.: Subtrochanteric Fractures of Femur Treated with Nail-Plate Devices: A Retrospective Study. Clin. Orthop., **131**:191–194, 1978.

641. Heiple, K. G.; Brooks, D. B.; Samson, B. L.; and Burstein, A. H.: A Fluted Intramedullary Rod for Subtrochanteric Fractures. J. Bone Joint Surg., **61A**:730–737, 1979.

642. Hibbs, R. A.: The Management of the Tendency of the Upper Fragment to Tilt Forward in Fractures of the Upper Third of the Femur. N. Y. Med. J., **75**:177–179, 1902.

643. Higinbotham, N. L., and Marcove, R. C.: The Management of Pathological Fractures. J. Trauma, **5**:792–798, 1965.

644. Kaufer, H.: Nonoperative Ambulatory Treatment for Fracture of the Shaft of the Femur. Clin. Orthop., **87**:192–199, 1972.

645. Koch, J. C.: The Laws of Bone Architecture. Am. J. Anat., **21**:177–298, 1917.

646. Kuderna, H.; Böhler, N.; and Collon, D. J.: Treatment of Intertrochanteric and Subtrochanteric Fractures of the Hip by the Ender Method. J. Bone Joint Surg., **58A**:604–611, 1976.

647. Leonidis, S., and Panagopoulos, N.: Surgical Treatment of Subtrochanteric Fractures. Injury, **6**:70–76, 1974–1975.

648. Mickelson, M. R., and Bonfiglio, M.: Pathological Fractures in the Proximal Part of the Femur Treated by Zickel-Nail Fixation. J. Bone Joint Surg., **58A**:1067–1070, 1976.

649. Mooney, V.: Fractures of the Shaft of the Femur. *In* Rockwood, C. A., and Green, D. P. (eds.): Fractures. Philadelphia, J. B. Lippincott, 1975.

650. Moore, M.: Treatment of Trochanteric Femoral Fractures

with Special Reference to Complications. Am. J. Surg., **84**:449–452, 1952.

651. Müller, M. E.; Allgöwer, M.; and Willeneger, H.: Manual of Internal Fixation. New York, Springer-Verlag, 1970.

652. Pankovich, A. M., and Tarabishy, I. E.: Ender Nailing of Intertrochanteric and Subtrochanteric Fractures of the Femur. J. Bone Joint Surg., **62A**:635–645, 1980.

653. Robey, L. R.: Intertrochanteric and Subtrochanteric Fractures of the Femur in the Negro. J. Bone Joint Surg., **38A**:1301–1312, 1956.

654. Russin, L. A., and Sonni, A.: Treatment of Intertrochanteric and Subtrochanteric Fractures with Ender's Intramedullary Rods. Clin. Orthop., **148**:203–212, 1980.

655. Sarmiento, A.: Functional Bracing of Tibial and Femoral Shaft Fractures. Clin. Orthop., **82**:2–13, 1972.

656. Sarmiento, A.: Unstable Intertrochanteric Fractures of the Femur. Clin. Orthop., **92**:77–85, 1973.

657. Schatzker, J.: Methylmethacrylate as an Adjunct in the Internal Fixation of Pathologic Fractures. Can. J. Surg., **22**:179–182, 1979.

658. Schatzker, J., and Waddell, J. P.: Subtrochanteric Fractures of the Femur. Orthop. Clin. North Am., **11**:539–554, 1980.

659. Schurman, D. J., and Amstutz, H. C.: Treatment of Neoplastic Subtrochanteric Fracture. Clin. Orthop., **97**:108–113, 1973.

660. Seinsheimer, F.: Subtrochanteric Fractures of the Femur. J. Bone Joint Surg., **60A**:300–306, 1978.

661. Shelton,, M. L.: Subtrochanteric Fractures of the Femur. Arch. Surg., **110**:41–48, 1975.

662. Taylor, G. M.; Neufeld, A. J.; and Nickel, V. L.: Complications and Failures in the Operative Treatment of Intertrochanteric Fractures of the Femur. J. Bone Joint Surg., **37A**:306–316, 1955.

663. Teitge, R. A.: Subtrochanteric Fractures of the Femur. J. Bone Joint Surg., **58A**:282, 1976.

664. Templeton, T. S., and Saunders, E. A.: A Review of Fractures in the Proximal Femur Treated with the Zickel Nail. Clin. Orthop., **141**:213–216, 1979.

665. Tronzo, R. G.: Surgery of the Hip Joint, pp. 576–582. Philadelphia. Lea & Febiger, 1973.

666. Velasco, R. U., and Comfort, T. H.: Analysis of Treatment Problems in Subtrochanteric Fractures of the Femur. J. Trauma, **18**:513–523, 1978.

667. Waddell, J. P.: Subtrochanteric Fractures of the Femur: A Review of 130 Patients. J. Trauma, **19**:582–592, 1979.

668. Watson, H. K.; Campbell, R. D.; and Wade, P. A.: Classification, Treatment and Complications of the Adult Subtrochanteric Fracture. J. Trauma, **4**:457–480, 1964.

669. Watson-Jones, R.: Fractures and Joint Injuries, Vol. 2, pp. 987–990. New York, Churchill Livingstone, 1976.

670. Winter, W. G., and Clawson, D. K.: Complications of Treatment of Fractures and Dislocations. *In* Epps, C.H. (ed.): Complications in Orthopaedic Surgery, Vol. I, pp. 439–441. Philadelphia, J. B. Lippincott, 1978.

671. Winter, W. G.; Combs, C. R.; Lewis, N. V.; and Brower, T. D.: Zickel Subtrochanteric Fracture Fixation. Orthop. Trans., **3**:256, 1979.

672. Zickel, R. E.: A New Fixation Device for Subtrochanteric Fractures of the Femur. Clin. Orthop., **54**:115–123, 1967.

673. Zickel, R. E.: An Intramedullary Fixation Device for the Proximal Part of the Femur. J. Bone Joint Surg., **58A**:866–872, 1976.

674. Zickel, R. E.: Subtrochanteric Femoral Fractures. Orthop. Clin. North Am., **11**:555–568, 1980.

675. Zickel, R. E., and Mouradian, W. H.: Intramedullary Fixation of Pathological Fractures and Lesions of the Subtrochanteric Region of the Femur. J. Bone Joint Surg., **58A**:1061–1066, 1976.

Dislocations and Fracture Dislocations of the Hip

676. Aggarwal, N. D., and Singh, H.: Unreduced Anterior Dislocation of the Hip. J. Bone Joint Surg., **49B**:288–292, 1967.

677. Allis, O. H.: The Hip. Philadelphia, Dornan Printer, 1895.

678. Amihood, S.: Posterior Dislocation of the Hip: Clinical Observations and Review of Literature. S. Afr. Med. J., **48**:1029–1032, 1974.

679. Amihood, S.: Anterior Dislocation of the Hip. Injury, **7**:107–110, 1975.

680. Armstrong, J. R.: Traumatic Dislocation of the Hip Joint. J. Bone Joint Surg., **30B**:430–445, 1948.

681. Aufranc, O. E.; Jones, W. N.; Turner, R. H.; and Thomas, W. H.: Fracture of the Acetabulum with Dislocation of Hip and Sciatic Palsy. Fracture of the Month. J.A.M.A., **201**:690–691, 1967.

682. Austin, R. T.: Hip Function After Central Fracture-Dislocation: A Long Term Review. Injury, **3**:114–120, 1971.

683. Banks, S. W.: Aseptic Necrosis of the Femoral Head Following Traumatic Dislocation of the Hip. J. Bone Joint Surg., **23**:753–781, 1941.

684. Barnes, S. N., and Stewart, M. J.: Central Fractures of the Acetabulum: A Critical Analysis and Review of Literature. Clin. Orthop., **114**:276–281, 1976.

685. Bigelow, H. J.: Luxations of the Hip Joint. Boston Med. Surg. J., **5**:1–3, 1870.

686. Bigelow, H. J.: On Dislocation of the Hip. Lancet, **1**:860–862, 1878.

687. Bigelow, H. J.: On Dislocation of the Hip. Lancet, **1**:894–895, 1878.

688. Bigelow, H. J.: On Dislocation of the Hip. Lancet, **1**:930–931, 1878.

689. Birkett, J.: Description of a Dislocation of the Head of the Femur, Complicated with its Fracture; with Remarks. Med. Chir. Trans. London, **52**:133–138,1869.

690. Bonnemaison, M. F. E., and Henderson, E. D.: Traumatic Anterior Dislocation of the Hip with Acute Common Femoral Occlusion in a Child. J. Bone Joint Surg., **50A**:753–756, 1968.

691. Brav, E. A.: Traumatic Dislocation of the Hip. J. Bone Joint Surg., **44A**:1115–1134, 1962.

692. Bromberg, E., and Weiss, A. B.: Posterior Fracture Dislocation of the Hip. South. Med. J., **70**:8–11, 1977.

693. Brown, R. F., and Simmonds, F. A.: An Unusual Dislocation of the Hip. Br. J. Surg., **59**:326–328, 1972.

694. Buchanan, J. J.: Reduction of Old Dislocations of the Hip by Open Incision. Surg. Gynecol. Obstet., **31**:462–471, 1920.

695. Buchanan, J. R.: Bowel Entrapment by Pelvic Fracture Fragments. Clin. Orthop., **147**:164–166, 1980.

696. Burman, M. S., and Feldman, T.: Fracture of Head of Femur with Dislocation of Hip. Bull. Hosp. Joint Dis., **20:**69–75, 1959.

697. Butler, J. E.: Pipkin Type II Fractures of the Femoral Head. J. Bone Joint Surg., **63A:**1292–1296, 1981.

698. Campbell, W. C.: Perineal Dislocation of the Hip. J.A.M.A., **78:**1115–1116, 1922.

699. Campbell, W. C.: Posterior Dislocation of the Hip with Fracture of the Acetabulum. J. Bone Joint Surg., **18:**842–850, 1936.

700. Canale, S. T., and Manugian, A. H.: Irreducible Traumatic Dislocations of the Hip. J. Bone Joint Surg., **61A:**7–14, 1979.

701. Carnesale, P. G.; Stewart, M. J.; and Barnes, S. N.: Acetabular Disruption and Central Fracture-Dislocation of the Hip: A Long-Term Study. J. Bone Joint Surg., **57A:**1054–1059, 1975.

702. Chakraborti, S., and Miller, I. M.: Dislocation of the Hip Associated with Fracture of the Femoral Head. Injury, **7:**134–142, 1975.

703. Choyce, C. C.: Traumatic Dislocation of the Hip in Childhood, and Relation of Trauma to Pseudocoxalgia: Analysis of 59 Cases Published up to January, 1924. Br. J. Surg., **12:**52–59, 1924.

704. Christopher, F.: Fractures of the Head of the Femur. Arch. Surg., **12:**1049–1061, 1926.

705. Connolly, J. F.: Acetabular Labrum Entrapment Associated with a Femoral-Head-Fracture-Dislocation: A Case Report. J. Bone Joint Surg., **56A:**1735–1737, 1974.

706. Cooper, A.: A Treatise on Dislocations and Fractures of the Joints, 2nd ed. London, Longman, Hurst, Rees, Orme, and Browne, 1823.

707. Coventry, M. B.: The Treatment of Fracture-Dislocation of the Hip by Total Hip Arthroplasty. J. Bone Joint Surg., **56A:**1128–1134, 1974.

708. Dall, D.; MacNab, I.; and Gross, A.: Recurrent Anterior Dislocation of the Hip. J. Bone Joint Surg., **52A:**574–576, 1970.

709. Dameron, T. B.: Bucket-handle Tear of Acetabular Labrum Accompanying Posterior Dislocation of the Hip. J. Bone Joint Surg., **41A:**131–134, 1959.

710. D'Aubigne, R. M.: Management of Acetabular Fractures in Multiple Trauma. J. Trauma, **8:**333–349, 1968.

711. Davis, J. B.: Simultaneous Femoral Head Fracture and Traumatic Hip Dislocation. Am. J. Surg., **80:**893–895, 1950.

712. Dehne, E., and Immerman, E. W.: Dislocation of the Hip Combined with Fracture of the Shaft of the Femur on the Same Side. J. Bone Joint Surg., **33A:**731–745, 1951.

713. DeLee, J. C.; Evans, J. A.; and Thomas, J.: Anterior Dislocation of the Hip and Associated Femoral-Head Fractures. J. Bone Joint Surg., **62A:**960–964, 1980.

714. Dencker, H.: Traumatic Dislocation of the Hip with Fracture of the Shaft of the Ipsilateral Femur. Acta Chir. Scand., **129:**593–596, 1965.

715. Derian, P. S., and Bibighaus, A. J.: Sciatic Nerve Entrapment by Ectopic Bone After Posterior Fracture-Dislocation of the Hip. South. Med. J., **67:**209–210, 1974.

716. Derian, P. S., and Purser, T., III: Intra-articular Small-Bowel Herniation Complicating Central Fracture-Dislo-cation of the Hip. J. Bone Joint Surg., **48A:**1614–1618, 1966.

717. Dingley, A. F., and Denham, R. H.: Pubic Dislocation of the Hip. J. Bone Joint Surg., **46A:**865–867, 1964.

718. Dowd, G. S. E., and Johnson, R.: Successful Conservative Treatment of a Fracture-Dislocation of the Femoral Head. J. Bone Joint Surg., **61A:**1244–1246, 1979.

719. Duncan, C. P., and Shim, S. S.: Blood Supply of the Head of the Femur in Traumatic Hip Dislocation. Surg. Gynecol. Obstet., **144:**185–191, 1977.

720. Dussault, R. G.; Beauregard, G.; Fauteaux, P.; Laurin, C.; and Boisjoly, A.: Femoral Head Defect Following Anterior Hip Dislocation. Radiology, **135:**627–629, 1980.

721. Ehtisham, S. M. A.: Traumatic Dislocation of the Hip Joint with Fracture of Shaft of Femur on the Same Side. J. Trauma, **16:**196–205, 1976.

722. Eichenholtz, S. N., and Stark, R. M.: Central Acetabular Fractures. J. Bone Joint Surg., **46A:**695–714, 1964.

723. Eisenberg, K. S.; Sheft, D. J.; and Murray, W. R.: Posterior Dislocation of the Hip Producing Lumbosacral Nerve-Root Avulsion. J. Bone Joint Surg., **54A:**1083–1086, 1972.

724. Elliott, R. B.: Central Fractures of the Acetabulum. Clin. Orthop., **7:**189–201, 1956.

725. Epstein, H. C.: Posterior Fracture-Dislocations of the Hip. J. Bone Joint Surg., **43A:**1079–1098, 1961.

726. Epstein, H. C. (Discussor with Harris, W. H.; Jones, W. N.; and Aufranc, O. E. Fracture of the Month: Fracture-Dislocation of the Hip), Grand Rounds at Massachusetts General Hospital. J.A.M.A., **186:**1160–1163, 1963.

727. Epstein, H. C.: Traumatic Anterior and Simple Posterior Dislocations of the Hip in Adults and Children. A.A.O.S. Instructional Course Lectures, **22:**115–145, 1973.

728. Epstein, H. C.: Traumatic Dislocations of the Hip. Clin. Orthop., **92:**116–142, 1973.

729. Epstein, H. C.: Posterior Fracture-Dislocations of the Hip: Long-Term Follow-up. J. Bone Joint Surg., **56A:**1103–1127, 1974.

730. Epstein, H. C.: Traumatic Dislocation of the Hip. Baltimore, Williams & Wilkins, 1980.

731. Epstein, H. C., and Harvey, J. P.: Traumatic Anterior Dislocations of the Hip. Orthop. Rev., **1:**33–38, 1972.

732. Epstein, H. C., and Harvey, J. P.: Traumatic Anterior Dislocations of the Hip. Management and Results. An Analysis of Fifty-five Cases. J. Bone Joint Surg., **54A:**1561–1562, 1972.

733. Fina, C. P., and Kelly, P. J.: Dislocations of the Hip with Fractures of the Proximal Femur. J. Trauma, **10:**77–87, 1970.

734. Funsten, R. V.; Kinser, P.; and Frankel, C. J.: Dashboard Dislocation of the Hip. J. Bone Joint Surg., **20:**124–132, 1938.

735. Garrett, J. C.: Epstein, H. C.: Harris, W. H.; Harvey, J. P.; and Nickel, V. L.: Treatment of Unreduced Traumatic Posterior Dislocations of the Hip. J. Bone Joint Surg., **61A:**2–6, 1979.

736. Ghormley, R. K., and Sullivan, R.: Traumatic Dislocation of the Hip. Am. J. Surg., **85:**298–301, 1953.

737. Gillespie, W. J.: The Incidence and Pattern of Knee Injury Associated with Dislocation of the Hip. J. Bone Joint Surg., **57B:**376–378, 1975.

738. Goetz, A. G.: Traumatic Dislocation of the Hip (Head of the Femur) into the Scrotum. J. Bone Joint Surg., **16:**718–720, 1934.

739. Gordon, E. J., and Freiberg, J. A.: Posterior Dislocation of the Hip with Fracture of the Head of the Femur. J. Bone Joint Surg., **31A:**869–872, 1949.

740. Göthlin, G., and Hindmarsh, J.: Central Dislocation of the Hip. The Prognosis with Conservative Managment. Acta Orthop. Scand., **41:**476–487, 1970.

741. Gregory, C. F.: Early Complications of Dislocation and Fracture-Dislocations of the Hip Joint. A.A.O.S. Instructional Course Lectures, **22:**105–114, 1973.

742. Griswold, R. A., and Herd, C. R.: Dislocation of Hip with Fracture of Posterior Rim of Acetabulum. J. Indiana State Med. Assoc., **22:**150–153, 1929.

743. Gupta, R. C., and Shravat, B. P.: Reduction of Neglected Traumatic Dislocation of the Hip by Heavy Traction,. J. Bone Joint Surg., **59A:**249–251, 1977.

744. Haddad, R. J., and Drez, D.: Voluntary Recurrent Anterior Dislocation of the Hip. J. Bone Joint Surg., **56A:**419–422, 1974.

745. Hamada, G.: Unreduced Anterior Dislocation of the Hip. J. Bone Joint Surg., **39B:**471–476, 1957.

746. Hammond, G.: Posterior Dislocations of Hip Associated with Fracture. Proc. R. Soc. Med., **37:**281–286, 1944.

747. Hampson, W. G. J.: Venous Obstruction by Anterior Dislocation of the Hip-Joint. Injury, **4:**69–73, 1972.

748. Hart, V. L.: Fracture-Dislocation of the Hip. J. Bone Joint Surg., **24:**458–460, 1942.

749. Haw, D. W. M.: Complication Following Fracture-Dislocation of the Hip. Br. Med. J., **1:**1111–1112, 1965.

750. Helal, B., and Skevis, X.: Unrecognized Dislocation of the Hip in Fractures of the Femoral Shaft. J. Bone Joint Surg., **49B:**293–300, 1967.

751. Henderson, M. S.: Old Traumatic Dislocation of the Left Hip. Surg. Clin. North Am., **10:**44–47, 1930.

752. Henderson, R. S.: Traumatic Anterior Dislocation of the Hip. J. Bone Joint Surg., **33B:**602–603, 1951.

753. Henry, A. K., and Bayumi, M.: Fracture of the Femur with Luxation of the Ipsilateral Hip. Br. J. Surg., **22:**204–230, 1934–1935.

754. Hirasawa, Y.; Oda, R.; and Nakatani, K.: Sciatic Nerve Paralysis in Posterior Dislocation of the Hip. Clin. Orthop., **126:**172–175, 1977.

755. Huckstep, R. L.: Neglected Traumatic Dislocation of the Hip. J. Bone Joint Surg., **53B:**355, 1971.

756. Hunter, G. A.: Posterior Dislocation and Fracture-Dislocation of the Hip. J. Bone Joint Surg., **51B:**38–44, 1969.

757. Ingram, A. J., and Turner, T. C.: Bilateral Traumatic Posterior Dislocation of the Hip Complicated by Bilateral Fracture of the Femoral Shaft. J. Bone Joint Surg., **36A:**1249–1255, 1954.

758. Jazayeri, M.: Posterior Fracture-Dislocations of the Hip Joint with Emphasis on the Importance of Hip Tomography in their Management. Orthop. Rev., **7:**59–64, 1978.

759. Jeffrey, C. C.: Fracture-Dislocation of the Hip with Displacement of Bone Fragment into Acetabulum During Closed Reduction. J. Bone Joint Surg., **39B:**310–312, 1957.

760. Judet, R.; Judet, J.; and Letournel, E.: Fractures of the Acetabulum: Classification and Surgical Approaches for Open Reduction. J. Bone Joint Surg., **46A:**1615–1646, 1964.

761. Katznelson, A. M.: Traumatic Anterior Dislocation of the Hip. J. Bone Joint Surg., **44B:**129–130, 1962.

762. Kelly, R. P., and Yarbrough, S. H.: Posterior Fracture-Dislocation of the Femoral Head with Retained Medial Head Fragment. J. Trauma, **11:**97–108, 1971.

763. Kelly, P. J., and Lipscomb, P. R.: Primary Vitallium-Mold Arthroplasty for Posterior Dislocation of the Hip with Fracture of the Femoral Head. J. Bone Joint Surg., **40A:**675–680, 1958.

764. King, D., and Richards, V.: Fracture-Dislocations of the Hip Joint. J. Bone Joint Surg., **23:**533–551, 1941.

765. Kirchner, P. T., and Simon, M. A.: Current Concepts Review: Radioisotopic Evaluation of Skeletal Disease. J. Bone Joint Surg., **63A:**673–681, 1981.

766. Kleiman, S. G.; Stevens, J.; Kolb, L.; and Pankovich, A.: Late Sciatic-Nerve Palsy Following Posterior Fracture-Dislocation of the Hip. J. Bone Joint Surg., **53A:**781–782, 1971.

767. Knight, R. A., and Smith, H.: Central Fractures of the Acetabulum. J. Bone Joint Surg., **40A:**1–16, 1958.

768. Kristensen, O., and Stougaard, J.: Traumatic Dislocation of the Hip: Results of Conservative Treatment. Acta Orthop. Scand., **45:**206–212, 1974.

769. Küntscher, G. B. G.: The Küntscher Method of Intramedullary Fixation. J. Bone Joint Surg., **40A:**17–26, 1958.

770. Lars-Olof, L.: Traumatic Dislocations of the Hip; Follow-up on Cases from Stockholm Area. Acta Orthop. Scand., **41:**188–198, 1970.

771. Larson, C. B.: Fracture-Dislocations of the Hip. Clin. Orthop., **92:**147–154, 1973.

772. Lasda, N. A.; Levinsohn, E. M.; Yuan, H. A.; and Bunnell, W. P.: Computerized Tomography in Disorders of the Hip. J. Bone Joint Surg., **60A:**1099–1102, 1978.

773. Letournel, E.: Surgical Repair of Acetabular Fractures More Than Three Weeks After Injury, Apart from Total Hip Replacement. Int. Orthop., **2:**305–313, 1979.

774. Levine, M. A.: A Treatment of Central Fractures of the Acetabulum. J. Bone Joint Surg., **25:**902–906, 1943.

775. Levy, M.: Hemipelvic Dislocation Complicated by Dislocation of the Ipsilateral Hip. Acta Orthop. Scand., **47:**67–69, 1976.

776. Liebenberg, F., and Dommisse, G. F.: Recurrent Post-Traumatic Dislocation of the Hip. J. Bone Joint Surg., **51B:**632–637, 1969.

777. Lipscomb, P. R.: Fracture-Dislocation of the Hip. A.A.O.S. Instructional Course Lectures **18:**102–109, 1961.

778. Litton, L. O., and Workman. C.: Traumatic Anterior Dislocation of the Hip in Children. J. Bone Joint Surg., **40A:**1419–1422, 1958.

779. Lowell, J. D.: Bursting Fractures of the Acetabulum, Involving the Inner Wall and Superior Dome. A.A.O.S. Instructional Course Lectures, **22:**145–158, 1973.

780. Lunt, H. R. W.: Entrapment of Bowel Within Fractures of the Pelvis. Injury, **2:**121–126, 1970.

781. Lutter, L. D.: Post-Traumatic Hip Redislocation. J. Bone Joint Surg., **55A:**391–394, 1973.

782. Lyddon, D. W., and Hartman, J. T.: Traumatic Dislocation

of the Hip with Ipsilateral Femoral Fracture. J. Bone Joint Surg., **53A:**1012–1016, 1971.

783. MacFarlane, J. A.: Anterior Dislocation of the Hip. Br. J. Surg., **23:**607–611, 1935.

784. MacGuire, C. J.: Fracture of the Acetabulum. Ann. Surg., **83:**718, 1926.

785. Markham, D. E.: Anterior Dislocation of the Hip and Diastasis of the Contralateral Sacro-Iliac Joint: The Rear-Seat Passenger's Injury? Br. J. Surg., **59:**296–298, 1972.

786. Maynard, R. L.: Reduction of Fractures of the Acetabulum with Penetration of the Head of the Femur into the Pelvis. Rhode Island Med. J., **23:**150–153, 1940.

787. M'Bamali, E. I.: Unusual Traumatic Anterior Dislocation of the Hip. Injury, **6:**220–224, 1975.

788. Meyerding, H. W., and Walker, H. R.: Fracture-Dislocation of the Acetabular Rim with Dislocation of the Hip and Traumatic Sciatic Paralysis. J. Int. Coll. Surg., **13:**539–548, 1950.

789. Meyers, M. H.; Telfer, N.; and Moore, T. M.: Determination of the Vascularity of the Femoral Head with Technetium 99 mm-Sulfer-Colloid: Diagnostic and Prognostic Significance. J. Bone Joint Surg., **59A:**658–664, 1977.

790. Miller, C. H.; Gustilo, R.; and Tambornino, J.: Traumatic Hip Dislocation, Treatment and Results. Minn. Med., **54:**253–260, 1971.

791. Moore, J. R.: Old Traumatic Dislocation of the Hip with Malunited Fracture of the Acetabulum. Surg. Clin. North Am., **33:**1551–1557, 1953.

792. Moore, T. M.; Hill, J. V.; and Harvey, J. P.: Central Acetabular Fracture Secondary to Epileptic Seizure. J. Bone Joint Surg., **52A:**1459–1462, 1970.

793. Morton, K. S.: Traumatic Dislocation of the Hip: A Follow-up Study. Can. J. Surg., **3:**67–74, 1959.

794. Nelson, C. L.: Traumatic Recurrent Dislocation of the Hip: Report of a Case. J. Bone Joint Surg., **52A:**128–130, 1970.

795. Nerubay, J.: Traumatic Anterior Dislocation of the Hip Joint with Vascular Damage. Clin. Orthop., **116:**129–132, 1976.

796. Nerubay, J.; Glancz, G.; and Katznelson, A.: Fractures of the Acetabulum. J. Trauma, **13:**1050–1062, 1973.

797. Newman, J. H.: Posterior Dislocation of the Hip with Ipsilateral Subcapital Fracture of the Neck of the Femur, Treated Conservatively: A Case Report. Injury, **5:**329–331, 1974.

798. Nicoll, E. A.: Proceedings and Reports of Councils and Associations: Traumatic Dislocation of the Hip Joint. J. Bone Joint Surg., **34B:**503–505, 1952.

799. Niloff, P., and Petrie, J. G.: Traumatic Anterior Dislocation of the Hip. Can. Med. Assoc. J., **62:**574–576, 1950.

800. Nixon, J. R.: Late Open Reduction of Traumatic Dislocation of the Hip; Report of Three Cases. J. Bone Joint Surg., **58B:**41–43, 1976.

801. Okelberry, A. M.: Fractures of the Floor of the Acetabulum. J. Bone Joint Surg., **38A:**441–442, 1956.

802. Palin, H. C., and Richmond, D. A.: Dislocation of the Hip with Fracture of the Femoral Head. J. Bone Joint Surg., **36B:**442–444, 1954.

803. Palmer, D. W.: Central Dislocation of the Hip. Am. J. Surg., **35:**118–121, 1921.

804. Paterson, I.: The Torn Acetabular Labrum. J. Bone Joint Surg., **39B:**306–309, 1957.

805. Patterson, F. P., and Morton, K. S.: Neurological Complications of Fractures and Dislocations of the Pelvis. J. Trauma, **12:**1013–1023, 1972.

806. Paus, B.: Traumatic Dislocations of the Hip: Late Results in 76 Cases. Acta Orthop. Scand., **21:**99–112, 1951.

807. Pearson, J. R., and Hargadon, E. J.: Fractures of the Pelvis Involving the Floor of the Acetabulum. J. Bone Joint Surg., **44B:**550–561, 1962.

808. Peet, M. M.: Fracture of the Acetabulum with Interpelvic Displacement of the Femoral Head. Ann. Surg., **70:**296–304, 1919.

809. Pennal, G. F.: Central Dislocation of the Hip. J. Bone Joint Surg., **40A:**1435, 1958.

810. Phemister, D. B.: Fractures of Neck of Femur, Dislocations of Hip, and Obscure Vascular Disturbances Producing Aseptic Necrosis of Head of Femur. Surg. Gynecol. Obstet., **59:**415–440, 1934.

811. Pipkin, G.: Treatment of Grade IV Fracture-Dislocation of the Hip. J. Bone Joint Surg., **39A:**1027–1042, 1197, 1957.

812. Poilly, J. N., and Hamilton, J. B.: Central Dislocation of the Hip Causing Mechanical Intestinal Obstruction. Injury, **5:**194–196, 1974.

813. Polesky, R. E., and Polesky, F. A.: Intrapelvic Dislocation of the Femoral Head Following Anterior Dislocation of the Hip. J. Bone Joint Surg., **54A:**1097–1098, 1972.

814. Potts, F. N., and Obletz, B. E.: Aseptic Necrosis of Head of Femur Following Traumatic Dislocation. J. Bone Joint Surg., **21:**101–110, 1939.

815. Pringle, J. H.: Traumatic Dislocation of the Hip Joint. An Experimental Study on the Cadaver. Glasgow Med. J., **21:**25–40, 1943.

816. Proctor, H.: Dislocations of the Hip Joint (Excluding 'Central' Dislocations) and Their Complications. Injury, **5:**1–12, 1973.

817. Putti, V.: The Treatment of Central Luxation of the Femur. Chir. Organi. Mov., **11:**530–538, 1927.

818. Putti, V.: The Treatment of Central Luxation of the Femur. Int. Abstr. Surg., **46:**134, 1928.

819. Rao, J. P., and Read, R. B.: Luxatio Erecta of the Hip: An Interesting Case Report. Clin. Orthop., **110:**137–138, 1975.

820. Reigstad, A.: Traumatic Dislocation of the Hip. J. Trauma, **20:**603–606, 1980.

821. Roeder, L. F., and DeLee, J. C.: Femoral Head Fractures Associated with Posterior Hip Dislocations. Clin. Orthop., **147:**121–130, 1980.

822. Rosenthal, R. E., and Coker, W. L.: Posterior Fracture Dislocation of the Hip. J. Trauma, **19:**572–581, 1979.

823. Rowe, C. R., and Lowell, J. D.: Prognosis of Fractures of the Acetabulum. J. Bone Joint Surg., **43A:**30–59, 1961.

824. Sarmiento, A., and Laird, C. A.: Posterior Fracture-Dislocation of the Femoral Head. Clin. Orthop., **92:**143–146, 1973.

825. Sauser, D. D.; Billimoria, P. E.; Rouse, G. A.; and Mudge, K.: CT Evaluation of Hip Trauma. Am. J. Roentgenol., **135:**269–274, 1980.

826. Scadden, W. J., and Dennyson, W. G.: Unreduced Ob-

turator Dislocation of the Hip. S. Afr. Med. J., **53**:601–602, 1978.

827. Scham, S. M., and Fry, L. R.: Traumatic Anterior Dislocation of the Hip with Fracture of the Femoral Head. Clin. Orthop., **62**:133–135, 1969.

828. Schoenecker, P. L.; Manske, P. R.; and Sertl, G. O.: Traumatic Hip Dislocation with Ipsilateral Femoral Shaft Fractures. Clin. Orthop., **130**:233–238, 1978.

829. Schwartz, D. L., and Haller, J. A.: Open Anterior Hip Dislocation with Femoral Vessel Transection in a Child. J. Trauma, **14**:1054–1059, 1974.

830. Scott, J. E., and Thomas, F. B.: Delayed Presentation of Post-traumatic Posterior Dislocation of the Hip with Acetabular Rim Fracture. Injury, **5**:325–326, 1974.

831. Scudese, V. A.: Traumatic Anterior Hip Redislocation. Clin. Orthop., **88**:60–63, 1972.

832. Seddon, H.: Surgical Disorders of the Peripheral Nerves. Edinburgh, Churchill-Livingstone, 1972.

833. Shirkhoda, B.; Brashear, H. R.; and Staab, E. V.: Computed Tomography of Acetabular Fractures. Radiology, **134**:683–688, 1980.

834. Skillern, P. G., and Pancoast, H. K.: Fracture of the Floor of the Acetabulum. Ann. Surg., **55**:92–97, 1912.

835. Slätis, P., and Latvala, A.; Irreducible Traumatic Posterior Dislocation of the Hip. Injury, **5**:188–193, 1974.

836. Smith, E. J. (for J. D. Buxton): Traumatic Anterior Dislocation of the Hip. Proc. R. Soc. Med., **27** (Part I):579–581, 1934.

837. Smith, G. R., and Loop, J. W.: Radiologic Classification of Posterior Dislocations of the Hip: Refinements and Pitfalls. Radiology, **119**:569–574, 1976.

838. Soreff, J.: Fracture-Dislocation of the Hip with Entrapment of the Femoral Head by Impaction Against the Acetabular Rim. Injury, **8**:127–128, 1976.

839. Speed, K.: Simultaneous Bilateral Traumatic Dislocation of the Hip. Am. J. Surg., **85**:292–297, 1953.

840. Steinke, C. R.: Recent Traumatic Dislocations of the Hip. Ann. Surg., **60**:617–621, 1914.

841. Stewart, M. J.: Management of Fractures of the Head of the Femur Complicated by Dislocation of the Hip. Orthop. Clin. North Am., **5**:793–798, 1974.

842. Stewart, M. J.; McCarroll, H. R.; and Mulhollan, J. S.: Fracture-Dislocation of the Hip. Acta Orthop. Scand., **46**:507–525, 1975.

843. Stewart, M. J., and Milford, L. W.: Fracture Dislocation of the Hip. J. Bone Joint Surg., **36A**:315–342, 1954.

844. Stewart, W. J.: Aseptic Necrosis of the Head of the Femur Following Traumatic Dislocation of the Hip Joint: Case Report and Experimental Studies. J. Bone Joint Surg., **15**:413–438, 1933.

845. Stimson, L. A.: A Treatise on Fractures. Philadelphia. H. C. Leas Son, 1883.

846. Stimson, L. A.: Five Cases of Dislocation of the Hip. N. Y. Med. J., **50**:118–121, 1889.

847. Stuck, W. G., and Vaughan, W. H.: Prevention of Disability After Traumatic Dislocation of the Hip. South. Surg., **15**:659–675, 1949.

848. Sullivan, C. R.; Bickel, W. H.; and Lipscomb, P. R.: Recurrent Dislocation of the Hip. J. Bone Joint Surg., **37A**:1266–1270, 1955.

849. Thompson, V. P., and Epstein, H. C.: Traumatic Dislocation of the Hip. J. Bone Joint Surg., **33A**:746–778, 1951.

850. Tipton, W. W.; D'Ambrosia, R. D.; and Ryle, G. P.: Central Fracture-Dislocation of the Hip: Comparison of Nonoperative Management Techniques. J. Bone Joint Surg., **57A**:135, 1975.

851. Tipton, W. W.; D'Ambrosia, R. D.; and Ryle, G. P.: Nonoperative Management of Central Fracture-Dislocations of the Hip. J. Bone Joint Surg., **57A**:888–893, 1975.

852. Townsend, R. G.; Edwards, G. E.; and Bazant, F. J.: Post-Traumatic Recurrent Dislocation of the Hip Without Fracture. J. Bone Joint Surg., **51B**:194, 1969.

853. Tronzo, R. G.: Surgery of the Hip Joint, pp. 451–454. Philadelphia, Lea & Febiger, 1973.

854. Upadhyay, S. S., and Moulton, A.: The Long-Term Results of Traumatic Posterior Dislocation of the Hip. J. Bone Joint Surg., **63B**:548–551, 1981.

855. Urist, M. R.: Injuries to the Hip Joint: Traumatic Dislocations Incurred Chiefly in Jeep Injuries in World War II. Am. J. Surg., **74**:586–597, 1947.

856. Urist, M. R.: Fracture-Dislocation of the Hip Joint: The Nature of the Traumatic Lesion, Treatment, Late Complications and End Results. J. Bone Joint Surg., **30A**:699–727, 1948.

857. Urist, M. R.: Fractures of the Acetabulum: The Nature of the Traumatic Lesion, Treatment, and Two-Year End-Results. Ann. Surg., **127**:1150–1164, 1948.

858. Wadsworth, T. G.: Traumatic Dislocation of the Hip with Fracture of the Shaft of the Ipsilateral Femur. J. Bone Joint Surg., **43B**:47–49, 1961.

859. Walker, W. A.: Traumatic Dislocations of the Hip Joint. Am. J. Surg., **50**:545–549, 1940.

860. Watkins, J. T.: Obturator Dislocations. J. Bone Joint Surg., **5**:243–259, 1923.

861. Watson, A. B.: A Note on the Treatment of Central Dislocation of the Hip-Joint. Br. J. Surg., **41**:9–11, 1953.

862. Watson-Jones, R.: Fractures and Joint Injuries, 5th ed., pp. 885–894. New York, Churchill-Livingstone, 1976.

863. Westerborn, A.: Central Dislocation of the Femoral Head Treated with Mold Arthroplasty. J. Bone Joint Surg., **36A**:307–314, 1954.

864. Whitehouse, G. H.: Radiological Aspects of Posterior Dislocation of the Hip. Clin. Radiol., **29**:431–441, 1978.

865. Whitman, R.: The Treatment of Central Luxation of the Femur. Ann. Surg., **71**:62–65, 1920.

866. Wilson, J. N.: The Management of Fracture Dislocation of the Hip. Proc. R. Soc. Med., **53**:941–945, 1960.

867. Wiltberger, B.R.: Mitchell, C. L.; and Hedrick, D. W.: Fracture of the Femoral Shaft Complicated by Hip Dislocation: A Method of Treatment. J. Bone Joint Surg., **30A**:225–228, 1948.

868. Winston, M. E.: Fractures of the Floor of the Acetabulum and Traumatic Central Dislocation of the Hip. Surg. Gynecol. Obstet., **113**:479–483, 1961.

869. Wright, P. E.: Dislocations. *In* Edmonson, A. S., and Crenshaw, A. H. (eds.): Campbell's Operative Orthopaedics, 6th ed., St. Louis, C. V. Mosby, 1980.

15

Fractures of the Shaft of the Femur

Vert Mooney
Bernd F. Claudi

Fractures of the femoral shaft represent a traumatic event so significant that it has "broken" the longest and strongest bone in the body. These injuries are usually serious and are frequently associated with severe blood loss, which can rapidly lead to shock and associated multiple organ failure. Many aspects of this severe injury may truly be life-threatening and deserve early and informed attention. Treatment of the fracture of the femoral shaft is a complex problem. The purpose of this chapter is to provide the fracture surgeon with as much information as possible so that the best judgement can be made.

Because of its length and ambulatory function, the femur must tolerate the most severe combination of axial loading and angulatory stresses. It is surrounded by massive musculature—the most powerful in the body. This musculature provides nearly unlimited blood supply and thus marvelous potential for healing. Consequently, the more significant problems related to fracture care of the femoral shaft are not so much those of bone healing as those related to returning the healing bone to sufficient strength to tolerate functional stress within a reasonable time.

Watson-Jones[232] in the early 1940s was able to report a consistent record of union in 142 consecutive femoral shaft fractures: "The fracture will surely unite if support is maintained long enough." But Sir James Paget,[160] nearly 50 years earlier, balanced this proposition with the admonition, "with the rest too long maintained, a limb becomes or remains stiff and weak and over-sensitive, even though there be no more of the process in it. . . . I

need hardly say that it may be sometimes difficult to decide the time at which rest after having been highly beneficial may become injurious."

The goal in expert care of these fractures is to use methods of treatment that offer the greatest potential for regaining early functional strength and use with the least threat of morbidity. Landmarks in the history of femoral fracture care are discoveries that offered means to stabilize the deformed limb segment and hasten the mobilization of the disabled patient.

HISTORICAL REVIEW

The ancients had a difficult time coping with the deforming gravitational and muscle forces, using the materials then available. The Arabs, two centuries ago, encased the fractured limb in a mound of plaster.[142] The Chinese and many Africans and Polynesians used wood or bamboo splints wrapped with sinews of leather or fibrous plants.[69,101] A method using pre-cut wooden strips is illustrated in Figure 15-1. Fabric stiffened with wax was described by Hippocrates.[2] Embalmer's bandage stiffened with gum was used by the Egyptians,[206] but in general these materials were too weak to give sufficient support to the fractured thigh. Fabric stiffened by albumin or gums was specifically described for the mobilization of patients with thigh fractures by Seutin[142] in 1849.

Mathysen[134] in 1852, using Seutin's method of encircling the limb with fabric strips, rediscovered

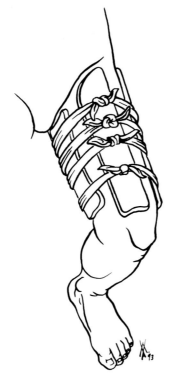

Fig. 15-1. A method of femoral fracture care advocated in modern Chinese medical literature based on immobilization techniques from many cultures. (Fang, H.; Chew, Y.; and Shang, T.: The Integration of Modern and Traditional Chinese Medicine in the Treatment of Fractures. Chin. Med. J., **83**:411–418, 1964.)

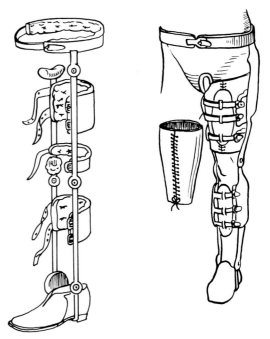

Fig. 15-2. The fracture brace (prosthesis) designed and used by Smith of Philadelphia for the ambulatory care of fractured femurs.

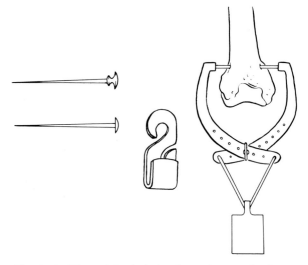

Fig. 15-3. The original skeletal traction method of Steinmann using two pins driven transversely into the femoral condyles. (Redrawn from Peltier, L. F.: A Brief History of Traction. J. Bone Joint Surg., **50A**:1603–1615, 1968.)

a method that the Egyptians had used centuries earlier and incorporated plaster of paris in the bandage. The efficacy of this method in treating the war-injured of Europe quickly made it popular. This composite material was strong enough for the fractured thigh.

External splinting devices and methods were apparently rudimentary in America in the 1850s. Patients were generally confined to bed with their deformities grossly corrected as well as possible, but no specific method was available to maintain correction.[205,208] The significant morbidity and mortality (50 percent, even for closed fractures) associated with this method at that time led Smith to give up completely on the injured limb and to construct a "prosthesis" to allow the early mobilization of the patient (Fig. 15-2). This method, to the surprise even of Dr. Smith, was successful in achieving union of all the fractures reported. Nevertheless, because of its complexity and the somewhat "irrational" concept of early mobilization of the

patient, it never found acceptance as a standard mode of fracture care.

Pressure for improved fracture stabilization came with the advent of radiography in the late 1890s.

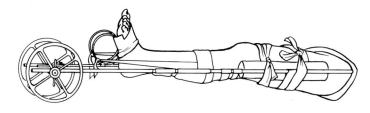

Fig. 15-4. The Thomas ring in the form used for the care and transfer of patients with a fractured femur. Traction was achieved by an adjustable track attached to spring steel hoops. Countertraction was by means of the ring at the root of the leg. (Redrawn from Peltier, L. F.: A Brief History of Traction. J. Bone Joint Surg., **50A**:1603–1615, 1968.)

The unfortunate status of the healing thigh bone buried beneath its cloak of muscles was now revealed for all to see. A review of consecutive femoral fracture cases at the Hospital of the University of Pennsylvania treated with Buck's skin traction from 1910 to 1920 labeled them "unsatisfactory in one-hundred percent of the cases."[170] An unfortunate corollary of this discovery was the potential that one might just treat an x-ray.

In 1907, Fritz Steinmann used two pins driven transversely from medial and lateral aspects into the distal femoral condyles as a method of improving on skin traction methods (Fig. 15-3).[215] He later adopted a through-and-through rod, but the name persists—Steinmann *pins*. Böhler improved upon Steinmann's original bow, modifying it to allow swivel action. In 1909, Kirschner introduced a principle of engineering—already applied to bicycle wheels—into orthopaedic practice.[110] He used a wire of small diameter, but obtained increased resistance to angulation by means of tension; thus, a smaller diameter wire could tolerate the traction forces. The current Kirschner traction bow, however, was not developed for another 25 years.[133] It is notable that Steinmann pins (rods) and Kirschner wires, in their present form and application, have been consistently used in fracture treatment since the 1930s.

One further aspect of the historic methods for stabilizing and mobilizing the patient with a fracture in his thigh should be noted. The Thomas splint was originally applied to fractured femurs to allow transfer and assisted home care.[222] At that time, before hospitalization for major trauma was commonplace and before the problems related to the full extension position of the fractured limb were identified by radiography, the caliper with the ring at the root of the leg was a major step forward. The simplicity of the device and its ready availability at the time of acute care of the femur have allowed variations of this design to be reapplied into current suspension splints. Probably no single device has had greater durability and long-term acceptance in clinical practice than the Thomas splint (Fig. 15-4).

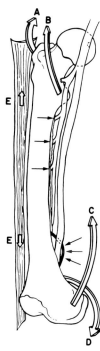

Fig. 15-5. Deforming muscle forces on the femur: (*A*) abductors, (*B*) iliopsoas, (*C*) adductors, (*D*) gastrocnemius origin. Medial angulating forces are resisted by the tension brace of the fascia lata (*E*). Sites of vascular threat are at the adductor hiatus and the perforating vessels of the profunda femoris.

SURGICAL ANATOMY

GROSS ANATOMICAL FEATURES

The features of significance for femoral fractures are related to its structural aspects, which are associated with stress concentration and the deforming forces of muscles and vascular aspects, as related to either trauma or surgery (Fig. 15-5).

STRUCTURAL ASPECTS

The shaft of the femur is roughly tubular, except for the contour of the linea aspera. From a mechanical standpoint, a tube is the mechanical structure that can resist angulation with the best weight-to-strength ratio. Because of the length of the femur and the lever arms involved, this is the chief structural requirement. However, a tube is not the best design to resist torsional forces.

The subtrochanteric area can be a site of stress concentration owing to the short radius of curvature at this site. When bone has insufficient opportunity for turnover and remodelling, as in metabolic bone disease, this may be a site of pathologic fracture. Although the widening distal diaphysis of a healthy femur is quite resistant to stress concentration and failure, with aging, slower bone turnover, and reduced resilience of skeletal structures, this area is more likely than the mid-shaft to shatter. The same is true of the supracondylar area.

The massive muscle attachments to the greater trochanter are a source of abduction deformity with fractures of the proximal femoral shaft. In addition, the attachment of a very large muscle complex—the iliopsoas—on the lesser trochanter, creates a flexion-external rotation deformity of the proximal fragment that may be impossible to control by longitudinal traction. The wide and extensive insertion of adductor musculature on the medial distal aspect forms a constant angulating force, which tends to create varus deformity in fractures of the mid-shaft. This tendency to deformity is accentuated by ambulatory loading, in that the forces of function are medial to the shaft of the bone. These deforming forces are resisted by the "tension braces" of the lateral thigh musculature and fascia lata.[105] However, this bracing action of the musculature may be considerably weakened by disuse and inactivity. Progressive weakening may be of considerable significance in the late mobilization of fractured femurs and their tendency to angulate or refracture.

The origin of the gastrocnemius on the distal femoral condyles is said to create a flexion force that causes deformity in the distal fragment.[171] In skeletal traction systems this is controlled by traction and knee extension, which brings the corrective balance of ligaments to bear.

Blood supply to the femur, like that of all tubular bones, is by the way of metaphyseal, periosteal, and endosteal supply. The periosteal blood supply is related to the multiple muscle origins from the shaft to the femur and thus is seldom in danger from fractures, except in the case of extensive stripping. Laing has specifically identified the nutrient artery blood supply in the femur.[119] The nutrient artery or arteries consistently perforate the

femoral shaft along the linea aspera. The arteries are derived from perforating branches of the profunda femoris artery. In most of his dissections in adults, there was but a single nutrient artery entering the proximal half, thus leaving a long descending branch in the intramedullary canal to supply the endosteum.

The perforating branches of the profunda femoris artery encircle the bone posteriorly and perforate the muscle attachments adjacent to the linea aspera aspect. There are usually four perforating branches. Injury to these vessels during surgical exposure may be a source of considerable exasperation, in that they will retract posteriorly and medially within the muscle, making ligation extremely difficult. The main femoral artery perforates anteroposteriorly at the adductor hiatus. This tether may be the location of vascular entrapment at the time of skeletal injury and thus, a suspected site of vascular injury.

Throughout most of its course in the thigh, the sciatic nerve is cushioned from the femur and, thus, is seldom involved in injury. The neurovascular supply of the vastus lateralis does emerge anteriorly in the proximal third of the rectus femoris and thus hinders a wide dissection of the femoral shaft anteriorly deep to the rectus (Henry approach).

SURGICAL APPROACHES

Because of the anatomical aspects identified above, access to the femoral shaft is relatively simple. The main vasculature is medial and posterior; the main nerve is free to move and is usually safely deep to the fracture site. In general the best surgical exposure is the safe and convenient lateral approach. The skin incision is along the line drawn from the greated trochanter distally to the lateral femoral condyle. The iliotibial band is split and the vastus lateralis dissected from the intermuscular septum. With appropriate retractors the large muscle mass may be swept anteriorly immediately to expose the entire length of the shaft. Perforating vessels are best secured with suture ligation, which will prevent the local complications and significant hematoma that can result from poorly controlled vasculature at this site. This approach may be used repeatedly without threat of achieving additional scarring or devascularization. The more anterior approach of Henry between the rectus and the lateralis is not favored because of its potential to scar the musculature. Certainly repeated use of this incision guarantees limited range of motion in the knee.

BLOOD SUPPLY OF THE FEMUR

With respect to microanatomy, there are several areas for consideration.[31] In healthy adult tubular bone, the relative contributions of the nutrient vascular system and the periosteal system remain controversial. The majority of evidence indicates that most of the cortical diaphyseal bone is supplied by the nutrient system with radial transverse branches supporting the cellular structure of most of the diaphysis.[119] Observations of blood flow *in vivo* have disclosed that the blood flow in the cortex is not completely centrifugal but returns to the venous sinusoids of the intramedullary canal.[181,211]

Knowing which contributes more to bone blood supply is, of course, important if one wishes to make a theoretical choice between stripping the periosteum for bone plating and destroying the intramedullary blood supply by nailing.[55] On a purely theoretical basis, intramedullary nailing seems to have the greatest potential for vascular destruction. Rhinelander has made a considerable contribution to our understanding of bone repair using microangiographic techniques.[31,182,183] The variations in repair associated with plating and rodding were analyzed. The conclusions of this work confirm that the intramedullary vessels are distributed to a greater portion of the normal cortex but nevertheless require their periosteal "neighbors" to function properly. Moreover, when the endosteal circulation is obliterated, periosteal blood supply can expand greatly in function, and most of the diaphysis can be supported by periosteal vasculature. When the intramedullary circulation is totally obliterated, indeed plugged, by a solid rod, total endosteal vascular obliteration occurs and healing is compromised. It is likely that healing failure occurs not so much from poor supply as from inefficient drainage. The high volume-low pressure flow of the venous sinusoids is obliterated. Judging from this evidence it is fortunate that no intramedullary device of tubular design has been developed that has the potential of completely obliterating and preventing the reformation of these conduits, the venous sinusoids of the intramedullary canal.

In dog studies, sites on the periosteum temporarily made avascular by periosteal stripping for plates rapidly revascularize by recruiting the endosteal supply and associated periosteal tissues.[11] Finally, because the periosteal blood supply is derived from a multitude of tiny vessels, none of which traverse the periosteum longitudinally, obliteration of blood supply to the bone by circumferential wire or suture material is impossible.

MECHANISMS OF INJURY

Femoral shaft fractures usually result from major violence, so these fractures are most common in young adults. This is not only because this age group is often more prone to violence, such as auto and motorcycle accidents and gunshot wounds, but also because the wider metaphyseal areas are frequently able to dissipate and transfer the stress force sufficiently before major fracture occurs. With any condition that retards bone turnover, the reorientation ability of the trabecular pattern to accept stress concentration is reduced. Aged bone is somewhat more brittle, and resilience of the trabecular pattern is lost so that unacceptable stress forces more easily produce a fracture. Thus, femoral shaft fractures are markedly less common to persons in the older age groups, who usually suffer fractures at the metaphyseal ends of the long bone.

Because fracture of the femoral shaft is frequently associated with violence, the energy of the impact may have been insufficiently dissipated by fracture of the long bone. Multiple comminution implies considerable expenditure of energy and thus considerable associated soft-tissue damage.[67,68]

CLASSIFICATION

As with all other fractures, it is necessary to distinguish between open and closed fractures of the femur. Open fracture from within suggests a higher degree of force and more injury and greater soft tissue tearing than an identical closed fracture. Open fractures also present a greater opportunity for contamination and thus have greater potential for infection. Open fractures associated with injuries from without usually show considerable necrosis from violence to the soft tissue and have great potential for infection.

Fractures may be classified as simple, butterfly fragment, and comminuted/segmental.[151] The simple fracture may be divided into three categories: (1) spiral; (2) oblique; and (3) transverse. The butterfly fragment type of fracture may also be divided into three categories: (1) with a single butterfly fragment; (2) with two fragments; and (3) with three or more intermediate fragments.

The most significant fracture, of course, is the comminuted/segmental fracture. This also can be divided into three categories, wherein the first is purely one segmental intermediate fragment, the second is that with short comminution, and the third is one with a large and significant length of comminution with multiple fragments.

Segmental fractures imply violent injury and dispersed areas of injury within the limb. There also must be moderate devascularization of the segments.[95] Problems of instability are magnified, obviously, and this makes internal fixation more complex, in that several areas must be stabilized.

From the standpoint of treatment, however, the most significant element in classification is geographic location along the limb. Fractures of the midshaft (that length of bone wherein the tube is relatively constant in diameter) are handled most easily by internal fixation with an intramedullary rod. Although usage has standardized the label, the device is best called a "medullary" rod rather than the redundant word, "intramedullary." Fractures of the midshaft also lend themselves very well to traction treatment, as the envelope of muscle tends to stabilize the fracture and the comminuted fragments. At either end, where the diaphysis widens into the metaphysis, treatment problems are different. Subtrochanteric fractures are excessively unbalanced by the hip flexor and abductor musculature, and thus are difficult to maintain in alignment. Although considerable trabecular bone at this site implies a rapid rate of healing (relatively more blood available), purchase on the bone by internal fixation devices is limited. Fracture of the distal quarter of the bone, which includes the supracondylar area, has problems similar to those of the subtrochanteric area.

Deforming muscle forces, in the form of multiple origins and insertions, may create deformities uncontrollable with simple longitudinal traction. In that these fractures are often associated with aging bone as described earlier, multiple areas of comminution may be expected, which further complicate the use of internal fixation devices.

Thus, in general, fractures of the shaft can be divided into those of the middle three fifths, which have relatively constant diameter, and those of the widening distal and proximal ends with poor cortical structure and deforming muscular attachments, which create problems of internal fixation and of maintaining position in traction.

SIGNS AND SYMPTOMS

Diagnosis of femoral shaft fractures is usually easy. Pain is usually significant, and shortening and deformity are readily notable. Angulation of midshaft fractures usually is anterior and lateral if deforming musculature is functioning. The patient is usually unable to move either his hip or his knee.

Usually the more significant signs or symptoms are caused by those injuries associated with the fracture. An expanding thigh indicates hemorrhage and a potential for shock. Pain at the hip may also indicate dislocation or fracture at the hip. Effusion at the knee should be tested for associated ligamentous instability. If there is any question, radiographic verification of ligament status by stress films is necessary.

Of course, nerve and vascular status should be observed. Physical findings relative to innervation may be misleading because of extreme, disabling pain and the patient's inability to cooperate in an examination. The evaluation of vascular status requires no patient cooperation, and the presence of distal arterial supply should be ascertained. The absence of palpable pulses does not necessarily mean that permanent vascular damage has occurred, but the fracture surgeon must maintain a high degree of concern for the vascular status. Doppler examination is necessary to establish pulsation and probably will need to be followed by arteriography. Consultation with a vascular specialist, if available, certainly can avoid catastrophe.

RADIOGRAPHIC FINDINGS

Radiographic findings are related to the signs and symptoms. Except for imminent fatigue fractures, there is seldom an opportunity for radiographic confusion over a femoral shaft fracture. A comminuted fracture may have fracture lines that are not notable in the two planes of view if the lines of fracture are not associated with any displacement. The comminuted fracture with multiple other undisplaced fracture lines may trap one into opting for internal fixation.

The significant x-rays may be those that were not taken at the time of initial injury. The fracture of the femoral neck or dislocated hip may be missed if the only view is mid-shaft or if the Thomas ring happens to obliterate the site of fracture. Fractures of the pelvis and tibia or knee may be easily passed over when one's attention is drawn to the unmistakable characteristics of the femoral shaft fracture.

METHODS OF TREATMENT

Fractures of the femoral shaft have an extensive history of many methods of care. This reflects the pressing need to avoid the severe disability that

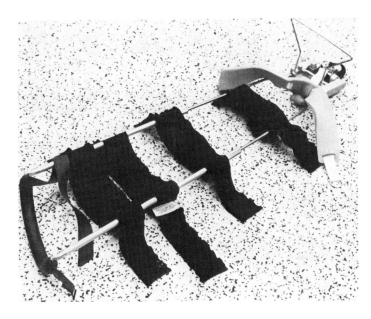

Fig. 15-6. Emergency-type splint using countertraction at the root of the leg, windlass traction for the foot, and stabilization using elastic Velcro closing straps.

results from insufficient or prolonged fracture care, the relatively common aspects of fracture of the thigh bone, and the interplay of surgical skills and engineering as related to improved fracture care. Each method discussed here has inherent advantages and disadvantages. Clinical opinion varies as to the role of each method, but there is a place for each in the armamentarium of the well-trained and informed fracture surgeon.

TRACTION

SKIN TRACTION

The concept of traction to the leg in extension for treatment of fractures in the thigh apparently was suggested by Guy de Chauliac nearly 500 years ago.[57] Although this idea had attractive aspects, the practical limitations of attaching traction to the limb delayed its effective clinical use. Traction to the foot and ankle could not be tolerated indefinitely.

By the time of the American Civil War, the practical aspects of attaching traction had been solved by the use of adhesive plaster, as described by Josiah Crosby. This method was advocated for military practice by Gurdon Buck and has since been known as Buck's extension.[36] It has severe limitations, of course. With the leg in full extension, there is little opportunity to control the deforming forces of muscles. The use of adhesive plaster extending high into the thigh and held in place by an encircling bandage offers an unhappy opportunity for tissue breakdown due to excessive shear

and compressive forces applied to the soft tissue. There is a definite limit to the amount of acceptable traction available by this method over a long period of time.

About the only practical application of the Buck's extension concept is the current variation applied in emergency transport splints. Here, traction is applied to the foot and ankle with countertraction in the groin. A good design using this concept in current practice is the emergency splint shown in Figure 15-6, wherein additional support and immobilization of the limb are achieved by easily adjustable straps with Velcrotype closure. The easy adjustability of this device makes it an admirable piece of equipment for the temporary needs of transport to the location of definitive care. Skin traction has only limited application to any form of adult femoral shaft care. It is best applied by the commercially available, adhesive-faced, sponge rubber devices that distribute the compressive forces of the stabilizing wrap over a broad area. Adhesive strapping alone is now chiefly of historic interest. If it is used, great care and attention to minute detail is necessary. The skin should be protected by a skin adhesive, such as tincture of benzoin. The edges of the wide adhesive strap should be cut at several places to allow smooth contouring and avoid concentration of tension to the skin.

One significant development in the history of skin traction for treatment of thigh fractures is the recognition that traction with the limb lying in extension is uncomfortable and associated with pain and muscle spasm. To correct this, the Australian surgeon, R. H. Russell, published his composite method in 1921.[194] With a continuous traction rope pulling vertically on a cuff at the distal thigh in an anterior direction and also axially at the leg, a force develops in the line of the femoral shaft but with the knee flexed. A direct quote from his article best indicates its present day application: "The house surgeon's duty will be to take the measurements at least every morning and evening and to inspect and adjust the pillows beneath the thigh and leg so that there may be no backward sagging at the seat of the fracture, and the heel should not be in contact with the bed. . . . This apparatus is far from being 'fool-proof' and cannot and will not look after itself." Time and the energies of the "house surgeon" have rather passed this method by. In general, its best application in skin traction form for adults is as a temporary means to provide comfort and support to the fractured limb until a definitive form of therapy is available. When skeletal traction is substituted for the surface methods, there are indeed advantages to its use.

SKELETAL TRACTION

Worldwide, skeletal traction still is the most common mode of early fracture care. Traction through the tibial tubercle with the limb suspended in some sort of hammock device is the usual mode.

The means of achieving skeletal traction has been alluded to earlier. From a mechanical standpoint, the most rational location of traction is in the distal femoral condyle, but this location is currently in disrepute because of a past history of associated stiffness of the knee joint, potential for infection at the knee through the suprapatellar pouch, and threat of introducing infection into the fractured thigh. With current techniques and a more enlightened attitude toward the time the patient should remain in traction, some of these objections have diminished. There is no reason not to apply traction to the distal condyle at the level of the adductor tubercle when it is necessary. The best case for use of skeletal traction in the distal femoral condyle is in the two-pin technique described by Stewart and associates[217] for fractures of the distal femur (see Chap. 16). It is essentially a variation on Russell's traction but uses discontinuous forces (split Russell's) so that the corrective traction on the distal femur can be separated from the longitudinal traction at the tibial tubercle. An inherent part of the two-traction-pin treatment is early active motion of the knee. As a result, in none of the cases reported by Stewart[217] was the use of the femoral traction pins associated with additional joint stiff-

ness. The femoral traction pin is used to control posterior angulation of the distal fragment. In general the application of the femoral traction pin can be delayed for 3 to 4 weeks. By that time it is recognized that the distal fragment remains uncontrolled. There is the advantage, however, of considerable resolution of fracture hematoma (and thus less threat of infection). At that time a greater amount of traction, perhaps one tenth of the patient's total weight, will be necessary to correct the plastic deformity.

The tibial tubercle is the most convenient site of skeletal traction. Its relatively subcutaneous location provides easy surgical access with no threat of creating neurovascular damage at the time of pin insertion. Considerable traction can be applied through the knee and is easily tolerated by the normal knee. No incidents of ligamentous knee complications have been reported related to normal tibial tubercle traction.

An alternative method to control the distal femoral angulation is the use of a Böhler-Braun frame with use of os calcis traction, as well as traction through the tubercle or the condyles. In general, this is a preliminary method of traction and should not be used as the definitive method of care because it severely restricts knee motion (Fig. 15-7 *top*).

Even though this is a common standard method of achieving skeletal traction, several errors in its application are notable. Neer, Grantham, and Shelton effectively pointed out these errors in their extensive study of supracondylar fractures of the femur.[153] The most common error in traction management is the varus internal rotation deformity enforced on the distal femoral fragment by the position of the skeletal traction. It should be remembered that the majority of the muscle forces on the proximal femoral shaft favor external rotation and slight flexion. The pull of the adductor magnus favors internal rotation of the distal fragment and varus. As in all traction procedures, it is necessary to try to match the uncontrollable (proximal) fragments by aligning the distal fragment.

One should recognize that the limb resting with patella pointing straight to the ceiling is a distinctly nonanatomical posture, and a more relaxed posture expects external rotation of the knee. Insertion of the skeletal traction should reproduce this same rotation at rest in an effort to provide balanced pull (Fig. 15-7 *bottom*). Thus, when traction is applied, the leg should lie in slight external rotation and allow the distal fragments to correspond more accurately to the alignment of the proximal fragments.

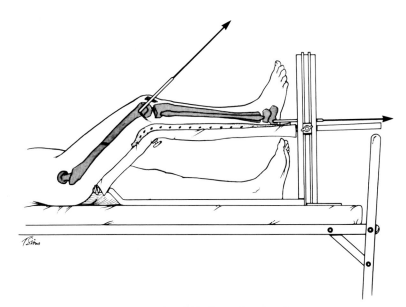

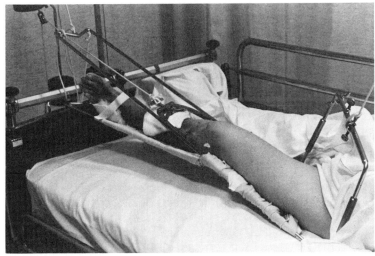

Fig. 15-7. (*Top*) Skeletal traction for femoral fractures on a Böhler-Braun frame. In conservative treatment of a fracture traction may be applied through a transcondylar pin. In distal femoral fractures it is advantageous to add an os calcis traction pin to prevent the distal femoral fragment from developing recurvatum. (*Bottom*) Skeletal traction and suspension for fracture of the distal femur demonstrating external rotation of the distal fragment and leg. This suspension device is the Harris-Aufranc design with Pearson attachment. Skeletal traction is by a Kirschner wire in the tibial tubercle.

The x-ray technician should be instructed to accept a slightly rotated posture of the limb as he takes his true anteroposterior view. Frequently, misjudgment as to the adequacy of traction is based purely on distortion of x-rays because true anteroposterior and lateral films were not obtained. This can happen because the technician expects the beam perpendicular to the floor to be the true anteroposterior of the femur and that parallel to the floor to be the true lateral of the femur. It is essential to obtain consistent and standardized views to avoid these misjudgments. Frequently, displacements of the fracture fragments disappear when the x-ray is taken in true anteroposterior and lateral position.

There are several important trade-offs to consider

in choosing the type of traction pin. The Steinmann pin inherently has more strength than the Kirschner wire. Its greater diameter, however, requires more soft-tissue destruction and a larger hole in the bone. In general, the only advantage to using a very large Steinmann pin for axial traction is to make purchase through osteoporotic bone, thus allowing a broader surface area for the bone to react against the significant stress concentrations of traction. The larger the diameter of the rod, however, the more effective torque concentration can be developed and the more likely the rod is to swivel within the bone. To a certain extent, the Böhler bow tries to counteract this if it is lubricated well.[20] This, unfortunately, is seldom the case, and some binding occurs as the device swivels. An alternative to this

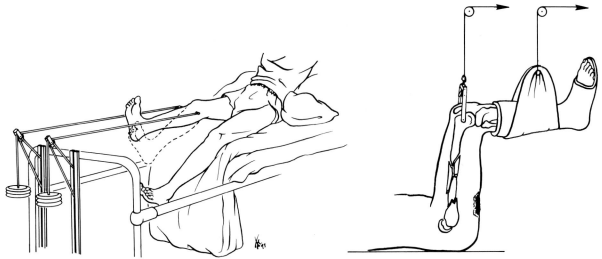

Fig. 15-8. (*Left*) Perkins split-weight traction system allows active knee motion once the fracture fragments have become stabilized. Angulatory correction can be achieved by varying medial or lateral weights. (Redrawn from Kirkaldy-Willis, W. H.; and Thomas, T. G.: Injuries to the Lower Limb. Edinburgh, E. & S. Livingstone, 1962.) (*Right*) 90-90 traction is especially applicable to fractures of the subtrochanteric area with associated wounds of the groin and buttock. Traction through the femoral condyles is most efficient, and it is not associated with stiffness at the knee. Suspension of the leg in a plaster cast is usually necessary.

problem is the use of two separate traction attachments that are self-lubricating. The method described by Perkins offers excellent control of the fracture by means of two independent traction systems.[109,172] Dynamic muscle activity is also encouraged by this system (Fig. 15-8 *left*). A recent report by Buxton from England indicates its persistent value and success.[40]

Another alternative to avoid motion of the rod within bone and soft tissues is to use a threaded Steinmann pin. Threading, of course, weakens the rod, and an even larger pin must be used. In general, a ³⁄₁₆-inch pin is the largest practical. Despite its size, it can sustain traction forces of 25 pounds or more.

A more reasonable traction device is the Kirschner wire with the appropriate spreader bow. Because the spreader bow must take very firm purchase on the wire, any motion of the bow is directly transmitted to the wire in contrast to the swivel effect of the Steinmann pin bow. Because of the thin diameter of Kirschner wires, however, this effect is seldom very significant. Threaded Kirschner wires have little advantage and probably some disadvantage because motion of the threaded device within the bone and skin interface is un-

avoidable, owing to the purchase of the traction bow. Also, the greater thickness necessary for the threaded wire makes attachment to the traction bow more difficult, and it is likely to slip. A Kirschner wire with the traction bow is, by and large, the most reliable method to achieve skeletal traction with the least chance of chronic problems after use.

Placement of skeletal traction pins must be accomplished under aseptic conditions. Insertion can be accomplished nicely under local anesthesia. The only sensible structures are the skin itself and the periosteum of the bone. Both the insertion location and the site where the pin emerges from the bone and through the skin must be blocked. Some pain is unavoidable during the insertion of skeletal traction pins under local anesthesia, for once the cortical bone is perforated, pressure equalization occurs with distention of the venous sinusoids in the intramedullary space, and sharp pain results. It is transitory, however, and a reasonable exchange for avoiding the logistical complications of general anesthesia.

Just as significant in the application of skeletal traction techniques as the traction pin itself is the suspension. Indeed, usually this is the problem of greatest concern and consumes the most time in the care of the patients with skeletal traction. The time-honored Thomas ring is the most common suspension method used. As discussed earlier, this device was originally designed not as a suspension method at all but rather as a countertraction system for extending the leg in axial traction. Only its ready availability has recommended it as a suspension system. To avoid the pressure concentration of the ring at the buttock and groin, the half Thomas ring is a better device. In this system, the superior portion of the ring remains rigid, while the hammock portion of fabric is soft and contours to the upper thigh.

But as every former house officer can recall, the tapering side calipers of the Thomas ring (or half ring) adjacent to the tapering thigh promote distal slipping of the fabric. This can be avoided by incorporating fabric into the ring itself. In this setting, a 6-inch, bias-cut stockinette makes an admirable hammock material that can be wound readily about the caliper rods of the suspension device, replaced after use, and custom fitted on each occasion to correspond to the weight of the limb. The usual materials, which depend on clips and pins, seem constantly to be displaced and misplaced. Soft fabric in 6-inch widths is a common hammock material. A length of felt at the interface between skin and fabric keeps the fabric hammock from riding back and forth.

As Russell[194] pointed out, the flexed knee is by far the more comfortable position and more adequately reduces muscular forces so that the limb may fall in line more easily by traction. Also, in contrast to earlier concepts in traction care, mobility of the knee joint is now looked on as an advantage not only to fracture healing, but as a method by which to avoid fibroarthrosis of the knee joint. Early muscle activity, as emphasized by DeLorme[59] and verified by Stewart,[216,217] has a very positive effect on muscle and joint function after the termination of traction. Thus, there is seldom a place for the fixed traction suspended splint, such as the Thomas ring alone. Dynamic methods to allow free muscle and joint functions offer far more potential for early union and good joint motion.

Another method of skeletal traction and suspension should be noted. This is the 90-90 traction as illustrated in Figure 15-8 *right*. It is especially appropriate for proximal fractures that allow the distal segment to match the flexed proximal fragment. Body weight is stable counter traction but, unfortunately, requires the patient to stay some-what fixed in bed. The flexed knee position at 90° is not generally a source of significant stiffness. Experience has demonstrated that flexion deformities are easily worked out once the patient is ambulatory but extension contractures are only worked out with great difficulty.

ROLLER TRACTION

The system that best offers the potential for free muscle and joint function, while at the same time providing an opportunity for traction to maintain alignment, is roller traction, which was designed by Alonzo Neufeld of Los Angeles.[136] This system "flows" with patient movements and in general is found to be quite comfortable. It incorporates suspension from a wheel on an overhead track and traction that is supplied in the usual manner, with weights and pulleys tied to the wheel assembly (roller) rather than to the patient himself. Because of the system's simplicity it is easily accepted by uninitiated house staff and nursing personnel. Also, because of its dynamic qualities it is ideally suited to the pediatric age group, whose usually restless behavior requires constant attention to maintain traction and order.[124,136,143]

The system can be applied immediately or, more realistically, within a day or so, after all factors related to the femoral fracture are clarified and a plan of treatment is established. If motion to the knee will not be disruptive to alignment, the system can be constructed so that the thigh and the shank portion are connected by a joint that will allow motion of the knee. But if early motion is ill advised due to precarious alignment, a long leg cast can be used initially. Often this is the best early approach because corrections of alignment can also be achieved by wedging the cast. In situations in which there is considerable instability of the distal femur, perhaps secondary to soft tissue loss, all of the early motion will occur at the fracture site, not at the knee, and thus the motion will be destructive to union (Fig. 15-9).

This is a skeletal traction method because initially the reduction is maintained by longitudinal traction while functioning muscles help to maintain alignment as they resist the distracting force. If this system is employed as the definitive method of care, a Steinmann pin should be used at the tibial tubercle; ultimately, the force transfer of the traction system will be transmitted to the skeletal system through this pin. A Kirschner wire is too thin to tolerate the transfer of force from the plaster to the bone. However, it should be recognized that if all

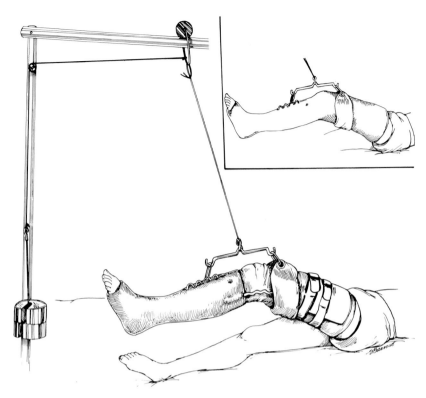

Fig. 15-9. Roller traction assembly demonstrating the traction and suspension system combined in one unit. The inset demonstrates the long leg cast configuration that later can be converted to an adjustable fracture brace system. A skeletal pin may be incorporated into the plaster.

other factors are equal (such as skill and experience of the surgeon, technique, and preparation of the skin, etc.), the use of the Kirschner wire, in comparison to the Steinmann pin, offers a lower incidence of overall infection.[189]

Once the pin has been placed in the usual manner, at the tibial tubercle (in unusual circumstances the pin can also be applied at the distal femoral condyle), then plaster application is appropriate. For fractures of the mid-shaft of the femur, knee motion probably will not be a problem, and thus from the beginning the brace can be in two sections. The traditional polycentric cast brace joints have the disadvantage of requiring parallel orientation so that they will function smoothly without binding. In a situation in which the thigh portion may be tightened to account for loss of thigh circumference secondary to reducing edema, hematoma, and muscle atrophy, single axis joints are not ideal. Hook and eye joints or plastic joints are more appropriate. It is important, however, initially to apply the thigh portion as firmly as possible because this seems to assist muscle activity.

Since initial thigh circumference usually is significantly enlarged, early muscle activity does have the benefit of not only providing early stability to the fracture, but also enhancing the rate of fluid

exchange, which encourages the loss of edema. Therefore, in simple fractures early motion should be encouraged even though initial total contact of thigh support is rapidly lost with the decreasing circumference. Initially, total contact support is not absolutely necessary because alignment can be achieved by the traction. No attempt is made to contour the rim of the cast proximally into a quadrilateral shape. The cast should extend as high into the groin as is comfortable. It is not possible to achieve ischial loading of a fracture brace; the function of the device is to encapsulate the limb sufficiently so that the femur can be made stable by active muscle forces and the hydraulic stability of the fleshy, cone-shaped thigh.

With the plaster in place, suspension hooks should be incorporated both in the thigh portion and the leg portion. These are attached by rope to the hook of the roller. A separate line runs from the roller to the pulley at the end of the bed and then to the weights. These are two separate lines: the one used to suspend the limb from the pulley system; and the one that transfers the force of the weights to the pulley. If motion at the knee is allowed, a spring can be substituted for a portion of the suspension line, allowing the patient to "jiggle" and thus start active muscle function. If

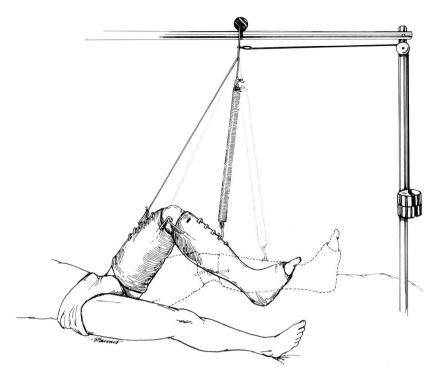

Fig. 15-10. Diagram of a patient in roller traction/suspension system. There are two separate lines—one for traction, and the other for suspension. Note the use of variable tensions created by changing hook placement.

the location of the suspension line along the row of hooks is changed, quadriceps function versus hamstring function can be favored (Fig. 15-10).

Once the patient is comfortable, he can be mobilized with partial weight bearing (toe touching). Usually, a pick-up walker is used. He should return to bed after the ambulatory activity, however, so that alignment can be restored by traction (Fig. 15-11). In addition, x-ray monitoring is necessary to assure maintenance of alignment and, when necessary, wedging of the cast is required to improve alignment.

When the fracture is stable (that is, it will not shorten or lose alignment when traction is removed), then discharge from hospital can be expected. At this time an adjustable plastic thigh portion may be substituted for the plaster (Fig. 15-12). This commercially available item is lighter and more comfortable, but may have the disadvantage of allowing insufficient water vapor evaporation in hot, humid climates. The thigh portion may also be constructed of various plaster substitute materials, which can also be made adjustable. At this point in treatment, patient compliance is necessary; various failures in treatment have resulted because the patient discontinued the thigh portion of the brace too early.

In our institution, the roller traction system has

supplanted all other traction suspension systems. The simplicity and self-correcting aspects of the device are appreciated by patients, nurses, and clinicians. It has also been used as the traction mobilization system for acetabular fractures, post hip arthroplasties, and severely comminuted fractures of the tibial plateau. The only unique piece of equipment is the roller running on the track attached to the overhead frame. These rollers are commercially available or may be constructed in local machine shops.

The system is extremely versatile and can be used in the full array of trauma problems. It has been advocated for the patient with multiple traumas because rapid mobilization is not hindered and the patient is able to sit up and achieve appropriate respiration.[34] In the pediatric group, for which internal fixation is inappropriate, it works well. Finally, in settings in which internal fixation is not available because of threat of infection, severe comminution, or lack of equipment and expertise, the system is satisfactory and safe. It can also be used as an adjunct to insufficient internal fixation.

Patients with a simple fracture can remove the traction themselves, usually within a week or so, begin partial, protected weight bearing, and then return back to the traction system after completion of ambulatory activities. In a recent consecutive

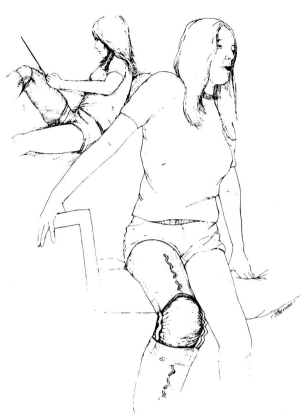

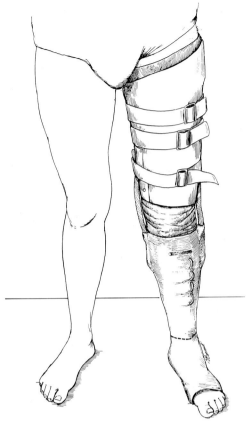

Fig. 15-11. Once the fracture is stable (when the patient is able to use his or her muscles comfortably) gradual mobilization may be accomplished. The patient should not be discharged from the hospital until the fracture is stable and a firm thigh support is available.

Fig. 15-12. The femoral fracture brace with adjustable plastic (or plaster substitute) thigh section. Hooks incorporated in shank plaster are for roller traction suspension. The dotted line at the ankle demonstrates where the foot section can be removed, which is possible as long as suspension of the thigh section is still available. (Note the plaster incorporated skeletal pin.)

series, the median time to hospital discharge was 25 days.[124] Discontinuation of traction can be achieved once static weight bearing on the injured limb is pain free, and the patient's limb has not been shown to shorten after being out of traction for a day.

Thus, in summary, roller traction has turned out to be the best combination of traction and brace systems in our experience. This relatively simple system can be used safely in situations in which skeletal internal fixation is either unavailable or inappropriate. It has been demonstrated to shorten hospitalization by approximately 2 weeks in comparison to the older traction and cast brace system, and, in fact, union can be expected to occur approximately 2 weeks sooner than suggested by previous experience.[124,143] However, roller traction does require a compliant patient and seldom results in a limb that presents perfectly normal alignment and length.

CAST BRACE

The cast brace was developed in reaction to long-term traction and spica care. Initially it was meant to be only a substitute for the spica. It was designed, however, to allow motion of the joints above and below the fracture, and to allow progressively more functional muscle activity. It was possible to demonstrate the positive effects of such a mobilization device in a series of 150 consecutive fractures in the distal half of the femur that were considered inappropriate for internal fixation at that time. All of these fractures united with an average healing time of 3½ months, and 80% of fractures were found to have a functional range of knee motion at the time of plaster removal (Fig. 15-13).[111]

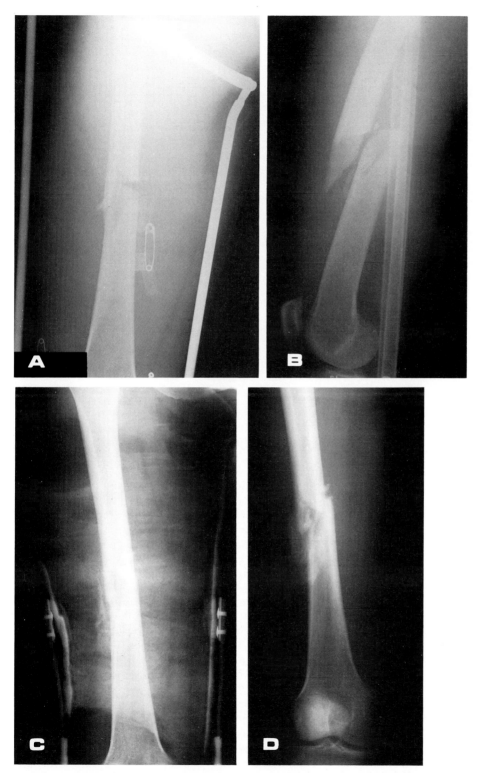

Fig. 15-13. Cast brace series. (*A,B*) Comminuted fracture at the mid- and distal shaft of the femur. (*C*) Position in cast brace 2½ months later. The brace had been applied 3½ weeks after fracture. The patient is fully ambulatory and ready for cast brace removal.

(*Continues on p. 1372.*)

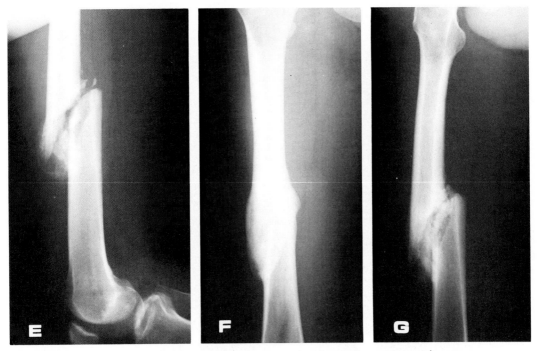

Fig. 15-13 (*Continued*). (*D,E*) After cast brace removal at 3 months postonset he was clinically sound. (*F,G*) Ten months postonset and 5 months out of brace.

Unfortunately, the more proximal the fracture and the more simple the fracture, the more difficult it is to maintain alignment because of the concentration of all angulatory forces at one location. Various maneuvers have been undertaken to maintain correction once the patient is ambulatory. Meggitt and associates[138] have demonstrated the use of a half-spica hip control brace technique with three-point fixation, which they have found successful.

If fracture bracing is a new concept to the operator, it is best used as a substitute for a spica cast and applied 5 to 7 weeks after injury (Fig. 15-14). Once one is confident using it, it can be applied far earlier, when the healing granuloma of fracture repair has achieved some degree of stability. This is evidenced by decreasing callus tenderness, lessening pain on activity in traction, and a decrease in swelling of the thigh. This may occur 1 to 4 weeks after injury, depending on the fracture's severity, comminution, and many other factors. Applying the cast brace in this early stage of healing, while the fracture is still quite loose, may have to be accomplished in the operating room on a fracture table with the patient in traction, under anesthesia if necessary. It is not necessary to apply the brace

joints at this time; they can be applied later in a two-stage, plaster cut-out method that avoids shortening, and thus, loss of alignment, at the fracture site.

Suspension of the cast brace is extremely important. If the plaster capsule slips distally, the support of the muscles is lost. For this reason, the shank and foot are incorporated and connected to the thigh portion of the cast brace by polycentric joints. Our own research studies indicate that this system can unweight the skeletal system by about 50% initially, but this rapidly falls to 10% to 20%. Thus, the cast brace is designed to maintain position, but it will not correct overriding or angulation. On occasion, we have maintained suspension and countertraction by leaving the tibial traction pin incorporated in the plaster and even returning the patient to traction when he is not walking. This serves well enough if the knee joints are aligned extremely well; otherwise, the stress forces on the traction pin site are rather severe and cause pain. We have used a molded plastic capsule about the thigh, suspended by a belt from the waist, with adjustable Velcro closures to maintain constant pressure on the thigh muscles. This procedure is appropriate only for firm fractures in an advanced

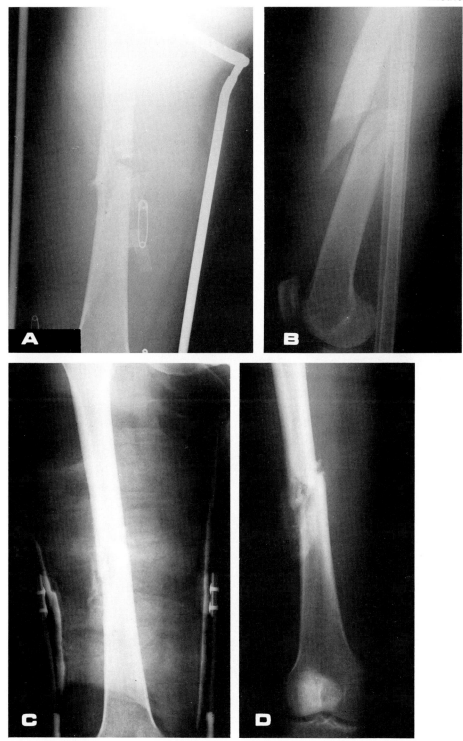

Fig. 15-14. The natural history of a femoral fracture treated with initial traction followed by cast brace application. (*A,B*) Initial position in traction. (*C*) The position in a plaster cast brace applied 4 weeks after onset. (*D*) The position at the time of removal of the cast brace. A total of 12 weeks postonset.

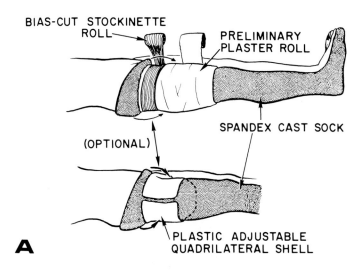

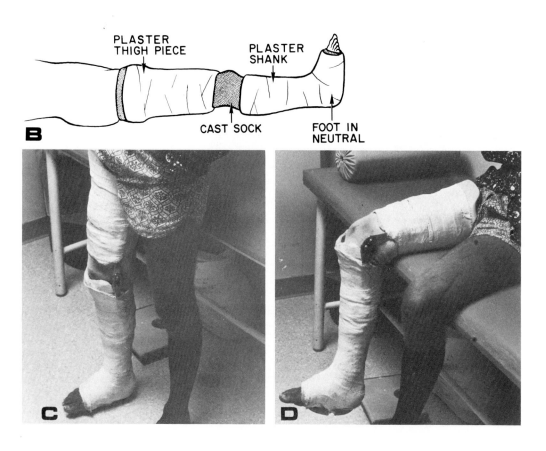

Fig. 15-15. (*A*) Diagrammatic representation of a cast brace application. (*B*) Total contact thigh cylinder with suspension by means of a leg cast with the foot included. The joints are to be added. (*C,D*) A cast brace on a patient with a fractured midshaft femur at time of removal.

stage of healing, but it demonstrates again the most significant aspect of cast brace program: the supplying of hydrodynamic support to the musculature of the thigh.

The application of joints to a total-contact cast is the only aspect of fracture brace care that may exceed the experience and confidence of the well-trained fracture surgeon (Fig. 15-15). Joints are available that have a polycentric design and can be attached to a special fixture to maintain the joints in parallel alignment. Metal joints have the advantage of considerable security. They will not allow anteroposterior or medial-lateral displacement, nor will they allow shortening. Thus, for fractures at the knee, they are critical. As time passes, it is reasonable to expect that plastic joints will eventually supplant the current metal devices.

The metal brace joints require some skill to position their axes to correspond to the complex anatomical axis of the knee. The joints should be positioned at the level of the adductor tubercle, which is usually about the level of the mid-patella. They also can be displaced approximately ½ inch posterior to the midportion of the leg, a position that more nearly reproduces the position of the anatomical axis at the knee.[144]

Because the fracture brace is meant to be a total-contact device, very little padding is necessary. Occasionally, relief is necessary over the fibular head and malleoli, if there is very little subcutaneous padding. The foot should be maintained in the position of neutrality in dorsiplantar flexion and at a slight valgus angle, if possible. As the brace is an ambulatory device, it should fix the foot flat for walking and should be able to tolerate ambulation. Initially a canvas cast shoe is used in ambulation; later, a walking heel applied to the plaster may allow younger, more vigorous patients to take longer strides.

Cast bracing is most applicable to comminuted fractures of the mid- or distal shaft, open fractures, and simple fractures in young patients. Its usefulness increases with the hazards posed by the alternative, operative approach.

Cast bracing is not appropriate for proximal shaft fractures, which should be fixed internally, if this is available, or maintained in traction until the fracture is firm. Supracondylar fractures, especially in older and osteoporotic persons, are good candidates for cast brace treatment following an initial period of skeletal traction with the knee in extension. Frequently, patients require the two-pin traction method of Stewart[217] to maintain the position of the distal fragment. The flexed-knee traction used for supracondylar fractures is inappropriate; as Neer, Grantham, and Shelton[153] pointed out, the extended knee does not flex the distal femoral fragment. Seldom will cuffs about the thigh control the distal fragment as well as a second traction pin does.

Once the leg is in a cast brace, the position of the fracture fragments can be corrected if angulation occurs by wedging of the plaster (Fig. 15-16). In our experience, no shortening has occurred greater than that accepted in skeletal traction. It must be recognized that if one chooses to treat the patient by skeletal traction, in all fractures except the anatomically reduced transverse fracture, he must accept a few millimeters of shortening. The shortening, however, helps early formation of a callus

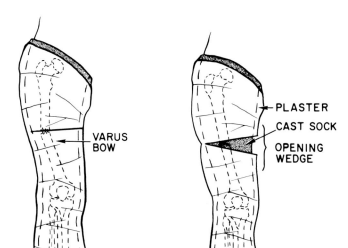

Fig. 15-16. Method of open wedging to achieve correction in the varus angulation that develops in proximal femoral fractures.

in that it provides a greater surface area over which the "weld" of new bone can be operative. The only way in which a femoral shaft fracture in traction can fail to unite is if the fracture fragments are maintained in distraction for a long time. Initial distraction to achieve the best alignment, followed shortly by ambulatory care does not result in nonunion. Even several manipulations to achieve best alignment do not threaten the result, as long as ambulatory cast brace care is available in the early phases of fracture healing. Closed manipulation of the fracture with the patient on a fracture table, under anesthesia if necessary, and maintenance in a total-contract cast, as described above, will correct most alignment problems.

EXTERNAL FIXATION

The percutaneous transfixion pin treatment of femoral fractures is a compromise maneuver between definitive skeletal traction and open reduction and internal fixation. A flurry of interest in this method began in the mid 1930s and reached its peak during World War II. Using techniques originally developed in veterinary medicine,[214] Roger Anderson of Seattle advocated multiple percutaneous pins that transversely fix the proximal and distal aspects of the fractured bone.[12,13] Immobilization was achieved by way of an outrigger beam attached to these protruding pins. This method frequently was successful in treating animals, and in the hands of advocates also had many outstanding clinical successes in humans. However, a critical review of the results of this method identified a failure rate of about 20%. The tendency to call the chronic pin tract infections "minor serous drainage" introduced the euphemism "Seattle serum" into orthopaedic vocabulary to indicate drainage at sites of infection. The rate of treatment failure with this method was so high that the Surgeon General himself ordered it to be discarded as a treatment for military personnel during World War II.

One of the sources of failure was the very rigid hardware that kept the bone ends distracted. This rigid hardware also concentrated stress at the skeletal attachment during muscle-or weight-bearing activities, which gradually loosened fixation. In addition, the pins easily worked loose, causing irritation at both the bone and skin interface. This chronic mechanical irritation, of course, was intolerable to living tissues and was the source of drainage.

In spite of the inglorious demise of this method in America, similar methods of transcutaneous

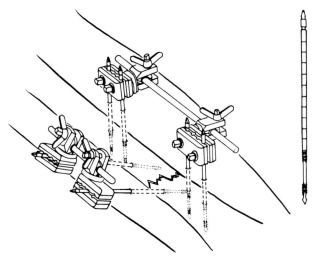

Fig. 15-17. Hoffmann's percutaneous skeletal fixation method.

external fixations for fracture remain popular in various parts of Europe. Adrey presented a series of experimental biomechanical studies confirming the stability of appropriately designed transcutaneous skeletal fixation systems.[4] A system developed by Raul Hoffmann, which uses specially designed threaded rods and external fixation by ball joints, is now marketed nearly all over the world. It is advocated for severely comminuted fractures with associated open wounds, drainage, chronic bone infections, and nonunions.[96] The successes reported by various authors have been ascribed to a well engineered, compatible system of hardware (Fig. 15-17).

The system for control of the femoral shaft suggested by Hoffmann has the disadvantage of perforating the anterior thigh musculature; the fixation of the fracture thus results in tethering and scarring. However, it was thought necessary to construct this multiplanar system to give stability to the fracture site.

An alternative system for external fixation of the femur is that designed by Wagner.[230] Originally used for leg lengthening, it was intended to cope with an inherent instability (the gradually lengthening femur). This system has been engineered so that it is extremely strong although it uses only a single lateral outrigger. Because there is a rigid bar laterally, there is no need to tether the quadriceps musculature (Fig. 15-18).

By and large, external fixation of femoral fractures is not usually indicated. The liberal use of these devices is not justified when some of the pecularities of femoral injuries are considered.[30] First, there is a basic difference in femoral fractures as compared to tibial fractures with regard to the protective soft tissues and vascular supply. The extensive muscle envelope that protects the femur usually allows for more generous consideration of internal fixation devices. This is especially true in open femoral fractures. Second, the anatomy of the thigh does not make the application of an external fixator as harmless as it should be. A through pin technique, which is most often performed for a frame fixation, is not feasible due to the limited space of the medial aspect of the thigh, as well as to the potential danger that the fixation pins may accidently injure the femoral vessels. The technique of pin placement for an external fixator through the quadriceps muscle causes severe impairment to the extensors of the knee joint because the muscle tethering from scar cannot be worked out in an early postinjury attempt to retain knee motion. Therefore, we favor the easier technique of half-pin fixation described below.

In general, we regard an external fixator only as a temporary, short-term device in femoral fractures. Definitive internal fixation should be accomplished as soon as possible. None of the most popular external fixator devices has a real chance to bring about a final result comparable to those of internal fixation. In addition, the higher incidence of problems related to instability, such as pin track infections, misalignment of fragments, malunion and nonunion, have to be anticipated, particularly when the external fixator has been kept in place over too long a period of time.[79]

In our institution the following are indications for using external fixators for femoral fractures: shotgun blast injuries causing excessive soft tissue damage, associated with marked bone loss; Grade III open fractures with extensive contamination of the soft tissues; ipsilateral fractures such as a combination of pelvic, femoral and tibial fractures, which are often associated with life-threatening injuries in polytraumatized patients. Further, we accept the use of an external fixator in those femoral fractures that are already infected at the time operative treatment is initiated. To repeat, external fixators in femoral injuries have been rare procedures since we almost always succeed in treating femoral fractures with a definitive internal fixation.

Two different devices have been mainly used in our institution. The Wagner[230] apparatus offers certain advantages over that devised by Roger Anderson,[12,13] although the latter's external fixator appears to be cheaper and therefore more useful

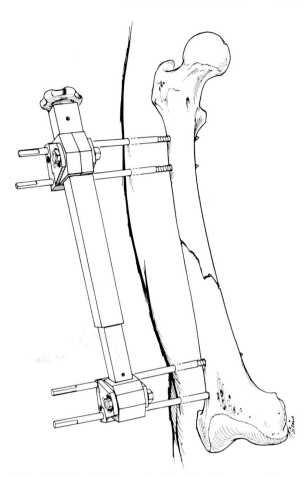

Fig. 15-18. The Wagner leg lengthening apparatus for lateral stabilization of femoral fractures.

financially to a county hospital system. The application of the Wagner apparatus is for the most part restricted to femoral fractures that come to our service for a delayed procedure and already present unacceptable shortening of the bone or infection. The options the Wagner apparatus offers for correcting shortening or malalignment or, as often necessary in infected fractures, maintaining the appropriate length of the bone makes it an extremely versatile and valuable instrument. In addition, its application as an initial fixation device for open femoral fractures in badly injured, polytraumatized patients is simple. A lengthy operative procedure is unnecessary. Since this device stays *in situ* only temporarily, certain recommendations concerning its application should be kept in mind.

Six-millimeter Schanz screws are used for fixation pins. The insertion of these screws always follows predrilling of the pin sites with a 3.5-mm

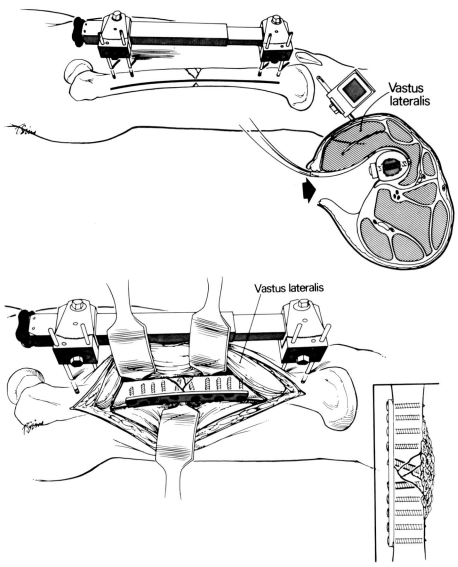

Fig. 15-19. (*Top*) The Wagner apparatus used as a temporary device before definitive plate fixation. (*Bottom*) Definitive stabilization of the fracture by means of a broad DCP. Note generous bone grafting opposite to the plate at the level of comminution. The Wagner apparatus is removed only after the plate has been applied.

drill bit over a drill guide. The length of the pin sites corresponds exactly to the length of the Schanz screws in their final position in the fixation clamps of the Wagner apparatus. To allow for a repeat operative procedure (*e.g.,* in the presence of an infection, as well as for definitive operative procedures such as internal fixation and bone grafting), the pins should be inserted in a more anterolateral-posteromedial direction. The pins must fully penetrate the medial cortex. Piercing the vastus lateralis musculature is less harmful than piercing the rectus

femoris muscle. When the goals of temporary fixation in the Wagner apparatus have been accomplished—restoration of length and axial alignment, cleansing of an infection, or improvement of the status of a multiply injured patient—definitive stabilization of the fracture is attempted.

We prefer when possible definitive fixation of the fracture with plates (broad dynamic compression plates [DCPs] or special lengthening plates) in combination with a generous autogenous cancellous bone grafting (Fig. 15-19). The more ventrally placed Schanz screws interfere neither with the usual lateral surgical approach nor with the placement of the plate, which ideally is done in such a way that the posterior edge of the plate lies parallel to the linea aspera. Most important is bone grafting of all bony defects opposite to the plate. The Wagner apparatus is not removed before internal fixation has been accomplished. For postoperative treatment we follow the same rules as already outlined for femoral fractures in general. Of course, a prolonged period of partial weight bearing postoperatively must be counted on. For more details see the studies of Wagner[230] and Hughes.[104]

The Wagner apparatus, unfortunately, is quite expensive and, on some occasions, unavailable. An alternative method of achieving external fixation for femoral fractures is Roger Anderson's device. This is a fairly inexpensive external fixation system and can be just as reliable as the Wagner apparatus when applied to femoral fractures. Typically, the type of fracture amenable to femoral external fixation is the shotgun blast with its considerable loss of soft and skeletal tissue. Under these circumstances, the bone defect has to be maintained in relatively normal anatomic alignment until bone grafting is available, and soft tissues have to be healthy with good granulation before bone grafting with autogenous cancellous graft is possible. With perfuse destruction of soft tissues and bone, however, often an abundant callus formation does occur and healing can be expected. Nevertheless, external fixation must be strong enough to be maintained for as long as 4 months. With appropriate understanding, even the less rigid system of Roger Anderson can be applied in this situation (Fig. 15-20A).

In our institution, the increased use of the Anderson device as an external fixator for femoral fractures has been mainly caused by financial considerations. Because the financial costs resulting from the loss of the Wagner apparatus (a certain percentage of our clientele never return, even with these costly Wagner implants still *in situ*) were considerable, we improved the techniques of the application of the Roger Anderson device. Relying on $\frac{3}{16}$ inch pins (for which the holding clamps have to be altered), we do the procedure according to the following steps, which were primarily learned from the management of the ASIF external fixator in femoral fractures:

1. The pin sites are predrilled with a 3.2 mm drill bit.
2. The pins are inserted by hand. All pins are inserted following the principles of the half-pin technique, and the topographic positioning of the pins is the same as that for the Schanz screws of the Wagner apparatus.
3. The two pins in each main fragment are widely spaced—one pin is inserted as close as possible to the fracture site and the other as far as possible away from the first pin.
4. The connecting bar is placed laterally and not tightened to the pins before prestressing the pins.
5. Prestressing of the pins is performed; thus, the bone-pin interface will be considerably strengthened, contributing to the stability of the fracture fixation.
6. The second connecting bar is added after the overriding pins beyond the first connecting bar are prestressed again (Fig. 15-20B).

This technique provides more rigidity to the system itself, but it has no direct influence on fracture stabilization. Since the Anderson device does not offer any mechanism by which distracting forces are applied, one has to watch carefully so that restoration of the bone length can be correctly done at the time of the first procedure. This shortcoming puts the device at a disadvantage in comparison to the Wagner, ASIF, or the Hoffmann systems. When the initial treatment proves successful and further procedures are considered, various secondary measures can be chosen to facilitate and secure final bone healing. Here the fracture type as well as the ability of a patient to cope with a given method of treatment are decisive factors in determining what type of consequential therapy is indicated. Full knowledge of both nonoperative and operative options allows the clinician to choose the most reasonable treatment in accordance with the pecularities of the fracture as well as the patient's situation.

PINS AND PLASTER

In America, Scudese has advocated a much simpler system specifically for femoral shaft fractures.[201] In this system, initial reduction and stabilization is achieved through the traditional skeletal traction and suspension method. Two to 3 weeks after injury, under general anesthesia, the proximal and distal fragments are fixed with $\frac{3}{16}$-inch threaded Steinmann pins transversely. With alignment of the fracture segments corrected and maintained by the tibial pin traction, a plaster thigh cylinder is wrapped incorporating the pins, which protrude through the skin. Two pins are used above the fracture fragments, and two below. The two pins

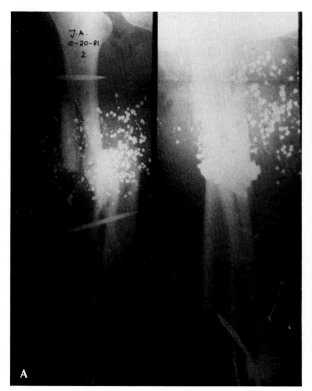
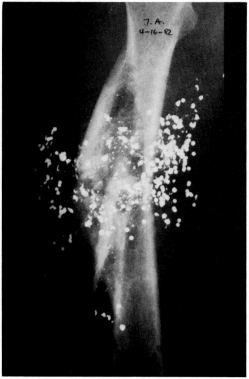

A

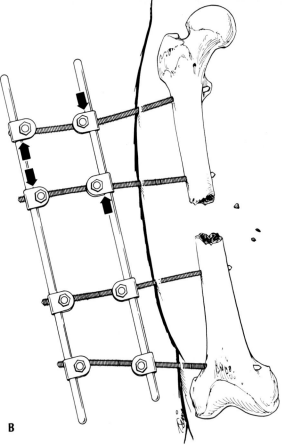

B

Fig. 15-20. (*A*) [*Left*] A gunshot wound to the thigh was an excellent opportunity for the application of external fixation. (*Right*) The fracture eventually united 6 months later. The external fixation pins maintained stability for the entire 6 months although alignment had to be changed on two occasions. (*B*) External fixation principles: (*1*) place pins laterally to tether least vital musculature. (*2*) Place pins as close to the fracture site as possible to gain maximum control. (*3*) Place pins with compressive load at pin-bone interface to ensure stability (prestressing). (*4*) Place fixation bar as close to the bone as possible. (*5*) Use double bar configuration to ensure that the external construction is torque resistant.

are used in each segment so that the bone will not swivel on the single axis of one Steinmann pin. To reduce skin problems, the skin is perforated on the medial aspect with only two of the pins; the other two pins perforate only the bone on the medial side (Fig. 15-21).

One problem with a system using pins and plaster is the potential for rapid loosening of the pin as the thigh circumference decreases. With the loss of circumferential support from the plaster, all the stress is placed on the pin-bone interface. To gain greater purchase in the bone an effort should be made to place thick threaded Steinmann pins (3/16 inch) into the greater trochanter in an oblique manner. One advantage to the use of pins and plaster is this system's ability to wedge the plaster into correct alignment. When nothing else is available this method still can provide an opportunity for mobilization of the patient without restricting the joints above and below. This is definitely a secondary method of fixation, but when nothing else is available, it can be made to work.[230] In addition, there are other methods for achieving external fixation, such as the use of epoxy-filled tubes as advocated by Murray.[176]

INTRAMEDULLARY FIXATION

Intramedullary nail fixation for the fractured femur has achieved a place of prominence and respect. Because a fixation device within the medullary canal is a load-sharing device that can transfer some of the stress to the bone, it is superior to all other types of implants. Although there had been some abortive attempts at intramedullary fixation with ivory, the first recorded attempt at internal fixation with a metal rod was by Hey-Groves in 1916.[90] He used nails of various designs, including a hollow steel tube with perforations. Owing to various complications, such as reactions to metal, infection, and metal failure, this method was abandoned. In 1940, Küntscher reported his experience with an intramedullary rod for the fractured femur.[115,116,117] His device was V-shaped, similar to the U-shaped nail used by Müller-Meernach for forearms in 1933. Küntscher recognized the advantages of intramedullary nailing for the femoral neck, a new method then only recently introduced. The femoral neck fixation was remarkable for its potential to mobilize patients previously incapable of ambulatory activity. Based on his experience with the femoral neck fixation nailing, he also recognized the advantages of radiographic control, as it allowed the surgeon to monitor fixation without opening the fracture site. For these reasons,

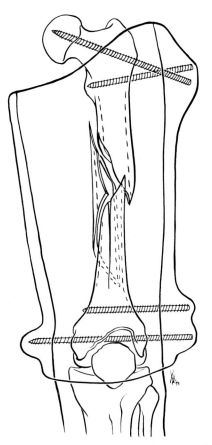

Fig. 15-21. The pins and plaster method for treating comminuted complex fractures of the femoral shaft.

from the very beginning Küntscher advocated a method of fixation of the femoral shaft fracture using a small incision at the greater trochanter and radiographically controlled placement of a guide wire over which the medullary cavity was reamed. Rigid fixation was expected by the matched fit of the nail within an extensively reamed intramedullary channel. Küntscher also took advantage of the recent developments of metallurgy to have the rod fabricated of stainless steel.

An alternative to stable rigid fixation as suggested by Küntscher was that first advocated in the United States by Leslie Rush. He used the dynamic fixation of a resilient, curved, thin rod to achieve three-point fixation. He first developed this system in 1938, and in 1968 reported on 30 years experience.[193] During that period there were only two cases of nonunion and no primary infections in 190 closed fractures of the femoral shaft. Unfortunately, this excellent experience has not been repeated by others.

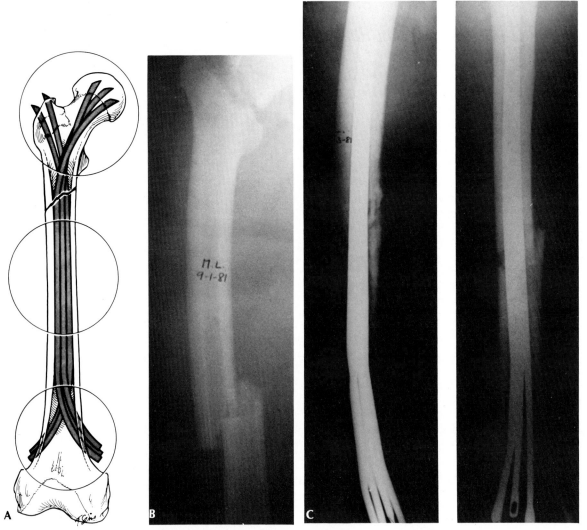

Fig. 15-22. The use of Ender's nails for stabilization of a femoral shaft fracture. (A) A three-point fixation has to be achieved for stability (*circles*). The nails should diverge in the femoral head, their tips ideally being placed in the subchondral bone. The medullary cavity should be tightly filled with an appropriate number of nails. The ends of the nails should lie flush with the flare of the condyles. In extremely wide medullary canals additional nails, inserted from the lateral condyles and anchored in the greater trochanter, might be indicated. (B) The x-ray of a polytraumatized 40-year-old woman with an oblique midshaft fracture and an intertrochanteric fracture of the femur. (C) Appropriate stabilization was achieved by four Ender nails that filled out the medullary cavity at the fracture level.

A somewhat similar system of maintenance of alignment that does not attempt a stable fixation is the use of Ender's pins, passed either antegrade or retrograde into the intramedullary canal.[66,161,180] This is a fairly simple procedure especially now with improved x-ray equipment. Ender's pins are flexible enough to account for variations in anat-omy by appropriate bending. The use of multiple Ender's pins (or even Rush rods) may be the only method available for maintaining alignment in the senile person with an extremely large medullary canal. Under these circumstances the multiple pins can be "stacked" to fill the canal. (Fig. 15-22).[86,162]

Because Rush rods and Ender's pins purposefully

lack rigid fixation, rod migration and unacceptable motion of the fracture fragments are frequent complications. Currently there are few surgeons who trust this method to control the severe mechanical stress placed on the fractured femur.

For stable fixation of the fractured femur there are four designs of femoral rod used in clinical practice today. The cloverleaf design of Küntscher (revised from the original V-shaped design) is the oldest and probably the most popular in general use. To use this device the femoral canal has to be reamed. Alternatives to the reaming method, especially in the absence of good x-ray control, are the designs of Schneider, and Hansen and Street. The double I-beam construct of Schneider has self-broaching edges at either end and therefore can be used both retrograde and antegrade for fixation of the femur by opening the fracture site. The diamond-shaped rod of Hansen and Street could be used either in a broaching manner or with reaming or, if thin enough, without any correction of intramedullary canal at all. Both these systems were designed to be used without guide-pins. The most recent basic design change is the Sampson rod, which is a tubular design with flutes circumferentially placed in order to achieve purchase on the bone. It was designed to offer greater strength than previous rods.[6] It was intended initially for situations in which there was severe comminution or nonunion and stress to the rod was expected to be prolonged and severe.

BIOMECHANICAL CONSIDERATIONS

The contribution of design to the biomechanical function of an intramedullary rod is a complex issue. Certainly the structural properties of the intramedullary device must be known. Fatigue failure in bending is the usual mode of failure, but unfortunately in the physiologic condition there is no accepted measure of fatigue strength. Usually fatigue strength is about one half of the static bending strength of the device.[241] Another extremely complex variable is the effective load transfer between bone segments and the nail itself. The rigidity of the nail may be a secondary problem if the load cannot be transferred from the bone to the nail.

Several studies have looked at the strength characteristics of femoral rods.[5,6] Three modes of failure were tested: bending strength, bending rigidity, and torsional rigidity. Under test conditions, torsional rigidity was weakest in the Küntscher nail (a cylinder is weakened by 50 times when a portion

of the wall is removed). The most resistant to torsion was the fluted cylinder rod. Allen and associates[6] have pointed out that the advantage of the fluted rod was even more significant when the analysis of resistance to torque was accomplished under standard conditions within reamed femurs. The fluted rod was nearly twice as resistant to break-away than the Küntscher rod under standard conditions. The next most successful rod was the double I-beam design of Schneider. These studies also pointed out that bending strength and bending rigidity were similar for all rod designs, and that the strongest rod other than the fluted rod was the Schneider rod. Nonetheless, even the fluted rod was 25% less stiff than the bone itself, which had a bending strength of 450 newton meters.

It must be recognized that the mechanical characteristics of the intramedullary device itself cannot be the only criterion for the successful choice of treatment. In human fracture care a very large part of the problem is the optimal distribution of load between the nail and the healing bone. Ideally, stress is initially tolerated by the intramedullary device but rapidly diminishes as the bone heals. Prolonged stress shielding of the fracture site must be avoided, and it is possible that the device and its fixation may indeed even be too stiff and too strong.

Another aspect of design is determining whether the intramedullary rod should more closely correspond to the gentle curve of the normal human femur or remain straight. Certainly it is realistic to expect that a better physiologic "working length" could be achieved if the intramedullary rod more accurately corresponded to the natural contour of the anterior bow of the femur. Flexible reamers are necessary to provide constant diameter to the reamed medullary canal and to provide a broader contact area (working length).

CHOICE OF NAIL AND TECHNIQUE

The most frequent technical complication of femoral rodding is choice of the wrong nail—too long, too short, too thin, or too thick. The nail too wide for the channel is particularly threatening in that it may become firmly incarcerated (especially with the use of a cloverleaf). The adventure of removing an incarcerated nail may require splitting the shaft, the use of a sterile hacksaw, vise grip pliers, sledge hammer, and even a diamond blade for the oscillating saw.[16] Extrusion of the nail guide reamer or the nail itself into the soft tissues (with potential neurovascular damage) is the most severe complication. It is more likely to occur with closed methods. Reaming the canal, as is necessary for Küntscher nailing, requires some skill in the use of the special instruments, and it has the potential for fracturing the femur even more. The closed method is unlikely to damage the hip joint, as the site of bone insertion in the medial aspect of the greater trochanter is chosen with great care. This complication may be possible in retrograde methods where the superior aspect of the neck is shattered as the nail explodes through. This can be avoided by predrilling with a long bit in a retrograde manner. The knee joint can be damaged by either method if the nail is too long or impacted too far. Essentially both methods require image intensification confirmation of the status of the knee joint during the operation.

The open method of internal fixation of femoral shaft fractures is still a common method. A major reason for this is the lack of appropriate x-ray and specialized table equipment necessary for the closed method as well as a lack of experienced teachers. This is indeed surprising when one remembers that the original Küntscher rodding described in the early 1940s was the closed method dependent on radiographic control. The lack of acceptance of the closed method of internal fixation of femoral fractures is partly due to the inability of the major teaching institutions to get appropriate equipment in the operating room. It is fair to say that sometimes political and territorial issues supersede valid medical priorities.

The open method of fracture care has a good success rate and little infection in well controlled institutions. Sage reported the Campbell Clinic experience using the open method, noting an infection rate of 6%.[195] A series by Stryker using the Schneider rod in over 200 cases showed an infection rate of less than 2%.[219] Both of the series reported are from teaching and training institutions and may not accurately reflect the general orthopaedic care in the community.

The choice of an intramedullary device must be made not only on biomechanical grounds, but economic factors must also be considered. The simplest system would use the self-cutting broach of the Schneider system in an open retrograde method. Such a system does not have great versatility but it is simple to use. The only extraordinary piece of equipment necessary with this system is a single extractor impactor device in addition to rods in multiple sizes.

However, as one proceeds in complexity to the closed method, using a flexible reamer to match the curved intramedullary rod, a huge array of equipment is necessary in addition to special tables and special x-ray equipment. At our institution, the cost of conversion to this method of care in 1978 was about $150,000. Moreover, as the procedure becomes increasingly complex, additional problems occur, potential for human error and lost equipment increases, and overall potential for frustration with the system intensifes. In situations in which the volume is sufficient, the equipment is adequate, and the surgeons have the skill and dedication, extremely high levels of success can be achieved using the closed system. The best series ever published on consecutive femur fractures, both open and closed, was done by Winquist and Hansen[241] using the closed method with radiographically controlled reaming and Küntscher rods.[86,87]

There is yet another system of intramedullary rods that must be discussed. These are rods with transfixing screw fixation that allows secure bone purchase at the proximal and distal ends. There are two examples of this type of design: the Huckstep nail[3,102] (Fig. 15-23) and the interlocking nail. These systems were originally designed for difficult fractures of the femoral shaft because their additional transfixing screws could control comminution and rotation, allow compression or distraction of the fracture site, and be strong enough to allow early weight bearing and mobilization. The Huckstep nail is designed for retrograde placement, currently comes in one diameter (12.5 mm), and uses an outrigger jig to allow the alignment of the transfixing screws within the rod. The rod is squared. In the Huckstep nail multiple screw holes placed at regular intervals along the quadrilateral "rod" give a wide range of fixation locations. The interlocking nail is more restricted in the location of screw holes but uses a standard rod design. Although the design suggests that stress concentration at the screws in the bone transfixing the rod may occur, early experience has not found this a problem.[103]

PLATING OF FEMORAL SHAFT FRACTURES

Despite the superiority of intramedullary nails, with their weight and load sharing design, there are situations in which plates may be of benefit. One must recognize that the plate is inherently a weight-bearing device (Fig. 15-24) and therefore must absorb, as compared to a rod, considerably more of the stress (perhaps up to 70%) that is supplied to the implant. Stress shielding may create a problem because the fracture may heal without functional stress being sufficiently supplied, resulting in the possibility of refracture at the time of plate removal. Therefore, a little loosening of the plate may in the long run be advantageous. Because open surgical approach is necessary for plate application, some devascularization of the femoral shaft must occur. All of these are relatively minor deterrents to the use of plates in comparison to the problem caused by anatomy: with significant comminution, in the presence of instability medially, unacceptable stress may have to be placed on the plate. In situations in which the medial comminution cannot be controlled, a significant amount of bone graft is necessary, and strict patient compliance to avoid loading the limb is necessary. In spite of all of these factors there are situations in which the plate may be the ideal solution. One example is the patient with multiple trauma, for whom fixation of the limb is necessary to achieve mobilization, but whose position on the operating table makes it difficult to use rod fixation. Frequently, an added factor to be considered in such a patient is a grade III open fracture of the femoral shaft. In this situation the disadvantage of devascularization of the open approach to fracture fixation is not a factor. Debridement of the wound is also necessary for grade III fractures, and in such a situation the plate fixation may accomplish exactly what is necessary: stabilization of the skeletal elements to allow appropriate soft tissue reconstruction and treatment.

Despite all of the biomechanical disadvantages plates present as fixation devices in weight-bearing bones, the fracture surgeon should be familiar with the techniques of proper application of plates.[8,130,151,192,224] There are also certain situations in which a plate may be the only device suitable for a given fracture. Third-degree open fractures should not be stabilized by means of a medullary device. In these fractures external blood supply usually is seriously compromised. Additional damage to the medullary blood supply, the result of medullary reaming, inevitably causes extensive bone necrosis. Other fractures such as distal and proximal femur fractures are sometimes more easily treated by plating than by successful nailing. Furthermore, there are still a number of institutions unable to perform medullary nailings due to lack of appropriate equipment and experienced surgeons. Most of the bad reputation plating acquired over the years is simply due to ill-advised indications for its use, technical mistakes made at the time of surgery, and ill-conceived postoperative rehabilitation.

Another application of plate fixation is the femoral shaft fracture in the growing child. If the fixation does not need to cross the epiphyseal line, deterrents to growth will not occur. Frequently the head-injured child shows profound spasticity and thrashing, so that maintenance in traction is impossible. In this situation, using a plate rather than allowing the fractured femur to tear its way through soft tissues and skin can salvage an otherwise disastrous situation.

TECHNIQUE OF PLATE APPLICATION

The operative procedure is done with the patient either in the supine or lateral position. The leg is fully prepped and draped, as is the adjacent pelvic area, to allow for a bone graft to be taken from the iliac crest. The fracture is approached through a straight lateral incision by which the vastus lateralis muscle is dissected from the intermuscular septum and anteriorly elevated. All perforating vessels are secured best by suture ligations. Once the fracture site has been reached any soft tissue stripping of the bone has to be limited to the *absolute necessity* for fracture reduction. Instead of rough manipulations, bone reduction clamps and holding forceps should be applied to minimize intraoperative damage. Larger butterfly fragments are fit in by means of lag screw fixation. Smaller fragments, particularly when completely devascularized, are better taken out and later replaced by bone grafting.

The implant of choice should be a broad compression plate such as the AO dynamic compression plate (DCP) of the appropriate length. The DCP allows for screw placement at different angles, improving the chance of holding butterfly fragments in anatomic position because the lag screw principle is applied whenever a plate screw crosses a fracture line. The plate should be applied to the lateral aspect of the femur, so that its posterior border lies flush with the linea aspera. The plate should be fixed with 8 to 9 cortices in each main fragment to provide enough stability. Bone grafting of all defects, particularly those opposite to the plate, must be done to protect the plate with bone. Any implant bridging an area with a contralateral cortical defect (Fig. 15-25) is prone to fatigue failure and breakage. Insufficient bony support due to neglected bone grafting is the most recognized cause of implant failure. For more technical details the principles outlined in the AO Manual should be thoroughly studied.[151] The wound is closed over a suction drainage, and the leg is placed without additional external support on a Böhler-Braun

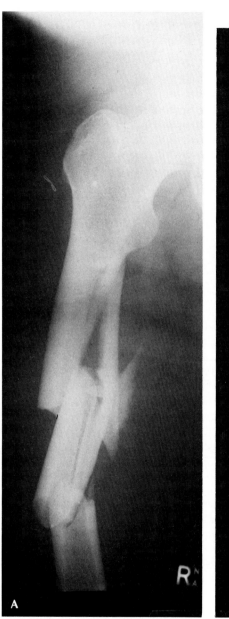

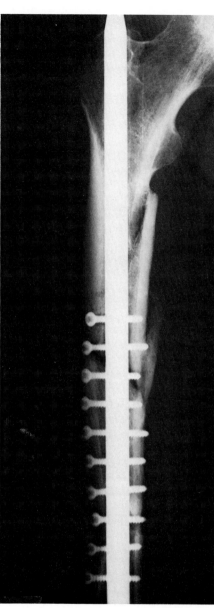

Fig. 15-23. (*A*) An example of the use of the Huckstep nail which uses interlocking screws through a quadralateral "rod" that must be placed in a retrograde manner. No reaming is necessary.

frame close to a 90-90 position for a few days (see Fig. 15-31).

POSTOPERATIVE MANAGEMENT

Postoperative treatment is similar to that outlined for nailed femoral fractures. The basic difference, however, is in the management of weight bearing. Toe touching is encouraged in the cooperative patient over the initial 4 postoperative weeks, followed by increased weight bearing, with a weekly increase of 10 to 15 pounds until full body weight is accomplished. Unfortunately, we are not always able to stick to this rehabilitation schedule because patients are unreliable. If it is obvious that a patient will not follow the treatment plan, we do not hesitate to temporarily keep him from bearing weight by using a well-padded, long leg cast with the knee in 90° flexion for 4 to 6 weeks. Of course,

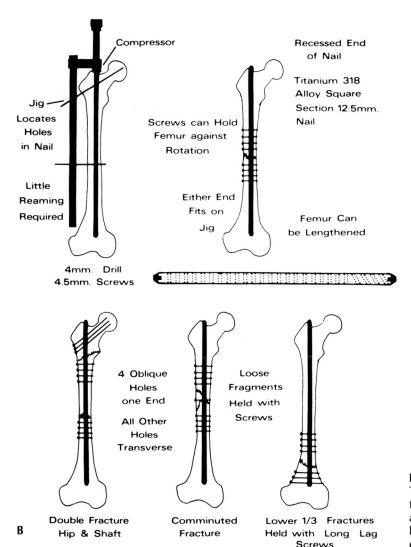

Rigid Strong Fixation With Compression

Compressor

Recessed End of Nail

Titanium 318 Alloy Square Section 12.5mm. Nail

Jig Locates Holes in Nail

Screws can Hold Femur against Rotation

Little Reaming Required

Either End Fits on Jig

Femur Can be Lengthened

4mm. Drill 4.5mm. Screws

4 Oblique Holes one End

All Other Holes Transverse

Loose Fragments Held with Screws

B   Double Fracture Hip & Shaft

Comminuted Fracture

Lower 1/3 Fractures Held with Long Lag Screws

Fig. 15-23 (*Continued*). (*B*) The Huckstep intermedullary femoral compression nail is applicable to multiple problems related to femoral shaft comminution and instability.

such treatment is in contradiction to our outspoken aims to do early functional follow-up of operatively treated fractures. However, as long as this remains the only measure preventing a patient from a series of complications, it seems to be more than justified.

Plate removal should not be allowed before 18 months after surgery, provided the fracture has securely united. After plate removal the bone undergoes a further remodeling, and the weakened cortex, lying immediately under the plate, gains further strength through normal bone stress due to body weight. It is extremely important to advise a patient to avoid any peak loading of the femur over

a period of 3 to 4 months after implant removal. We have frequently used an adjustable thigh cuff as an adjunctive support following plate removal. We have not felt it necessary to bone graft or drill the vacant screw holes. When refractures occur, they are almost always due to temporary overloading of the bone shortly after the implant removal. All patients undergoing treatment need to have this explained to them, although their understanding of treatment is very often limited. It is therefore better to control activity. Sports activities should not be started again before an interval of 4 to 6 months after plate removal.

The factors deciding whether a plate or a rod is best to use are various. In the older child, there is really little threat that passing a rod through the superior aspect of the base of the neck will cause any growth disturbance—as long as the distal epiphysis is not injured. As yet this is not usually standard practice in most communities, and growth disturbances related to trauma versus those related to surgery must be recognized. Of course, in the use of a plate in a midshaft fracture, there is no threat of injury to an epiphysis.

SPECIAL SITUATIONS

FRACTURES OF THE FEMORAL SHAFT ASSOCIATED WITH FRACTURES OF THE NECK OF THE FEMUR OR INTERTROCHANTERIC FRACTURES

The fracture combination of the femoral shaft and neck is not as unusual as one might expect. Quite often this serious injury is missed initially since inadequate x-ray examination does not allow for an early recognition. With regard to appropriate treatment one has to carefully evaluate the fracture pattern. We prefer to stabilize a true base of neck fracture associated with a proximal or a midshaft femoral fracture by a closed anterograde Küntscher nailing of the shaft fracture and screw fixation of the neck fracture. Three to four 6.5 mm cancellous screws of appropriate length are used. Half of them are inserted into the neck either ventrally or dorsally to the femoral rod.

An intertrochanteric fracture in combination with a midshaft or distal femoral shaft fracture may be amenable to a retrograde closed rodding inserting a short nail either through the intercondylar notch (with the knee in a flexed position) or through an opening in the lateral femoral condyle. The intertrochanteric fracture then may be fixed by means of a hip compression screw. Of course, there are other techniques that may result in acceptable treatments; one is the retrograde nailing technique with Ender's nails. So far, this technique has not produced problems in the fixation of the femoral shaft portion. Stabilization of the intertrochanteric or base of neck fracture always has been somewhat troublesome; it is difficult to correctly place a sufficient number of nails into the femoral head, thus guaranteeing enough rotational stability in the proximal fracture. These fractures are demanding with regard to the techniques of internal fixation. Since the later type of fixation almost always leaves some fracture instability, a prolonged period of

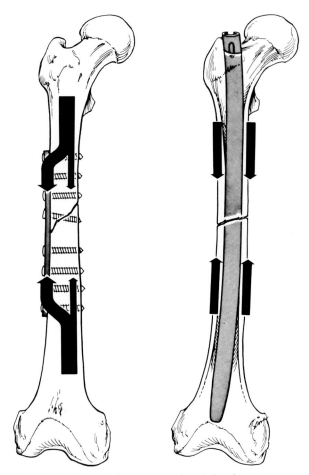

Fig. 15-24. Weight-bearing and weight-sharing implants in internal fixation of femoral fractures. (*Left*) A laterally placed broad DCP, stainless steel, absorbs more than 70% of all loading stresses applied to the fracture site. In this regard the plate becomes a weight-bearing device. (*Right*) An intramedullary rod serves as a splint. Almost all loading stresses are absorbed and transmitted by the bone, which enhances the process of "natural" fracture healing. Thus an intramedullary rod is regarded as a weight-sharing device.

nonweight bearing, probably 4 to 6 weeks, is strongly recommended. Afterward, a hinged cast or plastic brace device with a limited range of motion for the knee joint will prevent the fractures from peak loading for another 4 weeks.

COMMINUTED FRAGMENTS

Another controversial aspect of femoral fracture care is the method by which comminuted fragments should be handled. The amount of stress that the fixation device must tolerate is related directly to the stability of the fixation of the fracture fragments around it. There are essentially three methods by which comminuted fracture fragments may be stabilized in association with the primary fixation device: cerclage, screws and plates, and soft tissue. The most common method is by cerclage.[148,224] This system requires, of course, the visualization of the fracture fragments, the use of some safe system of wire passage, and an appropriate wire-tightening device. For the cerclage system to function adequately the wire has to be tightened sufficiently in order that interlocking of the fracture fragments can occur. Usually at least two cerclage wires are necessary so that a "toggle effect" will not occur. The earlier experience of Parham bands suggested that a cerclage system was an adverse environment for fracture healing. This is not true. The previous poor experience with Parham[164] bands was based largely on metalurgic factors, as well as a larger area of devascularization due to the width of the band. Certainly the minimal diameter of the wire used for cerclage is insufficient to devascularize the bony fragments.[54,74,164] Recently the use of nylon cerclage has been advocated by Partridge and Evans. This awaits general commercial availability, but it appears to be an appropriate type of material for diaphyseal stabilization.[165]

The second method for stabilization of an open site fracture is the use of screw fixation, especially if the fracture fragments are quite large. This is a dangerous maneuver because the use of screw fixation alone is not a safe system and requires that throughout the entire process of bone union stable fixation can be maintained by the screws. Screw fixation is strictly contraindicated in long spiral fractures as the primary method of care. With screw fixation, compression screw principles are necessary, and usually a neutralization plate is required to distribute the forces adequately. The AO principles of interfragmentary compression have proved to be the most appropriate guidelines to maintain stability using screws and plates.[151,152]

When there is an extreme amount of comminution it may be impossible to anatomically realign all of the fragments. Maintenance of alignment and length by internal fixation bridging the gap can be accomplished, but one must search for auxiliary stabilization from soft tissue as well. Thus, the use of an adjustable thigh corset may be necessary when a plate is used to bridge a severely comminuted defect. The use of interlocking nail systems also may represent bridging manuevers. Under all circumstances, however, stress to the healing area must be delayed until preliminary union of the comminuted fragments is achieved.

TIMING OF CARE

The timing of operative care for the fractured femur becomes an increasingly more significant issue when a method of treatment is chosen. The simple closed fracture in an otherwise healthy person does not require operative care. Treated with standard traction techniques, this fracture will heal quite well. The patient rapidly becomes comfortable and can escape any possibility of surgical care simply by spending time in bed in traction. Shortening and poor alignment may occur if the patient continues in the traction mode. All reports, however, suggest that very good function can be expected.

If we take the other end of the spectrum and look at the multiply injured patient, delay of aggressive fracture care offers significant disadvantages. It is now well established that prolonged recumbency in traction and body immobility enforced by multiple, unfixed fractures lead to greater mortality from respiratory death, as well as greater incidence of infection and chronic disability.[22] In the multiply injured patient or the patient with multiple systems involved, rapid mobilization is a necessity. Some system, either closed or open, must be found to allow the patient to sit up and move easily in bed.

At one time there was some thought that delay in fracture care offered a greater potential for fracture union because it was assumed that the periosteum was better prepared for fracture repair after a short delay.[49,53,209,210] Currently, however, there is no reason to support this theoretical view based on present clinical experience. Modern fracture series that choose to time a fixation strictly on the logistics of the situation and available operative time certainly have no deficiency in success rate as compared to the older studies.[86]

BONE GRAFTING

The need for bone grafting still remains somewhat controversial. In simple noncomminuted fractures with excellent fixation there is no major reason to attempt to speed the healing rate with the addition of autogenous graft, taken from another operative location such as the iliac crest, at the expense of time and additional operative morbidity. Recently, however, even fractures with minor comminution at the fracture site have been treated with little additional time and technical delay: when the

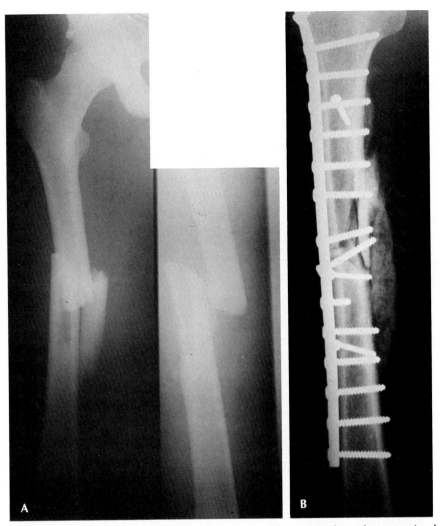

Fig. 15-25. Plating of femoral shaft fractures. (*A*) The x-ray of a polytraumatized 19-year-old man with a third degree open femoral fracture. Primary open reduction, internal fixation, and primary bone grafting were performed. (*B*) At 10 weeks postoperative an autogenous cancellous bone graft bridging bony defects opposite to the broad DCP was incorporated.

closed reaming system is used, the reamings are squeezed down into the fracture site before the nail is inserted. This technique has been demonstrated to speed the fracture healing rate.[35]

The severely comminuted fracture or delayed union with prolonged stress to the fixation device is a good reason to try to speed the healing process by the addition of autogenous graft. In general, the failure of fixation devices must be attributed to the inability of the rate of union to keep up with the rate of fatigue failure. This failure occurs as long as an implant is not prevented from sustaining cyclic load changes in the presence of instable fracture reduction and fixation. Thus it should be kept in mind that any implant should make use of the load-bearing capacity of bone. In case of a defect, particularly opposite to a plate, bone grafting has to be supplemented to provide the implant for bony support.

Even major defects have been demonstrated to be available for new bone formation with the addition of massive amounts of autogenous graft. Chapman[45] has shown that excellent blood supply in the presence of rigid fixation can allow building

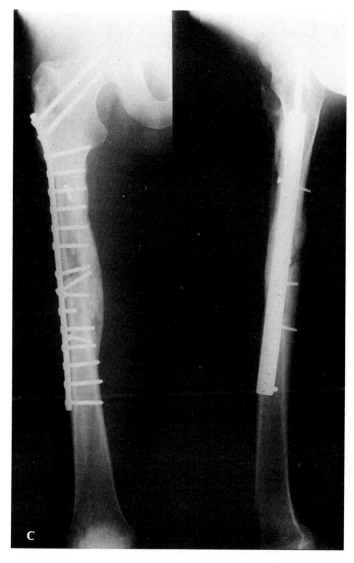

Fig. 15-25 (*Continued*). (*C*) At 1-year post-operative the fracture was securely united with the bone graft undergoing functional remodeling.

of new bone fairly rapidly. Certainly grafting is necessary to supplement the bone on the cortex opposite the plated femur with unstable fragments.

PROXIMAL AND DISTAL FRACTURES

The anatomical location of fractures along the femoral shaft creates progressively more complex problems related to fragmentation. The anatomical locations ideally suited for fixation of femoral rods are those locations where good fixation of the rods in the shaft can be achieved both proximal and distal to the site of the fracture. Thus, the subtrochanteric and supracondylar areas become progressively less favored locations for femoral rodding.

As the diaphysis expands to the metaphysis and the cortex gradually thins, fixation with a rod becomes less feasible. It is in these locations that screws and plates become necessary if internal fixation is to achieve anatomic stability.

SUBTROCHANTERIC FRACTURES

In the subtrochanteric area, the proximal fragment in the femoral neck and greater trochanter sometimes itself is comminuted.[73] Because the subtrochanteric area is a site of progressively greater uncompensated stress concentration in the aging skeleton, subtrochanteric fracture is most often seen in the elderly or associated with metabolic bone disease such as Paget's disease.[44,80] These points, therefore, complicate the biomechanical limitations peculiar to this site.[17] The average age of patients with subtrochanteric fractures is in the 70s. When the fracture site is 2 to 3 inches below the lesser trochanter, there is a very high rate of nonunion. Direct axial loading of the femur achieves a maximum stress concentration of about 1200 pounds per square inch at a site 1 to 3 inches distal to the lesser trochanter. (The tensile stress on the lateral aspect is less, and thus the failure tends to occur on the medial side.) Coupled with these potentials for comminution, the considerable muscle forces of the subtrochanteric area make fractures extremely difficult to treat (Fig. 15-26).[198]

An alternative method of achieving stability at the subtrochanteric area is the use of an interlocking device, which uses transfixing screws with the intramedullary rod to achieve proximal stability. The long, interlocking, oblique bolt applies significant rotational stability. It is usually not necessary to use the distal screws because firm purchase of the midshaft of the femur is available by the rod within the reamed canal. On occasion, additional stability by cerclage wires may be necessary.

Occasionally, fixation of the proximal shaft and subtrochanteric area has been recommended by the use of flexible rods (Ender's, Harris, or even Rush rods). Although successful use has been reported, in general, the lack of stability offered by these devices presents significant opportunity for shortening, rotational abnormality, and even delay in union. Therefore, when these small flexible devices are used, an auxiliary system to achieve reduced stresses such as roller traction for 3 to 4 weeks is highly recommended.

Metal fixation devices must withstand repeated, severe stress forces. To avoid litigation for failures several instrument manufacturers suggest in their brochures that nail-plate devices are not recommended for subtrochanteric fractures. Unfortunately, the anatomical location provides little fixation for an ordinary femoral rod in the proximal segment. To counteract this, an unusual design has been developed by Robert Zickel to answer this problem (Fig. 15-27).[246,248] The Zickel nail is a short intramedullary rod that provides purchase to the mid-shaft of the femur. The proximal aspect is perforated to allow transfixion by a nail into the femoral neck. A special locking mechanism at the superior end of the nail maintains a rigid relationship between the intramedullary rod and the nail in the femoral neck. This particular fixation device seems to be the most rational choice for the unusual and severe stress problems of the subtrochanteric area.

Blade plate fixation in the past has been frequently recommended for the proximal femoral fracture, but, as suggested above, in general practice it is seldom the ideal device. In the hands of experienced surgeons, however, the use of an angled blade has met with excellent results; the blade plate is applied as a tension band on the lateral aspect of the femur; and stability to the medial aspect is supplied by lag screw fixation and cerclage. Bone graft also is usually necessary. One of the problems in the use of the blade plate is that the craftsmanship must be very precise in the location of the initial blade so that the plate will follow the contours of the femur. To some extent this problem has been resolved by the use of the dynamic compression plate systems that are currently available. The proximal fixation device, a screw system, is allowed to swivel on the plate and thus precise location is not as necessary.

In all systems using blade plates, however, one must expect a lag before full loading is available. The patient should not bear weight and should expect to be on crutches and even in traction if compliance is in some question. The delay in loading the involved limb may be for as long as 6 weeks until preliminary union has occurred. The advantage, however, is the assurance of normal length and alignment that may not occur in the use of load sharing devices such as the Zickel nail.[247]

A more detailed discussion of subtrochanteric fractures is presented in Chapter 14.

SUPRACONDYLAR FRACTURES

Similar problems are related to the internal fixations of fractures of the distal third of the femur and supracondylar fractures.[9,33,200] In this case, getting purchase on the distal fragment by internal fixation methods is difficult. Bone frequently is porotic and may have several areas of fragmentation. The reports of internal fixation during the mid-1960s were very discouraging. In studies by Neer and colleagues[153] and by Stewart,[217] only about 50% of the cases treated by internal fixation could be considered as satisfactory results. The usual nail-plate or Rush rod combinations provided insufficient fixation. They gradually worked loose and caused delayed union, nonunion, infection, and other complications. In a survey of over 700 orthopaedic surgeons, most considered closed treatment as the method of choice in caring for the fractures of the supracondylar area.[185]

In dealing with comminuted distal femoral fractures, the method that offers the greatest opportunity for stability is the use of angled blade plates.

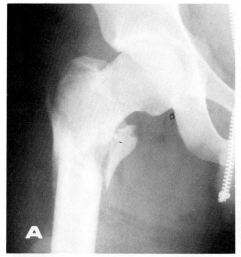

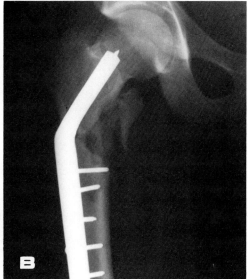

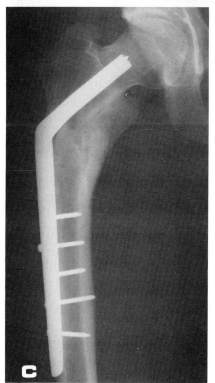

Fig. 15-26. Subtrochanteric fracture. (*A*) Severely comminuted subtrochanteric fracture in a young man. (*B*) Internal fixation with a nail-plate combination. Because of the patient's youth, the bone structure was quite strong. (*C*) Solid union in a slight varus position occurred before failure of the fixation device. Removal is indicated because eventually it will surely fatigue. This fixation device has been successful only because of the rapid rate of union and good purchase of the fixation devices in the skeletal structures.

Frequently it is not possible to achieve complete relocation of all fracture fragments due to severe comminution; the effort to do so would lead to additional devascularization. In these situations the plate must be considered a "bridging" device in which bone alignment and length are maintained until healing has developed at the fracture site; addititional bone grafting assists the process. The blade plate is quite demanding to use because

alignment along the shaft in relation to the femoral condyles must be completely accurate. A cancellous bone screw that fixes the condyles but allows correction of the plate relationship to the condyle may be somewhat easier to use but the fixation loses a little in stability. In situations in which "bridging" the comminuted site is the function of fixation, auxiliary support must be anticipated. A fracture brace that allows motion at the knee while enabling adjustments to be made that keep a firm encapsulation of the proximal thigh is ideal. For this reason the brace must be adjustable. In general the delay of full weight bearing in expectation of continued brace use should be for at least 2 months.

In the case of significant comminution and especially in situations in which the bone stock is weak, stable fixation may not be possible and the use of the principle of internal splinting may be the best solution. The device developed by Robert Zickel[249] is an ideal solution to the complex distal femoral fracture (Fig. 15-28). Technical demands in its application are not severe and early mobilization of the patient is possible. The technique is especially appropriate when the length of comminution in the distal third of the femur is significant. An alternative method of internal splinting is the use of Ender's pins, which may be inserted under radiographic control in an antegrade manner through the greater trochanter. To achieve some element of stability, however, the intramedullary canal has to be filled with an appropriate number of nails, which are bent in various positions to achieve fixation in both condyles. Due to the limited stability offered by the internal fixation device, roller traction for several weeks is appropriate, and then an application of supplementary bracing should be used until full ambulation is available. Here also an adjustable thigh section should be used postoperatively.

OPERATIVE VERSUS NONOPERATIVE TREATMENT

Many reports suggest that femoral shaft fractures can be treated with a high level of success by either nonoperative or operative means.[43] Advocates report 100% union and no infections with fractures treated either by internal fixation or by traction-and-plaster methods. If the same level of skills and equipment were necessary to implement either method, the only considerations would be how long the patient can afford to be disabled and out of work, and the prospects for long-term limitation of function.[131]

In a survey, Carr focused on that specific point and confirmed the somewhat traditional point of view that patients who had internal fixation spent less time in hospital (1½ months compared to 2½ months) and went back to work much sooner (9½ months compared to 13 months.)[41] Knee range of motion was about the same. In this series, which

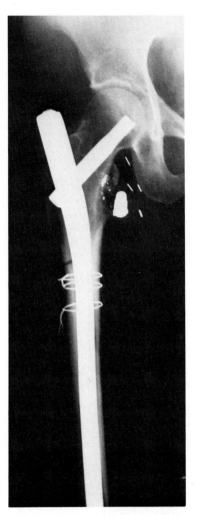

Fig. 15-27. The Zickel nail is ideally suited for application to the subtrochanteric area. Control of rotation and maintenance of alignment are the requirements for fixation at this level.

must be representative of community orthopaedic care in the late 1960s, there were fracture healing problems in at least 28% of those treated closed. This is about the same incidence of problems that Stryker identified (20%) from the military experience with the closed treatment of fractured femurs.[219] The average time of union was about 7½ months in this series, and only about 60% of Stryker's patients went back to duty. In the civilian series, about 19% of those with internal fixation had complications, of which four were deep infections and four were delayed union problems. Küntscher nails were used in these patients. (Stryker, using a Schneider rod, had a 2% infection rate.) Significantly, 96% of those Stryker treated by internal fixation went back to duty.

It must be recognized, however, that the percentage of fractures for which a closed method is chosen increases with the incidence of comminuted fractures. Usually, the simpler the fracture, the more likely it is to be treated primarily by internal fixation; the more comminuted the fracture is, the less likely internal fixation will be attempted.

The largest published series comparing various treatments is by Dencker, who recorded over 1000 femoral shaft fractures from Sweden during the early 1950s.[60,61] At this time the infection rate for internal fixation of closed fractures was 6% and for open fractures 21%. (Only 3% of open fractures treated closed became infected.) Although infection was the most serious complication in open methods, fracture healing problems were a consideration too. Sixteen percent of fractures fixed internally with the V-nail version of the Küntscher rod had union problems. When the encircling wire was the only fixation device, there were problems in 23%, while plate and screws had union problems in 7%. Delayed or nonunion occurred in 7% of those treated with traction. Those treated with traction alone (318 fractures) had minimal treatment complications. Three percent of the skeletal traction patients treated with a Kirschner wire through the tibia had problems related to the traction system itself (infection, cutting through, or nerve damage). When traction was applied through the distal femur at the adductor tubercle 9% of the patients had some sort of problem.

One consideration in the care of fractures of the femoral shaft, in addition to the morbidity of infection and the delay of union or knee disability, is the severest degree of morbidity—death associated with treatment. In the Dencker series, no deaths could be attributed to those treated by closed methods. There were seven deaths associated with or caused by open reduction and internal fixation. These are unfair statistics in that no series presented by an advocate of any specific method contains a mortality associated with that method. On the other hand, the Dencker series is a more realistic commentary on general fracture care in the hands of apparently qualified but not necessarily expert physicians.

An additional consideration when comparing the success rate of nonoperative versus operative methods of femoral shaft fracture care is the semioperative method of closed intramedullary nailing. This particular aspect was evaluated by Rokkanen in a series from Finland.[190] This series compared the care of 156 femoral shaft fractures treated by closed intramedullary nailing with a Küntscher rod with those treated by open methods and nonoperative methods. Again, the most severely comminuted fractures and the severest wounds were treated by nonoperative methods. No fracture in this series failed to unite but in all other variables the nonoperative method lagged behind. Those treated by nonoperative methods stayed in the hospital the longest and were delayed longest in returning to work or in walking unassisted. Those treated by closed nailing did slightly better than patients treated by open methods (the criteria being length of stay in hospital and length of time until they could walk without assistance). Moreover, in contrast to earlier experiences, no advantage was found in delaying closed nailing for several weeks. There was better joint range in those treated by closed nailing, and none were suffering disability at the end of 12 months.

The best results in the treatment of femoral shaft fractures in terms of rate of union, rate of infection, and ultimate function with preservation of length and alignment are seen in the Seattle series of Hansen and Winquist.[86] A closed rodding technique, extensive equipment, and the experience and dedication of personnel were responsible for the results. The AO group, using plates, reports similar excellent results with regard to union, infection, and function. In this series as well, equipment, personnel, and experience produced such results.[130,192]

Only a small portion of the extensive literature on this subject has been described here. It is evident that opinion has differed considerably as to the best method of handling a femoral shaft fracture.[7,13,28,29,40,50,75,107,131,149,234,236] A fair summary of the two points of view might be as follows: The traditional nonoperative method has insignificant danger of infection. Delayed union with closed traction methods may occur but is correctable by secondary procedures. Knee motion is usually satisfactory but may be limited when compared to the best internal fixation results. For severely comminuted fractures, the ones with severe soft-tissue damage, traction is unquestionably the safest and most reliable treatment. On the other hand, treatment by internal fixation clearly can be demonstrated to shorten hospitalization when compared to traditional traction care and in most series shortens total disability time.[228] It does carry a very small risk of infection. To achieve optimal results specialized skills, equipment, and training are required.

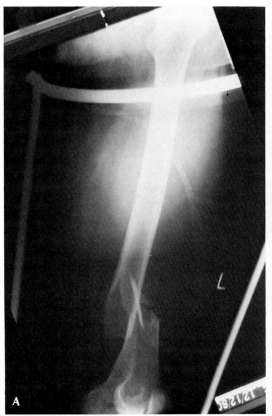 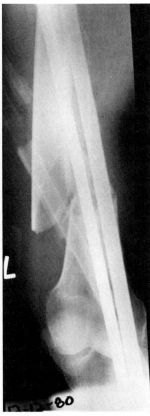

Fig. 15-28. (*A*) Two views of a comminuted distal femoral fracture in an osteoporotic 75-year-old woman. (*B*) Stable fixation and healing were achieved using the Zickel supracondylar device.

AUTHORS' PREFERRED METHODS OF TREATMENT

The optimum method of care should appropriate the best aspects of all methods of care and coordinate them into an ideal system based on past experience and a recognition of the skills of the competent fracture surgeon.

In contrast to the proponents of rest and prolonged rest to achieve fracture union, we take the view that early mobilization with return of physiologic function has been demonstrated to have unquestioned positive effects on rate of union, general patient morbidity, and degree of long-term disability.[125] Any method that can safely achieve mobilization and ambulatory function for the patient is to be favored.[12,37,55,141,208] This was early recognized in Delbet's designs for ambulatory spring-loaded devices[58] and Böhler's total-contact ambulatory plaster spicas.[20]

We are convinced that the function of muscles about and related to the fracture site promotes fracture repair by stimulating organization of collagen repair and local tissue metabolism. The hy-

drodynamic compressive effect of muscles in the thigh acts to stabilize the bones. These hydrodynamic effects of thigh function can be achieved with a patient in traction. Watson-Jones reported a 100% fracture healing rate in traction, but he suggested that the average time of traction should be 12 weeks.[231] This is totally unacceptable in today's social and economic structure.

Thus, although on many occasions skeletal traction and preliminary care is the appropriate form of reduction and stabilization of the fracture, it is certainly not the ideal method. It is usually appropriate to wait until "the dust settles" before a definitive method is identified so that the patient's metabolism can be stabilized for either operative care or mobilization.

In our program of fracture care, there is no place for long-term skeletal traction and spica care. The plaster spica, because it requires prolonged recumbency and frequently results in atrophy, joint fixation, and psychological stress, is not rational fracture care.

Alternative methods of fracture care have been reviewed in the previous section. There is no

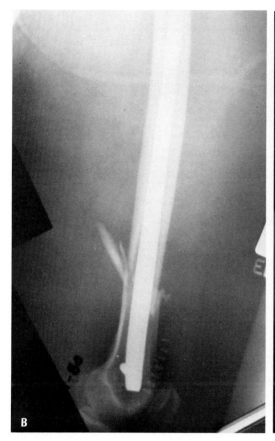
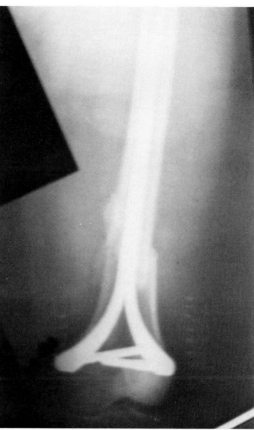

Fig. 15-28 (*Continued*).

question that skeletal traction with later application of some ambulatory device will offer a safe and, in general, reliable means of providing union and an infection-free course. However, with this method, one must not expect anatomical position as a final result. Skeletal traction must allow for some shortening. Varus position frequently occurs with cast brace care, and, by today's standards, probably no greater than 8° is acceptable. Even with that small amount of variation from normal, excessive stresses are placed on the knee, hip, and ankle. Long-term observation suggests that such stress may ultimately be a source of joint deterioration. Slightly more angulation from the lateral perspective (anterior bowing) is acceptable—perhaps 15° due to the compensation available from the knee joint. Some malrotation also is acceptable due to the compensation available at the hip (probably 15° internal and 20° external are acceptable). However, if an alternative to abnormal anatomic alignment is available, this should be the preferred method of care. With modern technology, operative skills, and

appropriate equipment, the closed rodding of femoral fractures can be made the standard of care. (The next section goes into some detail regarding the specific steps of this method of care.)

CLOSED MEDULLARY NAILING

Closed medullary nailing has the broadest application for the various problems of femoral shaft fractures. It can be used for fractures occurring perhaps 2.5 cm below the lesser trochanter to those 8 to 10 cm above the knee joint. It can be applied to simple as well as comminuted fractures. It can be done initially or after several weeks of traction. In fact, after several weeks of traction, there probably is enhanced proliferative bone response producing proliferative callus, although no study has definitely confirmed that delayed nailing speeds union. With this method infection and nonunion are rare complications (0.8% in the largest series).[242] However, unfortunately it takes extensive equipment, experience, and financial support to achieve these excellent results.

In a place where this extensive and expensive equipment is not available (*e.g.*, a small community hospital), early femoral rod care is still preferred to traction, fracture bracing, and long-term hospitalization in most patients. If techniques of closed rodding are not available, retrograde rodding using the open technique is certainly a reasonable substitute for the less complex femoral shaft fractures. In this method, probably the traditional methods described by Schneider[199] are quite appropriate. Under these circumstances, comminution may be dealt with using cerclage after antegrade approach. The open method of local bone devascularization has its price: some scarring of the musculature and a lateral thigh scar.

One other comment is necessary regarding the choice of intramedullary nailing. As we have discussed in preceding sections, there are many intermedullary devices, ranging from the flexible Rush rods and Ender's pins to the very stiff Sampson nail. Our choice is the prebent Küntscher nail with a tapered distal tip to allow easier insertion. This pre-bent nail has sufficient flexibility to be somewhat "forgiving" in the exact location of the entry site on the superior femoral neck. The location of the entry site may be the most critical aspect of closed rodding; if it is not in ideal position, a stiffer nail may cause fracture of the proximal shaft should it be placed either too far medially or laterally. A cloverleaf nail with appropriate reaming is strong enough to handle even the demands of a proximal femoral shaft fracture, and with fixation by interlocking screws, (discussed later in the section), rotation can be controlled very well. A multitude of other devices can do the job just as well, but it is our opinion, based on extensive experience with many devices, that this is the most broadly applicable intramedullary device, allowing treatment of the widest range of femoral shaft fractures without the need for an additional inventory of other devices.

PREOPERATIVE PLANNING

Before any type of open reduction and internal fixation, accurate preoperative planning has to be done. This includes appropriate x-ray documentation of the fractured femur itself and the adjacent hip and knee joints. The fracture pattern should be fully appreciated and, if necessary, drawn onto a comparison x-ray view of the noninjured side. Thus, a decision can be made as to what type and size of implant. All necessary equipment to perform a chosen technique must be at hand, and a reasonable array of implants of various sizes has to be available. Since operative procedures in femur fractures are demanding, an experienced surgeon's assistant should be available.

TECHNIQUE

INDICATIONS AND TIMING

Amenable to closed medullary nailing are almost all simple transverse and short oblique fractures of the femur extending from 2 cm to 3 cm below the lesser trochanter down to about 6 cm to 8 cm above the supracondylar area. Fractures with a single butterfly fragment are chosen for the closed technique as long as their reduction can be maintained due to sufficient apposition of the main shaft fragments. For more comminuted fractures the closed nailing may be accepted as long as fixation is done with an interlocking nail. This technique will be described in more detail later on. Postoperative traction will otherwise be necessary.

Closed medullary nailing has been the preferred method of internal fixation at our institution during the recent years. We are using the pre-bent Küntscher nailing in about 80% of all our femoral shaft fractures. We try to operate as early as possible. In patients with multiple trauma the fracture fixation is done on an emergency basis because we are convinced that early stabilization of multiple skeletal injuries improves the prognosis.[22,34] Isolated femoral fractures are operatively stabilized after a delay of 3 to 5 days (This is a commentary on the peculiarities of our institution—the operating room is often blocked because other trauma procedures are given high priorities). The femoral fracture is initially put in traction through a tibial tubercle pin. Placing one seventh to one tenth of the patient's body weight in traction usually guarantees adequate longitudinal traction. The extremity is placed in balanced suspension, which is applied by a short leg cast put on in the emergency room. Distal femoral pins are indicated in patients with concomitant knee or tibial plateau fractures.

If a complete stock of prebent Küntscher rods is available, the definitive determination of the length and size of the nail is done intraoperatively. It is, however, advisable for the sake of safety to carefully check the implants in stock. Appropriate size can be estimated from good quality x-rays; the width (on average, 2 mm larger than the radiographically measured width of the femoral isthmus) and length (taken from the tip of the greater trochanter to the condylar epiphyseal scar minus 10% due to magnification) of the nail need to be known. Information as to the degree of the femoral bow and the exclusion of concomitant hip or knee fractures or fracture dislocations must be available from the x-ray documentation. The appropriate nail size is determined preoperatively by one of several methods: clinical measurement of the contralateral femur; radiographic comparison of a nail of given length, taped to the non-injured thigh; or use of the Küntscher ossimeter. (This latter instrument shows two scales. The green one allows for a 10% magnification in measuring x-rays. The black scale gives an absolute reading of the actual nail size needed.) Preoperative traction, applied over a few days, should be radiographically checked and, if necessary, be corrected before the patient undergoes surgery.

POSITIONING OF THE PATIENT

While under general anesthesia the patient is placed on a traction table. The routine procedure is to place the patient in a straight lateral position, with the injured femur up and the non-injured side on the table. The hip, in slight adduction, may be flexed from 30° up to 90°, thus facilitating the approach to the greater trochanter. The knee joint may be straight, but should be flexed up to 90° if the hip is significantly flexed. Traction is maintained through a tibial or distal femoral pin. Usually the leg is internally rotated about 10° to 15°, which allows for correct rotational alignment (Fig. 15-29A). The noninjured limb is positioned in a way that does not interfere with the necessary movements of the image intensification x-ray unit. Sometimes it is advantageous to have the patient in a supine position, with the pelvis slightly tilted towards the noninjured side. This is especially helpful in the case of polytraumatized patients, for whom different procedures have to be done at the same sitting, or in the case of patients with bilateral femoral fractures. Reduction should be obtained under fluoroscopic control; it will be sometimes maintained only by means of supporting crutches. The procedure should not start until the reduction is achieved. Careful sterile prepping of the thigh and the adjacent parts of the pelvis is followed by draping. The thigh is prepared in case opening is necessary due to failure to achieve reduction or control comminution.

OPERATIVE PROCEDURE

A longitudinal incision is made over the tip of the greater trochanter, and the trochanteric fossa is approached by splitting the gluteus maximus and medius fibers. The fossa is where the base of the femoral neck joins the base of the greater trochanter. It is here where the ideal point of entrance, somewhat posterior to the midportion of the trochanter, is located. To meet this point exactly is crucial for the following procedure because eccentric reaming with weakening of the medial, anterior, or posterior cortex and subsequent malposition of the implant should be avoided. The tip of the awl is brought into the described position at the junction of the superior neck and trochanteric base and the cortex then gently perforated by manually twisting the awl until it finds its way into the medullary cavity (Fig. 15-29B). The positioning of the awl and the exact point of entrance are easily checked by the image intensifier. As long as no additional axial correction has to be done, the bulb-tipped reaming rod is inserted either by hand or gentle hammer blows until it comes down to the condylar epiphyseal scar. Again, this has to be fluoroscopically checked in two planes using the image intensification x-ray unit.

In case of uncorrected minor displacement at the fracture site it is advisable to slightly curve the distal 2 to 3 cm of the reaming rod, a technique facilitating passage into the distal fragment. In young and healthy people one often has to deal with very firm cancellous bone in the intertrochanteric region; even the placement of a 3-mm reaming rod might be impeded. The initial opening of the medullary cavity is made by sharp hand reamers, which come in different sizes 6 to 9 mm in diameter. If a major misalignment is present (ocurring particularly in proximal femoral shaft fractures), a short Küntscher rod 9-mm in diameter may be inserted into the proximal fragment. This procedure gives enough leverage to facilitate reduction. With the small nail in place it is then usually easy to place the guide rod into the distal fragment.

As soon as the exact placement of the reaming rod is confirmed, the exact length of the rod is determined by subtracting its overriding length from its total length. The amount of existing distraction of the fracture, still under traction at this point, as well as the necessary amount the nail finally should protrude from the point of insertion (approximately 1 cm), must be considered in order to make later nail removal somewhat easier. The preoperatively determined nail width now allows for rapid sterilizing of a few nails, all of which are similar in length and width.

Widening of the medullary cavity is performed

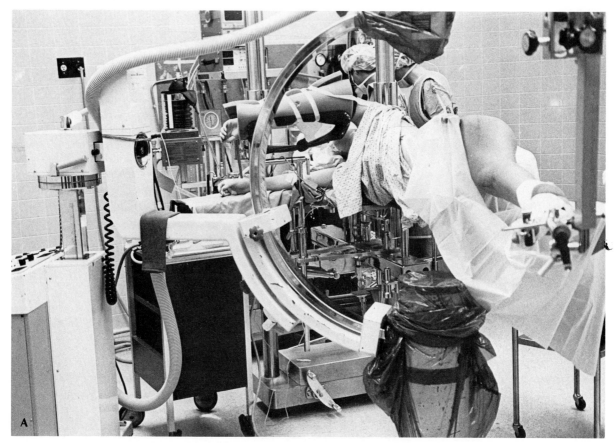

Fig. 15-29. (A) The position of a patient in preparation for closed rodding demonstrating slight flexion of the hip, slight adduction of the hip, and slight flexion of the knee. Skeletal traction is preferred if shortening is a problem preoperatively. Note the position of the ''C'' arm of the image intensifier x-ray equipment. This is necessary for the closed rodding technique.

with a set of *flexible* reamers driven by a compressed air power drill. Starting with a front-cutting, 9-mm reamer (Fig. 15-30), the medullary cavity is gradually reamed out at 0.5-mm increments. During all reamings it is of crucial importance to watch out for axial alignment of the fracture, thus guaranteeing correct placement of the medullary rod. Minor corrections of the fracture reduction are obtained by gentle pressure on that fragment which needs to have an improved position. When reaming strong bone, the fracture surgeon should always consider repeat cleansing of the reamer's heads, thus enabling them always to cut sharply when driven foward into the medullary cavity. Dullness or bluntness in reamer heads causes heat damage to the cortex and sometimes is the determining factor when a reamer is broken or a head is blocked in the medullary cavity. Reaming is usually pursued

until the reamer achieves good cortical contact (over 3 to 4 cm on either side of the fracture at least). This extension can only be determined by carefully evaluating the friction caused by the running reamer, which is transmitted through the air drill. We save the reamed bone cleaned from the reamers and pack it at the fracture site for bone graft before final insertion of the nail.[45]

After terminating reaming, the flexible, bulb-tipped reaming rod has to be replaced by a somewhat stronger, straight-tipped guide rod. Only when the guide rod is in an accurate position should the insertion of the nail, about 1 mm smaller in size than the last reaming performed, begin. The smaller width of the definitive nail helps to avoid troublesome incarceration and probable further comminution of the fracture site by simply splitting more bones apart. Correct alignment of the nail, with

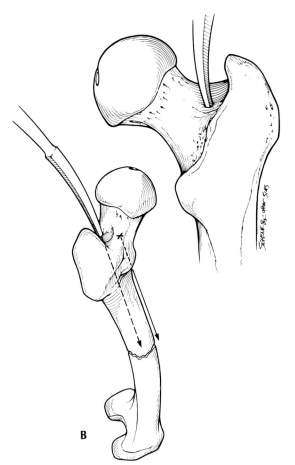

Fig. 15-29 (*Continued*). (*B*) Placement of the entry hole is critical. The tip of the awl should be at the base of the greater trochanter at the junction of the superior femoral neck. Placement (*right*) is slightly too medial and may cause a fracture of the medial cortex—especially if the rod is too stiff and a non-flexible reamer is used. Note the normal anterior bow physiologic to the femur which requires pre-bent nails and flexible reamers to achieve the best anatomical realignment of the fractured bone.

the slot pointing anteriorly, is a fundamental technical part in placing pre-bent femoral rods so that the chances of iatrogenic complications related to the technique of insertion are kept at a minimum. The clover-leaf shape allows for safe and solid impingement on the reamed medullary cavity. Extreme care has to be taken when the tip of the inserted nail is ready to pass the fracture site. Reduction must be optimal so that the nail can be driven into the distal fragment without overcoming any unusual resistance. The nail is inserted best by gentle hammer blows transmitted on the nail through

corresponding nail impacters. Once the nail is securely placed in the distal fragment (an insertion of 4 to 6 cm is adequate) the guide rod can be removed. At the same time traction may be released, but the original internal rotation of the leg of 10° to 15° should be maintained. Final impaction of the nail should allow for compression at the fracture site in normal rotatory alignment.

The trochanteric incision is closed finally in layers. With the patient in a supine position a final check of the rotational alignment is performed. While the patient is still in the operating room, operative results are documented by x-ray films in two planes. The anteroposterior plane film is taken in such a way that the fracture site as well as the hip joint are shown, thus allowing the fracture surgeon to judge whether the insertion has been properly made, and to see the trochanteric position of the selected nail. The lateral film includes the fracture site and the knee joint, thus demonstrating the position of the rod at the condyles.

POSTOPERATIVE MANAGEMENT

Rigidly nailed midshaft fractures do not need supplementary external support. To speed recovery of the range of knee flexion the leg may be placed on a frame in a 90°–90° position for several days (Fig. 15-31). Physical therapy should be initiated on the first postoperative day. For this purpose the patient is temporarily taken off the frame to straighten out the knee. The patient's active range of motion, supported by a temporary thigh cuff, is encouraged by the therapist with strengthening exercises for the thigh, especially the quadriceps muscles, given early in treatment. As soon as the patient has regained active muscle control, ambulation follows with weight bearing as tolerated. Stable medullary fixation in an anatomically restored fracture site allows for full weight bearing within a period of 2 weeks. Less stable fixation needs a somewhat longer period of partial weight bearing. Short-term use of either crutches or canes seems most helpful in any postoperative situation in patients with femoral fractures. The physical therapy should be pursued until the patient is able to fully extend the knee and flex it for more than 90°, which is usually achieved within the first postoperative month. X-ray control of fracture healing may be done with repeat films 6 to 12 weeks after surgery, provided the postoperative course has been uneventful. The return to previous activities is mainly determined by the patient's motivation. Full noncontact sport activities may be allowed within a period of 3 to 6 months, depending on the character of the fracture,

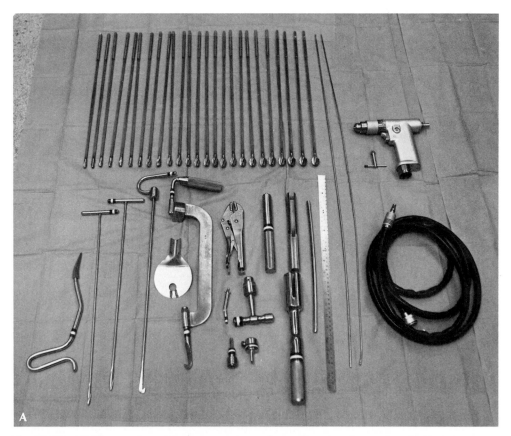

Fig. 15-30. (*A*) The equipment necessary to perform closed rod reaming. From top clockwise are an array of flexible reamers; two guide wires, the stiffer rod guide wire and the more flexible reaming guide wire with a slightly bent tip to assist in initial traverse across the fracture site; power drill equipment; a ruler for measuring; a 9 mm rod used to assist in alignment of the proximal fragment during placement of the flexible reaming guide rod; impacting equipment; extraction and tissue guard equipment; preliminary proximal shaft t-handle reamers; and the initial entry hole awl.

the quality of healing, and the type of sports the patient wishes to participate in. The return to previous professional nonathletic activities is anticipated somewhere between 4 to 8 weeks after surgery. In young patients we recommend implant removal somewhere between 18 to 24 months after injury. Further short-term protection of the femur after nail removal is not indicated as the bone will dispose at that time of full or even improved physiologic strength (a nail is a weight-sharing implant).

In less stable fixation, as is sometimes present in nailed proximal or distal femoral fractures, an additional external support over a period of 4 to 6 weeks may be advisable to maintain rotatory alignment. This is initiated with early postoperative roller traction, which is then followed by a customized long leg orthotic device. Partial weight bearing is allowed as tolerated. Repeat close clinical and radiographic controls usually have to be performed until approximately 5 to 6 weeks after surgery, when the danger of secondary misalignment has been surmounted by the progressed fracture healing.

COMPLICATIONS

Reflecting on the complications encountered in connection with femoral fractures one has to recall that these fractures often present life-threatening injuries. Most often associated with such injuries are hypovolemic shock and shock-related system failures, in the literature somewhat confusingly

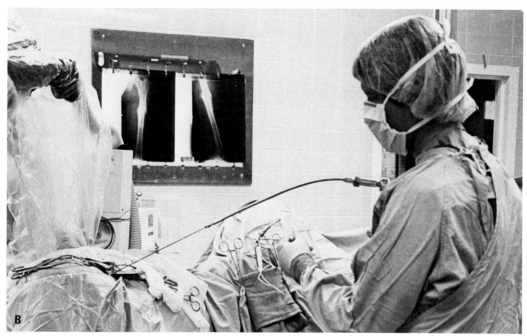

Fig. 15-30. (*Continued*). (*B*) The flexible reamer is placed over the bulb-tipped reaming guide rod, which is placed down the femoral canal to the site of the epiphyseal scar.

outlined as fat embolism syndrome, adult respiratory distress syndrome (ARDS), or simply shock lung syndrome. These conditions all probably have the very same etiologic factors; they all occur when initial shock treatment has not been managed properly.[22] Thus, early, aggressive shock treatment is necessary to successfully resuscitate and stabilize a patient with a femoral fracture.

Complications, particularly those associated with the technique of closed nailing, are most often related to technical errors done intraoperatively.[86,235] Improper placement of the point of entrance of the nail may be followed by eccentric reaming, which increases the chances of further comminution of the fracture site. Incorrect use of reaming and guiderods as well as careless handling of the reamers may end up in an iatrogenic vascular injury. Furthermore, negligence in the control of proper fracture alignment at the time the nail is passing the fracture site will lead to a series of complications at the fracture area, such as protrusion of the nail in the soft tissues; and impingement of the tip of the nail on the medial or lateral cortex will further fracture the bone. Incarceration of the nail is a common result of insufficient overreaming of the femur, which should be 1 mm more than

the size of the inserted nail. To release an incarcerated nail the respective fragment is best split longitudinally over a short distance by means of an oscillating saw. Overreaming is extremely important to match the shape of the nail with a significant anterior bow of the femur. Finally, the nail's length and width may be wrongly selected. Once the tension has been taken off the fragment the nail can be moved without major effort. All of these complications are mainly related to negligence of the basic principles, which have to be mastered; closed medullary nailing is a demanding, but potentially very successful technique.

Late complications such as shortening, angulation or rotational malalignment are usually the consequences of a badly selected nail, failure to appreciate the amount of comminution, or an ill-conceived postoperative treatment plan (*e.g.*, omitting a supplementary external support or traction during a necessary period). To avoid such complications, the fracture surgeon has to be fully aware of their potential until bone healing has occurred (Fig. 15-32).

If closed nailing has been selected as the method of choice for a fracture with bony defect, stability often cannot be achieved. Here one should gener-

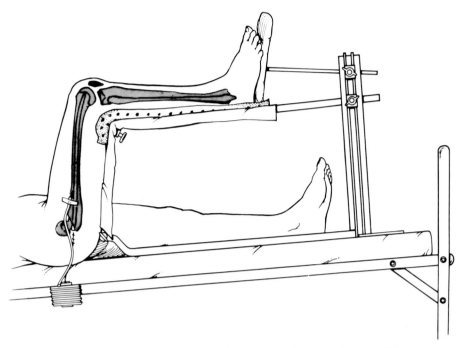

Fig. 15-31. Postoperative 90-90 position for operatively treated femoral fractures.

ously take advantage of the special technique of bone grafting as recommended by Chapman and others.[35,45] This is a closed technique of bone grafting, in which morselized, cancellous bone and the reaming material are placed at the fracture site through a specially prepared chest tube, which is placed into the medullary cavity with its tip ending at the level of the bone defect. This technique must be done before the definitive insertion of the medullary rod. So far we have encountered a few rapid fracture healings with this technique (Fig. 15-33).

TECHNIQUE OF OPEN MEDULLARY NAILING

INDICATIONS

Open nailing may be indicated when closed reduction cannot be accomplished.[235] In long spiral fractures or multifragmentary fractures, for which firm fixation with a nail alone cannot be obtained, additional cerclage wiring may be required to improve rigid fixation.

OPERATIVE TECHNIQUE

The patient is placed in a lateral or supine position, usually on an ordinary operative table or on a fracture table to maintain traction if that has already been preoperatively applied. The fracture site is approached through a straight lateral incision. The iliotibial band is split and the vastus lateralis gently stripped of the intermuscular septum by means of a sharp periosteal elevator. With the muscle anteriorly elevated and held by means of Hohmann or Bennett retractors, the fracture site is easily exposed. A set of appropriate reduction clamps facilitates the restoration of the fracture area. Larger butterfly fragments or long spiral fracture are held in place by cerclage wires that are usually 1.2 mm to 1.5 mm thick; these wires are applied using proper wire passers and tightening instruments. The reduced fracture site may then be secured by an additional semitubular plate of sufficient length placed temporarily on the anterolateral aspect of the femur, where it is held firmly by means of bone-holding forceps. If the proper reduction of the fracture site is not to be obtained because of extensive shortening over a couple of days, the result of insufficient preoperative traction, the use of a femoral distractor, as recommended by the AO group, should be considered. Instead of increasing skeletal traction over joints, it is wiser to exert disimpaction at the fracture site only where it is wanted. The nailing procedure itself follows the same sequential steps as those outlined for the

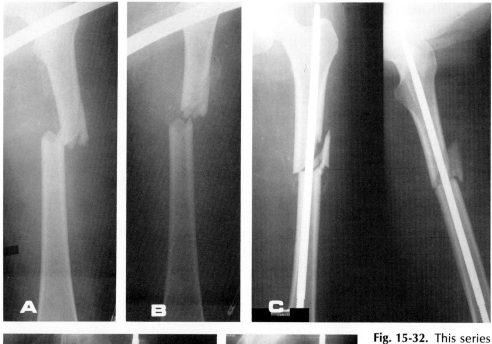

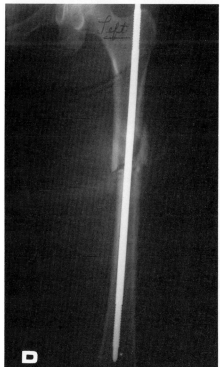

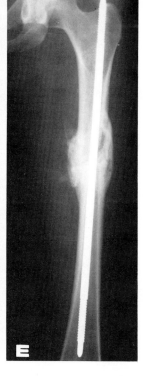

Fig. 15-32. This series of x-rays demonstrates the difference between adequate and excellent fracture care. (*A,B*) The fracture pattern demonstrated a proximal fracture with comminution. This type of fracture pattern is hard to control by closed methods, especially if control of both major fragments cannot be achieved. (*C*) The closed method was accomplished using a Schneider rod. A small rod and no reaming were used to maintain alignment. (*D*) Although rotation was correct at surgery, careful observation demonstrated that there was some malrotation that occurred postoperatively. (*B,E*) Comparatively, this was a very forgiving bone in which union occurred, the malrotation was accommodated by the hip, and ultimately the adequate result occurred. By today's standards this is not ideal care.

closed technique. Once the nail has been inserted, the plate is removed and the wounds are closed after careful cleansing with Ringer's lactate over suction drains. Since one usually deals with com-

minuted fractures, bone grafting should be supplemented whenever bony defects are encountered. For this purpose we usually preserve the reamings and take a few centimeters of cancellous bone out

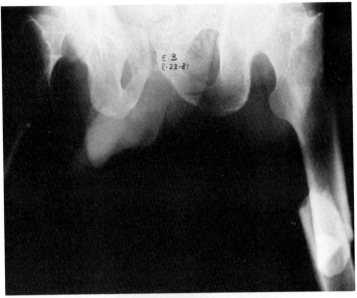

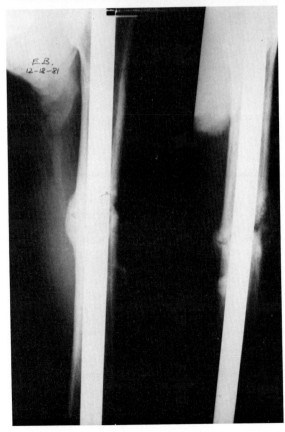

Fig. 15-33. Closed Küntscher nailing in femoral shaft fractures. (*Top*) A short oblique femoral fracture with little comminution. (*Bottom*) Stabilization with a prebent Küntscher rod, 16 mm in diameter, after reaming the medullary canal. Four months after injury uneventful fracture healing. Morselized bone grafting from the reamings was used to hasten union.

of the greater trochanter, which is harvested through the entrance hole for the nail; or, if indicated, we do not hesitate to take the necessary amount of bone graft from the ipsilateral iliac crest.

POSTOPERATIVE TECHINQUE

There is no basic difference between the postoperative management of open medullary nailing and that of the closed techniques. However, it must be kept in mind that due to the extent of the fracture and the associated soft tissue damage, fracture healing time is longer than in simple femoral fractures. Therefore, it is recommended to extend the postoperative period of partial weight bearing according to these considerations. We usually start ambulating with toe touching (about 10 pounds) for 2 to 4 weeks and then proceed with increasing loading. Full weight bearing is allowed about the end of the second postoperative month.

TECHNIQUE OF INTERLOCKING NAIL

Comminuted fractures as well as proximal and distal femoral fractures are not suitable for ordinary medullary nailings. Küntscher[115,117] and others[89,102,103] recommended for this fracture pattern the additional use of interlocking bolts. This method has been widely accepted, mainly in European countries,[111] as an appropriate technique for the fractures described above. An interlocking nail can be applied to serve as a static or a dynamic fixation device (Fig. 15-34). Inserted as a static device, both the proximal and distal fragments are secured by bolts, usually an oblique bolt in the proximal fragment and two transverse bolts in the distal fragment. The static interlocking nail becomes a weight-bearing device because the weight loads are translated through the nail. For a certain period of time, especially when comminuted fractures show a tendency to shortening early, the static nail is most preferable until healing of the fracture, usually after 6 to 8 weeks, makes transfer of the static mode of nail fixation into a dynamic system desirable. This is done by simply removing the bolt or bolts that are placed at the greatest distance from the fracture site. With ongoing weight bearing more physiologic stressing will be applied to the previous fracture area, which helps in rapidly increasing the bone healing process. With only one fragment held by a bolt, the very same nail is now able to act in its superior mechanical function, which is that of a weight-sharing device.

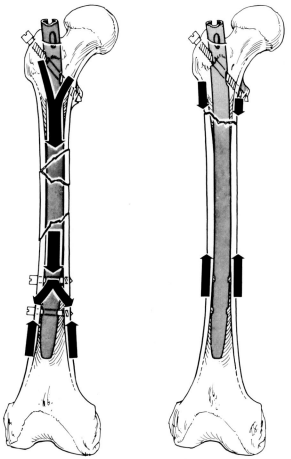

Fig. 15-34. Static and dynamic interlocking nailing in comminuted femoral shaft fractures. (*Left*) Both proximal and distal main fragments are held by interlocking bolts; thus an early collapse of the comminuted area will be prevented. Almost all of the loading stresses are absorbed by the proximal bolt, transmitted through the nail, and finally, reinserted into the femur at the level of the distal bolts. The distance between proximal and distal bolts remains constant. With this technique the nail is regarded as a weight-bearing device (static interlocking nail). (*Right*) Because only one main fragment is held by an interlocking bolt, either the proximal or distal fragment, loading stresses at the fracture site are almost totally transmitted to the bone (dynamic interlocking nail).

When applied as a dynamic interlocking nail, as ideally indicated in proximal or distal femoral fractures, the nail should have firm impingement at the midshaft portion of the femur. At this point, either the proximal or the distal fragment must be separately bolted. This technique secures rotatory stability, and the loading stresses can normally act on the fracture site. Actually, the interlocking nail that has been offered is 13 cm to 16 mm in diamater and 36 cm to 44 cm with 2 cm increments in length, separated for right and left femurs. It needs a few additional instruments to the basic nailing set for Küntscher nailing. The completeness of the appropriate instrumentation, however, is indispensable.

The operative procedure is done following the basic rules for closed nailing. The insertion of the interlocking bolts is relatively simple for the proximal oblique bolt because it is facilitated by the use of a corresponding jig (Fig. 15-35) The placement of the distal bolt has to be done under fluoroscopic control and is technically somewhat troublesome. Following the same postoperative management as that of simple closed nailings, the time when full weight bearing is initiated depends primarily on

the fracture pattern, the type of interlocking nail inserted (static or dynamic), and the patient's ability to cope with the needs of a rehabilitation plan. As mentioned earlier, the interlocking bolts should be removed from one of the main shaft fragments as soon as the status of fracture healing calls for it, which is usually between 6 to 8 weeks after initial surgery.

TREATMENT OF OPEN FEMORAL FRACTURES

In view of the differing positions in the literature concerning the role of internal fixation, particularly immediate internal fixation of open fractures in general, one has to remember some of the anatomical peculiarities of the femur.[10,45,188] An understanding of the femur makes it easier to comprehend

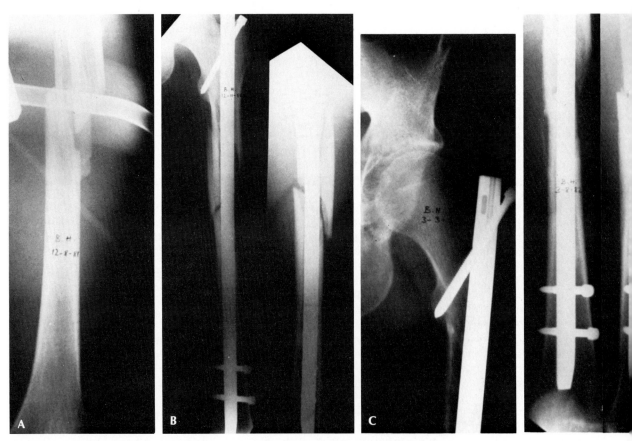

Fig. 15-35. (*A*) Closed comminuted fracture of the midshaft femur. (*B*) An interlocking nail was applied in the static mode to avoid shortening. Auxillary protection with the cast brace was also used to avoid peak loading to the fracture site. (*C*) The fracture was functionally united 4 months postonset with no shortening.

our approach to open femoral fractures, which is to stabilize these fractures quickly. In contrast to the tibia, the bone with the highest complication rate in early internal fixation, femoral fractures have an extensive blood supply as well as sound soft tissue protection by a thick muscle envelope. Even open femoral fractures present less problems related to technically sound internal fixation than do any other skeletal part. Because of fundamental anatomical differences a second-degree, open femur fracture cannot be compared to a second-degree, open tibia fracture when internal fixation is considered as method of choice in an early stage of treatment.

We are convinced that from the standpoint of clinical necessities (including facilitation of nursing care and prevention of multiple organ system failure) the early definitive stabilization of long bones is indeed advantageous for overall prognosis, particularly in a polytraumatized patient.[22] There is good evidence that early stabilization of open fractures presents the best prophylaxis against bone infection.[187] This point is controversial since the statistical data are mixed, regardless of the level of technical skills, pathophysiologic comprehension, and the bone in question.

In our institution we strive for an early fixation of all open femoral fractures. The busy emergency schedule and degree of contamination do not always allow the immediate stabilization of open fractures. Sometimes we perform a thorough debridement and irrigation as the initial step only, which is followed by skeletal traction and open wound treatment over a period of several days, until clean granulating soft tissues allow internal fixation. This procedure often presents the method of choice in first- or second-degree, open, isolated femoral fractures. In case of an immediate fixation we follow these rules:

1. All contused, contaminated, or dead soft tissue, as well as all devascularized bone fragments, is thoroughly debrided. This is done by a wide skin incision that includes existing soft tissue laceration, so that a later approach to the bone will not be hampered. Early cultures must be taken. For this first operative measure separate instruments have to be used. When enlargement of soft tissue damage by further skin incision is considered, it should be kept in mind that the usual approach for femoral fractures is a true lateral one because the vastus lateralis musculature is lifted off the intermuscular septum anteriorly. This approach is used even in situ-

ations in which part of the femoral fragments have caused a dissection or laceration of the ventral or medial portions of the quadriceps muscle.

2. Debridement is followed by extensive irrigation. We have been using a jet lavage system that uses a total of 6000 ml to 10,000 ml of pure Ringer's lactate solution without any additional antibiotics. We believe mainly in the mechanical effects of the irrigation.

3. Internal or external fixation then is done according to the needs and options of a given fracture. The guiding principle in any type of operative treatment of open fractures has to be kept in mind, which is achievement of the best possible stabilization of the fracture site. According to this principle, the decision is primarily what type of implant is feasible. The consideration of the biomechanical advantages of an implant follows in importance. Finally, the fracture surgeon must be aware that the pre-existing soft tissue damage is not worsened by the additional steps that are necessary to prepare the application or insertion of the chosen implant. With these factors in mind, we sometimes feel justified even in nailing the first- or second-degree open shaft fracture, provided the requirements mentioned above can be met. On the other hand, some fracture patterns in second-degree open fractures obviously do better with plating. Most of the third-degree open fractures can be managed by plating with the exceptions of those injuries which have extensive contamination, or those for which an external fixator is thought to do a better job over an initial period of time. The timing of bone grafting is not a simple problem. As long as the vascular supply of the protecting musculature remains unquestionably intact we do not hesitate to treat major bone defects by bone graft, regardless of the type of implant applied. With a questionable viability of soft tissue or bone left behind, we intend on a later, but early, bone grafting, which can be performed during repeat debridement or when the soft tissues are ready to be covered with a split-thickness skin graft.

4. A most important aspect of treatment is leaving all open wounds open with the intention of a delayed closure or a later skin grafting.

5. Systemic antibiotics are administered over a period of 48 hours and prolonged only when early onset of a local infection is proved. We aim at a simultaneous coverage for gram-positive and gram-negative bacteria.

6. In general, the postoperative treatment is the same as that outlined for closed femoral fractures. Positioning of the injured limb, physical therapy, and ambulation undergo only slight alterations that are strictly related to the particular situation of a patient with a given fracture.

It must be emphasized that all biologic and technical aspects of this aggressive operative procedure must be understood, and the procedure itself must be done well so that the soft tissues get the best care and the blood supply of the bone is well preserved.

POSTOPERATIVE CARE AND POSTFRACTURE REHABILITATION

As emphasized earlier, mobilization of the patient after his initial stabilization is a critical factor in attaining optimal results. Many of the complications of femoral fractures can be avoided by early mobilization.[154] Knee stiffness, refracture, muscle atrophy, and weakness all can be largely avoided if muscle and joint activity are resumed early.[184] Whether the method of care is internal fixation or skeletal traction followed by an ambulatory device, early muscle and joint activity are prerequisites to achieving the highest level of function possible with a given degree of injury. The likelihood of return to full normal activity varies inversely with the severity of damage to soft tissue. Nonetheless, specific efforts on behalf of mobilization are warranted.[47]

While the patient is in traction, he should be encouraged to use his muscles. It should be specifically pointed out to him that the relative motion of the fracture fragments is not an adverse event, as illustrated by fractures of the clavicle and ribs, which usually heal readily even though they cannot be completely immobilized. Pearson's attachment was a great advance in the care of the fractured femur because it made motion available at the knee, which must continue if fibroarthrosis is to be avoided. Any method of traction that allows functional activity of the muscles is of great benefit.

Once the healing process has begun to stabilize in those fractures treated in skeletal traction it is completely inappropriate to curtail muscle activity, once started, and to lock the tissues into a plaster spica. In every series in which this has been explored, the advantages of safety and security inherent in the skeletal traction system, when compared with the internal fixation systems, are lost because the tissues are allowed to languish

from the "cast disease" identified by the AO group. In the 1970 Stryker series from a Naval hospital, knee motion was limited considerably in over 50% of the patients treated with traction and spica but in only 7% of those treated with internal fixation.[219] Of course, these figures are biased by the fact that fractures with the severest soft tissue damage are, in general, not appropriate for internal fixation, while the simplest fractures are best suited for this maneuver. Nonetheless, it does emphasize expected long-term disability when the limb is locked in a plaster spica for 10 weeks, as was the case in Stryker's series.

A mode of ambulatory activity with crutch assist should be made available to all patients with fractured femurs as early as possible. If there is an upper extremity involved, a trough or strap should be provided on the crutches. If there is an amputation on the other side, plaster pylon temporary devices should be made available.

Frequently, good knee range and quadriceps function can be achieved more easily in the standing position than in a sitting position. It is unreasonable to prevent a patient from standing on his limb until his quadriceps is strong enough to hold the knee in full extension. Eighty percent of quadriceps strength is required to achieve the last 20° of extension. Weakened muscles are easily overwhelmed. They will not work when the demands placed on them exceed their immediate potential. Moreover, the sitting position is a flexed-hip posture, and postural reflexes may tend to inhibit the anterior horn cells of the quadriceps from maintaining a position of full extension at the knee (flexion versus extension patterns). On the other hand, appropriate proprioception reflexes in a standing position probably facilitate the anterior horn cells of the quadriceps and thus are more easily instructed by the cerebrum to function. Thus, weight bearing as tolerated on the fractured limb is the most natural maneuver for strengthening the weakened quadriceps. Active knee flexion and extension in a standing position by wobbling the knee with the foot lightly touching the floor (Fig. 15-36) is a far more natural exercise than those done in the more traditional sitting position, which extend the knee against weights. Finally, the sitting position is the one that exerts the greatest force on a fracture of the femoral shaft. Exercises in a sitting position should be restrained until the femur is competent to bear full weight on standing (Fig. 15-37).

Discomfort is an excellent indicator of the ability of the healing limb to tolerate incremental stresses,

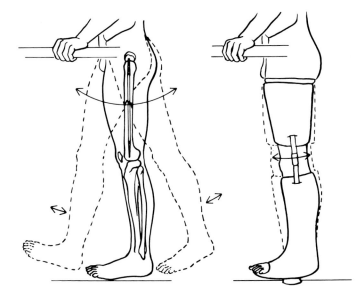

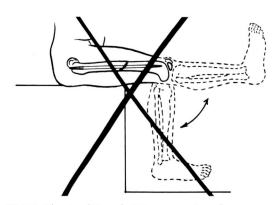

Fig. 15-36. Mobilization of the knee and strengthening of the quadriceps by the knee wobble technique.

Fig. 15-37. The traditional sitting exercises for strengthening of the quadriceps are contraindicated in the early rehabilitation of the fractured femur.

but it must be interpreted in the frame of the patient's personality. To a certain extent, the vigorous, athletic person should be cautioned and restrained from trying to go too fast. On the other hand, the frightened older person or the timid patient should be assured that they cannot hurt themselves and that a little discomfort is normal and harmless to their progress. Increasing pain at a fracture site is an unhappy sign and should be thoroughly investigated. Whether the patient has internal fixation or is ambulatory with an external support device, increasing pain is not the expected turn of events.

We think some attention to medication is reasonable in the rehabilitation phase for the fractured femur. Large amounts of tissue are being reorganized, and incompletely healed skeletal systems are being challenged; discomfort is to be expected. The patient should be given low levels of mild analgesics such as aspirin to assist him through the retraining period. These agents should be taken routinely (*e.g.,* two tablets with each meal) rather than as needed. Sedatives may be necessary for sleeping, but usually they are overused. Youthful patients may even store the pills and sell them on the street. Muscle relaxants are seldom warranted and are another special hazard for youthful patients, not only because tranquilizers may generate some personality aberrations but because habituation comes so easily.

For fractures that so severely limit normal function as those in the femur, it is reasonable to expect the need for some coaching in rehabilitation. Coaching in exercises and crutch walking by a physical therapist is usually of benefit and speeds the patient's progress. No one enjoys calisthenics or discomfort, and the intermittent reinforcement and guidance of a coach-therapist can convert the "motor moron"-type patient into a triumph of early function with limited disability.

PROGNOSIS

The prognosis for healing of femoral shaft fractures is, in general, excellent. Union is to be expected because of the magnificent blood supply around the femoral shaft. Infection should seldom be a threat if good judgment is used in choosing a method of internal fixation. Skeletal fixation should be the "right treatment for the right patient at the right time." Where the skills of the surgeon and the equipment of the institution are adequate, serious infections of fractures of the femoral shaft should be few. With the multiple techniques now available for early mobilization by external support even the early mobilization advantages of internal fixation are less. One should expect a union rate of 100% with good knee function and the patient to be able return to work by 6 months.[158]

COMPLICATIONS

In spite of the (theoretically) glowing prognosis in cases of fractured femur, a wide variety of complications can occur. Unfortunately, these are usually the result of poor judgment in management.

REFRACTURE

Probably the most embarrassing complication in the management of fracture is refracture of the limb once it has been declared or assumed to be sound.[202] Up until quite recently this has been a fairly frequent complication of fractures in the femoral shaft. Hartmann and Brav[88] reported an incidence of 9% in their military experience of the 1950s, and Stuck and Grebe[220] reported an incidence of about 15% in the mid-1940s.

The most effective measure against refracture is gradual application of incremental stresses to the fracture site until full functional stresses have been achieved while the fracture is still protected—either with internal fixation or with an external support. These stresses should be applied early, while the cells in the healing granuloma are still plastic. The "weld of callus" will refracture if its alignment has been random rather than according to the stresses of function that it must tolerate. Experimental work supports the view that connective tissue can be modified and oriented to the appropriate direction by means of the mechanical stresses applied to it.

Refracture after the removal of rigid skeletal fixation is also a problem. The other side of the coin from ideal and complete rigid fixation is new bone that has been totally protected from the stresses of function. Animal work shows that in even the most ideal fracture (transverse osteotomy), initial new bone that has developed directly from blood vessels without going through cartilaginous phase is oriented transversely to the longitudinal

alignment of the fracture.[158] This must be reoriented to the cortical alignment before it can tolerate the stresses of function. Thus, in a cortical fracture ideally and rigidly fixed, only the weld of new bone between the abutting cortices offers stability once the internal fixation device has been removed. Full realignment of the stresses must await the turnover of the osteones in related cortical tissue, and this may take years. Thus, the more ideally and rigidly the fracture has been internally fixed, the longer must be the delay before fixation can be removed. A fracture of the femoral shaft ideally fixed with a Küntscher rod after the entire channel has been reamed must properly wait 2 years before it is safe to remove the rigid internal fixation. Fortunately, plates and screws have a much greater concentration of stress forces and tend to loosen gradually. Thus, the stresses of function are applied gradually to the weld of new bone, and the new bone is reoriented according to the stresses it must tolerate. The plate applied to achieve rigid fixation cannot be removed for at least 1½ years.

In Carr's series refracture occurred in about 6% of femoral fractures treated by closed methods and in 1% of those treated by open methods.[41] All of these refractures occurred in the simplest fractures. This is because these fractures had the smallest open surface available to make a weld. Treating refracture generally is simpler than treating the initial fracture because it is only a simple stress fracture. Placement in an ambulatory cast brace is usually sufficient, but internal fixation with a rod may be necessary to improve anatomical alignment. Bone grafting is unnecessary.

COMPLICATIONS OF FIXATION DEVICES

Fracture of the fixation device has been a fairly common complication of femoral shaft care in the past. With better understanding of the function of the device (it is a temporary splint until skeletal union is achieved) and with improved metallurgy, it is a rare occurrence. Schneider reported one broken nail in 260 cases.[199] Breakage of plates is more common for several reasons. Unless the principles of the AO method are followed strictly, plates may indeed hold the fracture distracted, and, thus, the full stresses of function may be concentrated on the plate itself. Plates of the older Eggers and Sherman types have insufficient strength to tolerate stresses of function, yet they are frequently used in systems that retard the early formation of stress-oriented bone (*e.g.,* prolonged spica immobilization). Thus, when stresses of function were applied, they broke readily. If the plate is to be anything more than a temporary suture, it should be made according to the definitive engineering principles identified by the Swiss AO group.

Another complication of femoral nailing is the bent nail.[213] This is generally recognized radiographically before it presents itself clinically. It usually occurs because the patient is overloading the fracture site before the weld of new bone is strong enough to tolerate the stresses. It usually occurs in simple fractures, which have the smallest surface area for new bone formation. This problem can often be corrected by anesthetizing the patient on his side, supporting the knee on a very firm padded table, and gently bouncing on the thigh with the surgeon's buttock to straighten the nail. This is best accomplished with image-intensifier x-ray control. Once the alignment is corrected, a cast brace can be applied to help support the fracture site. Generally this is sufficient to buy time until new bone is strong enough to sustain the forces of function.

Another complication is migration of the nail. De Belder reported on a series with over 2,000 cases from a cumulative review of the literature. Migration occurred in approximately 1.5% of cases; one third of them migrated distally into the femoral condyle.[56] The cause of this complication is generally a loosening of the nail, frequently secondary to infection and often associated with osteoporotic bone. It was not a complication in any of Schneider's cases.[199] The most common reason for removal is discomfort at the greater trochanter related to the persistent nail protrusion from the greater trochanter. This problem occurs in approximately one third of the cases.

NERVE INJURY

Nerve damage seldom occurs at the time of initial injury, owing to the wide cushion of muscle between the bone and nerve. The most common nerve complication associated with femoral shaft fractures is peroneal nerve disability associated with traction. Prolonged and poorly managed traction with the leg in external rotation may place unacceptable pressure on the peroneal nerve at the head of the fibula before it rotates anteriorly. With poorly monitored suspension systems, flexion at the knee may not correspond to flexion in the suspension system, so that the Pearson attachment is displaced either proximal or distal to the knee. The only correction for this is attention. Adjustment of the suspension pulley system can usually correct the

problem. Padding at the head of the fibula is to be avoided in an effort to avoid direct pressure on the nerve. The most important maneuver to avoid this complication is moving about in the traction with as much freedom as possible, and the patient must be encouraged to do so. Frequent changes in position will avoid the constant pressures that are the source of peroneal nerve embarrassment.

VASCULAR INJURY

Vascular injuries associated with femoral shaft fractures may occur at the time of trauma or during treatment. Initial[62,63] vascular trauma may be a direct or a partial laceration; later vascular problems are false aneurysm or arteriovenous fistula formation, and contusion with injury to the intima and current or late thrombosis. Arterial vasospasm may be associated with compression by cast or by hematoma in trapped spaces. Major arterial occlusion or damage is a relatively uncommon complication of limb injury, occurring at the rate of about one in a thousand.[177] Because it is relatively rare in civilian practice, it may be overlooked. Acute embarrassment of the limb may result from blunt trauma or perforating injuries, such as gunshot or knife lacerations.[196] Gunshot injuries (shotgun excluded) in civilian practice are generally more likely to be low-velocity wounds and may not require extensive exploration and debridement, in contrast to war wounds.

If the mode of injury is blunt trauma, vascular injury in the popliteal area is likely to be a laceration due to tethering of the femoral artery at the adductor hiatus.[98] In the thigh, the femoral artery embarrassment would be due to thrombosis secondary to contusion.

Although cases have been reported in which the late vascular repair is available after resection of necrotic tissue, animal work suggests that 6 hours is the longest time that repair may be delayed before permanent necrotic changes of the muscle occur.[53] Usually 8 hours is available in humans before complications of necrosis begin to emerge. The vascular injury generally can be identified by arteriography and should be suggested by clinical signs of diminished blood supply in the distal limb.

Connolly confirmed the point suggested by the military experience—that it was not always necessary to perform internal fixation of the fracture at the time of arterial repair.[53]

In his series of 14 patients, six were treated with skeletal traction alone, following arterial repair. No patient who had traction exhibited impaired circulation secondary to the traction. Two patients whose popliteal arteries were repaired eventually required amputation because of failure of vascular repair. Both of these repairs had been done in conjunction with internal fixation for the femoral fractures. His series pointed out that the key determinants of extremity survival (besides the successful restoration of peripheral flow) included length of delay before repair, extent of disruption of the collateral circulation, and associated soft tissue damage and infection. Infection may come from the extensive dissection to achieve internal fixation. Skeletal traction can be effective in fracture management in these cases. The decision to use internal fixation should be based strictly on the fracture considerations and what is most appropriate for that particular problem. (Fig. 15-38).

Currently our institution has expert vascular surgeons who are readily available, and all patients with vascular injury are thoroughly evaluated with Doppler testing at least, and usually an arteriogram; even in questionable situations such as when a patient presents with gunshot wounds or stab wounds, there is no hesitation to pursue direct visualization of the vessels. Although it has been demonstrated that vascular repairs can survive in the setting of a nonfixed fracture, with today's armamentarium of stabilization devices available it seems much more appropriate to pursue internal or external fixation at the same time that vascular repair is accomplished. Certainly the soft tissues are better treated by a stable skeletal system, and the threat of infection is greatly diminished.[72] Generally, vascular repair is accomplished by team effort. The vascular surgeon restores peripheral blood flow by means of a temporary shunt, which may include venous flow as well. Then actual definitive stabilization can be formed without urgency. Following the fixation, either with external fixator or plate, vascular repair is performed.[184] Fasciotomies are frequently necessary, especially if the limb has been a prolonged time without perfusion.

Late cases of vascular embarrassment may be the result of a partially severed artery.[21] The resulting problem is either a gradual complete occlusion or

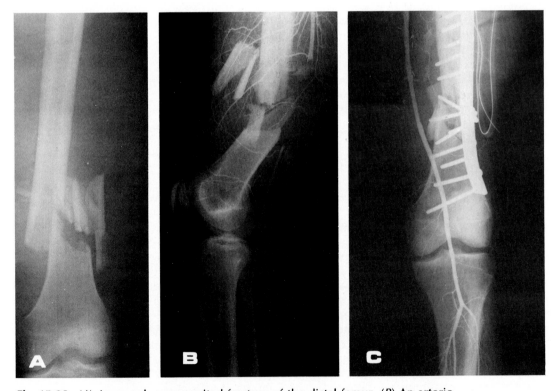

Fig. 15-38. (*A*) A severely communited fracture of the distal femur. (*B*) An arteriogram demonstrating vascular injury. (*C*) Vascular repair was accomplished and the bone was stabilized with plate fixation. This is an extremely difficult level to achieve stability if there is severe comminution.

a false aneurysm—frequently identified by a bruit audible on auscultation. Repair should be done immediately with either vein graft or direct anastomosis.

Vascular occlusion may occur later as a result of internal injuries at the time of skeletal injury or at the time of fracture manipulation and repair. Thus, initial identification of adequate distal pulses may not preclude later thrombosis due to intimal damage. Porter reported three cases of fractures of the femur in which this occurred and that later required resection of the segment. Later thrombosis or false aneurysm may occur in the course of fracture treatment as identified by Roper.[191] False aneurysm as a result of unnoted injury to perforating branches of the profunda femoris artery has been reported. Arteriography is diagnostic of the disability, and vascular repair is necessary.

Aside from technical problems associated with repair, infection is the crucial determinant for successful arterial repair. The most frequent cause of late disruption of vascular repair is infection. In none of the patients in Connolly's series was fracture instability the source of failure.[53]

Although venous embarrassment increases the danger of thromboembolism, this has not become a significant clinical problem in femoral shaft fracture care. Venous thrombosis is five times more common in patients over 40 years old than in younger persons and far more frequent in leg injuries. Nonetheless, the concern about thromboembolic problems should be tempered with the problems related to their treatment.[42] Although in all series available, those treated with anticoagulants had a lesser incidence of thrombosis and thromboembolic problems than the control group, there is some reasonable concern about the use of anticoagulants with fracture cases. The most reliable defense against thromboembolic problems is muscle activity and mobilization. Every effort should be focused at having the patient perform active muscle exercise, specifically in the calf, where evidence suggests that most thromboembolic disease begins.

One additional variation of vascular injury is the compartment syndrome. This has recently been reported by Onkey and colleagues[159] and Snowdy* as a rare complication of crush injuries to the thigh that is frequently associated with femoral shaft fractures. Awareness that this syndrome can occur, like compartment syndromes in other extremities, enables satisfactory treatment to be given. Pressure studies demonstrate increased fluid pressure within

the muscle mass, and fasciotomy, when accomplished, leaves tensely bulging musculature that eventually resolves and can be treated with secondary closure.

NONUNION

Nonunion of the femoral shaft fracture, in spite of considerably improved methods of femoral fracture care, have an incidence of 1%.[41] The majority of nonunions of the femoral shaft are due to factors within the control of the surgeon: incomplete fixation, insufficient or inappropriate mobilization, excessive traction, and—most important of all—prolonged overtraction-distraction.[24,27,221] Nonunions after internal fixation are related to wound infection and inadequate internal fixation.[233] Nonunion develops at one specific anatomical location, (*i.e.*, all other fracture sites unite, leaving the stress concentrated at the one site). Thus, nonunions generally present as relatively simple candidates for operation. The noncomminuted transverse fracture is both the easiest fracture to treat by internal fixation and usually the easiest type of nonunion to manage; for this reason, it is particularly well suited to internal fixation. The basic causes of the nonunion, insufficient blood supply and uncontrolled repetitive stresses, must be corrected by operation.

An intramedullary rod, which achieves firm stabilization of the fracture site, is an appropriate form of treatment.[122] Resection of the cartilaginous false joint is necessary, and usually bone graft is appropriate to "make a new game" out of the repair site. Frequently, sufficient bone graft can be obtained locally by petalling the fracture fragments to make available new blood vessels.

Because the nonunion is usually a simple transverse site, it is a good location for plate fixation if the bone is not too porotic. The solid medial buttress must be available to allow the plate to function as a tension band. When a strong fibrous union is present, it is usually neither necessary nor desirable to take down the nonunion. Rather, the proper application of a compression plate across the fracture site will ultimately convert the existing fibrous tissue and cartilage to bone (Fig. 15-39).[152]

Recently, enthusiasm has been growing for the use of electrical stimulation in the treatment of nonunion or delayed union. Most applications are for problems other than in the femur. One of the difficulties in the use of electrical stimulation is the threat of converting nonunion into malunion when electrical stimulation is used without the benefit of

---

*Snowdy, H. A.: Personal communication, 1983.

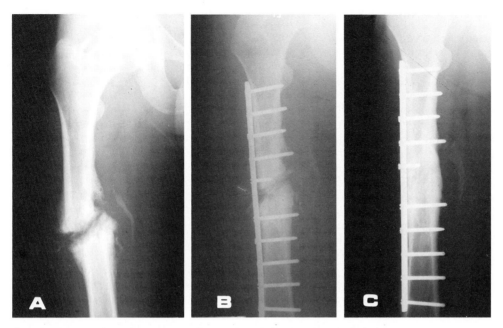

Fig. 15-39. (*A*) Infected nonunion, but with stability on the medial aspect. (*B*) Compression plate fixation with stability achieved owing to the firm medial buttress. (*C*) End result 3 years later.

surgical correction of alignment and surgical stabilization. In the case of the femur, once surgical correction and appropriate stabilization have been achieved the need for electrical stimulation seems remote. The only method that seems appropriate for electrical stimulation in the femur is the totally implanted system.[166] Very little experience has been published in the application of electrical stimulation to femurs. We are currently not using it for femur fractures at our institution.

MALUNION

A much more common phenomenon of fractures of the femur is malunion. Because of the unequal stress forces of muscle pull and gravity, a tendency towards angulation is quite common. The most frequent angulation is a varus bow created by the overpull of the adductors and insufficient lateral musculature associated with the medially placed center of gravity stress forces. Malunion is more often associated with fractures treated with skeletal traction and plaster immobilization. In those settings, especially where ambulatory devices are applied before the fracture is firm, angulation may occur. In that the fracture is still in a rubbery state, however, these can be corrected by wedging the

plaster device. Frequent survey of the fracture alignment status by radiography is thus extremely important. Where good fracture alignment cannot be obtained by skeletal traction even with the use of traction suspension, internal fixation may be indicated if all other factors favor a successful operative result. An anterior bow of 15° in the femoral shaft is acceptable, because it can be compensated well by knee and hip range. But a similar lateral bow is unacceptable because of the excessive stress forces it will later place on the knee. Angulation should be corrected with all feasible vigor; if it is identified while still in the healing phase, correction should be achieved by closed osteoclasis if possible.

Shortening of up to one-half inch is compatible with good function. An effort to achieve full normal anatomical length and alignment is not warranted if the potential for infection or nonunion is increased by this effort.

DELAYED UNION

Delayed union is a frequent complication of normal fracture care. Delayed union is better identified clinically than radiographically. It should be indicated by persistence of bone pain and tenderness

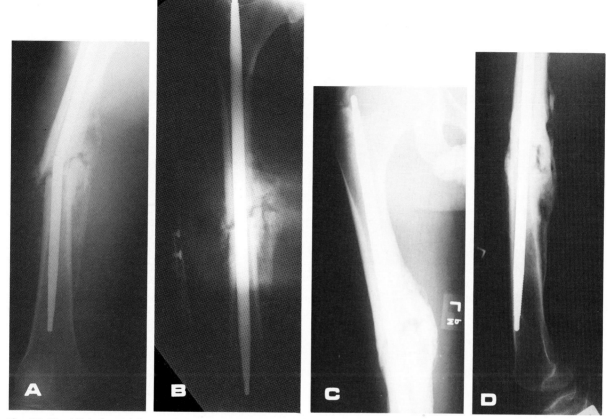

Fig. 15-40. (*A*) Infected femoral shaft fracture with delayed union and metal fatigue. (*B*) Debridement of fracture fragments with larger rod insertion and external supports applied by cast brace. (*C,D*) Eventual union occurred but chronic infection persisted.

past a reasonable period of healing consistent with the degree of skeletal and soft-tissue trauma. Three months is the upper limit for persistent bone pain in the normal healing of a femoral fracture. If pain persists and increases, the healing process is not proceeding normally, and some change in course must be taken.

The treatment for this usually is improved external support and realignment of the fracture fragments to approximate anatomical alignment as much as possible. Ambulatory care will generally resolve delayed union by allowing the hydrodynamic forces of muscle activity to enhance local blood supply and encourage the organization of the healing granuloma by allowing the stress forces to function. Fracture of the internal fixation device also indicates delayed union or associated infection (Fig. 15-40). Replacement with a stouter fixation device may be necessary, but ambulation with an external support may be sufficient to resolve the problem.

SKIN LOSS

Skin loss associated with femoral fractures may be severe and extensive, depending on the amount of trauma. In general, this is not a problem of acute concern and may be handled according to appropriate surgical principles while the wound is healing. Ambulatory activity of the thigh enhances tissue tone and muscle activity to such a degree that the initial size of the nonepithelialized tissue may be rapidly reduced during ambulation. Ambulation in a cast often decreases the size of the wound remarkably, so that considerably less split-skin grafting may be necessary than was anticipated initially (if any is needed at all). A granulating bed of tissue is extremely healthy and resistant to infection. Protection with any of the more commonly available skin dressings while in an external support device is all that is necessary for many weeks until the status of wound healing is stabilized. In general, mobilization and limb function are the most effective measures for reducing the complexities of skin coverage.

INFECTION

Although recently there have been many therapeutical improvements in treating infected fractures,[38,82,139,156] bone infections remain a serious problem. In the presence of an increasing number of operative procedures in fracture care there is a still growing incidence of early bone infections, mainly post-traumatic osteitis. There is no doubt that a high percentage of these infections is related to management failures at the time of the initial surgical treatment. Among these failures are a prolonged operating time; inappropriate handling of the soft tissues, including an unnecessary devascularization of bone fragments or of the main fracture site; an ill-conceived or failed technique of internal fixation; and serious mistakes in the postoperative fracture management. Since most of the infections occur in the early postoperative course it seems reasonable to outline the treatment guidelines for an infected femoral fracture. In an acute infection one first has to perform radical debridement of the infected area. Generous removal of dead bone and soft tissues has to be done regardless of the size of the defect that will be left behind. Thorough irrigation, best applied through a jet lavage system, enables evacuation of soft tissue pockets from debris and pus. In the presence of an implant the fracture surgeon must carefully check whether the device still guarantees stability of the fracture site or not. In case of maintained stability, proved by firm attachment of a plate to the bone, solid anchorage of the plate screws in the cortex, or lack of rotational movements in a nailed fracture, the implant *must* be kept *in situ*. Rittman's studies[187] and numerous other clinical evalutions in infected fractures[38,111,139] indicate that stability of the fracture site is the major prerequisite to achieve bony union. There is, however, only a rare chance of overcoming the infection at this point in time. Despite bony union, secretion from the fracture site usually continues until an implant removal can be performed, combined with a repeat debridement of the soft tissues, excision of fistulas, and thorough cleansing of the implant's bed. The wounds may be kept open and left behind for healing by sec-

ondary intention. When there is no doubt about the local character of an infection or its benign status, the wounds may be closed over a continuous suction irrigation system, and the infected area is irrigated with 3,000 to 5,000 ml of Ringer's lactate a day. If necessary, therapy is supplemented with antibiotics over a period of 8 to 10 days, until repeat cultures prove the efficacy of the initial treatment. As soon as the infection begins to heal, secondary procedures must be considered. The generous use of *cancellous bone* grafts, as described by Papineau,[163] to fill up any mechanically important bony defects is regarded of highest importance and priority. This surgical procedure can be done in a closed fashion, over a temporary continuous suction irrigation system or with open wound management (as described earlier).

In case of an unstable fixation, fracture stability must be secured. Removing the implant alone inevitably leads to increased fracture instability, enhancing the chances of maintaining and even increasing the severity of the infectious process. To achieve the necessary stability several options are available. For example, a loose plate should be removed, to be replaced either by a larger or a stronger plate, as long as this procedure is technically feasible. By no means should the replacement be done at the cost of an unacceptable further extension of the soft tissue dissection. If a simple plate replacement is not possible, one must consider the temporary application of an external fixator until the status of the infection allows reconsideration of an internal fixation device, usually an intramedually rod. Since the avoidance of initiating instability at the time of cleansing the infection is of utmost importance, most of the conservative measures such as casting or cast braces are of less appropriate value.

In case of an infected femoral rod presenting instability at the fracture site, restoring stability again comes first. This may be achieved by replacement of the rod with a larger one, or by a temporarily applied external fixator. Replacement of an unstable rod by a larger nail calls for another sequence of reamings of the medullary cavity, which enables the fracture surgeon to remove most of the infected medullary material. An additional placement of a medullary continuous suction irrigation system, administered through an in-flow tube all the way down the rod and an out-flow tube placed near the fracture site, or of its distal end, helps overcome the acute infection so that bony union may occur (Fig. 15-41).

In general the rules for rehabilitation in infected

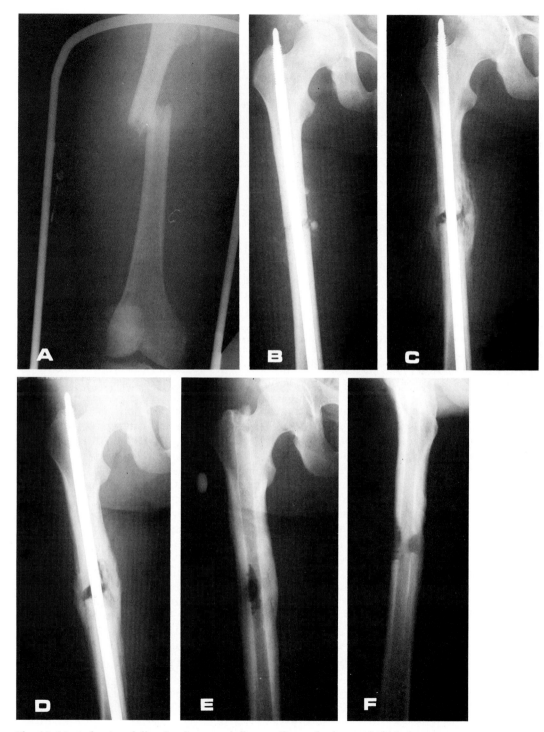

Fig. 15-41. Infection following intramedullary nailing of a femoral shaft fracture. (A) The fracture at onset. The patient was a good candidate for a femoral rod because of proximal location and simplicity of fracture fragments. (B) Postoperative position and alignment were excellent with early signs of healing 1 month after onset. (C) Three months after onset the area of bone destruction showed evidence of infection. (D) The fracture eventually healed with antibiotic treatment and local drainage. (E,F) Sequestrectomy and the nail removal 2 years post-onset. There has been no recurrence of drainage.

femoral fractures are the same as for noninfected fractures, with the exception that after-treatment with increased mobilization of the adjacent joints cannot be done too early, while the infection may still be in an active state. The chances that a post-traumatic infection will heal are limited as long as the implants are *in situ*. As soon as bony healing is secured one should attempt an early implant removal to eliminate the foreign material supporting the infection.

The systematic use of antibiotics (parenteral) for about 3 weeks after surgery is recommended. As long as all local cleansing of infection is properly done we do not see a need for long-term antibiotics during the healing of the infected fracture.[81,113] The choice of antibiotics is based on culture and sensitivities. If these are unavailable, the treatment course would be a combination of cephalosporins and aminoglycosides.[167] Almost all femoral infections have been successfully managed when the above principles have been used, and long-term, chronic osteomyelitis has been kept in check and the potential for occurrence of a late amputation has been minimized.

PATHOLOGIC FRACTURES

Pathologic fractures of the femur may be considered to result from two different processes. Most pathologic fractures are secondary to metastatic malignancy. (Carcinoma of the breast is the most frequent.) The fractures occur with a minimum of trauma, and in fact the pain of microscopic infraction may bring radiographic diagnosis before any significant displacement occurs. These fractures are well suited to closed nailing techniques. With no significant displacement, alignment problems are not significant and an appropriately sized intramedullary rod can be nailed into place under radiographic control without difficulty. On the other hand, the open method of internal fixation may be associated with an unusual amount of hemorrhage secondary to associated reactional vascularity. Ultimate prognosis is based on the lesion itself, but fracture union usually occurs.

A more complex form of pathologic fracture is that associated with metabolic bone disease such as Paget's and osteomalacia or osteoporosis. The femur is the bone most commonly fractured by patients with Paget's disease.[80] The two most common areas of infraction are the subtrochanteric area and the middle third. In Paget's disease, stress fractures occur at a convexity (*i.e.*, on the tension side of the deformity). The common deformity of the femoral shaft in Paget's disease is an extensive varus bow, resulting in increased tension stresses on the lateral aspect of the femoral shaft. The bow deformity, of course, creates a problem for internal fixation by intramedullary rod, and if the deformity is severe, the intramedullary canal cannot accommodate the straight rod. Under these circumstances, plates are the only feasible internal fixation device. Because the bone is extremely vascular, extensive hemorrhage is usually associated with attempts at internal fixation. Thus, when possible, nonoperative means are preferred. In fractures of the femoral shaft, the deformity can be corrected if one does not attempt to achieve anatomical reduction. In the case of subtrochanteric fractures, however, the deformity of the proximal fragment is severe and uncontrollable, and the only means of maintaining alignment is a short intramedullary rod. There is no evidence to indicate that fracture union is delayed by the disease.

In osteomalacia, the most frequent site of pathologic fracture of the femur is in the subtrochanteric area, where high stress concentration and excessive compressive stress loads are focused. Although the more common method of treating these fractures is a blade-plate combination, osteomalacic bone is of such poor quality that screw fixation is usually inadequate. Intramedullary nails, especially of the Zickel design, are a better fixation device. Patients with osteomalacia are not benefited by prolonged recumbency, so nonoperative measures are not recommended.

Another form of pathologic fracture, only on a different basis, is the fatigue fracture.[178,243] It occurs as a result of submaximal stresses repeated at a rate that exceeds the ability of the bone to realign the orientation of trabeculae and osteons. In undisplaced fractures, restricted physical activity is sufficient management, and union should occur without incident. Displaced fractures are simple and uncomminuted with minimal soft tissue damage. Good results may be expected from cooperative management or with intramedullary nailing. A fatigue fracture usually occurs when there is a rapid, consistent, and persistent increase in physical activity over the accustomed rate of the person. Thus, the most likely candidates for these fractures are military recruits and athletes in training camps.[25,78,146]

ASSOCIATED INJURIES

Dislocations and other fractures may be associated with a fracture of the femoral shaft.[1,99,114]

Dislocation of the hip and fracture of the femoral neck are infrequent, but severe complications in an already difficult fracture management problem.[127,197] These injuries generally occur when the femur is subjected to a severe, longitudinal force such as the dashboard injury. The severity of the force may not be expended purely by fracture of the femur and the force load extends more proximal to the hip. The severity of the femoral shaft fracture may be so significant that fragmentation of the bone may cause severe perforation of the musculature and may require operative repair on this basis alone.

The traumatic dislocation of the hip, of course, presents a complicated management problem. Without the handle on the hip of the thigh and knee, closed reduction is extremely difficult, although gentle traction *may* be successful in reducing the hip. Various maneuvers have been advocated to gain control of the proximal fragment, including intramedullary fixation of the fractured femur and then manipulation, various screws and hooks, and transfixing Steinmann pins in the greater trochanter. The basic principles of care are clear; however, the hip should be reduced as soon as possible, and fixation of the femoral shaft fracture may assist in the maintenance of position of the reduced hip.

Probably the most significant aspect of these types of injuries is the ease with which they can be mistreated. There are several cases in the literature in which the hip lesion had been overlooked for weeks. Thus, in femoral shaft fractures that are the result of considerable violence, one must be sure that the violence was dissipated only in the femoral shaft and has not proceeded more proximally.

The same concern should be focused on the knee. A severe transverse force sufficient to fracture the femur may also be sufficient to tear or avulse the collateral knee ligaments. Early diagnosis is, of course, difficult, because the false motion of the leg can certainly be accorded to the fracture of the femur.[203] The usual signs of ligamentous insufficiency—sudden effusion, discoloration, and ecchymosis—are not likely to occur. The ligament avulsion, in general, is not as severe as traumatic knee injuries, because a portion of the force has already been dissipated by the fracture of the femur and thus, the soft tissue eruption may be limited to the major ligaments only, but without any extensive disruption to the other soft tissues. As Pedersen has pointed out, internal fixation of the femur is a necessity before repair of the ligaments is possible.[169]

To avoid the problems that can result from delay in recognition of these associated injuries, it is imperative that the initial evaluation of a patient with a fractured femur include careful clinical and x-ray examination of the hip and knee.

REFERENCES

1. Abell, C. F.: Extrusion of Femoral Shaft Fragment by Trauma and Successful Replacement: A Case Report. J. Bone Joint Surg., **48A:**537–544, 1966.
2. Adams, F. (trans.): The Genuine Works of Hippocrates. Baltimore, Williams & Wilkins, 1939.
3. Adams, J. C.: Standard Orthopedic Operations, 2nd ed. Churchill-Livingston, London, 1980.
4. Adrey, J. (ed.): Hoffman's External Anchorage Coupled in Frame Arrangement: Biomechanical Survey of the Leg Fracture, 2nd ed. Paris, Gaed, 1971.
5. Allen, W. C., Piotrowski, G; Burstein, A. H.; and Frankel, V. H.: Biomechanical Principles of Intramedullary Fixation. Clin. Orthop., **60:**13–20, 1968.
6. Allen, W.; Heiple, K.; and Burstein, A.: A Fluted Femoral Intramedullary Rod: Biomechanical Analysis and Preliminary Clinical Results. J. Bone Joint Surg., **60A:**506–515, 1978.
7. Allgöwer, M.; Ehrsam, R.; Ganz, R.; Matter, P.; and Perren, S. M.: Clinical Experience with a New Compression Plate "DCP." Acta Orthop. Scand. **36**[Suppl.]:277–279, 1969.
8. Allgöwer, M.; Kinzl, L; Matter, P.; Perren, S. M; and Ruedi, T.: The Dynamic Compression Plate. New York, Springer-Verlag, 1977.
9. Altenberg, A. R., and Shorkey, R. L.: Blade-plate Fixation in Non-union and in Complicated Fractures of the Supracondylar Region of the Femur. J. Bone Joint Surg., **31A:**312–316, 1949.
10. Anderson, J. T., and Gustilo, R. B.: Immediate Internal Fixation in Open Fractures. Orthop. Clin., **11:**569, 1980.
11. Anderson, L. D.: Compression Plate Fixation and the Effect of Different Types of Internal Fixation on Fracture Healing. J. Bone Joint Surg., **47A:**191–208, 1965.
12. Anderson, R.: An Ambulatory Method of Treating Fractures of the Shaft of the Femur. Surg. Gynecol. Obstet., **62:**865, 1936.
13. Anderson, R. L.: Conservative Treatment of Fractures of the Femur. J. Bone Joint Surg., **49A:**1371–1375, 1967.
14. Bechtol, C. O.: The Principles of Fracture Fixation. A.A.O.S. Instructional Course Lectures, **11:**92, 1954.
15. Belder, K. R. J.: Distal Migration of the Femoral Intramedullary Nail. J. Bone Joint Surg., **50B:**324–333, 1968.
16. Bielejeski, L., and Garrick, J. G.: Method of Cutting *In Situ* Metallic Appliances. J. Bone Joint Surg., **52A:**585–587, 1970.
17. Böhler, J.: Results in Medullary Nailing of Ninety-five Fresh Fractures of the Femur. J. Bone Joint Surg., **33A:**670–678, 1951.
18. Böhler, J.: Percutaneous Internal Fixation Utilizing the X-ray Image Amplifier. J. Trauma, **5:**150–155, 1965.
19. Böhler, J.: Closed Intramedullary Nailing of the Femur. Clin. Orthop., **60:**51–67, 1968.

20. Böhler, L.: Treatment of Fractures (translated by E. W. Hey-Groves), 3rd ed. Bristol, John Wright & Sons, 1935.

21. Bonney, G.: Thrombosis of the Femoral Artery Complicating Fracture of the Femur. Treatment by Endarterectomy. J. Bone Surg., 45B:344–345, 1963.

22. Border, J. R.; LaDuca, J.; and Seibel, R.: Priorities in the Management of the Patient with Polytrauma. Prog. Surg., 14:84, 1975.

23. Boyd, H. B., and Anderson, L. D.: Management of Unstable Trochanteric Fractures. Surg. Gynecol. Obstet., 112:633, 1961.

24. Boyd, H. B., Anderson, L. D., and Johnson, D. S.: Changing Concepts in the Treatment of Non-union. Clin. Orthop., 43:37–54, 1966.

25. Branch, H. E.: March Fractures of the Femur. J. Bone Joint Surg., 26:387–391, 1944.

26. Brav, E. A.: Further Evaluation of the Use of Intramedullary Nailing in the Treatment of Gunshot Fractures of the Extremities. J. Bone Joint Surg., 39A:513–520, 1957.

27. Brav, E. A.: The Use of Intramedullary Nailing for Non-union of the Femur. Clin. Orthop., 60:69–75, 1968.

28. Brav, E. A., and Jeffress, V. H.: Fractures of the Femoral Shaft. A Clinical Comparison of Treatment by Traction Suspension and Intramedullary Nailing. Am. J. Surg., 84:16–25, 1952.

29. Brav, E.A., and Jeffress, V. H.: Modified Intramedullary Nailing in Recent Gunshot Fractures of the Femoral Shaft. J. Bone Joint Surg., 35A:141–152, 1953.

30. Brooker, A. F., and Edwards, C. C.: External Fixation: The Current State of the Art. Baltimore, Williams & Wilkins, 1979.

31. Brookes, M.; Elkin, A. C.; Harrison, R. G.; and Heald, C. B.: A New Concept of Capillary Circulation in Bone Cortex—Some Clinical Applications. Lancet, 1:1078–1081, 1961.

32. Brooks, D. B.; Burstein, A. H.; and Frankel, V. H.: The Bio-mechanics of Torsional Fractures. The Stress Concentration Effect of a Drill Hole. J. Bone Joint Surg., 52A:507–514, 1970.

33. Brown, A.; Brighton, C.; and D'Arcy, J. C.: Internal Fixation for Supracondylar Fractures of the Femur in the Elderly Patient. J. Bone Joint Surg., 53B:420–424, 1971.

34. Browner, B. D.; Kenzora, J. E.; and Edwards, C. C.: The Use of Modified Neufeld Traction in the Management of Femoral Fractures in Polytrauma. J. Trauma, 21,9:779–787, 1981.

35. Bucholz, R. W., and Mooney, V.: Fractures of the Femoral Shaft. In Evarts, C. M. (ed): Surgery of the Musculoskeletal System. New York, Churchill-Livingston, 1983.

36. Buck, G.: An Improved Method of Treating Fractures of the Thigh Illustrated by Cases and a Drawing. Trans. N.Y. Acad. Sci., 2:232–250, 1861.

37. Burri, C.: Posttraumatische Osteitis. Hans Huber, Verlag, Bern, Stuttgart, Wein, 1974.

38. Burstein, A. H.; Currey, J.; Frankel, V. H.; Heiple, K. G.; Lunseth, P.; and Vessely, J. C.: Bone Strength—The Effect of Screw Holes. J. Bone Joint Surg., 54A:1143–1156, 1972.

39. Burwell, H. N.: Internal Fixation in the Treatment of Fractures of the Femoral Shaft. Injury, 2:235, 1971.

40. Buxton, R. A.: The use of Perkins' Traction in the Treatment of Femoral Shaft Fractures. J. Bone Joint Surg., 63B:362–366, 1981.

41. Carr, C. R., and Wingo, C. H.: Fractures of the Femoral Diaphysis. A Retrospective Study of the Results and Costs of Treatment by Intramedullary Nailing and by Traction and a Spica Cast. J. Bone Joint Surg., 55A:690–700, 1973.

42. Castle, M. E., and Orinion, E. A.: Prophylactic Anticoagulation in Fractures. J. Bone Joint Surg., 52A:521–528, 1970.

43. Cave, E. F.: Fractures and Other Injuries. Chicago, Year Book Publishers, 1958.

44. Chalmers, J.: Subtrochanteric Fractures in Osteomalacia. J. Bone Joint Surg., 52B:509–513, 1970.

45. Chapman, M. W.: Closed Intramedullary Bone Grafting and Nailing of Segmental Defects of the Femur. J. Bone Joint Surg., 62A:1004–1008, 1980.

46. Chapman, M. W., and Mahoney, M.: The Role of Early Internal Fixation in the Management of Open Fractures. Clin. Orthop., 138:120, 1979.

47. Charnley, J.: Knee Movement Following Fractures of the Femoral Shaft. J. Bone Joint Surg., 29:679–686, 1947.

48. Charnley, J.: The Closed Treatment of Common Fractures, 3rd ed. Baltimore, Williams & Wilkins, 1961.

49. Charnley, J., and Guindy, A.: Delayed Operation in the Open Reduction of Fractures of the Long Bones. J. Bone Joint Surg., 43B:664–671, 1961.

50. Christensen, N. O.: Küntscher Intramedullary Reaming and Nail Fixation for Non-union of Fracture of the Femur and the Tibia. J. Bone Joint Surg., 55B:312–318, 1973.

51. Clawson, D. K.; Smith, R. F.; and Hansen, S. T.: Closed Intramedullary Nailing of the Femur. J. Bone Joint Surg., 53A:681–692, 1971.

52. Connolly, J., and King, P.: Closed Reduction and Immediate Cast-brace Ambulation in the Treatment of Femoral Fractures. J. Bone Joint Surg., 55A:1559–1580, 1973.

53. Connolly, J. F.; Whittaker, D.; and Williams, E.: Femoral and Tibial Fractures Combined with Injuries to the Femoral or Popliteal Artery: A Review of the Literature and Analysis of 14 Cases. J. Bone Joint Surg., 53A:56–68, 1971.

54. Coughlin, E.; Ellison, A.; and Fabriciasi, R.: The Use of Martin Barham Bands in Unstable Fractures of the Tibia and Fibula. J. Trauma, 4:692–701, 1964.

55. Danckwardt-Lilliestrom, G.: Reaming of Medullary Cavity and its Effect on Diaphysial Bone: Fluorochromic, Microangiographic and Histologic Study on the Rabbit Tibia and Dog Femur. Acta Orthop. Scand., 50[Suppl.]:128, 1969.

56. de Belder, K. R. J.: Distal Migration of the Femoral Intramedullary Nail. Report of Seven Cases. J. Bone Joint Surg., 50B:324–333, 1968.

57. de Chauliac, G.: Cyrugia Guidonis de Cauliaco; et Cyrugia Bruni; Teodoriei; Rolandi; Lanfranci; Rogerii; Bertapalie: 1.46ʳ Tract V, Doct I, Cap VII. Noviter Impressus. Ventiis: per Bernardinum Nevetum de Vitalibus, 1519.

58. Delbet, P.: Methode de Traitement des Fractures. Rev. Chir., 5:249–288, 1916.

59. DeLorme, T. L.; West, F. E.; and Schriber, W. J.: Influence of Progressive-Resistance Exercises on Knee Function

Following Femoral Fractures. J. Bone Joint Surg., **32A:**910–924, 1950.

60. Dencker, H.: Is the Length of Hospitalization for Patients with Femoral Shaft Fractures Shortened by Intramedullary Nailing? Acta Orthop. Scand., **35:**67–73, 1964.

61. Dencker, H.: Shaft Fractures of the Femur: A Comparative Study of the Results of Various Methods of Treatment in 1,003 Cases. Acta Chir. Scand., **130:**173–184, 1965.

62. Dickson, J. W.: False Aneurysm after Intramedullary Nailing of the Femur. J. Bone Joint Surg., **50B:**144–145, 1968.

63. Doporto, J. M., and Rafique, M.: Vascular Insufficiency Complicating Trauma to the Lower Limb. J. Bone Joint Surg., **51B:**680–685, 1969.

64. Drombrowski, E. T., and Dunn, A. W.: Treatment of Osteomyelitis by Debridement and Closed Wound Irrigation Suction. Clin. Orthop., **43:**215–231, 1965.

65. Duchenne, G. B.: Physiology of Motion: Demonstrated by Means of Electrical Stimulation and Clinical Observation and Applied to the Study of Paralysis and Deformities. Kaplan E. B., trans. and ed. Philadelphia, J. B. Lippincott, 1949.

66. Ender, J., and Simon-Weidner, R.: Fixierung trochanterer frakturen mit elastischen kondylennaegeln. Acta Chir., Austria, **1:**40, 1970.

67. Evans, F. G.: Stress and Strain in the Long Bones of the Lower Extremity. A.A.O.S. Instructional Course Lectures, **9:**264, 1952.

68. Evans, F. G.; Pedersen, H. E.; and Lissner, H. R.: The Role of Tensile Stress in the Mechanism of Femoral Fractures. J. Bone Joint Surg., **33A:**485–501, 1951.

69. Fang, H.; Chew, Y.; and Shang, T.: The Integration of Modern and Traditional Chinese Medicine in the Treatment of Fractures. Chin. Med. J. (Peking), **83:**411–418, 1964.

70. Fisk, G. R.: The Fractured Femoral Shaft—New Approach to the Problem. Lancet, **1:**659, 1944.

71. Frankel, V. H., and Burstein, A. H.: Load Capacity of Tubular Bone in Biomechanics and Related Bio-Engineering Topics. New York, Pergamon Press, 1965.

72. Fried, G.; Salerno, T.; Burke, D.; Brown, H. C.; and Mulder, D. S.: Management of the Extremity with Combined Neurovascular and Musculoskeletal Trauma. J. Trauma, **18:**481–485, 1978.

73. Froimson, A. I.: Treatment of Comminuted Subtrochanteric Fractures of the Femur. Surg. Gynecol. Obstet., **131:**465–472, 1970.

74. Funk, F. J.; Wells, R. E.; and Street, D. M.: Supplementary Fixation of Femoral Fractures. Clin. Orthop., **60:**41–49, 1968.

75. Funsten, R. V., and Lee, R. W.: Healing Time in Fractures of the Shafts of the Tibia and Femur. J. Bone Joint Surg., **27:**395–400, 1945.

76. Gant, G. C.; Shaftan, G. W.; and Herbsman, H.: Experience with the ASIF Compression Plate in the Management of Femoral Shaft Fractures. J. Trauma, **10:**458–471, 1970.

77. Garland, D. E.; Rothi, B.; and Waters, R. L.: Femoral Fractures in Head Injured Adults. Clin. Orthop. **156:**219–225, 1982.

78. Gilbert, R. S., and Johnson, H. A.: Stress Fractures in Military Recruits. A Review of Twelve Years' Experience. Milit. Med., **131:**716–721, 1966.

79. Green, S. A.; Complications of External Skeletal Traction: Causes, Prevention and Treatment. Springfield, Illinois, Charles C. Thomas, 1981.

80. Grundy, M.: Fractures of the Femur in Paget's Disease of Bone—Their Etiology and Treatment. J. Bone Joint Surg., **52B:**252–262, 1970.

81. Gustilo, R. B.: Use of Antimicrobials in the Management of Open Fractures. Arch. Surg., **114:**805, 1979.

82. Gustilo, R. B.: Management of Infected Fractures. *In* Gustilo, R. B. (ed.): Management of Open Fractures and their Complications, pp. 133–157. Philadelphia, W. B. Saunders, 1982.

83. Hahn, D.: Ischio-femoral Arthrodesis for Tuberculosis of the Hip. J. Bone Joint Surg., **45B:**477–482, 1963.

84. Hamilton, L., and Rodriguez, R. P.: Evaluation of the AO Compression Apparatus. J. Trauma, **7:**210, 1967.

85. Hampton, O. P.: Delayed Internal Fixation of Compound Battle Fractures in the Mediterranean Theatre of Operations. Ann. Surg., **123:**1–24, 1946.

86. Hansen, S., and Winquist, R.: Closed Intramedullary Nailing of the Femur: Kuntscher Technique with Reaming. Clin. Orthop., **138:**56–61, 1979.

87. Hansen, S. T., and Winquist, R. A.: Closed Intramedullary Nailing of Fractures of the Femoral Shaft. Part II. Technical Considerations. A.A.O.S. Instructional Course Lectures, **27:**90, 1978.

88. Hartmann, E. R., and Brav, E. A.: The Problem of Refracture in Fractures of the Femoral Shaft. J. Bone Joint Surg., **36A:**1071–1079, 1954.

89. Herzog, K.: Verlaengerungsosteotomie unter verwendung des percutan gezielt verriegelten marknagels. Monatsschr. Unfallheilk, **42:**226, 1951.

90. Hey-Groves, E. W.: On Modern Methods of Treating Fractures. Bristol, John Wright & Sons, Ltd., 1916.

91. Hicks, J. H.: The Relationship Between Metal and Infection. Proc. R. Soc. Med., **50:**842, 1957.

92. Hicks, J. H.: Internal Fixation of Fractures. *In* Clarke, R.; Badger, F. G.; and Sevitt, S.: Modern Trends in Accident Surgery and Medicine. London, Butterworth, 1959.

93. Hicks, J. H.: Fractures of the Forearm Treated by Rigid Fixation. J. Bone Joint Surg., **43B:**680–687, 1961.

94. Hilton, J.: Rest and Pain. Jacobson, W. H. A. (ed.). Philadelphia, J. B. Lippincott, 1920.

95. Hirsch, C.; Cavandias, A.; and Nachemson, A.: An Attempt to Explain Fracture Types. Experimental Studies on Rabbit Bones. Acta Orthop. Scand., **24:**8–29, 1955.

96. Hoffmann, R.: Osteotaxis, Osteosynthese Externe por Fiches et Rotules. Acta. Chir. Scand. **107:**72, 1954.

97. Hohl, M., and Luck, J. V.: Fractures of the Tibial Condyle. A Clinical and Experimental Study. J. Bone Joint Surg., **35A:**1001–1017, 1956.

98. Hoover, N. W.: Injuries of the Popliteal Artery Associated with Fractures and Dislocation. Surg. Clin. North Am., **41:**1099–1112, 1961.

99. Horwitz, T.: Ipsilateral Fractures of the Femoral Shaft and Neck Associated with Patellar Fracture and Complicated by Entrapment of a Major Intermediate Fragment within

the Quadriceps Muscle. A Report of Two Cases. Clin. Orthop., **83**:190–193, 1972.

100. Howland, W. S., Jr., and Ritchey, S. J.: Gunshot Fractures in Civilian Practice. An Evaluation of the Results of Limited Surgical Treatment. J. Bone Joint Surg., **53A**:47–55, 1971.

101. Hsien-Chih, F.; Ying-Ch'ing, C.; and T'ien-Yu, S.: The Integration of Modern and Traditional Chinese Medicine in the Treatment of Fractures. II. Treatment of Femoral Shaft Fractures. Chin. Med. J., **83**:411–429, 1964.

102. Huckstep, R. L.: Rigid Intramedullary Fixation of Femoral Shaft Fractures with Compression. J. Bone Joint Surg. **54B**:204, 1972.

103. Huckstep, R. L.: Early Mobilization and Rehabilitation in Orthopedic Surgery and Fractures. Aust. J. Surg., **47**:344, 1977.

104. Hughes, J. L., and Sauer, B. W.: Wagner Apparatus: A Portable Traction Device. In Seligson, D., and Pope, M. (ed.): Concepts in External Fixation. New York, Grune & Stratton, 1982.

105. Inman, V. T.: Functional Aspects of the Abductor Muscles of the Hip. J. Bone Joint Surg., **29**:607–614, 1947.

106. Johansson, O.: Internal Fixation by Wiring Fractures of Tibia. Treatment Results. Acta Chir. Scand., **101**:185–194, 1951.

107. Kennedy, R. H.: Traction-suspension Treatment in Fractures—Certain Commonly-Neglected Factors. J. Bone Joint Surg., **15**:320–326, 1933.

108. Kilfoyle, R. M.; Foley, J. J.; and Norton, P. L.: Spine and Pelvic Deformity in Childhood and Adolescent Paraplegia. J. Bone Joint Surg., **47A**:659–682, 1965.

109. Kirkaldy-Willis, W. H.; Hay, W.; and Thomas, T. G.: Injuries to the Lower Limb. *In* Principles of the Treatment of Trauma. Edinburgh, E. & S. Livingstone, 1962.

110. Kirshner, M.: Ueber Nagel Extension. Beitr. Klin. Chir., **64**:266–279, 1909.

111. Klemm, K., and Schellmann, W. D.: Dynamische und statische verriegelung des marknagels. Mschr. Unfallheilk, **75**:568, 1972.

112. Klemm, K.: Die stabilisierung infizierter pseudarthrosen mit verriege-lungsnagel. Langenbecks Arch. Chir., 334, 1973.

113. Kostuik, J. P., and Harrington, I. J.: Treatment of Infected Ununited Femoral Shaft Fractures. Clin. Orthop., **108**:90, 1975.

114. Kulowski, J.: Fractures of the Shaft of the Femur Resulting from Automobile Accidents. J. Int. Coll. Surg., **42**:412–420, 1964.

115. Küntscher, G.: Intramedullary Surgical Technique and its Place in Orthopaedic Surgery. J. Bone Joint Surg., **47A**:809–818, 1965.

116. Küntscher, G.: Practice of Intramedullary Nailing. Springfield, Charles C. Thomas, 1967.

117. Küntscher, G.: The Intramedullary Nailing of Fractures. Clin. Orthop., **60**:5–12, 1968.

118. LaFollett, A.; Griffith, T.; Roach, J.; and Albertson, C.: Management of Femoral Shaft Fractures and Cast Brace with Immediate Ambulation. A.A.O.S. Scientific Exhibit, San Francisco, 1979.

119. Laing, P. G.: The Blood Supply of the Femoral Shaft: Anatomical Study. J. Bone Joint Surg., **35B**:462–466, 1953.

120. Lam, S. J.: The Place of Delayed Internal Fixation in the Treatment of Fractures of the Long Bones. J. Bone Joint Surg., **46B**:393–397, 1964.

121. Laurence, M.; Freeman, M. A. R.; and Swanson, S. A. V.: Engineering Considerations in the Internal Fixation of Fractures of the Tibial Shaft. J. Bone Joint Surg., **51B**:754–768, 1969.

122. Laurent, L. E., and Langenskiold, A.: Osteosynthesis with a Thick Medullary Nail in Non-union of Long Bones. Acta Orthop. Scand., **38**:341–350, 1967.

123. Lee, M. L. H.: Intra-articular and Periarticular Fractures of the Phalanges. J. Bone Joint Surg., **45B**:103–109, 1963.

124. Lesin, B.; Mooney, V.; and Ashby, M.: Cast Bracing of Fractures of the Femur: A Preliminary Report of a Modified Device. J. Bone Joint Surg. **59A**:917–923, 1977.

125. Lucas-Championniere, J.: Dangers de l'Immobilisation des Membres. J. de Med. et Chir. Prat., **78**:81, 1907.

126. Lund, F. B.: The Parham and Martin Band in Oblique Fractures. Surg. Gynecol. Obstet., **23**:545–550, 1916.

127. Lyddon, D. W., Jr., and Hartman, J. T.: Traumatic Dislocation of the Hip with Ipsilateral Femoral Fracture. A Case Report. J. Bone Joint Surg., **53A**:1012–1016, 1971.

128. MacAusland, W. R.: Treatment of Sepsis after Intramedullary Nailing of Fractures of Femur. Clin. Orthop., **60**:87–94, 1968.

129. MacAusland, W. R., Jr., and Eaton, R. G.: The Management of Sepsis following Intramedullary Fixation for Fractures of the Femur. J. Bone Joint Surg., **45A**:1643–1650, 1963.

130. Magerl, F.; Wyss, A.; Brunner, C.; and Binder, W.: Plate Osteosynthesis of Femoral Shaft Fractures in Adults. Clin. Orthop., **138**:63, 1979.

131. Magnuson, P. B.: Fundamentals Versus Gadgets in the Treatment of Fractures. Surg. Gynecol. Obstet., **62**:276–286, 1936.

132. Mahorner, H. R., and Bradburn, M.: Fractures of the Femur—Report of 308 Cases. Surg. Gynecol. Obstet., **62**:1066–1079, 1936.

133. Mathews, S. S.: A Simple Wire Pin Skeletal Traction Apparatus. J. Bone Joint Surg., **13**:595–597, 1931.

134. Mathysen, A.: Du Bandage platre et de son application dans le Traitement des Fractures, 1854. Liege. [A second and amplified edition of the pamphlet published at Harlem in 1852 in which he first described the method.]

135. Matter, P.; Brennwald, J.; and Perren, S. M.: The Effect of Static Compression and Tension on Internal Remodelling of Cortical Bone. Helv. Chir. Acta Suppl. **12**:1975.

136. Mays, J., and Neufeld, A. J.: Skeletal Traction Methods. Clin. Orthop., **102**:141–151, 1975.

137. McNeur, J. C.: The Management of Open Skeletal Trauma with Particular Reference to Internal Fixation. J. Bone Joint Surg., **52B**:54–60, 1970.

138. Meggitt, B. F.; Juett, D. A.; and DerekSmith, S. J.: Cast Bracing for Fractures of the Femoral Shaft; A Biomechanical and Clinical Study. J. Bone Joint Surg., **63B**:12–23, 1981.

139. Meyer, S.; Weiland, A.; Willenegger, H.: The Treatment

of Infected Non-union of Fractures of Long Bones. J. Bone Joint Surg., **57A**:836, 1975.

140. Modlin, J.: Double Skeletal Traction in Battle Fractures of the Lower Femur. Bull. U.S. Army Med. Dept., **4**:119–120, 1945.

141. Moll, J.: The Cast-brace Walking Treatment of Open and Closed Femoral Fractures. South. Med. J., **66**:345–352, 1973.

142. Monro, J. K.: The History of Plaster-of-Paris in the Treatment of Fractures. Br. J. Surg., **23**:257, 1935.

143. Montgomery, S., and Mooney, V.: Femur Fractures: Treatment with Roller Traction and Early Ambulation. Clin. Orthop., **156**:196–201, 1981.

144. Mooney, V.: Cast Bracing. Clin. Orthop., **102**:159–166, 1974.

145. Mooney, V., Nickel, V. L.; Harvey, J. P.; and Snelson, R.: Cast-brace Treatment for Fractures of the Distal Part of the Femur. J. Bone Joint Surg., **52A**:1563–1578, 1970.

146. Morris, J. M., and Blickenstaff, L. D.: Fatigue Fractures: A Clinical Study. Springfield, Illinois, Charles C. Thomas, 1967.

147. Mubarak, S., and Owen, C. A.: Compartmental Syndrome and its Relation to the Crush Syndrome: A Spectrum of Disease. Clin. Orthop., **113**:81–89, 1975.

148. Muhr, G.; Tscherne, H.: Trentz, O.; and Haas, N.: Die Osteosynthese mit Marknagel und Zusaetzlichen Drahtumschlingungen bei Oberschenkelschaftbruechen. Akt. Traumatoloi, **6**:387, 1976.

149. Müller, M. E.: Internal Fixation for Fresh Fractures and for Non-union. Proc. R. Soc. Med., **56**:457, 1963.

150. Müller, M. E.: Treatment of Non-unions by Compression. Clin. Orthop., **43**:83–90, 1966.

151. Müller, M. E.; Allgöwer, M.; Schneider, R.; and Willenegger, H.: Manual of Internal Fixation. New York, Springer-Verlag, 1979.

152. Müller, M. E.; Allgower, M.; and Willenegger, H.: Technique of Internal Fixation of Fractures. New York, Springer-Verlag, 1965.

153. Neer, C. S. II; Grantham, S. A.; and Shelton, M.: Supracondylar Fracture of the Adult Femur. A Study of 110 Cases. J. Bone Joint Surg., **49A**:591–613, 1967.

154. Nichols, P. J. R.: Rehabilitation after Fractures of the Shaft of the Femur. J. Bone Joint Surg., **45B**:96–102, 1963.

155. Nicoll, E. A.: Quadricepsplasty. J. Bone Joint Surg., **45B**:483–490, 1963.

156. Norden, C. W.: Osteomyelitis. *In* Mandell, G. L.; Douglas, R. G.; and Bennett, J. E. (ed.): Principles and Practice of Infectious Disease, pp. 950–955. New York, John Wiley & Sons, 1979.

157. Olerud, S.: Operative Treatment of Supra-condylar-condylar Fractures of the Femur. J. Bone Joint Surg., **54A**:1015–1032, 1972.

158. Olerud, S., and Danckwardt-Lilliestrom, G.: Fracture Healing in Compression Osteosynthesis in the Dog. J. Bone Joint Surg., **50B**:844–851, 1968.

159. Onkey, R. G., and Brannan, J. J.: The Anterior Thigh Syndrome. J. Bone Joint Surg., **47A**:855–856, 1965.

160. Paget, J.: Clinical Lectures and Essays. London, Longmans Green, 1879.

161. Pankovich, A. M.: Adjunctive Fixation in Flexible Intramedullary Nailing of Femoral Fractures. A Study of Twenty-six Cases. Clin. Orthop. **157**:301, 1981.

162. Pankovich, A. M.; Goldflies, M. L.; and Pearson, R. L.: Closed Ender Nailing of Femoral Shaft Fractures. J. Bone Joint Surg., **61A**:222–232, 1979.

163. Papineau, L. J., Alfageme, A.; and Dalcourt, J. P.: Osteomyelite honique: Excesion et greffe de spongieux à l'air libre aprés mises à plat extensive. Int. Orthop., **3**:165, 1979.

164. Parham, F. W.: Circular Constriction in the Treatment of Fractures of the Long Bones. Surg. Gynecol. Obstet., **23**:541–544, 1916.

165. Partridge, A. J., and Evans, P. E. L.: The Treatment of Fractures of the Shaft of the Femur Using Nylon Cerclage. J. Bone Joint Surg., **64B**: 910–914, 1982.

166. Patterson, D. C.; Lewis, G. N.; and Cass, C. A.: Treatment of Delayed Union and Non-union with an Implanted Direct Current Stimulator. Clin. Orthop. **148**:117–128, 1980.

167. Patzakis, M. J.; Harvey, J. P.; and Tyler, D.: The Role of Antibiotics in the Management of Open Fractures. J. Bone Joint Surg., **56A**:532, 1974.

168. Pearson, M. G., and Drummond, J.: Fractured Femurs: Their Treatment by Caliper Extensions. London, Oxford University Press, 1919.

169. Pedersen, H. E., and Serra, J. B.: Injury to the Collateral Ligaments of the Knee Associated with Femoral Shaft Fractures. Clin. Orthop., **60**:119–121, 1968.

170. Peltier, L. F.: The Impact of Roentgen's Discovery upon the Treatment of Fractures. Surgery, **33**:579–586, 1953.

171. Peltier, L. F.: A Brief History of Traction. J. Bone Joint Surg., **50A**:1603–1615, 1968.

172. Perkins, G.: Fractures and Dislocations. London, The Athlone Press, 1958.

173. Perren, S. M.; Huggler, A.; Russenberger, M.; Allgöwer, M.; Mathys, R.; Schenk, R., Willenegger, H.; and Müller, M. E.: The Reaction of Cortical Bone to Compression. Acta Orthop. Scand., **36**[Suppl.]:125, 1969.

174. Perren, S. M.; Huggler, A.; Russenberger, M.; Straumann, F.; Müller, M. E.; and Allgöwer, M.: A Method of Measuring the Change in Compression Applied to Living Cortical Bone. Acta Orthop. Scand., **36**[Suppl.]:125, 1969.

175. Perren, S. M., Russenberger, M.; Steinemann, S.; Müller, M. E.; and Allgöwer, M.: A Dynamic Compression Plate. Acta Orthop. Scand., **36**[Suppl.]:125, 1969.

176. Pontarelli, W. R.: External Fixation of Fractures. Iowa Orthop. J., **2**:80–88, 1982.

177. Porter, M. F.: Delayed Arterial Occlusion in Limb Injuries. A Report of Three Cases. J. Bone Joint Surg., **50B**:138–140, 1968.

178. Provost, R. A., and Morris, J. M.: Fatigue Fracture of the Femoral Shaft. J. Bone Joint Surg., **51A**:487–498, 1969.

179. Putti, V.: Un nuovo Metodo di Osteosintesi. Clin. Chir. (Milano), **22**:1021–1024, 1914.

180. Raugstad, T. S.; Molster, A.; Haukeland, W.; Hestenes, O.; and Olerud, S.: Treatment of Pertrochanteric and Subtrochanteric Fractures of the Femur by the Ender Method. Clin. Orthop., **138**:231, 1979.

181. Rhinelander, F. W.: The Normal Microcirculation of Diaphyseal Cortex and its Response to Fracture. J. Bone Joint Surg., **50A:**784–800, 1968.

182. Rhinelander, F. W., and Baragry, R. A.: Microangiography in Bone Healing. I. Undisplaced Closed Fractures. J. Bone Joint Surg., **44A:**1273–1298, 1962.

183. Rhinelander, F. W.; Phillips, R. S.; Steel, W. M.; and Beer, J. C.: Microangiography in Bone Healing. II. Displaced Closed Fractures. J. Bone Joint Surg., **50A:**643–662, 1968.

184. Rich, N. M.; Metz, C. W.; and Hutton, J. E., Jr.: Internal vs. External Fixation of Fractures with Concomitant Vascular Injuries. J. Trauma, **11:**463, 1971.

185. Riggins, R. S.; Garrick, J. G.; and Lipscomb, P. R.: Supracondylar Fractures of the Femur. A Survey of Treatment. Clin. Orthop., **82:**32–36, 1972.

186. Riska, E. B.; von Bonsdorff, H.; Hakkinen, S.; Jaroma, H.; Kiviluoto, O.; and Paavilainen, T.: Prevention of Fat Embolism by Early Internal Fixation of Fracture in Patients with Multiple Injuries. Injury, **8:**110, 1976.

187. Rittman, W. W., and Perren, S. M.: Cortical Bone Healing after Internal Fixation and Infection. In Biomechanics and Biology. New York, Springer-Verlag, 1974.

188. Rittman, W. W.; Schibli, M.; Matter, P.; and Allgöwer, M.: Open Fractures: Long Term Results in 200 Consecutive Cases. Clin. Orthop., **138:**132, 1979.

189. Rohan, N. J., and Miller, W. E.: Pin Tract Osteomyelitis. South. Med. J., **62:**1316–1319, 1969.

190. Rokkanen, P., Slates, P.; and Vankka, E.: Closed or Open Intramedullary Nailing of Femoral Shaft Fractures? A Comparison of Conservatively Treated Cases. J. Bone Joint Surg., **51B:**313–323, 1969.

191. Roper, B. A., and Provan, J. L.: Late Thrombosis of the Femoral Artery Complicating Fracture of the Femur. J. Bone Joint Surg., **47B:**510–513, 1965.

192. Ruedi, T., and Luescher, N.: Results after Internal Fixation of Comminuted Fractures of the Femoral Shaft with DC Plates. Clin. Orthop., **138:**74, 1979.

193. Rush, L. V.: Dynamic Intramedullary Fracture-fixation of the Femur. Reflections on the use of the Round Rod after Thirty Years. Clin. Orthop., **60:**21–27, 1968.

194. Russell, R. H.: Theory and Method in Extension of the Thigh. Br. J. Med., **2:**637–638, 1921.

195. Sage, F. P.: The Second Decade of Experience with the Küntscher Medullary Nail in the Femur. Clin. Orthop., **60:**77–85, 1968.

196. Saletta, J. D., and Freeark, R. J.: The Partially Severed Artery. Arch. Surg., **97:**198–205, 1968.

197. Schatzker, J., and Barrington, T. W.: Fractures of the Femoral Neck Associated with Fractures of the Same Femoral Shaft. Canad. J. Surg., **11:**297, 1968.

198. Scheuba, G.: Selection of Osteosynthesis Procedure for Pertrochanteric Fractures. Arch. Orthop. Unfallchir., **68:**172–174; 204–218, 1970.

199. Schneider, H. W.: Use of the Four-flanged Self-cutting Intramedullary Nail for Fixation of Femoral Fractures. Clin. Orthop., **60:**29–39, 1968.

200. Scuderi, C., and Ippolito, A.: Non-union of Supracondylar Fractures of the Femur. J. Int. Coll. Surg., **17:**1–18, 1952.

201. Scudese, V. A.: Femoral Shaft Fractures, Percutaneous Multiple Pin Fixation, Thigh Cylinder Plaster Cast and Early Weight Bearing. Clin. Orthop., **77:**164–178, 1971.

202. Seimon, L. P.: Refracture of the Shaft of the Femur. J. Bone Joint Surg., **46B:**32–39, 1964.

203. Shelton, M. L.; Neer, C. S. II; and Grantham, S. A.: Occult Knee Ligament Ruptures Associated with Fractures. J. Trauma, **11:**853, 1971.

204. Slatis, P., Ryöppy, S.; and Huittinen, V. M.: AOI Osteosynthesis of Fractures of the Distal Third of the Femur. Acta Orthop. Scand., **42:**162–172, 1971.

205. Smith, D. G.: The Development of Fracture Bracing. Resident Papers, Rancho Los Amigos Hospital, 1969.

206. Smith, G. E.: Ancient Egyptians and the Origin of Civilization. London, Harper, 1923.

207. Smith, H.: Medullary Fixation of the Femur. Radiology, **61:**194–199, 1953.

208. Smith, H.: On the Treatment of Ununited Fractures by Means of Artificial Limbs which Combine the Principle of Pressure and Motion at the Seat of Fracture and Lead to the Formation of an Ensheathing Callus. Am. J. Med. Sci., **29:**102–119, 1855.

209. Smith, J. E. M.: Internal Fixation in the Treatment of Fractures of the Shafts of the Radius and Ulna in Adults. J. Bone Joint Surg., **41B:**122, 1959.

210. Smith, J. E. M.: The Results of Early and Delayed Internal Fixation of Fractures of the Shaft of the Femur. J. Bone Joint Surg., **46B:**28–31, 1964.

211. Sofield, H. A.: Anatomy of Medullary Canals. A.A.O.S. Instructional Course Lectures, **8:**8, 1951.

212. Solheim, K., and Vaage, S.: Operative Treatment of Femoral Fractures with the AO Method. Injury, **4:**54–60, 1972.

213. Soto-Hall, R., and McCloy, N. P.: Cause and Treatment of Angulation of Femoral Intramedullary Nails. Clin. Orthop., **2:**66, 1953.

214. Stader, O.: Preliminary Announcement of a New Method of Treating Fractures. North Am. Veterinarian, **18:**37, 1937.

215. Steinmann, F. R.: Eine neue extensions methode in der Frakturenbehandlung. Zbl. Chir., **34:**938–942, 1907.

216. Stewart, M. J.: Athletic Injuries, Particularly to the Ligaments of the Knee: Diagnosis, Repair and Physical Rehabilitation. Am. J. Orthop., **3:**52–55, 1961.

217. Stewart, M. J.; Sisk, T. O.; and Wallace, S. L.: Fractures of the Distal Third of the Femur. J. Bone Joint Surg., **48A:**787–807, 1966.

218. Street, D. M.: One Hundred Fractures of the Femur Treated by Means of the Diamond-shaped Medullary Nail. J. Bone Joint Surg., **33A:**659–669, 1951.

219. Stryker, W. S.; Russell, M. E.; and West, H. D.: Comparison of the Results of Operative and Nonoperative Treatment of Diaphyseal Fractures of the Femur at the Naval Hospital, San Diego, Over a Five-year Period. J. Bone Joint Surg., **52A:**815, 1970.

220. Stuck, W. G., and Frebe, A. A.: Complications of Treatment of Fractures of the Shaft of the Femur. South. Surg., **14:**735–754, 1948.

221. Taylor, L. W.: Principles of Treatment of Fractures and

Non-union of the Shaft of the Femur. J. Bone Joint Surg., **45A**:191–198, 1963.

222. Thomas, H. O.: Disease of the Hip, Knee and Ankle Joints. Liverpool, T. Dobb & Co., 1875.

223. Thunold, J.: Fractura Cruris. Acta Chir. Scand., **135**:611–614, 1969.

224. Tscherne, H., and Trentz, O.: Operationstechnik und Ergebnisse bei Mehrfragment und Truemmerbruechen des Femurschaftes. Unfallheilkunde, **80**:221, 1977.

225. Vesely, D. G.: Use of the Single and Double Split Diamond Nail for Fractures of the Femur: 1957–1964. South. Med. J., **59**:394–399, 1966.

226. Vesely, D. G.: Technique for use of the Single and the Double Split Diamond Nail for Fractures of the Femur. Clin. Orthop., **60**:95–97, 1968.

227. Vesely, D.G.: The Single and Double Split Diamond Femoral Intramedullary Nail. Clin. Orthop., **92**:235–238, 1973.

228. Viljanto, J., and Paananen, M.: Return to Work after Femoral Shaft Fracture. Ann. Chir. Gynaec. Fenn., **62**:30–35, 1973.

229. Wade, P. A.: ASIF Compression has a Problem. J. Trauma, **10**:513–518, 1970.

230. Wagner, H.: Technik und indikation der operativen verkuerzung und verlaengerung von ober-und unterschenkel. Orthop., **1**:59, 1972.

231. Watson-Jones, R.: Fractures and Joint Injuries, Vol. 2, 4th ed. Baltimore, Williams & Wilkins, 1960.

232. Watson-Jones, R., and Coltart, W. D.: Slow Union of Fractures. Br. J. Surg., **30**:260, 1943.

233. Weber, B. G., and Cech, O.: Pseudarthroses, Pathophysiology, Biomechanics, Therapy and Results. Hans Huber, Verlag, 1976.

234. Weil, G. S.; Kuehner, H. G.; and Henry, J. P.: The Treatment of 278 Consecutive Fractures of the Femur. Surg. Gynecol. Obstet., **62**:435–441, 1936.

235. Weller, S.; Kuner, E.; and Schweikert, H.: Medullary Nailing According to Swiss Study Group Principles. Clin. Orthop., **138**:45, 1979.

236. Wickstrom, J.: Current Concepts in Management of Trauma: An Assessment. Clin. Orthop., **44**:99–107, 1966.

237. Wickstrom, J., and Corban, M. S.: Intramedullary Fixation for Fractures of the Femoral Shaft. J. Trauma, **7**:551, 1967.

238. Wickstrom, J.; Corban, M. S.; and Vise, G. T., Jr.: Complications following Intramedullary Fixation of 325 Fractured Femurs. Clin. Orthop., **60**:103–113, 1968.

239. Willenegger, H., and Roth, W.: Die antibakterielle spueldrainage als behandlungspringzip bei chirurgischen infektionen. Dtsch. Med. Wschr. **87**:1485, 1962.

240. Wilson, J. N.: The Management of Infection after Küntscher Nailing of the Femur. J. Bone Joint Surg., **48B**:112–116, 1966.

241. Winquist, R., and Hansen, S. T.: Segmental Fracture of the Femur Treated by Closed Intramedullary Nailing. J. Bone Joint Surg., **60A**:934–939, 1978.

242. Winquist, R. A., and Hansen, S. T.: Comminuted Fractures of the Femoral Shaft Treated by Intramedullary Nailing. Orthop. Clin., **11**:633–648, 1980.

243. Wolfe, H. R. I., and Robertson, J. M.: Fatigue Fracture of Femur and Tibia. Lancet, **2**:11–13, 1945.

244. Wright, D. B., and Stanford, F. D.: Supracondylar Fractures of the Femur. Clin. Orthop., **12**:256–267, 1958.

245. Young, R. H.: Prophylaxis and Treatment of the Stiff Knee Following Fracture of the Femur. Proc. R. Soc. Med., **35**:716, 1942.

246. Zickel, R. E.: A New Fixation Device for Subtrochanteric Fractures of the Femur. A Preliminary Report. Clin. Orthop., **54**:115–123, 1967.

247. Zickel, R. E.: An Intramedullary Fixation Device for the Proximal Part of the Femur. J. Bone Joint Surg., **58A**:866, 1976.

248. Zickel, R. E.: Fractures of the Adult Femur Excluding the Femoral Head and Neck: A Review and Evaluation of Current Therapy. Clin. Orthop. **147**:93–114, 1980.

249. Zickel, R. E.; Fietti, V. G., Jr.; Lawsing, J. F. III; and Cochran, G. V. B.: A New Intramedullary Fixation Device for the Distal Third of the Femur. Clin. Orthop., **125**:185–191, 1977.

16

Fractures and Dislocations of the Knee

Mason Hohl
Robert L. Larson
Donald C. Jones

Part I: FRACTURES ABOUT THE KNEE

Mason Hohl

FRACTURES OF THE DISTAL FEMUR

Fractures in the distal femur have posed considerable therapeutic challenges throughout the history of fracture treatment. Difficulties in obtaining and maintaining reduction, whether by closed or open means, have led to better traction methods and more efficient metallic devices for internal fixation, and have thus effected a gradual improvement in results. The problems of reduction and restoration of function are compounded when the fracture extends between the femoral condyles into the knee joint.

Powerful muscles about the lower thigh and knee produce characteristic fracture deformities, which are often difficult to reduce by closed means. Skeletal traction using one or two pins and any of a variety of knee flexion angles has been used, followed by a spica cast that stays on until the fracture is solidly united. A specially molded long-leg cast or cast brace applied after a preliminary traction period has offered the patient earlier mobility.

Open reduction techniques, on the other hand, have been difficult, exacting, and far from uniformly successful in producing good results. Straight plates proved unsatisfactory, but blade plates such as the Blount, Elliott, and Jewett have been more suc-

cessful. The AO compression system, because of the more secure internal fixation it provides, seems to be an improvement over other methods. Medullary devices, such as Rush pins, split nails, and medullary rods, have been employed in these fractures, but rigid fixation is seldom obtained. Supracondylar fractures require careful therapeutic management to obtain good cosmetic and functional results.

HISTORICAL REVIEW

The early literature did not separate the treatment of fractures involving the distal femur from the treatment of other fractures in the femoral shaft. Since Hippocrates, fractures of the femur had been treated with the leg straight,[60] and splints were developed to maintain the lower extremity in extension. Desault, early in the 19th century, designed a long-leg splint that was commonly used for femoral shaft fractures.

Physick, in the United States, modified the Desault splint to apply isometric traction also.[60] Hugh Owen Thomas, in the 19th century, described his ring splint, also to be used with isometric traction.[80] Treatment remained unchanged until Percival Pott introduced a new concept in fracture management. He realized that most fracture deformities result from the pull of the surrounding muscles and that this pull produces the displacement and interferes with the reduction. He concluded that the fractured extremity should be placed in the position in which the surrounding muscles are most relaxed. For the femur this meant flexion of the hip and knee.

Frank Hastings Hamilton, a leading 19th century American authority on fractures, published results from treatment in all types of fractures. In the final edition of his fracture tables, he reported on 80 fractures of the femoral shaft. Only nine were considered to have a perfect result.[32,34,35,36] Because of the continued poor results following treatment of femoral fractures, new techniques were developed, centering primarily around overcoming the deforming forces of the large thigh muscles. Isotonic traction was then substituted for isometric traction. Gurdon Buck, in 1861,[11] reported on the use of skin traction in treatment of femoral shaft fractures. This later became known as Buck's extension. R. Hamilton Russell, in 1921, described a method of using isotonic skin traction together with positioning the limb in hip and knee flexion.[65,66]

In 1907, Steinmann[75,76] described a method of applying skeletal traction by means of a pin placed through the femoral condyle. Two years later, Martin Kirschner introduced a method of skeletal traction using smaller wires and a tension bail.[47] Skeletal traction subsequently became popular, and reports of improved results appeared. Mahorner and Bradburn, in 1933, reported on 308 fractures of the femur with poor results using Russell's apparatus and satisfactory results with skeletal traction.[52] In this series, 31 fractures involved the distal femur and had the highest percentage of poor results. Open reduction and internal fixation for Y-condylar and single condylar fractures using screws was also mentioned.

Frederick J. Tees, in 1937,[79] devoted a paper entirely to the problems inherent in management of supracondylar fractures. As in most papers, the primary concern was with the relative lack of control over the distal fragment and its tendency to assume a flexed position.

In 1945, John Modlin[53] of the Army Medical Corps, described a technique of double-pin skeletal traction using the standard proximal tibial pin, but adding a pin in the distal femoral fragment to correct its flexed position. This technique was used when standard skeletal traction failed to obtain adequate reduction. The results in 23 cases were "encouraging, with more accurate reduction and earlier motion resulting in a more rapid recovery." Hampton, in 1951,[39] and Wiggins, in 1953,[88] also reported good results with this method of treatment.

Reports of results following open reduction and internal fixation are few. Umansky, in 1948,[82] and Altenberg and Shorkey,[1] in 1949, all reported satisfactory results following open reduction and internal fixation using the reverse Blount plate.

In 1956, White and Russin[87] wrote that supracondylar fractures "should be regarded in the same category as intertrochanteric fractures in which internal fixation is the standard method of treatment." However, in the analysis of their cases, poor results occurred in 25%.

Watson-Jones, in 1955,[84] in discussing supracondylar fractures, believed that most could be managed by standard proximal tibial skeletal traction, adjusting knee flexion to control the distal fragment. He did not recommend the two-pin technique, and stated that open reduction and internal fixation were probably better than risking perforation of the femoral artery with the distal femoral pin.

Lorenz Böhler, in 1935,[6] described a technique of skeletal traction through the proximal tibia combined with a Braun splint, the angle of which was moved proximally and placed at the fracture site rather than behind the knee. In 1956[7] he reported success in controlling posterior angulations in every one of over 100 personal cases. This technique was also advocated by Smillie,[74] who stated, "those who deny the efficiency of this procedure have failed to master the technique." Charnley, in 1961,[14] also advocated a similar method of closed treatment.

Wertzberger and Peltier reported on 45 supracondylar fractures in 1967.[86] Sixteen of them were treated by open reduction using Rush pins. These were the more comminuted, unstable fractures, which they felt were better controlled by adequate fixation with Rush pins, also allowing early range of motion without weight bearing.

Stewart, Sisk, and Wallace, in 1966,[78] reported on 442 fractures of the distal femur. In those treated by closed methods, 67% had good results while 33% had poor outcomes. In the group treated with open reduction, 54% had good results while 46% had poor results. It was their conclusion that simple nonoperative methods of treatment produced good results in the majority of these fractures and should therefore be the method of choice. The two-pin skeletal traction technique previously described by Modlin[53] was advocated. A year later Neer, Grantham, and Shelton reported on 110 supracondylar fractures.[58] They suggested a classification based on the type of displacement of the distal fragment and described the common errors in traction management. They also concluded that operative treatment should be limited to the debridement of open fractures and that internal fixation should be attempted only in rare cases of arterial injury or some other unusual problem in the management of associated injuries.

More recently Connolly,[16] Moll,[54] Mooney,[55] and Rockwood[61] have advocated the use of the cast brace in the ambulatory care of femoral shaft fractures and fractures about the knee. Reported advantages are shorter traction time, early knee motion, early ambulation, and therefore decreased hospital time.

Many devices and techniques for open reduction and internal fixation have previously been used and recommended.[1,3,4,27,28,29,29a,31,42,44a,49,50,57, 59,67,68,72,72a,73,86,90].

Schatzker and colleagues[67] noted that supracondylar fractures, rigidly fixed, obtained 75% good to excellent results by operative means. Schatzker and Lambert[68] in a sequel to the previous study had 71% good to excellent results with rigid fixation. They noted that with less than rigid fixation of intra-articular extension the fractures did much less well. In older individuals in their sixth decade or above, osteoporosis rendered rigid fixation much more difficult. Tscherne[81] advocates a variety of fixative devices in the attempt to gain rigid fixation. Good to excellent results were obtained in 67%.

Seligson and Kristiansen[72] used the Wagner apparatus in five supracondylar fractures with associated severe soft tissue injuries, noting that such external fixation worked well in controlling the fracture. Benum[4] reported the use of adjunctive bone cement with internal fixation in elderly patients with healing in 12 or 14 patients despite early mobilization.

ANATOMY*

The supracondylar region is considered to extend from the femoral condyles proximally to the junction of the metaphysis with the femoral shaft (Fig. 16-1). Supra- and intercondylar fractures represent more severe involvement when fracture lines extend into the knee joint.

Displacement of fractures in this area is partially predictable with posterior angulation and posterior displacement of the distal fragment (Fig. 16-2). The powerful thigh muscles tend to cause shortening, external rotation of the femoral shaft (by adduc-

* A more detailed discussion of knee anatomy is found in the section on ligamentous injuries, Part 2. Only specific anatomical points as they relate directly to fractures about the knee are presented in the section on fractures.

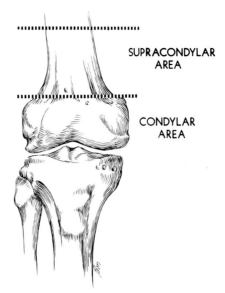

Fig. 16-1. The supracondylar and condylar areas of the femur.

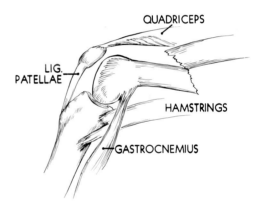

Fig. 16-2. Typical fracture displacement in the supracondylar region showing the muscles that are responsible.

tors), and posterior displacement of the condylar fragment (by quadriceps, hamstrings, and gastrocnemius). Muscle attachments to the respective femoral condyles tend to produce rotational malalignments with intercondylar fractures that are difficult to control with traction or even at surgery. Fractures of a single condyle displace from the trauma or the muscle forces acting across the knee joint.

MECHANISMS OF INJURY

Severe varus or valgus stress forces with axial loading, and rotational forces produce the majority of these fractures. Most occur from high-velocity

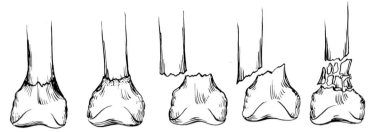

Undisplaced Impacted   Displaced   Comminuted

Fig. 16-3. Types of supracondylar fractures.

vehicular injury, but falls from heights are also a frequent cause. In the older age group with metaphyseal osteoporosis an impacted fracture may be caused by a fall onto the flexed knee.

SUPRACONDYLAR FRACTURES OF THE FEMUR EXCLUDING INTRA-ARTICULAR FRACTURES

CLASSIFICATION

Supracondylar fractures of the femur are classified as either undisplaced, impacted, or displaced. Displaced fractures are frequently transverse or oblique and occasionally comminuted (Fig. 16-3). Open fractures from within are not uncommon, as the distal femur is driven through the skin of the lower thigh, usually in the region of the suprapatellar pouch.

SIGNS AND SYMPTOMS

A history of trauma is followed immediately by painful swelling and often deformity in the supracondylar region of the femur. Findings of false motion and crepitus are the rule, except in impacted or undisplaced fractures. Vascular or neural impairment, although uncommon, is devastating when unrecognized and must be considered before definitive treatment is begun and for several days thereafter. Proximity of the neurovascular elements to the fracture area makes damage to these structures a definite possibility.[5,43,48] Unusual and tense swelling in the popliteal area, as well as the usual signs evident in the lower leg, such as pallor and pulselessness, should suggest rupture of a major vessel in the fracture area, which demands prompt surgical repair.

RADIOGRAPHIC FINDINGS

The fracture configuration and displacement is well defined in the two standard radiographic views—anteroposterior and lateral. Visualization of the entire femoral shaft and hip joint prevents missing other serious injuries, such as a fracture of the femoral neck or a dislocated hip. On occasion several other radiographic views may be necessary to determine whether the fracture extends into the knee joint.

METHODS OF TREATMENT

Closed or open treatment methods are available in supracondylar fractures. Closed methods begin with traction, followed at some interval by either a contoured long-leg, weight-bearing cast, a cast brace, or a spica cast until union is assured. Open treatment involves the use of metallic implants to secure and maintain reduction, followed either by immobilization in plaster or early active knee movement (Fig. 16-4).

Casts

Most impacted supracondylar fractures may be treated with a well-molded, long-leg cast or spica cast for several weeks until union is established. There is a danger when using cast treatment in undisplaced fractures, because the powerful thigh muscles can cause angulation or displacement. A preliminary period in light traction is advisable for these fractures.

Traction

The most commonly used treatment for supracondylar fractures is skeletal traction with the pin placed through the proximal tibia in the region of the tubercle with the thigh, knee, and leg supported in suspension with some knee flexion (Fig. 16-5). Initial traction weight is 15 to 20 pounds; thereafter it is reduced gradually. A common error in management is to flex the knee excessively in traction. A few degrees is usually sufficient. Manipulative reduction under anesthesia, preferably using the image intensifier, is advisable when accurate reduction cannot be obtained by traction alone. Traction can be used to maintain position until bone healing is well established (usually a period of 8 to 12 weeks), or a cast or cast brace may be

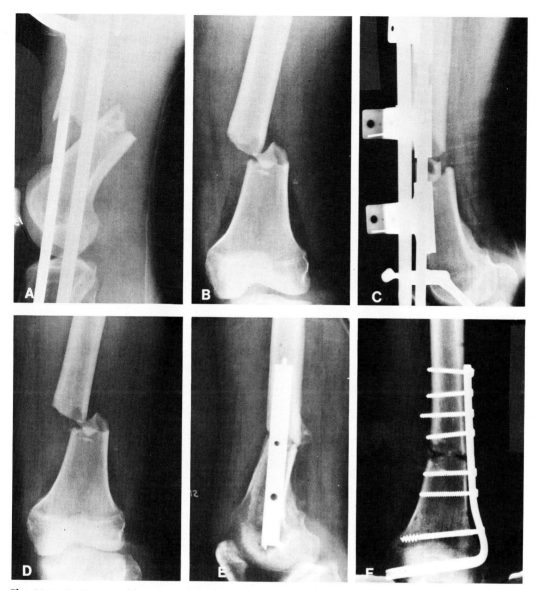

Fig. 16-4. A 28-year-old man sustained a supracondylar fracture of the femur in a motorcycle accident. (*A, B*) X-rays made soon after injury showed the typical fracture displacement. (*C, D*) X-rays made after 2 weeks in traction showed some improvement in reduction but with distraction. (*E, F*) X-rays made 2 months after open reduction and internal fixation.

applied somewhat earlier after the fracture becomes "sticky." Knee movement during the period of traction is encouraged by those who feel that this helps to prevent adhesions of the quadriceps to the fracture area and also speeds fracture union. It is most important to avoid overpulling the fracture to avoid delayed union or nonunion.

The two-pin traction method adds a traction pin through the distal femur to aid in accurate reduction and maintenance of fracture reduction and to permit early movement in the knee.[78] Whenever a second traction pin is added, the risks of vascular injury from pin insertion or infection in the fracture area must be considered (Fig. 16-6).

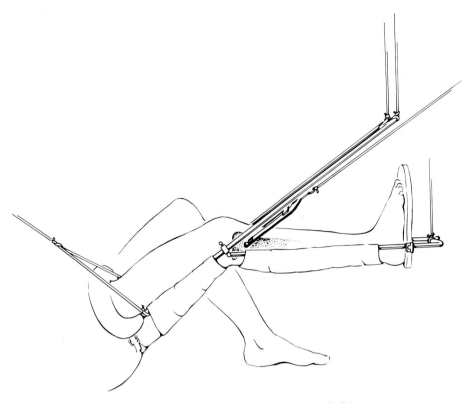

Fig. 16-5. Method of skeletal traction through the proximal tibia.

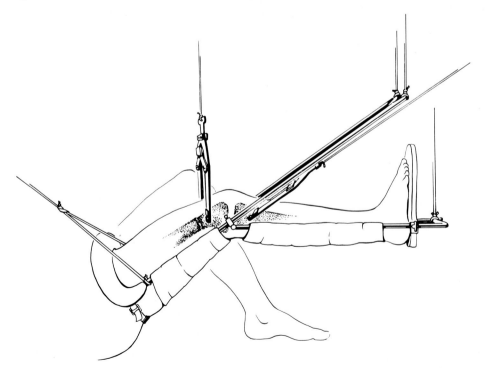

Fig. 16-6. Method of two-pin traction. Note the pin through the distal femur.

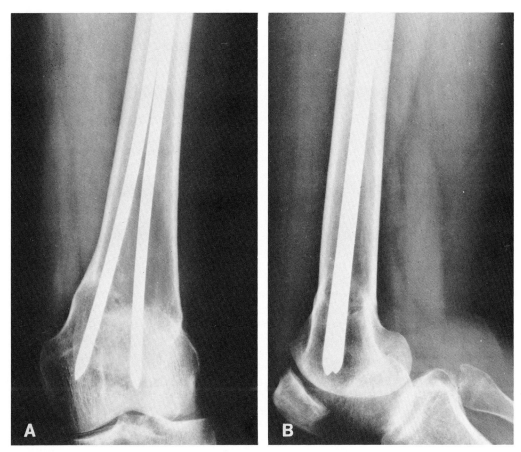

Fig. 16-7. A 50-year-old man sustained a fracture through the middle third of the femur as well as the supracondylar region. Internal fixation by the Street split nail led to good union of both fractures.

Open Reduction

The major reasons for unsatisfactory results by closed treatment are limited knee motion, residual varus, and internal rotation deformity.[58] Most proponents of open reduction propose early motion (to obviate the limited movement problem) and accurate reduction with good fixation (to avoid deformities). However, the contours of the distal femur make accurate insertion of a blade plate quite difficult.[57]

Open reduction techniques are of two basic types: (1) medullary fixation with Rush pins, split nail, or medullary nails, and (2) blade plates such as the Elliott, Jewett, and AO (Fig. 16-7). Internal fixation devices that do not provide rigid fixation such as the medullary nails usually necessitate suspension, traction, or cast support during the healing phase to prevent loosening of the metal with loss of reduction and fixation. The more solid fixation devices, including the blade plates, tend to produce varus or valgus angulation when inserted improperly. Meticulous attention to technical detail is necessary to prevent these complications. Refinements in the immediate postoperative care after open reduction, such as wound suction and positioning the hip and knee at right angles for a few days, have been helpful in restoring a good range of active motion early.

INDICATIONS FOR OPEN AND CLOSED TREATMENT

Open reductions are best used early after injury under ideal conditions (*i.e.*, minimal soft tissue trauma—as after ski injuries—undamaged skin, and an experienced team using the available strong internal fixation devices). The exception may be the use of rigid fixation in selected open fractures to permit optimal soft tissue injury management. When skin or other soft tissue damage is considerable, wound complications are frequent, and it may be advisable either to use closed methods for fracture management or external fixation.[72] Open fractures tend to have more soft tissue injury and a greater propensity for later wound infection. Careful debridement of the open wound must be carried out. A decision is then needed as to whether rigid internal fixation or external fixation can be carried out. If this is possible and is performed well, recent studies of open wounds suggest that a lesser incidence of wound and bone complications may be expected. If such rigid fixation is not possible traction remains a good option.

Open reduction also may be required after failure of reduction by traction methods. If internal fixation is elected, it should be carried out using rigid buttress blade- or screw-plate, and screw combinations, grafting bone defects with iliac bone. Comminution of the fracture is not necessarily a deterrent to internal fixation but may necessitate modification of the optimal early mobilization postoperative regime.

Closed treatment is almost universally applicable and can produce a high percentage of acceptable results (Stewart[78] had 67%; Neer,[58] 84%). It is necessary to achieve and maintain an adequate fracture reduction, if necessary by using a second traction pin located in the distal femur. Overpull and distraction of the fracture delay union. It is better, in general, to accept slight shortening of the leg than to risk delayed union or nonunion. The advantages of closed treatment are the avoidance of operative complications, but there is also a definite morbidity in closed treatment, which includes the possibility of pin tract infections, knee stiffness, and the complications of prolonged confinement to bed.

AUTHOR'S PREFERRED METHOD OF TREATMENT

I prefer closed treatment in many of these fractures, especially those in older people, and use open treatment for ideal conditions, as previously defined, or for those cases where adequate closed reduction cannot be obtained or maintained.

Whenever closed reduction is used, good fracture position and opposition are considered mandatory. A second pin is placed in the distal femur at the level of the adductor tubercle if reduction is not successful after a day or two of single-pin traction. Active movement of the knee throughout the traction period is felt to be important in obtaining a good functional result and in hastening the rate

of fracture callus formation. After several weeks in traction a decision can be made about the use of supplementary support for the fracture based on the amount and quality of callus and clinical fracture stability. I favor the use of a cast brace after 4 to 6 weeks in traction in order to mobilize the patient and his fracture and shorten the hospital stay. The cast brace is maintained until solid union is present by x-ray.

When I elect to do open reduction, the goal is rigid fracture fixation using buttress blade- or screw-plates, and screws. Fracture defects are filled with cancellous grafts, and after surgery the knee is flexed to 90° for a few days. As in all joint fractures I believe the key to a good result is early motion to lessen stiffness and adhesions, both intra- and extra-articular.

CARE AFTER REDUCTION OR OPERATION

Traction is maintained either until good callus is radiographically evident or until clinical stability is determined to be present. The use of spica cast or cast brace for a few weeks more—until the callus is stronger—is common practice, and it is advisable.

After open reduction, wound healing is the most important consideration. It is aided by wound suction and positional drainage, as suggested by Müller and colleagues.[57] Early mobilization of the knee is one of the advantages of open reduction and should be encouraged, if it does not compromise wound healing, and provided that internal fixation is strong and secure.

PROGNOSIS

Most supracondylar fractures heal within 3 to 4 months. Delayed unions are not infrequent and are usually successfully treated by a further period of immobilization. Limitation of knee motion is managed by therapeutic active exercises in the months following immobilization. Many patients have some permanent restriction of knee flexion.

COMPLICATIONS

Immediate complications encountered after fracture of the distal femur include open fracture as the femur penetrates the skin or impairment of blood or nerve supply to the limb from direct injury.

Open fractures usually occur from severe trauma and produce varying degrees of skin and muscle damage. Careful wound cleansing and debridement must be carried out as soon as practicable and decision made regarding the advisability of rigid internal or external fixation. The additional dissection and trauma of such fixation has proved in some trauma centers to actually favor uncomplicated wound healing. Closure of the skin wound, however, is not done primarily but instead later as a delayed primary or secondary closure. The incidence of infection after older methods of internal fixation persuaded most surgeons to use traction and delay needed internal fixation until wound healing was complete.

Vascular integrity of the limb must be assured before definitive treatment of the fracture, for in the event of damage to the femoral or popliteal artery, early repair is mandatory.[5,48] Unusual popliteal swelling may indicate vascular damage and should alert the surgeon. Arteriography should be carried out if there is suspicion of arterial damage, but obvious arterial injury should be operated upon promptly, with or without arteriography. Continued attention to the circulation of the foot, especially in the few days following fracture, is important. Vascular repairs require much operating time and good judgment. No internal fixation, or suboptimal fixation, such as Rush rods or threaded pins followed by more traction, may be considered against more lengthy and definitive internal fixation to avoid additional wound complications.

Nerve injuries from supracondylar fractures are usually of the stretch type and are thus best treated by watchful waiting. Return of function may be expected after 3 to 4 months for most patients.

During the early phase of treatment the occurrence of fat embolism is not infrequent, and later the danger of phlebitis with pulmonary embolism must be considered. Measures to reduce venous stasis and blood coagulability are helpful in reducing this danger (see Chapter 4).

A supracondylar fracture that is not healing or becoming clinically solid after 3 to 4 months is a delayed union, and a further period of immobilization is indicated. Cast bracing may be a useful stimulus to union in some patients. When it is apparent that clinical motion persists and union has failed, it is usually necessary to perform internal fixation with a strong plate using the compression-immobilization principle supplemented by bone grafting and a period of postoperative immobilization.

Later complications include malunions with valgus-varus and rotational deformity producing cosmetic impairment and limited knee motion (Fig. 16-8). Late corrective osteotomy may help to restore alignment. Late deformity is not necessarily eliminated by open reduction, since it may be very difficult to be exact in the insertion of internal fixation devices. Traction treatment has the virtue of adjustability up to the time of bone union, although prolonged and repeated changes in position to achieve better reduction may result in delayed union or nonunion. Because of proximity of the fracture to the quadriceps mechanism and the damage to soft tissue, some limitation of knee motion is virtually inevitable. The extent of this impairment can be minimized by knee movement and quadriceps exercises early in traction or by the use of strong and solidly placed internal fixation devices with emphasis on early active motion in the postoperative period.

SUPRACONDYLAR AND INTERCONDYLAR FRACTURES OF THE FEMUR (INTRA-ARTICULAR FRACTURES)

Involvement of the femoral condyles and knee joint with a supracondylar fracture creates a very complex therapeutic problem. Results of treatment vary, depending on the extent of articular surface damage and the success in restoring congruity to the femoral condyles and the patellofemoral gliding surfaces.

CLASSIFICATION

The supracondylar portion of the fracture is often oblique or comminuted with a fracture line or lines extending into the joint, causing a variety of patterns of condylar involvement. These frequently are called T- or Y-fractures. Neer's classification is most frequently accepted (Fig. 16-9).[58]

SIGNS AND SYMPTOMS

In addition to the deformity produced by the supracondylar fracture, swelling and widening of the knee are apparent. Crepitus on attempted active or passive knee motion is also present.

RADIOGRAPHIC FINDINGS

X-rays taken in the anteroposterior and lateral projections may not be sufficiently accurate to portray the extent, severity, and displacement of the fracture. Oblique projections are often helpful in these determinations. Congruity of the patellofemoral and tibiofemoral articulations is important in the determination of definitive treatment.

METHODS OF TREATMENT

Both closed and open methods are useful, depending on the particular problem presented by the fracture. Often a displaced fracture lines up satisfactorily with skeletal traction through a pin in the proximal tibia (Fig. 16-10). Accurate placement of the pin is important to prevent rotational and

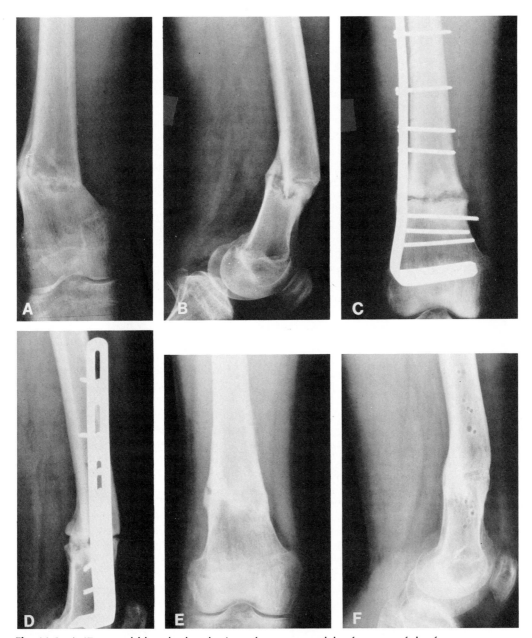

Fig. 16-8. A 17-year-old boy had malunion of a supracondylar fracture of the femur. (*A, B*) The malunited fracture was evident with varus and anterior bowing. (*C, D*) Views after an osteotomy and internal fixation were performed. (*E, F*) Note improved alignment 7 months after osteotomy and removal of hardware.

angular deformities.[58] Adjustments in the angle of pull and knee flexion may aid considerably in reduction, but closed manipulation may occasionally be necessary to align the fracture fragments. When malrotation of the femoral condyles is present, closed reduction and percutaneous pin fixation may be helpful in achieving improved condylar position. Open reduction may be comprehensive, fixing the condyles and the supracondylar fracture, or limited, fixing just the condyles, leaving the patient in traction for treatment of the supracondylar portion of the fracture.[91]

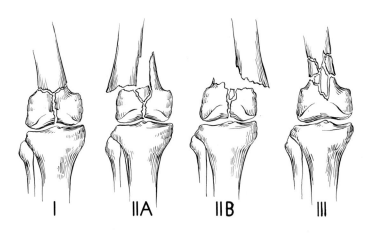

I   IIA   IIB   III

Fig. 16-9. Classification of supra- and intercondylar fractures (Neer, C. S.; Grantham, S. A.; and Shelton, M. L.: Supracondylar Fractures of the Adult Femur. J. Bone Joint Surg., **49A**:592, 1967.)

Initially, patients with supra- and intercondylar fractures are placed in skeletal traction with a proximal tibial pin, allowing continuing observation of the circulatory status in the lower leg. Fifteen to 20 pounds is adequate at the outset until check films determine the need for adjustments of the traction angle or amount (Fig. 16-11). During the first 24 hours, one or more films may be required to assure that any displacement is reduced promptly. Stewart[78] does not hesitate to add another traction pin on the second or third day through the adductor tubercle of the distal femur—even through the fracture, if necessary—to gain better control of the distal femoral fragment. Maintenance of reduction in traction is monitored by x-rays until bridging callus develops. Traction weight can be reduced gradually during this period.

In the event of repeated failure of the condyles to fall into alignment in traction, although the supracondylar fracture reduces well, consideration should be given either to closed reduction with percutaneous pinning of the condyles (which may be very difficult) or to a limited open reduction, using minimal dissection, and one or two lag screws or bolts to hold the condyles together and in alignment. This technique is especially useful in open fractures, when the additional dissection of intact soft tissues must be minimized. After fixation of the condyles, traction is used to treat the supracondylar fracture.

Internal fixation is advocated by some authors as the best solution to the treatment of this difficult fracture. However, open reduction requires considerable dissection and is unwise in the presence of extensive soft-tissue damage. It is most useful in those fractures sustained in falls or twisting injuries, seen and treated early. Accurate anatomical restoration of the fracture fragments is not easy but is necessary to avoid postoperative angular deformities. One of the reasons for failure with open reduction has been the types of fixation devices available (Fig. 16-12). Recent developments, including the AO system, with its blade plates and compression screws, produces better anatomical and functional results than earlier techniques.[59,67,68,73] If the AO implants are used, strict adherence to the operative techniques described in the AO manual[56] is recommended. One of the advantages of rigid internal fixation is the opportunity it affords for early active mobilization of the knee, which limits the development of intra- and extra-articular adhesions (Fig. 16-13). Open reduction loses much of its appeal if confinement in plaster is necessary during the first few weeks after surgery.

INDICATIONS FOR CLOSED AND OPEN REDUCTION

Regardless of what treatment is selected it is important that the intra-articular relationships of the knee be re-established. Open reduction may be necessary to accomplish this.

As in supracondylar fractures, closed methods of treatment are applicable in the majority, since with traction the condyles generally reduce to acceptable position and the supracondylar portion usually realigns. Early knee motion in traction is helpful in restoring function and at times in hastening the rate of formation and quality of fracture callus. After a trial period in traction, if reduction is not acceptable, open reduction is advisable, if skin condition permits. Open reduction in patients under 40 years of age without extensive soft tissue damage, done soon after fracture, produces the most satisfactory results.

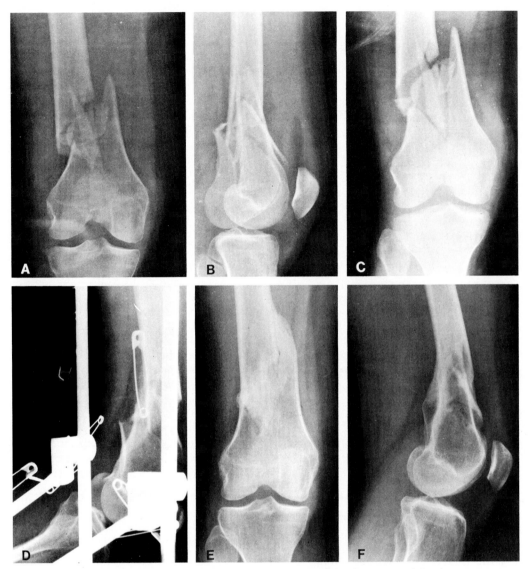

Fig. 16-10. A 56-year-old woman had supra- and intercondylar fractures of the femur treated in traction. (*A, B*) Views after injury showed some comminution and mild displacement. (*C, D*)) Some improvement in position was noted in traction. (*E, F*) Nine months after fracture there was solid evidence of healing. Knee motion was recovering well.

AUTHOR'S PREFERRED METHOD OF TREATMENT

I prefer an initial period of single-pin traction, which often achieves adequate restoration of alignment. If reduction is successful with traction, certainly there is no reason to consider internal fixation. However, when initial traction does not restore condylar congruity, internal fixation is likely to improve the final result. When open reduction is performed, a strong blade plate is used as internal fixation to permit early active knee movement. Primary open reduction is not used without at least a few hours of skeletal traction to judge the adequacy of the reduction.

CARE AFTER REDUCTION

Traction is maintained with gradual lessening of weight until there is radiographic evidence of clinical fracture stability and callus. This takes a min-

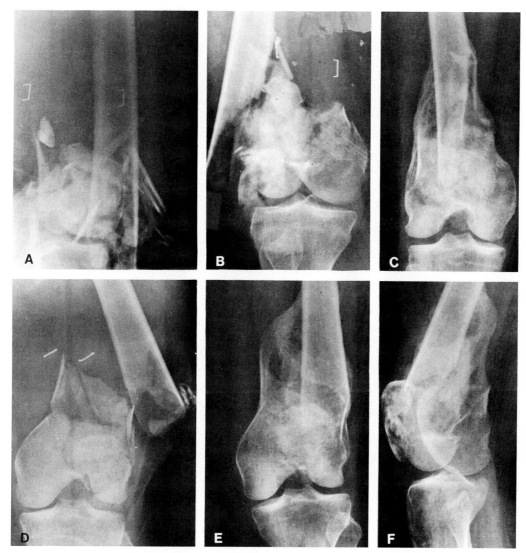

Fig. 16-11. A 30-year-old woman sustained open supra- and intercondylar fractures of both femurs, which were treated by debridement, closure, and traction. (*A, B*) Original x-rays of the right lower femur. (*C*) The healed fracture at 6 months. (*D*) Original anteroposterior x-ray of the left lower femur. (*E, F*) The position in which the fracture healed as seen at 6 months.

imum of 6 weeks, but often as long as 12. Transfer of the patient into a cast or a cast brace for a period sufficient to strengthen the union is indicated. Rehabilitation of strength and motion begins in a cast brace. After all external fixation is removed, active muscle and knee motion exercises are indicated.

PROGNOSIS

Results after supra- and intercondylar fractures are not nearly as satisfactory as those after fractures

without joint involvement. More intra-articular and quadriceps adhesions are anticipated, resulting in slower and less complete return of motion. For these reasons final motion will be improved if movement can be started early in traction or early after rigid internal fixation. Valgus or varus angulations at the knee are more frequent with the Y- or T-fracture configurations.[28a]

COMPLICATIONS

The complications are similar to those of the su-

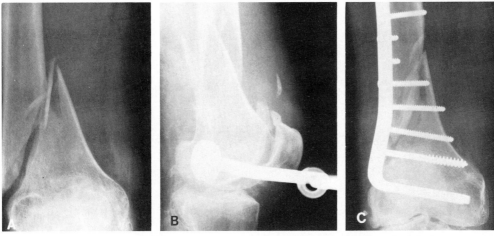

Fig. 16-12. (*A, B*) A 73-year-old woman had an arthritic knee and a closed oblique supracondylar fracture which was treated with an AO condylar blade-plate. (*C*) A postoperative view showed reduction and internal fixation that permitted gentle postoperative mobilization without external fixation.

pracondylar fracture, but return of motion is slower. Early active exercises help lessen these complications.

FRACTURES OF THE FEMORAL CONDYLES

Isolated fractures of the femoral condyles are not common, but they do demand careful attention to prevent the complications of malunion and subsequent impairment of knee function.

Hyperabduction or adduction forces with axial loading from weight bearing may split off the entire femoral condyle or a portion of it.

The condyles are precise mechanical structures that demand accurate fracture reduction. Incongruity and deformity result from healing in malposition, which in turn leads to early and disabling traumatic arthritis of the knee.

CLASSIFICATION

Fractures of several types occur: (1) sagittal, with part or all of the condyle split off; (2) coronal, usually with the posterior portion of the condyle displaced; and (3) a combination of sagittal and coronal (Fig. 16-14).

SIGNS AND SYMPTOMS

Following injury to the knee, pain and swelling are noted. The patient is unable to walk. Instability, crepitus, and hemarthrosis of the knee are noted.

RADIOGRAPHIC FINDINGS

Special tangential or oblique x-rays may be necessary to portray accurately the extent and displacement of the fractured condyle. It is important that enough views be taken to establish the location of the fracture, in order to plan appropriate treatment.

METHODS OF TREATMENT

There is a temptation to treat the relatively undisplaced condyle fracture in a long-leg cast. However, valgus and varus motion occur within the average long-leg cast, frequently producing displacement and unpredictable results. The patient with a short, large thigh is especially vulnerable to loss of fracture position. A spica cast, a cast brace, or traction is more appropriate in the treatment of undisplaced fractures.

If the fracture is displaced, skeletal traction through the upper tibia at times aids in reduction of displacement, especially in the vertical fractures. Maintenance of the reduction in traction is possible, as a rule, and is especially useful when the patient has other injuries that require bed care or skin problems that prevent open reduction.

Open reduction and internal fixation is the only reliable method of insuring accurate articular surface restoration and retention of this reduction. Accurate reduction of the fracture, restoring articular surface congruity with internal fixation by bolts or cancellous screws, is the key to a good

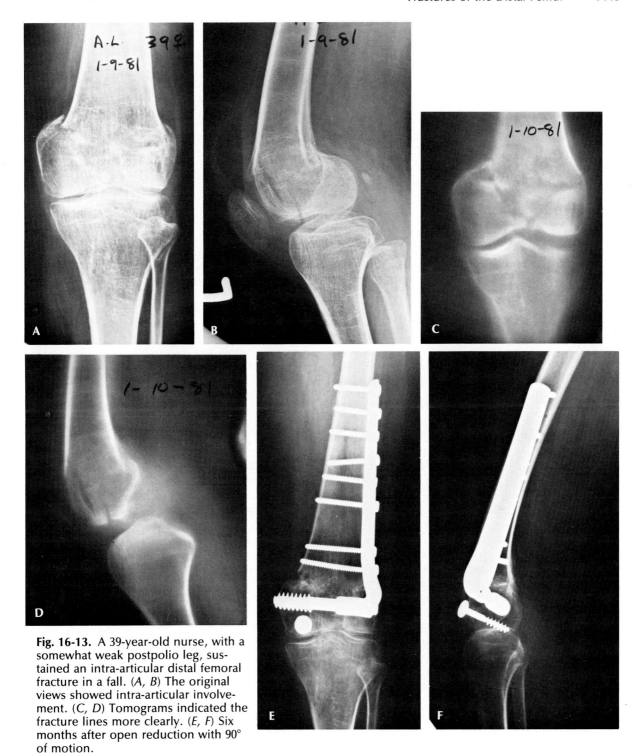

Fig. 16-13. A 39-year-old nurse, with a somewhat weak postpolio leg, sustained an intra-articular distal femoral fracture in a fall. (*A, B*) The original views showed intra-articular involvement. (*C, D*) Tomograms indicated the fracture lines more clearly. (*E, F*) Six months after open reduction with 90° of motion.

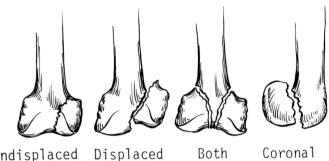

Undisplaced   Displaced   Both condyles   Coronal

Fig. 16-14. Types of femoral condylar fractures.

result (Fig. 16-15). The ability to start knee motion early makes open reduction an especially attractive choice.

AUTHOR'S PREFERRED METHOD OF TREATMENT

I prefer open reduction and internal fixation with cancellous screws or bolts in single condyle fractures of the femur, in order to produce a more predictable result and to facilitate return of function through early active knee motion.

CARE AFTER REDUCTION OR OPERATION

If the fracture has been treated by traction, it is important to continue traction until callus is evident before applying a cast. A cast is used until union is secure. Thereafter, active range of motion exercises are started.

The first priority in postoperative care is to insure primary wound healing by appropriate compression dressings during the early period, and then, provided the internal fixation by cancellous screws or bolts is secure, active motion of the knee and gentle quadriceps strengthening is begun. Weight bearing is delayed until complete union is well established.

PROGNOSIS

Results after femoral condyle fractures generally are good, provided healing occurs in anatomical position and mobility of the knee is begun sufficiently early to prevent the formation of intra-articular adhesions.

When accurate reduction is not obtained, union is delayed, and angular deformity of the knee quite likely will occur, and probably degenerative changes later. Marginal fracture from the posterior condyles may have a poor end result, because the fragment is deprived of blood supply, resulting in the rapid onset of degenerative change.

COMPLICATIONS

Failure to obtain reduction of the condyles suggests the urgent need for open reduction. Delayed union or nonunion is unusual after open reduction, but with traction or cast treatment union may tend to be delayed. Prompt recognition of this is important, so that internal fixation and grafting can be performed to avoid prolonged immobilization.

FRACTURES OF THE PATELLA

Fractures of the patella constitute about 1% of all skeletal injuries[107] and occur in all age groups. The mean age for these fractures is reported to be between 40 and 50 years.[107,189] Men predominate in a ratio of nearly 2:1. No predominance has been noted in the involved side, and bilateral fractures are uncommon.

FUNCTION

The importance of the patella in the action of the extensor mechanism is not universally agreed on. Brooke,[109] Hey-Groves,[151] and Watson-Jones[235] believed the patella inhibited the action of the quadriceps tendon and that the efficiency of the knee was improved with patellectomy. Others such as DePalma,[129] Jensenius,[157] McKeever,[175] Haxton,[146] and more recently Kaufer[158] have felt that the patella is an important functional unit in the extensor mechanism and that excision results in altered mechanics and a weakened quadriceps mechanism.

Three functions of the patella are to increase the mechanical advantage of the quadriceps tendon, to aid in nourishment of the articular cartilage of the femur, and to protect the femoral condyles from injury.

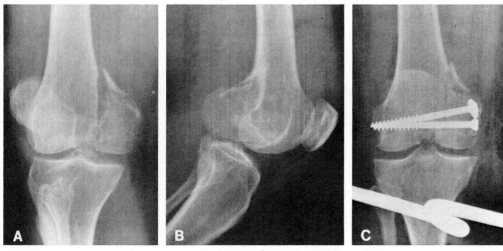

Fig. 16-15. A 60-year-old woman was struck by an automobile and sustained a fracture of the medial femoral condyle. (*A, B*) The original x-rays showed some proximal displacement of the medial condyle. (*C*) A postreduction view showed restoration of stability and alignment. Cancellous screws were used.

ANATOMY

The patella, the largest sesamoid bone in the body, lies within the quadriceps tendon. The ossification center usually appears at age 2 to 3, but it may appear as late as age 6. Occasionally anomalies of ossification occur, usually evidenced by the presence of an accessory ossification center located at the superolateral corner of the patella, the so-called bipartite patella. If a similar lesion is present in the opposite knee, the diagnosis is clear. However, if not, special x-rays may be necessary to differentiate it from an old, unhealed fracture.

The normal patella is triangular, with the apex directed distally. The superior border receives the insertion of the rectus femoris, vastus medialis, vastus lateralis, and vastus intermedius. The medial and lateral margins receive fibers from the vastus medialis and vastus lateralis, respectively. Distally, the apex provides the origin of the patellar tendon, which inserts into the tibial tubercle. A thin layer of quadriceps tendon passes over the anterior surface of the patella, joining the patellar tendon distally.[142]

The cartilaginous surface articulates with the anterior surface of the femoral condyles. The area of contact between the patella and the femur varies according to the position of the knee. With the knee extended, only the lower portion of the patella is in contact with the femur. Increasing flexion brings first the middle then the upper portion of the patella into contact. The articular surface itself is divided into seven articular facets. A longitudinal ridge divides the surface into medial and lateral portions. Each has an upper, an intermediate, and a lower facet. The seventh is a thin longitudinal strip on the medial aspect of the patella, the medial facet.

The medial and lateral extensor retinacula, or "expansions," are composed of longitudinal fibers of the vastus medialis and vastus lateralis, and, together with some fibers of the fascia lata, they bypass the patella and insert directly into the upper tibia. If these lateral expansions are preserved after the extensor mechanism is injured, it is still possible to extend the knee joint actively, a fact that is important in both diagnosis and treatment.

The blood supply to the patella is from a patellar plexus composed of branches from the superior, medial, and inferior genicular arteries.[125,210] The primary blood supply from this plexus enters in the central portion and at its distal pole. This fact is important for understanding avascular necrosis as a sequela of transverse fractures. Scapinelli, in 1967,[210] described 41 cases of avascular necrosis, mostly in the proximal pole, following transverse fractures.

MECHANISMS OF INJURY

Patellar fractures occur by either direct or indirect forces.[176] An indirect force fractures the patella when its intrinsic strength is exceeded by the pull of the musculotendinous units attaching to it, and typically occurs in the act of stumbling or partially falling. Although falling often follows such an injury, the patella was already fractured before the fall and was unable to maintain strength in the knee. After the bony patella fractures, continuing quadriceps muscle pull tears the medial and lateral quadriceps expansions to some degree. The extent of separation of the proximal and distal poles depends on the degree of quadriceps expansion tearing (Fig. 16-16). The typical fracture that occurs by indirect force is transverse and may show some comminution.

Since the patella is subcutaneous, it is subjected to direct trauma, as in striking a solid object such as the dashboard. An abrasion or open wound may mark the area of direct injury. The fractures resulting are incomplete or undisplaced, stellate or comminuted. There is usually little or no separation of the fragments, because the medial and lateral quadriceps expansions are not torn. The patient may be able to demonstrate active knee extension against gravity.

Combined direct and indirect injuries occur and are characterized by evidence of direct trauma to the skin, but in addition, there is considerable fragment separation indicative of medial and lateral quadriceps expansion tearing.

CLASSIFICATION

Most classifications of patellar fractures use the terms transverse or oblique, stellate or comminuted, longitudinal or marginal (Fig. 16-17).

Transverse and oblique fractures are the most common types in reported series, constituting anywhere from 50% to 80% of the fractures. Stellate and comminuted fractures account for 30% to 35% in the same series, while longitudinal fractures make up 12% to 27%.

SIGNS AND SYMPTOMS

Diagnosis of fracture is usually made from the history and examination and confirmed by radiography. The history of direct violence, such as the knee striking the dashboard followed by painful swelling and weakness, suggests fracture. Another type of history is that of a mis-step followed by collapse of the knee with painful swelling, suggesting the mechanism of indirect violence. At times a patient looks at or feels the knee immediately after the trauma and notices two patellar fragments and the defect between them.

As the patella lies in a subcutaneous position, it lends itself to examination by palpation. Its general outline, point of maximum tenderness, and a defect or separation of fragments can usually be detected.

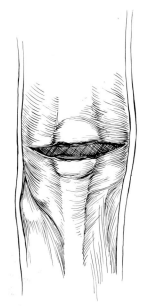

Fig. 16-16. Tearing of the retinaculum with fracture of the patella.

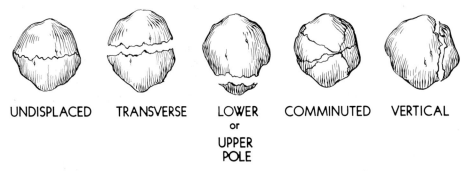

UNDISPLACED   TRANSVERSE   LOWER or UPPER POLE   COMMINUTED   VERTICAL

Fig. 16-17. Types of patellar fractures.

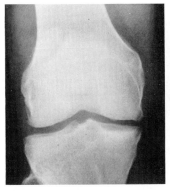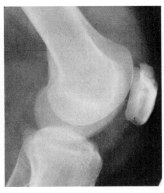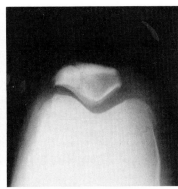

Fig. 16-18. A bipartite patella was discovered in a routine x-ray examination of the knee in a 35-year-old man with a torn medial meniscus. Note the characteristic position of the fragment in the superior lateral pole of the patella.

Undisplaced fractures may show only moderate swelling and normal anatomy, point tenderness over the fracture being the only impressive finding.

Regardless of the mechanism of injury, it is important to determine the ability of the patient to actively extend the knee completely. This ability depends on continuity of the quadriceps mechanism, which when not present indicates the need for surgical restoration of continuity.

A hemarthrosis results from most fractured patellae, but blood may escape into the adjacent subcutaneous tissue planes. Considerable tissue tension may develop and require aspiration for relief.

RADIOGRAPHIC FINDINGS

Two views are routinely used in the diagnosis of patellar fractures, but at times other special views may be indicated and helpful.

The anteroposterior view, even though superimposed on the distal end of the femur, may indicate sufficient detail to diagnose stellate fracture and may facilitate diagnosis of transverse fracture. The lateral view, however, is most helpful, because it profiles the patella and shows fragment displacement as well as the congruity of the articular surface.

For the injured patient with direct patellar soreness and no diagnostic findings in the routine views, a skyline or axial view is helpful for ruling out vertical fractures, which are usually undisplaced.

Bipartite patella is at times a confusing entity following injury to the knee (Fig. 16-18). It is usually present as a developmental ossicle of moderate size at the superior lateral patellar margin.[92,195]

If the same configuration is found in the other knee, the diagnosis is quite certain, but if the lesion is only on the injured knee, laminagrams may be needed to determine the sharpness of the bony margins to differentiate an old condition from a new fracture.

TREATMENT

The aim of treatment in patellar fractures is to ensure or provide continuity of the quadriceps mechanism by closed or open methods, in order to restore function and strength to the knee.

EARLIER CONCEPTS OF TREATMENT

Up until 1870 fractures of the patella were generally treated by splinting the extremity in an attempt to relax the quadriceps muscle by placing the knee in extension with the hip flexed. Bed rest, elevation, and massage were part of the treatment regimen. Fibrous union was the usual result and some degree of permanent disability was expected. In efforts to obtain bone union and to improve results, surgeons began exploring different methods of treatment. Most attempted to grasp the two fragments from above and below (usually with pins) and, using loops of leather or metal, to bring them together and hold them until union was accomplished. Malgaigne[179] devised a clamp that grasped each fragment by two sharp hooks that pierced the skin. The two pairs of hooks were approximated with a screw mechanism. These methods were abandoned because they produced infection and joint sepsis.

In March of 1877, Sir Hector Cameron of Glasgow, Scotland performed the first open reduction of a patellar fracture.[113] In October of the same year, Joseph Lister performed a similar operation.[169] Both inserted silver thread through drill holes. The first open reduction in Germany was performd by Trendelenburg in 1878.[231] Dennis, in 1885,[127] reported on 49 open reductions and believed that arthrotomy and open reduction with metal sutures was the ideal method of treatment at that time. Stimson,[224] in 1898, also agreed that with open reduction the period of convalescence and rehabilitation was much less and a good result more certain, but he added that when failures did occur they were often disastrous.

By 1900 open reduction had become popular. With the development of antiseptic and later aseptic surgery, the chief objection to open reduction—infection—had been overcome.

As open reduction became accepted, attention was directed to various types of suture material. Some of the materials that were employed for this purpose were catgut, kangaroo tendon, silver thread, aluminum thread, and bronze thread. Then stainless steel wire became popular.

Techniques of suturing also varied. Berger (1892) and Thiem[227] (1905) recommended cerclage (*i.e.,* encircling the patella); Cameron[113] and Lister[169] pierced the fracture fragments. Quénu[200] (1898) described a technique of fixation with wire passed through a transverse hole in one fragment and encircling the other. He called this hemicerclage. Payr[197] (1917) and later Magnuson[177] (1936) described passing the wire through longitudinal holes.

Thompson,[228] in 1935, introduced partial patellectomy, retaining one large fragment. McKeever,[175] in 1955, reported on use of a patellar prosthesis for acute fractures, including comminuted fractures, and showed good results.

CURRENT CONCEPTS OF TREATMENT

Nonoperative Treatment

Nonoperative treatment is recommended by several authors for undisplaced fractures with preserved extensor mechanism.[106,107,129,219] Indications for this form of treatment are that the fragments are not displaced, the articular surface is not severely disrupted, and the quadriceps apparatus (*i.e.,* the medial and lateral retinacula) is not torn. J. Böhler accepted 2 mm to 3 mm of separation. Boström[107] acceptd 3 mm to 4 mm with a 2 mm to 3 mm step in the articular surface. If a tense hematoma is present, aspiration is recommended by DePalma,[129] Smillie,[219] and Boström.[107]

A cylinder cast is recommended almost universally, but there is some disagreement about the advisability of full weight bearing. DePalma recommended partial weight bearing, while J. Böhler, Smillie, and Boström allowed full weight bearing with crutches for support. Quadriceps exercises with straight leg raising are begun a day or two after injury. Most authors recommend removal of the cast in 4 to 6 weeks, while Smillie prolonged this to 8 weeks.

Operative Treatment

Operative treatment has been recommended in cases in which the fracture separation exceeds 4 mm,[107] in comminuted fractures with displacement of articular surface, in osteochondral fractures with displacement into the joint, and in marginal or longitudinal fractures with displacement. Open and closed fractures should be operated on as soon as the patient's condition permits. Open contaminated wounds should have debridement; depending on the condition, definitive treatment is carried out at the same time or delayed until the open wound has healed thoroughly.

Cerclage (circumferential wire loop) was first described by Berger in 1892 and is still being used by many. Wire through longitudinal drill holes as described by Payr[197] and Magnuson[177] was also recommended by Anderson in 1971.[97] Hemicerclage is also a current method, as is wire through transversely drilled holes. Screw fixation is recommended by DePalma,[129] Müller,[185] and Smillie.[219]

The AO group uses a unique form of internal fixation in transverse fractures of the patella, so-called tension band wiring.[185] This technique differs from the usual cerclage wiring in that the fracture fragments are united with a wire passed through the insertions of the quadriceps and patellar tendons onto the patella (*i.e.,* on the anterior aspect of the bone rather than circumferentially). This results in a gap between the fracture fragments posteriorly at the time of surgery, but the compressive force of the quadriceps closes this gap during the postoperative period. Thus, active motion of the knee is not only allowed after this technique; it is actually advisable. Their biomechanical studies have demonstrated the markedly increased strength of fixation when the wire is placed on the tension side of the bone, as compared with the usual circumferential wiring. Recently, due to some problems with tension band wiring, two Kirschner wires have been used from superior to inferior to hold the patellar alignment and to provide proximal and distal anchors for the tension band wire.

Postoperative plaster immobilization is used by all, except after AO tension band wiring. Length of immobilization varies from 3 to 8 weeks.[106,107,129,219] The position of the knee during plaster immobilization varies from full extension[129] to 5° or 10° of flexion.[107,239]

Repair of the extensor mechanism retaining one large fragment has been recommended in transverse fractures where there is difficulty obtaining a smooth articular surface or when one large fragment and small polar fragments exist. The smaller piece is excised. In comminuted fractures similar partial patellectomy is advised if one large fragment can be saved.[97,99,106,129,219]

When patellectomy is indicated most authors advise excision of the lower pole.[97,99,129,228] Based on his studies of vascular supply, Scapinelli[210] recommended preservation of the lower pole and its fat pad with excision of the upper pole to avoid avascular necrosis.

Attention to suturing the remaining tendon close to the articular surface of the retained fragment and not near the anterior portion is important in order to prevent tilting of the fragment with subsequent chondromalacia and degenerative arthritis.[99,135]

Longitudinal or marginal fractures should be excised "to prevent osteoarthritis," according to some.[128,192,211] Others feel that rarely are such fragments symptomatic and only those that are need excision.[104,163]

Total patellectomy has been recommended in comminuted fractures where no large fragment remains. Brooke[109] reported results following total patellectomy for fracture and showed that good mobility results. The advocates of patellectomy cite the advantages of shorter immobilization, less complicated operative technique, and earlier mobilization and return to work.

Haxton[146] (1945) and Kaufer[158] (1971) advised preserving the patella where possible after demonstrating that the patella improves function of the knee joint in respect to extension and serves a protective function. Boström[107] stated, "Total excision of the patella never seems to be the treatment of choice but is recommended in exceptionally severe cases; i.e., open, comminuted fractures or when other methods of treatment have failed."

Whichever procedure is indicated, it is essential that the extent of injury to the medial and lateral retinacula is recognized and repaired anatomically, in order to obtain satisfactory results.

Management following patellectomy is much the same for most authors. A thorough rehabilitation program is considered important after any type of treatment that immobilizes the knee.

AUTHOR'S PREFERRED METHOD OF TREATMENT

Undisplaced Fractures

Nonoperative treatment likely will produce a good result in patellar fractures that have no more than 1 mm to 2 mm of displacement, a smooth articular surface, and a quadriceps mechanism capable of extending the knee against gravity.

Initial application of compressive bandage and ice help to minimize swelling; however, aspiration of the hemarthrosis may be necessary to relieve swelling and pain and to reduce intra-articular tension. A cylinder cast is the most reliable method of immobilization and should be applied from groin to ankle with the knee in full extension but not hyperextended. Weight bearing and exercises for the quadriceps muscle are begun early and continued throughout the period of cast immobilization. Depending on the extent and severity of fracture, the cast is worn for 3 to 6 weeks with some form of knee bandage support thereafter.

Displaced Fractures

Displaced fractures, even with quadriceps expansion tears, do heal by scar tissue, and return of some function is seen occcasionally in a patient whose multiple injuries prevented treatment of the patellar injury. In the weeks following injury this patient does regain some knee extension; however, significant quadriceps weakness and extension lag are to be expected. Therefore, to avoid these problems operative treatment offers the best likelihood of restoring good quadriceps function. Articular surface incongruity is an indication for surgery, because persistence of irregularity results in traumatic degenerative changes.

The optimal time for surgery is as soon as the patient's condition and skin permit. Certainly for the patient it is best to perform the surgery within a week after injury. When fresh, clean skin abrasions occur at the time of injury, indicated operative treatment is best performed within a few hours, but if this is not possible, delay is necessary until skin conditions are optimal, in other words, until the abrasions have healed.

Transverse fractures often occur through the middle or distal pole, and excision of the smaller fragment with suturing of the patellar tendon to the remaining fragment and repair of the quadriceps expansions is indicated (Fig. 16-19). When the distal pole is the major intact fragment, it may be

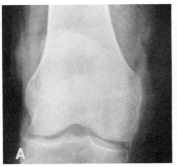
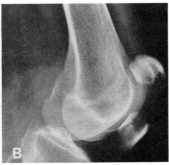
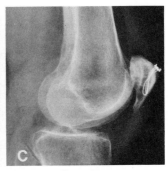

Fig. 16-19. An active 72-year-old woman sustained a transverse patellar fracture. At open repair the distal pole was markedly comminuted and was excised with repair of the patellar tendon to the proximal pole. (*A, B*) The original x-rays showed the patellar fracture. (*C*) At 3-year follow-up the knee lacked 10° of full flexion, but had strong active extension, and the patient had no symptoms.

left and the quadriceps tendon sutured into its superior border, provided that at least 50% of the original articular surface does remain.

Transverse fractures through the mid-portion of the articular surface are treated by apposition of both fragments and some means of internal fixation. Any method that ensures good alignment of the articular surface and apposition of the cancellous bone is satisfactory (Fig. 16-20). I prefer a positive means of keeping the articular surface accurately reduced and still permitting early knee motion. Therefore, I use either two Kirschner wires or a screw between the fragments plus tension band wiring between the patellar and quadriceps tendons.

Comminuted fractures, unless virtually undisplaced, are best treated by excision of the multiple fragments—shelling them out of the quadriceps and patellar tendons—and re-establishing the quadriceps mechanism by suturing the expansions. Continuity between the quadriceps and patellar tendons is provided either by imbrication or by direct suture. Attention to operative detail obviates many of the sequelae of complete patellectomy, mainly the loss of strength in the quadriceps mechanism and extension lag (Fig. 16-21).

CARE AFTER REDUCTION OR OPERATION

Cast immobilization is indicated after definitive treatment of these fractures unless excellent fixation is obtained with tension band wiring. The length of cast time should vary, depending on the type of healing that must take place. When bone-to-bone healing is required a minimum of 3 weeks' immobilization is suggested, followed by protection in a knee splint thereafter until bone union is identified by radiography. Quadriceps isometric exercises and gentle active, not passive, movements may be used to prevent adhesions and retain quadriceps muscle tone.

Repair requiring tendon healing to bone should be protected for at least 3 to 4 weeks, and the repair of tendon to tendon, as in total patellectomy, for a minimum of 4 weeks, after which active knee movements are used with protection between exercise sessions. Passive stretching does not help to restore mobility, and it may actually harm the repair. Active exercises seem to promote stronger tendon-to-bone union. Several months of continuing effort is necessary to produce maximum range of motion and strength.

PROGNOSIS

The prognosis for healing and restoration of function in patellar fractures is generally good. Articular fractures do result in articular cartilage destruction and chondromalacic changes, which may progress to the classic traumatic arthritis with spur formation and eburnated bone. Despite such changes, function may continue to be good if pain is not a serious problem.[99,136,242]

Motion is usually well restored but full flexion is often not regained after patellectomy or hemipatellectomy in many cases. Extension lag does occur occasionally, but with good patient effort and cooperation it should be uncommon.

Full function in the knee following treatment of fracture of the patella does not return until 6 to 12 months after operation.[135]

Complaints are reported by most patients fol-

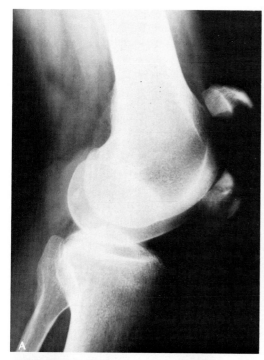

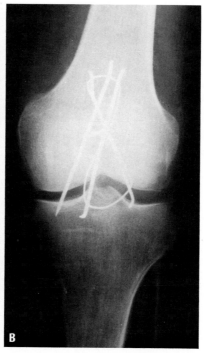

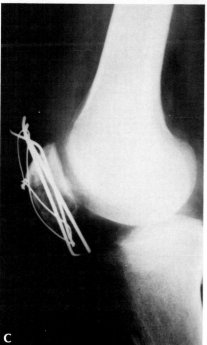

Fig. 16-20. A 49-year-old man sustained a somewhat comminuted transverse patellar fracture. (*A*) Note wide fragment separation. (*B, C*) Tension band wiring using Kirschner wires to maintain reduction. Immediate motion was encouraged and 90° movement was present at 2 weeks. The wires were too long and required removal at 3 months.

lowed through an adequate length of time. Crenshaw and Wilson[124] suggested that the follow-up needs to include 1 year in order to assess the complaints. About 70% of patients have some complaint.[99,136,198,225] The majority of patients can walk without difficulty and are unaware of a significant weakness in the extremity. Weakness in climbing stairs, walking downhill, and kneeling are

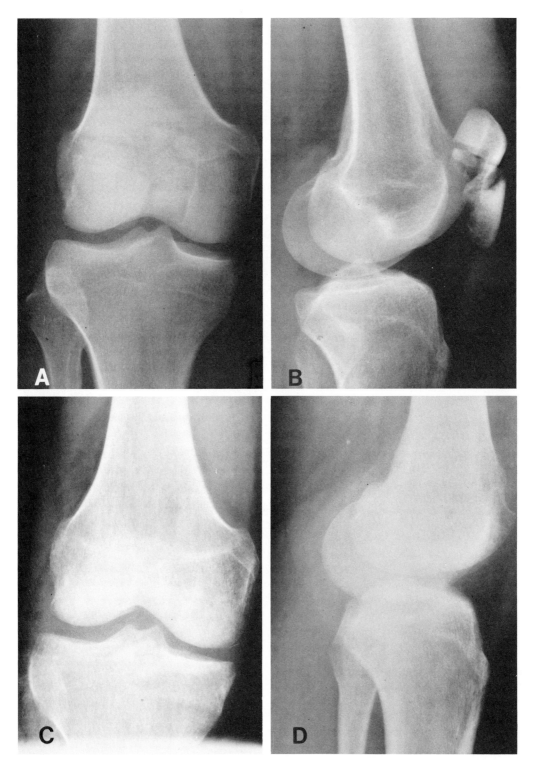

Fig. 16-21. A 58-year-old man sustained a dashboard injury with comminution of the patella. (*A, B*) Original views showed the extent of patella articular damage. (*C, D*) X-rays made after complete excision of the patella and repair of the quadriceps mechanism.

common symptoms. The greatest difficulty in the above functions involved patients who had total patellectomy. Range of motion is generally good following all procedures, but it tends to be best after total patellectomy.[198,225,242]

Degenerative arthritis is common following both conservative and operative treatment.[107,216]

COMPLICATIONS

Early complication of fracture fragment separation or dehiscence of the fracture repair is uncommon, but it generally results from inadequate internal fixation, or in some cases from an inadequate period of postoperative support of the joint.

Postoperative infection does occur but in closed wounds without skin problems the incidence should be low. Refracture is reported to be rare in nearly all series; the incidence varies from less than 1% to 5%. Rather than being a true refracture, some interpret this to be the disruption of a fibrous union.

Avascular necrosis is reported by most authors to be rare; however, Scapinelli[210] reviewed 162 transverse fractures, of which 41 showed evidence of partial necrosis. Thirty-eight of these involved the proximal fragment. This represented a 25% incidence. Radiographically, avascular necrosis becomes evident 1 to 2 months after fracture; the peak contrast between the two fragments appears after 2 to 3 months. When followed, it was generally asymptomatic, and revascularization occurred spontaneously within 2 years.

It is generally unwise to manipulate a knee to regain movement after a patellar fracture, because strength of union is questionable and the structures under stress (including tendon and bone), are generally not strong and so may fracture or separate.

Open fractures require immediate treatment with cleansing, debridement, repair, and closure, unless the wound is older or contaminated, in which case the skin and subcutaneous tissues may be left open. However, it is best to repair the quadriceps mechanism at the time of open wound debridement.

FRACTURES OF THE PROXIMAL TIBIA

Fractures of the proximal tibia are either articular or nonarticular, but knee joint function must be considered in the management of both. Little is accomplished if the fracture heals anatomically but knee function is poor. The articular fractures consist of the various types of tibial condylar fractures and present all of the serious and thought-provoking problems of a fracture in a major weight-bearing joint. The nonarticular fractures include those of the tibial spine and intercondylar eminence, the tibial tubercle, and the subcondylar area.

ANATOMY

The upper tibia flares from the shaft proximally in the subcondylar area, providing contours and bony prominences for ligament and tendon attachments, a small articulation for the proximal tibiofibular joint, and relatively flat articular surfaces to support the femoral condyles (Fig. 16-22). Depression of the weight-bearing portion of the tibial condyles results in some degree of valgus or varus change at the knee (Fig. 16-23).

The intercondylar eminence of the proximal tibia is a nonarticular region between the tibial condyles that provides attachments from anterior to posterior of the anterior cruciate ligament, medial semilunar cartilage, lateral semilunar cartilage, and the posterior cruciate ligament. The ligamentous structures are enclosed by the synovial lining of the knee and thus are extraarticular. Two bony prominences, the medial (anterior) spine and the lateral (posterior) spine, are located at the edge of the intercondylar region. The anterior cruciate ligament and the posterior cruciate ligament do not attach to the tibial spines but rather to the adjacent intercondylar nonarticular bone.

FRACTURES OF THE PROXIMAL TIBIAL ARTICULAR SURFACE

Articular fractures of the proximal tibia have been treated by a variety of methods. Surgical restoration of the articular surface seemed to be a sensible approach, but the earlier advocates grew disillu-

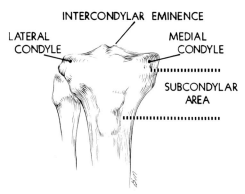

Fig. 16-22. The regions of the upper tibia.

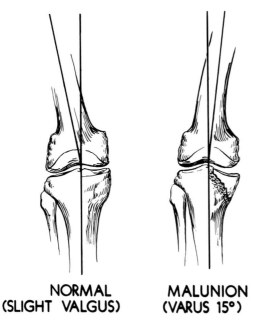

**NORMAL
(SLIGHT VALGUS)**   **MALUNION
(VARUS 15°)**

Fig. 16-23. Normal valgus and malunion with varus deformity due to loss of medial tibial condyle elevation.

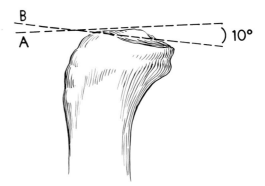

Fig. 16-24. Representation of the correct projection (10° caudal) to see the upper tibial articular surface.

sioned as it became abundantly clear that the added surgical insult produced inferior functional results in too many instances. A wave of enthusiasm for traction treatment did improve functional results but left a significant number of knees with residual instability or angular deformity. A good result provides the patient with a strong, stable, nearly fully movable knee with normal or nearly normal alignment. Long-term result studies suggest that progress is being made in the salvage of more good knees by the use of newer techniques in properly selected cases.[262,264,293,320,356,359,371,379,382]

Many authors base the selection of treatment to some extent on the amount of condylar depression measured on the x-ray. However, this is only accurate on special anteroposterior tibial condylar views taken with a tube angulation of approximately 10° caudad in relation to the long axis of the tibia to conform with the anatomical configuration of the proximal tibia.[357] Correct projection avoids exaggerating posteriorly located depressions (Fig. 16-24).

MECHANISMS OF INJURY

Historically, tibial condylar fractures have been referred to as "bumper" or "fender" fractures, but it has always been known that falls from a height or a twisting fall are also common causes of these injuries. A study by the author of mechanisms of

injury in more than 900 cases cites 52% caused by auto-pedestrian injuries, 17% in falls from heights, and the remainder from miscellaneous causes.[320]

Forces of vertical compression, as in a fall, produce characteristic fracture configurations, usually of the T- or Y-type. Pure varus or valgus forces tend to cause ligament tearing injuries rather than condylar fractures,[327,334,406] but when body weight (axial loading) is on the knee, various types of compression fractures may occur. Twisting forces also produce a variety of fracture configurations.

The location, and to some extent the amount, of depression in a compression fracture depends on the flexion angle of the knee at the moment of injury. With the knee in full extension, the compression force is exerted anteriorly on the tibial condyles. The intercondylar notch of the distal femur begins to impinge on the intercondylar eminence of the tibia after only a few millimeters of articular compression, thereby resisting further compression. However, with the knee in flexion there is no such restraint on the extent of compression. The middle or posterior portion of the condyle is involved as the flexed knee is injured.

Collateral ligament injuries occur more frequently in some fracture types, as continuing valgus, varus, or twisting forces produce a combination of bone and ligament injuries.

CLASSIFICATION

Any classification of proximal tibial articular fractures cannot possibly encompass the enormous variety seen in clinical practice. Through the years clinicians have used a number of classifications for the purposes of the promotion of better therapeutic judgments and promulgation of knowledge by comparative study of results. Evolution of newer and better classifications is to be anticipated in the future.

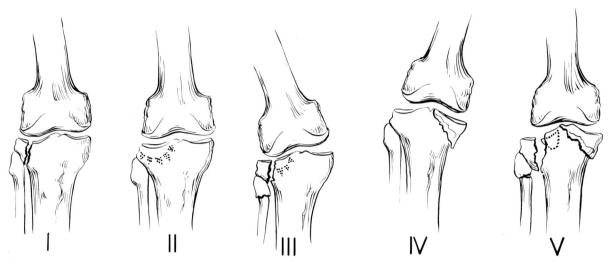

Fig. 16-25. Classification of plateau fractures. (I) Minimally displaced; (II) local compression; (III) split compression; (IV) total condylar depression; and (V) bicondylar. (Redrawn from Hohl, M.: Tibial Condylar Fractures. J. Bone Joint Surg., **49A**:1456, 1967.)

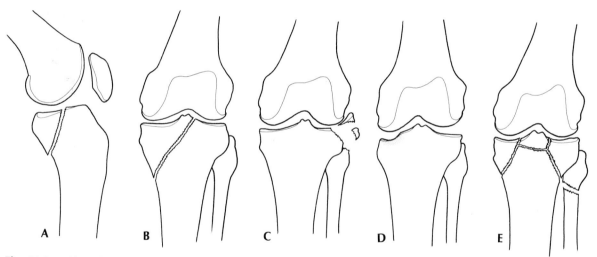

Fig. 16-26. Classification of fracture-dislocations of the knee. (A) Split fracture; (B) entire plateau fracture; (C) rim avulsion; (D) rim compression; (E) four-part fracture. (Redrawn from Hohl, M., and Moore, T. M.: Articular Fractures of the Proximal Tibia. *In* Evarts, C. M. (ed.): Surgery of the Musculoskeletal System. New York, Churchill Livingstone, 1983.)

Recently, Moore[355] developed a new classification of proximal tibial articular fractures dividing them into plateau fractures and fracture-dislocations. The plateau fractures are the well-known compression, split-compression, total condylar, and bicondylar types, in which usually the major problem involves the bone injury. The fracture-dislocations are injuries in which soft tissue lesions produce instability and require operative treatment in the majority of patients. These knees are unstable, and despite adequate treatment often the patient has less than satisfactory results.

Though a step in the right direction, this classification may not endure. Plateau fracture without and with ligament injury (collateral or cruciate) may become the most useful classification. I offer Moore's concept as the best available therapeutic classification (Figs. 16-25 and 16-26).

Plateau fractures consist of minimally displaced fractures with less than 4 mm of depression or condylar widening encompassing about 25% of proximal tibial articular fractures. Displaced fractures are compression fractures (local or split type), total condylar fractures, and bicondylar fractures.

Compression fractures are divided into two distinct subtypes, each having different treatment considerations. The local compression fracture is a depressed condylar fracture shaped like the femoral condyle that produced it. The articular surface may assume a mosaic type of articular surface compression, or a section of it may be depressed. The split-compression fracture is characterized by compression in the middle of the articular surface as well as a peripheral split-off fragment on which there is intact articular cartilage and cortex.

The total depression fracture may involve either condyle but frequently involves the medial with the fracture line entering the articular surface near the intercondylar eminence on the same side as the fracture. The articular surface is undamaged except for this area.

Bicondylar fractures involve both articulating condyles in a wide variety of configurations often combining elements of compression or a split compression fracture on one condyle with a total condylar on the other.

Fracture-dislocations of the knee are divided into five types, depending on the radiographic appearance. The types are split fracture, entire plateau fracture, rim avulsion, rim compression, and four-part fracture (Fig. 16-26).

The split fracture was classified previously by the author as type V, a coronal plane fracture, usually medial and posterior, which has a characteristic anteroposterior double horizon appearance and is best shown by tomography. In knee flexion the femoral condyle articulates with the split fragment and reduction of the fracture is sometimes possible in extension. Ligament injury is almost always associated.

The entire plateau fracture differs from the total condylar fracture in that the fracture line enters the opposite compartment of the knee and the fragment includes both cruciate ligament attachments. Collateral ligament injury is very frequently associated and must be tested for by stress x-rays.

Rim avulsion fractures indicate capsular and ligamentous disruptions as a large or small fragment is pulled from the periphery of the articular surface.

Rim compression fractures occur on either condyle and result only if the collateral ligaments and capsule have ruptured, allowing the femoral condyle to produce the characteristic fracture defect.

The four-part fracture is literally a loose bag of bones and is very unstable because of the loose intercondylar fragment with the cruciate attachments.

SIGNS AND SYMPTOMS

Knee injury is followed by painful swelling and hemarthrosis. Patients may be aware that the knee was deformed at the time of injury. A knee effusion is present in most cases, but at times the capsule is torn and the hemorrhage drains spontaneously into the tissues. Tenderness is present over the fracture and may be noted in the area of the medial ligament, suggesting the possibility of disruption of the medial ligament. As a rule, limited knee motion is caused by pain and hemarthrosis. Stress testing of the knee usually demonstrates some instability in valgus or varus. This is most frequently due to fracture displacement, but it may represent ligamentous instability. Stress x-rays offer the best documentation of whether the ligaments are intact.

RADIOGRAPHIC FINDINGS

Routine anteroposterior and lateral x-rays demonstrate the presence of the vast majority of tibial condylar fractures. Fortunately, other projections and techniques are available that are capable of accurately defining the extent of fracture and its displacement. Oblique projections often help in localizing a fracture but tomograms are excellent for portraying the depth of depression and its location.[299,302,361,380] The 10° caudal plateau view also gives an accurate determination of depth of depression.[357]

It is important to attempt to classify the fracture type accurately on the basis of the original injury films. Areas of ligament attachment, such as the medial and lateral femoral condyles, the intercondylar eminence, and the fibular head, should be scrutinized for possible avulsion fragments. The initial x-rays of a lateral tibial condyle fracture may demonstrate widening of the medial cartilage space, which is indicative of medial ligament damage.[350]

Valgus and varus stress films are recommended in fracture types known to have a higher frequency of ligament injuries. The rim avulsion and rim compression fractures described by Moore are examples. The split-compression fracture and the minimally displaced fracture are also good candidates for stress studies. Stress films are most accurate and revealing when taken with the patient under anesthesia, preferably regional or general, in order to eliminate pain.[306,319,324,386] Valgus and varus stresses are applied to the knee in full extension and in approximately 15° of flexion with x-ray

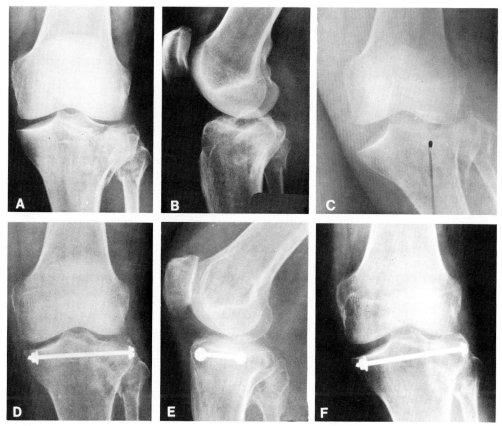

Fig. 16-27. A 42-year-old man with a split compression-type fracture of the lateral tibial condyle and rupture of the medial ligament and capsule underwent operation for bone repair and ligament damage. (*A, B*) Original x-rays demonstrated the fracture. (*C*) A stress film taken in surgery reproduced the deformity assumed by the knee at the time of injury. Note widening of the medial cartilage space and the intrusion of the lateral femoral condyle into the fracture. (*D, E*) Postoperative views showed restoration of support for the femoral condyle. (*F*) A stress film 4 months after open reduction and ligament repair showed improved stability.

recording the findings (Fig. 16-27). Patients who are to undergo surgical repair of the condylar fracture should have the stress films made after anesthesia is induced in surgery and before skin preparation has begun. Arthrography may also help to delineate traumatic capsular and ligamentous defects.

METHODS OF TREATMENT

Many treatment alternatives are available for tibial condyle fractures, including soft dressings, cast, traction, closed reduction, and open reduction. The decision to use one or more of these modalities is based on a wide variety of considerations, including the patient's age, general condition, skin condition, associated injuries, type and severity of fracture,

and the quality of knee function required by the patient.[321]

One important objective of treatment is to produce a knee that extends fully and flexes through a range of at least 120°. Achievement of full extension is most certain when initial treatment maintains the knee in extension, as with a cast or a traction apparatus that returns the knee to full extension at rest. Recovery of knee movement and strength is more rapid and complete when begun within 3 to 4 weeks after injury.

Some degree of angular deformity is a frequent sequela of tibial condylar fractures.[320,323] Restoration of normal condylar level and maintenance of this level in the post-fracture period does the most to insure restoration of normal knee alignment.

Instability of the knee may result from unrepaired ligament injury or residual depression of a tibial condyle.[324] Obviously many ligament injuries are of the avulsive type in the age group of the patient with condylar fracture. Such ligament avulsions tend to heal well and give rise to little or no residual instability, which accounts for the little instability found in some late follow-up studies.[358] Restoration of normal or nearly normal articular level and ligament repair are both important in preventing late instability.

Minimally Displaced Fractures

Minimally displaced fractures have been treated in a wide variety of ways, including an elastic bandage and early motion, traction, and a long-leg cast. Almost regardless of the treatment used, end results are good, provided that the supporting ligamentous structures were not injured at the time of the original trauma.[320,325] Very few of these fractures tend to displace further. Thus, with reliable patients, soft supports are generally sufficient. Traction is used frequently when bed confinement of the patient is otherwise required, but the most frequently used treatment is a cylinder- or a long-leg cast. Following a short period of immobilization, knee motion generally recovers well, but the longer the cast is used, the slower and less complete the return of movement will be.[312]

It is important in minimally displaced tibial condylar fractures to ascertain the integrity of the supporting ligamentous structures by stress testing. When a ligament is demonstrated to be torn, repair is advisable.[319,324]

Author's Preferred Method of Treatment. In reliable patients with no ligament damage I prefer a few days of splinting in a Jones dressing or plaster splint followed by active knee movement, if follow-up x-rays show that no change in position has occurred. Weight bearing should be delayed until fracture healing is evident. In patients who are not reliable a long-leg cast is satisfactory for a few weeks.

Active exercise should be carried out to ensure continued strength of the quadriceps mechanism. Within 3 to 4 weeks at least 90° of motion is ordinarily present. When x-rays show evidence of healing, in the case of fractures involving the tibial articular surface, weight bearing may be started. Where a minimally displaced central compression fracture is present, assessment of healing by x-rays is not possible, but these fractures are in cancellous bone and tend to heal quite rapidly, so that it is possible to begin light weight bearing within 6 to 8 weeks (Fig. 16-28).

Prognosis. The prognosis of minimally displaced fractures is generally good, except when ligament injuries are not diagnosed initially and thus are not repaired.[324]

Complications. Complications of minimally displaced fractures include the possibility of gradual varus or valgus angulation resulting from progressive deformity of the fracture occurring in the first few weeks. This is noted most frequently in fractures extending from the intercondylar area to the medial or lateral tibial cortices.[323] It is important to reexamine patients clinically and radiographically in the early period after fracture to detect loss of position and institute corrective measures promptly.

Local Compression Fractures

Selection of proper treatment for local compression fractures requires mature clinical judgment. In general, patients accept mild valgus or varus knee angulations resulting from fracture. A few millimeters of depression results in minimal angular change. With depression of 8 mm or more, a further decision is necessary, because of the frequency of distressing angular deformities. Clinical evaluation of the knee may be quite helpful in determining which patients can benefit from surgery. For instance, a test of knee stability in extension and near extension helps to indicate what the knee will be like in the future without operation. If the knee is stable in these positions the chances are very good that the final result will be acceptable. However, if there is instability with stress testing, open reduction should be seriously considered.[371] Posteriorly located depressions do not show much instability on this clinical test and thus should not be as strongly considered for open reduction as those located in the middle or anterior portions of the condyle.

Nonoperative Treatment. Nonoperative management is uncomplicated, since local compression fractures have sustained maximum bone deformation at the time of initial trauma, and no significant further depression is anticipated, with or without the use of a cast or another external fixation method. Closed reduction has no place in the treatment of these fractures, because manipulation cannot result in elevation of the depressed articular fragments. Most patients are more comfortable after aspiration of the hemarthrosis. A Jones-type com-

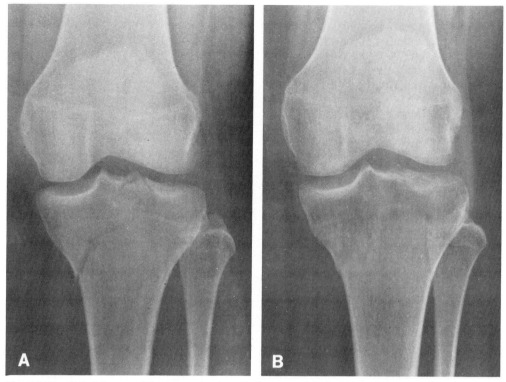

Fig. 16-28. This 21-year-old woman had an undisplaced fracture extending from the intercondylar area to the medial upper tibia. It was treated in a cast for 8 weeks. (*A*) In the original film, note the good position of the fracture. (*B*) Four months later the fracture was well healed.

pressive dressing or cast is used for a period of a few days to a maximum of 3 weeks.

Buck's traction is useful, especially when other injuries confine a patient to bed. A week or two in traction with active knee motion is comfortable for the patient and is a simple way to regain movement. Active exercises may be used from the outset if the patient is cooperative and comfortable.

Operative Treatment. Open reduction techniques involve the creation of a defect in the tibial condylar lateral cortex, in order that the depressed fragments can be pressed up to normal condylar level under direct vision with an impactor or periosteal elevator.

Although it is not difficult to restore good condylar level, it is difficult to maintain it. Many fixation techniques are available, ranging from the use of multiple Kirschner wires into the elevated fragments to packing cancellous grafts or a cortical graft under the elevated fragments. Replacement of a badly damaged articular surface with ilium or

patella has been successful in a number of cases, but this technique is seldom required.[307,332a,342]

Author's Preferred Method of Treatment. I use open reduction most often when articular depression exceeds 8 mm. Open reduction is also used with lesser depressions when clinical stress testing demonstrates 5° or more instability in extension. A plaster cylinder cast or postoperative knee splint is used with lesser depressed fractures after aspiration of the knee. Soreness usually lasts only a few days, and then active knee movement and exercises are begun.

Open reduction is done preferably the day of injury or after a few days when the initial tissue tension has begun to subside. Approach to the lateral condyle is made with the knee flexed about 90°. I begin the surgical incision just distal to the area of the femoral condylar attachment of the collateral ligament, incising anteriorly and crossing the joint line lateral to the patellar tendon, turning distally down to the tibial crest (Fig. 16-29). Thus this incision can be extended distally to obtain a cortical tibial graft from the lateral tibial surface when necessary. The fibers of the iliotibial band may be split near the joint line and reflected distally, exposing the capsule. Since the meniscus itself is frequently found undamaged, sometimes only detached peripherally, I feel that it should be preserved. The coronary ligaments holding the meniscus to the tibia are divided anterolaterally and laterally to permit visualization of the tibial condyle. When posterior exposure is necessary the meniscus is freed posterolaterally, along with the lateral collateral ligament (Fig. 16-30). With varus stress this opens the lateral space, giving excellent tibial articular exposure as the meniscus is reflected with the femoral condyle. Of course, when the knee is closed the coronary ligaments are resutured[414]; if it is divided, the collateral ligament is repaired. The local compressed area is well visualized, and the condylar level is restored by gentle impactor pressure from below through a tibial window. Although many surgeons have been successful in using cancellous grafts to support these multiple depressed articular fragments, I have found the use of a cortical graft to provide better support. This graft is driven through a window in the condyle about 1 cm below the articular surface medially into intact cancellous bone. There is usually sufficient support to permit early movement of the knee after operation. This graft is obtained from the lateral surface of the upper tibia through a linear extension of the

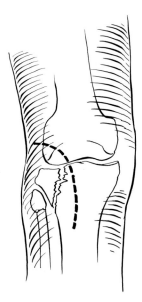

Fig. 16-29. An extensile skin incision for open reduction of lateral tibial condylar fractures.

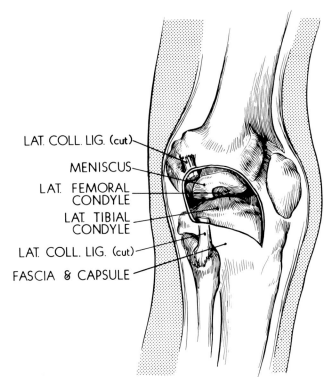

LAT. COLL. LIG. (cut)
MENISCUS
LAT. FEMORAL CONDYLE
LAT. TIBIAL CONDYLE
LAT. COLL. LIG. (cut)
FASCIA & CAPSULE

Fig. 16-30. Approach to the lateral knee compartment is shown reflecting the meniscus with the femoral condyle after severing the coronary ligaments and lateral collateral ligament.

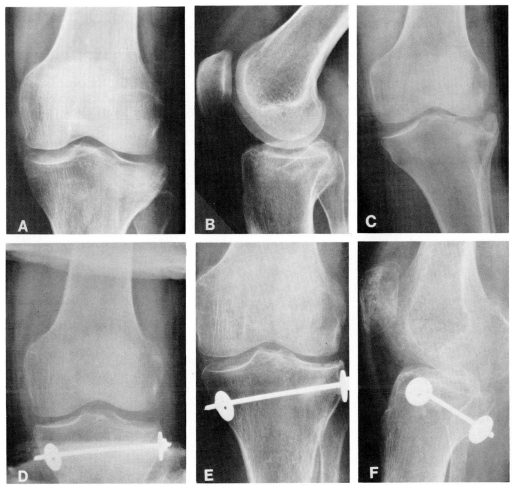

Fig. 16-31. A 70-year-old active woman with a local compression fracture of the lateral condyle was treated by open reduction, bone grafting, and a cast brace. (A, B) The original x-rays demonstrated a local compression fracture of the lateral tibial condyle. (C) A stress film demonstrated very little medial space widening. (D) A postoperative film in cast brace. Varus stress was applied with the cast brace, and weight bearing was begun 10 days after surgery. (E, F) Anteroposterior and lateral views made 4 months after surgery. Note healing of the central depression fracture without change from the postoperative position.

same incision. On occasion, especially in the elderly, the upper tibial cancellous bone does not provide sufficient support for the graft, and a tibial bolt is inserted just below, which provides good fixation. An x-ray is taken at surgery before closure to ensure that complete and satisfactory reduction has been obtained. Wound suction helps in postoperative comfort, as does a temporary Jones dressing. Active movement of the knee is encouraged from the outset; weight bearing is delayed until healing and strengthening of the articular surface is complete.

Postoperative Care and Rehabilitation. The postoperative care and rehabilitation of local compression fractures can be a problem, because the pressure of the femoral condyle tends to redepress the elevated fragments. A well-molded, long-leg cast may give slight assistance in avoiding this pressure, but the cast brace seems the best means of relieving the operated tibial condyle (Fig. 16-31). Protection of this articular surface is necessary for several weeks, until the articular fragments are incorporated in callus. If a cast has been used, motion is begun in 3 weeks. When a cast brace is used, light weight bearing and movement may be started immediately. Protected weight bearing without support is generally permitted at 2 to 3 months, with full weight bearing at 3 to 5 months.

Prognosis. The prognosis for recovery of strength and motion is good, but due to ever-present avascular necrosis of some elevated fragments and the damage to the articular surface, mild residual depression is frequently observed with resulting mild angular deformity.

Complications. Complications of treatment of the fracture include redepression, despite articular surface restoration. In my experience this has occurred most frequently when cancellous grafts have been used to bolster the elevated fragments and rarely when Kirschner wire fixation with grafting or cortical grafting has been used. Traumatic and degenerative changes occur with some regularity in the years following such an injury, although a mild valgus angular deformity is tolerated well.

Split Compression Fractures

These fractures have a mosaic depression similar to local compression fractures on the weight-bearing surface, but in addition there is a bone fragment with articular cartilage peripherally. Whereas local compression fractures are not amenable to closed reduction, the split compressions may well be, because very adequate stability and function result if the split fragment can be repositioned to support the femoral condyle. Thus, either closed or open reduction has potential use in the treatment of this fracture. The relative frequency of ligament injuries makes stress films important for proper care. Demonstrably torn ligaments should be repaired.

Mechanisms of Injury. As the split compression fracture occurs, the femoral condyle strikes against the tibial surface with force, splitting off a fragment and continuing into the more central articular surface, creating a defect shaped like the femoral condyle. Frequently, as the force is dissipated, elasticity of the structures may bring the split fragment back into acceptable position. At times, however, a bone fragment is driven distally like a wedge between the upper tibia and the split fragment, holding it in a displaced position (Fig. 16-32).

Methods of Treatment. Methods of treatment include the use of a cast, in cases of minimal displacement, and some type of manipulative or open reduction for moderate or severe displacements. Traction is not especially useful in these fractures, but when it is used it should be of the skeletal type. After 2 to 4 weeks traction, a cast-brace may be used until union of the fracture is assured. Whenever traction is used, movement of the knee should be encouraged to at least 90°.

A cast, cast-brace, or traction may be used when the split fragment is well positioned under the femoral condyle.[382]

Closed Reduction. Manipulative reduction under anesthesia may be useful in some patients with displaced split fragments. Strong application of traction with impaction of the split fragment using hand pressure, a giant nutcracker, or a Böhler clamp often produces a satisfactory reduction. This, of course, leaves a depression in the midportion of the tibial condyle, but the reduced split fragment provides adequate support for the femoral condyle.

A more sophisticated reduction technique is known as the traction-compression reduction.[330,415] This method uses anesthesia, preferably spinal; with the patient positioned on a fracture table, 30 to 60 pounds of skeletal traction are applied through a distal tibial pin. The knee is aspirated and wrapped in an Esmarch or Martin bandage for gentle compression. Check x-rays are taken to ascertain the position of the split fragment. Should it need elevation, a padded mallet is used to bring it to proper articular level. After this has been done, impaction of the fragment against the remainder of the articular surface is carried out using a Böhler clamp. Traction is reduced to 20 pounds, and the patient is transferred to bed in an exercise traction apparatus that permits at least 90° of passive or active exercise (Fig. 16-33). Exercise for range of motion and muscle strength is begun the first week. Decreasing traction is required for a minimum of 4 weeks, and intermittent use of a splint thereafter. This method is preferred in severely comminuted fractures of the proximal tibia but is also useful in the split compression type.

Open Reduction. Open reduction techniques are designed to restore stability to the split fragment by fixing it strongly in place by internal fixation, such as tibial bolts or cancellous compression screws. As with local compression fractures, the joint is best entered distal to the meniscus through the coronary ligament, reflecting the meniscus with the femoral condyle. In this fracture the coronary ligament is frequently torn, leaving the peripheral portion of the meniscus loose and allowing it to be reflected similarly. Repair and resuture are carried

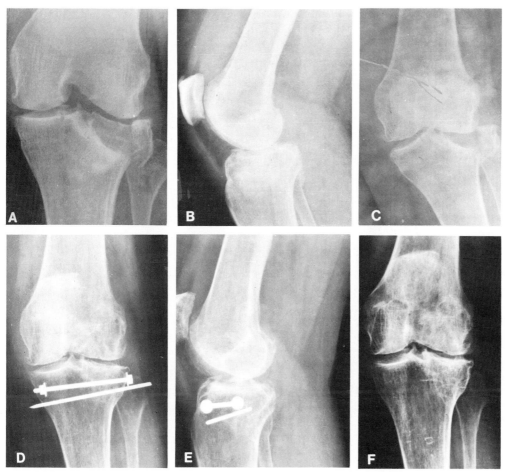

Fig. 16-32. A 58-year-old woman with a split compression fracture of the lateral tibial condyle was treated by open reduction. (*A, B*) On the original anteroposterior and lateral views, note the severe compression of the central articular surface and the split fragment. (*C*) A stress film demonstrated an intact medial capsule. (*D, E*) Note restoration of the articular surface 7 months after operation. (*F*) Considerable traumatic arthritis was noted 2 years after operation.

out later as the wound is closed, leaving the meniscus in place. The split fragment is identified and a decision is made as to whether the depressed articular fragments can be restored to condylar level. Although this restoration is usually possible, on occasion the damage is so great that it is advisable to excise some of the depressed and loose fragments rather than permitting them to be free in the joint. After excision of the fragments, reshaping of the fracture area permits the split fragment to be positioned well under the femoral condyle. The repositioned split fragment is held by a tibial compression bolt or bolts, and occasionally a contoured side plate is necessary to avoid redisplacement of the fragment. This is most commonly necessary in

porotic bone, when the fragment has been completely displaced from the tibia, or in the presence of a subcondylar fracture (Fig. 16-34).

Indications for Closed and Open Treatment. Nonoperative treatment is applicable if there is less than 8 mm true depression and if the split fragment is in good position. If the split fragment is displaced outward, so that the femoral condyle lacks support, manipulative reduction should be considered to bring the fragment into reduction. Retention of this reduction in traction rather than in a cast is advisable. When depression is in excess of 8 mm, traction-compression closed reduction is useful in the presence of a large split fragment. With smaller

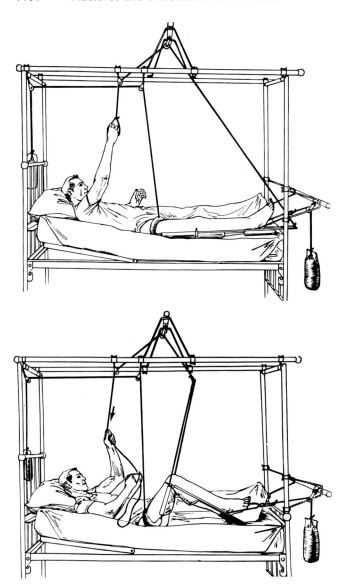

Fig. 16-33. A traction method for tibial condylar fractures allowing 90° of knee movement. (Hohl, M.: Tibial Condylar Fractures. J. Bone Joint Surg., **49A:**1460, 1967.)

split fragments or greater depressions open reduction provides the opportunity for more accurate restoration of the condylar anatomy, rigid internal fixation, and early knee movement.[379]

Author's Preferred Method of Treatment. I use nonoperative treatment when the split is situated properly supporting the femoral condyle at normal articular level. The depressed part of the fracture in these less major injuries does not need elevation. A long-leg plaster cast for 3 weeks followed by cast bracing works well. Since the goal of treatment is to have the split fragment support the femoral condyle, operative reduction is needed in two thirds of these fractures and must include

rigid interval fixation using cancellous screws, a buttress plate, or tibial bolts. Rigid fixation will permit knee motion as soon as wound healing is assured. Manipulative reduction, such as the traction-compression method is useful when skin or the patient's condition does not permit open reduction.

Prognosis. The prognosis for this fracture is for recovery of good motion and stability; however, as a rule, some traumatic arthritic changes in the affected compartment appear over the years.

Complications. Complications unique to this fracture involve inaccurate or inadequate internal

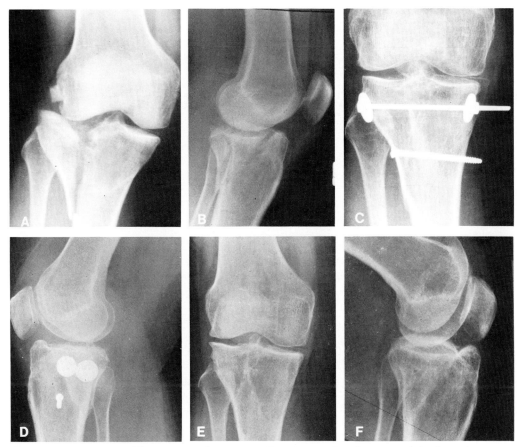

Fig. 16-34. A 52-year-old woman with severe split compression fracture of the lateral tibial condyle was treated by open reduction. (*A, B*) Note avulsed fragment near the lateral femoral condyle in these x-rays made after the injury. (*C, D*) Six months after surgery, healing had occurred in fairly good alignment. (*E, F*) Five years after fracture, some post-traumatic changes were seen in the lateral compartment. Function was good.

fixation at surgery with resultant angular deformity or loss of reduction. Although the surgeon may consider that he has fairly good visualization of the intra-articular anatomy, there is no substitute for an intraoperative x-ray to prove it. Screws used to hold the split fragment are not as strong or secure as a tibial bolt or bolts. Sufficient internal fixation should be used to permit knee movement without necessitating postoperative cast support. A buttress plate is useful when there is comminution of the split fragment or poor interdigitation of the cortical fracture margins.

Total Condyle Depression Fracture

A fracture of the total condyle depression type leaves the major portion of the articular surface undamaged, with the fracture line beginning between the tibial spines or just in the involved compartment, passing obliquely distalward, intersecting the cortex at or near the flare of the tibia. Most of these fractures involve the medial condyle. Attachments of the medial capsule and ligament to the fractured condyle render reduction in most cases quite simple. Emergency splinting of the leg may at times effect reduction. Retention of the reduction is the problem. Loss of reduction in a long-leg cast does occur frequently even after manipulative reduction, indicating that a long-leg cast does not provide adequate protection against displacement.[338]

Methods of Treatment. Nonoperative, manipulative reduction and open techniques are all useful in the treatment of these fractures. Nonoperative methods are indicated when minimal displacement of the fracture is present (*i.e.*, less than 4 to 6 mm).

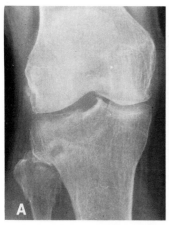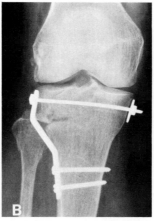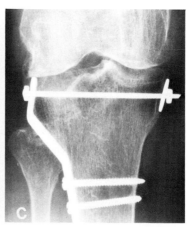

Fig. 16-35. A 71-year-old woman with a total condylar depression fracture of the lateral condyle was treated by open reduction to permit early mobilization of the knee and the patient. (*A*) Initial anteroposterior view. (*B*) In the postoperative view, note the contoured plate and tibial bolt supporting the lateral condyle. (*C*) Six years later good function and stability were preserved.

More displacement is tolerated on the lateral condyle than on the medial. The tendency of the fracture to displace further must be stopped by the use of traction or a cast brace. However, in some cases a long-leg cast may be satisfactory, if frequent check x-rays are taken. Any change in position should signal the need for alteration in treatment to traction, manipulation, or open reduction.

Manipulative reduction is usually very successful for medial condyle fractures and somewhat less rewarding for the lateral condyle. On the lateral side, gentle upward pounding of the fractured condyle may be necessary to obtain reduction. Recurrence of displacement is quite frequent, except when traction is used after reduction.

Cast-bracing with appropriate stressing to reduce pressure across the knee on the involved condyle seems to be a reasonable approach to holding this difficult fracture against subsidence into varus. Nonetheless frequent x-rays and a willingness to take off the cast-brace and perform open reduction for slippage must be part of the management program.[322]

Open reduction is especially helpful in total condylar depression fractures but internal fixation must effectively prevent fracture displacement. If there is an accurate interdigitation of the cortical portion of the fracture, cancellous screws or tibial bolts will suffice. However, if the cortices are weak or comminuted it is advisable to use a contoured side plate or buttress plate (Fig. 16-35).

Author's Preferred Method of Treatment. Lateral condyle fractures with depression or displacement less than 5 or 6 mm can be treated in traction for a few days, followed by cast-bracing until the fracture is healed. As a rule, the result will be satisfactory with minimum added valgus deformity. Greater depressions and displacements are treated by open reduction using rigid fixation methods including a buttress plate.

Medial condyle fractures, although displaced or depressed only a few millimeters, are managed by open rigid fixation to prevent the all-too-frequent fracture migration. Early motion of the knee is then encouraged.

Traction with early motion works well with fractures of either condyle if the patient is otherwise confined to bed.

Prognosis. The prognosis is excellent for restoration of knee motion and strength. Degenerative changes occur mainly when treatment has resulted in residual varus deformity of the knee. An objective of treatment in this type of fracture, therefore, is to restore normal knee alignment to prevent this serious problem.

Complications. Complications of treatment occur when the surgeon is unaware of the propensity of this fracture to displace and healing takes place in malposition (Fig. 16-36). This may require subcondylar or condylar osteotomy, and it should be

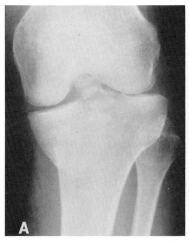 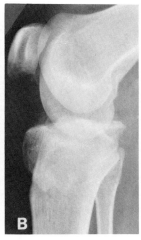 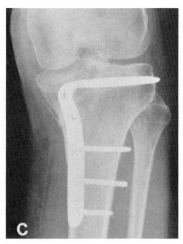

Fig. 16-36. A 20-year-old woman with a total condylar fracture of the medial condyle as well as an intercondylar eminence fracture. Open reduction with a blade-plate failed to achieve adequate reduction. (*A, B*) Initial views of the knee showed the intercondylar eminence fracture and the total condyle depression fracture of the medial condyle. (*C*) The postoperative view showed a blade-plate stabilizing the fracture in malposition. Intraoperative x-rays should have been taken and the malposition corrected at that time.

done early, before degenerative changes have occurred. Another problem is the use of internal fixation that is insufficient to prevent loss of reduction.

Bicondylar Fracture

Bicondylar fractures present an ominous appearance because of often tremendous distortion of both tibial condyles. However, many realign amazingly well after the application of skeletal traction, and they recover with good alignment and motion.[374] Too often, ill-conceived surgical procedures doom the knee to a less satisfactory result. There are skilled surgeons who can reconstruct the proximal tibia by fixing it internally, so that a badly displaced fracture is converted into an undisplaced fracture and is thereafter treated accordingly.[375] The mainstay of management of this fracture, however, will probably remain traction, with manipulative reduction when required. It is important to monitor circulation to the leg and to the anterior compartment, because vascular injury does occur in tibial condylar fractures and most often in the bicondylar type. Observation of foot pulses and tension or pain in the anterior compartment is necessary early after this injury.

Methods of Treatment. The single most useful method of treatment for bicondylar fractures of the tibial condyle is skeletal traction with a pin through the distal tibia or the os calcis.[249] Fifteen pounds of traction will realign the upper tibia in most patients. Check x-rays taken after a few hours should show improved position and indicate whether more weight is required or a change to another method of treatment is necessary. If the traction produces acceptable alignment, it should be continued with the institution of passive and active motion as soon as discomfort and swelling permit (Fig. 16-37). Generally, bone healing is sufficiently advanced within 4 to 6 weeks to permit removal from traction. The use of a splint is advisable; it is removed several times daily for exercises.

Reduction may not be possible in traction alone, and manipulative reduction should be considered. This is best performed under anesthesia with x-ray or image intensifier control. The patient is returned to traction thereafter. A better alternative in severe cases is the traction-compression reduction described in the section on split compression fractures (p. 1462). More controlled and accurate reduction is possible with the added advantage of impaction of the fracture at the conclusion of the procedure. Traction must be used after manipulation, to avoid loss of reduction. A cast will not likely maintain reduction until such time as healing produces fracture stability. Even in minimally displaced comminuted fractures, treatment in a long-leg cast may result in angular deformity later.[338,377]

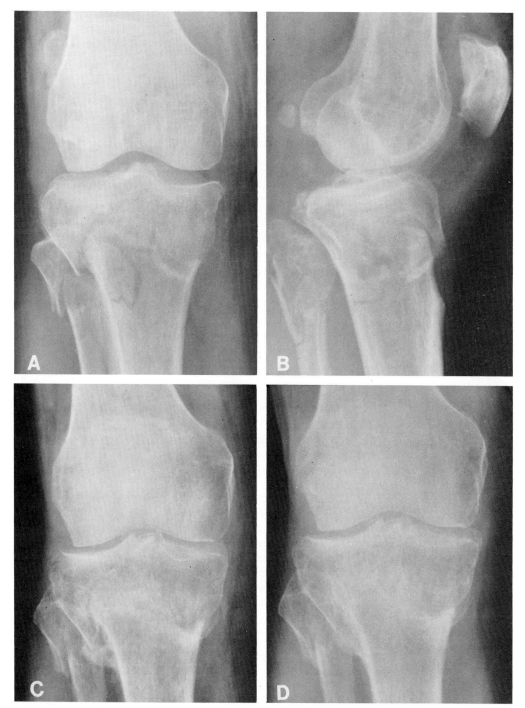

Fig. 16-37. A 65-year-old man with a bicondylar fracture of the upper tibia and a subcondylar fracture of the tibia as well. This fracture was treated in skeletal traction with early motion of the knee. (*A, B*) Initial views demonstrated little fracture displacement. (*C*) Early healing was seen 10 weeks after fracture. (*D*) One-year postfracture the knee functioned well, and the fracture was well healed.

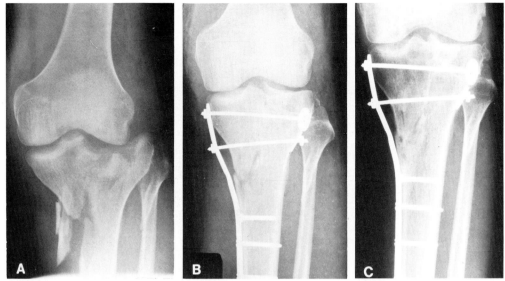

Fig. 16-38. A 29-year-old man sustained a severe bicondylar fracture of the upper tibia, which was treated by open reduction. (*A*) The initial view demonstrated severe articular damage laterally and gross damage to the proximal tibia. (*B*) In the postoperative view, note fixation by a single sideplate, two tibial bolts, and numerous screws to fix the plate. (*C*) Six months after operation the fracture had healed well, and knee function was improving.

Open reduction should only be used by those experienced in comprehensive approaches to the knee and in effective methods of internal fixation (Fig. 16-38).[375,379] Limited open reduction, however, to replace a split fragment, for instance, and continuing traction treatment thereafter may have its value in some cases. In general, the objective of open reduction is to convert the fracture into a stable, undisplaced fracture, and this likely will require one or two side plates with tibial bolts and screws, or the equivalent. Should the fixation be inadequate, return to traction is indicated. One does well to begin movement early but to defer weight bearing until consolidation of the fracture.

Author's Preferred Method of Treatment. I prefer to institute skeletal traction through the distal tibia and observe the degree of restoration of the tibial condyles. If reduction is not acceptable, a decision is then made as to whether traction-compression reduction or open reduction would be the best. This decision depends on a number of factors. Skin condition must be optimal for open reduction. Risk of sepsis is great with the extensive exposure, dissection, and time required to complete the procedure, and open reduction should never

be done except under optimal conditions. Closed reduction may be done with minimal risk.

Exposure of both condyles may be done through separate incisions but this leads to problems in fracture visualization and reduction. A comprehensive anterior approach is best, using a Y-skin incision with 120° between the limbs of the incision and the dividing point just lateral to the tibial tubercle. Rarely is it necessary to divide the patellar tendon to obtain needed exposure of both condyles simultaneously. At times two buttress plates are required, but because of the bulk of the metal if rigid fixation can be secured through the use of a single plate and cancellous screws, the chances of wound complications are lessened (Fig. 16-39).

I prefer to treat most comminuted fractures nonoperatively in traction. Early knee motion is used regardless of treatment method.

Care After Reduction or Operation. Posttreatment care begins by ensuring good skin condition and wound healing by use of a Jones compressive dressing until swelling begins to subside. Then movement of the knee is begun passively and actively with the objective of 90° of motion in 4 weeks. When clinical stability is present with

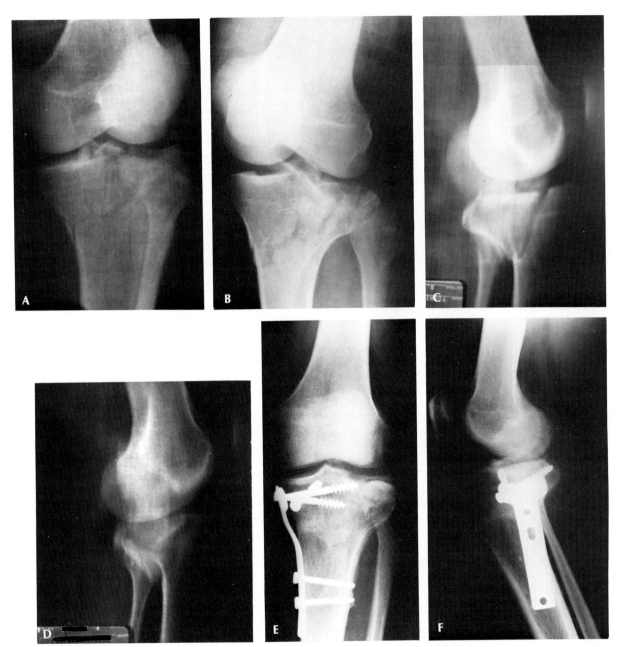

Fig. 16-39. This 35-year-old skier sustained a comminuted bicondylar fracture of the left proximal tibia. (*A, B*) Original oblique projections showed part of the fracture complexity. (*C, D*) Original lateral tomograms portrayed the exact medial split-type fracture and lateral compression fracture. (*E, F*) Four months postoperative after wearing a cast brace for 2 months.

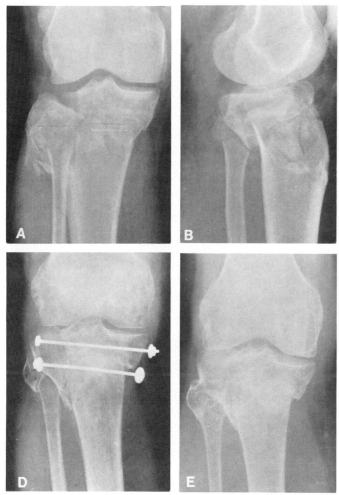

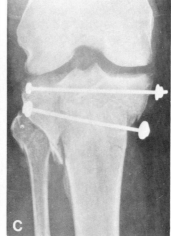

Fig. 16-40. A 53-year-old man with a bicondylar fracture of the proximal tibia was treated by insufficient internal fixation. (*A, B*) Initial views of the fracture. (*C*) Immediately postoperative there was good general alignment. (*D*) Four months later collapse was apparent along the medial condylar area with loss of normal knee valgus. (*E*) After removal of hardware, a subcondylar osteotomy was indicated.

callus about the fracture, traction may be discontinued in favor of a part-time splint. This requires from 4 to 6 weeks in traction.

Prognosis. Prognosis after this fracture is reasonably good with treatment as outlined. Knee strength, alignment, and motion should be acceptable in most cases. The extensive damage to the articular surface leads to traumatic arthritic changes, but with restoration of good alignment the effect of the changes probably will not seriously affect function of the knee.

Complications. Complications include loss of reduction and limitation of motion. Angular deformities are treated by subcondylar osteotomy; the surgeon should plan for a slight degree of overcorrection (Fig. 16-40). Loss of motion in the

knee is treated by continued active exercise. Manipulation to regain movement is seldom helpful. Open lysis of adhesions rarely produces more than a few degrees of additional motion. Whenever practical, therefore, early knee movement should be insisted on to prevent this complication.

FRACTURE-DISLOCATIONS

Split Fracture

The split fracture is uncommon but has quite distinctive characteristics. Most frequently the posterior or anterior articular margin of the medial condyle is fractured and displaced distally. This fracture is similar to the posterior malleolar fracture of the ankle. Closed reduction techniques are seldom useful, but it should be observed that many of the fractures off the posterior margin reduce (or nearly so) when the knee is in full extension and displace when the knee is flexed. In fact, the femoral condyle tends to dislocate onto the split fragment in most cases. Stress testing to determine integrity of the cruciate and collateral ligaments is important with repair of these if they are demonstrated to be torn.

Methods of Treatment. Treatment of the split fracture is usually open reduction and internal fixation when more than minimal displacement is present initially. Percutaneous fixation by several threaded wires may be a useful technique in those cases where the fragment reduces in full extension. At open reduction, lag screws or threaded pins are used for internal fixation with early motion advocated only for those patients in whom solid internal fixation has been achieved. Otherwise, external immobilization is used for 6 weeks.

Author's Preferred Method of Treatment. I prefer open reduction in order to obtain accurate reduction and strong fixation to allow early and rapid return of knee function (Fig. 16-41). In patients with other injuries that preclude surgery the percutaneous method is most useful.

Prognosis. Prognosis is good if reduction is achieved and if motion is started soon after surgery. Complications of persistent knee subluxation with loss of motion and deformity may be the price of healing in the displaced position.

Entire Plateau Fractures

Entire plateau fractures may be quite unstable because of associated ligament injury and the inclusion of cruciate ligament attachment with the fracture fragment (see Fig. 16-26). Although fracture reduction may be fairly easy with traction, retention of reduction may be difficult, especially in fractures involving the medial condyle. Diagnosis of the full extent of ligament injury may require stress films, especially if the fracture is mildly displaced. Moderate or severe displacement would only be possible with complete collateral ligament rupture or avulsion and this should be evident in the original x-ray.

Methods of Treatment. The majority of these fractures are best managed by open reduction and fixation of the fracture and repair of the ligament damage. If the fracture surfaces interdigitate accurately, cancellous screws should be sufficient fixation, but without strong fracture surfaces a buttress plate will serve best and perhaps fixed by a tibial bolt.[355] Postoperative support for ligament repair should be used for 4 to 6 weeks. Manipulation under anesthesia may permit accurate reduction of the fracture; however, it is often difficult to hold the reduction in a cast or cast brace. If either of these is elected, frequent check films to detect fracture redisplacement are important.

Author's Preferred Method of Treatment. I prefer to use open reduction with rigid fixation as obtained often by cancellous screws, a tibial bolt, or buttress plate. Closed methods are only used when skin condition does not permit open surgery without undue risk. In these instances a cast brace with frequent check x-rays usually provides a satisfactory result.

Prognosis. When accurately maintained in reduction, these fractures may show some instability, especially of the lateral ligament, but otherwise knee function usually is reasonably good.

Complications. The major fracture complication is gradual redisplacement with closed treatment or often inadequate internal fixation, especially when the major fragment involves the medial condyle. Frequent check x-rays are important, together with a willingness to change treatment should redisplacement occur.

Rim Avulsion Fractures

The rim avulsion fracture occurs with severe valgus or varus stress when the bone avulses instead of the ligament tearing. Such injuries are most often seen on the lateral side of the knee and are associated with avulsion fractures of the fibular head or Gerdy's tubercle (Fig. 16-42). Occult ruptures of the cruciate ligaments are occasionally noted.[243a]

Methods of Treatment. These rim avulsion fractures are almost always displaced and because of their capsular attachments cannot be reduced by closed means. Open replacement of these fragments is advocated with fixation by screws or pins, depending on fragment size. Associated ligament injury should be repaired at the same time.

Author's Preferred Method of Treatment I prefer open reduction of the avulsed bony fragment, fixing it with a screw. Torn capsule and ligamentous structures are repaired, and the knee is supported for 4 to 6 weeks in a long-leg cast.

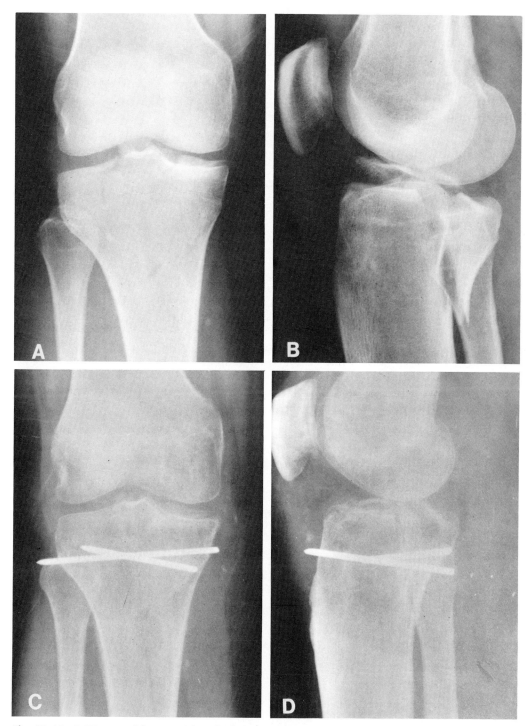

Fig. 16-41. A 35-year-old man with split fracture of the medial tibial condyle as well as an intercondylar eminence fracture treated by open reduction. (*A*) The initial anteroposterior view showed a double shadow of the medial condyle suggestive of a split fracture. (*B*) The initial lateral view confirmed the fracture of the posterior margin. (*C, D*) Five months postoperative views showed good reduction and healing.

Prognosis. Prognosis of these fractures is good for return of function. The residual problems relate to late instability from ligament insufficiency or from other complications.

Complications. Complications observed have been a high incidence of peroneal nerve stretch injury and occasional popliteal artery rupture.

Rim Compression Fractures

Rim compression fractures are caused by the impact of the femoral condyle after the contralateral ligament integrity has been compromised. The bone injury resembles a localized compression of the articular margin or a small depressed marginal split fracture. Assessment of the ligament injury and its repair is vital to successful management of this fracture (Fig. 16-43).

Methods of Treatment. Closed management is likely to result in an unstable knee and should rarely be considered. Moore, in eight medial rim compressions, found fibular styloid avulsion in five, anterior spine avulsion in one, and occult anterior cruciate injuries in three. In eight lateral rim compressions there were five avulsion fractures of the anterior spine and six complete medial collateral ligament ruptures;[355] consequently, open manage-

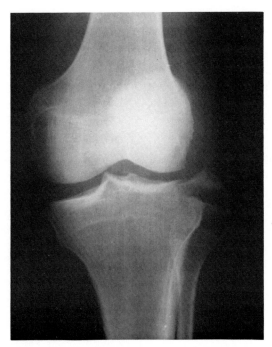

Fig. 16-42. A 38-year-old male motorcyclist with a lateral rim avulsion fracture. Note the large avulsion fracture involving a portion of the articular surface.

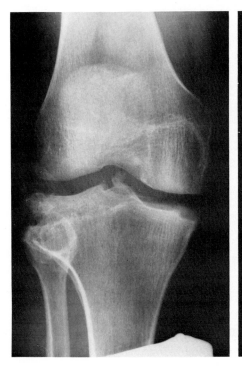

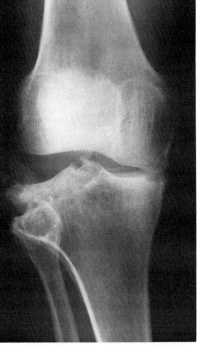

Fig. 16-43. A 45-year-old man who was struck by an automobile sustained rim compression and rim avulsion fractures. (*Left*) Note defect at the medial articular margin and evidence of cruciate injury in the intercondylar region. (*Right*) Stress view demonstrated widening of the lateral cartilage space and rim avulsion fracture. The lateral injuries especially required open repair.

ment is generally required following stress testing in the operating room. The rim compression may need repair and stabilization but the ligament injuries demand repair. Postoperative management in plaster immobilization is necessary until ligament healing is complete.

Author's Preferred Method of Treatment. I prefer to examine the knee under anesthesia with documentation by stress x-ray. The unstable knee should be opened and the rim compression corrected and the torn cruciate and collateral ligaments repaired. Plaster immobilization is used for 4 to 6 weeks. The stable knee is treated by a cast for 4 to 6 weeks.

Prognosis. Despite optimal management of both the bone and ligament injury, some degree of residual instability is anticipated. The goal of treatment is to minimize this instability and maximize knee strength and function.

Complications. When involving the medial condyle, these fractures are associated with peroneal nerve stretch injury on occasion and infrequent arterial injury. Late complications involve knee instability, which requires bracing or reconstructive procedures.

Four-Part Fractures

Four-part fractures are a variety of bicondylar fracture in which the intercondylar eminence and the cruciate attachments are separated from the tibia. The collateral and capsular ligaments remain attached to the condylar fragments, but these condylar fractures render the knee markedly unstable. The incidence of neurovascular complications is high, so that initial and repeated evaluations for vascular status become very important.

Methods of Treatment. Most four-part fractures are best managed by open reduction and accurate restoration of articular surfaces fixing the intercondylar eminence. A buttress plate and cancellous screws provide solid fixation in the majority of fractures. Closed methods may be used, but when there is no associated fibular fracture, varus deformity is the likely outcome. Traction with early motion is a reasonable treatment method if the fracture realigns well.

Author's Preferred Method of Treatment. I prefer to place these fractures in skeletal traction to observe how well reduction can be obtained. If

the reduction is satisfactory, traction is used until callus develops, when a cast brace is applied. Very often, however, adequate reduction is not obtained in traction, and I prefer to openly secure the intercondylar eminence to the condyles using a buttress plate and cancellous screws. Rigid fixation may then permit careful early knee movement.

Prognosis. The major problem after these fractures is neurovascular injury. If this can be properly managed and the fracture maintained in good position until healed, eventual function should be satisfactory.

Complications. Aside from neurovascular problems, important complications are late knee deformity or instability if accurate articular reduction has not been maintained.

FRACTURES OF THE TIBIAL SPINE

Fractures of either the tibial spines or the intercondylar eminence indicate probable alteration of the cruciate ligament stability in the knee. Blocking of full knee extension may be caused by displacement of bone fragments and may require surgical correction.

MECHANISMS OF INJURY

Tibial spine or intercondylar eminence fractures occur from violent twisting or abduction-adduction knee injuries and some probably from direct contact with the adjacent femoral condyle. Hyperextension of the knee may avulse the tibial attachment of the posterior cruciate ligament with a bone fragment. Additional ligament or bone injuries are usually seen with these fractures.[418,419,420,425]

CLASSIFICATION

Either or both tibial spines may be fractured. Fractures of the intercondylar eminence are classified by degree of displacement. This is important as it pertains to the proper selection of treatment (Fig. 16-44).[420] A type I fracture is tilted up only on the anterior margin. In type II the anterior portion is lifted completely from its bed with only some posterior apposition. In type IIIA the intercondylar fragment is not in contact with the tibia, and in type IIIB it is rotated.[420,421] Zaricznyj has suggested an additional category for comminution of the eminence.[425]

SIGNS AND SYMPTOMS

The patient gives a history of knee injury, usually abduction and rotation, followed by painful swelling. Examination may show some effusion and a block to full extension. The anterior and posterior drawer signs should be tested and may be intact, although aspiration of a hemarthrosis may be necessary to obtain a valid examination. The finding of associated ligament injuries, especially to the collateral ligaments, is frequently noted and must be examined for and considered in the determination of treatment.

RADIOGRAPHIC FINDINGS

Routine knee views for injury usually reveal the fracture, but an intercondylar or tunnel view is helpful and should be obtained. Isolated spine fractures or one of the types of intercondylar eminence fractures shown in Figure 16-44 may be seen. Careful inspection of the joint margins and areas of ligament attachment should be made to rule out avulsion fractures.

METHODS OF TREATMENT

The primary objective of treatment in tibial spine fractures is to restore the full mobility and stability of the knee. Isolated fractures of one or both spines are immobilized in plaster in nearly full extension for 4 to 6 weeks to permit associated soft-tissue injuries to heal. Type I or II intercondylar eminence fractures may reduce in part with closed manipulation under anesthesia, thus permitting the knee to extend fully. If good fracture reduction has been obtained (as demonstrated by x-rays), immobilization of the knee in plaster for 5 to 6 weeks is indicated.

Open reduction with anatomical reduction of a displaced fracture provides the best opportunity for acccurate restoration of the bony and ligamentous architecture of the knee. Often the fracture fragment can be reduced into its bed and held in place by suture. Elaborate pull-out sutures are seldom necessary to hold these fragments in reduction, but external casting to allow healing is advisable for several weeks (Fig. 16-45).

Arthroscopic techniques are sometimes useful in repositioning displaced fractures and assessing associated intra-articular problems.[419a]

Indications for Closed and Open Treatment

Closed treatment is indicated when the fractures are in good position and examination indicates that the ligamentous structures are intact. Collateral ligament injuries must be recognized and repaired if damaged. An attempt at closed reduction is indicated in knees that lack full extension. The result should be checked by x-rays while the patient

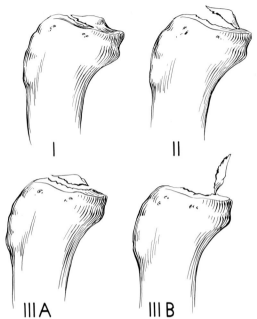

Fig. 16-44. Classification of intercondylar eminence fractures. (Redrawn from Meyers, M. H., and McKeever, F. M.: Fractures of the Intercondylar Eminence of the Tibia. J. Bone Joint Surg., **52A:**1677–1684, 1970.)

is still anesthetized. If successful reduction is not obtained, open reduction should be carried out immediately.

Primary open reduction is indicated in type III fractures to restore bone apposition or where ligament stability is significantly impaired.[420,422]

Author's Preferred Method of Treatment

I prefer an attempt at closed reduction in all cases where there appears to be a chance of success. The manipulation is gentle and basically brings the knee into full extension. If the x-ray confirms good position a cast is applied within a few degrees of full extension. If good position is not obtained or if the block to extension is not relieved, arthrotomy is performed, cleansing the joint and replanting the fragment in its bed and holding it by simple suture if possible.

POSTOPERATIVE CARE

Regardless of the method of treatment, cast immobilization in nearly full extension for a period of 5 to 6 weeks is advisable. Thereafter, active exercise programs to restore motion and strength are indicated.

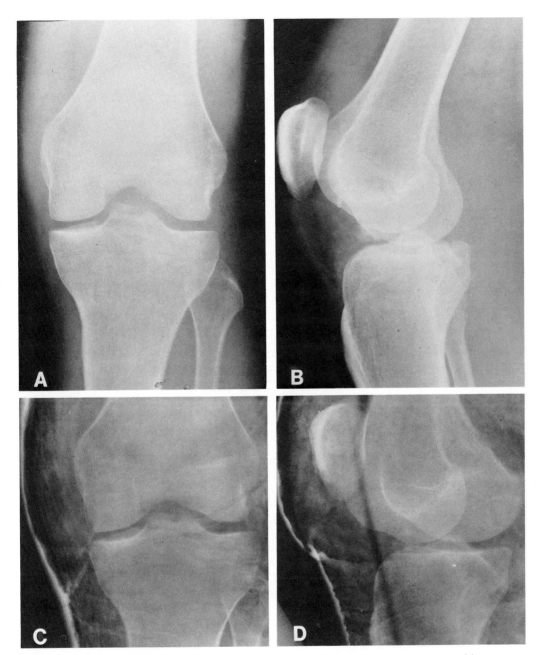

Fig. 16-45. A 31-year-old man with an intercondylar eminence fracture was treated by open reduction. (*A, B*) Initial views demonstrated the fracture displacement. This was a type III-A fracture. (*C, D*) Postoperative views showed the fragment in place.

PROGNOSIS

The results after fractures of the intercondylar eminence in adults are rarely perfect. Usually there is some residual discomfort or instability of the knee in the anteroposterior plane, despite the choice of treatment.[420,421]

COMPLICATIONS

Problems have arisen in closed reductions with further fragment displacement, perhaps related to excessive force on manipulation. The late complication of a bony ossicle representing a fracture fragment partially loose in the joint and causing intermittent blocking suggests the need to remove the fragment.

FRACTURES OF THE TIBIAL TUBERCLE

Fractures of the tibial tubercle are very uncommon isolated injuries, but they are found more often in association with comminuted fractures or subcondylar fractures of the proximal tibia. Since the tibial tubercle provides insertion for the quadriceps mechanism through the patellar tendon, it is important that the fracture fragment heals strongly and in good position.

MECHANISM OF INJURY

Fractures of the tibial tubercle usually occur from indirect violence with the knee flexed and the quadriceps violently resisting further flexion. The tubercle avulses and displaces proximalward. The diagnosis should be suspected after a history of injury, especially as described, and findings of local swelling and tenderness in the tubercle area, with pain on attempted extension. Incomplete active extension may be possible with the patellar retinaculum intact.

METHODS OF TREATMENT

Treatment by closed means is not satisfactory, and open reduction is the treatment of choice, because it provides the opportunity for accurate reduction and internal fixation. Most physicians who write or talk about these fractures (including me) use screws or staples to secure the torn periosteum and tendinous attachments.[418] Cast support with the knee extended is used until the tubercle unites; a period of 6 weeks. Some quadriceps exercise is begun during the period of immobilization with further rehabilitative exercise after cast removal.

COMPLICATIONS

The major complication of treatment is loss of fixation of the tubercle with redisplacement. It is best to reoperate and reattach the tubercle before healing and contracture takes place in the displaced position.

SUBCONDYLAR FRACTURES OF THE PROXIMAL TIBIA

MECHANISM OF INJURY

The region of the proximal tibial metaphysis is injured by severe angular or rotatory stress. The fractures produced are transverse or oblique and seldom are significantly displaced. Most often lines extend from the subcondylar fracture into the knee joint, or the fracture occurs in combination with one of the tibial condylar fractures. Such a fracture is often termed a comminuted fracture of the proximal tibia and treated by traction until consolidation occurs.

METHODS OF TREATMENT

Treatment of subcondylar fractures is predominantly closed. A long-leg cast is most commonly used in the stable transverse fractures until healing occurs, usually within a period of about 8 weeks. Closed reduction may be required to correct displacement or angular deformity, usually holding the reduction in a cast. Open reduction is rarely indicated and only when reduction cannot be obtained closed or when there is an associated fracture of the tibial condyle that requires open reduction. It is then best to open both fractures and fix the subcondylar fracture with a contoured side plate to permit early motion of the knee.

FRACTURES OF THE PROXIMAL END OF THE FIBULA

Fractures of the proximal end of the fibula are relatively unimportant. Their presence, however, should alert one to the possibility of associated problems. These include peroneal nerve injury or biceps tendon injury—either by contusion or traction, lateral instability from associated ligament rupture, injury to the anterior tibial artery leading to thrombosis, and avulsion of the fibular styloid, which may be pulled upward and trapped in the joint.

There are three mechanisms of injury: direct blow, twisting injury at the ankle, or varus (adduction) stress to the knee. A fracture of the fibular head resulting from a direct blow is usually comminuted and not displaced. A fracture below the head of the fibula should make one suspicious of an associated fracture at the ankle joint, usually due to an external rotation injury (see Chapter 18).

Isolated fractures of the proximal fibula have been called the silent fractures in parachute injuries, because they produce so few symptoms. They are often misdiagnosed as muscle strains.

ANATOMY

See Knee Anatomy (p. 1480) and Dislocation of the Proximal Tibiofibular Joint (p. 1508).

MECHANISM OF INJURY

More important than those fractures of the proximal fibula caused by a direct blow or rotational injury of the ankle are the fractures of the fibular head produced by varus strain to the knee (Fig. 16-46). If it is a severe injury, the lateral ligaments may be ruptured or the common peroneal nerve may be stretched or torn.

"Lateral compartment syndrome of the knee"[430] and "ligamentous peroneal nerve syndrome"[428] are names that have been coined to describe the association of an adduction stress to the knee, rupture of the lateral capsular and ligamentous structures, and a peroneal nerve injury. Platt[428] described the condition in association with an avulsion fracture of the fibular head in 1928. This condition is discussed on page 1537, Acute Lateral Ligament Injuries. It suffices to say that when an avulsion-type fracture of the fibular head is diagnosed, the knee should be checked for damage to the lateral supporting structures and for evidence of peroneal nerve injury.

Watson-Jones,[431] in 1931, reported a case of avulsion of the fibular styloid, which became trapped in the lateral joint compartment of the knee. There was an associated peroneal nerve injury. The surgical procedure necessary to free the entrapped fragment showed that the fibular collateral ligament and part of the biceps tendon were still attached to the fragment.

Fractures of the head of the fibula may be associated with lateral tibial condyle fractures from a valgus stress.

METHODS OF TREATMENT

The fibula bears no weight. The fracture itself, therefore, may not require any treatment other than protection to avoid discomfort. Conditions associated with the fracture may require treatment.

Rupture of the lateral supporting structures of the knee and tendon attachments need repair if instability is present (see p. 1534).

Peroneal nerve injury as a result of traction by the adduction force to the knee may result in

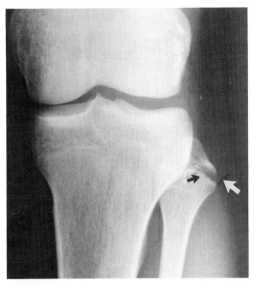

Fig. 16-46. X-ray of a 21-year-old football player who was struck on the inner side of the left knee. No instability and no neurologic signs were present. *Arrows* show the partial avulsion of the fibular styloid produced by this varus stress.

neurapraxia, axonotmesis, or neurotmesis. Return of function depends on the extent of injury and the time interval between injury and repair. Towne and colleagues,[430] Novich,[427] and Smillie[429] have recommended early exploration with definitive repair as soon as possible. White[433] recommends exploration if there is no evidence of recovery within 3 months.

If ligament repair is required, the nerve should be explored and repaired if necessary or feasible. When the torn nerve cannot be approximated at the initial surgery, the ends are tagged for later repair. The prognosis with extensive resection of the damaged nerve, anastomosis, or homografts is poor. Neurapraxic lesions begin to show recovery after 3 months.

Part II: DISLOCATIONS AND LIGAMENTOUS INJURIES OF THE KNEE

Robert L. Larson
Donald C. Jones

The knee, because of its anatomical structure, its exposed position, and the functional demands of use, is one of the areas most vulnerable to injury. This is particularly true in athletes. Nicholas[434] lists five basic components of knee movement: precision (balance) at rest, walking, running, jumping, and kicking. These basic movements allow the knee "(1) to provide support and balance for a wide range of movements from stance to speed; (2) to act as a propulsive and restraining mechanism; (3) to provide a stable pedestal for power of body movements; (4) to adapt to sudden changes in movement to forces transmitted from the ground, from unusual surfaces, or from trunk and upper extremity movements (throwing hard); (5) to provide means for rapid change in direction, acceleration, and deceleration."

Restoration of a knee to its normal and full use is the goal after any injury. Any of these basic movements may be compromised by loss of motion, loss of stability, decreased muscle strength, or pain.

The age of the patient and the functional demands of the knee after rehabilitation may influence the type of treatment. The early results of treatment may not be the final result. Excess wear of the joint from incongruous articulations, from deformity, or from laxity may occur with the passage of time and the demands of use. A rational approach is to consider all factors—age, use, laxity, motion, incongruity, chances of successful treatment, degeneration, strength, capabilities, later reconstructive measures, and other circumstantial influences—before deciding on the method of treatment.

ANATOMY*

This chapter deals with many injuries about the knee, including fractures as well as ligamentous injuries and injuries of the quadriceps mechanism. In order to understand knee injuries and the complexities of knee motion, it is important to have a basic understanding of normal knee anatomy. Rather

* This section was written in conjunction with one of our associates, Dr. Stanley L. James, from material given by us in Instructional Course Lectures for the American Academy of Orthopaedic Surgeons.

than providing a detailed anatomy section with each particular type of injury, which would require much repetition, this section deals with the general anatomy of the knee. Each section has amplification of the anatomy germane to that particular injury.

The present discussion stresses those components important in functional stability. Trauma to the knee that disrupts the integrity of these structures destroys their stabilizing function. A good foundation in normal knee anatomy is necessary in order to surgically reconstruct these stabilizing structures as closely to their previous anatomical state as possible.

THE OSSEOUS STRUCTURES

The osseous structures of the knee consist of three components: the patella, the distal femoral condyles, and the proximal tibial plateaus. The knee is described as a hinge joint, but actually it is more complicated than a hinge joint because, in addition to flexion and extension, it also has a rotatory component to its motion. The knee joint may really be considered three joints in one, with a joint between the patella and the femur and between each tibial condyle and femoral condyle.

FEMORAL CONDYLES

The femoral condyles are two rounded prominences, eccentrically curved, the anterior portion being part of an oval and the posterior portion a section of a sphere. Thus, the condyles are more broadly curved anteriorly than posteriorly. Anteriorly, the condyles are somewhat flattened, the lateral slightly more than the medial condyle. This provides a greater surface area for contact and weight transmission. The condyles project very little in front of the femoral shaft but markedly behind. The groove that runs anteriorly between the condyles is the patellofemoral groove, or trochlea, which accepts the patella. Posteriorly the condyles are separated by the intercondylar notch. The articular surface of the medial condyle is longer than the lateral condyle, but the lateral condyle is wider. The long axis of the lateral condyle is oriented essentially along the sagittal plane; the medial condyle is usually at about a 22° angle to the sagittal plane.

TIBIAL PLATEAU

The expanded proximal end of the tibia is formed by two rather flat surfaces, or condyles, which articulate with the femoral condyles. They are separated in the midline by the intercondylar eminence with its medial and lateral intercondylar tubercles. Anterior and posterior to the intercondylar eminence are the intercondylar areas that serve as attachment sites for the cruciate ligaments and menisci. The posterior lip of the lateral tibial condyle is rounded off where the lateral meniscus slides posteriorly with flexion of the knee.

THE PATELLA

The patella is a somewhat triangular sesamoid bone, wider at the proximal pole than at the distal pole. The articular surface of the patella is divided by a vertical ridge that creates a smaller medial and a larger lateral articular facet, or surface. Wiberg[498] described three patellar configurations. A type I

patella has equal medial and lateral articular surfaces that are slightly concave. A type II patella has a smaller medial surface and a larger lateral surface, both being slightly concave. The type III has a very small medial facet. Baumgartl[441] has expanded these descriptions and lists six basic types of patellae (Fig. 16-47). The patellar shape is best assessed by a tangential x-ray of the patellofemoral joint taken with the patient prone and the knee flexed 55° (Fig.16-48). This technique has been described by Hughston.[459] The type II patella is the most common variety.

With the knee in extension, the patella actually rides above the superior articular margin of the femoral groove. In extension the distal portion of the lateral patellar facet articulates with the lateral femoral condyle, but the medial patellar facet barely articulates with the medial femoral condyle until complete flexion is approached. At 45° of flexion, contact moves proximally to the midportion of the articular surfaces. In complete flexion, the proximal

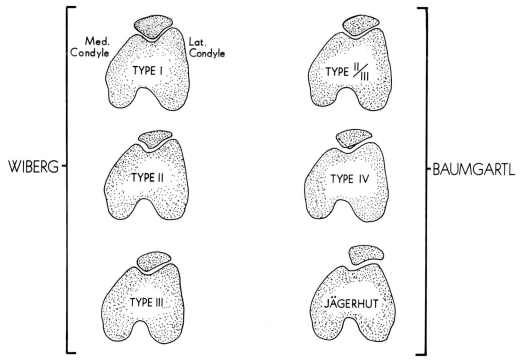

Fig. 16-47. Patellar configurations as described by Wiberg[498] and Baumgartl.[441] Type I has equal facets that are slightly concave. Type II has a smaller medial facet; both facets are concave. Type III has a smaller medial facet but a convex surface. Type II/III has a flat medial facet. Type IV has a very small medial facet or none. Type V (Jägerhut) has no medial facet, no central ridge, and shows lateral subluxation. Stresses are well distributed on types I and II. The other types are prone to unequal stresses to the patellar articular surfaces.

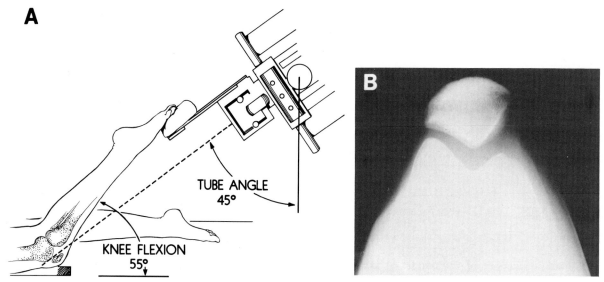

Fig. 16-48. (A) Hughston's[607] method for a tangential infrapatellar view. The knee is flexed 55°. The tube is tilted 45° from the vertical. (B) In a x-ray obtained by this method, the configuration of the bony contour of the patella, the shape of the patellofemoral groove, and the height of the femoral condyles can be ascertained.

portions of both facets are in contact with the femur. During flexion and extension the patella moves some 7 cm to 8 cm in relation to the femoral condyles. With complete flexion, more pressure is applied to the medial facet.

QUADRICEPS TENDON

The quadriceps tendon inserts into the proximal pole of the patella. The four components of the quadriceps mechanism form a trilaminar quadriceps tendon attaching to the patella (Fig. 16-49). The tendon of the rectus femoris flattens immediately above the patella and becomes the anterior lamina, which inserts at the anterior edge of the proximal pole. The tendon of the vastus intermedius continues downward as the deepest lamina of the quadriceps tendon and inserts into the posterior edge of the proximal pole. The middle lamina is formed by the confluent edges of the vastus lateralis and vastus medialis. The fibers of the medial retinaculum, formed from the aponeurosis of the vastus medialis obliquus, insert directly into the side of the patella to help prevent lateral displacement of the patella during flexion. The patellar tendon takes origin from the apex, or distal pole, of the patella and inserts distally into the tibial tubercle.

MECHANICS

If the shaft of the femur is held vertically, the medial condyle projects farther distally than the lateral; however, in a normal upright posture, this is not true. This is because the mechanical axis and the anatomical axis of the femur do not coincide (Fig. 16-50). The anatomical axis passes through the center of the knee joint and along the femoral shaft, inclining laterally. The mechanical axis, on the other hand, passes from the center of the knee joint through the center of the hip joint and is more vertical. The angle between the mechanical axis and the anatomical axis is approximately 6°.

Because of disparity between the lengths of the articular surface of the femoral condyles and the tibial condyles, two types of motion during flexion and extension are noted in relation to the tibial and femoral condyles. The first is a rocking motion in which points equidistant on the tibia come into contact with points that are equidistant on the femoral condyles. The second type of motion is a gliding motion in which a constant point on the tibia comes into contact with ever-changing points on the femur. It is believed by many that the first 20° of flexion of the knee consist of a pure rocking motion[493]; however, Lindahl and Movin[476] have disputed this and state that during the first 20° to 30° of flexion there is, rather, a combined rocking and gliding motion. After the first 20° to 30° of flexion a pure gliding motion ensues. Because of the eccentricity of the femoral condyles, the transverse axis of rotation constantly changes position (instant center of rotation)[448] as the knee progresses from extension into flexion.

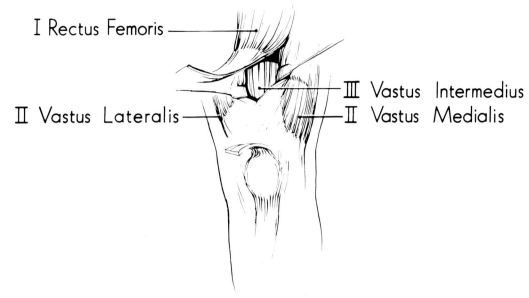

Fig. 16-49. The quadriceps tendon forms a trilaminar structure. The outer layer is in the tendon of the rectus femoris; the middle layer, the confluence of the fascia of the vastus lateralis and vastus medialis; and the deepest layer is the tendon of the vastus intermedius.

The vertical axis for rotation is described as passing medial to the medial tubercle of the intercondylar eminence. The medial side of the knee joint is more securely anchored than the lateral (see below) so that in flexion the lateral tibial condyle can sweep through a greater arc of rotation than the medial condyle does. If the medial ligaments are disrupted, the axis of rotation shifts laterally. The knee has little or no rotation when it is in complete extension, but rotation is increased in flexion. The amount of rotation available has been studied by a number of investigators[454] with varying conclusions. One of the problems, of course, is in finding a neutral position from which to measure internal and external rotation of the tibia on the femur.

MEDIAL ASPECT OF THE KNEE

The major structures on the medial aspect of the knee are the medial retinaculum, the tibial collateral ligament, the medial capsular ligament, and the pes anserinus, which consists of the tendinous expansions of the sartorius, gracilis, and semitendinosus (Fig. 16-51).[434]

Warren and Marshall[495] have described the major structures of the knee as lying in three distinct layers. Layer I is composed of the deep fascia or crural fascia. Layer II consists of the superficial

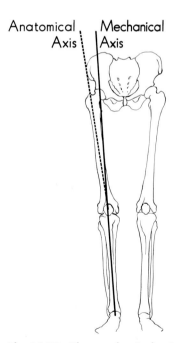

Fig. 16-50. The mechanical axis of the leg passes along the line of weight bearing from the middle of the hip joint to the middle of the talus. This projected line usually falls near the center of the knee joint unless a genu valgum or varum is present. The anatomical axis of the femur inclines laterally along the femoral shaft.

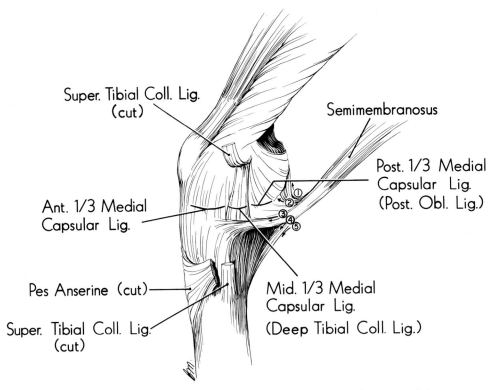

Fig. 16-51. The medial supporting structures of the knee. The midportion of the tibial collateral ligament (superficial tibial [medial] collateral liagment) has been removed. The posterior trailing edge of the tibial collateral liagment often blends into the posterior medial capsular ligament (posterior oblique liagment). For a description of expansions of semimembranosus see p. 1485. (Modified from Slocum, D. B.; Larson, R. L.; and James, S. L.: Late Reconstruction Procedures used to Stabilize the Knee. Orthop. Clin. North Am., **4**:679–689, 1973.)

medial collateral ligament (tibial collateral ligament), various structures anterior to this ligament, and the posterior medial corner. The capsule of the knee and the deep medial ligament make up the third layer.

MEDIAL RETINACULUM

The medial retinaculum is a distal expansion of the vastus medialis obliquus aponeurosis. This fascial layer attaches along the medial border of the patella and patellar ligament with an insertion into the periosteum of the tibia. The sartorius inserts into this network of fibers and does not have an isolated tendon like the gracilis and semitendinosus.

The function of the medial retinaculum is to guy the patella medially. It covers and may blend into the anterior medial capsular ligament; however, the medial retinaculum can be dissected free from the tibial collateral ligament. Contraction of the vastus medialis helps to tighten the anterior portion of the medial capsular ligament.

TIBIAL COLLATERAL LIGAMENT

The tibial collateral ligament (superficial tibial [medial] collateral ligament) is the outermost component of the medial supporting structures of the knee. This ligament is covered superficially by fascia extending distally from the vastus medialis to the superior edge of the fascia of the pes anserinus (medial retinaculum). The distal attachment of the tibial collateral ligament to the tibia is directly beneath the anterior medial portion of the pes anserinus group of tendons. This ligament is a well-delineated, bandlike structure inserting proximally into the medial femoral epicondyle and about a hand's breadth distally below the joint line onto the medial aspect of the tibia. It glides forward in extension and posteriorly with flexion. Warren and

Marshall[495] attribute considerable importance to the long fibers of the superficial tibial collateral ligament as the primary stabilizers of the medial side of the knee against valgus and rotary stress. Their work contradicts that of Kennedy and Fowler,[470] who found that with a combination of valgus and external rotation forces the medial ligaments were torn sequentially as follows: (1) the medial capsular ligament; (2) the superficial tibial collateral ligament; and (3) the anterior cruciate ligament. The former work also disputes the importance of the posterior oblique ligament as described by Hughston and Eilers[459] (see below).

MEDIAL CAPSULAR LIGAMENT

Deep to the tibial collateral ligament is the medial capsule of the knee. This capsule has been divided into three anatomical regions. The anterior portion of this capsule is a very thin layer reinforced by the patello-epicondylar ligament and the patello-tibial ligament. Separated from the tibial collateral ligament by a bursa, the mid-medial capsule (deep capsular ligament, deep tibial [medial] collateral ligament) is a thicker portion of the capsule with vertically oriented fibers consisting of a meniscofemoral and meniscotibial component. The meniscofemoral portion is the strongest and longest portion of the deep capsular ligament. This ligament may be a discrete structure throughout its length or may tend to merge with the overlying tibial collateral ligament near its proximal attachment. The meniscotibial ligament (coronary ligament) is routinely independent of the tibial collateral ligament. The third portion of the medial capsule is the posterior capsular ligament. The term "posterior oblique ligament of the knee" was coined by Hughston and Eilers.[459]

This ligament is described as a thickening of the capsular ligament attached proximally to the adductor tubercle of the femur and distally to the tibia and posterior aspect of the capsule. Three arms compose the distal attachment: (1) the prominent central or tibial arm that attaches to the edge of the posterior surface of the tibia close to the margin of the articular surface and central to the upper edge of the semimembranosus tendon; (2) the superior or capsular arm that is continuous with the posterior capsule and the proximal part of the oblique popliteal ligament; and (3) the poorly defined inferior or distal arm that attaches distally both to the sheath covering the semimembranosus tendon and to the tibia just distal to the direct insertion of the semimembranosus tendon. This complex is an important stabilizing structure, particularly against rotatory instability. It is tightened by contracture of the semimembranosus muscle during knee flexion and provides dynamic and static stabilization.

PES ANSERINUS

The conjoined tendons of the sartorius, gracilis, and semitendinosus form the pes anserinus, inserting along the proximal medial aspect of the tibia. These muscles help protect the knee against rotary and valgus stress. They are primarily flexors of the knee and secondarily internal rotators of the tibia.

POSTERIOR ASPECT OF THE KNEE

The important stabilizing structures of the posterior aspect of the knee are (1) the posterior capsule, (2) the ramifications of the semimembranosus tendon, (3) the oblique popliteal ligament, which is an expansion of the semimembranosus, (4) the arcuate ligament, (5) the popliteus muscle, and (6) the ligaments of Wrisberg and Humphrey (Fig. 16-52).

SEMIMEMBRANOSUS MUSCLE

The semimembranosus is especially important as a stabilizing structure around the posterior aspect of the knee. It has five distal expansions (see Fig. 16-51). The first is the oblique popliteal ligament (1), which passes from the insertion of the semimembranosus on the posterior medial aspect of the tibia, obliquely and laterally upward toward the insertion of the lateral gastrocnemius head. It acts as a very important stabilizing structure of the posterior aspect of the knee. The semimembranosus helps tighten this structure with contraction. When the oblique popliteal ligament is pulled medially and forward, it tightens the posterior capsule of the knee. This maneuver is used to tighten the posterior capsule and the posterior medial corner of the knee in surgical repair.

A second tendinous attachment is to the posterior capsule and posterior horn of the medial meniscus (2). This tendinous slip functions to help tighten the posterior capsule and pull the medial meniscus posteriorly with knee flexion. The anterior or medial tendon (3) continues medially along the flare of the tibial condyle and inserts beneath the superficial tibial collateral ligament just distal to the joint line.

The direct head of the semimembranosus attaches to the infraglenoid tubercle (4) on the posterior aspect of the medial tuberosity of the tibia, just

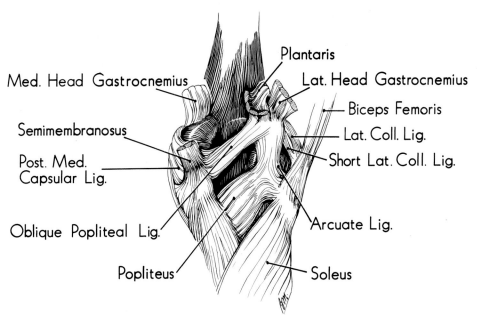

Fig. 16-52. The posterior aspect of the knee. The oblique popliteal ligament is the lateral expansion of the semimembranosus. The arcuate ligament reinforces the posterolateral corner of the knee. (Modified from Slocum, D. B.; Larson, R. L.; and James, S. L.: Late Reconstruction Procedures used to Stabilize the Knee. Orthop. Clin. North Am., **4**:679–689, 1973.)

below the joint line posteriorly. This tendinous attachment provides a firm point in which sutures can be anchored in posteromedial capsule repair.

The distal portion of the semimembranosus tendon continues distally to form a fibrous expansion over the popliteus and fuses into the periosteum of the medial tibia (5).

Functionally, the semimembranosus muscle acts as a flexor and internal rotator of the tibia. It retracts the posterior rim of the medial meniscus posteriorly in flexion, and through the oblique popliteal ligament it tenses the posterior capsule. All branches of this muscle act as a major stabilizer for the posteromedial aspect of the knee. Contraction of this muscle tenses the posterior capsular ligament (posterior oblique ligament) producing kinetic and static stability.

POPLITEUS MUSCLE

The popliteus muscle is unusual in that it has three proximal tendinous origins, and the fleshy muscle belly attaches to the tibia on its posterior aspect distally. The first origin is that which attaches to the lateral femoral condyle just below the attachment of the lateral collateral ligament. The second tendinous origin is to the posterior aspect of the

fibular head, and the third tendinous origin is to the posterior horn of the lateral meniscus. Basmajian and Lovejoy[440] have described these three tendinous origins as forming a Y-shaped ligament, the arms being joined together by the capsule and the meniscal origin. This linkage over the anterior portion of the popliteus muscle is called the arcuate ligament. The insertion of the popliteus is by its muscle belly into the posterior aspect of the tibia.

The tendinous origin from the lateral femoral condyle passes through the popliteal hiatus, which is an opening bordered medially by the body of the lateral meniscus. Cohn and Mains[445] obtained measurements of the hiatus and found its length to be 1.3 ± 0.1 cm. Tears of the lateral meniscus frequently occur in this region. Knowledge of the normal popliteal hiatal length will allow interpretation of lateral meniscal pathology and therefore prevent needless meniscectomies.

The contour of the popliteus bursa on arthrogram can also provide useful information. Narrowing, compression, or complete absence of the popliteus bursa is associated with tears of the lateral menisci and with discoid menisci. Absence of this bursa can also be indicative of adhesive capsulitis or a rare congenital anomaly.

The function of the popliteus is primarily internal rotation of the tibia on the femur. It also pulls the posterior horn of the lateral meniscus posteriorly with flexion of the knee providing rotary stability by preventing forward dislocation of the tibia on the femur during flexion. Further stability is provided by the attachments of the tendon laterally and by the extensions of the posterior horn of the lateral meniscus to the ligaments of Wrisberg and Humphrey, which attach anteriorly and posteriorly to the femoral attachment of the posterior cruciate ligament.

LIGAMENTS OF WRISBERG AND HUMPHREY

The ligament of Wrisberg lies behind the posterior cruciate ligament and runs from the posterior aspect of the lateral meniscus to the inner side of the medial femoral condyle. The ligament of Humphrey lies in front of the posterior cruciate and attaches to the posterior horn of the lateral meniscus and runs to the inner side of the medial femoral condyle. Both of these ligaments function to draw the posterior arch of the lateral meniscus in a medial direction as internal rotation of the tibia occurs with flexion of the knee and simultaneous contraction of the popliteus. As mentioned above, this action in concert with the contracting popliteus provides stability to the tibia and prevents abnormal forward motion.

THE POSTERIOR CAPSULE

The posterior capsule in extension is pulled tightly around the femoral condyle and helps to stabilize the knee in extension. When the posterior capsule is intact, the knee will be stable to valgus stress in extension, even with all other stabilizing structures cut. With the knee in flexion, the posterior capsule relaxes, and loss of integrity of the cut medial structures can be demonstrated. As mentioned in the section above regarding the semimembranosus muscle, the oblique popliteal ligament through the semimembranosus contraction helps to tighten the posterior capsule with flexion of the knee.

LATERAL ASPECT OF THE KNEE

The important stabilizing structures on the lateral aspect of the knee are (1) the iliotibial tract, (2) the lateral (fibular) collateral ligament, (3) the short collateral ligament (fabellofibular ligament), (4) the biceps tendon, (5) the popliteus tendon, and (6) the extension of the vastus lateralis (Fig. 16-53).

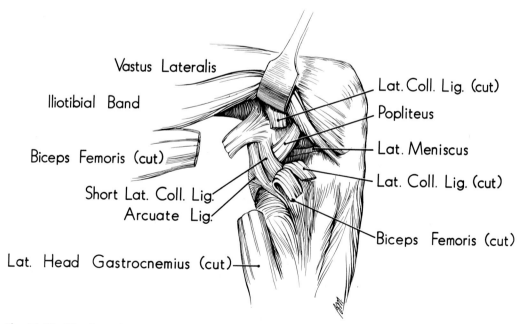

Fig. 16-53. The lateral supporting structures of the knee. The iliotibial band and vastus lateralis have been reflected anteriorly to show the deeper lateral structures. See text.

ILIOTIBIAL TRACT

The iliotibial tract inserts proximally into the lateral epicondyle of the femur and distally into the lateral tibial tubercle. If forms an additional ligament contiguous anteriorly with the vastus lateralis and posteriorly with the biceps. The iliotibial band moves forward in extension and backward in flexion but is tense in both positions. With flexion the iliotibial band, popliteus tendon, and lateral collateral ligament cross each other, thus enhancing lateral stability. During flexion, the iliotibial band and biceps tendon remain parallel to each other, as in extension, and enhance lateral stability.

LATERAL COLLATERAL LIGAMENT

The lateral (fibular) collateral ligament is separated from the lateral meniscus, unlike the medial capsular ligament, which is intimately associated with its peripheral attachment to the medial meniscus. The lateral collateral ligament is inserted into the lateral femoral epicondyle proximally and the fibular head distally. When viewed in the coronal plane it is located more posteriorly than the midportion of the medial capsular ligament (deep medial collateral ligament). This ligament provides lateral stability, particularly when the knee is in extension. As the knee goes into flexion, the lateral collateral ligament relaxes to permit rotation.

SHORT COLLATERAL LIGAMENT

The short collateral ligament lies deep to the lateral collateral ligament. When a fabella is present, it attaches to it and is then called the fabellofibular ligament. It runs parallel to the lateral collateral ligament and attaches to the fibular head posterior to the tendon of the biceps. Its action is to reinforce the posterior capsule and also to contribute to the lateral stability of the knee.

BICEPS TENDON

The biceps tendon inserts in the fibular head lateral to the insertions of the lateral and short collateral ligaments. It is a strong flexor of the knee with simultaneous strong external rotation of the tibia.

POPLITEUS TENDON

The popliteus has been discussed above under Popliteus Muscle (p. 1486). It is located on the lateral side of the knee between the lateral collateral ligament and the femoral condyle and, as previously mentioned, functions as a stabilizer of the knee in flexion.

EXTENSION OF THE VASTUS LATERALIS

The extension of the vastus lateralis lateral retinaculum attaches to the iliotibial tract and helps to tense this tract as the knee extends and the iliotibial tract moves forward. The vastus lateralis functions not only in extension of the knee but also contributes toward lateral stability.

QUADRUPLE COMPLEX

Kaplan[467] has described the stabilizing structures of the lateral side of the knee. These he calls the quadruple complex, which include the iliotibial tract, the lateral collateral ligament, the popliteus tendon, and the biceps muscle. According to Kaplan, stability and nearly normal function are maintained, in spite of loss of any two of these four structures. In flexion, the biceps muscle, iliotibial tract, and popliteus tendon are the chief lateral stabilizers. The lateral collateral ligament provides its stabilizing action when the knee is in extension.

LATERAL CAPSULAR LIGAMENT COMPLEX

As described by Johnson[464] the lateral capsular ligament complex has both a vertical and horizontal component. The vertical division attaches to bone, ligament, and tendon, including the iliotibial tract. The horizontal division attaches to the lateral meniscus and to the ligamentous structures in the posterior and intercondylar areas of the knee.

The vertical component of this complex has a thick central portion that blends into the lateral retinacular structures. This complex attaches to the femur, fibula, tibia. The femoral insertion has a reflection onto the lateral head of the gastrocnemius while the fibular attachment has a reflection onto the biceps femoris tendon with an extension around the popliteus sheath. The attachment to the lateral aspect of the tibia is a strong ligamentous structure.

Johnson believes that the lateral capsular complex plays a significant role in stabilizing the lateral aspect of the knee against rotary stresses. The acute avulsion fracture of the lateral ligament with soft tissue remaining intact as described by Wood,[500] and Johnson[464] suggests that this structure is much stronger than previously appreciated.

INTERNAL KNEE ANATOMY

MENISCI

The following characteristics have been attributed to the menisci: nutrition around the joint, shock absorption, stability (deepen joint), control of motion, enlargement of contact area, and lubrication of the joints. (These characteristics are discussed in more detail on p. 1549). The menisci have definite motions during flexion and extension of the knee. They are displaced forward with extension by the action of the patellomeniscal ligaments, which are expansions of the extensor retinaculum, and by the rolling action of the femoral condyles. With flexion the menisci move posteriorly, owing to muscle action of the popliteus on the lateral meniscus and the semimembranosus on the medial meniscus as well as the rolling action of the femoral condyles. The lateral meniscus is more mobile. The medial meniscus has a more firm peripheral attachment to the medial capsular ligament. Motion with flexion and extension occurs between the menisci and the femur. Rotary motion of the knee occurs between the menisci and the tibia.

CRUCIATE LIGAMENTS

The cruciate ligaments function in both anteroposterior and rotary stability. With external rotation of the tibia on the femur, the cruciates unwind. With continued external rotation, the anterior cruciate ligament is wrapped around the medial side of the lateral femoral condyle and limits further external rotation. With internal rotation, the cruciate ligaments twist on each other and limit internal rotation. Owing to the oblique insertions on the femoral condyles, a torsional effect is placed on the cruciates with flexion and extension. This arrangement maintains some fibers of the cruciates taut at all times. (Further detailed discussion of cruciate anatomy is on p. 1540.)

DISRUPTION OF THE EXTENSOR MECHANISM

Four injuries around the knee may disrupt the extensor mechanism and interfere with its normal function. These are quadriceps tendon rupture, fractures of the patella, patellar tendon ruptures, and avulsion of the tibial tubercle. The mechanism of injury—other than direct laceration or direct blow to the patella or tendons—is the same (*i.e.,* sudden violent contraction of the quadriceps against the body weight with the knee flexed). The age of the patient and inherent weakness in a particular unit of the quadriceps mechanism determines which segment is injured by the overload.

McMaster[522] has shown that normal tendon does not rupture under stress. Linear tension on a musculotendinous unit causes disruption at the musculotendinous junction, in the muscle belly, or at the tendinous insertion into bone. He showed that even with 75% of the tendon fibers severed, normal activity did not cause rupture. Rupture of tendinous tissue is, therefore, associated with some pathologic process. (This concept has been questioned by Barfred,[505] who explained the osseous failure of tendon insertions in laboratory animals by decreased bone strength, due to their inactivity.) Predisposing factors include tendinous calcification, arthritis, acute infectious disease, systemic lupus erythematosus, syphilis, tubercular tenosynovitis, old fractures, tumor, fatty degeneration, and metabolic diseases. Cases of rupture of apparently normal tendon may be due to microscopic damage to the vascular supply to tendons. Steroid injections into tendinous tissue have been implicated as a causative factor in tendon rupure.[516,538]

Age appears to play a very important role as to whether the patellar tendon ruptures or the quadriceps tendon tears. A review of the literature from 1880 until 1978 revealed 117 cases in which the age of the patient was given.[532] Eighty-eight percent of the quadriceps tendon ruptures occurred in patients who were 40 years old or older, while 80% of the patellar ligament ruptures occurred in patients who were younger than forty years.

Symptoms of extensor tendon rupture about the knee are pain, crepitation, and loss of function. When the continuity loss is in the quadriceps tendon a defect is present, and the anterior femur can be palpated easily. If the tear occurs below the patella, the patella shifts upward. Late or neglected cases of either condition are recognized by extensor weakness, difficulty in climbing stairs, or lack of stability when walking or running.

The objectives of treatment for disruptions of the extensor mechanism are apposition of the ruptured parts and restoration of quadriceps muscle power. Treatment choices are nonoperative immobilization or operative restoration of continuity. In nearly all cases, the surgical approach is recommended to insure firm healing of so important a structure.

In late cases, Conway[85] has listed four factors that determine successful treatment. These are (1) ablation of all old cicatricial tissue, (2) restoration of the continuity of the tendons, (3) rehabilitation of the quadriceps, and (4) absence of any intra-articular complications.

RUPTURE OF THE QUADRICEPS TENDON

Few conditions have such an illustrious list of early contributors to the literature as does rupture of the quadriceps tendon. Reports begin with Galen's description of the condition, and include Lister's report of his first attempt at surgical repair, and McBurney's study,[520] who was the first to publish his technique of surgical repair in the American literature in 1887.[509] The latter used catgut to approximate the tendon to the patella, followed by silver wire attached through drill holes in the patella to reinforce the repair.

Although it would seem to be an injury easily recognized, Ramsey and Müller[525] reported a series of 17 cases, only ten of which were recognized within the first week. The other seven went unrecognized and untreated for from 14 days to a year.

SURGICAL ANATOMY

(See Knee Anatomy, p. 1482.)

MECHANISM OF INJURY

The usual mechanism is a sudden violent reflex contraction of the quadriceps against the weight of the body, as when attempting to avoid a fall from a sudden slip or stumble. This mechanism often fractures the patella, detaches the patellar tendon (particularly in the adolescent), or produces a supra- or dicondylar fracture of the femur. Rupture of the quadriceps tendon is seen more frequently in the sixth and seventh decades of life, when the tendon may be weakened. With the knee in the semi-flexed position, the patella is held firmly over the anterior aspect of the femur buttressed by the medial and lateral femoral condyles as it sits in the patellofemoral groove. Failure of the extensor mechanism occurs at the weakest point as determined by pre-existing pathology. Factors that contribute to the quadriceps tendon weakness include obesity, fibrotic changes in the tendon from arteriosclerosis, old injuries, lues, or other degenerative conditions. Rupture of this tendon has been reported in association with diabetes mellitus, nephritis, gout, and hyperparathyroidism.

PATHOLOGY OF THE TEAR

Tears begin in the central portion anteriorly, and extend into the medial and lateral fibers; the extent of tearing depends on the duration and amount of force. The proximal margin usually retracts 2 cm to 5 cm. Partial tears usually involve only the superficial layer of the quadriceps tendon. Complete tears involve the entire three layers of this tendon. Ruptures often occur at different levels of the three layers of the quadriceps; the deeper layers tear at a higher level than the superficial layer. The synovial membrane of the suprapatellar pouch is commonly torn in complete tears.

When any of the associated conditions mentioned above are present, pathological changes in the tendon may be seen. These include fibrinoid necrosis, chronic inflammatory reaction that may accompany chronic tophaceous synovitis, as well as the fatty degeneration often seen in the obese. McLaughlin and Francis biopsied fresh ruptures and routinely demonstrated "a decrease in collagen in the tendon fibers and marked loss of nuclei with fibrotic degeneration."[521] In Ramsey and Müller's[525] series all adults with rupured quadriceps tendons showed radiographic evidence of degenerative joint disease and some degree of obesity.

SIGNS AND SYMPTOMS

The history of injury of the mechanism is as described and is associated with a sudden knifelike pain. After the intense initial pain, which lasts only a few minutes, subsequent pain may be minimal. Some return of quadriceps function may occur after several weeks without treatment. The patient continues to note frequent episodes of buckling of the knee and inability to climb stairs or inclines without support.

The most obvious complaint and physical finding is the inability to extend the knee or maintain the passively extended knee against gravity. If the rupture is incomplete, lack of complete extension may be confused with an internal derangement of the knee. The diagnosis may be missed, because the knee may have little swelling or the patient, little pain. Evaluation may reveal no evidence of ligamentous laxity, and x-rays show no fracture. The condition then may be misdiagnosed as a sprain. Testing for the integrity of the quadriceps mechanism by having the patient actively extend the knee is an essential part of a knee examination.

Physical findings include a palpable soft tissue defect proximal to the superior pole of the patella. The patella may be noted to sit lower on the femoral condyles on the injured side when compared with the opposite knee when standing. The patella can be moved easily from side to side. A large hemarthrosis or subcutaneous ecchymosis may be present. If the synovial membrane has been ruptured, hemarthrosis is not present. If complete rupture has occurred, standing is possible, but walking is not. When seen later (after several weeks) contraction of the quadriceps may be noted easily. Late fibrosis developing in the rectus femoris primarily, and to a lesser extent in the vastus medialis, vastus lateralis, and vastus intermedius, may produce some return of quadriceps function.

X-rays may reveal the more distal position of the

patella or fragments of bone from the superior pole of the patella detached along with the tendinous insertion.

METHODS OF TREATMENT

Early repair gives a better result in complete or significant tears. This is clearly demonstrated in the series of Siwek and Rao.[532] Immediate repair of quadriceps tendon ruptures in 30 patients were all graded excellent or good. All patients in the group had knee motion of 120° or more after physical therapy. Although the number of patients was smaller, the results of late repair were far less gratifying. Six patients were reviewed, and three were graded as good and three as unsatisfactory. Only one patient regained more than 90° of knee flexion. Persisting quadriceps atrophy was the rule and not the exception.

If there has been only a partial tear with an extensor deficiency of only a few degrees, a cylinder cast with the knee in full extension can be used for 5 to 6 weeks. We lean toward surgical repair unless the general condition of the patient contraindicates surgery or the weakness of full extensor power is compatible with the activity level of the patient. Those patients with more extensive tearing and loss of voluntary quadriceps contraction require surgical reapproximation of the tendon.

After the exposure of the torn tendon one must ascertain if the tear extends into the knee joint. If so, synovial membrane closure must first be accomplished. If the tear is at the suprapatellar region, fixation to the patella through drill holes is best. Repair of the tendinous substance requires reapproximation of the decussating fibers of the vastus medialis and lateralis. Restoration of the rectus femoris layer is then done. Careful placement of sutures is necessary, both for secure apposition of tissue and to avoid obstructing the blood vessels found in the tendinous substance.

Several methods have been described to minimize the difficulty of approximating ragged tissue end-to-end. Kangaroo tendon has been used as a suture in the past. Quadriceps-plasty with insertion of the quadriceps tendon into a bone trough on the superior patella can be done, if enough mobilization of the quadriceps is available.

Acute Injuries

For fresh ruptures, debridement of shredded portions of the tendon and approximation by mattress sutures with the knee in full extension is used. Because degenerative processes within the tendon are present in most ruptures, a reinforcement of

the suture line by turning a triangular flap of quadriceps tendon distally as described by Scuderi[528] is recommended. A Bunnell pull-out wire, pulling the quadriceps distally to take tension off the suture line, can be added for increased security. McLaughlin and Francis[521] used a tibial bolt through the patella. The wires passing through the quadriceps tendon are tied to the bolt on each side of the patella to reduce tension on the suture line (see Rupture of the Patellar Tendon, p. 1494). Ramsey and Müller[525] have used a Kirschner wire through the distal end of the proximal side of the repair, incorporating this in the cast for fixation.

Late Repair

When repair is done late, approximation of the edges may be impossible. A lengthening of the quadriceps tendon by the method of Codivilla[528] can be used. Often a fascia lata strip is preferable as suture material to provide some bulk and increased strength to the suture line. Buttner[507] described a method of taking strips from the vastus medialis and vastus lateralis to reinforce a free fascia lata graft for an old tear with wide separation.

Ramsey and Müller[525] used a transverse incision rather than the longitudinal incision described by Scuderi.[528] We likewise use the transverse incision and find this to be very satisfactory, although a longitudinal incision does, indeed, also give you adequate exposure. They further stated that a pull-out wire is not necessary if repair is done within the first week. Care must be exercised so as not to shorten the quadriceps mechanism, particularly in the younger active person. When this occurs the normal glide of the patella through the femoral groove may be excessively tight and may produce patellar symptoms. A skier whom one of us (R. L. L.) examined had sustained a quadriceps tendon rupture with repair 1 year earlier. Her patellar symptoms were disabling enough to prevent her from skiing competitively, although she did have full extensor power.

AUTHORS' PREFERRED TREATMENT

Surgical repair of the acutely torn quadriceps tendon is the treatment of choice unless the tear is partial or the patient's general condition is unstable. As mentioned earlier, we debride the shredded portions of the tendon and approximate the tendon with mattress sutures. A triangular flap of quadriceps tendon is turned distally to reinforce the suture line. We recommend the use of suture line tension sparing techniques as described by McLaughlin.[521] Remember that the quadriceps tendon is a trilaminar structure and may extend into the synovium and retinaculum medially or laterally. This often needs to be repaired.

In the late repair of the quadriceps tendon, do not approximate the tendon under undue tension. Because of possible patellar problems, lengthening of the quadriceps tendon by the method of Codivilla[528] is preferred.

POSTOPERATIVE CARE

A plaster cylinder with the knee in full extension is worn for 6 weeks. The pull-out wires may be removed after 3 weeks. Weight bearing is allowed with the cast on. After removal of the cast, supervised active exercise to regain motion and strength is started. During the first few weeks of active use, the knee should be protected to prevent inadvertent forced flexion. We use a postoperative knee brace with surrounding stays that can be removed for exercise periods and bathing. As soon as motion to 60° of flexion and extension of the knee with 20 pounds of weight can be accomplished, the splint is discontinued.

PROGNOSIS

Ramsey and Müller[525] report that maximum improvement is obtained within the first 6 months. The best results are found in those patients who had an early repair. Those repaired late rarely regain full extension power, although good knee motion and stability are present.

COMPLICATIONS

Weakness of extension or lack of flexion may occur and are more likely in late repairs. Recurrent rupture can occur if too violent an activity is allowed too soon. The degenerative processes that allowed the rupture to occur remain. Preventive measures (such as weight reduction in the obese) should be instituted if possible.

Excessive shortening of the quadriceps mechanism may produce patellar compression problems in an active athletic person doing excessive and repeated deep flexion of the knee.

Calcification or ossification of ruptured tissues may occur in missed or neglected quadriceps tears (Fig. 16-54).

RUPTURE OF THE PATELLAR TENDON

The continuation of the quadriceps tendon distal to the patella has been called tendon by some and ligament by others. Though it attaches to bone proximally and distally, the patella is merely a sesamoid bone in the common tendinous structure of the quadriceps.

Rupture of the patellar tendon is the least common injury producing extensor mechanism disruption. Disruption through the substance of the tendon is particularly rare; most occur at the tendon insertions proximally and distally. McMaster[522] in reviewing the literature in 1933 did not find any cases of rupture through the patellar tendon. A study at the Mayo Clinic[504] of 54 quadriceps disruptions found that about one third involve the patellar tendon, but the authors did not state which portion of the tendon is involved.

SURGICAL ANATOMY

Proximally the tendon attaches to the inferior border of the patella on both its superficial and deep surfaces. Beneath the proximal part of the tendon is the infrapatellar fat pad, which separates the tendon from the synovial membrane. The importance of the fat pad is that it carries the vascular supply to the tendon. Disruption of this fat pad or overly generous surgical dissection in this region may cause necrosis of the tendon.

The distal attachment is to the tibial tubercle. The lower portion of the tendon is separated from the tibia by the deep infrapatellar bursa. A certain number of fibers extend downward from the quadriceps tendon and into the patellar tendon but do not insert directly or indirectly into the tibial tuberosity. These attach to surrounding fascia. This becomes clinically important with tibial tubercle fracture, because only partial loss of function occurs if these fibers are still intact.

Overlying the tendon is a thin fascial membrane—the tendon sheath—continuing from the extensor retinaculum above. This membrane can often be used to cover suture lines after surgical repair.

MECHANISM OF INJURY

The mechanism for patellar tendon rupture is basically the same as for the other injuries of the extensor mechanism. The unexpected stretch of the quadriceps along with a forceful quadriceps contraction produces a dynamic overload on the extensor system. This injury is most likely to occur in a young adult athlete with a strong quadriceps muscle whose tibial epiphyses have closed. According to Kelikian and colleagues[517] the tendon commonly avulses from the inferior pole of the patella, often with a small ossicle from the bone. Studies[516,538] have suggested that injections of steroids into tendinous tissue lessen its tensile strength

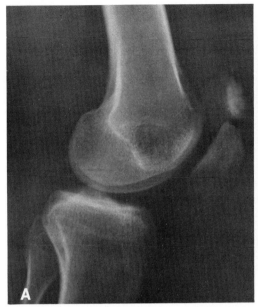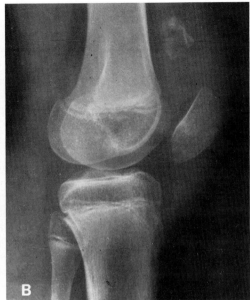

Fig. 16-54. A 13-year-old boy involved in a bicycle accident sustained massive swelling and stiffness about the knee. Subsequently he slipped on two occasions and the knee collapsed under him. Two months later he slipped, heard a loud snap in front of the knee, and was unable to straighten the leg actively. Surgical exploration 3 months after the original injury showed that the entire medial quadriceps mechanism was torn and the quadriceps retracted. There was considerable calcification in the quadriceps tendon. The quadriceps mechanism was reattached surgically to the proximal patella. (*A*) X-ray 2 months after original injury, 10 days after last injury. There was calcific plaque proximal to the patella, which sat farther distally than normal. The patient was unable to actively extend the knee. (Courtesy of O. N. Jones, M.D., Hillsboro, Oregon.) (*B*) X-ray 4 years after original injury. The patient complained of patellar pain with activity. The patella was in a more distal position than normal.

and predispose the tendon to rupture with vigorous activity. Bilateral rupture has been reported in patients with systemic lupus erythematosus.[527,538]

SIGNS AND SYMPTOMS

Discomfort and inability to extend the knee suggest disruption of the extensor mechanism. An abnormally high patella with increased mobility from side to side and a palpable defect at the patellar tendon site indicates the site of extensor mechanism inadequacy (Fig. 16-55). Occasionally swelling and hematoma over the patellar tendon may mask the defect. In late or neglected cases, weakness of the extensor mechanism may be manifest by difficulty climbing stairs or inability to run. Thigh muscles may feel weak and tight, and some atrophy of the quadriceps musculature may be evident.

X-rays may show a small fragment of bone from the inferior pole of the patella or from the tibial attachment, which is pulled loose with the tendinous attachment. The pathognomonic sign, with or without bone avulsion, is an upward shift of the patella, which can be noted clinically and verified by lateral x-rays.

METHODS OF TREATMENT

Acute Injuries

Surgical reapproximation of the torn tendon ends is necessary to reestablish the extensor mechanism. The capsule on either side of the tendon may also be torn and should be repaired. Those cases with only partial tear should also be repaired, unless a contraindication exists. Surgical treatment provides a quicker and more certain end result.

Tears from the inferior border of the patella can be reattached to the patella through drill holes. Detachments from the tibial attachment should also be attached directly to the tibia. When suturing the

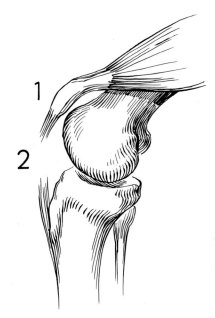

Fig. 16-55. Disruptions of the patellar tendon are diagnosed by the abnormally high patella (*1*) and a palpable defect in the patellar tendon (*2*).

tendon substance, care should be exercised so that blood supply to the tendon is not obstructed. McMaster[522] has shown in animal experiments that the blood supply is through the substance of the tendon rather than its sheath. Repair of the sheath is important to reduce adhesion to overlying tissue.

To take the tension off the healing tissue, one of several methods can be used. These are (1) use of a Kirschner wire through the patella incorporating it into the cast to hold the patella downward; (2) a Bunnell pull-out wire; (3) McLaughlin's[521] technique using a circular wire with a pull-out loop around the superior pole of the patella with each end secured distally to a tibial bolt passed transversely through the tibial tuberosity; or (4) the method of Chandler[508] using a circular wire through a proximal transverse drill hole in the patella and a transverse drill hole at the tibial tuberosity.

Late Repair

Late repair of patellar tendon rupture is more difficult because of quadriceps contraction. Often it is necessary to use preliminary skeletal traction through the patella for several weeks to allow enough stretching of the quadriceps for repair.

Two methods of late repair are described in *Campbell's Operative Orthopaedics*.[502] One method uses a strip of fascia lata inserted through a trans-verse hole in the distal third of the patella and woven distally through the proximal patellar tendon, across the defect and into the distal fragment of the patellar tendon.

The second method is as described by Kelikian, Riashi, and Gleason.[517] The first stage requires a simple surgical release of adhesions of the quadriceps-patellar tendon, followed by skeletal traction with active quadriceps exercise. After quadriceps contraction is overcome, the second operation is done. The semitendinous tendon is detached proximally at its musculotendinous junction and left attached distally. Its free end is passed through a drill hole in the tibial tuberosity from medial to lateral. The tendon end is then passed proximally and threaded laterally to medially through a drill hole in the distal third of the patella. The tendon end is sutured to itself distally, or, if it is not long enough, to the gracilis tendon on the medial side of the knee. Postoperatively, the Kirschner wire used previously for traction is incorporated with a traction bow in a long-leg cylinder cast in extension to relieve tension on the suture lines.

AUTHORS' PREFERRED TREATMENT

In acute tears of the patellar tendon, approximation of the torn tendon is most desirable. If the tear is located at the distal patellar pole-tendon interface, reattachment of the tendon to the patella through drill holes is performed. We prefer the technique of McLaughlin,[521] which takes the tension off of the healing tissue. In late repairs, the two stage procedure of Kelikian[57] is our treatment of choice.

POSTOPERATIVE CARE

A long-leg cylinder cast with the knee in extension is used postoperatively. Quadriceps setting exercises are started as soon after surgery as the patient can tolerate them. Six weeks of immobilization allows the tissues to heal. Following the cast, the patient should be afforded some protection by a postoperative knee brace until quadriceps power has returned, to prevent any unexpected collapse of the knee. Vigorous activity requiring strong quadriceps contraction should be restricted until quadriceps strength has returned.

McLaughlin and Francis[521] believed that firm fixation was produced by the pull-out wire technique. Balanced suspension after 72 hours was started and knee flexion to 30° was allowed. After mobilization, a cylinder cast in extension was used. Ambulation with weight bearing was permitted in 2 to 4 weeks postoperatively, depending on the severity of the injury. At 8 weeks the cast and pull-out wire and tibial bolt were removed. A cast brace with a hinge constructed to limit knee flexion to 30°, we believe, would be a satisfactory modification of this regimen.

PROGNOSIS

Fresh tendon ruptures repaired early give satisfying results. In the series by Siwek and Rao,[532] 20 patients with immediate repair of the patellar ligament were graded as having excellent results. All of these patients regained a full range of motion and normal strength of the quadriceps muscle. Four patients were graded as good because of the limitation of full knee motion. Like the atrophy often present in other muscles after tendon repair, persistent quadriceps atrophy may be noticed. Late repair is less satisfactory and the likelihood of regaining full extension is less.

COMPLICATIONS

In the repair of the patellar tendon, it is important to be mindful of the patellofemoral mechanism. If the patellar tendon is excessively shortened, a low-lying patella (patella baja) may be produced. This situation increases patellar compression and may produce cartilaginous erosion of the patellar articular surfaces. A test for full flexion of the knee and observation of the position of the patella with flexion at the time of operation will help to allow proper repair with the right amount of tendon tension.

TRAUMATIC DISLOCATION OF THE PATELLA

Review of the literature on acute traumatic dislocation of the patella impresses one with the rarity of this condition as compared to recurrent dislocations and subluxations of the patella. Though a recurrent dislocation had an initial episode when it was the first dislocation, the frequency of recurrence and the associated finding of a congenital deficiency of the extensor mechanism makes one mindful of the relative stability of the normal patellofemoral relationship. Indeed, if a normal patellofemoral configuration is present, the supporting muscles are normal, and the alignment of the knee mechanics is adequate, a relatively severe injury is necessary to produce a dislocation. It is our impression that more problems arise from a patella that is too tight and produces too much pressure in its gliding action in the patellofemoral groove than from one that is too loose.

SURGICAL ANATOMY

The osseous anatomy of the patella has been covered in the section on knee anatomy (see pp. 1480–1482). The vastus medialis and medial retinaculum act to guy the patella medially. The lateral retinaculum has a similar function laterally. Thickenings of the lateral and medial retinacula pass from the patellar margins to the femur (patellofemoral ligaments) as well as a distal expansion medially and laterally from the patella to the tibia (patellotibial ligaments). This complex of guy bands direct the patella in its path through the patellofemoral groove.

Because the mechanical axis of the femur and its anatomical axis do not coincide (see Anatomy, p. 1482) the direction of the pull of the quadriceps tendon is not in the same alignment as the patellar tendon. The patella sits at the apex between the two (called the Q-angle; Fig. 16-56). Though this situation produces an inherent tendency toward lateral luxation, this is more than normally compensated for in the normal knee by the triangular shape of the patella, the depth of the patellofemoral groove, and the guy action mentioned above. If there is a deficiency or inadequacy of one of the above factors, predisposition toward subluxation, dislocation, or recurrence is present.

MECHANISM OF INJURY

The usual mechanism for dislocation is a powerful quadriceps contraction or a direct blow to the patella when the knee is flexed. In athletic activity, when a runner is cutting to the direction opposite the planted foot, a valgus knee force and external rotation of the leg adds to the vectors acting to force the patella laterally out of its groove.

Some of the predisposing abnormalities that enhance the trauma are (1) a more laterally inserted patellar tendon, (2) an excessive external tibial torsion (often related to 1), (3) internal femoral rotation that acts functionally as 1, (4) femoral neck anteversion with internal rotation of the femoral condyles (often seen with external tibial torsion), (5) abnormally high patella (patella alta),[555] (6) insufficient height of the lateral femoral condyle with a resultant shallow patellofemoral groove,[554] (7) weakness of the anteromedial retinaculum, (8) dystrophy or weakness of the vastus medialis muscle, (9) genu valgum (congenital or acquired), (10) genu recurvatum, producing a general laxity of the extensor mechanism and loss of general buttressing action of the lateral femoral condyle, and (11) hypermobility of the patella due to poor muscle tone.

A rare type of patellar dislocation—intra-articular dislocation of the patella—occurs from a direct blow over the partially flexed knee, which forces the patella from its superior and anterior moorings into the intra-articular space.

CLASSIFICATION

Afflictions of the patellofemoral integrity may be classified as follows:

A. Acute dislocation
  1. Lateral
     a. With congenital abnormality
     b. Without congenital abnormality
  2. Intra-articular (variously called downward dislocation, horizontal luxation, intercondylar dislocation)
  3. Vertical (Watson-Jones[678] described such a case in which the patella was pushed proximally and locked over osteophytes on the anterior surfaces of the femoral condyles)
  4. Intercondylar (associated with fracture of the femoral condyles)
B. Recurrent dislocation (always associated with congenital abnormality or acquired deficiency of the patello-femoral extensor mechanism)
C. Subluxations (Hughston[607] believes this condition is always associated with a predisposing congenital deficiency of the extensor mechanism)
D. Habitual dislocations (the patella dislocates every time the knee is flexed, and is associated with quadriceps contracture. Differential point from recurrent dislocations is that if the patella is held forcibly in the midline, the knee cannot be flexed more than 30°. Further flexion is possible only if the patella is allowed to dislocate.)

Though medial dislocation of the patella can occur with the proper magnitude and direction of force, we have never seen it as an acute condition. It does, however, occur as a complication of a patellar tendon transplant for correction of recurrent lateral dislocations.

SIGNS AND SYMPTOMS

It is surprising to us how many patients who have a dislocated patella or have had one that reduced spontaneously are unaware of the problem. Often

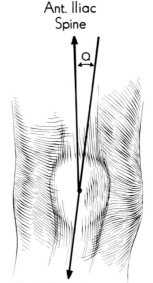

Fig. 16-56. The Q-angle is the angle formed between a line from the anterior superior iliac spine to the center of the patella and a line from the center of the patella to the center of the tibial tubercle with the foot held straight up. (The illustration shows the right knee from the front.) This angle may be increased in those people who are predisposed to dislocation.

the injury is masked by trousers, and the patient relates that the knee "went out of joint" or that it "popped" (often twice—once when it went out and once when it spontaneously reduced with extension of the leg).

If the patella is still dislocated when examined, the deformity and prominence lateral to the lateral femoral condyle are easily discernible (Fig. 16-57). When reduction occurs spontaneously, as is often the case, it sometimes becomes difficult to tell if the patient sustained a meniscal tear or a patellar dislocation. The knee is swollen, often with a bloody effusion. If seen early, the tenderness along the medial aspect of the patella and over the lateral femoral condyle can be detected. Some say that the defect in the medial retinacula from the tearing of this tissue can be palpated. (We have never been so fortunate.) There is often tenderness on the undersurface of the patella and discomfort with compression. One helpful sign is easily elicited by pushing the patella laterally—the Fairbank's test. The patient will anxiously grab at the knee, because this reproduces the feeling that whatever slipped out before is about to slip again. This sign is variously called the grab sign, panic sign, and the anxiety or apprehension sign.

The patient is often seen some time after the initial dislocation or only after several recurrences. After reduction has occurred, the discomfort is minimal and only if there is considerable swelling does the symptom of tightness occur. This may be the patient's chief complaint. When seen late, the pain is often nondescript and poorly localized. The patient gives a history of locking, popping, or giving out.

A patient with subluxation gives a similar history. The catching is due to the slipping of the patella into the patellofemoral groove at the moment during walking or running when the weight-bearing leg begins to extend from the flexed position (*i.e.,* between mid-stance and takeoff). It is, therefore, a disorder of acceleration. Hamstring spasm may occur, producing a limitation of extension. Acute dislocation may occur after recurrent subluxation.

Either the acute dislocation or recurrent dislocation or subluxation may be confused with a torn medial meniscus. Each occurs in a similar fashion on a flexed valgus knee with strong quadriceps contraction. We are particularly careful with female patients to rule out patellar pathology before diagnosing a meniscal lesion. Arthrograms are helpful in this differential.

The intra-articular dislocations are recognized by the prominence at the joint line anteriorly and the defect immediately above the prominence. The knee cannot be extended, even passively. Either the superior pole is pointed posteriorly with the articular surface inferiorly or the inferior pole is pointed posteriorly with the articular surface pointing superiorly. The superior pole pointing posteriorly is by far the most common.

A condition frequently associated with patellar dislocations is an osteochondral fracture (see Fig. 16-60). This occurs to the lateral femoral condyle or medial patellar facet as the patella snaps back into the patellofemoral groove. When this injury has occurred, hemarthrosis is certain to be present. The fracture fragment may produce signs of internal derangement (causing further difficulty in differentiating from a meniscal tear). The fragment may or may not be visible on x-rays. When a fragment is visible in a chronic knee problem, one should be mindful of patellar dislocation as its cause. Rarely, the force during reduction may be severe enough to result in a comminuted fracture of the patella.[543]

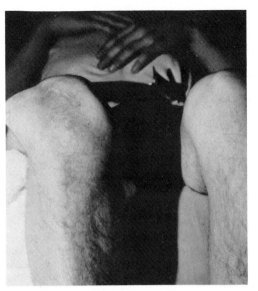

Fig. 16-57. Appearance of the knee with a dislocated patella.

RADIOGRAPHIC FINDINGS

An x-ray should be taken, even if the diagnosis is evident, to determine if osteochondral fractures are present (Fig. 16-58). It is preferable to get an x-ray before and after reduction, because osteochondral fragments are often difficult to see or are obscured by overlying shadows.

When evaluating the patella, multiple views are needed. No single view clearly demonstrates all of the retropatellar surface or is pathognomonic of a patient's predisposition to further dislocation or subluxation because of patellofemoral dysplasia. A "patella survey" consisting of a standing anteroposterior view including both knees, a lateral view with the knee flexed 30°, a lateral view with the knee flexed 90°, a tangential view taken by the Hughston method, and a Merchant's view,[646] which includes both knees, is recommended. Oblique projections with the leg rotated inward and outward 45° allow unobstructed visualization of the patellar margins and can be added when an osteochondral fracture is suspected.

The anteroposterior view shows the position of the patella in relation to the femoral sulcus and the joint line. If technique is proper, the contour of the patella can be evaluated and fractures of the margins or body ascertained. One should be mindful of the possibility of a bipartite patella and closely correlate clinical and radiographic findings.

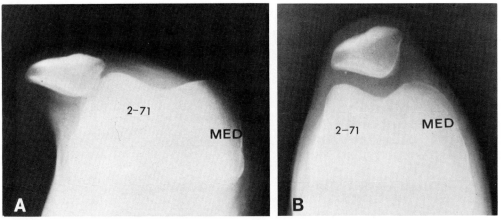

Fig. 16-58. A 17-year-old boy sustained a dislocated patella while playing handball. He had had no previous problems. He suffered a recurrence 3 years later while skiing. It reduced spontaneously. (*A*) Initial injury showed the lateral dislocation of the patella. (*B*) Postreduction view. Note the patellar configuration (Jägerhut) and the decreased height of the lateral femoral condyle.

On the anteroposterior film, two observations can be made with respect to patellofemoral relationship. The inferior pole of the patella normally lies at the level of the joint line. If, however, the inferior pole is proximally diplaced greater than 20 mm, one should suspect patella alta. On the perfectly aligned standing anteroposterior view, the patella should be centered over the femoral sulcus. If this is not the case, lateral subluxation is a possibility.

A lateral view of the knee with 30° of flexion is helpful in assessing the relationship of the patella to the femoral sulcus. In 1938, Blumensaat described a method of determining patella alta. Blumensaat's line is drawn through and parallel to the bony cortical roof of the intercondylar notch of the femur (Fig. 16-59). Patella alta was thought to exist if the inferior tip of the patella lay above this line. However, Brattstrom[555] evaluated 100 randomly selected patients and found an average variance of between 27° to 60° in the angle formed by Blumensaat's line and the longitudinal axis of the femur. Jacobson and Bertheussen concluded that the normal patella can be up to 30 mm above Blumensaat's line and not exhibit patella alta.

Because of the inexact nature of Blumensaat's line, Insall proposed another means of determining patella alta. The simplicity and applicability of Insall's[617] ratio of length of the patella to the length of the patellar tendon to the routine lateral radiograph makes this method attractive. The normal ratio is approximately 1:1. More than 20% variation

indicates an abnormal patella position, and a ratio of 0.8:1 or less indicates patella alta.

A lateral x-ray taken with the knee flexed 90° may also be used to help diagnose a high riding patella. Labelle and Laurin[626] noted that a line extending down the anterior aspect of the shaft of the femur passes over the superior pole of the patella in 97% of normal knees. Patella alta is present if the patella is above this line.

Merchant[646] described an x-ray that is taken with the knee flexed 45° over the end of the table. This view is designed to demonstrate the relationship of the patella to the femoral sulcus in a tangenital fashion. The congruence angle is calculated by bisecting the sulcus angle to establish the 0 reference line. A second line is then projected from the apex of the sulcus angle through the lowest point on the central articular ridge of the patella. The angle measured between these two lines is the congruence angle. If the apex of the patellar articular ridge is lateral to the 0 reference line, then a positive value is assigned to the congruence angle. If the apex is medial to the 0 line, the congruence angle is considered to be negative. A congruence angle of greater than +16° is abnormal.

Laurin[633] described a tangential patellar view that is taken with the knee flexed 20° to 30°. The calculation is simple; however, this view is technically difficult, as the knee is flexed only 20°.

The Hughston view[607] is also very helpful in determining the status of the patellofemoral joint (Fig. 16-60). If subluxation or previous dislocation

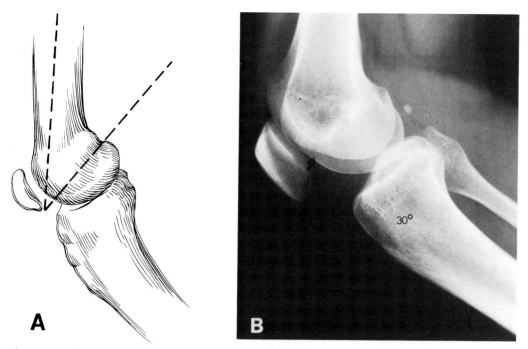

Fig. 16-59. Blumensaat's line (*A*) is a line projected through and parallel to the dome of the intercondylar fossa. (*B*) It is identified on a lateral x-ray by the increased density of cortical bone at the roof of the fossa (*arrow*).

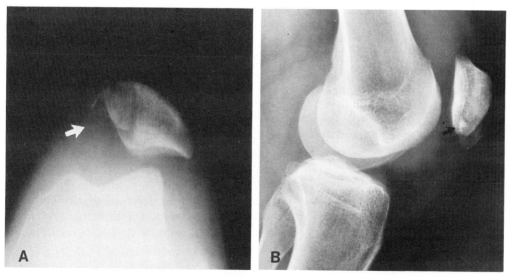

Fig. 16-60. A 21-year-old woman sustained a dislocated kneecap while running. She had a history of two previous dislocations and many subluxations. The present dislocation was reduced by the patient but subsequently developed hemarthrosis. (*A*) A Hughston view showed the fracture of the medial side of the patella. Note the persistent lateral subluxation. (*B*) A lateral view showed the fracture to be on the inferior portion of the medial edge, which is the common site for osteochondral fractures of the patella associated with dislocation.

is suspected, this view is carefully evaluated for (1) tilting of the patella (noted by increased joint space between the medial facet and groove in reference to the lateral joint space); (2) subluxation when the lateral edge of the patella lies laterally to the rim of the lateral femoral condyle and the apex of the patella is lateral to the deepest part of the patellofemoral groove; (3) patellar configuration and classification according to Wiberg and Baumgartl (see Figs. 16-47 and 16-58, and Anatomy, p. 1481); (4) the depth of the patello-femoral groove and deficiency of the lateral femoral condyle; and (5) osteochondral fractures (Fig. 16-60).

Evaluation of intra-articular dislocation is best made by the lateral view. Whether the articular surface of the patella faces inferiorly or superiorly indicates which pole of the patella is trapped in the joint. When the articular surface points distally, the superior pole of the patella is pointing posteriorly.

As is obvious by now, it is seldom that a single view provides the treating physician with enough information to diagnose a spontaneous reduction of an acute dislocation or demonstrate all of the patellofemoral joint characteristics that predispose to recurrent dislocations. Therefore, a systematic radiographic approach and correlation with the clinical history and physical findings must be used.

METHODS OF TREATMENT

Reduction of the laterally dislocated patella is usually accomplished easily with extension of the knee as gentle pressure, directed medially from the lateral side of the patella, is applied. If marked apprehension or guarding interferes with this maneuver, a short-acting general anesthetic can be given. Care should be taken to avoid forceful reduction, which might produce an osteochondral fracture.

After reduction, a cylinder cast with the knee in extension is applied and worn for 6 weeks. While the knee is in the cast, quadriceps tone is maintained by daily quadriceps setting exercises. Quadriceps tightening is initiated immediately and done as pain allows. As soreness recedes, four-point shrug exercises and progressive resistance exercises are begun. The four-point shrug exercise is:

1. Tighten the quadriceps muscle as strongly as possible.
2. Without relaxing, tighten some more.
3. Without relaxing, lift the leg and tighten the muscle some more.
4. Without relaxing, lower the leg and tighten the quadriceps some more.

Patients are told that this is like pulling all the slack out of a rope as it is wound around a winch. They are instructed to do this exercise before meals and at bedtime, working up to where they can do it 50 times at each sitting (four times a day).

Should early surgical repair of acute patellar dislocations be considered? There is not a universally accepted answer to this problem. The success of conservative treatment of patellofemoral dysfunction is well documented. DeHaven and colleagues[567] reported a success rate of 82% in young athletes with patellofemoral syndromes treated conservatively. Henry and Crosland[601] reported that 76% of their patients with patellofemoral subluxation improved with nonoperative care. Palumbo[651] has described a dynamic patellar brace that is thought beneficial in patellar subluxation in growing children, in patients with mild or occasional subluxation, and patients with acute subluxation, or persons with dislocation or subluxation in which surgery is contraindicated or must be delayed. However, it does not appear that the success of conservative care for the less catastrophic patellofemoral dysfunction syndromes can be transferred to the patients with acute patellar dislocations. A recent report by Cofield and Bryan[559] demonstrates a 42% failure rate for nonsurgical treatment of acute patellar dislocations. This high rate of recurrence is extremely bothersome. Because of residual problems following dislocations, numerous authors advocate immediate surgical repair for acute dislocations.[574,649,654,662,665,668] O'Donoghue[649] feels that surgical repair of the medial retinaculum after an acute dislocation achieves better apposition of torn tissue, and hence better healing with less inelastic scar. If surgical repair is decided upon care should be taken to correct any condition that predisposes to recurrence and to check for osteochondral fracture of the patella and edge of the lateral femoral condyle.

Cotta,[670] in 1959, reviewed 137 different operations for patellar dislocations. Others have been added since. Three basic types of procedures or combinations are used: (1) those involving soft tissue—tightening, release, transfer; (2) those involving bone tissue; and (3) those that include a patellectomy.

AUTHORS' PREFERRED TREATMENT

In a nonathlete with a first-time dislocation of the patella, we prefer immobilization alone if a defect in the medial retinaculum cannot be readily palpated and there is no radiographic evidence of an associated osteochondral fracture. With recurrent dislocations, however, a soft tissue procedure consisting of a formal lateral retinacular release and medial retinaculum plication are performed unless an abnormal Q angle is present. In the skeletally mature person with an abnormal Q angle, a bony procedure is also added. Our bony procedure of choice is the patellar tendon transplant done in the manner of Elmsie-Trillat[676] (Fig. 16-61). Great care is taken not to advance the patellar tendon distally but to merely shift it medially so that it is aligned with the anatomical axis of the femur. During either soft tissue procedures or bony procedures, it is wise to open the synovium and check for chondral fractures from the lateral femoral condyle or the retropatellar surface.

The competitive athlete with an acute first time dislocation of the patella presents a somewhat different problem. A rapid return to sporting activities and thus high demands on the knee necessitate a somewhat different approach. In these individuals we choose to examine the patient under anesthesia and to perform immediate arthroscopy. While performing the examination under anesthesia and arthroscopy, we evaluate the retropatellar surface, the lateral femoral condyle, the menisci, and the cruciate ligaments. If the medial retinaculum is torn, a medial plication and lateral retinacular release is undertaken. However, when the medial retinaculum is simply attenuated, we choose to perform a transarthroscopic lateral retinacular release alone. It is very seldom that we choose to perform a bony procedure. Only if extreme deficits exist in the extensor mechanism alignment do we also perform a tibial tubercle transplant.

If an osteochondral fracture is present, an arthrotomy is peformed to remove the fragment, or if it is large and involves the articular surface, to reattach it. Up to one third of the patellar facet can be removed without dysfunction. If the fragment is removed from the articular surface, the defect is shaved and drilled to allow fibrocartilaginous healing to occur. Postoperatively a cylinder cast with the knee in extension is applied. If desired, a bulky cotton compression dressing with a posterior plaster splint can be used. When swelling has subsided, the cylinder cast can be applied and worn for 6 weeks. Weight bearing is allowed when tolerated, and quadriceps exercises are begun as described above.

Intra-articular dislocations are very difficult to reduce. If reduction cannot be accomplished easily, immediate open reduction is recommended. Brady and Russell[553] recommend open reduction because

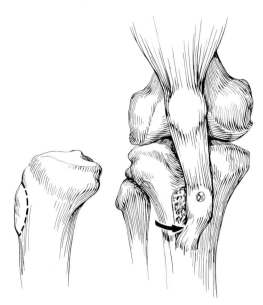

Fig. 16-61. Elmsie-Trillat method of patellar tendon transplant. The tibial tubercle is shifted medially to align the patellar tendon with the anatomical axis of the femur. Knee flexion is checked prior to seating of the screw to make certain the knee can be flexed fully and that the patella does not shift medially with flexion. (From Slocum, D. B.; Larson, R. L.; and James, S. L.: Late Reconstruction of the Medial Compartment of the Knee. Clin. Orthop., **100**:23–55, 1974.)

of the terrific force necessary for a successful closed reduction. The taut quadriceps mechanism retains the patella in its intra-articular position, acting as a bowstring in conjunction with the patellar tendon. Adequate relaxation to allow reduction is difficult to obtain, even with flexion of the hip and extension of the knee. This maneuver may be necessary along with a direct anterior pull on the patella during open reduction to extract the patella from the joint. Damage to the proximal or distal ligament attachments is generally not present, although there may be some periosteal elevation of the distal pole of the patella or elevation of the quadriceps tendon from the superior pole of the patella. After reduction has been accomplished, cylinder cast immobilization is continued for 4 to 6 weeks. Quadriceps exercises are also started as early as they can be tolerated.

PROGNOSIS AND COMPLICATIONS

Prognosis following an acute traumatic dislocation depends on several factors. If a deficiency of the extensor mechanism exists, the incidence of recurrence is very high. Andersen[541] stated that 75% of all patellar dislocations are associated with dysplasia of the patella or patellofemoral groove. Damage to the cartilaginous articular surfaces of the patella or femoral condyles or groove cannot be ascertained by x-rays. If considerable roughening has occurred, a prolongation of knee discomfort and patellofemoral joint deterioration are likely.

Surgical repair of patellar dislocations, either acute or recurrent, can produce postoperative complications. These include chondromalacia, degenerative joint disease, diminution in quadriceps strength, and medial dislocation of the patella.

DISLOCATION OF THE KNEE

Dislocation of the knee is a true surgical emergency. Notwithstanding its rarity and the differences of opinion about treatment of the ligamentous problems, there is unanimity of opinion that the vascular insult caused by such a severe injury requires immediate and respectful attention. The position of the joint when first seen cannot be considered an accurate indication of popliteal artery injury, because the immediate displacement caused by the violent force may have been much greater than can be appreciated at initial examination. In a series collected at Massachusetts General Hospital[728] between 1940 and 1968, 10 of 26 cases (38%) had vascular damage. Kennedy[715] reported a 32% incidence of vascular involvement in 22 cases. Peroneal nerve involvement brings the incidence of neurovascular involvement to 54% and 50% in each of the above series.

Accidents in motor vehicles are the most common mode of injury; athletic injuries probably rank second. Though violence is the usual cause, knee dislocations have been reported from lesser types of injuries, such as stepping into a hole or falling down steps.

SURGICAL ANATOMY

The section on the ligamentous anatomy of the knee should be reviewed, if necessary, for a proper appreciation of the structures involved in knee dislocation. The neurovascular anatomy needs amplification at this point.

The popliteal artery is fixed both proximally and distally. It originates at the tendinous hiatus of the adductor magnus muscle, which firmly attaches it to the femoral shaft. Distally it passes beneath the tendinous arch of the soleus muscle, which also holds it firmly to the bone. Such an arrangement causes the artery to bowstring across the popliteal space and allows little tolerance for skeletal distortion.

Though the popliteal artery gives off five arterial branches in the popliteal space, the collateral circulation is particularly vulnerable. This is because of scant soft-tissue protective covering and the likelihood of tearing of the delicate communicating arteries of the superior and inferior geniculate rings when displacement of the skeletal structures occurs.

The nerves of the popliteal area, the tibial and the common peroneal, do not have such a firm fixation as the popliteal artery and are therefore less likely to be injured. Nerve injury is usually a traction type in which the peroneal nerve is stretched around the posterior femoral condyle.

CLASSIFICATION

Dislocation of the knee is classified by the relationship of the tibia to the femur (Fig. 16-62). A tibia that is anterior to the femur is an anterior dislocation. The five major types of dislocation are anterior, posterior, lateral, medial, and rotary. The rotary dislocations are further classified by some into anteromedial, anterolateral, posteromedial, and posterolateral.

The dislocation can also be described as open or closed and as a pure dislocation or a fracture-dislocation.

MECHANISM OF INJURY

Anterior dislocation is by far the most common type. This type comprises one third to one half of most reported series of a significant number. Considerable violence is generally the common factor in this injury. The patient is often unable to give a description of the mechanism. Quinlan and Sharrard in a paper on posterolateral dislocations describe a severe abduction-medial rotation violence on the flexed leg bearing no weight as the mechanism of anterior dislocation.

Kennedy,[727] in a study on cadaver extremities, showed that anterior dislocation was produced by hyperextension of the knee with tearing of the posterior capsule and cruciate ligament. The posterior capsular tear usually occurred at about 30° hyperextension, followed by stretching and tearing of the posterior cruciate ligament. Girgis and associates[833] stated that their anatomical studies showed that the posterior cruciate ligament acted

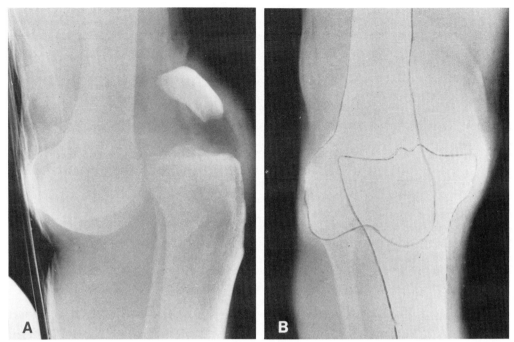

Fig. 16-62. Anterior dislocation of the knee. A 62-year-old man sustained an anterior dislocation of the left knee when 30 sacks of seed grain fell on his left knee. At surgical repair 9 days after injury, he had detachment of both gastrocnemius heads, rupture of medial ligaments, both cruciate ligaments, and posterior capsule. Initially distal pulsations were poor but improved after reduction. No vascular or neurologic problems developed. (*A*) Lateral view. Classification of knee dislocation is based on the relationship of the tibia to the femur. (*B*) Anteroposterior view.

as a check to hyperextension only after the anterior cruciate ligament was torn.

A posterior dislocation was found by Kennedy to be difficult to produce experimentally because the extensor mechanism acted as a tether, preventing the tibia from dislocating posteriorly. When posterior dislocation did occur, rupture of the patellar tendon was found.

Attempts at producing medial and lateral dislocations commonly caused a tibial plateau fracture or a supracondylar fracture.

Kennedy's clinical observations of his 22 reported cases suggested the following:

a. Anterior dislocations occur from trivial to violent injuries with hyperextension of the knee.
b. Posterior dislocations occur from crushing injuries.
c. Medial and lateral dislocations occur with extreme forces, usually with a lateral and rotary stress.

Anterior dislocations have the higher rate of

vascular problems. Hyperextension of the knee that causes this type stretches the popliteal artery. Damage may be rather extensive, producing thrombosis and transverse lacerations. Internal damage caused by the stretching may be undetectable by external examination of the artery.

Vascular damage associated with posterior dislocation is usually a rupture of the popliteal artery at one or two points caused by the sudden posterior displacement of the tibia.

Posterolateral dislocation is the type most likely to produce severe nerve damage. The peroneal nerve is stretched over the lateral femoral condyle in anterior dislocations, whereas the backward force on the tibia in posterolateral dislocation may cause actual tearing of the nerve.

The posterolateral dislocation has been called the irreducible dislocation. Reduction may be prevented by the medial femoral condyle being trapped in a buttonhole rent in the medial capsule and invagination of the medial ligament into the joint. An open reduction is necessary to free the medial ligament and capsule from the joint, after which reduction is easily achieved.

There is often no correlation between the type of dislocation and the amount of damage done to the ligamentous structures. In anterior and posterior dislocations one or both cruciates may be torn and the collateral ligaments merely stretched. The posterior capsule is always ruptured. Laceration of the skin posteriorly is often prevented by the forward slip of the tibia, which relieves the tension produced by the initial hyperextension.

SIGNS AND SYMPTOMS

Prior to reduction, the deformity is quite obvious. Because of the ease of reduction of many of these dislocations, the deformity often has been corrected at the scene of the accident or before examination by the physician. Indeed, because of the vascular problems produced by the bony distortion, immediate reduction by the person who gives first-aid is recommended, particularly if there are no distal pulses.

Kennedy[715] feels the reported rarity of this condition is due to the fact that many are reduced at the scene of the accident and are not recorded, and many go unrecognized immediately because of other injuries associated with the initial violence.

Because of the high incidence of vascular complications, initial evaluation should be directed toward the circulatory status. Palpation for the dorsalis pedis pulse, warmth of the foot skin, and sensation of the foot should be noted. A warm foot with no cyanosis is not a dependable sign of popliteal artery continuity.

The neurologic status of the extremity should be checked carefully. It is often difficult to ascertain whether sensory disturbance and paralysis are from concomitant injury of the tibial and peroneal nerves or the result of ischemia. Loss of cutaneous sensation, particularly over the digits, suggests critical ischemia. Identifying a pure nerve lesion may be easier than differentiating a combined arterial and neural lesion from a pure arterial injury.

If the knee is being examined for laxity after a suspected dislocation, care must be exercised to avoid further injury to vascular or neural structures posteriorly. Hyperextension of even 15° was found by Kennedy in his cadaver experiments to stretch the peroneal nerve. Excessive varus opening on testing for lateral ligament stability may stretch the peroneal nerve, and such testing should be done very carefully.

With anterior dislocation, excessive passive hyperextension is always present, owing to the rupture of the posterior capsule and usually the posterior cruciate ligament. Hughston and his associates have found the most reliable test for posterior cruciate rupture is medial joint opening on valgus stress with the knee fully extended or hyperextended. We feel, however, that with a torn posterior capsule such instability can be present even with an intact posterior cruciate ligament. The laxity demonstrated would be less than if the posterior cruciate were also torn.

With posterolateral dislocation the medial femoral condyle is prominent and easily palpable anteriorly beneath the skin. Distal to this protrusion the skin is puckered and drawn into a deep transverse groove. The posterior tibia is palpable in the popliteal fossa.

Clinical findings in the other types of dislocations also relate to easy palpation of the tibia in its displaced location.

Other findings associated with knee injuries, such as swelling, effusion, ecchymosis, and tenderness, are inconsequential in view of the marked pathology. Lack of significant swelling in the knee itself merely indicates the presence of a complete capsule tear, which allows blood and joint fluid to extravasate into the surrounding soft tissues. A marked fullness or puffiness in the popliteal area should alert one to the possibility of popliteal vessel injury.

Probably the most common error in knee evaluation made by the unskilled is to call the obvious deformity of a dislocated patella "a dislocated knee" (see Fig. 16-57). We have even been called to the emergency room by a physician for a dislocated knee, only to find the deformity produced by the patella sitting laterally. The familiarity of patients with the terms *knee, deformity,* and *dislocation* often brings about this mistake in terminology.

RADIOGRAPHIC FINDINGS

Time should not be wasted obtaining x-rays of a knee dislocation, particularly if there is any question of circulatory embarrassment of the extremity. Even though a fracture around the knee may be suspected, if circulation is impaired, traction should be instituted to restore alignment and to possibly relieve pressure on vital arterial channels.

The position of the tibia in relation to the femoral condyles is used to classify the dislocation (Fig. 16-63). Both anteroposterior and lateral views are necessary to evaluate this position. X-rays should always be taken, even if reduction has been accomplished, to ascertain if there are any associated fractures.

The posterolateral dislocation may be more de-

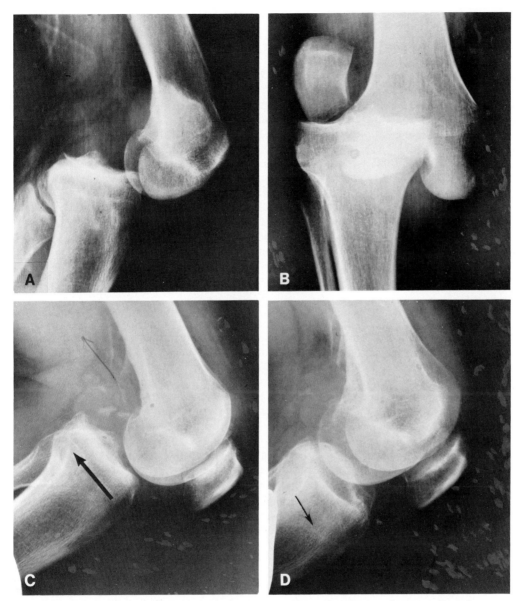

Fig. 16-63. Posterior dislocation of the knee. A 29-year-old military pilot was ejected from a plane going 250 m.p.h. after it was hit by gunfire. Reduction took place 5 to 6 hours after injury. There were no neurovascular problems. He was treated initially with a cast; knee reconstruction was done 9 months after injury for marked laxity. (*A*) Lateral view. (*B*) Anteroposterior view. (*C*) Posterior and (*D*) anterior stress views (taken 6 months after injury) showed the posterior displacement of the tibia.

ceptive in its radiographic interpretation. The medial femoral condyle may be trapped in a capsular rent medially and the degree of displacement may not be easily recognized. Since this is a rotary type of dislocation, posterior displacement of the lateral tibial condyle is usually not marked. On the anteroposterior view, lateral displacement of the lat-

eral tibial condyle on the femur is never more than a quarter the width of the condyle, according to Quinlan and Sharrard.[727] The medial femoral condyle, because of tibial rotation, appears to project medially to a greater extent than the tibia does laterally.

It may be well, at this point, to mention arteriograms in assessment of popliteal artery injury. There are some who question their value, some who believe the procedure can contribute to arterial spasm, and some who believe they delay necessary operative intervention. Arteriography should be done only if the surgeon is prepared to follow through with immediate exploration and repair, if necessary. The study is of value in localizing the injured area of the artery and determining the extent of collateral circulation. If such a diagnostic procedure is to be used, it should be done quickly, preferably in the operating room while the patient is being prepared for surgery. If there is any doubt as to the patency of the popliteal artery, open exploration should be undertaken. As many have emphasized, watchful expectancy, procrastination, equivocation, temporizing, or wishful thinking because of a warm foot may prove disastrous.

METHODS OF TREATMENT

IMMEDIATE TREATMENT

Closed reduction should be attempted as quickly as possible. Kennedy recommends that the reduction be done under spinal anesthetic, because this gives good relaxation and provides a lumbar sympathetic block that increases circulation to the leg. Prompt reduction helps restore circulation and lessens the chance of nerve injury from prolonged stretching.

Anterior dislocation is usually easily reduced by longitudinal traction followed by lifting the femur into the reduced position. Care is taken to avoid pressure in the popliteal area during reduction and to avoid hyperextending the knee. Pushing the proximal tibia posteriorly also produces reduction, but because of the ruptured capsule and cruciate ligaments, one must be particularly careful not to cause hyperextension by this method of reduction. Injury to the popliteal vessels could occur.

Reduction of a posterior dislocation is accomplished by longitudinal traction while extending the knee and lifting upward on the proximal tibia. Lateral and medial dislocations are similarly reduced by longitudinal traction and appropriate pressure on the tibia and femur.

Closed reduction may be blocked by interposed soft tissue. Failure of closed reduction most often occurs in posterolateral dislocation due to either infolding of the medial capsule and collateral ligament or to a buttonhole tear in the medial capsule, which traps the medial femoral condyle.

After reduction, the knee should be immobilized in 15° of flexion on a posterior plaster splint. It is best to avoid circular plaster casts in the first week or two, so that the circulation of the foot and leg can be observed constantly.

INDICATIONS FOR OPERATIVE TREATMENT

There are three situations for which immediate surgical intervention is indicated: (1) an open dislocation, (2) an irreducible dislocation, and (3) injury to the popliteal artery.

Open dislocation requires immediate cleansing and debridement. Soft tissue damage is often extensive, and sepsis may occur as a complication. In the Massachusetts General Hospital series of 26 dislocations, nine were open dislocations. Two of these required amputation because of infection. Irrigation with an antibiotic solution and systemic antibiotic coverage is recommended.

Careful interpretation of the x-rays after closed reduction, particularly the posterolateral type, is necessary. If there is any suggestion of widening of the joint space or doubt that full reduction has been achieved, open reduction is necessary. The approach is directed toward the area blocking reduction. Extraction of the trapped soft tissue or extension of the buttonhole and freeing the femoral condyle allows easy realignment of the joint surfaces. When open reduction is required, ligament repair should be done at the same operation, unless other factors preclude this.

Postreduction assessment of circulation to the extremity distal to the knee is of paramount importance. Lack of pulse in the dorsalis pedis or posterior tibial arteries, inability to move the toes, or the presence of tenseness in the popliteal region are grave signs of developing vascular problems. These findings may be noted even though the foot remains warm. Such findings are indications for popliteal arteriography. If there is any doubt about the competence of the popliteal artery, surgical exploration is warranted. Many feel arteriography is an unnecessary step. Certainly if it is not immediately available, or if the surgeon is not prepared to take the necessary steps for arterial surgery, the procedure should be omitted.

The management of the arterial injury varies from simple thrombectomy to vein graft or crimped tube prosthesis. Consultation by a vascular surgeon should be obtained, but if such is not readily available, standard texts on arterial surgery should be consulted by the surgeon unfamiliar with these procedures. Ligation of the popliteal artery is contraindicated. The time interval between injury and surgical repair is the main factor in limb salvage after arterial injury. Six hours seems to be the point after which success of surgical repair begins to diminish markedly.

The question arises whether immediate repair of the damaged ligaments should be attempted. In an injury so severe, ligament tissue does not escape injury. Kennedy, however, has shown that anterior dislocation can occur with only partial disruption of major ligaments. The marked instability in the dislocated position is often mistakenly interpreted to be due to ligament disruption. The knee may be stable after reduction except for the posterior laxity due to posterior capsular tear. Bonnin[722] has noted that the collateral ligaments are often torn from their attachments to the femoral condyles. When reduction was accomplished, surrounding soft tissues approximated the torn tissues. Ruptures near the midoint of the collateral ligaments are less apt to provide a stable knee after healing.

Many reports attest to good functional results and minimal instability with the nonoperative treatment of a dislocated knee.[739] It would seem, however, that the work of O'Donoghue[722] (showing the superior end results of early surgical repair of major ligamentous injuries to the knee as compared to conservative treatment) cannot be ignored. Meyers and colleagues[720] reviewed the results of 33 dislocations of the knee and believed that surgical repair was indeed superior to conservative care.

Postreduction evaluation of the vascular status of the lower extremity in a serial manner is of paramount importance. During the evaluation, several facts should be remembered: (1) A popliteal pulse may be present initially despite injury to the popliteal artery due either to transmission of the pulse or nonocclusive internal damage; (2) evaluation of ischemic pain and neurologic changes may be difficult because of associated direct nerve trauma; (3) intact distal pulses may be present early, only to have delayed arterial thrombosis occur at varying intervals; (4) one should never attempt to explain the absence of pulses on vascular spasms or the presence of local spasm; and (5) it is not satisfactory to judge capillary filling alone as evidence of adequate circulation.

Since dislocations of the knee are asociated with a high incidence of popliteal artery damage, and arteriography is associated with low morbidity, some authors recommend arteriography in all knee dislocations. If signs of arterial injury appear clearcut, however, arteriography may be omitted and immediate surgical exploration undertaken without delay. When the treating physician does not feel that initial arteriography is needed, close observa-tion for pulse change, neurologic variation, and positive stretch signs or progressive swelling in the popliteal space should alert him to consider this procedure.

Although results of revascularization have been most successful when the popliteal artery occlusions have been less than 6 hours,[725] there is no exact period after which direct repair of the vessel is no longer feasible. Ischemic tolerance is variable and depends on multiple factors such as the patient's age, the amount of collateral circulation about the knee, the amount of popliteal artery occluded, and the amount of soft tissue damage. Doporto and Rafique[697] successfully revascularized a young man's leg 36 hours after a knee dislocation had caused complete occlusion of the popliteal artery. Mac-Gowan[718] resected and replaced a segment of damaged popliteal artery 4 days after traumatic occlusion occurred. Therefore, although time is of the utmost importance, an A-K amputation should not be prematurely contemplated when revascularization may still be possible.

The management of the arterial injury varies, depending on the extent of damage to the popliteal artery. For this reason, expertise in the area is essential. The orthopedic surgeon should obtain a consultation from a vascular surgeon. Seldom is end-to-end anastomosis of the artery satisfactory unless there is an isolated laceration. According to O'Donnell,[723] isolated thrombectomy alone will fail in all instances. Ligation of the popliteal artery also is now considered doomed to failure. The popliteal artery is a critical vessel. Although there is an isolated report of limb salvage despite popliteal artery ligation following knee dislocations,[706] this is not the recommended treatment of choice; in World War II, most arterial injuries were managed by ligation and 364 of 502 legs were amputated.[695] During the Korean and Vietnam wars, restablishment of popliteal artery blood flow resulted in a decrease in the amputation rate from 73% to 32%.[729]

The use of a reversed saphenous vein graft is now used to reanastomose the damaged artery in a high percentage of cases. Associated popliteal vein damage should also be looked for and repair accomplished if possible. In combined injuries, fasciotomy should be readily used.

AUTHORS' PREFERRED TREATMENT

Our preference for treatment of a closed dislocated knee is immediate reduction and immobilization with a posterior splint in 15° of knee flexion. This is followed by a 1-week period of observation to ascertain the circulatory status. (Developing thrombosis in an artery with damage to the intima may not become apparent for several days following injury.) If, however, repair of a damaged popliteal artery is acutely necessary, we do attempt to repair whatever structures can be exposed through the incision used by the vascular surgeon.

We feel that immediate repair of the torn ligaments is secondary to establishing that a satisfactory vascular status is present. When it is established there are no vascular problems or other injuries contraindicating surgery, a surgical repair to correct instability is carried out.

We choose to perform this surgery under tourniquet control once the vascular status has been deemed satisfactory. If, however, there is any question concerning the vascular status or there is massive soft tissue swelling at the time of repair, we attempt to perform this procedure without tourniquet control.

If the anterior or posterior cruciate ligament is avulsed with a fragment of bone, surgical attachment can be done after an appropriate period of observation. These ligament *avulsion* injuries will heal well. Cruciate ligaments torn in their fibrous substance have less chance of healing satisfactorily because of the very scant blood supply to these ligaments. Even with the knowledge that the repaired ligament may be less than satisfactory, we do not choose to add the associated trauma of intra-articular or extra-articular cruciate ligament augmentation procedures. If proper muscle rehabilitation measures fail to restore functional stability, surgical reconstruction measures may be used on an elective basis to compensate for the residual laxity.

CARE AFTER REDUCTION OR OPERATION

Six weeks of immobilization to allow healing is required after either conservative treatment or surgical repair of the injured ligaments. After the first week in the posterior splint, a long-leg cast is applied in the same position. Quadriceps setting exercises are started early, followed by active leg lifting exercises when the patient is able to tolerate them. When the cast is removed the usual rehabilitative exercise programs to restore motion and muscle strength are begun. More detailed convalescent care is given in the section on acute ligamentous injuries.

PROGNOSIS AND COMPLICATIONS

Limited motion and ligament laxity with resultant instability are the usual problems associated with a less-than-satisfactory result. Many report better results with conservative treatment; others feel operative treatment gives the best chance of a stable knee. We agree with the latter unless the laxity is so minimal or the functional demands of the patient do not warant surgical intervention.

It is difficult to compare treatment groups in knee dislocation because of the wide varieties of injury and the presence of associated problems such as arterial injury, nerve injury, and fracture.

Most series report an incidence of arterial injury in 20% to 35% of the cases. Should arterial damage occur, other complications may result. These include acute renal tubular necrosis associated with prolonged muscle ischemia and the release of myoglobin and related blood pigments, gangrene, trophic skin changes, hyperalgesia, claudication, recurrent ulceration, and ischemic contracture of muscles. Amputation is, of course, the end result if ischemic residuals are severe. The number of amputations correlates closely with the number of cases with arterial injury. Amputations were required in nine of 14 knee dislocations in Hoover's[710] series; five of Kennedy's[713] 22 cases; five of Shields'[737] 26; four of Jonasch's[728] 39; six of Nikolai's 33; and none in 15 dislocations reported by Reckling and Peltier.[728]

Nerve problems occur in 25% to 35% of the cases, often in association with arterial injuries. Sensory disturbances and motor paralysis may be secondary to the ischemia of arterial injury. Injuries to the nerves are usually traction injuries from which recovery may occur. Late repair may be done if recovery does not ensue (see p. 1537).

Any injury to a joint increases the chance of that joint developing degenerative changes. The more stable the joint, the greater the chances of minimizing or delaying the onset of degenerative changes. This is why we feel that after the acute problem of limb survival has been resolved, attention should be directed toward providing as stable a joint as possible. Generally a surgical repair offers the best chance of achieving this goal.

DISLOCATION OF THE PROXIMAL TIBIOFIBULAR JOINT

The upper end of the fibula has been called a poor relation of the knee. Dislocation of the proximal fibula was first described by Nélaton in 1874.[745] It is a rare condition ascribed almost exclusively to parachute injuries. The recent popularity of sky diving and hang gliding may increase its incidence. It has also been called the horseback rider's knee.

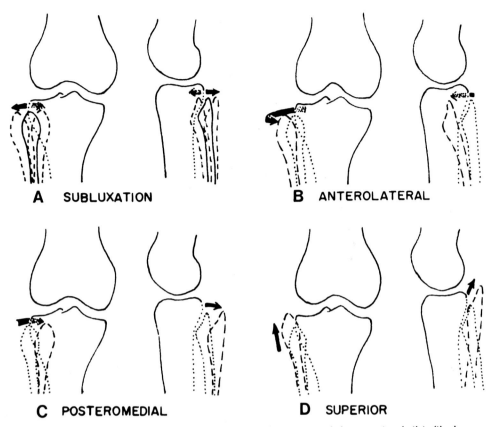

Fig. 16-64. Classification of subluxation and dislocations of the proximal tibiofibular joint. (Ogden, J. A.: Subluxation and Dislocation of the Proximal Tibiofibular Joint. J. Bone Joint Surg., **56A:**145–154, 1974.)

The fibular head may be bumped against the gatepost as the rider rides through, causing a posterior dislocation of the fibular head.

SURGICAL ANATOMY

The proximal tibiofibular joint is an arthrodial joint composed of two oval surfaces, surrounded by a synovial membrane and a joint capsule attached to the margins of the articular surfaces.

Anteriorly it is reinforced by the anterior tibiofibular ligament consisting of three broad bands extending from the head of the fibula to the tibia and extensions of the biceps tendon. The posterior tibiofibular ligament is a single broad band extending obliquely upward and reinforced by the tendon of the popliteus muscle. Superior support is provided by the fibular collateral ligament.

The inclination of the joint varies. Its motion is proximal-distal translation and axial rotation. The ease of dislocation is related to the joint inclination and to the strength of the supporting structures.

The peroneal nerve, which winds around the neck of the fibula just distal to the head, is vulnerable to injury as it comes from the posterior aspect to the anterolateral position. Injury to the nerve is more likely to occur with posterior dislocation.

CLASSIFICATION

There are three types of acute traumatic dislocations of the proximal tibiofibular joint (Fig. 16-64): (1) Anterior dislocation (anterolateral) is twice as common as posterior. (2) Posterior dislocation (posteromedial) is usually from direct violence to the flexed knee. It is a more serious injury and is associated with recurrent subluxation and peroneal nerve injury. (3) Superior dislocation is nearly always associated with superior dislocation of the lateral malleolus. Such an injury must suffer interosseous membrane damage.

Subluxation, as described by Ogden,[749] is excessive and symptomatic anteroposterior motion without frank dislocation.

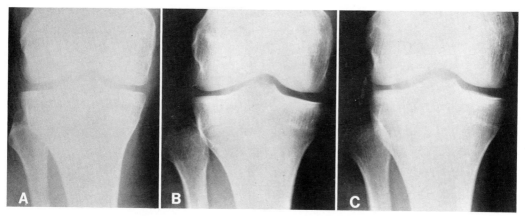

Fig. 16-65. (A) Anteroposterior view of the uninjured right knee. Note the overlap of the fibular head and the lateral margin of the tibia. (B) Anteroposterior view of the injured left knee. The entire fibular head was lateral to the tibial condyle. This indicated an anterior dislocation of the fibular head. (C) Postreduction x-rays showed improvement in the position of the fibular head.

MECHANISM OF INJURY

The mechanism for anterior dislocation is adduction of the lower leg with flexion of the knee. In the parachute landing position the knees are flexed and the feet are kept together. In this position the fibular collateral ligament and the biceps are relaxed. A sharp inversion of the ankle causes peroneal muscle tension as reflex contraction of the muscle resists the forced ankle inversion. A lateral twist of the trunk is transmitted to the tibia. This may cause a tear of the posterior tibiofibular ligament, which allows the proximal fibula to be pulled forward, hinging on the intact anterior tibiofibular ligament.

Posterior dislocation is either by direct violence (horseback rider's knee) or due to a twisting injury that tears the capsule and ligaments. This, associated with a strong biceps femoris muscle contraction, pulls the loosened fibular head posteriorly.

Superior dislocation can occur only when the entire fibular shaft displaces superiorly. This is associated with an ankle injury, causing a severe force resulting in disruption of the distal tibiofibular joint and displacement of the lateral malleolus superiorly.

SIGNS AND SYMPTOMS

After the injury, on arising the patient may feel the knee "out of joint." He may be unable to walk, or there may be minimal symptoms.

Examination and palpation shows the fibular head to be protruding in comparison with the opposite knee. The biceps tendon stands out in abnormal relief. There is little swelling or ecchymosis, because the area is relatively avascular. Inversion-eversion motion of the ankle may produce knee pain. Laxity of the fibular head may be demonstrated manually. Rarely, the peroneal nerve is injured and numbness of the lateral side of the foot or foot drop may be present.

RADIOGRAPHIC FINDINGS

Comparison of the normal knee with the injured one is helpful in diagnosis. A normal anteroposterior view of the knee shows an overlap of the fibular head and the lateral margin of the tibial condyle (Fig. 16-65A). In a normal lateral view, the fibular head is just slightly visible behind the tibia.

An anterior dislocation shows the entire fibular head lying lateral to the tibial condyle (Fig. 16-65B). The lateral view shows the fibular head sitting forward, overlapped by the tibia.

Similar differences in comparison with the normal side occur with posterior and superior dislocations.

METHODS OF TREATMENT

Anterior dislocations are nearly always reducible by direct manipulation. Anesthesia adequate to allow muscle relaxation is necessary. The knee is flexed to 90° to relax the biceps tendon; the foot is strongly inverted to provide peroneal muscle pull; and direct pressure is applied to the fibular head in the appropriate direction to produce reduction. Reduction usually occurs with an audible snap and is generally quite stable.

Posterior and superior dislocations are reduced in the same manner as anterior dislocations, except for the direction of pressure on the fibular head. Posterior and superior dislocations are more likely to be unstable and recur.

Immobilization after closed reduction varies from simple support with an elastic bandage to cast immobilization. The type of immobilization does not appear to affect the recurrence rate. We prefer a soft dressing. Crutches are used initially with graduated weight bearing as tolerated. Crutches are used for 1 to 2 weeks, chiefly to protect the patient against twisting strains at the ankle, which would stress the proximal tibiofibular joint. Activity should be regulated for an additional 3 weeks, after which full activity may be resumed including sports activity. The ankle injury associated with a superior dislocation of the fibula usually requires cast immobilization.

If closed manipulation is unsuccessful or if dislocation recurs, open reduction is indicated. The fibular head may become trapped in front of the tibial condylar flare and be held by a tight fibular collateral ligament.

Several methods of operative treatment have been described. Arthrodesis, resection of the proximal head of the fibula, and screw fixation have been used. None are recommended for acute dislocations. Arthrodesis prevents rotation of the fibula that normally occurs with dorsiflexion and inversion-eversion motions of the foot. With resection of the proximal fibula, restoration of the lateral supporting structures that attach to the head of the fibula is required. With screw fixation, bone absorption with loosening may occur.

When open reduction is necessary, we prefer the method recommended by Parkes and Zelko[751] of stabilization after reduction with two smooth Kirschner wires and repair of the torn capsule and ligaments. The pins are removed under local anesthesia at the end of 6 weeks. After open reduction and fixation, a short-leg cast is used to prevent ankle motion and minimize motion at the proximal joint. The cast is removed at the same time as the wires.

AUTHORS' PREFERRED TREATMENT

In acute dislocation of the proximal tibiofibular joint, adequate anesthesia is required prior to closed reduction. With adequate anesthesia, the posterior, superior, and anterior dislocations are frequently reducible by direct manipulation. If, however, the closed manipulation is unsuccessful, open reduction is indicated. With open reduction, we prefer the method of Parkes and Zelko.[751] The reduction is stabilized with two smooth Kirschner wires and the torn capsule and ligaments are repaired. This is followed by cast immobilization for 6 weeks.

PROGNOSIS AND COMPLICATIONS

The chances of residual problems are minimal in acute dislocations treated adequately. Peroneal nerve palsies, according to Lyle,[748] occur in 5% of cases.

Neglected cases may result in instability of the joint and eventual erosion of joint surfaces and cystic degeneration from the torn capsule.

Owen[750] reported spontaneous recurrent dislocation of the superior tibiofibular joint in young patients, usually under 18 years of age. Such dislocations are fleeting episodes that occur without injury and are often associated with little pain. The condition usually occurs in girls and resolves with conservative treatment and with maturity.

Dennis and Rutledge[744] reported a case of bilateral spontaneous recurrent dislocation with peroneal nerve palsy. Bilateral resection of the fibular heads resolved the problem and allowed return to sports.

Degenerative changes at the joint can be treated by resection of the fibular head or arthrodesis. We favor joint resection to preserve normal knee and ankle motion.

CHONDRAL AND OSTEOCHONDRAL FRACTURES

Persistent symptoms involving the knee after injury without a definitive diagnosis should make one suspect a chondral or osteochondral fracture. O'Donoghue[776,777] states that osteochondritis dissecans, chondromalacia (particularly of the patella), joint mouse, idiopathic synovitis with effusion, chronic sprain, and "in fact many other lesions of the knee not initially diagnosed may well have originated as a chondral fracture."

Early arthrotomy for ligament and meniscus injury has sometimes revealed associated fresh chondral or osteochondral fractures. There has in recent years been an increasing awareness of these fractures as a source of persistent and prolonged knee disability after injury. With time it becomes increasingly difficult to differentiate—by history, examination, radiographs, and even surgical exploration—chondral or osteochondral injury from

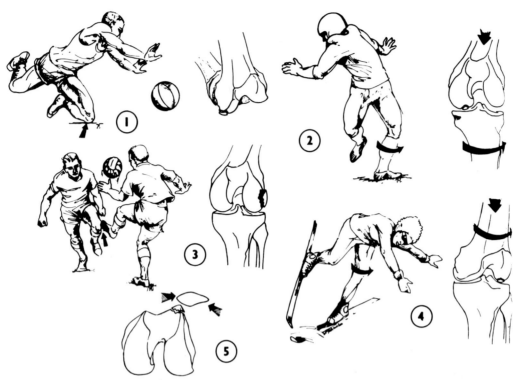

Fig. 16-66. The mechanisms of injury in osteochondral fractures: (*1*) direct shearing force on the medial condyle; (*2*) rotary compression force on the medial epicondyle; (*3*) direct shearing force on the lateral condyle; (*4*) rotary compression force on the lateral condyle; (*5*) action of the patella on the lateral condyle in dislocation or reduction. (Kennedy, J. C.; Grainger, R. W.; and McGraw, R. W.: Osteochondral Fractures of the Femoral Condyles. J. Bone Joint Surg., **48B**:437–440, 1966.)

chondromalacia, osteochondritis dissecans, or other types of cartilage defects.

A chondral fracture involves only the articular cartilage and would not, therefore, be visible radiographically by usual techniques. An osteochondral fracture carries, with the articular cartilage, underlying subchondral bone which can be seen on the x-rays. Often the layer of bone is very thin and difficult to see.

In 1904 Kroner[763] first reported a patellar dislocation in which the osseous portion reduced itself, leaving the cartilage surface of the patella dislocated laterally. Since this paper, osteochondral fractures about the patella and lateral femoral condyle have been reported with increasing frequency, particularly since World War II when more attention was directed toward this lesion. Ambroise Paré described the removal of loose bodies from a joint in 1558.[763] One wonders if these were indeed osteochondral fractures.

A study by the Army Air Force of 186 loose bodies in the knee found 21 due to osteochondral fracture, either of the femur or of the patella.[755]

MECHANISM OF INJURY AND CLASSIFICATION

Injury to the articular surfaces may be caused by direct impact to the joint (exogenous) and those resulting from indirect sources and muscular contraction (endogenous). The mechanism of these fractures can further be grouped into those caused by compaction or compression forces, shearing forces, or avulsion injuries at the sites of ligament or tendon insertions (Fig. 16-66).

There are six major sites of injury: medial and lateral femoral condyles, medial and lateral tibial condyles, the patella, and the intercondylar notch area.

Considering these factors—mechanism of injury, forces involved, and site of injury—a classification of these fractures can be evolved (Table 16-1).

Table 16-1. Classification of Chondral and Osteochondral Fractures of the Knee

Site	Type	Mechanism
Patella	Exogenous Endogenous	Direct impact 1. Shearing force related to patellar dislocation or reduction 2. Avulsion by quadriceps tendon, medial retinaculum, or patellar tendon
Femoral condyles 1. Lateral	Exogenous Endogenous	Direct impact—compression or shearing force 1. Rotation and compression 2. Shearing related to patellar dislocation and reduction
2. Medial	Exogenous Endogenous	Direct impact—compression or shearing force Rotation and compression
Tibial condyles 1. Lateral	Exogenous Endogenous	Direct impact Rotation and compression by femoral condyle
2. Medial	Exogenous Endogenous	Direct impact Rotation and compression by femoral condyle
Intercondylar	Endogenous	1. Avulsion of tibial attachment of anterior cruciate 2. Avulsion of femoral attachment of posterior cruciate

Modified from Kennedy, J. C.; Grainger, R. W.; and McGraw, R. W.: J. Bone Joint Surg., **48B**:437–440, 1966.

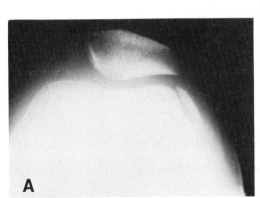 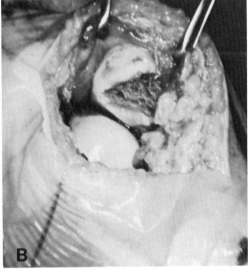

Fig. 16-67. A 15-year-old girl sustained a dislocated patella. (*A*) Sunrise (tangential) view showed a large osteochondral fragment lying lateral to the lateral femoral condyle (endogenous shearing). (*B*) Surgical exploration revealed the fragment to be a large osteochondral defect from the articular surface of the medial facet of the patella. View is from an anterior medial incision into the knee joint.

Those fractures that occur with patellar dislocation are the most frequent of the osteochondral fractures. When the patella dislocates, it may become trapped by the lateral edge of the lateral femoral condyle. As the vastus medialis obliquus muscle contracts in the flexed knee, a tangential force is exerted through the patella. The resulting fracture produced can occur to the medial patellar facet (Fig. 16-67) or to the lateral femoral condyle, or to both. Rosenberg[781] feels that if both surfaces fracture, the fractures do not occur at the same instant but may occur with a single injury. He further stated that in his series of 15 lateral femoral fractures, a dislocation was not essential for the injury to occur. Besides the mechanism described above, which causes the fracture at the time of reduction, the lateral patellar margin can act as a chisel into the lateral femoral condyle or the patella's articular surface as a sledge into the femoral articular cartilage. These latter injuries can occur as the dislocation occurs or without an actual dislocation. The degree of flexion, according to Rosenberg, probably determines whether the lateral edge of the patella or its articular surface produces the fracture.

Landells' studies[768] have shown that injured articular cartilage tends to tear along the junction of calcified and uncalcified cartilage (tidemark), leaving the osteochondral junction undisturbed. The adolescent has little calcified cartilage, and so the tangential forces are directed to the subchondral region. This factor, along with the elasticity of young cartilage and ligaments, accounts for the high incidence of osteochondral fractures in adolescents. Adults are more likely to sustain chondral fractures when exposed to similar forces.

If the femoral fragment remains undisplaced, necrosis of the underlying bone may occur, giving the same radiographic appearance as osteochondritis dissecans. Fragments that do displace become chondral free bodies with calcified centers—indistinguishable either radiographically or microscopically from those of osteochondritis dissecans.[781] This cycle of separation of cartilage from the underlying matrix (whether undisplaced or displaced), necrosis of the attached subchondral bone, and regeneration is the same as in osteochondritis dissecans. The hyaline cartilage covering the articular surface of the fragment does not become necrotic because of the nourishment received from the synovial fluid. In some cases separation of the fragment from its bed may never occur, and healing ensues. The marked similarities to the classic description of osteochondritis dissecans lead O'Donoghue[776,777] to conclude and Rosenberg[781] to suggest that the etiology of osteochondritis dissecans is, in many instances, trauma.

SIGNS AND SYMPTOMS

Those chondral and osteochondral fractures that occur with a dislocation of the patella have the signs and symptoms of the dislocation. In addition the patient may feel and hear a painful snap. The joint distends rapidly and when aspirated the effusion is found to be blood filled with fat droplets (see Fig. 16-60). In undisplaced fractures this hemarthrosis may be minimal or absent. Locking may occur. Tenderness is present over the area of fracture if this can be palpated. Tenderness around the medial retinaculum and medial patellar bordr is present if the retinaculum has torn or if there is injury to the medial edge of the patella. In a fresh patellofemoral injury, the patient may be unable to hold the knee actively extended or to activate the quadriceps mechanism.

Ahstrom[754] found hypermobility of the patella in nearly all of those patients who had osteochondral fractures associated with patellar dislocation. Hypermobility was defined as the ability to passively push the patella, so that its inferior angle or apex was even with or lateral to the lateral edge of the lateral femoral condyle with the knee relaxed and extended.

When a patellar dislocation has not occurred, there is a history of a direct blow to the flexed knee or a violent twist on the flexed knee (Fig. 16-68). With the rotational forces, a loud snap is heard and felt. Hemarthrosis, often joint locking, and tenderness are found on examination.

When not recognized early, intermittent locking, recurrent effusion, persistent pain, and crepitation is noted.

These signs may lead to an erroneous diagnosis of meniscus tear. If the fracture is not radiographically evident the differentiation may indeed be difficult. A careful assessment of the mechanism of injury, signs of patellar hypermobility, and arthrography will be helpful. As O'Donoghue[777] states, "in any case in which the symptoms seem worse than the recognizable findings . . . one should suspect chondral damage."

RADIOGRAPHIC FINDINGS

A careful inspection of high quality x-rays—often with a bright spotlight—is necessary. In addition to the routine anteroposterior and lateral views, one should obtain right and left oblique views, notch (tunnel), and patellar views. Tangential views of the patella in different degrees of knee flexion (sunrise and Hughston views, see Fig. 16-48) help to assess the patella more accurately.

The x-rays may reveal flake fractures or a defect of the lateral femoral condyle, bone fragments along the medial border of the patella, avulsion fractures of the area around the medial tibial spine, or the femoral attachment of the posterior cruciate ligament, depressions of the femoral condyles, or loose fragments within the joint.

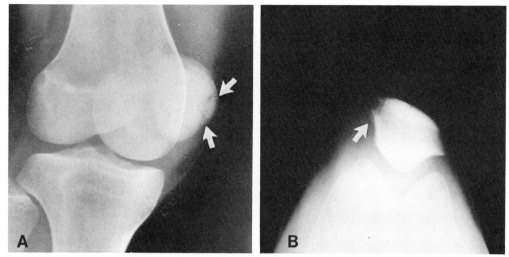

Fig. 16-68. A 25-year-old woman fell and struck her flexed left knee on a curb. (A) The oblique view showed the osteochondral fracture of the medial edge of the patella (exogenous—direct impact). (B) A Hughston view showed the fracture along the medial edge. Note the adequate patellofemoral groove and type II patella. Compare with Figure 16-67A, which shows an endogenous shear-type fracture associated with dislocation.

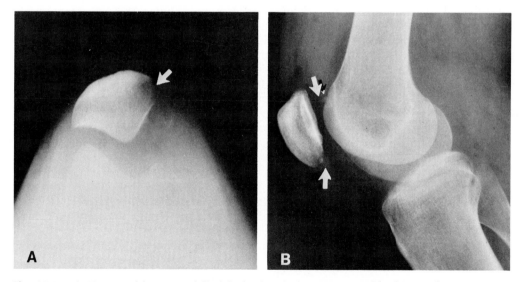

Fig. 16-69. A 22-year-old woman fell, felt the knee "pop out," and had immediate swelling. Blood was aspirated from the joint. She gave a history of two previous episodes of the knee "going out." (A) In the Hughston view, note the abrupt, irregular medial border of the patella with calcification in the tissue immediately beneath this edge. (B) The lateral view showed a loose bone fragment in the proximal portion of patellofemoral groove (*arrow*) and a fragment near the distal pole of the patella (*arrow*). At surgery a 1-cm osteochondral fracture from the inferior surface of the patella was found. The patellar tendon was partially avulsed on the medial aspect of its attachment. Some scuffing of the lateral femoral condyle was noted.

Avulsion fragments of the patella occur from a pull of the quadriceps insertion proximally or the patellar tendon distally (Fig. 16-69). (These are discussed on pp. 1489 and 1492.)

Osteochondral fractures of the patella associated with dislocation occur at the inferior medial border. This is in contrast to bipartite patella, which usually involves the superior lateral margin of the patella. Occasionally, an osseous defect of the articular surface of the patella can be seen on a lateral or tangential view.

It is sometimes difficult to determine if the osteochondral fracture occurred with the present dislocation or earlier. Hughston[765] found six of 74 knees studied for subluxation and dislocation to have associated osteochondral fractures.

Osseous fragments from the curved distal end of the femur may project on the x-ray as either a curved line or two lines with their ends overlapping. This, according to Milgram,[773] is pathognomonic of an osteochondral fracture of the distal femoral condyle and is often seen best on the anteroposterior view.

Detection of depression or of defects in the femoral condyles requires close inspection of lateral, anteroposterior, and oblique views (Fig. 16-70). They are often best seen on the anteroposterior view, on which projection there is no overlap of condyles. Comparison with similar views of the normal knee may be helpful.

A cleft lesion may be produced by a violent twist or pivot (Fig. 16-71). These lesions involve the middle and more posterior surfaces of the femoral condyle. They occasionally may be seen on x-rays as a small pencil line shadow or notch in the subchondral plate of the femoral condyle.

Special radiographic techniques may be necessary to diagnose or rule out chondral and osteochondral fractures. Tomograms may reveal small flakes obscured by overlying bone shadows. Arthrograms may show articular defects of the joint surfaces. The craters present are often so shallow that identification is usually difficult.

ARTHROSCOPY

Arthroscopy provides a method of evaluation of the inside of the knee. After an acute injury when such pathology is suspected, particularly where no bone is radiographically visible with the fragment, arthroscopy can be a very useful tool. Where appropriate, removal of fragments may be accomplished by arthroscopic methods. This prevents the need for arthrotomy and the possible increased morbidity associated with the latter.

METHODS OF TREATMENT

Once the diagnosis of a chondral or osteochondral fracture has been made, the treatment is operative if the patient is an adult. In a child or young adolescent, an undisplaced osteochondral fracture (osteochondritis dissecans) may be treated conservatively. This may involve immobilization and a period of no weight bearing.

If there is locking, a foreign body in the joint, or an acute condylar defect, there is little justification for delaying operation. Conservative treatment is undesirable for several reasons: a larger area of weight-bearing surface may be present than is recognized by x-rays; internal derangements resulting from fragments left in the joint may occur; delayed surgery—even after only 10 days—makes fitting the free fragment into the defect difficult should this be indicated.

In most instances, the chondral or subchondral fragment can be removed and discarded (Fig. 16-72). When the defect involves the weight-bearing surface, its edges should be trephined until all fragments or undermined cartilage are removed. O'Donoghue[776,777] emphasized that the defect edge should not be tapered. Regeneration, whether from the bony bed or from the margins, has less defect to fill in a trephined hole than in a beveled one. He states that articular cartilage does regenerate. Though it may not be true hyaline cartilage, the regenerated tissue in the filled defect is indistinguishable from hyaline cartilage.

Replacement of the osteochondral defect has been used by Smillie.[782] Most feel that when the defect is small or does not involve the weight-bearing surface, the fragment should be removed. Though Kennedy and colleagues[766] suggest replacement of large, weight-bearing, fresh fractures, they reported that seven of eight cases of large osteochondral fractures that were removed had good results after an average follow-up of 6 years.

Ahstrom[754] and Rosenberg[781] also report good results after fragment removal. If the fracture occurs concomitantly with patellar dislocation, patellar instability needs correction to assure a satisfactory result. Rosenberg[781] states that untreated patients with a history of injury during adolescence, osteochondral loose bodies, and lateral condyle defects showed surprisingly little degenerative changes in their knee joints 3 or 4 decades later. This is particularly true if the loose bodies became attached

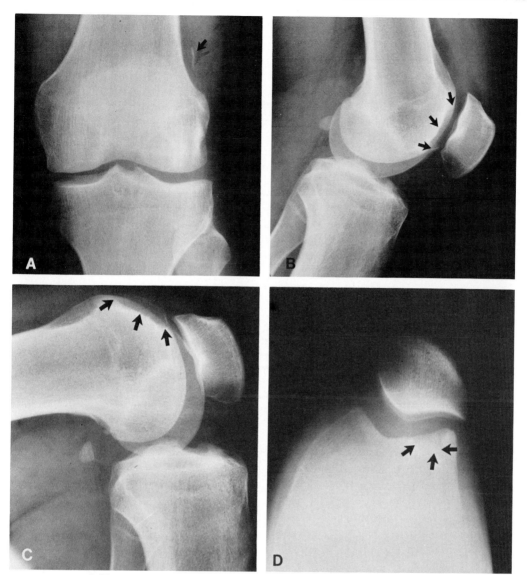

Fig. 16-70. A 16-year-old boy injured his knee on the long jump in track. His knee went into hyperextension. No immediate swelling was present. He noticed a lump on the medial side of the patella and subsequently had catching. He was first seen 1 month after injury. (*A*) The anteroposterior view showed a thin bone fragment just superior to the lateral femoral condyle. (*B*) A lateral view with the knee at 30° flexion showed a defect of the lateral femoral condyle (*arrows*) directly beneath the patella. There was a small flake of bone at its distal margin. (*C*) A lateral view with the knee flexed to 90° showed the lateral femoral defect (*arrows*) in better relief just proximal to the proximal pole of the patella. (*D*) A Hughston view showed slight lateral subluxation of the patella. The defect in the lateral femoral condyle can be seen (*arrows*). This was a type II/III patellar configuration.

to the synovium in a position that did not allow impingement and if the extensor mechanism was normal. The condylar defect did not cause late arthritis when the fragment had been excised.

Should one choose to replace the fragment, care should be taken so that pins are not left projecting into the joint where they may cause synovial irritation, pannus formation, and joint stiffness.

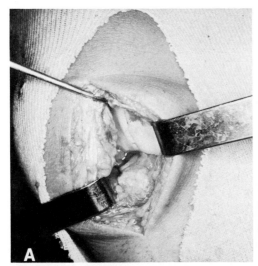
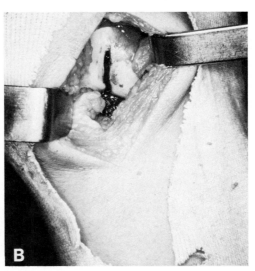
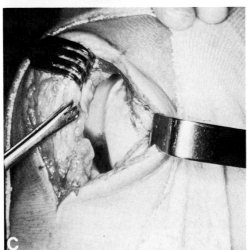

Fig. 16-71. A 22-year-old man was struck on the front of the knee while playing soccer. Seen 10 days after injury, he complained of a pressure pain with activity and no push-off power with running. The knee developed some catching. X-rays were negative. The preoperative diagnosis was medial meniscus tear. (A) A paramedial incision was made into the knee joint. A vertical split of the articular cartilage of the midportion of the medial femoral condyle can be seen. (B) The surgical procedure was to trim the loose edges perpendicular to the subchondral bone and multiple drill holes in the osseous bed. (C) Arthrotomy was performed 21 months later for a loose body after another injury. The previous articular cartilage split had completely filled in and was difficult to see. This is a view of the medial femoral condyle through a paramedial incision.

Milgram[772] advocates elevation of depressed femoral condyle fractures. A staple is used to realign the outer table. Weight bearing is prohibited until the dead space beneath the compressed area fills in.

Osteochondral fragments avulsed by cruciate attachments (*i.e.,* femoral attachment of the posterior cruciate or tibial attachment of the anterior cruciate) should be replaced surgically. Small fragments are removed and the ligament is reattached to the bony bed through drill holes, as described by O'Donoghue.

Fragments that are entirely cartilage are replaced and pinned by some, particularly if they involve a weight-bearing surface. O'Donoghue[776,777] feels these are best discarded and the defect trephined. Pinning requires immobilization and no weight bearing. Removal allows regeneration of articular cartilage, which is encouraged by active function. After trephining active use with weight bearing is encouraged. When a well-defined defect has been created by trephining, no actual weight is borne on the regenerating cartilage until the defect is filled. If an especially large defect on the femoral condyle is present, O'Donoghue[776,777] recommends full activity but not full weight bearing.

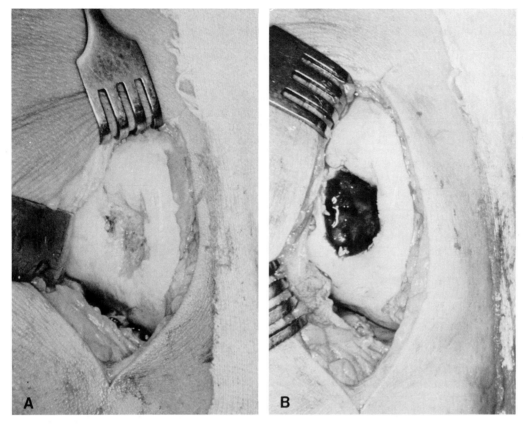

Fig. 16-72. Operative views of the case shown in Figure 16-70. (*A*) Anterolateral incision showed the defect in the lateral femoral condyle. (*B*) The defect was trephined, and the osseous bed was drilled.

AUTHORS' PREFERRED METHOD OF TREATMENT

Our preference has always been to remove the fragment, trephine the crater, and to make multiple drill holes in the osseous bed with a small Stein-mann pin. This is done to allow better vascularity and, it is hoped, better healing. It is important to remove articular cartilage that is undermined and not actually attached to the underlying bone. If left, this cartilage may break off, producing more loose bodies in the joint. It is sometimes difficult to determine where to stop trimming the edges of the cartilage. There may be a surrounding soft area of cartilage. This is more likely to be seen in chondromalacia than in acute chondral or osteo-chondral fractures. In either case, if there is no separation, the cartilage is left in place rather than removed, which would create a large defect.

Fractures along the patellar edge are, of course, removed. If the patellar edge is roughened, one can do a partial facetectomy of the patellar border. Up to one third of the patella, either medially or laterally, can be removed without dysfunction or deformity.

When patellar dislocation has occurred, the remaining articular cartilage on the patella may be abraded, contused, or split. Should the area show enough damage, it too should be treated as a chondral fracture. Removal of cartilage debris, by trephining, shaving, or facetectomy may be necessary. If complete disruption of the patellar surface has occurred, it may be necessary to consider patellectomy. In the younger patient, patellar shaving to subchondral bone would be preferable. Unless patellectomy as a possible treatment was discussed with the patient prior to surgery, we would not do it at the original surgery. It is prudent to mention this possibility, particularly to those who have had long-standing patellar symptoms prior to their osteochondral fracture.

POSTOPERATIVE CARE

If simple removal of the fragment with trephining of the cartilage and drilling of the crater is done, the postoperative care is the same as that after arthrotomy. A bulky cotton dressing (modified Jones compression dressing) is applied for 3 or 4 days, until the reaction of surgery has subsided. Quadriceps setting and straight leg raising exercises should be instituted on the first day after the operation. The bulky dressing is replaced by a light elastic wrap, which can be discontinued when swelling is no longer a problem.

Active motion is begun after the bulky dressing has been removed. Crutches are used, and protected weight bearing is allowed on the first or second postoperative day. Protected weight bearing is continued until the quadriceps strength is sufficient to protect the knee in walking. This is arbitrarily stated to be when the patient can lift 15 to 30 pounds ten times. The required weight to be lifted before crutches are discarded depends on the size of the individual and what activities we can anticipate he will be doing, once crutches are discarded.

We have had no experience with the replacement and pinning of chondral and osteochondral fractures. Smillie[782] recommends an initial 2-week period of mobilization of the joint with no weight bearing. A cylinder cast is then applied with a caliper for a period of 3 months. Later, removal of the nails is suggested.

PROGNOSIS

Removal of the free fragments protects the joint from undue scuffing and wear. The defects, which are usually small, do not produce significant disability.

Ahstrom[754] reported 18 patients with osteochondral fractures of the patella or lateral femoral margins related to patellar dislocation and reduction. All were treated surgically. The one poor result was due to a persistent chronic patellar dislocation. He recommends extensor realignment when patellar hypermobility is present.

A good prognosis can be expected with early surgical treatment. Undiagnosed or neglected cases may ultimately develop a chronic condition leading to joint deterioration, recurrent effusion, chronic pain, intermittent locking, and possibly, as suggested by O'Donoghue,[776,777] chondromalacia and osteochondritis dissecans.

COMPLICATIONS

Complications relate more to the untreated cases as mentioned above. Other complications are the same as for other surgical procedures on the knee.

Recurrent loose bodies may occur if articular cartilage separates from the margins of condylar defects.

If large condylar defects fill incompletely, producing irregular articular surfaces, one would expect symptoms of joint irritation. Clinical complaints have been reported to be surprisingly few, even with degenerative changes seen secondary to an osteochondral fracture.

INJURIES OF THE LIGAMENTS OF THE KNEE

Ivar Palmer,[938] in 1938, wrote:

> For the main theme, which I hope will be clear to the reader, is that the recent distortion injuries of the knee joint should be diagnosed with greater precision and, in the serious ligamentous injuries, operative action aimed at anatomic restitution should be taken into consideration while the injury is still acute.

Anatomical studies have demonstrated that the knee is stabilized through its range of motion by a complex of bones, ligaments, and muscle actions. These studies have helped to give an appreciation of the type of laxity that interferes with normal knee use, both in walking and running. The number of contributors to this basic understanding is great. Their clarifications of the normal and pathologic anatomical concepts have helped to devise better methods of repair of acute ruptures around the knee, as well as more sophisticated reconstructive techniques for knee stabilization.

Early surgical repair of ligamentous ruptures about the knee has been generally accepted as producing a better functional result than either conservative care by cast immobilization or late reconstructive measures. The aim of the surgical approach is to restore the ligaments to their previous anatomical position and tension. Variations in degree and type of ruptures, condition of the tissues involved, and blood supply of the ruptured ligaments often necessitate alterations or additions of basic repair to include some of the reconstructive techniques used in late repair. Familiarity with these reconstructive techniques is most helpful to the surgeon faced with repair of markedly disrupted and frayed ligament tissue in adult injuries.

Experimental studies on dogs showed the rapid onset of proliferative and degenerative changes in knee joints after surgical section of the anterior cruciate ligament. Marshall[905] found proliferative changes and osteophyte formation as early as 26 days after operation. In another study, Marshall and Olsson[907] studied the long-term proliferative and degenerative changes in dogs whose anterior cruciate was cut. These changes were increasingly severe for about 1 year. Because of thickening of the joint capsule with time, instability gradually lessened.

The large number of ligament injuries of the knee sustained in athletic endeavors, the high degree of proficiency of knee function necessary for an athlete to return to his chosen sport, and the realization that a knee that is functional in a sedentary or walking activity is not necessarily functional for athletic activities have provided an impetus to develop improved surgical techniques for ligament repairs about the knee. O'Donoghue,[931-935] Hughston,[853-858] Slocum,[957-959] Nicholas,[918-921] Kennedy,[875-879] MacIntosh,[902] and many others have made significant contributions to providing the surgical methods to restore knee stability necessary for athletic endeavor. Continued study and research in problems relating to knee stability, including recent developments of a ligament prosthesis, indicate an even brighter future for those who sustain serious ligamentous disruption about the knee.

SURGICAL ANATOMY

(See Anatomy, p. 1483)

MECHANISM OF INJURY

The stability of the knee is derived primarily from its surrounding soft-tissue structures. Its inherent instability is owing to the flat articular surface and the combination of flexion-extension and rotation in knee motion. The knee is most stable in extension. Forceful activity, such as running, lifting, jumping, is accomplished with a flexed knee.[869] In running, full extension of the knee occurs only in the trailing leg, which bears no weight. The ligaments of the knee must function as dynamic stabilizers as the knee flexes and rotates through the helicoid of its action.

Palmer[939] demonstrated the functional overlap of the supporting ligamentous structures. His description of the two-fold function of the ligaments is most interesting. One is a guiding rein of the complex knee movements. Their second function as a stabilizer against "unphysiologic movements" works in two ways. The ligaments are innervated by myelin-free nerve fibers. Tension in the ligaments produces an increase in tonicity of the musculature functionally connected with the ligament—ligamentomuscular reflex. Should the muscles fail or be overstretched, the ligaments act as mechanical stabilizers through their firm inelastic tissue.

Most ligamentous injuries of the knee occur in athletic activities, particularly football. Other sports, such as skiing, soccer, basketball, gymnastics, and wrestling, take their toll, with industrial, home, and motorized accidents providing the remainder.

The medial side of the knee most frequently sustains ligamentous injury. This is because in the act of running and cutting to the opposite direction, a valgus stress is applied to the knee. If the foot catches—a trapped cleat, an opposing player, an impaled ski—as the person is turning away from the other leg, increased valgus stress as well as rotary stresses are placed on the medial supporting structures. In football, enhancement occurs as the tackler or blocker strikes the outer side of the knee. When such forces exceed the tensile strength of the ligaments, rupture occurs. The degree of force, the position of the knee, and the muscle strength resisting the force determines the degree of injury.

Injuries to the lateral aspect of the knee occur through a varus stress, usually associated with an inward rotation of the tibia on a flexed knee. Since blows to the inner side of the knee are relatively uncommon, the injury is likewise comparatively rare. Such an injury can occur when, in the act of running, the participant attempts to change direction toward the weight-bearing leg by crossing over with the opposite extremity. If the foot becomes fixed or trapped, a varus inward rotation stress of the tibia on the femur results. As with a severe valgus stress, cruciate ligament rupture may also occur with this injury. Usually the anterior cruciate ruptures as the cruciates tighten with internal rotation of the tibia.

The mechanisms of so-called isolated cruciate injuries—if they do occur—are inward rotation of the tibia causing anterior cruciate rupture, hyperextension injuries causing anterior or posterior cruciate rupture, or a posteriorly directed blow to the proximal tibia on a flexed knee producing posterior cruciate rupture. (These will be discussed on p. 1539.)

Wall[976] believes an isolated anterior cruciate tear can occur from a forceful contraction of a powerfully developed quadriceps when the tibia is fixed and knee extension is prevented. According to his studies this injury occurs without contact with no hyperextension and no rotatory torque at the knee.

SPRAIN AND RUPTURE

The forces applied and the resistance against them may be such that only a minor sprain occurs. The *Standard Nomenclature of Athletic Injuries*[785] defines three degrees of sprain. First degree is mild, with mild point tenderness, minimal hemorrhage and swelling, no abnormal motion, and little disability. There is little if any tearing of ligament fibers. Second degree is defined as a moderate sprain with more loss of function than in first degree, localized tenderness, more joint reaction (*i.e.,* effusion), slight abnormal motion, and partial tearing of the ligamentous tissues. Third degree denotes marked abnormal motion, indicating a complete tear of the ligament.

Our preference for designation of ligament injuries of the knee is to use *sprain* only when there is no demonstrable instability. Sprains without instability do occur with varying degrees of pain, reaction, and disability and can therefore be classified as mild, moderate, or severe.

Rupture of ligaments can be of increasing severity (Fig. 16-73). Mild or Grade I rupture involves a minimal amount of ligament tissue damage with mild instability. Grade II rupture signifies more instability because of more extensive ligament tearing. Grade III rupture indicates a significant loss of joint stability and ligament disruption, often involving many components of structural stability. The components of structural stability are closely interrelated. Studies by electron scan of transmitted light show ligaments with considerable intimal destruction due to stretching may appear intact on direct visualization. Indeed, isolated injuries of the ligaments—anterior cruciate or others—may merely reflect our inability to demonstrate these invisible lesions. Grade I instability is more severe than any degree of sprain by our definition, and usually requires a surgical repair. Sprains, on the other hand, are always treated conservatively.

It is interesting to consider Nicholas'[918] study of looseness and tightness of the joints of football players in relation to knee injuries. He reports the chances of ligament rupture are seven times greater if the person is able to perform three or more of his five indices for looseness.

CLASSIFICATION

We prefer to classify injuries to ligaments of the knee as follows:

A. Sprains—mild, moderate, severe (no instability present)
B. Ruptures—Grade I (mild instability)
    Grade II (moderate instability)
    Grade III (severe instability)

When instability is determined by stress testing—often this can only be assessed with an anesthetic—the type of instability should be ascertained. These types can be categorized as follows:[855,856,876]

I. One-plane instabilities
   A. Medial
   B. Lateral
   C. Anterior
   D. Posterior
II. Rotatory instabilities
   A. Anteromedial rotatory instability (AMRI)
   B. Anterolateral rotatory instability (ALRI)
   C. Posteromedial rotatory instability (PMRI)
   D. Posterolateral rotatory instability (PLRI)
III. Combination instabilities
   A. Anterolateral-posterolateral rotatory instabilities
   B. Anterolateral-anteromedial rotatory instabilities
   C. Anteromedial-posteromedial rotatory instabilities

It is sometimes difficult, yet important, to determine what type of instability is present. Should this not be clearly determined prior to surgical repair, the functional deficit may not be adequately corrected. In an acute injury, tenderness at the sites of rupture and points of hemorrhage noted at surgery are helpful clues. Such clues are not, however, 100% accurate. Tenderness may be diffuse and not well localized. Hemorrhage may spread in the tissues, and areas of relative avascularity may be torn without significant ecchymosis. The final assessment of the type of instability depends on stress testing of the knee in its various parameters to see if excess motion occurs. This stress testing includes rotary testing as well as valgus-varus and anterior-posterior stress. Hallen and Lindahl[840] showed that the maximum amount of rotation occurs in the normal knee at 60° of flexion. They suggest that the knee be in this degree of flexion to produce the more sensitive test for diagnosis of isolated ligament injuries. With a Grade I instability there may be only anteromedial laxity, detected by

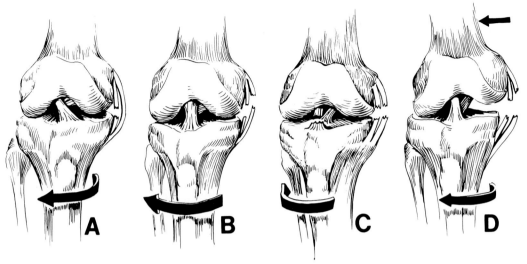

Fig. 16-73. The degrees of rupture of the medial side of the knee. Each successive layer involved in the injury produces a greater degree of clinical instability. (*A*) Rupture of the capsular ligament only. (*B*) More extensive rupture involving the capsular ligament and the tibial collateral ligament. (*C*) Still more extensive rupture with the medial capsular ligament, tibial collateral ligament, and anterior cruciate ligament involved. (*D*) Valgus and external rotation forces produce ligamentous rupture more quickly than external rotation alone. (Redrawn from Slocum, D. B.: Early Degenerative Arthritis Following Meniscal or Ligamentous Injury. *In* A.A.O.S. Symposium on Sports Medicine. St. Louis, C. V. Mosby, 1969.)

excessive anterior external rotation of the medial tibial condyle as forward stress is applied on the proximal tibia with the foot rotated externally. This may indicate that the deep portion of the capsular ligament has been torn. With more excessive tears involving the superficial tibial collateral ligament, more marked joint laxity can be demonstrated, particularly with a valgus stress.

SIGNS AND SYMPTOMS

The history of a twisting or inward or outward stress to the knee is always related. In some situations (such as an auto accident or a pile-up in football) it may be difficult to define the mechanism. Pain is felt at the time of injury. It is, however, significant that pain often subsides quickly in grade III ruptures. In sprains or lesser tears, there may be considerably more pain. Hughston[854] and Andrews,[786] in a study of 50 severe tears of the medial joint compartment, found that 76% of patients were able to walk off the field and into the doctor's office unaided and without crutches.

The patient may relate a feeling of giving way in the knee, a sensation of tearing, or he may hear a pop at the time of injury. Instability is often masked in the early stages by muscle spasm and tightness of the knee due to swelling.

It is important to ascertain when the swelling or joint effusion occurred. Immediate swelling indicates hemorrhage into the joint from torn tissues or osteochondral fractures. Effusion that occurs after 12 to 24 hours is suggestive of synovial fluid accumulation because of irritation, as in a sprain. The absence of intra-articular swelling does not rule out ligament rupture. If the capsule tear is complete, the fluid can escape into the surrounding tissues and may not be readily apparent.

Tenderness is present at the site of the tear and is helpful in localizing the tear. If there has been extensive ligament disruption, tenderness may be diffuse. Tenderness well localized along the joint line may indicate a meniscal tear, and any associated joint laxity should be evaluated with care. It is often helpful at this point in the examination to see whether stress or compression of the joint elicits more discomfort. Stress on a sprained or torn ligament elicits pain, whereas compression of that side of the joint may produce pain with a meniscal tear.

There may be localized edema at the site of injury. This edematous fluid may contain blood, indicating the site of tear.

Tests for Instability

The *sine qua non* of examination in ligament injuries is the clinical tests for instability. When the knee is examined immediately after the injury, as by the team physician at a football game, the presence or absence of joint laxity may be reliably determined. With time, as swelling occurs and muscle spasm ensues, the evaluation becomes increasingly difficult. This is particularly true in the athletic, well-muscled person. Often the first stress when the patient is relaxed is the only clue the examiner has that laxity is present at that particular examination. Subsequent testing meets with increasing muscular resistance. Examination with an anesthetic should be done if there is a question as to the presence of laxity. When the tenderness is well localized, we often use local anesthetic infiltration and obtain enough relaxation and relief of pain to make a reliable evaluation possible. If not, a general or regional anesthetic is required. The patient is prepared for surgery and he is told that we will proceed with a surgical repair if instability is found.

The method of testing for joint laxity is important. The uninjured knee is tested first, both to relax the patient and to ascertain the degree of physiologic laxity of the patient's ligaments. Particularly in adolescents is unusual joint laxity found. A study of 285 English school children showed excessive joint laxity in at least four pairs of joints in 7%.[800] Of 235 adult orthopaedic outpatients tested, six had hypermobility of the knees.[966]

The valgus (abduction) stress test is done first to evaluate the status of the medial ligament of the knee. This should be done gently and with as much relaxation of the leg as possible. The examiner either supports the leg or rests the thigh on the examining table. Stress is first applied with the knee in 30° flexion and the foot externally rotated. (The external rotation is done to tighten the medial capsular ligament for a more reliable test.) Extending the hip may help relax the hamstrings. With the foot cradled in the examiner's axilla, a valgus stress is applied to the knee with one hand. Palpation of the medial side of the knee with the other hand is helpful. If it is a particularly large leg, it may be necessary to use one hand to support the calf. A gentle swinging motion rather than a sudden forceful thrust often allows evaluation of laxity without producing reflex muscle spasm. Excessive

abduction of the knee and tactile evaluation of opening of the joint space indicates a positive test. The presence or absence of instability is more important than its grade. The test is graded as 1+, 2+, or 3+. An opening of less than 0.5 cm is 1+, 0.5 to 1 cm opening is 2+, and greater than 1 cm distraction of the medial joint line is 3+.

The valgus test is then done with the knee in full extension. If hyperextension greater than that in the opposite knee occurs, anterior cruciate rupture may be suspected. If medial joint compartment opening occurs with the knee in extension, a posterior capsule—and possibly a posterior cruciate—tear is present.

Varus (adduction) testing of the knee is carried out in a similar manner: first at 30° flexion with the foot in internal rotation, and then in extension. With the knee in full extension, the lateral collateral ligament is tight, and varus stress tests the integrity of this ligament. If the knee goes into recurvatum with excessive external rotation due to subluxation of the lateral tibial condyle posterolaterally, a posterolateral laxity has been demonstrated. Injury to the popliteus tendon, lateral collateral ligament, and arcuate ligament allows for this instability.

The Lachman test is probably the most sensitive test for anterior cruciate instability.[970] This test is done while the patient is supine and his knee is in approximately 15° of flexion, with the foot resting on the ground or table. The distal femoral condyle is gripped with one hand to stabilize the femur. The other hand grips the proximal tibial condyle on its posterior aspect and applies an anterior directed force in an attempt to produce a forward translation of the tibia on the femur. An anterior displacement of more than a few millimeters without a firm end point is a positive Lachman test. It is also helpful as this test is done to view the contour of the knee from the lateral aspect. Loss of the normal slightly concave slope of the patellar tendon also is confirmatory of a positive Lachman's test.

Anteroposterior instability of the knee is checked next. This is done with the knee flexed 60° to 90° and the foot resting on the examining table. The examiner sits on the foot to stabilize the leg in neutral rotation. The hands are placed on each side of the knee to feel for relaxation of the hamstrings and to allow a push and pull to the proximal tibia. A drawer test is performed in the usual manner.

Controversy exists as to the reliability of the anterior drawer sign. Girgis and colleagues[833] demonstrated in their study that the bulk of the anterior cruciate ligament is relaxed in flexion. There is, however, an anteromedial band of the cruciate that tightens with flexion. Whenever this band was cut, an anterior drawer sign was present. Block to an anterior drawer test, even with an injured anterior cruciate, can occur owing to muscle spasm, torn menisci, blocking cruciate stumps, and loose bodies.

An increased posterior drawer sign is always present when the posterior cruciate ligament is ruptured, according to Girgis and colleagues.[833] Andrews[786] and Hughston[854] state that the posterior drawer sign is not a valid test for acute posterior cruciate tear. They report nine of 18 cases with a negative test (checked under anesthesia) in which the posterior ligament was ruptured. Moore and Larson[915] found that no one test was 100% accurate for acute posterior cruciate injury. The posterior drawer was the most predictive, being positive in 12 of 18 knees (67%). One can only conclude that when the posterior drawer sign is positive, there is rupture of the posterior cruciate, but a negative test does not rule out such a lesion.

It may be difficult, in assessing anteroposterior laxity of the knee, to determine whether it is excessive anteriorly or posteriorly, or both. The contour of the anterior aspect of the knee in the testing position should be checked. Loss of the normal prominence of the tibial tubercle or flattening of the front of the knee may indicate the proximal tibia is sagging posteriorly (Fig. 16-74). Lateral x-rays with anterior and posterior stress help to resolve this uncertainty.

In the same position rotary instability is evaluated. Sixty degrees of knee flexion may be used, as suggested by Hallen and Lindahl.[840] The important thing is to check both knees in the same degree of flexion. The instability is evaluated first with the foot rotated internally 30°. This tightens the lateral structures of the knee and a forward-backward thrust on the knee tests their integrity. The foot is then placed in 15° external rotation to tighten the medial structures. Again, a forward-backward thrust is done to see if excessive external rotation of the medial tibial plateau is occurring.

The "lateral pivot shift," as described by MacIntosh,[902] or "jerk test" evaluates anterolateral instability. MacIntosh believes this instability results from loss of the stabilizing effect of the anterior cruciate. The test is done with the foot in neutral or internal rotation and the knee in extension. The knee is then flexed, maintaining a valgus stress. As the knee is brought to 15° to 30° flexion, a thud or jerk is felt. This is produced by the lateral tibial plateau reducing to its normal position beneath the lateral femoral condyle. In extension, the lateral tibial condyle rotates forward and inward, allowing the lateral femoral condyle to slide posteriorly on the sloping posterior lateral tibial condyle into a position of subluxation. Maintaining the valgus stress as the knee is flexed accentuates the thud or jerk of reduction as flexion occurs.

During the examination one must be mindful of a combination of the types of instability mentioned or an additional instability of the patellofemoral mechanism. The mechanism that produced a medial collateral ligament tear may also disrupt the medial retinaculum and vastus medialis obliquus and allow the patella to subluxate or dislocate laterally.

RADIOGRAPHIC FINDINGS

Though the examination of the ligaments under stress usually gives the diagnosis, x-rays should be made. They indicate associated fractures or osteo-

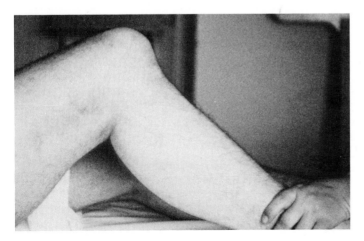

Fig. 16-74. Obvious posterior sag of the proximal tibia and loss of normal tibial tubercle contour indicate loss of posterior cruciate integrity.

chondral fractures. Stress films, particularly in the adolescent, should be exposed to determine if the abnormal laxity is due to epiphyseal opening. Lateral push-pull films are helpful in determining whether the tibia is moving too far posteriorly or anteriorly, and to see if any bone fragments of the cruciate attachments are present. If such fragments are seen radiographically, the site of tear and the repair technique necessary at surgery can be pre-determined.

Arthrography of the knee may be helpful for full evaluation of the knee after injury. If done early the area of the tear can be localized. Associated meniscal injury can be diagnosed, particularly of the posterior horns, which are difficult to visualize when inspecting the joints. Liljedahl and colleagues[895,896] believed that arthrography was particularly valuable as a diagnostic aid for anterior cruciate ligament injury. If the anterior cruciate was not seen or if the continuity was doubtful, an examination under anesthesia was done. Their criteria for rupture were excessive anterior mobility or abduction instability in hyperextension.

A formal arthrogram requires proper positioning of the x-ray tube, so that it is exactly perpendicular to the joint line to properly assess the status of the menisci. This often requires special techniques, such as image intensification, to assure this localization. In an acute injury the primary concern is the status of the ligamentous structures rather than the menisci. For the study of ligament integrity one can inject 25 ml of Hypaque Meglumine (60%) or Renografin (60%) and 5 ml of Lidocaine. Tongue and Larson[969] had an accuracy rate of 82% in diagnosing anterior cruciate and medial collateral ligament integrity doing such a limited arthrographic study. Four views are taken: two anteroposterior views, one of these with appropriate varus or valgus stress, and two lateral views, one with an anterior stress to the tibia. The anteroposterior view shows leakage of dye if there is a rent in the capsular layer, and the lateral view aids in assessing the integrity of the cruciate ligaments. The lateral view taken with an anterior stress to the tibia is important, because the synovial covering overlying the ligament, if intact, may be confused with an intact cruciate. Anterior stress helps to obliterate this shadow or narrows it markedly, if the anterior cruciate is torn.

Recently the use of CT scans to detect tears of the menisci and cruciate ligaments, also done with arthrography, has determined that such lesions of these soft tissues can be diagnosed.[825] Glick and colleagues[834] were able to determine the status of

18 anterior cruciate ligaments in 21 knees. They stated gross tears of the menisci could be detected in most instances but experience suggests that subtle tears were not easily determined.

ARTHROSCOPY

Over the past decade, fascination with the arthroscope in the orthopaedic community has led to ever-increasing proficiency in its use and application. With few exceptions, it is now accepted as a valuable aid in diagnosis and treatment of the "acute knee" and the "chronic problem knee." DeHaven and Collins[811,812] increased their diagnostic accuracy from 78% to 94% with the aid of the arthroscope. Its value in facilitating needed procedures and preventing unnecessary arthrotomies is pointed out by Jackson and Dandy.[867] In reviewing 614 cases that would have undergone arthrotomy if the arthroscope were not available, the authors found that 196 (32%) patients avoided an open procedure and the treatment was modified in another 165 (27%).

During the earlier periods of arthroscopy, the value of this procedure in the acute knee injury was questioned because of poor visualization (Jackson[866] and Casscells[801]). Improved equipment and irrigation techniques have eliminated this concern. The problem of when the acute knee should be arthroscoped is now more of a concern.

Evaluation of the acute knee injury by clinical examination is often very difficult due to effusion, protective splinting, and reflex muscle spasm. Additional information can occasionally be gained following aspiration and injection of local anesthetic into the joint space.

Arthrography has long been recognized as a valuable tool in investigation of possible pathology within the knee. DeHaven and Collins[811] demonstrated an overall arthrographic accuracy of 78% in a prospective study of 100 patients. The accuracy of arthrography varies in different series; however, several constants are present. The medial compartment accuracy is greater than the lateral compartment accuracy, and if an error occurs, it is usually a false negative and not false positive.

Using arthroscopy in conjunction with arthrography has provided a means to demonstrate all anatomical areas of concern following acute knee injuries. Whereas the arthrogram demonstrates the menisci and the continuity of the capsular ligaments and cruciates, the arthroscope allows visualization of the articular surface, the intercondylar notch, and popliteus tendon, as well as the menisci and cruciates.

We believe that arthroscopy should be used when its findings will influence the treatment plan in the early stages of an injury. The diagnosis of a meniscal tear within the first few days is not always critical. However, some orthopaedists desire very early evaluation of the anterior cruciate ligaments. Both Noyes and colleagues[924] and DeHaven[809] have pointed out that 75% of knees which develop a hemarthrosis within the first 24 hours following trauma are associated with anterior cruciate pathology. Demonstration of anterior cruciate incompetence during the first few days following injury is often difficult by clinical examination for laxity. This is clearly emphasized in a study which depicted only 4% of patients who eventually developed anterior cruciate laxity were initially diagnosed as having this problem.[925] DeHaven[810] found in 35 consecutive cases of proven, acute, "isolated" anterior cruciate tears, the classical anterior drawer test was positive without anesthesia in only 10%. With examination under anesthesia, this test was clearly positive in only 50%. The Lachman test was the most valuable, finding positive results in 80% of patients without anesthesia and 100% under anesthesia.

Not all acute ligamentous knee injuries need or should be arthroscoped. When gross laxity makes a clinical evaluation of significant ligamentous description evident, arthroscopy should not be done or done with extreme care. Cases have been reported of the irrigation fluid used in arthroscopy spilling out into the surrounding tissue allowed by the disruption. This may produce pressure on the neurovascular structures with dire consequences when not recognized.[810]

Judicial use of arthroscopy, which has low morbidity, as well as examination of the knee while the patient is under anesthesia, greatly improves the accuracy of diagnosis in the acute knee.

METHODS OF TREATMENT FOR COLLATERAL LIGAMENT INJURIES

NONOPERATIVE TREATMENT

Injuries to ligaments that do not produce instability should be treated conservatively. Sometimes a tear of the meniscus is associated with these injuries. In the early stages, the meniscal injury may not be recognized. Swelling, soreness, and limitation of motion may preclude an adequate examination to determine if there is meniscal injury. If one is certain that no ligament instability is

present, the knee can be treated conservatively and followed for evidence of meniscal tear.

Conservative care varies with the severity of the injury. Mild sprains may need no treatment other than immediate icing and compression to minimize swelling. Activity is allowed commensurate with tolerance. Quadriceps exercises should be instituted immediately to retain muscle tone and to speed recovery.

Moderate to severe sprains without laxity may require immobilization, either by splint or cast, for protection of stretched or partially torn tissues. Crutches may be necessary until walking is comfortable. Quadriceps exercises are particularly important. These can be isometric early to retain muscle strength. Restriction of vigorous activity that might put strain on the injured structures should be continued until tenderness is resolved and quadriceps strength is nearly normal. Our regimen is to have quadriceps strength regained to within 90% of that of the uninjured leg before the patient returns to contact sports.

A cast-brace for those patients in whom immobilization is felt necessary is particularly valuable for the nonoperative treatment of acute knee injuries. A cast-brace with a hinge with a limited arc of 40° extension to 70° flexion protects the ligaments from stretching. Motion with a full arc hinge can be used in the second stages of treatment to prevent a severe valgus or varus stress to the knee as later stages of healing occurs. If it is felt necessary to limit rotation, the foot should be included in the initial cast. The foot piece can be removed and partial weight bearing begun as symptoms subside, tenderness resolves, and strength returns.

When the knee is unstable, surgical repair is usually indicated. There are two exceptions. If the ligament detachment is confined to the femoral attachment of the tibial collateral ligaments with no evidence of other ligament tear, the application of a cast will suffice. Injuries of this type usually show minimal instability. The ecchymosis and tenderness are well localized to the femoral epicondyle. These tears are well approximated at this site, and surgical intervention cannot improve the situation. The second exception must take into consideration the age of the patient, the functional demands for use of the injured knee, and the degree of instability. An elderly patient whose only activity is going to be walking and whose laxity is grade I is best treated by simple casting for 6 weeks. A middle-aged athletic person with a similar amount of laxity must be carefully evaluated for an anterior cruciate injury. If associated medial collateral ligament injury and anterior cruciate injury is present, surgical repair will provide the best chance of a stable knee. Without the associated anterior cruciate deficiency, nonoperative treatment may suffice if it is felt that healing will occur without significant lengthening of the involved ligament.

Though the early literature emphasizes the use of casts for the treatment of ligament rupture, recent writers are almost unanimous that, with few exceptions, early surgical repair is the treatment of choice. O'Donoghue, who has pioneered this concept, states, "The surgery will never be easier than immediately after injury."

OPERATIVE TREATMENT

Acute Rupture of Medial Collateral Ligaments

The patient is placed on the operating room table so that the foot of the table can be dropped, allowing the knee to flex beyond 90°. We use a triangular bolster on which to rest the distal thigh (Fig. 16-75). The patient is placed so that 6 cm of space is present between the block and the popliteal crease. This protects the posterior structures and allows the surgeon to get to the posterior aspect of the knee through either the lateral or medial incision. After preparation and draping, the foot is dropped so that the knee is in 90° of flexion.

The medial incision begins just above the medial femoral epicondyle, extends anteriorly to the medial side of the patella at its midportion, thence distally along the medial border of the patellar tendon to the level of the lower border of the pes anserinus (Fig. 16-76A). The skin flap is reflected posteriorly so that the entire medial aspect of the knee can be inspected from the patella and patellar tendon anteriorly to the popliteal space posteriorly (Fig. 16-76B). If one is certain there are no posterior elements to the tear, the midportion of the incision can be used. We strongly recommend, however, that the full incision be used, so that testing for ligament laxity under direct vision can be done. This is done in the same manner as previously described, but it allows better determination of where the laxity is. The site of rupture is often indicated by hematoma or ecchymosis, which is best detected after the superficial fascia has been incised.

When torn ligaments are easily identified, simple repair is done to restore the ligament to a state as near normal as possible. Often the posterior portion of the superficial tibial collateral ligament is torn along with the posterior medial capsule (posterior oblique ligament). One should determine the extent

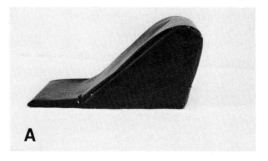

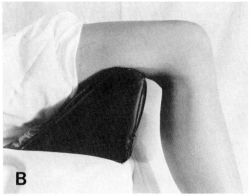

Fig. 16-75. (*A*) A bolster is used to allow knee flexion past 90°. (*B*) Positioning on the bolster. Note the space between the top edge of the bolster and the popliteal crease, which allows room to approach the posterior aspect of the knee through either medial or lateral incisions.

of the tear of the capsular ligament, since it may go past the posterior medial corner and into the posterior structures in the back of the knee.

Often there is so much disruption of the tissues that it is difficult to identify layers or define planes. We prefer to identify the lower edge of the pes anserinus and incise this edge, but leave the semitendinosus insertion on the tibia intact until it is determined whether this tendon might be used for augmentation of an anterior cruciate ligament repair (see Anterior Cruciate Injuries). If the latter is not a possibility or if a pes anserine transfer is contemplated, the lower two thirds of the pes anserine attachment can be detached and elevated to facilitate identification of the distal attachment of the superficial tibial collateral ligament. The plane between the pes anserine group superficially and the superficial collateral ligament, which is deep to the pes, is followed from below upward. This makes it much easier to determine the site of rupture and to prevent incising portions of the tibial collateral ligament that remain intact. The

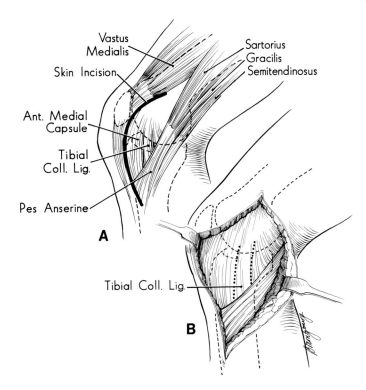

Fig. 16-76. (*A*) Medial skin incision and underlying medial structures (see text). (*B*) A posterior skin flap allows visualization of the medial side of knee from the patellar tendon to the posterior medial corner. (Slocum, D. B.; Larson, R. L.; and James, S. L.: Late Reconstruction of the Medial Compartment of the Knee. Clin. Orthop., **100**:23–55, 1974.)

upper margin of the pes anserine is identified and the fascia proximal to this is divided to trace the superficial tibial collateral ligament more proximally. The proximal one third of the pes anserine attachment is left attached to the tibia at this stage, so that a pes-plasty may be done, if desired.

It is important to identify tears in the capsular ligament lying deep to the superficial tibial collateral ligament. These tears may involve elements of the anterior third of the capsule, the mid-third, the posterior medial capsular oblique ligament (posterior oblique ligament), or extensions into any part of this capsular half-sleeve. The condition of the capsular layer in its meniscofemoral and meniscotibial portions should be determined (see p. 1558). If the meniscus is intact and if its attachment to the capsular layer is sound, the capsule can be reattached to the area from which it was torn—femur or tibia. There is sometimes enough of a tag left at the bone site to allow direct repair of this layer. If not, the layer can be sutured into drill holes in the bone, or sutures may be passed through parallel drill holes across the tibia or femur and tied on the opposite side.

The importance of the meniscus as a functional unit of the knee has received considerable attention in recent literature (see Meniscal Injuries). The

consensus is now that as much of a stable, symmetrical rim of meniscal tissue as possible should be preserved. Peripheral tears should be reattached. If the entire body of the meniscus is shredded and so damaged that its presence will provide a detriment to knee function, the meniscus then requires removal. If there is a sufficient tag of meniscofemoral or meniscotibial portion of the deep capsular ligament present, its reattachment should certainly be accomplished.

Inspection within the joint should be done after an assessment of ligament damage. If the medial joint structures are markedly disrupted, the joint can be easily opened to ascertain the integrity of the menisci and cruciate ligaments. When the ligament tears are less revealing, an anterior incision medial to the patellar tendon is utilized. Through this incision, the medial and lateral menisci can be inspected and probed with a small hook, and the integrity of the cruciates can be ascertained. If any meniscal tissue is torn in the body, this can be removed in the attempt to preserve as much of a stable, symmetrical rim as possible. If the cruciates are torn, they should be repaired as described by O'Donoghue.[931] (More will be said of the cruciates in a later section of this chapter.) A probe passed to the posterior medial corner of the knee through the anterior incision helps to identify a rent in the capsular ligament that may be difficult to visualize because of overlying tissue.

Particular attention should be directed to the posterior medial corner for possible tears of the posterior medial capsular ligament (posterior oblique ligament). Fibers of this portion of the deep capsular ligament, according to Hughston and Eilers,[857] incur the greatest degree of disruption in acute ligament tears. Restoration of the integrity of the postero-medial corner of the knee is extremely important to prevent residual rotary instability (Figs. 16-77 and 16-78).

What does one do when the medial components are so disrupted that identification of layers and a neat repair looms as an impossibility? After the

brow is wiped, a search is made for other structures on the medial side of the knee to replace or reinforce damaged tissue. Several structures can be used (Fig. 16-79).

If the posterior medial corner is in a bad state of disarray, the medial one third of the medial head of the gastrocnemius tendon can be detached from the posterior femoral condyle. It is split downward from the remaining tendon to allow this free end to be swung medially and anteriorly where it is reattached to the medial femoral condyle. This provides some tissue of substance to which frayed ligament tissue can be reattached.

The semimembranosus complex can also be used (Fig. 16-78). The tendon sheath is carefully incised to expose the proximal portion of the tendon. By

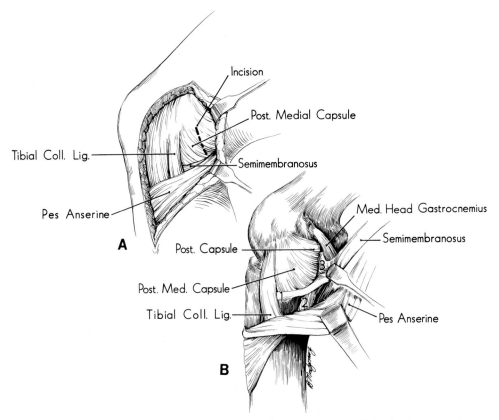

Fig. 16-77. (*A*) The elective incision to inspect the posterior medial joint is through the soft area behind the strong oblique band that forms the trailing edge of the posterior medial capsular ligament (posterior oblique ligament). (*B*) Posterior medial structures: posterior medial capsule, posterior capsule, and three of the tendons of the semimembranosus. (*1*) Anteromedial tendon; (*2*) the direct head inserting into the posterior tubercle of the tibia; (*3*) the lateral expansion, which becomes the oblique popliteal ligament. (Slocum, D. B.; Larson, R. L.; and James, S. L.: Late Reconstruction of the Medial Compartment of the Knee. Clin. Orthop., **100**:23–55, 1974.)

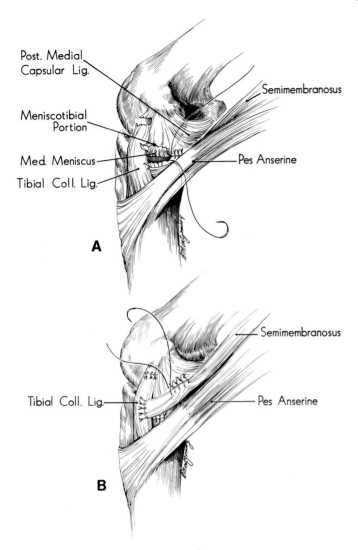

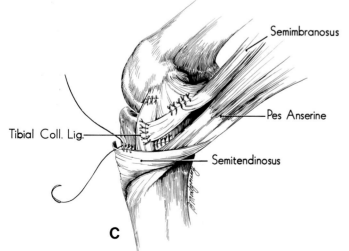

Fig. 16-78. A 20-year-old football player was struck on the outer side of the right knee by a blocker. Immediate testing for stability revealed valgus laxity with the knee at 30° flexion. Surgical exploration showed a tear of the posteromedial capsule (meniscotibial portion) and a tear of the femoral attachment of the tibial collateral ligament. The medial meniscus and anterior cruciate ligament were intact. (*A*) At repair of the meniscotibial portion of the posterior capsular ligament (posterior oblique ligament), the meniscus was left in place. (*B*) Repair of the posteromedial capsule and reinforcement with advancement of the semimembranosus (see text). (*C*) A pes anserine transplant was done to help control excessive external rotation during active running and cutting.

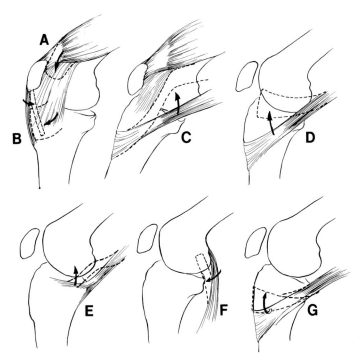

Fig. 16-79. Structures that can be used for reinforcement in acute ligament repairs of the medial side of the knee. For anterior medial capsule reinforcement: (*A*) distal advancement of the vastus medialis obliquus, and (*B*) split patellar tendon and anterior advancement of the anterior medial capsule. For tibial collateral ligament reinforcement: (*C*) advancement of the sartorius, and (*D*) pes anserine as a patch over deficient tissue. For posterior medial capsule reinforcement: (*E*) anterior proximal advancement of the semimembranosus, and (*F*) medial anterior reattachment of the medial half of the tendinous medial head of the gastrocnemius. For anterior cruciate deficiency and rotary laxity: (*G*) pes anserine transplant.

bringing this tendon medially, anteriorly, and proximally, leaving its distal attachments intact, one can reinforce the posteromedial capsule by suture of this tendon to this area (posterior oblique ligament) or trailing edge of the superficial tibial collateral ligament. It is necessary to incise the fascia that connects the semimembranosus and medial head of the gastrocnemius tendon in order to shift the semimembranosus tendon adequately. It should be noted that the semimembranosus is not detached distally but merely shifted into its new position, with the direct tendon insertion of the semimembranosus as its pivot point. The anteromedial attachment, which passes beneath the superficial tibial collateral ligament, is detached and reattached superficial to the tibial collateral ligament so that it lies in a direct line with its proximal muscle fibers (Fig. 16-78*B*). This allows a more direct pull when the semimembranosus contracts, a broader area of fixation, and increased efficiency in stabilization of the posteromedial corner.

The pes anserinus group of muscles have in the past been used as a patch over a defect of the medial collateral ligament complex. These may have to be used as such. More efficient use of these muscles can be obtained by using their dynamic strength in other ways. We are thinking particularly of their use in pes anserine transplant, as described by Slocum and Larson[957] (Fig. 16-78*C*).

For reestablishing anterior support, Slocum modified the pes-plasty by advancing the sartorius anteriorly and suturing it to the posteromedial edge of the vastus medialis obliquus proximally, leaving its distal attachment to the tibia (Fig. 16-80). The tendon and muscle of the sartorius are thus aligned with the anterior edge of the superficial tibial collateral ligament, providing a dynamic support over the medial side of the knee. Care must be exercised in mobilizing the muscle proximally to protect the sartorial branch of the saphenous nerve and to prevent its entrapment. The semitendinosus and gracilis are reflected upward and attached to the medial edge of the patellar tendon in the manner described for pes anserine transfer.

When disruption of the anteromedial tissues is such that repair is difficult, two other structures are available. The vastus medialis can be mobilized proximally and advanced downward. A small tag of tendinous cuff is left attached to the muscle edge to give firm tissue in which to anchor sutures. Mobilization both laterally and medially allows the muscle to be pulled distally 1.2 cm to 2.5 cm. It is sutured to the retinacular tissue at this level, or if the pes anserinus has been reflected proximally as a patch over the medial joint, the vastus medialis edge can be sutured to it. This provides a dynamic tightener of the capsule of the medial side of the knee.

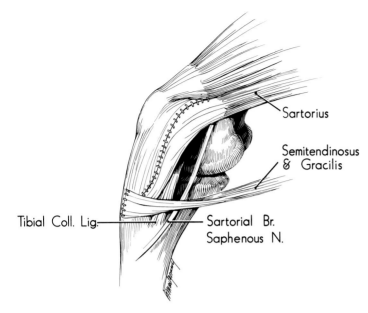

Sartorius

Semitendinosus & Gracilis

Tibial Coll. Lig.

Sartorial Br. Saphenous N.

Fig. 16-80. Sartorius advancement. The tibial collateral ligament can be reinforced by mobilizing the sartorius and suturing it along the anterior border of the tibial collateral ligament and into the distal edge of the vastus medialis fascia. The distal insertion of the sartorius is left attached. Care is taken in mobilizing the muscle to protect the sartorial branch of the saphenous nerve. The remaining two components of the pes anserine—the semitendinosus and gracilis—are reflected proximally and attached to the medial border of the patellar tendon, as in the usual pes anserine transfer. (Slocum, D. B.: Personal communication.)

During inspection of the medial side of the joint after an acute tear, the vastus medialis should be examined. If a tear of the muscle or its retinaculum is found, this should be repaired, thus restoring its stabilizing function to the patella.

Another structure that can be used to reinforce the anterior medial aspect of the knee is the patellar tendon. Slocum and colleagues[960] have used the medial one third to one half of this tendon (Fig. 16-81). This section of the tendon is detached distally. The gap created is closed by advancing the anterior medial capsule to the medial edge of the remaining attached portion of the patellar tendon. This serves to tighten the medial capsular sleeve. After it is split the patellar flap is swung medially from the remaining attached lateral portion of the patellar tendon. The medial flap is reattached under appropriate tension to the anterior proximal tibial condyle through a small periosteal slit. The underlying bone is roughened to enhance a firm attachment. This partial tendon transfer also provides a medial guying action to the patella, should medial retinacular laxity be a concern.

Occasionally the posterior capsule is torn. It should be inspected and repaired if ruptured. Suture of the torn edges is done if possible. When the capsule is torn from its posterior tibial attachment, drill holes can be made in the tibial condyle and the sutures in the capsule passed through the holes to snug the capsule into the posterior aspect of the tibia (Fig. 16-82).

We very frequently reinforce acute repairs by

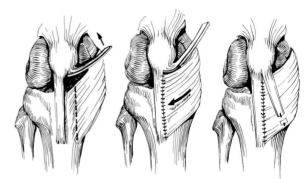

Fig. 16-81. Method to reinforce the anterior medial corner of the knee by splitting the patellar tendon. (*Left*) The patellar tendon is split and the medial half is reflected proximally. (*Center*) The anterior medial capsule is advanced laterally to the edge of the attached portion of the patellar tendon. (*Right*) The split end of the patellar tendon is reattached medially to the tibia to reinforce the anterior medial corner. (Modified from Slocum, D. B.; Larson, R. L.; and James, S. L.: Late Reconstruction of the Medial Compartment of the Knee. Clin. Orthop., **100:**23–55, 1974.)

one of the above methods. The frayed, hemorrhagic ruptured tissue often makes the security of the repair suspect. Because it is difficult to repair the torn ligaments to make them as tight as they were prior to rupture, the addition of a dynamic stabilizer further helps to provide firm support.

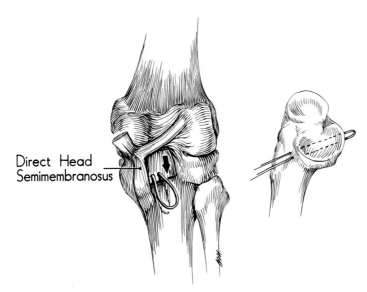

Direct Head
Semimembranosus

Fig. 16-82. The posterior capsule should be repaired if it is torn. When detached from the posterior tibia it can be reattached through drill holes in the proximal tibia placed lateral to the direct head of semimembranosus. (From Slocum, D. B.; Larson, R. L.; and James, S. L.: Late Reconstruction of the Medial Compartment of the Knee. Clin. Orthop., **100**:23–55, 1974.)

Authors' Preferred Treatment. We use all procedures mentioned above as single methods of repair or in combination. Our aim is to provide a functional, stable knee joint. To do so requires individualization with the procedures chosen depending on the age of the patient, the structures involved, and the degree of instability at the time of examination under anesthesia. The procedure, or the combination of procedures to be used, can only be determined by the surgeon. Familiarity with the above mentioned procedures provides sound surgical principles on which to proceed.

Acute Rupture of the Lateral Supporting Structures

Acute lateral instability of the knee is not only less common but is less frequently recognized when present than medial instability. The stabilizing structures of the lateral side of the knee are the iliotibial tract, popliteus tendon, biceps tendon, and the lateral capsule and lateral (fibular) collateral ligament (see Fig. 16-53).

Functional instabilities resulting from injuries to one or more of these structures include simple varus instability, alone or in combination with either anterior or posterior luxation of the lateral tibial condyle. One must first determine by appropriate stress testing (see p. 1524) the type of lateral instability.

Nicholas[919] feels that simple varus instability with no significant rotary laxity, either anterior or posterior, can be treated conservatively, either with cast or brace, and produce excellent functional results. The immobilization or protection is contin-

ued for 4 to 6 weeks. The reason for the good results of conservative care with a simple varus instability is that little varus stress is placed on the knee in usual activity. It is a valgus stress that the knee is continually called on to resist.

When marked varus instability is present, or when anterolateral or posterolateral instability is present, operative repair gives the best chance for good functional recovery.

Positioning, preparation, and draping of the patient is the same as with repair of the medial structures. The incision begins just above the lateral femoral epicondyle and extends anteriorly to the distal lateral edge of the patella, and then distally along the lateral side of the patellar tendon. Its distal end can be swung slightly posteriorly below the joint line to aid in exposure of the fibular head area. A posterior flap is developed allowing visualization of the lateral side of the joint from the patella, the patellar tendon, and the tibial tubercle anteriorly to the posterior lateral aspect of the knee.

Visual inspection for areas of ecchymosis and stressing the knee as points of laxity are assessed visually helps determine what areas require repair.

Kennedy and Fowler[877] stressed cadaver specimens, but were unable to show any sequential yielding of lateral compartment structures when forces of varus and internal rotation were applied.

Methods used for reconstruction for lateral instability may be necessary for adequate functional recovery (Fig. 16-83). It is advantageous for the surgeon to be aware of these reconstructive techniques should he need to use them to reinforce the acute repair.

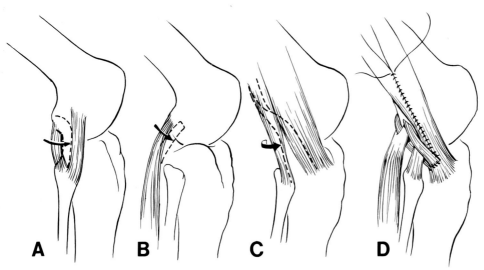

Fig. 16-83. Structures used to repair and reinforce the lateral side of the knee. (*A*) Advancement of the lateral edge of the arcuate ligament and posterior capsule to the lateral capsule and the posterior edge of the lateral collateral ligament. (*B*) Lateral anterior reattachment of the lateral half of the tendinous lateral head of the gastrocnemius. (*C*) Transplantation of the biceps tendon, either by detaching and proximally advancing the lower three fourths of its insertion on the fibular head or by detaching its attachment completely and reattaching it to the anterior lateral tibial condyle. (*D*) Detaching a strip of iliotibial band for reinforcing the lateral side of the knee (see text).

Identification of the iliotibial band, biceps tendon, and lateral collateral ligament or their remnants is first accomplished for orientation. Inspection of the joint through the rent of the lateral side is done if possible. If necessary, an anterolateral incision through the capsule is made for adequate inspection of the cruciates and both lateral and medial menisci. Appropriate measures for damage within the knee—repair of the cruciates, repair of the torn menisci, or removal of the torn portion of menisci—are first accomplished. If cruciate repair is necessary, the techniques of O'Donoghue[931] are used. Tying of the cruciate repair is delayed until the lateral structures are repaired.

Augmentation of cruciate repairs is often done to enhance the tensile strength of the repair (see Cruciate Ligament Ruptures). When an anterior cruciate ligament injury is present, a lateral pivot shift phenomenon may be present (see pp. 1524–1525). When such an instability is present, the operative creation of a check rein to prevent forward displacement of the lateral tibial condyle might be appropriate. Several methods to achieve this have been described.[820] The iliotibial band is useful for reinforcing the lateral side, if that is necessary.

MacIntosh,[902] in stabilizing an anterior luxation of the tibia (which he believes is due to anterior cruciate deficiency), detaches a 2- to 4-cm-wide strip of the iliotibial band proximally, for a distance of 15 to 20 cm, leaving its distal attachments intact. The free end of the fascia is passed posteriorly beneath the lateral collateral ligament and woven through the intermuscular septum posteriorly for a distance. An alternate to this procedure is, after passing it beneath the lateral collateral ligament, to attach the fascia at the posterolateral corner or to the lateral edge of the gastrocnemius insertion, or to pass it through a drill hole in the posterior lateral femoral condyle, and to bring the remainder of the fascia distally, suturing it to itself and to the intact tibial attachment of the iliotibial tract. This maneuver controls anterior slipping of the tibia on the femur and reinforces the lateral aspect of the knee (Fig. 16-83*D*).

Ellison[819] detaches the iliotibial band at Gerdy's tubercle and reroutes it beneath the fibular collateral ligament. The anterior limb of the biceps tendon is also rerouted around the fibular collateral ligament for additional dynamic support to prevent anterior subluxation of the lateral tibial plateau.

Our preference for the use of the iliotibial band in this situation is discussed in the following section on Cruciate Ligament Rupture.

Anatomical restoration of the lateral structures is the aim of acute repair. Repair is done with the flexed knee held in valgus and external rotation to restore the posterolateral corner as snugly as possible when varus and anterolateral instability are the components being corrected.

Should the tissues be so disrupted that suture placement is difficult, a strip of fascia lata may be used as a suture. It is taken from the lateral thigh with a fascial stripper. This strip, sutured with a Gallie needle, provides bulk to allow the suture to hold without pulling through the attenuated tissue. The posterolateral capsule is plicated and advanced to the posterior edge of the lateral collateral ligament. The arcuate ligament, which is the lateral edge of the posterior capsule and the confluence of the popliteus tendon origins, when intact, provides a firm anchor to which the middle third of the capsule and posterior edge of lateral collateral ligament can be attached.

It was previously recommended that lateral meniscectomy be done when advancing and imbricating the posterolateral structures. Because of the investigative studies indicating the importance of the menisci to continued knee use, such a recommendation is no longer made. Meniscal mobility after these repairs should be visualized. If congruent joint motion is present without meniscal entrapment, no problems should arise. If an abnormality of meniscal motion is produced, an alteration of the repair may be in order.

It may be necessary to mobilize the lateral head of the gastrocnemius to reinforce the posterolateral corner when marked disruption has occurred. Gastrocnemius advancement tightens the upper portion of the posterior capsule and provides muscle support to the posterolateral corner, thereby decreasing the tendency for anterior or posterior luxation of the tibia.

When the femoral attachment of the popliteus tendon or lateral collateral ligament has been torn loose, reattachment with proximal advancement will help tighten these structures. Attachment to bone can be accomplished either with drill holes or barbed staples. The tibia should be rotated externally and pushed backward to provide as much tightening as possible as the ligaments are repaired.

If both anterior advancement of the gastrocnemius and posterior capsule and proximal advancement of the lateral collateral ligament and popliteus tendon are done, the gastrocnemius is attached over the popliteus-lateral collateral ligament fixation.

The biceps femoris may also be used to reinforce the repaired tissue. The biceps femoris can be transplanted by detaching the lower three fourths, rolling it over on itself for a distance of 6 cm to 8 cm and suturing the distal posterior edge to the distal margin of the iliotibial band. Its tendinous insertion may also be detached from the fibular head and reinserted immediately behind the attachment of the iliotibial band to the lateral tubercle of the tibia (tubercle of Gerdy). The contiguous edges of the biceps and iliotibial band are sutured for additional support. The transplant of the biceps femoris gives active support to the lateral side of the knee and decreases the posterior pull on the fibular head. Its anterior reattachment also helps control anterior and internal luxation of the tibia on the femur.

Posterolateral instability[858] is present if there is excessive posterior rotation of the fibular head, excessive dropping back or external rotation of the posterolateral corner of the knee as the knee is extended holding the heel in the hand, a posterior drawer sign, or excess varus instability with recurvatum. Repair of the ligament disruption should be done with the tibia in internal rotation, valgus, and with the tibia held forward on the femur. This position is difficult to maintain. Transfixion by a tibiofemoral pin can be used to immobilize the knee in this position. Alternatively, percutaneous pins in the proximal tibia can be incorporated in the postoperative cast and removed when healing has occurred.

Reapproximation of the structures at the posterolateral corner is necessary when the injury has involved these structures. The lateral collateral ligament and popliteus tendon are identified. The posterior capsule and lateral attachment of the gastrocnemius tendon are inspected. One must ascertain if the posterior cruciate ligament is intact or stretched. When the condition of the above structures has been determined, repair can begin. Posterior cruciate reattachment or repair by O'Donoghue's method[931] is the first step. Next, mobilization of the lateral head of the gastrocnemius and posterior capsule is done. (If the acute tear does not involve the posterior capsule or posterior cruciate, the above steps are not necessary.) Anterior advancement of the lateral head of the gastrocnemius and posterior capsule, as explained previously, may be necessary to reconstitute the posterolateral corner. The distal portion of the posterior capsule is fixed beneath the posterior edge of the lateral tibial condyle through drill holes. Suturing the posterior capsule to the upper border of the popliteus fascia may also provide fixation, if good purchase with the sutures is possible.

The popliteus tendon, if torn, should be advanced proximally and anteriorly for reattachment. The arcuate ligament, the posterior edge of the lateral collateral ligament, and the transplanted gastrocnemius head can be sutured together to reinforce the posterolateral corner. As these structures are tightened by suturing, care must be taken to see that extension of the knee and flexion can be accomplished. Some slight limitation at extremes of these motions is permissible, because the repaired tissue usually stretches with use. It is best to have a tight repair, so that the patient does have to stretch the tissue after immobilization has been discontinued. We have not found regaining of motion to be a problem, although it may take several months to achieve maximum motion.

As a further dynamic reinforcement for posterolateral instability, a pes anserine transplant can be added. This helps stabilize the tibia against excessive external rotation and reinforces the internal rotation effect of the popliteus. A pes anserine transplant should not be done if the posterior cruciate has been torn, because this is the axis about which the dynamic rotation by the transplanted pes occurs.

Another structure that bears scrutiny at the time of lateral ligament repair is the peroneal nerve. It may be stretched, or in severe cases even ruptured. Platt[947] called the association of severe adduction injury and peroneal nerve paralysis "ligamentous peroneal nerve syndrome." It has also been called "lateral compartment syndrome of the knee."[971] The injury is due to traction and varies from a mild neurapraxia to complete disruption of the nerve. It should be suspected in any adduction injury to the knee with signs of damage to the lateral ligament and capsular structures. Towne and colleagues[971] and Novich[923] recommend early exploration of the peroneal nerve with definitive repair as soon as possible. White[981] recommends exploration if there is no evidence of recovery after 3 months. If extensive resection is necessary at repair, the prognosis is not favorable.

Authors' Preferred Treatment. Again, a preferred approach to the repair of torn lateral knee structures cannot be undertaken. We at one time

or another choose to use one or a combination of all of the above procedures.

POSTOPERATIVE CARE

Cast immobilization with the knee in the position of flexion and rotation that best takes the strain off the repaired tissue is provided. The amount of flexion used for immobilization varies from 30° to 60°. The latter is used when a posterior capsule repair has been done. A web strap is incorporated into the proximal anterior end of the cast, which can be buckled to a pelvic band to help decrease the weight of the cast on the leg (Fig. 16-84).

Immobilization is continued for 6 to 8 weeks. During this time exercises are done; quadriceps and hamstring tightening are done regularly. When acute reaction has subsided, leg lifts with hip flexion, abduction, and extension are done to preserve muscle tone. The cast is changed when necessary if it becomes loose.

Swedish investigators determined, by suturing divided ligaments of the knee with elastic suture on cadaver specimens, that there was no pull on the ligatures in the 30° to 60° range of knee motion. They have incorporated a hinged cast with stops to allow knee motion in this range. We routinely use such a hinged cast with stops at 40° and 70°. (This allows a slight safety factor in preventing the knee going past 30° in the cast). This is applied at 7 to 10 days postoperatively. Some believe that when anterior cruciate repair and augmentation are necessary, a longer period of protection should be provided. Paulos and colleagues[943] do not apply the hinged cast when intra-articular surgery has been done until approximately 4 weeks postoperatively.

Some concern about the adequacy of immobilization provided by a cast is necessary if one reviews the work of Krackow and Vetter.[888] They found on cadaver studies that casts applied over minimal or no padding allowed significant varus-valgus, anteroposterior, and rotatory motion of the knee when manipulated manually. They suggest that the risk of significant stretch or disruption of the repair is present even in the cast. This study further amplifies the necessity for an adequate and firm repair and the importance of dynamic reinforcement.

The motion provided by the hinged cast may well support Dehne's[813] spinal adaptation concept. Dehne and Torp[814] proposed that the degree of joint motion permissible after fracture or ligament

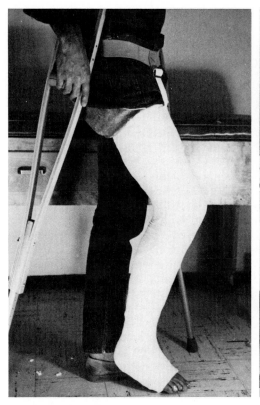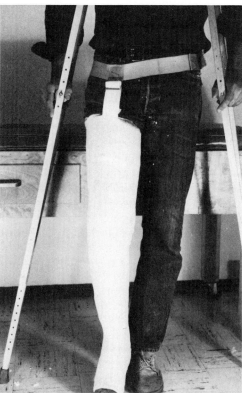

Fig. 16-84. A web strap incorporated into the proximal cast and buckled to a pelvic band helps decrease the weight of the cast on the leg.

repair is determined by the rate of decrease of inflammatory signs, and later by their continued absence. Stabilization is held to the minimum necessary to protect against noxious stimuli. The concept of spinal adaptation is that repair is an adaptive process sensitive to adverse external stimuli and responsive to regulated feedback exposure.

The limited hinge cast is changed to a cylinder cast with a full motion hinge at approximately 6 to 8 weeks. Motion is gradually obtained and partial weight bearing instituted, starting with 10% weight and working upward each week through 25%, 50%, and then 75% of full weight-bearing capacity. Full weight bearing is allowed when muscle strength has returned to appropriate levels. When anterior cruciate repair and augmentation has been done, weight bearing is instituted by keeping the knee in the flexed position and bearing weight on the ball of the foot to prevent the knee from extending, placing additional stress on the repaired cruciate ligament (see Cruciate Ligament Injuries).

USE OF BRACES

The use of a brace with a dial that can be preset through certain arcs of motion can be used instead of a cast. This allows tightening of the brace during the rehabilitation period and more easily accomplishes wound care. When such braces are used, the same criteria as mentioned in the previous section, that is, motion between a limited arch of motion between 40° and 70° is used during the early stages of healing and changed to a full range arch of motion at approximately 6 weeks.

After the cast has been removed, regulated and supervised muscle and joint rehabilitation is begun. No attempt is made to force extension or flexion, except by active exercises. A corset-stay knee support or commercial postoperative knee splint is used after the cast is removed, until muscle tone and strength allow adequate support to handle the leg. Crutches are continued until the patient can lift a given amount of weight with an isometric contraction of the quadriceps with the knee at 45° flexion. The amount of weight is determined by the build of the patient. Generally, we require women to lift 15 to 20 pounds ten times. For a husky athletic man the requirement is 30 pounds ten times. These figures, though arbitrary, give the patient a goal; we feel that this amount of quadriceps strength develops enough support to the knee that unprotected weight bearing can be started without undue stress on the knee. Nicholas[920] recommends the use of a derotational knee brace to protect the knee until full power and motion are restored. These braces can be fitted to help control valgus or varus stress and internal or external rotation. (The appropriate brace must be ordered for the side of the knee that needs protection.)

CRUCIATE LIGAMENT INJURIES

Rupture of the cruciates in association with other ligament injuries has been discussed in the section on acute ligament injuries. Because of the controversies that still exist about isolated cruciate injuries, further discussion is necessary. That there is a condition, such as isolated tear of the anterior cruciate ligament, is denied by some; others are skeptical, and yet another group are certain it exists. The controversy does not end there. Accepting its existence, surgery for repair of the isolated tear is deemed necessary by some and unnecessary by others. This latter dilemma is not to be construed to mean that acute repair should be neglected if surgical repair of other ligaments or meniscectomy is necessary.

The predicament is stoked by many factors. The blood supply to the cruciates is so tenuous that healing after repair is sometimes poor or absent. (Kennedy and colleagues[879] in an anatomical study stated that "the vascular supply though not profuse . . . was by no means sparse . . . and appeared to be adequate for healing of the ligament. . . .") The structural complexity of the cruciate ligaments is just beginning to be appreciated.[833,844,878,879,926] Even though structural continuity can be established, the restoration of their dynamic action remains difficult. Finally, there are those persons, on whom knee surgery is done, who are found to have anterior cruciate ruptures of long standing. Functionally, they have seemingly managed in vigorous activity quite effectively.

On the first premise—that isolated cruciate injuries do or do not occur—one must again consider the work of Palmer.[939] As he indicated, the ligaments do not work independently. There need be only minor insufficiency—"partial injury" to one of the components—for the functional loss of the other to be clinically evident. His cadaver experiments were expressed as (1) CS + (KS) for lateral rocking and (2) KS + (CS) for a drawer sign, where CS is collateral ligament injury, KS cruciate ligament injury, and parentheses denote a partial or overstretching lesion. He believed that cruciate ligament injuries are not isolated. Hawkins and Kennedy[844] found that the anterior cruciate ligament stretched considerably before it actually tore. These studies were done using the Instron Tension Analyzer after mercury strain gauges were sutured onto the ligament.

Plastic deformation of stretched ligaments may not be detectable by direct inspection. Also, with other ligament injuries, stretching or internal damage to the cruciates may be undetectable by visual examination.

Studies have shown[816,833,889,895,896,905,907,939,946] the tendency for degenerative changes, recurrent effusion, and stability problems to be manifest with anteroposterior instability. Since the cruciates, in addition to their stabilizing function, act with other ligaments to guide the knee through its normal balance of motion, loss of this function increases meniscal and articular cartilage wear. We therefore feel that acute anterior cruciate ligament rupture should be repaired, along with correction of other functional deficiency. Augmentation of the repaired cruciate ligament is also believed to be of benefit in most instances of anterior cruciate tear.[891]

Acute posterior cruciate rupture should also be repaired. A study by Moore and Larson[915] revealed early diagnosis, complete ligament repair, and dynamic reinforcement when indicated provide the best prognosis for long-term functional stability.

ISOLATED CRUCIATE INJURY

Injuries do occur of which the predominant feature is anterior or posterior cruciate rupture. As mentioned, they are, in our opinion, associated with some other ligament injury that may not be clinically detectable. Most reported series of cruciate ligament injuries to the knee attest to the high number of associated injuries. O'Donoghue[934] reported the results of 82 operations for ligament injuries; 62 involved the cruciate ligaments. Seven were considered isolated cruciate ruptures—three anterior, three posterior, and one combined. Liljedahl and colleagues[895] in a series of 43 operative cases verified anterior cruciate injuries (33 complete ruptures and ten partial ruptures) reported 13 isolated injuries. The remainder had concomitant injuries, most (24) to the medial collateral ligament. Pickett and Altizer[946] had a series of 129 knee ligament injuries, of which they reported 59 involved only the anterior cruciate ligament. Fifty of these, however, had an associated meniscal tear. They reported three isolated posterior cruciate tears and two combined anterior and posterior cruciate injuries. Solonen and Rokkanen[964] reported 90 cases of ligament injuries to the knee. Twelve of the injuries are listed as anterior cruciate only, three as posterior cruciate only, and one a combination of the two. It is our feeling, even after review of these excellent studies, that a concomitant injury is present, though it may not produce a recognizable clinical finding. The predominant or clinically evident instability is what demands treatment.

There is good reason for the smaller number of posterior cruciate tears as compared to anterior cruciate injury. Hawkins and Kennedy,[844] reporting on tension studies of knee ligaments, found the posterior cruciate to be nearly twice as strong as the anterior cruciate.

ANATOMY

Each cruciate has two functional parts. The bulk of the anterior cruciate is loose in flexion but has an anterior medial portion that is tight. In extension, both parts are tense. The posterior cruciate has the bulk of the ligament taut in flexion, but a posterior portion is loose in this position. With extension the posterior portion tenses, and the bulk of the ligament is loose (Fig. 16-85). When one accepts these findings of Girgis and colleagues[833] it can be seen that the anterior drawer sign is not present unless the anterior medial portion of the anterior cruciate is ruptured; that a posterior drawer sign is not elicited unless the bulk of the posterior cruciate is ruptured; that slight hyperextension occurs when the anterior cruciate is severed in its entirety; and that marked hyperextension occurs only when the posterior portion of the posterior cruciate is also ruptured with the anterior cruciate (Table 16-2).

The middle geniculate artery provides the major vascular supply to the anterior cruciate ligament.[879] A branch of this artery, the tibial intercondylar artery, passes along its dorsal surface. Histologic studies of the anterior cruciate ligament by Kennedy and colleagues revealed an irregular arrangement of fasciculi separated by spaces containing loose connective tissue, tortuous blood vessels, and nerve fibers.[879]

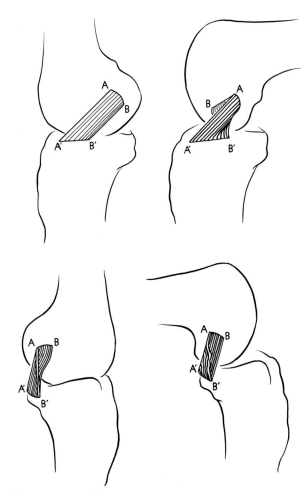

Fig. 16-85. Attachments of the cruciate ligaments. (*Top*) Anterior cruciate. Note that in extension both components are tight. With flexion the anteromedial fibers (A-A') remain tight, while the bulk of the ligament relaxes (B-B'). (*Bottom*) Posterior cruciate. In extension the posterior fibers (A-A') are tight, and the bulk of the ligament relaxes (B-B'). With flexion, the posterior fibers relax, and the anterior bulk becomes tense. (Girgis, F. G.; Marshall, J. L.; and Al Monajem, A.R.S.: The Cruciate Ligaments of the Knee Joint. Anatomical, Functional and Experimental Analysis. Clin. Orthop., **106**:216–231, 1975.)

MECHANISM OF INJURY

There has been some confusion as to the mechanism of injury that produces "isolated" cruciate ruptures.

Kennedy and associates[879] applied stress to a cadaver knee joint with three mechanisms: abduction-external rotation, anterior dislocation by hyperextension, and an anteriorly directed force to

Table 16-2. Tenseness of Cruciate Ligaments in Flexion and Extension

	Anterior Cruciate		Posterior Cruciate	
	Anterior Medial Portion	Bulk	Bulk	Posterior Portion
Flexion	Tight	Relaxed	Tight	Loose
Extension	Tight	Tight	Loose	Tight

Modified from Girgis, F. G., Marshall, J. L.; and al Monajem, A. R. S.: The Cruciate Ligaments of the Knee Joint. Anatomical, Functional, and Experimental Analysis. Clin. Orthop., **106**:216–231, 1975.

the posterior tibia. In none of these could they be certain that only the anterior cruciate ligament ruptured.

Definite associated capsular and ligament injury was evident in the first two mechanisms. Their attempts to produce an isolated anterior cruciate injury with internal rotation of the tibia failed to produce such an injury before either the tibia or femur fractured. In spite of failure to produce such a lesion in the laboratory, they feel internal rotation of the tibia was the mechanism for an isolated anterior cruciate tear in six of 50 patients found to have anterior cruciate rupture at arthrotomy. They relate a high incidence of meniscal injuries with isolated anterior cruciate rupture. A quick deceleration—twisting injury to the knee, often associated with a pop—is the mechanism as described by Feagin and colleagues.[821] Hyperextension has been described by others as the chief mechanism.

Wall[976] has described a mechanism of injury for an isolated anterior cruciate tear to be a forceful contraction of the quadriceps when the tibia is fixed. No hyperextension and no rotatory torque occurred in his analysis of the game films of players who sustained such an injury.

Kennedy and Grainger[878] state: "Avulsion of the tibial attachment of the posterior cruciate ligament was such a consistent finding in hyperextension experiments on the knee that this phenomenon must be considered a major etiological factor in producing lesions of the posterior cruciate." Girgis and colleagues[833] challenged this finding with their conclusions that the posterior cruciate is a check to hyperextension only *after* the anterior cruciate is severed. The meticulous anatomical descriptions of the anterior and posterior cruciate ligaments lend credence to their statement.

Lack of uniformity of opinion relative to the mechanism of isolated cruciate tear helps deny its existence. These authors' opinions are as follows:

Injuries can occur in which the predominant

clinical feature is a cruciate instability. Their occurrence is rare. They are associated with other lesions of the knee. The possible exceptions are stress that is purely internal rotation, anteroposterior, or hyperextension. In the latter, portions of both cruciates are either stretched or torn. Kennedy[875] showed on cadaver experiments that the posterior capsule gave way before the posterior cruciate ligament in hyperextension stress.

Posterior instability produced by hyperextension requires an anterior cruciate stretch or tear.

If a valgus stress produces a medial joint opening in extension or hyperextension, the posterior capsule is probably torn as well as the posterior or anterior cruciate.

If acute cruciate injury is diagnosed, surgical repair is indicated as with other acute ligamentous injuries of the knee.

CLASSIFICATION

Cruciate injuries can be classified as "partial" (overstretching or rupture of only one functional segment) or complete. They can also be classified as to the site of rupture—femoral attachment, tibial attachment, or in the substance or body of the ligament (Fig. 16-86).

It has been our observation that the majority of cruciate injuries associated with major disruptions of the collateral ligaments due to rotational forces are ruptures near the femoral insertion. These often extend into the midsubstance. The tibial stump of cruciate tissue is usually the major portion. This is particularly true when the anterior cruciate rupture is associated with a medial collateral ligament injury. Anterior cruciate deficiency may occur in an adolescent when the tibial spine and the adjacent intercondylar attachment of the anterior cruciate is fractured. This mechanism is usually from an acute forceful flexion of the knee. The tight anteromedial portion of the anterior cruciate pulls off its bony attachment to the tibia. Femoral insertion detachments rarely are associated with bone fragments.

Kennedy and colleagues[879] reported a series of 50 anterior cruciate ruptures verified at arthrotomy. The midportion of the ligament was the most common site of rupture (72%). These were described as being in the middle 2 cm of the 4-cm ligament.

Evaluation by gross inspection of the extent of ligament disruption, elongation, or damage to its blood supply is unreliable. Partial ligament disruption or an overstretched ligament noted on inspection is also unsatisfactory in the determination of total ligament injury. Experimental work by Noyes

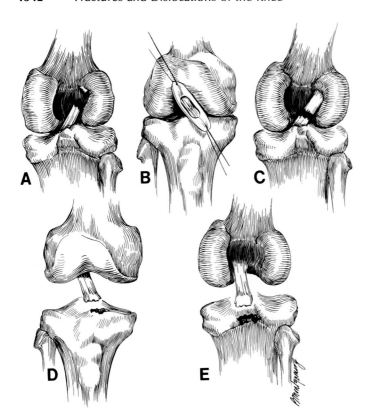

Fig. 16-86. Common areas of cruciate ligament tears. (*A*) Anterior cruciate from the femoral attachment (posterior view). (*B*) Subsynovial tears (stretching) of the anterior cruciate (seen only after synovial covering has been incised; anterior view. (*C*) Midportion tear of the anterior cruciate (posterior view). (*D*) Tear of the tibial attachment of the anterior cruciate. This sometimes carries the bony attachment to the tibia (anterior view). (*E*) Detachment of the bony insertion of the posterior cruciate to the tibia (posterior view).

and colleagues[926] suggested that fast-rate deformation produced greater elongation than did slow rate deformation.

SIGNS AND SYMPTOMS

The history of a mechanism in which the stresses are by internal rotation, an anteroposterior direction, or hyperextension should alert one to the possibility of a predominant cruciate injury. A report of "isolated anterior cruciate injuries" in athletes alleges that the injury occurs during running with a twisting, noncontact strain (excessive internal rotation of the tibia) or a forceful quadriceps contraction against a fixed tibia. A pop is usually heard; the person is unable to continue to play. A tense effusion develops, and often "pseudolocking" is present.

Posterior cruciate ligament rupture should be suspected when the mechanism of injury is a forceful posterior displacement of the proximal tibia on the flexed knee. It should be noted that the anteromedial portion of the anterior cruciate is taut at this position and may be stretched or torn with this mechanism of injury. Abrasions or contusions over the front of the proximal tibia or ecchymosis or hematoma in the popliteal area should suggest

the possibility of posterior cruciate tear. The bleeding in the back of the knee is often due to the detached bony tibial insertion of the posterior cruciate. When such an injury has occurred it is important to look especially for posterior capsule rupture or detachment and for rupture or stretching of the medial capsular ligament. These injuries should also be repaired at the time of cruciate repair.

Anterior or posterior instability may be evident. Anterior instability may be masked by muscle spasm, torn menisci, blocking cruciate stumps, loose bodies, or excessive joint hemorrhage or effusion. If there is excessive joint hemarthrosis, this should be aspirated to allow a more reliable test. The anterior drawer sign cannot occur, acccording to Girgis[833] without a tear of the anterior medial fibers of the anterior cruciate.

Posterior instability is not affected by muscle spasm. The patient flexes his knee with the foot supported on the table. If the proximal tibia is seen to drop backward, producing a concavity to the contour of the anterior knee from the tibial tubercle to the patella rather than its normal flat or convex appearance, posterior instability is evident. Comparison with the opposite side is helpful.

RADIOGRAPHIC FINDINGS

Routine radiographic studies may show a bone fragment at the site of cruciate insertion. These are nearly always from the tibial attachment of the cruciates if they are seen. It should be mentioned that the tibial spines are not the attachments of the cruciate ligaments. Consequently, tibial spine fractures do not connote cruciate ligament injury, although their presence suggests the elevation of the adjacent intercondylar bone to which the cruciate attaches.

Arthrograms are particularly helpful in diagnosing cruciate ligament tears. Liljedahl and colleagues,[570] as mentioned previously, felt examination under anesthesia was indicated if cruciate ligament continuity was absent or doubtful on arthrograms. When arthrography fails to show the anterior cruciate ligament (the same would hold true for posterior cruciate) and an examination under anesthesia shows increased sagittal mobility, arthrotomy is indicated.

It must be remembered that the cruciate ligaments are extrasynovial. The synovium is invaginated from the posterior aspect into the notch area during development. The cruciates have an anterior synovial layer. It is possible for the anterior cruciate to be ruptured beneath this synovial layer (see Fig. 16-86). This produces two possible sources for error. With arthrography, the synovial band may be interpreted as an intact cruciate. At surgery, if anterior cruciate disruption is suspected and not seen, the overlying synovial layer, if still intact, must be split to visualize the substance of the cruciate tissue adequately.

A less formal arthrogram, as described in the preceding section on radiographic findings in ligamentous injuries, is helpful for assessing cruciate integrity.

Pavlov and colleagues[944] reported an accuracy of 94% in interpreting an anterior cruciate cause in both chronic and acute cases of anterior cruciate tear. The anterior surface of the anterior cruciate as seen on the arthrogram was evaluated. The cruciate was normal if this surface was straight. If the surface was bowed, wavy, or absent, the anterior cruciate ligament was torn or absent.

METHODS OF TREATMENT

Complete rupture requires surgical repair. The methods described by O'Donoghue[931] serve well for reattachment of the cruciate ligament. Instruments designed to aid in proper placement of the drill holes from the femoral condyles to the inter-condylar notch are most helpful. Several such drill guides are available.

It is well to consider the femoral and tibial attachments of the cruciate ligaments. The femoral attachment of the anterior cruciate lies well back on the inner side of the lateral femoral condyle. The most frequent error is reattaching it too far forward in the notch area. Such an attachment may limit full flexion or cause stretching of the ligament. We feel a careful attempt should be made to re-establish the normal position of insertion. The femoral attachment is slightly oblique anteriorly from the vertical. The attachment is broad; therefore, two drill holes spaced the approximate width of the normal attachment should be used. Girgis and colleagues[833] found this width to average 23 mm. Though the ideal is normal anatomical reattachment, this goal is often difficult to achieve because of frayed tissue ends, the confined area of the notch, which makes accurate suture placement difficult, and the difficulty of visualization for the placement of drill holes. One can only keep the anatomical points in mind and strive for as near perfection as is possible under the circumstances that prevail.

The same principles hold true when reattaching the posterior cruciate to the inner side of the medial femoral condyle in the intercondylar notch. This attachment is slightly more anterior than the femoral attachment of the anterior cruciate, but it is still past the midline posteriorly in the notch. Its attachment is more horizontally oriented and averages 32 mm in width. Reattachment to the inner side of the medial femoral condyle is technically less difficult than reattachment of the femoral attachment of the anterior cruciate. When the body of the ligament is intact it should be snugged up firmly to its femoral insertion to prevent or minimize posterior displacement of the tibia on the femur.

The tibial attachment of the anterior cruciate usually presents no problem with reattachment to its normal bed. Often a piece of bone allows good fixation for the suture.

The tibial detachment of the posterior cruciate provides problems with exposure relative to its repair. There is often a fragment of bone avulsed from the tibia. If this is the only injury of major significance, some advocate a posterior approach as described in *Campbell's Operative Orthopaedics*[796] and by O'Donoghue.[933] This certainly makes reattachment easier but does not allow adequate visualization of the joint to see if any other problems exist.

Brennan[793] uses two incisions—an anteromedial and a posteromedial—to repair the tibial avulsion of the posterior cruciate. We prefer to use the medial skin incision as described in the previous section on operative repair of the medial ligaments. The joint can be opened anteromedially for inspection and posteromedially to visualize the tibial attachment of the posterior cruciate ligament. The posteromedial incision into the fascia extends vertically from the vastus medialis above to the sartorius below (see Fig. 16-77). The posterior aspect of the joint is entered through the thin part of the capsular sleeve. This is found by palpating the relatively thick trailing edge of the medial capsule posteriorly until the thin tissue is identified. Posterior to this the palpating finger can feel the heavier tissue of the posterior capsule. The capsular incision is from the medial femoral epicondyle distally toward the posterior capsule to the semimembranosus tendon complex.

Sutures through the detached ligament or over the avulsed bone can be brought through drill holes through the proximal tibia by the O'Donoghue method. Should the posterior capsule be detached or relaxed, snugging of this can be accomplished at the same time as described in the previous section on medial ligament repair (see Fig. 16-82). This is often necessary, because the posterior capsule is often torn or stretched with the posterior cruciate rupture.

Ruptures through the body of either cruciate ligament are most difficult to approximate. Again the method of O'Donoghue—pulling one section of the fibers proximally by suture through drill holes and the other section distally so that they overlap—can be used. To avoid strangulation of the blood supplies care should be taken so that the ligament is not under too much tension. This type of tear probably gives the least chance of satisfactory healing. Some believe the chances of functional healing are so remote that the surgical time necessary for this type of repair is not warranted.

Solonen and Rokkanen[964] have reinforced anterior cruciate repair with a distally based fascial graft to act as its core. Some of the tissues used for anterior cruciate substitution are various portions of the patellar tendon,[872,889] the ilotibial band transferred into the intercondylar notch,[836,934] the semitendinosus[790,] of gracilis[816] tendon, and meniscus.[977] There are various extra-articular procedures to correct anteroposterior instability.

Posterior cruciate substitution has used the gracilis,[816] the patellar tendon,[790] the semitendinosus,[878,965] the medial portion of the medial head of the gastrocnemius tendon, the popliteus tendon,[791] and the transferred meniscus.

O'Donoghue does not advocate anterior cruciate reconstruction in the acute injury, even though the cruciate ligament is irreparable. Kennedy and Grainger[878] believe that major reconstructive operations to supplement acute repair should not be encouraged routinely in posterior cruciate rupture. They did, however, state that such was indicated in very occasional situations and described a method using the semitendinosus.

Kennedy's[879] most recent study on anterior cruciate injuries showed good or excellent results in 77% in which repair was not done and similar results in 84% in which the repair was done. These, however, are short-term results. Other studies have shown an increased incidence of degenerative changes, effusion, and meniscus wear with sagittal laxity.

AUTHORS' PREFERRED METHOD OF TREATMENT

Augmentation of a repaired anterior cruciate ligament has three advantages: (1) The augmentation will provide a scaffolding for the cruciate fibers and hopefully will enhance the tensile strength of the repair. (2) The fibers of the torn anterior cruciate will provide increased vascularity to the augmentation. (3) The augmentation will help provide a stent and help stabilize the repaired ligaments.

Our present preference is to use the semitendinosus as the structure for augmentation. This tendon is detached proximally at its musculotendinous junction and delivered distally where it is left attached to the tibia. We previously reattached the proximal musculotendinous rim of the semitendinosus to the remaining gracilis. This required either extending the incision proximally or using an accessory incision over the posterior medial aspect of the thigh. Lipscomb[897] has recently shown that by not reattaching the semitendinosus and allowing it to heal where it will attach has caused only a 7% reduction in pes anserine strength after 1 year.

A drill hole is made in the proximal tibia beginning just medial to the patellar tendon above the semitendinosus attachment into the notch entering just medial to the medial tibial spine just behind the tibial attachment of the remaining anterior cruciate stump (Fig. 16-87). The free end of the semitendinosus is passed through the drill hole into the notch. If an adequate stump of anterior cruciate is present for several sutures, such sutures are passed through the cruciate stump from medial to lateral. Three or four such sutures from proximal to distal area are passed through the stump. Each

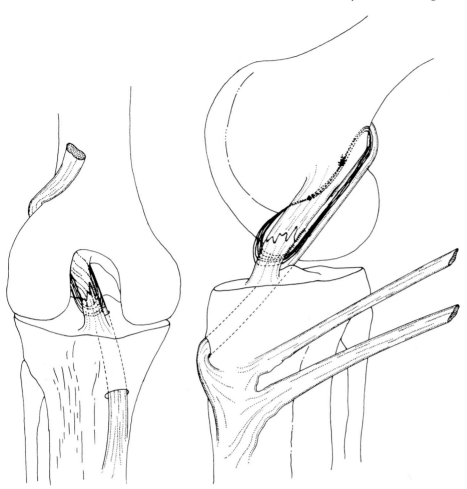

Fig. 16-87. (*Left*) Anterior view of the semitendinosus tendon passing through a drill hole in the proximal tibia and over the top of the lateral femoral condyle. Sutures have been passed through the stump of the anterior cruciate from lateral to medial. The lateral bundle of sutures is passed through a drill hole in the lateral femoral condyle and the medial bundle is taken over the top with the semitendinosus tendon. (*Right*) Cut away lateral view of the placement of the semitendinosus tendon. The medial sutures and the lateral sutures are tied individually over the intervening block of bone (see text). (Larson, R. L.: Acute Disruptions Around the Knee. *In* Straub, L. R., and Wilson, P. D. Jr. (eds.): Clinical Trends in Orthopaedics. New York, Thieme-Stratton, 1982.)

end of the suture is identified so that they can be tied individually when they are brought out laterally. (We use knots in the ends of the sutures [no knots for the most proximal suture], one knot in each end for the second sutures, and so forth). If the anterior cruciate stump is not long enough to provide a repair, the remaining stump ends are sutured to the semitendinosus so that they will be pulled toward the femoral stump as the semitendinosus tendon is pulled out over the top of the lateral femoral condyle.

If the cruciate sutures are used, the medial bundle will be passed through the posterior lateral aspect of the notch over the top of the lateral femoral condyle and the lateral bundle of fibers will be passed out a drill hole that will be made 1 cm distal and 1 cm anterior to the point where the sutures penetrate the posterior lateral capsule as they come over the top of the lateral femoral condyle. By passing the lateral bundle of sutures through the drill hole in the lateral femoral condyle, and the medial bundle of sutures through the posterior orientation, a restoration of the normal twist of the anterior cruciates is provided. The bundle of sutures and the semitendinosus are passed together through the notch penetrating the posterolateral capsule and over the lateral femoral condyle. After semitendinosus tendon and sutures have been passed the sutures are tied individually, starting with the proximal suture and tying it over the intervening bone between the drill hole and the exit over the lateral femoral condyle. The semitendinosus tendon is then fixed to the lateral femoral condyle area, either by suturing to the intermuscular septum, by stapling, or by directing the tendon into a small drill hole and fixing it with a staple or sutures. A final step in this procedure is to detach the infrapatellar fat pad proximally, leaving it attached at a broad base distally. A suture is passed through its free proximal tip and is delivered out over the top in the same direction as the semitendinosus. The suture is tied to the soft tissues laterally. This provides a fat-pad covering for the repaired and augmented tissues, to enhance its vascular supply and to help protect the repair and transplanted tissue from the fibrolytic action of the synovial fluid.

When it is felt that an extra-articular reinforcement is necessary, one of the procedures of transferring the iliotibial band to a more posterior orientation can be done (see preceding section on Operative Treatment). We prefer to incise the iliotibial tract approximately 1 cm posterior to its anterior edge, beginning at Gerdy's tubercle to a point just above the lateral femoral condyle. The stump of the semitendinosus is then delivered through a slit in the iliotibial band at a point that approximates the area of attachment of the linea aspira. The soft tissues on the posterior portion of the lateral femoral condyle just distal to this attachment of the linea aspira are stripped from the region and the bone roughened. A second slit is then made in the iliotibial band approximately 1 cm anterior and 1 cm distal to the first slit. The semitendinosus is then passed through this slit, first superficially then deep. The semitendinosus is then pulled into the same drill hole through which the lateral sutures in the cruciate stump had been passed. When this lateral reconstruction is done, a quarter-inch drill hole in the lateral femoral condyle is necessary to accommodate the tendon end. The tendon end can be secured by passing a suture through it and passing this suture into the drill hole as the tendon is pulled into the drill hole, securing the suture anteriorly. This, of course, has to be done before the fat pad is pulled into the

notch. Additional sutures are placed in the semitendinosus laterally, where it penetrates the iliotibial band for additional fixation.

This latter procedure provides fixation of the iliotibial band in the posterior orientation as the knee extends and is a constraint to the anterior displacement of the lateral tibial condyle. This type of iliotibial band transfer is a modification of that described by Hughston and Andrews.[856]

When posterior instability is the problem, tightening of the posterior capsule may help. If dynamic protection is desired, we would transfer the medial third of the tendinous portion of the medial gastrocnemius through the back of the intercondylar notch and thence through a drill hole in the medial femoral condyle. The hole is drilled so that it enters the notch near the normal femoral attachment of the posterior cruciate ligament. The medial third of the medial gastrocnemius tendon is split distally from the remainder of the tendon to its muscle belly after it is detached proximally from the back of the medial femoral condyle. It is then passed through the back of the capsule into the joint, thence through the drill hole in the medial femoral condyle. If there is not enough length to bring it to the surface where it can be sutured, a small drill hole is directed obliquely into the larger drill hole, one suture is pulled through this, and the sutures are tied over the intervening block of bone for fixation of the transplanted tendon.

If, after anterior cruciate repair, there is still some laxity present, we use a pes anserinus transplant. Though this does not control anteroposterior laxity, it does provide more internal rotation power for running and cutting activities. With this increased rotary power and proper quadriceps development the anterior cruciate deficiency does not become a functional problem. It must be remembered that firm lateral stabilizing structures should be used, as well as an intact posterior cruciate ligament to preserve the normal axis of rotation, in order that the transplanted pes anserinus functions efficiently.

Avulsion injuries of the tibial spine, which often carry with them the intercondylar bone to which the anterior cruciate attaches to the tibia, are discussed previously. We would only reiterate here that if accurate reduction is not obtained or if marked anteroposterior instability is evident, open reduction and fixation provides the best chance of restoring stability.

POSTOPERATIVE CARE

The postoperative care is the same as that for collateral ligament injuries. As mentioned, a limited hinged cast is applied at 7 to 10 days for joint mobilization and hence lubrication to stimulate healing. Tension of some segment of the cruciate ligaments is present, no matter what the degree of flexion or extension of the knee. When a posterior capsule repair is done, the knee is immobilized at 60° to take the strain off this repair.

Some studies[943] have shown that large forces are produced on the anterior cruciate ligament through the range of 30° of flexion to full extension (0°). These forces were found to be highest at full extension and increased by one or two times by the addition of a 7 pound foot weight. It thus seems prudent to minimize the risk of stress to the repaired and augmented anterior cruciate by omitting exercises through this range of motion in the early phases of rehabilitation. The limited hinge cast (a 40° to 70° hinge is provided to allow a slight safety factor) helps prevent extension past 30° in the early phases of healing. When a full hinge is applied 8 to 16 weeks after surgery, progressive limited weight bearing is allowed. Weight bearing is started by walking on the ball of the foot to prevent extensor stresses. Animal studies suggest that even after 12 weeks, ligament strength is less than 50% of normal maximum strength.[556] When full weight bearing begins at the 12- to 16-week period, full extension with weight bearing is started. During the period in which the patient is in the cylinder cast with the full hinge, a gradual program of active and passive extension with no excessive stress to the joint is allowed.

REHABILITATION AFTER KNEE LIGAMENT REPAIRS

We routinely use isometric exercises initially following removal of the cast. This is done because knee motion is inadequate, at first, to provide a good range of motion exercise and also to protect the joint from an overzealous isotonic exercise program. If there are degenerative changes in the articular surfaces of the patellofemoral or tibiofemoral joints, isotonic exercise regimes may cause joint irritation.

Active range of motion exercises are important. Vigorous passive stretching should be omitted during the first few months of the exercise program.

Internal tibial rotation exercises are begun early after the cast is discontinued. This can be done as an isometric exercise by placing the feet together, with the knees flexed, separating the heels and pushing inward against the sides of the forefoot— one foot resisting the other. Both clenched fists

held side by side between the knees stabilize the knees in the correct position for this isometric exercise. Maximum resistance is maintained for 6 seconds and repeated ten times as part of the daily exercise program.

As muscle strength improves and joint mobility increases, a graduated program of activity is added. Many methods of muscle strengthening are described. Nearly any training program done regularly with sufficient intensity, duration, and frequency increases muscle strength and endurance. After acute knee ligament repair, supervision of the chosen rehabilitation program should be provided so that the activity level does not produce undue stress to the repaired ligaments. Full strength of the supporting musculature of the knee should be required before vigorous programs are allowed. Research studies[835] attest to the effectiveness of quadriceps and hamstrings contraction in limiting excess abduction and adduction of the knee.

Development of maximum strength usually requires at least 6 months of an intense exercise program. Studies have shown that even at 1 year postoperative, 50% of the operated extremities had not regained 90% strength of the unoperated leg.[967] Since the first 4 to 6 months of rehabilitation require a moderation in exercise and activity, it is not until 9 to 12 months later that advanced rehabilitation, including running, can be started. The rapidity with which a complete return to activities can be made is determined by evidence that the knee has full motion, at least 90% of strength and power of the normal leg, and no evidence of joint reaction such as swelling. The use of a protective brace during this period, and when the patient returns to vigorous activity should also be considered.

One deficiency often noted after a knee rehabilitation program is that the quadriceps has been strengthened well, but the other muscles of the leg have been neglected. For total rehabilitation of the injured limb, hip extension, abduction, and flexor strength are necessary. Hamstring strength must be back to normal. Gastrocnemius and supporting muscles of the ankle should be fully strengthened.

The West Point Program[864] for regaining endurance, agility, and coordination is good for the later stages of rehabilitation. This provides for lateral mobility, sudden starts and stops, back-pedaling, cutting, and other activities that require full muscle use of the extremity. Their program also includes the athlete's awareness of lower extremity positioning with activity. Individual counseling is given, so that the athlete understands the present and future effects of his injury and can develop realistic goals for sports and occupational activity.

COMPLICATIONS

Surgical repair of torn and damaged tissue is not without risk.

The immediate postoperative complication to be concerned with is hematoma. A tourniquet is used routinely during the surgical repair to allow better identification of tissue landmarks. It should be released before skin closure and a careful hemostasis should be accomplished. Several small plexuses of vessels are encountered both medially and laterally, which should be cauterized or sutured prior to wound closure. Even after these larger vessels are clamped, there is often considerable oozing from the large amount of involved tissue. It is, therefore, important to use suction drainage to minimize serosanguineous accumulations. Our practice is to continue suction drainage until the 24-hour total is less than 30 ml. The drain (or drains, if necessary) is removed usually at 48 hours after surgery.

Wound breakdown and postoperative infection are closely akin to hematoma formation. Preventing them is best done by preventing this hematoma from developing. It is our routine to irrigate the wound before closure with an antibiotic solution. Once the hematoma has developed, antibiotics are not carried into it by the bloodstream. Intravenous antibiotics are, therefore, given during the surgical procedure through the intravenous drip. At tourniquet release, an intravenous push of the antibiotic is given. Four subsequent intravenous doses by push at 6-hour intervals are administered, after which the intravenous infusion and antibiotics are discontinued.

If a surgical infection does occur, opening of the surgical wound, evacuation of the hematoma, and removal of nonabsorbable sutures are necessary. The wounds are left open to heal from within, like other deep-seated infections.

Intra-articular infection is rare. If it does occur, treatment is carried out as for any infective arthritis.

Thrombophlebitis does not spare the knee patient. Its incidence after major ligament disruption is, however, surprisingly low. It is somewhat disquieting to review the work of Cohen and colleagues[807] who found by postoperative venography 20 patients with deep venous thrombosis on the operated limb among 35 patients who had surgery for arthritis of the knee. Of the 21 venograms on the non-operated leg, only one venous thrombosis was reported.

Should this complication occur, appropriate medical management is begun immediately. The casted leg presents some problem, for both diagnosis and management. If necessary, the cast can be bivalved, and the posterior portion can be used until ambulation is allowed. At this time a full-leg cast can be reapplied.

There are several problems relating to nerves about the knee after surgery. Temporary peroneal palsy may occur when excessive retraction of the soft tissue in back of the knee is necessary. This condition may also occur from cast pressure over the fibular head. If the latter is recognized early and the cast is softened, windowed, or padded at the area around the fibular head, peroneal nerve function returns.

Two other nerves subject to injury on the medial side of the knee are the sartorial branch and the infrapatellar branch of the saphenous nerve. The latter is routinely sectioned with the medial incision used. Its loss is of no clinical importance. If it is preserved and receives excessive traction or heals in scar tissue, an infrapatellar nerve neuroma may result. This produces a localized tender area just medial to the tibial tubercle. Treatment is excision of the neuroma.

The sartorial branch of the saphenous nerve may be damaged by the inital injury or by the surgical procedure. Its loss produces a numb area of the skin overlying the anteromedial aspect of the calf to the level of the medial malleolus. The nerve is identified and protected during a pes anserine transplant or sartorius muscle advancement. It should be mobilized enough with these procedures to prevent its entrapment when these structures are shifted to their new locations. This nerve can be involved in neuroma formation, scar-tissue fixation, or pressure from the overriding tendons of the reflected pes.

Loss of motion of the knee can occur after any knee surgery, particularly after injury where ligamentous tissues and the joint are involved. The severity of the injury and the development of fibrous bands within the knee joint have some relationship to its occurrence. The aim of a surgical repair of ligamentous tissue is to produce firm stabilization. Often a period of stretching and active exercise is necessary to regain full motion. If the tibial collateral ligament binds to the tissues so that its normal posterior glide with flexion cannot occur, flexion may be limited.

Slowness in recovering complete extension may occur after prolonged immobilization. This may be due, in part, to the ligament repair, which needs to be gradually stretched. Maximum motion may require 6 months of exercise and use. If a persistent contracture develops, a period of Russell's traction with the sling behind the calf rather than at the knee or a gentle manipulation under anesthesia is used. The use of an extension-desubluxation hinge incorporated into cylindrical thigh- and lower-leg casts can be used for the gradual extension of knees with marked flexion contracture. Correction to within 15° of extension can be obtained with gradual adjustment of the hinges.

Residual laxity after repair of acute ligament rupture may persist. No ligament repair will provide tissue as firm and elastic as that present prior to its rupture. Adequate immobilization to prevent stress on healing tissue, protection to avoid excess use of the casted leg, muscle exercise programs in the cast, and proper rehabilitation after cast removal are necessary steps to obtaining as good a result as possible. Omission or short cuts in the normal postoperative and convalescent regimen may adversely affect an otherwise adequate surgical procedure.

PROGNOSIS

The tissue and the degree of damage with ligament injury, the many methods used when surgical repair is accomplished, and the newer concepts of knee repair and reconstruction make the task of specifying prognosis difficult. The prognosis for a chronically unstable knee is meniscus wear and progressive joint deterioration. The degree of wear and timing of onset of clinical symptoms relates to the amount of residual instability and the use to which the knee is put.

With early diagnosis and proper treatment, satisfactory results can be anticipated. Most reports on surgical repair[937,946,964] of injured ligaments give 50% to 60% good to excellent results in those cases treated early. Less satisfactory figures are given for late repairs. Hughston and Eilers[857] report nearly 100% return to athletic activities after acute surgical repair when special attention is given to proper recognition and repair of the posterior oblique ligament (posterior medial capsular ligament). Oster[937] reported that 20% of athletes gave up their sport after medial ligament repair but that all patients were working.

A study of results of anterior cruciate repair and augmentation showed that 88% of patients had good or excellent results 1 to 3 years after surgery.[874] It was encouraging to note that the results did not seem to deteriorate over the 3-year period of observation. A continuation of evaluation of even longer term results after cruciate repair is still required to determine the ultimate effectiveness of the intra-articular repair and augmentation of anterior cruciate ligament ruptures.

Poor results may be attributed to failure to correct all components of instability, unsatisfactory healing of repaired ligament tissues, persistent cruciate insufficiency, failure to develop full muscle support to the extremity, or development of one of the complications associated with this injury.

In summary, the prognosis depends on the ability to return the knee to its normal stability and power. Factors interfering with this goal increase the chances of a poorer prognosis.

MENISCUS INJURIES

The frequency of injury to the meniscus, the belief that loss of the meniscus has little effect on joint function, the ease of meniscectomy, and the rarity of serious postoperative problems make removal of the meniscus one of the most popular surgical procedures of the orthopaedist. In World War II the most frequent noncombat injury to military personnel was to the meniscus, and the most frequent orthopaedic operation was meniscectomy.[1191]

The confusion of mechanical disorders preventing normal knee joint motion was categorized in 1784 by William Hey, who coined the phrase, internal derangement of the knee joint.[1133] The surgical approach to correct such a condition was introduced by Paré, who reported in 1558 the first removal of a loose body within the joint. The removal of a torn meniscus as a mechanical impediment to joint motion was first accomplished by Annandale of Edinburgh in 1877.[1133,*]

Though the diagnosis of a torn meniscus is becoming more accurate with the use of arthrography and arthroscopy, the degree of functional loss and the late results in a knee deprived of its meniscus remains unresolved.

The importance of the meniscus in the normal knee is now well recognized. No longer is this structure considered a vestigial organ without a function. Various functions of the menisci include:

1. Shock absorption. The important weight-bearing function of menisci has been suspected as

---

* Helfet,[552] citing the same article as Murdoch (cited above) writes, "In November 16, 1883, Thomas Annandale (1885) performed the first recorded operation for displaced semilunar cartilage. . . . He did not excise the cartilage but cured his patient by drawing the cartilage forward and stitching it to its former attachment."

early as 1948 when Fairbank[1042] discussed the radiographical changes in knees following meniscectomy. Walker and Erkman[1203] have demonstrated that the intact lateral meniscus carries the majority of the lateral compartment load of the extended knee. On the medial side of the knee, approximately one half of the load is transmitted through the meniscus. Krause[1101] showed a two- to three-fold increase across the joint when the menisci are absent.

2. Nutrition. The synovial fluid provides nutrition for the articular cartilage. The meniscus helps to distribute a thin film of synovial fluid over the surface of the articular cartilage.

3. Stability. The meniscus acts as a joint spacer and compensates for the incongruity of the femoral and tibial articulating surfaces by providing a deepening effect, thereby changing the upper tibial plateau into a modified socket. It also aids in the complex rotatory mechanics of the knee joint by participating in stabilization of the knee during the screw home mechanism of knee extension.

SURGICAL ANATOMY

A brief discussion of meniscus anatomy has been given in the section on knee anatomy. Amplification for understanding of the mechanics of injury is necessary.

The medial meniscus is a C-shaped structure attached by the anterior horn to the articulating surface of the tibia and to the lateral meniscus by the ligamentum transversum. The posterior horn is attached to the excavation just posterior to the intercondylar tubercle of the tibia.

The lateral meniscus is more circular and covers more of the articulating surface of the tibia. The peripheral synovial attachment is interrupted by a groove for the popliteus tendon. The lateral collateral ligament is separated from the meniscus by the inferior lateral geniculate vessels.

The inner three fourths of the meniscus is essentially avascular. The more peripheral fibrous zone contains capillaries and fuses into the parameniscal zone, which is the vascular connection between the capsule and the meniscus. The blood supply to the meniscus is not uniform. Even the outer one third, where most of the vascularity is, shows avascular areas.[1160]

The microstructure of the menisci has been well outlined through the work of Bullough[1008] and Cameron and colleagues.[1012] The alignment of the fibers in both the medial and lateral meniscus are similar. The collagen fibers of the menisci are predominantly oriented in two planes. The body of the meniscus is composed primarily of collagen bundles oriented in the longitudinal axis of the meniscus. Grouped over the tibial surface and to a lesser extent over the femoral surface of the meniscus, radially arranged fibers are noted throughout the meniscal body. These radially arranged fibers function to resist the splitting force along the longitudinal fibers.

Arnoczky and Warren[993a] have recently demonstrated that the blood supply to the human menisci predominantly comes from the lateral, medial, and middle genicular arteries. The normal tensile stresses on the menisci are in the longitudinal axis. Because the predominant fiber pattern is in this plane, tears are not unusual. The small number of peripheral radial collagen bundles is inadequate to prevent longitudinal tears when the force is substantial. Likewise, horizontal cleavage tears occur because of the paucity of vertically oriented fibers. Once these few fibers have been disrupted either from trauma or degeneration, there is no internal splinting to prevent the development of horizontal splitting of the body of the meniscus.

Both the lateral and medial menisci have firm attachments at their anterior and posterior horns. The elastic fibrous structure of the menisci and their peripheral attachments cause them to return to their peripheral position after displacement with joint motion. An uncontrolled flexion or extension movement with a block to the normal rotation, which takes place with this action, may trap the meniscus between the condyles of the tibia and femur. The tension produced by the peripheral attachments to the joint capsule and the fixed meniscus attempting to return to its normal position may cause a tear when the tolerance of either the cartilaginous substance of the meniscus or its fibrous attachments to the capsule are exceeded. Helfet,[1065] Kronner,[1160] and Smillie[1185] attribute the tear to violent stretching of the meniscus; Konzetzny and Schaer[1160] explain the tear by the crushing action of the femoral and tibial condyles acting as a pair of pliers, tearing the meniscus longitudinally and displacing the torn portion toward the intercondylar notch. The more frequent medial meniscus tears are explained by the first group to be due to the more firmly attached peripheral border. The lateral meniscus, because of its loose capsular attachments, has greater mobility and is subjected to fewer tension forces. Konzetzny relates the difference to the contour of the articular surface of the tibia. The medial plateau is somewhat concave, favoring displacement of the meniscus into the joint, while the lateral tibial articular surface is slightly convex.

Transverse tears are produced by excessive stretching of the concave inner border of the meniscus. The mechanisms previously mentioned (or, according to Smillie,[1185] a direct blow to the periphery of the lateral meniscus) may tend to straighten its concave edge and cause both a transverse tear and degeneration of the cartilage.

Degeneration of the meniscus is not limited to the older age group. Fowler and Brock[1044] reviewed 117 adolescent patients under 17 years of age who underwent meniscectomy. One half of these patients had histological studies on the removed menisci. Despite the young age, all but two of the patients demonstrated degenerative changes in these structures.

Factors other than trauma may increase the susceptibility of a person to meniscal injury. The number of persons with the history of two or more meniscectomies suggests that constitutional factors play a part in the vulnerability of menisci to injury. Congenital anomalies of the meniscus may predispose to a tear with minimal trauma. The most common congenital meniscal anomaly is the discoid meniscus. This abnormality is almost always found in the lateral compartment of the knee and tears of this structure occur more frequently than in a normal lateral meniscus. Abnormal mechanics of the knee joint as the result of ligamentous injury also leads to early meniscal degeneration and a greater incidence of disruption. Congenital or acquired varus or valgus malalignment may result in altered joint mechanics and lead to early meniscal problems. Persons with laxity of the meniscal attachments to the capsule, poor fibrocartilage, periarticular muscle weakness, obesity, and ligamentous laxity of the joint may be at risk for meniscal tear.

Fractures of the tibial plateau may be associated with meniscal injury due to direct violence. Concomitant injuries have been reported in 70% in one series and in 80% to 90% in another.

CLASSIFICATION

Classification of tears of the meniscus can be made with reference to etiology (*i.e.,* degenerative, traumatic), type of tear, mechanism of injury, and so forth. The usual classification as to type—bucket-handle, parrot-beak, peripheral, transverse, horizontal cleavage, pedunculated—does little but catalog a list of pathologic variations. One is left with the problem of trying to fit a meniscus with a combination of types into the most nearly appropriate category.

More meaningful, in our opinion, is the classification of Groh.[1160]

1. Spontaneous detachment (primary degeneration)
2. Fresh traumatic tear
3. Late changes after a traumatic tear (secondary degeneration)
4. Late changes after ligament damage (pseudo-primary degeneration)

In the spontaneous detachment type, primary degeneration leads to changes in the cartilage substance, which then predisposes to tears. Abnormal stresses encountered in occupations that require squatting or kneeling could produce such degenerative changes. The wear and tear of joint use with aging could do likewise. When the degenerative changes of the meniscus have developed, often a trivial, common motion may lead to the spontaneous detachment. Such degenerative tears, according to Smillie,[1185] are usually horizontal. The horizontal cleavage tear he so aptly describes is such a lesion.

Traumatic tears have the highest incidence. The history is usually clear-cut. The tear is often longitudinal—either bucket-handle or along the periphery. These tears are the lesions of youthful athletes. These tears or those produced by later changes most often produce joint locking.

Late changes after a traumatic tear is a classification very useful to explain the early minor symptoms after knee injury followed by locking in the later stages. A healthy meniscus does not tear easily. Often the first injury produces only a partial tear or detachment. If the tear is at the periphery, healing may be incomplete. With continued mechanical stress, the tears may become enlarged or the torn part of the meniscus may become degenerated. Minimal injury or even just continued use produces further tearing and joint symptoms and locking.

Late changes after ligament damage are the result of the increased wear to the meniscus as the result of joint laxity. Often the posterior horn of the medial meniscus develops secondary degenerative changes from anterior medial joint laxity.[1182] The posterior horn of the lateral meniscus often shows similar changes with anterior lateral laxity.

To this classification could be added tears of regenerated menisci. Bruce and Walmsley[1042] showed in dog experiments that regeneration of excised menisci was progressing and not yet complete, even after 5 months. The regenerated meniscus is thinner and narrower than normal. It is more fibrous, whiter, and has a less sharp concave edge and a dense peripheral attachment with no obvious demarcation as does normal meniscus and capsule.[1185]

SIGNS AND SYMPTOMS

The meniscus does not have sensory nerve endings.[1160] Symptoms are produced by tear and irritation near the joint capsule and by the mechanical interference with joint motion. Other post-traumatic conditions of the knee produce symptoms mimicking those of a torn meniscus. Diagnosis often becomes difficult, particularly immediately after injury when associated ligament sprain or effusion prevents adequate examination of the joint and when there has not been joint use to produce some of the symptoms associated with this condition.

A history is most important. A sudden uncontrolled rotary motion or a sudden flexion or extension of the knee in such a way that the normal tibial external rotation of extension, or the internal rotation of flexion, is blocked is significant. In an athlete, the moment of injury may be quite clear, when he feels the pop, catch, or lock when twisting or cutting on the leg. The activity may be a trivial movement such as squatting, stumbling, or a twist in bed. In the latter situations, a spontaneous detachment or a secondary tear from an older meniscus or ligament injury should be considered. The patient should be questioned about what position he normally assumes at work and about the history of previous injury to the knee.

The presence of joint effusion and the timing of its occurrence are significant. A rapidly distended joint indicates hemorrhage, which would more likely suggest ligament damage, synovial rupture, or osteochondral fracture. An effusion that develops more slowly over a 6- to 12-hour period is more suggestive of a minor ligament sprain or a meniscal tear with joint irritation. Often meniscal tears from degenerated menisci produce no effusion.

The classical symptom associated with meniscus tear is locking. True locking, when the patient cannot fully straighten the knee, relieved by rotation and passive extension, is almost pathognomonic of a meniscal tear, provided a loose body in the joint has been ruled out by x-rays.

Unfortunately, this symptom occurs infrequently and usually only with longitudinal tears. Smillie[1185] reviewed 1,000 cases with surgically proven torn menisci and found only 30% to have true locking.

More significant is the lack of full extension, sometimes not appreciated by the patient.

The history of giving way, "something slipping in the joint," clicking, or momentary catching may be present in less extensive tears. These symptoms, however, are also found in other conditions such as subluxation of the patella, ligamentous instability, cruciate tears, loose bodies, and chondromalacia.

The triad of pain, swelling, and locking was said by Lipscomb and Henderson[1114] to be present in at least 70% of those with meniscus tears.

The most helpful finding on clinical examination, in our opinion, is tenderness along the joint line on the involved side. Irritation of the capsule and synovium from the malfunction of the torn meniscus most likely produces this finding. Occasionally, even this finding is absent in a patient who you are almost certain has a torn meniscus. The question arises as to which meniscus is causing the problem. This is when arthrography is most helpful. We have been impressed by the fact that when localizing signs are absent it is often the lateral meniscus that is injured.

The second most helpful diagnostic test in our examination is to have the patient squat, first with the feet in internal rotation and then with the feet in external rotation. With the feet in internal rotation, squatting produces increased pressure on the medial joint compartment or produces a painful pull on the lateral meniscus as it is displaced into the joint. The pressure or tension on the irritated tissue often elicits pain at the site of injury. Squatting with the feet externally rotated does the same to the opposite sides of the joint. Many times pain is elicited no matter which way the feet are directed, but usually to the same joint compartment.

Many types of maneuvers are used to produce pain or tenderness or a cartilage click or snap in the knee. These include the second Steinmann's sign, Bragard's sign, Böhler's sign, Payr's sign, first Steinmann's sign, Merke's sign, McMurray test, Fouche's test, and the Apley test. There are probably others. All are manipulative tests to elicit the area of pain or tenderness along the peripheral edge of the meniscus by compression or tension or to trap the torn fragment in the joint by forcing the meniscus toward the center of the joint. One should decide which tests or signs he is going to use and use them routinely, because experience in their use increases their value as diagnostic aids. Of the above, we prefer the Apley test and use it routinely. The above tests (except for Fouche's sign[1038]) are nicely described in *Meniscus Lesions—Practical Prob-*

lems of *Clinical Diagnosis, Arthrography, and Therapy* by Ricklin, Ruttiman, and Del Buono.[1160]

Mention should be made of the increased likelihood of diagnostic error in women thought to have meniscus tears. Powers[1155] reports a 23% error in diagnosis in women, whereas the reported error rate in men ranges from 4% to 13%. Smillie[1185] reviewed 8,000 meniscectomies; 981 were in women. The overall diagnostic error rate was 4%, while in the 981 women the error rate was 15%. The lesson is to be particularly precise in evaluating women with knee joint problems. Meniscectomy should not be done unless established pathologic findings are demonstrated. Arthrography as a diagnostic aid is most helpful in this total evaluation.

RADIOGRAPHIC FINDINGS

The use of routine views of the knee should be done, even though the meniscus is not radiographically visible. We routinely use four views of the knee; a standing anteroposterior view of both knees on one plate, a lateral view with the knee in 30° flexion, a notch view, and a modified Hughston view (see Fig. 16-48).

The joint should be assessed for any recent bone injuries or lesions such as osteochondritis, degenerative joint changes, or loose bodies. More rare conditions such as calcification of the menisci, calcification of the infrapatellar or dorsal fat pads, bone tumors, or cystic lesions of the bone may be seen.

The patellar views are particularly helpful in leading to the suspicion of patellar subluxation or dislocation as a cause of the joint malfunction.

ARTHROGRAPHY

Mention has been made of arthrography. It is in the diagnosis of meniscal lesions that it is most frequently used. Many excellent articles have been written on its use and interpretatioin.[1140,1146,1160]

We have surmised that the surgeon's use of arthrography can be divided into four groups: those who never use them; those who use them routinely; those who use them in the more difficult diagnostic problems; and those who use them primarily to assure the patient and themselves that a meniscal tear is not present. It is with the limited use of arthrography that we feel problems may arise. Experience in interpretation comes from reviewing negative as well as positive studies. One can rely

on the radiologist for interpretative readings; however, we feel more value is obtained by a review of the radiologist's readings, a reading by the surgeon himself, and a correlation with the history and physical examination as well as the surgical findings. We are using this evaluation more and more as a routine in the work-up of a meniscus lesion. The exception is when the acute findings are so clear-cut (*e.g.,* a locked knee) and the scheduling with the radiologist would delay the necessary surgical procedure.

The arthrogram is not only helpful in diagnosis of the immediate problem; it may detect lesions in the opposite joint compartment not recognized by clinical examination. It is also most helpful in assessing lesions of the posterior horns of the meniscus, an area that cannot be visualized adequately at the time of arthrotomy. It is comforting to know as the meniscus is being removed that arthrograms showed a lesion in the posterior horn.

Familiarity with the radiologist and the technique employed makes one more assured of his interpretation. We find it most difficult to read arthrograms done by radiologists we do not know and by techniques with which we are unfamiliar.

Arthrography does not replace the history and physical examination in the diagnosis of meniscal tears. A negative arthrogram has a greater chance of error than a positive one. If there is a conflict in diagnosis, the surgeon's clinical evaluation must still outweigh the x-ray tube in the final assessment. The posterolateral corner of the knee, because of dye in the popliteal recess, remains an area difficult to interpret. Small peripheral collections of dye or overlapping bursa shadows may falsely be misinterpreted as tears or obscure regions where tears are located. Technical errors may make interpretation difficult. If the examination is unsatisfactory or if symptoms persist, repeat arthrography can be done if a meniscus tear is strongly suspected.

The accuracy of diagnosis in those fully experienced with the procedure has been reported to be 95% with medial meniscus injuries and 85% with lateral meniscus injuries.[1146]

ARTHROSCOPY

Meniscal tears are one sort of lesion that can be identified through the arthroscope. Arthroscopy is particularly helpful in a group of conditions called "meniscal mimes" by Jackson.[1678] These are conditions that frequently present as a torn meniscus and may sometimes result in the harmful removal of a normal meniscus.

ARTHROSCOPIC SURGERY

Although arthroscopy has many applications in knee surgery, there is now a strong focus on its use in diagnosing and treating meniscal lesions. Such an emphasis is well warranted. The arthroscope, however, merely extends one's visual perception of a small area and must be combined with an intelligent interpretation of what is seen and, if pathologic, how that pathology was produced. Arthroscopic skills take a long time to master. One should develop the motor skills necessary to perform a thorough, diagnostic examination before attempting actual intra-articular procedures. When the entire knee can be visualized and the examiner has developed interpretive diagnostic skills to recognize lesions when present, one can then progress to the elementary transarthroscopic surgical procedures. Skill will only come with persistence and patience while these techniques are being learned.

Arthroscopic Versus Traditional Meniscectomy

With the advent of arthrography, and then arthroscopy, we have greatly enhanced our ability to evaluate the meniscus. Studies of meniscal function and the better results seen in those patients who had only partial meniscectomies, when no other lesion was present in the remainder of the meniscus, have caused opinion to shift towards preserving as much meniscus as possible. Evaluations by Jackson and Rouse[1080] have shown that the area beneath the meniscal tissue is usually protected better even in those with degenerative menisci. The preservation of as much meniscal tissue as possible and the use of partial meniscectomy has been one of the major advances of meniscal surgery. The concept of arthroscopic surgery and partial meniscectomy through the arthroscope does not mean that arthrotomy is unwarranted.

The surgical exercise of arthroscopic removal of the meniscus can be a frustrating experience. Not everyone has the opportunity to develop the surgical skill and technique necessary for arthroscopic meniscectomy, which requires special equipment and many hours devoted to developing the necessary skills. The volume of patients may not be great enough to enable the orthopaedist to develop the skills. If arthrography and diagnostic arthroscopy are used to confirm the diagnosis of meniscal pathology, often only a small incision is required to remove torn meniscal tissue. If such an incision is made, these patients can be treated as if they have had an arthroscopic meniscectomy, with immediate exercise and activity as tolerated by the patient.

There are several techniques that can be used to enhance knee function after an arthroscopic meniscectomy. One is to infiltrate the skin incision as well as the joint with 0.25% Marcaine and epinephrine to minimize the pain resulting from the incision and to allow immediate muscle contraction. The second is the use of galvanic electrical simulation to provide quadriceps contraction immediately following surgery. If motion of the knee and muscular strength is maintained, then arthroscopic meniscectomy or arthrotomy as a method of meniscectomy should have the same morbidity. Whether the meniscus is removed by arthroscopy or arthrotomy, 6 months after surgery the results will be the same. The critical factor in long-term results will be the amount of meniscal tissue that will have to be removed.

Though all menisci probably *could* be removed through the arthroscope, *should* all meniscal lesions be removed through the arthroscope? There are several situations in which arthroscopic removal may not be worth the time or effort. Anatomical obstructions within the knee, such as an excessively large fat pad, a large ligamentum mucosa, or a discoid type of meniscus may present surgical problems that would lengthen the time required for removal of the meniscus to the point that it is not warranted.

Even though the fat pad or mucosal tissue can be shaved away, the procedure is often time consuming and may produce bleeding and perhaps adhesions. The results may be a disservice rather than a benefit to the patient. The patient may have a tight knee, which makes it difficult to get the instruments between the articular surfaces without producing articular damage. As Casscells[1014] has warned, "The longer the operating time the greater the likelihood of damage to the articular cartilage. Repeated passages of instruments inside the joint increase the likelihood of doing damage here." If, after a half hour, and certainly by an hour, progress has not been made and considerable difficulty either in visualization or meniscal removal is demonstrated, arthrotomy for the removal of this pathologic meniscus is certainly justified.

A final situation deserves special emphasis. In many knees, the meniscal tear results from underlying instability that allows the meniscus to tear secondarily. There is sometimes a tendency for arthroscopic surgeons to focus on a meniscus tear, which they eagerly envision removing through the arthroscope. All aspects of knee function should be kept in perspective. If the meniscal lesion is secondary to instability, removal of the meniscus is very likely to enhance this laxity. Consideration needs be given to improving the function of the knee, which may require other surgical procedures that cannot be accomplished through the arthroscope. If instability such as anterior medial rotatory laxity is increased following meniscectomy, perhaps tightening by imbrication of the posterior oblique ligament or pes anserine transfer is in order.

Hughston and Terry have indicated that a single lesion within the knee is "exceedingly rare." They believe that after meniscectomy the stability of the knee joint must be evaluated while the patient is still under anesthesia. If significant laxity can be detected, then appropriate surgical shortening of the attached ligament structures is necessary to restore the dynamic and capsular ligament stability of the knee.

Types of Meniscal Tears

As outlined in Lanny Johnson's text, *"Diagnostic and Surgical Arthroscopy,"* multiple types of tears are amenable to surgical resection (Fig. 16-88). The medial parrot beak tear is perhaps the most simple meniscal lesion to resect. This usually occurs in the anterior or medial portion of the medial meniscus, is easily incised with a knife blade, and removed with forceps.

The transverse tear is usually seen in the mid-third of the meniscus and is best treated with circumferential saucerization about the tear. This tear can be complete or incomplete. When incomplete, it should be completed and the marginal portion of the meniscus removed.

The flap tear is usually based medially or at the posterior horn of either the medial or lateral meniscus. This can be simply excised at its base and removed. The remainder of the meniscus should be inspected for an associated transverse or complex component.

The bucket handle tear is one of the most frequent and more amenable types of meniscus tears for arthroscopic removal. The bucket handle is first detached at its anterior detachment, grasped with a forcep from the opposite portal, and then detached from its posterior attachment.

Various authors have described the exact techniques for removal of various types of tears, and it would be well for those considering removal by arthroscopic means who are unfamiliar with these techniques to review them before attempting this type of surgery. One should take care to inspect the remaining rim after the bucket handle has been removed since a second bucket handle may be

Parrot beak

Flap

Peripheral

Transverse

Bucket handle

Complex

Longitudinal

Horizontal cleavage

Fig. 16-88. Types of tears of the meniscus (see text for description). (Johnson, L. L.: Diagnostic and Surgical Arthroscopy. St. Louis, C. V. Mosby, 1981.)

present or additional transverse tears may require dissection.

Complex combination tears also occur. They require a complete resection of the torn tissue while attempting to leave as much of the stable rim as possible. All mobile tissue should be removed with the meniscus cutter or basket forceps so that the remainder of the tissue can be easily visualized and any vertical, horizontal, or flap tears removed. The remaining tears are saucerized so as to leave as smooth and congruous a rim as possible.

One should consider the possibility of reattaching a peripherally torn meniscus if the body of the meniscus is still intact. Meniscorhesis, as it has been termed, has been demonstrated to be both practical and beneficial for long term knee function.

Instruments for Arthroscopy

Various brands of arthroscopes, both in size and angulation of the lens, are available. For routine arthroscopic work, we prefer the 4-mm 30° angle scope with 5-mm sheath. Larger scopes are available but infrequently used. Though the needle scope was popular originally it is now used only occasionally for visualization of tight knees.

Television Camera and Monitor. Though television is not a must for arthroscopic visualization or arthroscopic surgery, it does have many advantages. Its chief advantage is allowing the operative assistants to visualize what is going on and to anticipate what instrumentation will be necessary as the procedure develops. It also allows the surgeon to remain in one position. This is a definite advantage over the various contortions necessary when using direct visualization through the arthroscope. Its use allows the surgeon freedom of his hands, since one of the assistants can control the arthroscope and the TV camera. An additional benefit is that the procedure can be recorded for later visualization by both the surgeon and the patient and can be used as a teaching aid.

One does have to adjust to using the camera since a different orientation results. The surgeon is not looking into the knee but at a television screen, and the camera must be oriented as though he were looking into the knee directly. If the camera is rotated, the image projected on the screen may be completely opposite as to what the surgeon thinks he is visualizing and may produce confusion until proper orientation is reestablished.

Leg Holder. The use of a leg holder is a benefit in manipulating the knee into valgus and varus

positions and to maintain its position during arthroscopic surgery. There are some, however, who do not feel a leg holder is necessary.

Surgical Instruments. The surgical instruments used for arthroscopic surgery should include the following: (1) The probe, which is the most important instrument in the set of arthroscopic tools, acts as an extension of the surgeon's fingertips and allows intra-articular palpation. They range in design and size, and each surgeon must determine which works best for him. (2) Grasping instruments also vary in size and angulation. Preferences are usually developed as one does arthroscopic surgery. These are used for holding and manipulating tissue while it is being cut. (3) Scissors and various types of basket forceps are also available, along with small meniscal knives, which allow cutting of the pathologic tissue. (4) An intra-articular shaver is an aid in arthroscopic surgical procedures. In addition to its use in removing pathologic tissue, it can also be used to resect obstructing tissue such as the synovium and fat pad for the purposes of visualization.

Surgical Technique

The knee is first examined, after an anesthetic has been given, to test for any instability that may be present. Following this, the knee is placed in the knee holder and the leg prepped and draped in the usual manner as one would for an arthrotomy (Fig. 16-89). Because of the large amount of irrigation fluid used throughout the procedure, water resistant drapes are preferable. A tourniquet is usually used; however, if the procedure is being done prior to reconstructive of ligamentous repairs, the arthroscopy can be done without the tourniquet to preserve tourniquet time for the additional surgery.

Many portals of entry have been prescribed for evaluation of the interior of the knee. One usually develops a preference for a particular portal. We prefer to begin with an anterolateral portal and use as many additional portals as necessary as the procedure progresses both for instrumentation and visualization.

Proper placement of the arthroscope to allow the best visualization of the knee is one of the first and most important techniques to be learned. The portal, as described by Gillquist, is defined by palpating the area where the curve of the anterolateral femoral condyle meets the lateral edge of the junction of the patella and the patellar tendon. The scope is inserted at this point. This allows the scope to be above the fat pad for better visualization.

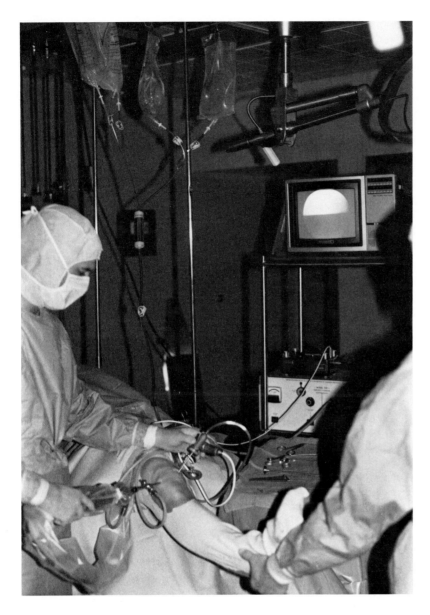

Fig. 16-89. Arthoscopic equipment set-up.

Before the arthroscope is introduced, a large bore needle (we prefer to use the trocar and sheath of the intra-articular shaver) is introduced through a stab wound at the level of the medial superior border of the patella. This introduces the needle into the suprapatellar pouch area and allows distention of the joint with the saline solution. It is necessary to make certain that the needle is in the pouch by moving it distally and proximally. Two 3-liter bags of saline, suspended above the knee, are then used to maintain distention (note the precautions that should be followed in evaluation of an acute knee by arthroscopic means as described on page 1527). With the knee distended, a small stab wound is made into the portal of entry and is carried into the capsular layer. The blunt trocar and sheath can then be introduced with less likelihood of scarring the articular surfaces. The outflow tube is then connected to the stop cock on the arthroscope, maintaining a continual flow of fluid through the joint.

With the knee in extension, the suprapatellar pouch area is first inspected and the condition of the synovium noted. The scope is drawn distally so that the retropatellar surface and trochlear groove can be inspected. The knee can be flexed so that the entrance of the patella into the trochlea can be determined. As the knee is carried in 30° of flexion, the scope is swept over the medial condyle to inspect the medial recess. It then enters the medial compartment for visualization of the medial meniscus.

In most instances, the medial meniscus can be visualized by moving the scope from anterior to posterior in the compartment and applying appropriate valgus or varus stress and at the same time internally-externally rotating the tibia on the femur. When a 30° angled scope is used, rotation of the scope so that its lens changes posteriorly to anteriorly allows visualization of the meniscus with relatively little side-to-side motion of the scope. The examination should include the use of a probe, which is introduced through the anteromedial portal, to palpate the articular surfaces as well as the meniscus and to see if any excess meniscal mobility is present. The scope is then carried into the lateral joint compartment while the knee is placed in the varus position. It is often helpful to bring the foot into a "number four position," which opens up the lateral joint and allows nearly complete visualization of the lateral meniscus from its anterior to posterior aspect. Again, probing the meniscus as well as the articular surface is of benefit.

After examining the medial and lateral compartment, the scope is moved into the intercondylar notch as the knee is flexed to 45°. The visualization is frequently difficult particularly in old cruciate injuries. If there is a copious amount of synovium, one can use the intra-articular shaver to debride the redundant synovium or obstructive fat pad. Once the anterior cruciate ligament is identified, the probe is again used for palpation of the anterior cruciate. While this is being done, the anterior drawer test is placed on the knee to help determine the status of this structure.

Introduction of the scope into the posteromedial compartment can be accommplished through the notch area. This is carried along the medial edge of the anterior cruciate and the medial edge of the bony notch until it is pushed into the posterior compartment, which usually occurs with a slight pop.

The 30° scope allows visualization of the posterior medial compartment, where the meniscus attaches to the capsule, and visualization of the edge of the posterior cruciate ligament. The use of the 70° scope allows better visualization of the posteromedial compartment. The scope can then be introduced into the posterolateral compartment by going laterally to the anterior cruciate ligament and into the posterolateral compartment.

In a study of 100 knees, Baldwin found that by using the Gillquist approach, the posteromedial compartment could be visualized through the notch in 98% of the cases and the posterolateral compartment visualized in 93% of the cases through this portal. In those knees in which it is impossible to introduce the scope through the notch, the posteromedial and posterolateral portal may be used. The techniques are somewhat more difficult, and reference to appropriate arthroscopic literature would be of benefit before these portals of entry are tried.

After completion of the arthroscopic evaluation and any arthroscopic surgery required, the joint is thoroughly irrigated. Thirty cubic centimeters of 0.25% Marcaine and epinephrine is then instilled into the joint and into the small incisional portals of entry. The wounds are appropriately closed with suture or steri-strip, and compressive dressings are applied.

METHODS OF TREATMENT

Once a meniscal tear is identified through a careful history and physical examination and the use of arthrography or arthroscopy, a plan of treatment must be formulated. Depending on the age of the patient, the desired level of activity, and the type of meniscal tear, the choice between nonsurgical and surgical treatment must be made.

NONSURGICAL TREATMENT

If a knee is locked secondary to a bucket handle tear of the meniscus and cannot be released by conservative methods, there is no doubt that operative treatment is the wisest choice. Likewise, if a patient has a documented tear of the meniscus causing symptoms that prevent comfortable participation in daily activities, nonsurgical treatment is usually not reasonable.

However, the importance of the meniscus in the normal biomechanical function of the knee is no longer questioned. These structures should be saved if possible. Fortunately, certain meniscal lesions will heal, as first demonstrated in animal experiments by King in 1936.[1093] He documented that first, a tear limited to the substance of the meniscus probably never heals; second, a peripheral tear through the synovial attachments of the meniscus is capable of healing; and third, a complete transverse or oblique tear that extends to the synovium may heal. Therefore, if a tear of the synovial meniscal attachment can be identified through arthrography or arthroscopy and this vascularized portion of the meniscus can be held reduced and immobilized, healing is possible.

Even if a tear develops in the meniscal body and does not heal, this in itself is not an indication for meniscectomy. If such a tear does not cause a mechanical block to the movement of the knee and the symptoms are minor, one should consider the experimental data of Cox and Cordell[1021] before recommending total meniscectomy. In dogs, it was found that animals exposed to total meniscectomy developed severe degenerative changes while, in contrast, experimentally created meniscal lesions did not erode the articular surface as long as they did not interfere with knee motion.

If the tear is minor or peripheral, conservative care can be instituted with the realization that surgical intervention can be considered at a later date if failure is obvious. Rehabilitation of the knee is an integral part of conservative treatment.

SURGICAL TREATMENT

As Cassidy and Shaffer[1015] point out in their work on repairs of peripheral meniscus tears, a torn meniscus presents a real dilemma to the orthopaedic surgeon. First, the orthopaedic community has been told that leaving a torn meniscus in place will precipitate more degenerative change within the knee joint.[1185] Jackson and Dandy[1028] also concluded that damaged menisci have an adverse effect on condylar articular cartilage and recommended early diagnosis and meniscectomy. However, Casscells[1014] presented data that did not seem to support the much repeated statement that a torn meniscus is the primary cause of unicompartmental osteoarthritis. And Cox and Cordell[1021] demonstrated in experimental animals that outside of the entrapped bucket handle tear and free floating flap tear, degenerative changes within the knee are more severe following meniscectomy than with leaving the torn meniscus.

Numerous authors conclude that removing the meniscus will precipitate more rapid degenerative changes within the joint,[1019,1083,1084,1101,1148] while others report that meniscectomy will protect the knee against further damage.

Can a torn meniscus be repaired? Cassidy and Schaffer[1015] reviewed the results of 27 patients with 29 repairs of tears in the peripheral one third of the meniscus. Their results demonstrate that repair of a peripheral tear is possible. Stone[1192] showed that repair of peripheral meniscal tears gives satisfactory results. Price and Allen[1156] reported that

25 of 26 patients examined an average of 2.7 years after meniscoplasty showed no evidence of meniscal derangement. Hughston[1071] reported saving the medial meniscus in 68 of 100 consecutive surgically treated medial compartment tears without a single subsequent tear; the average follow-up time was 4 years.

More intriguing than the peripheral tear is the inner body tear. It is known that the inner two thirds of the meniscus is avascular, which leads one to wonder if healing can occur. In animal studies, Cabaud and colleagues[1011] demonstrated that surgical lacerations of the body of the meniscus will heal when the meniscal laceration is contiguous with the synovium. The surgical lesions were sutured with Dexon and these menisci were shown to heal by fibrovascular scar in 94% of the animals. Heatley[1063] also demonstrated that in rabbits transverse lacerations of the menisci will heal from cells derived from the synovium. This healing mechanism has not been clinically demonstrated in man, although cases of natural healing of transverse tears have been reported.[1183] It must be emphasized that both experiments used laboratory animals and do not prove or disprove that such repairs will prevent or delay late instability and degenerative changes.

When the decision is made for meniscectomy, the next question is whether a partial or complete meniscectomy should be performed. The function of the normal meniscus and reasons for a concentrated effort to prevent its removal have been outlined. The advantages of a partial meniscectomy have been supported by both clinical and experimental evidence.[988,1001,1013,1027,1044,1079,1119,1195] The best results in partial meniscectomy occur when the tear is either a bucket handle tear or a flap tear. These tears can be resected by a trained endoscopist using the arthroscope and arthroscopic equipment. One must be cognizant of the need to leave a stable balanced rim of meniscal tissue when doing a partial meniscectomy. Leaving a frayed edge along the remaining rim does not appear to be a problem as repeat arthroscopy has demonstrated that the edges will smooth out. However, in the bucket handle tear, be aware of the double longitudinal tear.

The advantages of partial meniscectomy are shorter hospitalization, less trauma to the joint, and a much more rapid rehabilitation. The long-term benefits of partial meniscectomy are only speculative at this point. Only after these patients have been evaluated 20 years after surgery will we know if such a procedure passes its hoped-for benefit of maintaining joint stability and preventing degenerative joint disease.

AUTHORS' PREFERRED METHOD OF TREATMENT

If the previously stated criteria for partial meniscectomy can be met, this procedure is most desirable. Preferably, this should be done with the use of the arthroscope; however, even if an arthrotomy is needed because of technical problems, only the torn portion of the meniscus should be removed. When a peripheral tear of the meniscus is identified in an isolated case or along with a ligament injury, repair is attempted over the choice of total meniscectomy.

A total meniscectomy is still performed in patients with complex tears. The patient should not be subjected to a second procedure if it is obvious that the remaining portion of the meniscus will not provide sound mechanical function. In these cases, care should be taken in dissection at the meniscal capsular border. The soft spot between meniscus and capsule can be palpated with the knife edge, and this line of cleavage is developed. This produces the best conditions for regeneration of the meniscus.

If the total medial meniscus cannot be removed through an anteromedial incision, an accessory posteromedial incision is made to recover the posterior horn. In making this incision care is taken to restore the integrity of the posterior medial capsule (posterior oblique ligament) with closure of the wound.

A more oblique anterolateral incision is used for removal of the lateral meniscus. This is to allow the deeper incision to be in line with the fibers of the iliotibial tract, thus preserving its function in lateral stability. A torn lateral meniscus may be found after inspection of the joint through an anteromedial incision. The anterior portion of the lateral meniscus can be detached through this incision and a second posterolateral incision is used to detach and remove the remainder of the meniscus. The posterolateral incision is made posterior to the lateral collateral ligament. Care is taken to identify and protect the popliteus tendon. Closure is accomplished by reattaching the arcuate ligament to the posterior edge of the fibular collateral ligament.

POSTOPERATIVE CARE

We prefer to use a bulky cotton dressing after arthrotomy. This provides compression to the joint as well as immobilization. It is removed on the fourth or fifth day after operation and replaced with a light dressing and an elastic wrap. Cast immobilization does not decrease the incidence or degree of effusion once mobilization is begun.[1007]

Quadriceps setting exercises are started on the first day after operation, and straight leg raising exercises when the patient is able. Four-point shrug exercises are also initiated (see p. 1500). The patient is allowed crutch walking on the first or second day after operation, with touch-only weight bearing.

The usual quadriceps exercises are instituted. We favor isometric-type exercises in the early weeks of knee rehabilitation to avoid joint irritation. This is done as a progressive resistive exercise in the manner described by Leach and colleagues.[1111] The single maximum weight that can be lifted by the leg in an isometric manner is first determined. Using 5 pounds less as the starting weight, leg lifts are done for ten repetitions. Five pounds is removed, and a second ten repetitions are done. Another 5 pounds is removed, and a third set of ten repetitions are done. The above should be done with the knee at 45° flexion and at full extension—the weight to be used is determined independently at each position. Should the weight that can be lifted at this initiation of the exercise program be less than 10 pounds, the second set of repetitions can be done with half the original weight, and the third set with the weight of the leg only. Every 2 or 3 days another 1 or 2 pounds of weight are added to the starting weight. When quadriceps strength has returned enough to protect the knee, crutches are discontinued. This is arbitrarily designated at ten repetitions with 30 pounds in an athlete. Females and less muscular individuals are required to lift less weight. Rehabilitation of the total extremity is necessary as with other injuries around the knee (see p. 1547).

COMPLICATIONS

The two most common complications of meniscus surgery are postoperative hemarthrosis and recurrent synovitis with effusion.

HEMARTHROSIS

If hemarthrosis is great enough to be painful, aspiration can be done. If minimal, we usually protect the joint and allow normal absorption to occur. Some advocate suction drainage of the joint or a synovial puncture in the suprapatellar pouch at surgery[1007,1113] to prevent fluid from accumulating in the joint. Bryan and colleagues[1007] did not find the benefit of suction drainage significant enough to warrant its use. We have not found hemarthrosis to be enough of a problem to use drainage or synovial puncture. On rare occasions it is necessary to aspirate the joint for hemarthrosis. Because of the proximity of the inferior lateral geniculate vessels to the joint line, bleeding and subsequent hemarthrosis may be more of a problem with lateral meniscectomy.

SYNOVITIS WITH EFFUSION

Synovitis with effusion is usually the result of too early and too vigorous use of the joint postoperatively. Joint use should be regulated by muscle power. Minor effusions are treated by compression, joint protection, and muscle exercises. Joint swelling is indicative of joint irritation. It is unwise to continue a strong exercise program while the joint is swollen. If certain degrees of joint tension are reached, a reflex inhibition of quadriceps activity occurs,[1181] and a vicious cycle of continued irritation and effusion begins. Initial rest and a slow and graduated program of exercises to increase muscle tone are necessary. If effusion is pronounced enough to cause bulging of the incisional wound, aspiration can be done. This may help prevent a synovial sinus from developing.

SYNOVIAL SINUS

Rarely a synovial sinus may develop from excess joint fluid forcing its way through the synovial incision.[1139] Quadriceps contraction and knee flexion may actually cause the synovial fluid to squirt through the sinus tract. If no infection develops, immobilization with the leg straight and compression dressings usually allow healing in 7 to 10 days. If the sinus persists after 2 weeks, excision of the tract and repair of the synovium and capsule are required.

TECHNICAL ERRORS

Technical errors in meniscectomy may also be considered among the complications. These include damage to articular cartilage; incomplete removal of the meniscus with meniscal remnants causing continued joint impingement; failure to follow the natural cleavage planes at the periphery of the meniscus (which may cause capsule damage or irregular scar tissue of the regenerated meniscus, or may prevent development of a regenerated meniscus); and failure to properly close the capsule incisions, either anterior or posterior but particu-

larly the latter, thus allowing increased rotational laxity.

Injury to the popliteal vessels may occur with the blind dissection required of the posterior horns of the menisci. When it occurs, diagnosis is no problem, as the blood wells up within the joint. Consultation with a vascular surgeon and immediate repair are required.

Another complication is the meniscus removed in error. This is well described by Murdoch.[1133,1134] A certain percentage of error is inevitable for any surgeon doing meniscectomies. Mention has already been made of error rates in men reported to be between 4% and 13%. Errors in diagnosis in women are higher, reported as 15%[1185] and 23%[1155] in two studies. Careful evaluation and diagnostic studies help to minimize the error rate.

PROGNOSIS

Degenerative joint changes are the enigma of the pre- and postmeniscectomy knee. Are the changes initiated by the irritation to the articular surfaces by the torn meniscus or are the degenerative changes hastened by its removal?

Fairbank[1042] listed the radiographic changes that occur after meniscectomy to include osteophytic ridge formation, narrowing of the joint space, and flattening of the femoral condyles. He believed that the menisci share in weight bearing, and their loss results in a relative overloading of the articular surfaces on that side of the joint with increasing compression of the articular cartilage.

When the mechanical impediment of a torn meniscus is removed, the early results are uniformly good. Should other joint pathology be present, the results are less satisfactory. Lipscomb and Henderson[1114] reported 77% excellent results after meniscectomy and an additional 15% who were improved. Other studies have reported 60% to 90% satisfactory results.[1082]

Johnson and colleagues[1082] and Tapper and Hoover,[1195] reporting late results, state that approximately 50% of patients have either excellent or poor results, while the other 50% have varying degrees of symptoms and disability.

Tapper and Hoover state further that about 40% of patients who had uncomplicated meniscectomies have normally functioning knees, and 10% have a bad outcome.

Johnson and colleagues[1082] report in their study (with an average follow-up of 17.5 years) that 39.4% of the knees that had meniscectomy showed degenerative changes on x-ray; only 6.1% of the opposite knees showed any degenerative changes. Of 147 athletes reviewed by Sonne-Holm and colleagues[1187] only 45% of the patients were asymptomatic after an average follow-up period of 4.25 years. The primary problem was a feeling of instability and pain on weight bearing. Fifteen percent of the patients had to give up sporting activity, and 12% had to restrict their chosen sporting activity following meniscectomy.

Meniscectomy in children is not a benign procedure. Zaman and Leonard[1210] reviewed 49 children with a history of meniscectomy and an average follow-up of 7.5 years. The results of the series were disappointing. Less than half of the patients had good results at follow-up. Most disturbing were the results among young women, 70% of whom were symptomatic at follow-up. Furthermore, only 27% of patients had normal x-rays and the preoperative diagnosis was correct in only 65% of the cases.

In the older population, the results of meniscectomy are varied. Lotke and colleagues[1115] reviewed 66 patients with an average age of 55.6 years. They found that good to excellent results were found in 90% of patients with no preexisting degenerative joint disease, 63% of patients with meniscal joint changes, and only 21% in those patients with moderate or marked disease. Therefore, meniscectomy should not be considered in elderly patients with knee pain unless the pain is caused by the tear in the meniscus, and not associated with degenerative joint disease.

Factors that may influence the long-term results include ligament laxity (particularly in those patients with a positive anterior drawer sign and rotary instability), a long duration of symptoms and greater frequency of reinjury, the sex of the patient, and which meniscus was removed.

The final prognosis may very likely involve unmeasurable factors, such as the remaining stability of the knee after meniscectomy, the development and efficiency of a regenerated meniscus, and constitutional factors that predispose a person to degenerative joint changes.

REFERENCES

Fractures About the Knee

Fractures of the Distal Femur

1. Altenberg, A. R., and Shorkey, R. L.: Blade-Plate Fixation in Non-Union and in Complicated Fractures of the Supracondylar Region of the Femur. J. Bone Joint Surg., **31A:**312–316, 1949.
2. Aufranc, O. E.; Jones, W. N., and Harris, W. H.: Comminuted Intercondylar and Supracondylar Femoral Fracture. J.A.M.A., **187:**293–295, 1964.
3. Baijal, E.: A Method of Internal Fixation of Supracondylar Fractures of the Femur. Injury, **11:**115–122, 1979.
4. Benum, P.: The Use of Bone Cement as an Adjunct to Internal Fixation of Supracondylar Fractures of Osteoporotic Femurs. Acta Orthop. Scand., **48:**52–56, 1977.
5. Bergan, F.: Traumatic Intimal Rupture of the Popliteal Artery with Acute Ischemia of the Limb in Cases with Supracondylar Fractures of the Femur. J. Cardiovasc. Surg., **4:**300–302, 1963.
6. Böhler, L.: The Treatment of Fractures. 4th ed. Bristol, Wright, 1935.
7. Böhler, L.: Treatment of Fractures. New York, Grune & Stratton, 1956.
8. Bonney, G.: Thrombosis of the Femoral Artery Complicating Fracture of the Femur. Treatment by Endarterectomy. J. Bone Joint Surg., **45B:**344–345, 1963.
9. Borgen, D., and Sprague, B. L.: Treatment of Distal Femoral Fractures with Early Weightbearing. A Preliminary Report. Clin. Orthop. **111:**156–163, 1975.
10. Brown, P. E., and Preston, E. T.: Ambulatory Treatment of Femoral Shaft Fractures with a Cast-Brace. J. Trauma, **15:**860–868, 1975.
11. Buck, G.: An Improved Method of Treating Fractures of the Thigh Illustrated by Cases and a Drawing. Trans. New York Acad. Med., **2:**232–250, 1861.
12. Cave, E. F.; Nicholson, J. T.; West, F. E.; MacAusland, W. R. Jr.; Sullivan, C. R.; Lipscomb, P. R.; Evans, R. G.; Cobb, C. A.; and Hillman, J. W.: Symposium on Fractures about the Knee. A.A.O.S. Instructional Course Lectures, **18:**73–91, 1961.
13. Charnley, J.: Knee Movement Following Fractures of the Femoral Shaft. J. Bone Joint Surg., **29:**679–686, 1947.
14. Charnley, J: The Closed Treatment of Common Fractures. 3rd. ed. Edinburgh, E. & S. Livingstone, 1961.
15. Chiron, H. S.; Tremoulet, J.; Casey, P.; and Müller, M.: Fractures of the Distal Third of the Femur Treated by Internal Fixation. Clin. Orthop., **100:**160–170, 1974.
16. Connolly, J. F.: Dehne, E.; and Lafollette, B.: Closed Reduction and Early Brace Ambulation Treatment of Fractures. Part II. Results in One Hundred and Forty-Three Fractures. J. Bone Joint Surg., **55A:**1581–1599, 1973.
17. Connolly, J. F., and King, P.: Closed Reduction and Early Cast Brace Ambulation Treatment of Fractures. Part 1. A Quantitive Analysis of Immobilization in Skeletal Fracture and a Cast Brace. J. Bone Joint Surg., **55A:**1559–1580, 1973.
18. Cooper, A. P.: A Treatise on Dislocations and Fractures of the Joints. Philadelphia, Lea & Blanchard, 1844.
19. Crenshaw, A. H. (ed.): Campbell's Operative Orthopeadics, 4th ed. St. Louis, C. V. Mosby, 1963.
20. Crenshaw, A. H. (ed.): Campbell's Operative Orthopaedics, 5th ed. St. Louis, C. V. Mosby, 1971.
21. Crock, H. V.: The Arterial Supply and Venous Drainage of the Bone of the Human Knee. Anat. Rec. **144:**149–217, 1962.

22. Crosby, J.: The Application of Extension in Fractures by Means of Adhesive Plaster. New Hampshire J. Med., **1**:65, 1850.

23. Crosby, J.: On the Application of Extension in Fractures by Means of Adhesive Plaster. New York J. Med., 2nd Series, **6**:137–138, 1851.

24. Daniell, W. C.: Method of Treating Fracture of the Thigh Bone. Am. J. Med. Sci., **4**:330–333, 1829.

25. Della Torre, P.: Results of Rigid Fixation in 54 Supracondylar Fractures of the Femur. Arch. Orthop. Trauma Surg., **97**:177–183, 1980.

26. DePalma, A.: The Management of Fractures and Dislocations. Philadelphia, W. B. Saunders, 1959.

27. Djoric, L.: Repair of Supracondylar Fractures of the Femur with Two Intramedullary Nails. Srpski. Arh. Celok. lek., **84**:176–186, Feb., 1956.

28. Elliot, R. B.: Fractures of the Femoral Condyles: Experiences with a New Design Femoral Condyle Blade Plate. South. Med. J., **52**:80–95, 1959.

28a. Egund, N., and Kolmert, L.: Deformities, Gonarthrosis and Function after Distal Femoral Fractures. Acta Orthop. Scand., **53**:963–974, 1982.

29. Gallannaugh, S. C.: Supracondylar Fractures of the Femur in the Elderly: Treatment by Internal Fixation. Injury, **5**:259–264, 1974.

29a. Giles, J. B.; DeLee, J. C.; Heckman, J. D.; and Keever, J. E.: Supracondylar–Intercondylar Fractures of the Femur Treated with a Supracondylar Plate and Lag Screw. J. Bone Joint Surg., **64A**:864–870, 1982.

30. Griswold, R. A.: Fractures and Dislocations Involving the Knee Joint. *In* Bancroft, F. W., and Murray, C. R. (eds.): Surgical Treatment of the Motor-Skeletal System, Vol. 2. Philadelphia, J. B. Lippincott, 1945.

31. Hall, M. F.: Two-plane Fixation of Acute Supracondylar and Intracondylar Fractures of the Femur. South Med. J., **71**:1471–1479, 1978.

32. Hamilton, F. H.: Fracture Tables Showing the Results of Treatment in One Hundred and Thirty-Six Cases. Buffalo, Jewett, Thomas, 1849.

33. Hamilton, F. H.: Fracture Tables. With a Supplement Compiled from Dr. Hamilton's Notes by John Boardman, A. B., Comprising in All an Analysis of 461 Cases of Fractures. Buffalo, Jewett, Thomas, 1853.

34. Hamilton, F. H.: Deformities After Fractures. Part 1. Trans. Am. Med. Assoc., **8**:347–444, 1855.

35. Hamilton, F. H.: Report on Deformities After Fractures. Part 2. Trans. Am. Med. Assoc., **9**:69–232, 1856.

36. Hamilton, F. H.: Report on Deformities After Fracture. Part 3. Trans. Am. Med. Assoc., **10**:239–454, 1857.

37. Hamilton, F. H.: A Practical Treatise on Fractures and Dislocations. Philadelphia, Blanchard & Lea, 1860.

38. Hamilton, W. C.; Canale, S. T.; Snedden, H. E.; and Stewart, W. B.: Supracondylar Fracture of the Femur in the Elderly Patient. J. Bone Joint Surg., **45B**:491–495, 1963.

39. Hampton, O. P.: Wounds of the Extremities in Military Surgery, St. Louis, C. V. Mosby, 1951.

40. Hand, F. M.: Fractures into and near the Knee Joint. A.A.O.S. Instructional Course Lectures, **1**:165–180, 1943.

41. Hippocrates: The Genuine Works of Hipprocrates. Adams, F. (trans.) Baltimore, Williams & Wilkins, 1939.

42. Holt, E. P., Jr.: Blade-Plate Internal Fixation of Supracondylar Fractures of the Femur. South. Med. J., **52**:1331–1336, 1959.

43. Hoover, N. W.: Injuries of the Popliteal Artery Associated with Fractures and Dislocations. Surg. Clin. North Am., **41**:1099–1112, 1961.

44. Jones, R.: Orthopedic Surgery of Injuries, Vol. 1. London, Oxford Medical Publications, 1921.

44a. Joseph, F. R.: Evaluation of the Zickel Supracondylar Fixation Device. Clin. Orthop., **169**:190–196, 1982.

45. Kelly, R.: Treatment of Knee Joint Fractures. A.A.O.S. Instructional Course Lectures, **2**:402–407, 1944.

46. Kennedy, R. H.: Treatment of Fractures of the Shaft of the Femur. An Analysis of 120 Cases. Ann. Surg., **107**:419–437, 1938.

47. Kirschner, M.: Ueber Nagelextension. Beitr. Klin. Chir., **64**:266–279, 1909.

48. Klingensmith, W.; Oles, P.; and Martinez, H.: Arterial Injuries Associated with Dislocation of the Knee or Fracture of the Lower Femur. Surg. Gynecol. Obstet., **120**:961–964, 1965.

49. Laros, G. S.: Symposium. Rigid Internal Fixation of Fractures. Supracondylar Fractures of the Femur: Editorial Comment and Comparative Results. Clin. Orthop., **138**:9–12, 1979.

50. Laskin, R. D., and Zimmerman, A. J.: The Displaced Intercondylar T-fracture of the Distal Femur: A Simplified Method of Internal Fixation. Orthop. Rev., **4**:49–51, 1975.

51. McKeever, F. M.: Fracture of the Shaft of the Femur in Adults. J.A.M.A., **128**:1006–1012, 1945.

52. Mahorner, H. R., and Bradburn, M.: Fractures of the Femur. Report of 308 Cases. Surg. Gynecol. Obstet., **56**:1066–1079, 1933.

52a. Mize, R. D.; Bucholz, R. W.; and Grogan, D. P.: Surgical Treatment of Displaced, Comminuted Fractures of the Distal End of the Femur. J. Bone Joint Surg., **64A**:871–874, 1982.

53. Modlin, J.: Double Skeletal Traction in Battle Fractures of the Lower Femur. Bull. United States Army Medical Department, **4**:119–120, 1945.

54. Moll, J.: The Cast Brace Walking Treatment of Open and Closed Femur Fractures. South. Med. J., **66**:345–352, 1973.

55. Mooney, V.; Nickel, V. L.; Harvey, J. P.; and Snelson, R.: Cast-Brace Treatment for Fractures of the Distal Part of the Femur. J. Bone Joint Surg., **52A**:1563–1578, 1970.

56. Müller, M. E.; Allgöwer, M.; and Willenegger, H.: Technique of Internal Fixation of Fractures. New York, Springer-Verlag, 1965.

57. Müller, M. E.; Allgöwer, M., and Willenegger, H.: Manual of Internal Fixation. New York, Springer-Verlag, 1970.

58. Neer, C. S.; Grantham, S. A.; and Shelton, M. L.: Supracondylar Fractures of the Adult Femur. J. Bone Joint Surg., **49A**:591–613, 1967.

59. Olerud, S.: Operative Treatment of Supracondylar-Con-

dylar Fractures of the Femur. J. Bone Joint Surg., **54A:**1015–1032, 1972.

60. Peltier, L. F.: A Brief History of Traction. J. Bone Joint Surg., **50A:**1603–1617, 1958.

61. Rockwood, C. A., Jr.; Ryan, V. L.; and Richards, J. A.: Experience with Quadrilateral Cast Brace [Abstr.]. J. Bone Joint Surg., **55A:**421, 1973.

62. Rosenberg, N. J.: Osteochondral Fractures of the Lateral Femoral Condyle. J. Bone Joint Surg., **46A:**1013–1026, 1964.

63. Rowe, C. R.: The Management of Fractures in Elderly Patient is Different. J. Bone Joint Surg., **47A:**1043–1059, 1965.

64. Rush, L. V.: Atlas of Rush Pin Techniques. Meridian, Mississippi, Berivon, 1955.

65. Russell, R. H.: Theory and Method on Extension of the Thigh. Br. Med. J., **2:**637–638, 1921.

66. Russell, R. H.: Fracture of the Femur: A Clinical Study. Br. J. Surg., **11:**491–502, 1924.

67. Schatzker, J.; Home, G.; and Waddell, J.: The Toronto Experience with the Supracondylar Fracture of the Femur, Injury, **6:**113–128, 1974.

68. Schatzker, J., and Lambert, D. C.: Supracondylar Fractures of the Femur. Clin. Orthop., **138:**77–83, 1979.

69. Schmiesser, G., Jr.: A Clinical Manual of Orthopaedic Traction Techniques. Philadelphia, W. B. Saunders, 1963.

70. Scuderi, C., and Ippolito, A.: Nonunion of Supracondylar Fractures of the Femur. J. Int. Coll. Surg., **17:**1–18, 1952.

71. Seinsheimer, F.: Fractures of the Distal Femur. Clin. Orthop., **153:**169–179, 1980.

72. Seligson, D., and Kriansen, B. A.: Use of Wagner Apparatus in Complicated Fractures of the Distal Femur. J. Trauma, **18:**795–799, 1978.

72a. Shelbourne, K. D., and Brueckmann, F. R.: Rush-Pin Fixation of Supracondylar and Intercondylar Fractures of the Femur. J. Bone Joint Surg., **64A:**161–169, 1982.

73. Slatis, P.; Ryöppy, S.; and Huittinen, V.: AO. Osteosynthesis of Fractures of the Distal Third of the Femur. Acta Orthop. Scand., **42:**162–172, 1971.

74. Smillie, I. S.: Injuries of the Knee Joint, 4th ed, pp. 246–259. Baltimore, Williams & Wilkins, 1971.

75. Steinmann, F. R.: Eine neue Extensionsmethode in der Frakturenbehandlung. Zentralbl. Chir., **34:**938–942, 1907.

76. Steinmann, F. R.: Die Nagelextension. Ergeb. Chir. Orthop., **9:**520–560, 1916.

77. Stewart, M. J.: Twenty-five Years of Progress in Treatment of Fractures. Am. Surg., **22:**485–504, 1956.

78. Stewart, M. J.; Sisk, T. D.; and Wallace, S. L., Jr.: Fractures of the Distal Third of the Femur. A Comparison of Method of Treatment. J. Bone Joint Surg., **48A:**784–807, 1966.

79. Tees, F. J.: Fractures of the Lower End of the Femur. Am. J. Surg., **38:**656–659, 1937.

80. Thomas, H. O.: The Treatment of Deformities, Fractures and Diseases of Bones in the Lower Extremities. London, H. K. Lewis, 1890.

81. Tscherne, H.: Long term Results of the Distal Femoral Fracture and its Special Problems. Zentralbl. Chir., **102:**897–904, 1977.

82. Umansky, A. L.: Blade-Plate Fixation for Fracture of the Distal End of the Femur. Bull. Hosp. Joint Dis., **9:**18–21, 1948.

83. Wade, P. R., and Okinaka, A. J.: The Problem of the Supracondylar Fracture of the Femur in the Aged Person. Am. J. Surg., **97:**499–512, 1959.

84. Watson-Jones, R.: Fractures and Joint Injuries, 4th ed. Baltimore, Williams & Wilkins, 1956.

85. Weil, G. C.; Kuehner, H. G.; and Henry J. P.: The Treatment of 278 Conservative Fractures of the Femur. Surg. Gynecol. Obstet., **62:**435–441, 1936.

86. Wertzberger, J. J., and Peltier, L. F.: Supracondylar Fractures. J. Kansas Med. Soc., **68:**328–332, 1967.

87. White, E. H., and Russin, L. A.: Supracondylar Fractures of the Femur Treated by Internal Fixation with Immediate Knee Motion. Am. Surg., **22:**801–820, 1956.

88. Wiggins, H. E.: Vertical Traction in Open Fractures of the Femur. U.S. Armed Forces Med. J., **4:**1633–1636, 1953.

89. Wright, P. B., and Stanford, F. D.: Supracondylar Fractures of the Femur. Clin. Orthop., **12:**256–267, 1968.

90. Zickel, R. E.; Fietti, V. G.; and Lawsing, J. F.: A New Intramedullary Fixation Device for the Distal Third of the Femur. Clin. Orthop., **125:**185–191, 1977.

91. Zimmerman, A. J.: Intra-articular Fractures of the Distal Femur. Orthop. Clin. North Am., **10:**75–80, 1979.

Fractures of the Patella

92. Adams, J. D., and Leonard, R. D.: A Developmental Anomaly of the Patella Frequently Diagnosed as Fracture. Surg. Gynecol. Obstet., **41:**601–604, 1925.

93. Alameda, J. C.; Feddis, R.; and Hull, D. I.: Management of Injuries to the Extensor Mechanism of the Knee. Med. Bull. US Army, Europe, **11(S):**187–190, 1954.

94. Albee, F. H.: Bone Graft for Fracture of the Patella. Int. Clin., **2:**224–226, 1928.

95. Allen, A. W.: Fractures of the Patella. J. Bone Joint Surg., **14:**640–648, 1934.

96. Anderson, F.: Transverse Fracture of the Patella. Scalpel, **3:**820, 1898.

97. Anderson, L. D.: In Crenshaw, A. H. (ed.): Campbell's Operative Orthopaedics, 5th ed. St. Louis, C. V. Mosby, 1971.

98. Anderson, R.: An Ambulatory Method of Treating Fractures of the Patella. Ann. Surg., **101:**1082–1090, 1935.

99. Andrews, J. R., and Hughston, J. C.: Treatment of Patellar Fractures by Partial Patellectomy. South Med. J., **70:**809–813, 1977.

100. Austin, H. W.: Longitudinal Fracture of the Patella, Fragments Removed, Recovery. Annual Report. Superv. Surg. Mar. Hospital, Washington, 123, 1887.

101. Baker, L. D., and Saubel, H. J.: Operative Treatment of Fracture of the Patella. North Carolina Med. J., **4:**382–385, 1943.

102. Bechtol, C. O.: Muscle Physiology. A.A.O.S. Instructional Course Lectures, **5:**181–189, 1948.

103. Bertwistle, A. P.: Notes on Fractured Patella. Lancet, **1:**1349–1351, 1929.

104. Black, J., Jr., and Conners, J.: Vertical Fractures of the Patella. South. Med. J., **62:**76–77, 1969.

105. Blodgett, W. E., and Fairchild, R. D.: Fractures of the Patella. Results of Total and Partial Excisions of the Patella for Acute Fracture. J.A.M.A., **106**:2121–2125, 1936.

106. Böhler, J.: Behandlung der Kniescheibenbruche. Osteosynthese, Teilexstirpation, Exstirpation. Dtsch. Med. Wochensch. **86**:1209–1212, 1961.

107. Boström, A.: Fractures of the Patella. Acta Orthop. Scand., **143** (Suppl.):1–80, 1972.

108. Boucher, H. H.: Patellectomy in the Geriatric Patient. Clin. Orthop., **11**:33–40, 1958.

109. Brooke, R.: The Treatment of Fractured Patella by Excision. A Study of Morphology and Function. Br. J. Surg., **24**:733–747, 1936–37.

110. Brooke, R.: Fractured Patella. An Analysis of 54 Cases Treated by Excision. Br. Med. J., **1**:231–233, 1946.

111. Bruce, J., and Walmsley, R.: Excision of the Patella. Some Experimental and Anatomical Observations. J. Bone Joint Surg., **24**:311–325, 1942.

112. Bull, W. T.: The Results of Treatment of Fracture of the Patella Without Operation. Med. Rec., **37**:313–318, 1890.

113. Cameron, H. C.: Transverse Fracture of the Patella. Glasgow Med. J., **10**:289–294, 1878.

114. Campbell, W. C.: Fractures of the Patella. South. Med. J., **28**:401–408, 1935.

115. Cargill, A. O.: The Long Term Effect on the Tibiofemoral Compartment of the Knee Joint of Comminuted Fractures of the Patella. Injury, **6**:309–312, 1975.

116. Cave, E. F., and Rowe, C. R.: The Patella: Its Importance in Derangement of the Knee. J. Bone Joint Surg., **32A**:542–553, 1950.

117. Chiroff, R. T.: A New Technique for the Treatment of Comminuted, Transverse Fractures of the Patella. Surg. Gynecol. Obstet., **145**:909–912, 1977.

118. Clein, L. J., and Rostrup, O.: An Investigation into Clinical and Experimental Patellectomy with the Use of a New Prosthesis. Can. J. Surg., **7**:88–92, 1964.

119. Cohn, B. N. E.: Total and Partial Patellectomy. An Experimental Study. Surg. Gynecol. Obstet., **79**:526–536, 1944.

120. Cokkinis, A. J.: Fractures of the Patella. Practitioner, **127**:185, 1931.

121. Corner, E. M.: Figures About Fractures and Refractures of the Patella, Ann. Surg., **52**:707–709, 1910.

122. Corrigan, F. P.: A Method for Immediate Treatment of Fractured Patella. J.A.M.A., **87**:408–409, 1926

123. Crenshaw, A. H.: Campbell's Operative Orthopaedics, 4th ed, pp. 426–430. St. Louis, C. V. Mosby, 1963.

124. Crenshaw, A. H., and Wilson, F. D.: The Surgical Treatment of Fractures of the Patella. South. Med. J., **47**:716–720, 1954.

125. Crock, H. V.: The Arterial Supply and Venous Drainage of the Bones of the Human Knee Joint. Anat. Rec., **144**:199–218, 1962.

126. DeNio, A. E., and Hudson, O. C.: An End Result Study of Patellectomy. Am. J. Surg., **94**:62–64, 1957.

127. Dennis, F. S.: Treatment of Fractured Patella by the Metallic Suture. NY State J. Med., **43**:372–377, 1886.

128. DePalma, A. F.: Diseases of the Knee Joint. Philadelphia, J. B. Lippincott, 1954.

129. DePalma, A. F.: The Management of Fractures and Dislocations. Philadelphia, W. B. Saunders, 1959.

130. DePalma, A. F., and Flynn, J. J.: Joint Changes Following Experimental Partial and Total Patellectomy. J. Bone Joint Surg., **40A**:395–413, 1958.

131. DeTarnowsky, G.: Compound Fractures of the Patella. Am. J. Surg., **27**:229, 1913.

132. Detmar, S. J.: The Treatment of Patella Fractures. Arch. Chir. Neerl., **18**:109–118, 1966.

133. Dobbie, R. P., and Ryerson, S.: The Treatment of Fractured Patella by Excision. Am. J. Surg., **55**:339–373, 1942.

133a. Dowd, G. S. E.: Marginal Fractures of the Patella. Injury, **14**:287–291, 1982.

134. Due, G., and Brighenti, G. M.: Vertical Fracture of the Patella. Arch. Orthop., **69**:373–387, 1956.

135. Duthie, H. L., and Hutchinson, J. R.: The Results of Partial and Total Excision of the Patella. J. Bone Joint Surg., **40B**:75–81, 1958.

136. Einola, S.; Aho, A. J.; and Kallio, P.: Patellectomy After Fracture. Long-term Follow-up Results with Special Reference to Functional Disability. Acta Orthop. Scand., **47**:441–447, 1976.

137. Eliason, E. L., and Hinton, D.: Fractures of the Patella. *In* Whipple, A. O. (ed.): Nelson's Loose Leaf Living Surg, 3rd ed., 372–374, 1927.

138. Frankel, V. H., and Burstein, A. H.: Orthopaedic Biomechanics. Philadelphia, Lea & Febiger, 1970.

139. Gallie, W. E., and LeMesurier, A. B.: The Late Repair of Fractures of the Patella and of Rupture of the Ligamentum Patella and Quadriceps Tendon. J. Bone Joint Surg., **9**:47–54, 1927.

140. Geckeler, E. O., and Quaranta, A. V.: Patellectomy for Degenerative Arthritis of the Knee. Late Results. J. Bone Joint Surg., **44A**:1109–1114, 1962.

141. Gem, W.: Probable Cause of Nonunion of the Fracture of the Patella. Br. Med. J., **2**:431, 1883.

142. Gray, H.: Anatomy of the Human Body. Goss, C. M., (ed), 28th ed. Philadelphia, Lea & Febiger, 1966.

143. Griswold, Arthur S.: Fractures of the Patella. Clin. Orthop., **4**:44–56, 1954.

144. Haggart, G. E.: Fractures of the Patella. Surg. Clin. North Am., **12**:773, 1932.

145. Hawley, G. W.: Fractures of the Patella. Surg. Gynecol. Obstet., **67**:1074–1078, 1937.

146. Haxton, H.: The Function of the Patella and Effects of Its Excision. Surg. Gynecol. Obstet., **80**:389–395, 1945.

147. Heineck, A. P.: The Modern Operative Treatment of Fractures of the Patella. Surg. Gynecol. Obstet., **9**:177–248, 1909.

148. Henderson, M. S.: The Use of Beef Bone Screws in Fractures and Bone Transplantation. J.A.M.A., **74**:715, 1920.

149. Hertzler, A. E.: A Pin Method for the Approximation of the Fragments in Fractured Patella. Surg. Gynecol. Obstet., **32**: 273, 1921.

150. Hey-Groves, E. W.: Material and Technique of Wire Suture of Bone. Lancet, **2:**945–947, 1912.

151. Hey-Groves, E. W.: A Note on the Extension Apparatus of the Knee-Joint. Br. J. Surg., **24:**747–748, 1937.

152. Higgins, R. E.: Fracture of the Patella. Surg. Clin. North Am., **6:**327, 1926.

153. Higgins, T. T.: Fracture of Both Patellae by Muscular Action. Br. Med. J., **1:**1006, 1925.

154. Hipps, H. E.: Surgical Repair of Patellar Fractures, Am. J. Surg., **101:**198–207, 1961.

155. Hollinshead, W. H.: Anatomy for Surgeons, Vol. 3, 2nd ed. Back and Limbs. New York, Hoeber-Harper, 1969.

156. Horwitz, T., and Lambert, R. C.: Patellectomy in the Military Service. A Report of 19 Cases. Surg. Gynecol. Obstet., **82:**423–426, 1946.

157. Jensenius, H.: On Results of Excision of Fractured Patella. Acta Chir. Scand., **102:**275–284, 1951.

158. Kaufer, H.: Mechanical Function of the Patella. J. Bone Joint Surg., **53A:**1551–1560, 1971.

159. Ketenjian, A. Y., and Shelton, M. L.: Primary Internal Fixation of Open Fractures: A Retrospective Study of the Use of Metallic Internal Fixation in Fresh Open Fractures. J. Trauma, **12:**756–763, 1972.

160. Key, J. A., and Conwell, H. E.: The Management of Fractures, Dislocations, and Sprains. St. Louis, C. V. Mosby, 1934.

161. Kleinberg, S.: Vertical Fractures of the Articular Surface of the Patella. J.A.M.A. **81:**1205–1206, 1923.

162. Langvad-Neilsen, A.: Treatment of Fracture of Patella. Acta Chir. Scand., **101:**143–150, 1951.

163. Lapidus, P. W.: Longitudinal Fractures of the Patella. J. Bone Joint Surg., **14:**351–379, 1932.

164. Leavitt, P. H.: Fascial Strips in Patella Fractures. N. Engl. J. Med., **203:**728, 1930.

165. Le Boutillier, W. G.: Excision of Patella in Extensive Wound of Knee. Ann. Surg., **37:**945, 1903.

165a. Leung, P. C.; Mak, K. H.; and Lee, S. Y.: Percutaneous Tension Band Wiring; A New Method of Internal Fixation for Mildly Displaced Patella Fracture. J. Trauma, **23:**62–64, 1983.

166. Lewis, R. C., and Scholz, K. C.: Cruciate Repair of the Extensor Mechanism Following Patellectomy. J. Bone Joint Surg., **48A:** 1221–1222, 1966.

167. Lieb, F. J., and Perry, J.: Quadriceps Function. An Anatomical and Mechanical Study Using Amputated Limbs. J. Bone Joint Surg., **50A:**1535–1548, 1968.

168. Lima, B.: Longitudinal Fracture of the Patella and its Treatment. Brasil Med., **41:**1281, 1927.

169. Lister, J.: A New Operation for Fracture of the Patella. Br. Med. J., **2:**850, 1877.

170. Loomis, L.: Internal Fixation of Fractures of the Patella, with Cotton Suture Material. Surgery, **15:**602–605, 1944.

171. Lotke, P. A. and Ecker, M. L.: Transverse Fractures of the Patella. Clin. Orthop., **158:**180–184, 1981.

172. Ludloff: Resection of the Patella for Better Function. Zentralbl. Chir., **52:**786–788, 1925.

173. MacAusland, W. R.: Total Excision of the Patella for Fracture: Report of Fourteen Cases. Am. J. Surg., **72:**510–516, 1946.

174. McFarland, B.: Excision of the Patella for Recurrent Dislocation of the Knee Joint. J. Bone Joint Surg., **30B:**158–160, 1948.

175. McKeever, D. C.: Patellar Prosthesis. J. Bone Joint Surg., **37A:**1074–1084, 1955.

176. McMaster, P. E.: Fractures of the Patella. Clin. Orthop., **4:**24–43, 1954.

177. Magnuson, P. B.: Fractures, 2nd ed. Philadelphia, J. B. Lippincott, 1936.

178. Magnuson, P. B., and Coulter, J. S.: Fractured Patella, Int. Clin., **2:**148–173, 1936.

179. Malgaigne, J. F.: Dennis System of Surgery, Vol. I. Philadelphia, Lea Brothers, 1895.

180. Martin, E. D.: Results of Work Done on Fractures of Patella for Past 26 Years with Conclusions. New Orleans Med. Surg. J., **84:**846–849. 1931.

181. Meekison, D. M.: Hitherto Undescribed Fracture of the Patella. Br. J. Surg., **25:**64–65, 1937.

182. Mehriz, M. M.: Simple Fracture of Patella Treated by Removal of Fragments. Lancet, **1:**91, 1939.

183. Michele, A. A., and Krueger, F.: Patella Fractures: A Method of Wiring. Surgery, **24:**100–102, 1948.

184. Moberg, E.: On the Operative Therapy and Prognosis in Fracture of the Patella. Acta Chir. Scand., **90:**295–316, 1944.

185. Müller, M. E.: Allgöwer, M.; and Willenegger, H.: Manual of Internal Fixation. Technique Recommended by the AO-Group, pp. 175–177. New York, Springer-Verlag, 1970.

186. Murphy, J.: Bilateral Fracture of the Patella. Br. Med. J., **1:**725, 1943.

187. Murray, P. D. F.: Bones. New York, Cambridge University Press, 1936.

188. D'Netto, D. C.: Fractures of the Patella. Postgrad. Med., **39:**83–85, 1963.

189. Nummi, J.: Fracture of the Patella. A Clinical Study of 707 Patellar Fractures. Ann. Chir. Gynaecol. Fenn., **179** (Suppl.): 1–85, 1971.

190. Ober, F. R.: A New Operation for Fracture of the Patella. J. Bone Joint Surg., **14:**640–642, 1932.

191. O'Donoghue, D. H.: The Place of Patellectomy in the Treatment of Fractures of the Patella. South Surg. **15:**640–655, 1949.

192. O'Donoghue, D. H.: Treatment of Fractures of the Patella. Northwestern Med., **57:**1592–1600, 1958.

193. O'Donoghue, D. H., and Hays, M. B.: The Patella: Basic Considerations. J. Okla. State Med. Assoc., **45:**248–250, 1952.

194. O'Donoghue, D. H.; Tompkins, F.; and Hays, M. B.: Strength of Quadriceps Function After Patellectomy. West. J. Surg. Gynecol. Obstet., **60:**159–167, 1952.

195. Oetteking, B.: Anomalous Patellae. Anat. Rec., **23:**269–278, 1922.

196. Parham. F. W.: Fracture of the Patella. Surg. Clin. North Am., **2:**1307–1312, 1922.

197. Payr, E.: Zur Operativen Behandlung der Kniegelenksteife nach langdauernder Ruhigstellung. Zentralbl. Chir. **44:**809–816, 1917.

198. Peeples, R. E., and Margo, M. K.: Function after Patellectomy. Clin. Orthop. **132:**180–186, 1978.

199. Powers, C. A.: The Question of Operative Interference

in Recent Simple Fractures of the Patella. Ann. Surg., **28:**67–107, 1898.

200. Quénu, E.: Bull. Mém. Soc. Chir (Paris). T., **24:**242. (Quoted by Thiem).

201. Rapp, Ira H.: The Use of Patellectomy. South. Med. J., **47:**720–728, 1954.

202. Roberts, J. B.: Bony Union of Transverse Fracture of Both Patellae Without Operative Suture. Ann. Surg., **64:**116–117, 1916.

203. Roberts, J. B.: Subcutaneous Fixation of Transverse Fractures of the Patella. Ann. Surg., **74:**105–106, 1921.

204. Rogers, C. C.: Removal of the Patella for Ununited Comminuted Fracture. Illinois Med. J., **13:**648–652, 1908.

205. Rowe, C. A.: Refracture of the Patella Following Partial Patellectomy. West. J. Surg., **60:**404–405, 1952.

206. Salerno, D. J.: Fractures of the Patella: Closed and Open Repair Versus Patellectomy. J. Am. Osteopath. Assoc., **74:**538–541, 1975.

207. Salmond, R. W. A.: The Recognition and Significance of Fractures of the Patellar Border. Br. J. Surg., **6:**463–465, 1918–1919.

208. Sanderson, M. C.: The Fractured Patella: A Long-term Follow-up Study. Aust. N.Z. J. Surg., **45:**49–54, 1975.

209. Scannell, D. D.: Compound Fracture of the Patella. Report of Unusual Case. Tabulation of all Fractures in the Boston City Hospital in Forty-two Years. Boston Med. Surg. J., **155:**568–573, 1906.

210. Scapinelli, R.: Blood Supply of the Human Patella. Its Relation to Ischaemic Necrosis After Fracture. J. Bone Joint Surg., **49B:**563–570, 1967.

211. Schmier, A. A.: Excision of the Fractured Patella. Surg. Gynecol. Obstet., **81:**370–378, 1945.

212. Schopp, A. C., and Fellhauser, C. M.: Plastic Operation in Fracture of the Patella. J. Missouri Med. Assoc., **47:**179–183, 1950.

213. Scott, J. C.: Fractures of the Patella. J. Bone Joint Surg., **31B:** 76–81, 1949.

214. Scudder, C. L.: Comminuted Fracture of Each Patella. Excision of One Patella, Wiring of the Other Patella. Recovery with Useful Knees. Boston Med. Surg. J., **138:**231, 1896.

215. Scudder, C. L., and Miller, R. H.: Certain Facts Concerning the Operative Treatment of Fractures of the Patella. Boston Med. Surg. J., **175:**441–442, 1916.

216. Seligo, W.: Fractures of the Patella. Treatment and Results. Wiederherstel. Chir. Traum., **12,** 84–102, 1971.

217. Shorbe, H., and Dobson, C. H.: Patellectomy. Repair of the Extensor Mechanism. J. Bone Joint Surg., **40A:**1281–1284, 1958.

218. Smillie, I. S.: Injuries of the Knee Joint, 2nd ed. Baltimore, Williams & Wilkins, 1951.

219. Smillie, I. S.: Injuries of the Knee Joint, 4th ed. Edinburgh, E. & S. Livingstone, 1970.

220. Sorensen, K. H.: The Late Prognosis After Fracture of the Patella. Acta Orthop. Scand., **34:**198–212, 1964.

221. Speed, K.: A Textbook of Fractures and Dislocations. Philadelphia, Lea & Febiger, 1928.

222. Steinke, C. R.: Simultaneous Fractures of Both Patellae. Ann. Surg., **58:**510–525, 1913.

223. Stewart, S. F.: Frontal Fractures of the Patella. Ann. Surg., **81:**536–539. 1925.

224. Stimson, L. A.: Treatment of Fracture of the Patella. Ann. Surg., **28:**216–228, 1898.

225. Sutton, F. S.; Thompson, C. H.; Lipke, J.; and Kettlekamp, D. B.: The Effect of Patellectomy on Knee Function. J. Bone Joint Surg., **58A:**537–540, 1976.

226. Tait, D.: Fractured Patella. J.A.M.A., **35:**253, 1900.

227. Thiem, C.: Ueber die Grösse der Unfallfolgen bei der blutigen und unblutigen Behandlung der einfachen (subcutanen) Querbruche der Kniescheibe. Verh. Dtsch. Ges. Chir. **34:**374–393, 1905.

228. Thompson, J. E. M.: Comminuted Fractures of the Patella. Treatment of Cases Presenting One Large Fragment and Several Small Fragments. J. Bone Joint Surg., **17:**431–434, 1935.

229. Thompson, J. E. M.: Fracture of the Patella Treated by Removal of the Loose Fragments and Plastic Repair of the Tendon. A Study of 554 Cases. Surg. Gynecol. Obstet., **74:**860–866, 1942.

230. Todd, J.: The End-Results of Fracture of the Patella. J. Bone Joint Surg., **32B:**281, 1950.

231. Trendelenburg: Verh. Dtsch. Ges. Chir., 1878. (Quoted by Thiem).

232. Wakeley, C. P. G.: Fractures of the Patella and Their Treatment. Practitioner, **122:**238–245, 1929.

233. Wass, R.: Treatment of Fractures of the Patella. Med. Press Circular, **210:**87–90, 1943.

234. Watson-Jones, R: Fractures and Other Bone and Joint Injuries. Edinburgh, E. & S. Livingstone, 1939.

235. Watson-Jones, R.: Excision of Patella [Correspondence]. Br. Med. J., **2:**195–196, 1945.

236. Watson-Jones, R.: Fractures and Joint Injuries, Vol. 2, 3rd ed. Edinburgh, E. & S. Livingstone, 1946.

237. Watson-Jones, R.: Fractures and Joint Injuries, 4th ed. London, E. & S. Livingstone, 1952–1955.

238. Weber, M. J.; Janecki, C. J.; McLeod, P.; Nelson, C. L.; and Thompson, J. A.: Efficacy of Various Forms of Fixation of Transverse Fractures of the Patella. J. Bone Joint Surg., **62A:** 215–244, 1980.

239. West, F. E.: End Results of Patellectomy. J. Bone Joint Surg., **44A:**1089–1108, 1962.

240. West, F. E., and Soto-Hall, R.: Recurrent Dislocation of the Patella in the Adult. End Results of Patellectomy with Quadricepsplasty. J. Bone Joint Surg., **40A:**386–394, 1958.

241. Wight, J. S.: Fractures of the Patella. Int. Clin., **3:**155–187, 1905.

242. Wilkinson, J.: Fracture of the Patella Treated by Total Excision: A Long Term Follow-up. J. Bone Joint Surg., **59B:**352–354, 1977.

243. Willis, W. M.: Report of a Case of Excision of the Patella Given Before the Nottingham Medico-Chirurgical Society. Lancet, **2:**1689, 1907.

Fractures of the Proximal Tibia

243a. Abdalla, F.; Tehranzadeh, J.; and Horton, J.: Avulsion of the Lateral Tibial Condyle in Skiing. Am. J. Sports Med., **10:**368–370, 1982.

244. Ahern, G. S., and Lipscomb, P. R.: Fracture of the Tibial

Plateau: Report of Case. Proc. Staff Mayo Clin., **23**:288–290, 1948.

245. Anderson, P. W.; Harley, J. D.; and Moslin, P. V.: Arthrographic Evaluation of Problems with United Tibial Plateau Fractures. Radiology, **119**:75–78, 1976.

246. Anderson, R., and Loughlen, I.: Fractures of the Tibial Plateau. Clin. Orthop., **4**:10–23, 1954.

247. Anger, R., et. al.: Etude critique du traitement des fractures articulaires de l'extremite superieure du tibia. Rev. Chir. et rep. de l'Appareil Moteur, **54**:259–274, 1968.

248. Apley, A. G.: Fractures of the Lateral Tibial Condyle Treated by Skeletal Traction and Early Mobilization. J. Bone Joint Surg., **38B**:699–708, 1956.

249. Apley, A. G.: Fractures of the Tibial Plateau. Orthop. Clin. North. Am., **10**:61–74, 1979.

250. Aufranc, O. E.: Fracture of the Lateral Tibial Plateau. J.A.M.A., **176**:676–679, 1961.

251. Aufranc, O. E.; Jones, W. N.; and Harris, W. H.: Depressed Lateral Tibial Plateau Fracture. J.A.M.A., **178**:835–837, 1961.

252. Badgley, C. E., and O'Connor, S. J.: Conservative Treatment of Fractures of The Tibial Plateau. Arch. Surg., **64**:506–515, 1952.

253. Bakalim, G., and Wilpulla, E.: Fractures of the Tibial Condyles. Acta Orthop. Scand., **44**:311–322, 1973.

254. Barr, J. S.: The Treatment of Fracture of the External Tibial Condyle (Bumper Fracture). J.A.M.A., **115**:1683–1687, 1940.

255. Barr, J. S., and MacAusland, R., Jr.: Injuries Involving the Knee Joint. In Cave, E. F. (ed.): Fractures and Other Injuries. Chicago, Year Book Publishers, 1958.

256. Barrington, T. W., and Dewar, F. P.: Tibial Plateau Fractures. Can. J. Surg., **8**:146–152, 1965.

257. Bezouglis, C., and Eliopoulos, C.: Perkutane Osteosynthese der Tibiakopffrakturen und sofortige Mobilisierung des Knies. Z. Orthop., **110**:983–985, 1972.

258. Bick, E. M.: Fractures of the Tibial Condyles. J. Bone Joint Surg., **23**:102–108, 1941.

259. Blackburn, J. E.: Maintenance of Reduction of Tibial Plateau Fractures with Charnley Compression Devices. Clin. Orthop., **123**:112–113, 1977.

260. Böhler, L.: The Treatment of Fractures, 5th ed. New York, Grune & Stratton, 1958.

261. Bömler, J. et al.: Resurfacing of Depression Fractures of the Lateral Tibial Condyle. A Report of 5 Cases. Acta. Orthop. Scand., **52**:231–232, 1981.

262. Bowes, D., and Hohl, M.: Tibial Condylar Fractures. Evaluation of Treatment and Outlook. Clin. Orthop., **171**:104–108, 1982.

263. Bradford, C. H.; Kilfoyle, R. M.; Kelleher, J. J.; and Magill, H. K.: Fractures of the Lateral Tibial Condyle. J. Bone Joint Surg., **32A**:39–47, 1950.

264. Brown, G. A., and Sprague, B. L.: Cast Brace Treatment of Plateau and Bicondylar Fractures of the Proximal Tibia. Clin. Orthop. **119**:184–193, 1976.

265. Buckner, H. T.: Bumper Fractures of the Tibia. Northwest. Med., **37**:102–105, 1938.

266. Buckner, H. T.: Fractures of the Upper End of the Tibia with Lateral Displacements. Am. J. Surg., **51**:707, 1941.

267. Burri, C.; Bartzke, G.; Coldewey, J.; and Muggler E.: Fractures of the Tibial Plateau. Clin. Orthop., **138**:84–93, 1979.

268. Burrows, H.: Fractures of the Lateral Condyle of the Tibia. J. Bone Joint Surg., **38B**:612–613, 1956.

269. Buttermann, F.: Klinik det Tibiakondylenbruche. Arch. Clin. Chir., **190**:580, 1937.

270. Caldwell, E. H.: Fractures of the Condyles of the Tibia. Surg. Gynecol. Obstet., **63**:518–522, 1936.

271. Campbell, O. J.: Bumper Fractures of the Tibia. Minnesota Med., **19**:593, 1936.

272. Cave, E. F.: Fractures of the Tibial Condyles Involving the Knee Joint. Surg. Gynecol. Obstet., **86**:289–294, 1948.

273. Cave, E. F.: Fractures and Other Injuries. Chicago, The Year Book Publishers, 1958.

274. Chuinard, E.: Fractures of the Condyles of the Tibia. Clin. Orthop., **37**:115–129, 1964.

275. Clarke, H.; Fripp, A.; Stamm, T.; and Fairbank, H.: Discussion on Fractures of the Tibia Involving the Knee Joint. Proc. R. Soc. Med., **28**:1035–1050, 1935.

276. Collert, S.: Tibiakondylfrakturer—Operation och omedelbar mobilisering. Nord. Med. **79**:263–264, 1968.

277. Cooper, A.: A Treatise on Dislocations and on Fractures of the Joints. Boston, Wells & Lilly, 1825.

278. Cornell, C. M., and Hardy, R. C.: Plateau Fractures of the Tibia. Surgery, **28**:735–743, 1960.

279. Cotton, F. J.: Fender Fractures. Surg. Gynecol. Obstet., **62**:442–443, 1936.

280. Cotton, F. J., and Berg, R.: Fender Fracture of the Tibia at the Knee. N. Engl. J. Med., **201**:989–995, 1929.

281. Courvoisier, E.: Les fractures intraarticulaires de l'extremite superieure du tibia. Helv. Chir. Acta, **32**:257–263, 1965.

282. Cubbins, W. R.; Conley, A. H.; Callahan J. J.; and Scuderi, C. S.: Fractures of the Lateral Condyle of the Tibia: Classification, Pathology, and Treatment. Surg. Gynecol. Obstet., **59**:461–468, 1934.

283. Cubbins, W. R.; Conley, A. H.; and Seiffert, G. S.: Fractures of the Lateral Tuberosity of the Tibia with Displacements of the Lateral Meniscus between the Fragments. Surg. Gynecol. Obstet., **48**:106–108, 1929.

284. Daniel, E., and Rice, T.: Valgus-Varus Stability in the Hinged Cast used for Controlled Mobilization of the Knee. J. Bone Joint Surg., **61**:135–136, 1979.

285. Danielsson, L. G., and Hernborg, J.: Clinical and Roentgenological Study of Knee Joints with Osteophytes. Clin. Orthop., **69**:302–312, 1970.

286. d'Aubigne, R., and Mazar, F.: Formes anatomiques et traitement des fractures de l'extremite superieure du tibia. Rev. Chir. Orthop., **46**:289–318, 1960.

287. Dehelly, M.: Ecrasement du plateau tibial. Reconstitution de ce plateau par greffons osteoperiostiques. Bull. Soc. Nat. Chir., **53**:1296–1299, 1927.

288. Dejour, H.; Chambat, P.; Caton, J.; and Melere, G.: Les fractures des plateaux tibiaux avec lesion ligamentaire. Rev. Chir. Orthop., **67**:593–598, 1981.

289. Diamond, B.: Tibial Plateau Fractures. Med. Trial Tech. Q., **11**:1–13, 1965.

290. Dickson, J.: Fractures of the Knee Involving the Tibia. Am. J. Surg., **38**:700–705, 1937.

291. Dobelle, M.: A New Method of Closed Reduction of Fractures of the Lateral Condyle of the Tibia. Am. J. Surg., **53**:460–462, 1941.

292. Dorrance, F. S.: An Unusual Fracture of the Upper End of the Tibia. Can. Med Assoc. J., **31**:184–185, 1934.

293. Dovey, H., and Heerfordt, J.: Tibial Condyle Fractures. A Follow-up of 200 Cases. Acta. Chir. Scand., **137**:521–531, 1971.

294. Drennan, D. B.; Locher, F. G.; and Maylahn, D. J.: Fractures of the Tibial Plateau. Treatment by Closed Reduction and Spica Cast. J. Bone Joint Surg., **61**:989–995, 1979.

295. DuParc, J., and Ficat, P.: Fractures articulaires de l'extremite superieure du tibia. Rev. Chir. Orthop., **46**:399–486, 1960.

296. Edeland, H. G.: Open Reduction of Central Compression Fractures of the Tibial Plateau. Preliminary Report of a New Method and Device Arrangement. Acta Orthop. Scand., **47**:686–689, 1976.

297. Edeland, H. G.: A Method for Treatment of Rim Fractures of the Tibial Condyle. Description of a New Surgical Technique and a New Fracture Fixation Device. Acta Orthop. Belg., **44**:393–396, 1978.

298. Eliason, E. L., and Eberling, W. W.: Non-Operative Treatment of Fractures of the Tibia and Femur Involving the Knee Joint. Surg. Gynecol. Obstet., **57**:658–667, 1933.

299. Elstrom, J.; Pankovich, A. M.; Sasson, H.; and Rodriguez, J.: The Use of Tomography in the Assessment of Fractures of the Tibial Plateau. J. Bone Joint Surg., **58A**:551–555, 1976.

300. Enneking, W. F., and Horowitz, M.: The Intra-articular Effects of Immobilization on the Human Knee. J. Bone Joint Surg., **54A**:973–985, 1972.

301. Eucher, L.: Deux Cas de Fracture des Plateaux Tibiaux Traites par Griffe de Rotule. Acta. Chir. Belg., **60**:804–816, 1961.

302. Fagerburg, S.: Tomographic Analysis of Depressed Fractures Within the Knee Joint, and of Injuries to the Cruciate Ligaments. Acta Orthop. Scand., **27**:219–227, 1958.

303. Fairbank, T. J.: Condylar Fractures of the Knee-joint. Proc. R. Soc. Med., **48**:95–96, 1954.

304. Foged, J.: Operative Treatment of Fracture of a Tibial Condyle. Ugeskr. Laeger, **105**:451, 1943.

305. Foged, J.: Osteosynthesis of the Tibial Condyle. Acta. Chir. Scand., **91**:143–160, 1944.

306. Forster, E.; Mole, L.; and Coblentz, J.: Etude des lesions ligamentomes dans les fractures du plateau tibial. Ned. T. Geneesk, **105**:2173–2181, 1961.

307. Freehafer, A.; Goldman, S.; and Chapman, K.: Stubbins' Arthroplasty for fractures of the Tibial Condyle. Clin. Orthop., **90**:140–145, 1973.

308. Fripp, A. T.: Fractures of the Tibia Involving the Knee-Joint. Clin. J., **65**:20–23, 1936.

309. Fryjordet, A., Jr.: Operative Treatment of Tibial Condylar Fractures. Acta. Chir. Scand., **133**:17–24, 1967.

310. Fyshe, T. G.: Fractures of the Condyles of the Tibia

311. Immobilized by the Stader Splint. Can. Med. Assoc. J., **67**:103–107, 1952.

311. Garrison, L. E., and Garrison, M.: The Use of Periosteal Sutures in Open Fixation of Fractures of the Tibial Condyle. J. Bone Joint Surg., **20**:498, 1938.

312. Gausewitz, S. H., and Hohl, M.: The Significance of Early Motion in the Treatment of Tibial Plateau Fractures. Orthop. Trans., **7**:68–69, 1983.

313. Gerard-Marchant, P.: Fractures des plateaux tibiaux. Rev. Orthop., **26**:499–546, 1939.

314. Gossling, H. R., and Peterson, C. A.: A New Surgical Approach in the Treatment of Depressed Lateral Condylar Fractures of the Tibia. Clin. Orthop., **140**:96–102, 1979.

315. Gottfries, A.; Hagert, C. G.; and Sorensen, S. E.: T- and Y-Fractures of the Tibial Condyles. A Follow-up Study of Cases Treated with Closed Reduction and Surgical Fixation with a Wire Loop. Injury, **3**:56–63, 1971.

316. Goylling, U., and Lindholm, R.: Fractures of the Tibial Condyle. Ann. Chir. Gynecol. Fenn., **42**:229–235, 1953.

317. Haldeman, K. O.: The Healing of Joint Fractures. A Clinical and Experimental Study. J. Bone Joint Surg., **20**:912–922, 1939.

318. Heerfordt, J., and Mouritzen, V.: Follow-up on 50 Cases with Fractures of the Lateral Tibial Condyle Treated Predominantly by Operation. Acta Orthop. Scand., **42**:430–431, 1971.

319. Hohl, M.: Tibial Condylar Fractures. J. Bone Joint Surg., **49A**:1455–1467, 1967.

320. Hohl, M.: Tibial Condylar Fractures: Long Term Follow-up. Tex. Med., **70**:46–56, 1974.

321. Hohl, M.: Treatment Methods in Tibial Condylar Fractures. South. Med. J., **68**:985–991, 1975.

322. Hohl, M.: Management of Tibial Condylar Fractures. *In* Evarts, C. M. (ed.): A.A.O.S. Symposium on Reconstructive Surgery of the Knee. St. Louis, C. V. Mosby, 1978.

323. Hohl, M: Complications of Fractures and Dislocations of the Knee. *In* Epps, C. H. (ed.): Complications in Orthopedic Surgery. Philadelphia. J. B. Lippincott, 1978.

324. Hohl, M., and Hopp, E.: Ligament Injuries in Tibial Condylar Fractures (abstr.). J. Bone Joint Surg., **58A**:279, 1976.

325. Hohl, M., and Luck, J. V.: Fractures of the Tibial Condyles. A Clinical and Experimental Study. J. Bone Joint Surg., **38A**:1001–1018, 1956.

326. Hohl, M., and Moore, T. M.: Articular Fractures of the Proximal Tibia. *In* Evarts, C. M. (ed.): Surgery of the Musculoskeletal System. New York, Churchill Livingstone, 1983.

327. Hulten, O.: Uber die Indirekten Bruche des Tibiakopfes Nebst Batragen zur Rontgenologie des Kniegelenks. Acta. Chir. Scand., **66**, (Suppl):167, 1929.

328. Hymbert, R.: Contribution a l'etude du traitement des fractures. Suisse Romande, **59**:641–646, 1939.

329. Ibsen, J., and Mossing, N.: Conservative Treatment of Tibial Condylar Fractures. Acta Orthop. Scand., **42**:431–432, 1971.

330. Ilfeld, F. W., and Hohl, M.: Closed Reduction Treatment of Tibial Condylar Fractures (abstr.) J. Bone Joint Surg., **42A**:534–535, 1960.

331. Inclan, A.: El tratamiento quirurgico de las fracturas

grave de las tuberosidades de la tibia. Chir. Orthop. Traumatol. (Havana), **5:**32, 1937.

332. Jackson, D.: The Use of Autologous Fibula for a Prop Graft in Depressed Lateral Tibial Plateau Fractures. Clin. Orthop., **87:**110–115, 1972.

332a. Jacobs, J.: Patellar Graft for Severely Depressed Comminuted Fractures of the Lateral Tibial Condyle. J. Bone Joint Surg., **47A:**842–847, 1965.

332b. Jacobsen, A.: Operative Treatment of the Lateral Tibial Condyle Fractures. Acta Orthop. Scand., **23:**34–50, 1953.

333. Jensenius, H.; Jensen, I.; and Nielsen, F. K.: Tibiakondylfrakturc. Nord. Med., **66:**1573–1579, 1969.

334. Kennedy, J. C., and Bailey, W. H.: Experimental Tibial-Plateau Fractures. J. Bone Joint Surg., **50A:**1522–1534, 1968.

335. Kennedy, W. R.: Fractures of the Tibial Condyles. A Preliminary Report on Supplementary Fixation with Methyl Methacrylate. Clin. Orthop., **134:**153–157, 1978.

336. Key, J. A., and Conwell, H. E.: Fractures, Dislocations, and Sprains, 6th ed. St. Louis, C. V. Mosby, 1956.

337. Knight, R. A.: Treatment of Fractures of the Tibial Condyles. South. Med. J., **38:**246–255, 1945.

338. Krackow, K. A., and Vetter, W. L.: Knee Motion in a Long Leg Cast. Am. J. Sports Med., **9:**233–239, 1981.

339. Landelius, E.: Die operative Behandlung der Spaltbruche des proximalen Tibiaendes. Acta Chir. Scand., **82:**90–97, 1939.

340. Leadbetter, G. W., and Hand, F. M.: Fractures of the Tibial Plateau. J. Bone Joint Surg., **22:**559–568, 1940.

341. Lee, H.: Fractures of the Tuberosities of the Tibia. N. Engl. J. Med., **204:**583–594, 1931.

342. Lee, H.: Osteoplastic Reconstruction in Severe Fractures of the Tibial Condyles. Am. J. Surg., **94:**940–944, 1957.

343. Lindholm, R. V.: Treatment of Fractures of the Tibial Condyles by Active Movement Therapy. Acta Orthop. Scand., **23:**320–323, 1954.

344. Lippman, R. K.: Surgical Treatment of Depressed Fractures of the Plateau. J. Mt. Sinai Hosp., **17:**761–768, 1951.

345. Lucht, U., and Pilgaard, S.: Fractures of the Tibial Condyles. Acta Orthop. Scand., **42:**366–376, 1971.

346. Luck, J. V.: Response of Joints to Trauma. Presented at the Annual Meeting of The American Academy of Orthopaedic Surgeons, New York, 1950.

347. Luck, J. V.: Traumatic Arthrofibrosis. Bull. Hosp. Joint Dis., **12:**394–403, 1951.

348. Maatz, R., et. al.: Grenzen der Seitenkongruenz der tibialen Gelenkflachen. Chirurg, **43:**522–524, 1972.

348a. MacAusland, W. R., Jr.: Fractures of the Tibial Plateau. In Reynolds, F. C. (ed): A.A.O.S. Instructional Course Lectures, **18:**87–91, 1961.

349. Maisel, B., and Cornell, N. W.: Conservative Treatment of Fractures of the Tibial Condyles. Surgery, **23:**591–598, 1948.

350. Martin, A. F.: The Pathomechanics of the Knee Joint. I. The Medial Collateral Ligament and Lateral Tibial Plateau Fractures. J. Bone Joint Surg., **42A:**13–22, 1960.

351. Mauer, I., and Friedman, A.: Hinged Casts in the Treatment of Tibial Plateau Fractures. Bull. Hosp. Joint Dis., **20:**61–68, 1959.

352. Metz, A. R.; Householder, R.; and DePree, J. F.: Impaction of Fractures by Large Pressure Tongs. Am. J. Surg., **59:**447–449, 1943.

353. Mikkelsen, O.: Intraartikulare Frakturen des obersten Tibiaendes. Acta Chir. Scand., **73:**1–42, 1934.

354. Milch, H.: Cortical Avulsion Fracture of the Lateral Tibial Condyle. J. Bone Joint Surg., **18:**159–164, 1936.

355. Moore, T. M.: Fracture-Dislocation of the Knee. Clin. Orthop. **156:**128–140, 1981.

356. Moore, T. M.: Management of Tibial Plateau Fractures. In Moore, T. M. (ed.): A.A.O.S. Symposium on Trauma to the Leg and its Sequelae. St. Louis, C. V. Mosby, 1981.

357. Moore, T. M., and Harvey, J. P., Jr.: Roentgenographic Measurement of Tibial Plateau Depression due to Fracture. J. Bone Joint Surg., **56A:**155–160, 1974.

358. Moore, T. M.; Meyers, M. H.; and Harvey, J. P.: Collateral Ligamentous Laxity of the Knee: Long Term Comparison Between Fractures and Normal. J. Bone Joint Surg., **58A:**594–598, 1976.

359. Müller, M. E.; Allgöwer, M.; Schneider, R.; and Willenegger, H.: Manual of Internal Fixation. New York, Springer-Verlag, 1979.

360. Neviaser, J. S., and Eisenberg, S. H.: Diagnostic and Therapeutic Obstacles Encountered in Tibial Plateau Fractures. Bull. Hosp. Joint Dis., **17:**48–57, 1956.

361. Newberg, A. H., and Greenstein, R.: Radiographic Evaluation of Tibial Plateau Fractures. Radiology, **126:**319–323, 1978.

362. O'Donoghue, D. H.: Treatment of Injuries to Athletes. Philadelphia, W. B. Saunders, 1962

363. Olaussen, T.: Intraarticular Fractures in the Upper End of the Tibia and Lower End of the Femur. Acta Chir. Scand., **94:**407–428, 1946.

364. Olerud, S.: Osteotomy on the Tibial Tuberosity in Fractures of the Tibial Condyle. Acta Orthop. Scand., **42:**432–435, 1971.

365. Palmer, I.: Compression Fractures of the Lateral Tibial Condyle and Their Treatment. J. Bone Joint Surg., **21:**674–680, 1939.

366. Palmer, I.: Fractures of the Upper End of the Tibia. J. Bone Joint Surg., **33B:**160–166, 1951.

367. Perey, O.: Depression Fractures of the Lateral Tibial Condyle. Acta Chir. Scand., **103:**154–157, 1952.

368. Porter, B.: Crush Fractures of the Lateral Tibial Table. J. Bone Joint Surg., **52B:**676–687, 1970.

369. Poulsen, J. O., and Tophj, K.: The Conservative Treatment of Tibial Plateau Fractures. Nord. Med., **82:**1243–1246, 1969.

370. Rasmussen, P. S.: Lateral Condylar Fracture of the Tibia. Acta Orthop. Scand., **42:**429, 1971.

371. Rasmussen, P. S.: Tibial Condylar Fractures. J. Bone Joint Surg., **55A:**1331–1350, 1973.

371a. Rasmussen, P. S.: Tibial Plateau Fractures as a Cause of Degenerative Arthritis. Acta Orthop. Scand., **43:**566–575, 1972.

372. Reibel, D. B., and Wade, P. A.: Fractures of the Tibial Plateau. J. Trauma, **2:**337–352, 1962.

373. Rinonapoli, E., and Aglietti, P.: Comparison of Treatment by Open and Closed Reduction of Comparable Cases of

Articular Fractures of the Proximal Tibia. Ital. J. Orthop. Traumatol. [Suppl.], **3**:99–116, 1977.

374. Roberts, J. M.: Fractures of the Condyles of the Tibia. J. Bone Joint Surg., **50A**:1505–1521, 1968.

375. Rombold, S.: Depressed Fractures of the Tibial Plateau. J. Bone Joint Surg., **42A**:783–797, 1960.

376. Salter, R. B.; Simmonds, D. F.; Malcolm, B. W.; Rumble, E. V.; Macmichael, R.; and Clements, N. D.: The Biological Effect of Continuous Passive Motion on the Healing of Full-thickness Defects in Articular Cartilage. J. Bone Joint Surg., **62A**:1232–1251, 1980.

377. Sarmiento, A.; Kinman, P. B.; and Latta, L. L.: Fractures of the Proximal Tibia and Tibial Condyles: A Clinical and Laboratory Comparative Study. Clin. Orthop., **145**:136–145, 1979.

378. Schatzker, J., and Schulak, D. J.: Pseudoarthrosis of a Tibial Plateau Fracture: Report of a Case. Clin. Orthop., **145**:146–149, 1979.

379. Schatzker, J.: McBrown, R.; and Bruce, D.: The Tibial Plateau Fracture. The Toronto Experience. Clin. Orthop., **138**:94–104, 1979.

380. Schioler, G.: Tibial Condylar Fractures with a Particular View to the Value of Tomography. Acta Orthop. Scand., **42**:462, 1971.

381. Schulak, K. F., and Gunn, D. R.: Fractures of the Tibial Plateaus. A Review of the Literature. Clin. Orthop., **109**:166–177, 1975.

382. Scotland, T.: The Use of Cast-bracing as Treatment for Fractures of the Tibial Plateau. J. Bone Joint Surg., **63B**:575–582, 1981.

383. Scudder, C. L.: Treatment of Fractures, 3rd ed. Philadelphia, W. B. Saunders, 1902.

384. Sever, J. W.: Fracture of Tuberosities of the Tibia. A Report of Three Cases. Am. J. Orthop. Surg., **14**:299–302, 1916.

385. Sever, J. W.: Fractures of the Tibial Spine Combined with Fractures of the Tuberosities of the Tibia. Surg. Gynecol. Obstet., **35**:558–564, 1922.

386. Shelton, M. E.; Neer, C. S., II; and Grantham, S. A.: Occult Knee Ligament Ruptures Associated with Fractures. J. Trauma, **11**:853–856, 1971.

387. Shires, P. R.: Tibial Condylar Fractures. The Late Results of Conservative Treatment. Postgrad. Med. J., **40**:543–548, 1964.

388. Shybut, G. T., and Spiegel, P. G.: Tibial Plateau Fractures. Clin. Orthop., **138**:12, 1979.

389. Slee, G. C.: Fractures of the Tibial Condyles. J. Bone Joint Surg., **37B**:427–437, 1955.

390. Smillie, I. S.: Injuries of the Knee Joint, 3rd ed. Baltimore, Williams & Wilkins, 1962.

391. Solonen, K. A.: Fractures of the Tibial Condyles. Acta Orthop. Scand., [Suppl.] **63**:32, 1963.

392. Speed, J. S.: Fractures and Dislocations, 2nd ed. Philadelphia, Lea & Febiger, 1928.

393. Speed, J. S., and Smith, H. (eds.): Campbell's Operative Orthopaedics, 3rd ed. St. Louis, C. V. Mosby, 1956.

394. Spigelman, L.: Positive Pressure in the Reduction of Fractures of the Tibial Condyle. A Preliminary Report. J. Bone Joint Surg., **35A**:696–700, 1953.

395. Stern, W. G., and Papurt, L. E.: Healing of the Newer

396. Stimson, L. A.: Fractures and Dislocations. Philadelphia, Lea Brothers, 1899.

397. Swett, P.; McPherson, S.; and Pike, M.: Fracture of the Tibia into the Knee Joint. New Engl. J. Med., **204**:749–756, 1931.

398. Thamhayn, C.: Interesanter Bruch des Condylus Tibiae. Z. Deutsch. Chir., **6**:327–329, 1852.

399. Thiele, K.: Schienbeinkopfbruche, Hefte Unfallheilk., **95**:1–126, 1968.

400. Turner, V. C.: Fractures of the Tibial Plateaus. J.A.M.A., **169**:923–926, 1959.

401. von Bahr, V.: Depressed and Comminuted Fractures of the Lateral Tibial Tuberosity. Acta Chir. Scand., **92**:139–149, 1945.

402. Watson-Jones, R.: Fractures and Joint Injuries, 4th ed. Baltimore, Williams & Wilkins, 1955.

403. Waddell, J. P.; Johnston, D. W.; and Neidre, A.: Fractures of the Tibial Plateau: A Review of 95 Patients and Comparison of Treatment Methods. J. Trauma, **21**:376–381, 1981.

403a. Watson-Jones, K.: Fractures and Joint Injuries, 4th ed. Baltimore, Williams & Wilkins, 1955.

404. Webb, R. C.: Fractures of the Upper End of the Tibia Involving the Knee Joint. Minnesota Med., **18**:186–187, 1935.

405. Weber, W. L.: Fractures of the Tibial Condyles. Calif. West. Med., **60**:96–98, 1944.

406. Weis, E. B. Jr.; Pritz, H. B.; and Hassler, C. R.: Experimental Automobile-Pedestrian Injuries. J. Trauma, **17**:823–828, 1977.

407. Weissman, S., and Herold, Z.: Fractures of the Tibial Plateau. Clin. Orthop., **33**:194–200, 1964.

408. White, J. C.: T- and Y-Fractures of the Tibial Condyles. Injury, **3**:56–63, 1971.

409. Wilppula, E., and Bakalim, A.: Kiel Bone in Tibial Condylar Fractures. Acta Orthop. Scand., **43**:62–67, 1972.

410. Wilppula, E., and Bakalim, A.: Ligamentous Tear Concomitant with Tibial Condylar Fracture. Acta Orthop. Scand., **43**:292–300, 1972.

411. Wilson, P. D.: Experience in the Management of Fractures and Dislocations. Philadelphia, J. B. Lippincott, 1938.

412. Wilson, P. D., and Cochrane, W. A.: Fractures and Dislocations. Philadelphia, J. B. Lippincott, 1925.

413. Wilson, W. J., and Jacobs, J. E.: Patellar Graft for Severely Depressed Comminuted Fractures of the Lateral Tibial Condyle. J. Bone Joint Surg., **34A**:436–442, 1952.

414. Wirth, C. R.: Meniscus Repair. Clin. Orthop., **157**:153–160, 1981.

415. Wise, R.: Combined Traction Compression Method for Treatment of Bicondylar Tibial Fractures. Surg. Gynecol. Obstet., **72**:778–780, 1941.

416. Wittebol, P.: Treatment of Fractures of the Tibial Condyles. Arch. Chir. Neerland, **23**:253–267, 1968.

417. Wolf, M. D., and White, E. H.: Depressed Fractures of the Tibial Plateau. Surg. Gynecol. Obstet., **116**:457–462, 1963.

417a. Zenker, H., and Springer, H.: Das Posttraumatische Kniegelenk (Bandverletzung und Tibiakopfbruch) Lebensversicherungsmedizin Heft, **9:**202–203, 1982.

Fractures of the Tibial Spine

418. Hand, W. L.; Hand, C. R.; and Dunn, A. W.: Avulsion Fractures of the Tibial Tubercle. J. Bone Joint Surg., **53A:**1579–1583, 1971.

419. Levi, J. H., and Coleman, C. R.: Fracture of the Tibial Tubercle. Am. J. Sports Med., **4:**254–263, 1976.

419a. McLennan, J. G.: The Role of Arthroscopic Surgery in the Treatment of Fractures of the Intercondylar Eminence of the Tibia. J. Bone Joint Surg., **64B:**477–480, 1982.

420. Meyers, M. H., and McKeever, F. M.: Fractures of the Intercondylar Eminence of the Tibia. J. Bone Joint Surg., **51A:**209–222, 1959.

421. Meyers, M. H., and McKeever, F. M.: Fractures of the Intercondylar Eminence of the Tibia: Follow-up Note. J. Bone Joint Surg., **52A:**1677–1684, 1970.

422. Roberts, J. M., and Lovell, W. W.: Fractures of the Intercondylar Eminence of the Tibia. J. Bone Joint Surg., **52A:**827, 1970.

423. Sever, J. W.: Fractures of the Tibial Spine Combined with Fractures of the Tuberosities of the Tibia. Surg. Gynecol. Obstet., **35:**558–564, 1922.

424. Smillie, I. S.: Injuries of the Knee Joint, 3rd ed. Baltimore, Williams & Wilkins, 1962.

425. Zaricznyj, B.: Avulsion Fracture of the Tibial Eminence: Treatment by Open Reduction and Pinning. J. Bone Joint Surg., **59A:**1111–1114, 1977.

Fractures of the Proximal End of the Fibula

426. Lord, C. D., and Coults, J. W.: A Study of Typical Parachute Injuries Occurring in 250,000 Jumps at the Parachute School. J. Bone Joint Surg., **26:**547–557, 1944.

427. Novich, M. M.: Adduction Injury of the Knee with Rupture of the Common Peroneal Nerve. J. Bone Joint Surg., **42:**1372–1376, 1960.

427. O'Donoghue, D. H.: Treatment of Injuries to Athletes, 2nd ed. Philadelphia, W. B. Saunders, 1970.

428. Platt, H.: On the Peripheral Nerve Complications of Certain Fractures. J. Bone Joint Surg., **10:**403, 1928.

429. Smillie, I. W.: Injuries of the Knee Joint, 4th ed. Baltimore, Williams & Wilkins, 1971.

430. Towne, L. C.; Blazina, M. E.; Marmor, L.; and Lawrence, J. F.: Lateral Compartment Syndrome of the Knee. Clin. Orthop., **76:**160–168, 1971.

431. Watson-Jones, R.: Styloid Process of the Fibular in the Knee Joint with Peroneal Palsy. J. Bone Joint Surg., **13:**258–260, 1931.

432. Watson-Jones, R.: Fractures and Joint Injuries, 4th ed. Baltimore, Williams & Wilkins, 1956.

433. White, J.: The Results of Traction Injuries to the Common Peroneal Nerve. J. Bone Joint Surg., **50B:**346–350, 1968.

Dislocations and Ligamentous Injuries of the Knee

434. Nicholas, J. A.: Glossary of Sports Maneuvers in which the Knee is Immediately Involved. Presented at A.A.O.S. Postgraduate Course, "The Injured Knee in Sports. Special Reference to the Surgical Knee." Eugene, Oregon, July 23–25, 1973.

Anatomy

435. Abbott, L. C.; Saunders, J. B.; Bost, F. C.; and Anderson, C. E.: Injuries to the Ligaments of the Knee Joint. J. Bone Joint Surg., **26:**503–521, 1944.

436. Ahmad, I.: Articular Muscles of the Knee: Articularis Genus. Bull. Hosp. Joint Dis., **35(1):**58–60, 1975.

437. Andreassi, G., and Ronzoni, P.: On the Morphology and Function of the Plica Synovialis Infrapatellaris in the Human Knee Joint. Verh. Anat. Ges., **62:**313–316, 1967.

438. Arial, G.: The Effect of Knee-joint Angle on Harvard Step-Test Performance. Ergonomics, **12(1):**33–137, 1969.

439. Barrie, H. J.: The Pathogenesis and Significance of Menisceal Cysts. J. Bone Joint Surg., **61B(2):**184–189, 1979.

440. Basmajian, J. V., and Lovejoy, J. V.: Functions of the Popliteus Muscle in Man. J. Bone Joint Surg., **53A:**557–562, 1971.

441. Baumgartl, F.: Das Knieglenk. Berlin, Springer-Verlag, 1944.

442. Beauchamp, P., and Laurin, C. A.: Anterior Cruciate Ligament: Current Concepts. Union Med. Can., **105:**1380–1386, 1976.

443. Brantigan, O. C., and Voshell, A. V.: The Mechanics of the Ligaments and Menisci of the Knee Joint. J. Bone Joint Surg., **23:**44–66, 1941.

444. Brantigan, O. C., and Voshell, A. F.: The Tibial Collateral Ligament: Its Function, its Bursae, and its Relation to the Medial Meniscus. J. Bone Joint Surg., **25:**121–131, 1943.

445. Cohn, A. K., Mains, D. B.: Popliteal Hiatus of the Lateral Meniscus. Am. J. Sports Med., **7:**221–226, 1979.

446. Didio, L. J.; Zappal'a, A.; Cardoso, A. D.; and Diaz, R. A.: Musculus Articularis Genus in Human Fetuses, Newborn and Young Individuals. Anat. Anz. **124:**121–132, 1969.

447. Duparc, J., and Massara, C.: Radiological Measurement of the Angular Deviation of the Knee in the Frontal Plane. Ann. Radiol., **10:**635–656, 1967.

448. Frankel, V. H.; Burstein, A. H.; and Brooks, D. B.: Biomechanics of Internal Derangement of the Knee. Pathomechanics as Determined by Analysis of the Instant Centers of Motion. J. Bone Joint Surg., **53A:**945–962, 1971.

449. Furman, W.; Marshall, J. L.; and Girgis, F. G.: The Anterior Cruciate Ligament. J. Bone Joint Surg., **58A:**179–185, 1976.

450. Girgis, F. B.; Marshall, J. L.; and Al Monajem, A. R. S.: The Cruciate Ligaments of the Knee Joint. Anatomical, Functional and Experimental Analysis. Clin. Orthop., **106:**216–231, 1975.

451. Gray, D. J., and Gardner, E.: Prenatal Development of the Human Knee and Superior Tibiofibular Joints. Am. J. Anat., **86:**235–287, 1950.

452. Grenier, R.: Patella and the Extensor System of the Knee. 1. Anatomic, Physiologic and Clinical Considerations. Union Med. Can., **105:**34–38, 1976.

453. Grodecki, J., and Steinig, D.: Organogenetic Analysis of the Variation of Insertions of the Fibular Collateral Ligament and the Biceps Muscle at the Knee. Bull. Assoc. Anat. (Nancy), **59:**885–888, 1975.

454. Hallen, L. G., and Lindahl, O.: Rotation in the Knee

Joint in Experimental Injury to the Ligaments. Acta Orthop. Scand., **36**:400–407, 1965.

455. Harty, M.: Anatomic Features of the Lateral Aspect of the Knee Joint. Surg. Gynecol. Obstet., **130**:11–14, 1970.

456. Helfet, A. J.: Mechanism of Derangements of the Medial Semilunar Cartilage and their Management. J. Bone Joint Surg., **41B**:319–336, 1959.

457. Heller, L., and Langman, J.: The Meniscofemoral Ligaments of the Human Knee. J. Bone Joint Surg., **46B**:307, 1964.

458. Hildebrand, R.: Muscular Variant in the Region of the Popliteal Fossa. Folia Morphol. (Praha), **28**:156–158, 1980.

459. Hughston, J. C., and Eilers, A. F.: The Role of the Posterior Oblique Ligament in Repairs of Acute Medial (Collateral) Ligament Tears of the Knee. J. Bone Joint Surg., **55A**:923–940, 1973.

460. Hunter, L. Y.; Louis, D. S.; Ricciardi, J. R.; and O'Conner, G. A.: The Saphenous Nerve. It's Course and Importance in Medial Arthrotomy. Am. J. Sports Med., **7**:227–230, 1979.

461. Jacobsen, K.: Area Intercondylaris Tibiae: Osseous Surface Structure and its Relation to the Soft Tissue Structures and Applications to Radiography. J. Anat., **117**:604–618, 1974.

462. James, S. L.: Surgical Anatomy of the Knee. Fortschr. Med., **96**:141–146, 1966.

463. Jelaso, D. V.: The Fascicles of the Lateral Meniscus: An Anatomic-Arthrographic Correlation. Radiology, **114**:335–339, 1975.

464. Johnson, L. L.: Lateral Capsular Ligament Complex: Anatomical and Surgical Considerations. Am. J. Sports Med., **7**:156–160, 1979.

465. Kapandji, I. A.: The Physiology of Joints: Lower Limb, 2nd ed. reprint. London, Churchill Livingstone, 1970.

466. Kaplan, E. B.: Factors Responsible for the Stability of the Knee Joint. Bull. Hosp. Joint Dis., **18**:51–59, 1957.

467. Kaplan, E. G.: Some Aspects of Functional Anatomy of the Knee Joint. Clin. Orthop., **23**:18–29, 1962.

468. Karpf, P. M.: Anatomic Principles as a Prerequisite for the Diagnosis of Knee-Ligament Injuries in Skiing. Fortschr. Med., **95**:191–194, 1977.

469. Kaufer, H. Mechanical Function of the Patella. J. Bone Joint Surg., **53A**:1551–1560, 1971.

470. Kennedy, J. C., and Fowler, P. J.: Medial and Anterior Instability of the Knee. An Anatomic and Clinic Study Using Stress Machines. J. Bone Joint Surg., **53A**:1257–1270, 1971.

471. Kennedy, J. C.; Weinberg, W. H.; and Wilson, A. S.: The Anatomy and Function of the Anterior Cruciate Ligament. As Determined by Clinical and Morphological Studies. J. Bone Joint Surg., **56A**:223–235, 1974.

472. Lahla'idj, A.: Morphological Value of Posterior Insertion of the External Meniscus in the Human Knee. Rev. Chir. Orthop., **57**:593–600, 1971.

473. Last, R. J.: The Popliteus Muscle and the Lateral Meniscus. J. Bone Joint Surg., **32B**:93–99, 1950.

474. Laurence, M., and Strachan, J. C.: The Dynamic Stability of the Knee. Proc. R. Soc. Med., **63**:758–759, 1970.

475. Lieb, F. J., and Perry, J.: Quadriceps Function. An Anatomical and Mechanical Study using Amputated Limbs. J. Bone Joint Surg., **50A**:1535–1548, 1968.

476. Lindahl, O., and Movin, A.: The Mechanics of Extension of the Knee Joint. Acta Orthop. Scand., **38**:226–234, 1967.

477. Mains, D. B.; Andrews, J. G.; and Stonecipher, T.: Medial and Anterior Posterior Ligament Stability of the Human Knee, Measured with a Stress Apparatus. Am. J. Sports Med., **5**:144–153, 1977.

478. Maquet, G.; Pelzer, G.; and de Lamotte, F.: Mechanical Aspects of Knee during Walking. Acta Orthop. Belg., (Suppl.) **41**:119–132, 1975.

479. Marshall, J. L.; Girgis, F. G.; and Zelko, R. R.: The Biceps Femoris Tendon and its Functional Significance. J. Bone Joint Surg., **54A**:1444–1450, 1972.

480. Mcleish, R. D.: Standing with a Bent Knee. Nature, **233**:278, 1971.

481. Menschik, A.: Mechanics of the Knee Joints (author's transl). Z. Orthop., **112**:481–495, 1974.

482. Moschi, A., and Zingoni, S.: Biomechanics of the Knee. Ital. J. Orthop. Traumatol., (Suppl) **3**:7–20, 1977.

483. Mordgren, B.: Anthropometric Measures and Muscle Strength in Young Women. Scand. J. Rehabil. Med., **4**:165–169, 1972.

484. Norwood, L. A., Jr., and Cross, M. J.: The Intercondylar Shelf and the Anterior Cruciate Ligament. Am. J. Sports Med., **5**:171–176, 1977.

485. Oxnard, C. E.: Tensile Forces in Skeletal Structures. J. Morphol., **134**:425–435, 1971.

486. Palmer, I.: On Injuries to the Ligaments of the Knee Joint. A Clinical Study. Acta Chir. Scand., (Suppl.) **81**:3, 1938.

487. Pavlov, H., and Goldman, A. B.: The Popliteus Bursa: An Indicator of Subtle Pathology. Am. J. Roentgen., **134**:313–321, 1980.

488. Pfeil, E.: Transverse Ligament of the Knee Joint. Beitr. Orthop. Traumatol., **19**:268–273, 1972.

489. Pool, J.; Binkhorst, R. A.; and Vos. J. A.: Some Anthropometric and Physiological Data in Relation to Performance of Top Female Gymnasts. Int. Z. Angew. Physiol., **27**:329–338, 1959.

490. Ribot, C.: Adaptation of Ligaments to Sliding, Pressure and Flexion. Arch. Anat. Histol. Embryol. (Strasb.), **52**:233–311, 1969.

491. Schilling, H.: The Meniscus from Embryonal and Functional Points of View (author's transl.). Munch. Med. Wockenschr., **117**:977–980, 1975.

492. Schmitt, O., and Mittelmeier, H.: The Biomechanical Significance of the Vastus Medialis and Lateralis Muscles (author's transl.). Arch. Orthop. Trauma Surg., **91**:291–295, 1978.

493. Steindler, A. L.: Kinesiology of the Human Body under Normal and Pathologic Conditions. Springfield, Illinois, Charles C. Thomas, 1955.

494. Walker, P. S.; Dowson, D.; Longfield, M. D.; and Wright, V.: Boosted Lubrication: In Synovial Joints by Fluid Entrapment and Enrichment. Ann. Rheum. Dis., **27**:512–520, 1968.

495. Warren, L. F., and Marshall, J. L.: The Supporting

Structures and Layers on the Medial Side of the Knee. J. Bone Joint Surg., **61A:**56–62, 1979.

496. Warren, L. F.; Marshall, J. L.; and Girgis, F.: The Prime Static Stabilizer of the Medial Side of the Knee. J. Bone Joint Surg., **56A:**665–674, 1974.

497. Weingart, G.: Subcutaneous Connective Tissue Structures and Fasciae of the Knee Region. Gegenbaurs Morphol. Jahrb., **119:**897–920, 1973.

498. Wiberg, G.: Roentgenographic and Anatomic Studies on the Femoropatellar Joint. Acta Orthop. Scand., **12:**319–410, 1941.

499. Wilson, A. S.; Legg, P. G.; and McNeur, J. C.: Studies on the Innervation of the Medial Meniscus in the Human Knee Joint. Anat. Rec., **165:**485–491, 1969.

500. Wood, W.: Lateral Capsular Sign: X-Ray Clue to a Significant Knee Instability. Am. J. Sports Med., **7:**27–33, 1979.

501. Zivanoviʻo, S.: Menisco-meniscal Ligaments of the Human Knee Joint. Anat. Anz., **135:**35–42, 1974.

Disruption of the Extensor Mechanism

502. Anderson, L. D.: Affections of Muscles, Tendons and Tenson Sheaths. *In* Crenshaw, A. H. (ed.): Campbell's Operative Orthopaedics, Vol. 2, 5th ed. St. Louis, C. V. Mosby, 1971.

503. Anderson, L. D.: Affections of Muscles, Tendons and Tendon Sheaths. *In* Crenshaw, A. H. (ed.): Campbell's Operative Orthopaedics, Vol. 2, 6th ed. St. Louis, C. V. Mosby, 1980.

504. Anzel, S. H.; Covey, K. W.; Weiner, A. D.; and Lipscomb, P. R.: Disruption of Muscles and Tendons. An Analysis of 1014 Cases. Surgery, **45:**4–6, 414, 1959.

505. Barfred, T.: Experimental Rupture of the Achilles Tendon. Comparison of Experimental Ruptures in Rats of Different Ages and Living under Different Conditions. Acta Orthop., Scand., **42:**406–428, 1971.

506. Böhler, L.: The Treatment of Fractures, Vol. 5. New York, Grune & Stratton, 1958.

507. Buttner, A.: Clinical Aspects and Evaluation of Quadriceps Tendon Ruptures. Beitr. Klin. Chir., **179:**247–272, 1950.

508. Chandler, F. A.: Patellar Advancement Operations. A Revised Technic. J. Int. Surg., **3:**433, 1940.

509. Conway, F. M.: Rupture of Quadriceps Tendon with Report of Three Cases. Am. J. Surg., **50:**3–16, 1940.

510. Dalal, V. C., and Whittam, D. E.: Bilateral Simultaneous Rupture of the Quadriceps Tendon. Br. Med. J., **2:**1370, 1966.

511. Ecker, M. L.; Lotre, P. A.; and Glazer, R. M.: Late Reconstruction of the Patellar Tendon. J. Bone Joint Surg., **61A:**884–886, 1979.

512. Galen: De usu partium corpus huminis librae. Interprete Basileae, Nicolas Reggio, 1533.

513. Gallie, W. E., and LeMesurier, A. B.: The Late Repair of Fractures of the Patella and of Rupture of the Ligamentum Patellae and Quadriceps Tendon. J. Bone Joint Surg., **9:**47–54, 1927.

514. Gilcreest, E. L.: Ruptures and Tears of Muscles and Tendons of the Lower Extremity. J.A.M.A., **100:**153–160, 1933.

515. Graney, C. M.: Bilateral Rupture of Quadriceps Femoris Tendons with Six Year Interval between Injuries. Am. J. Surg., **61:**112–116, 1943.

516. Ismail, A. M.; Balakrishnan, R.; and Rajakumar, M. K.: Rupture of the Patellar Ligament after Steroid Infiltration. J. Bone Joint Surg., **51B:**503–505, 1969.

517. Kelikian, H.; Riashi, E.; and Gleason, J.: Restoration of Quadriceps Function in Neglected Tear of the Patellar Tendon. Surg. Gynecol. Obstet., **104:**20–204, 1957.

518. Levin, P. D.: Reconstruction of the Patellar Tendon using a Dacron Graft. Clin. Orthop., **118:**70–72, 1976.

519. Levy, M.; Seelenfreund, M.; Moor, P.; Fried, A.; and Lurie, M.: Bilateral Spontaneous and Simultaneous Rupture of the Quadriceps Tendon in Gout. J. Bone Joint Surg., **53:**510–513, 1971.

520. McBurney, Charles: Suture of the Divided Ends of a Ruptured Quadriceps Extensor Tendon with Perfect Recovery. Ann. Surg., **6:**170, 1887.

521. McLaughlin, H. L., and Francis, K. C.: Operative Repair of Injuries to the Quadriceps Extensor Mechanism. Am. J. Surg., **91:**651–653, 1956.

522. McMaster, P. E.: Tendon and Muscle Ruptures. Clinical and Experimental Studies on the Causes and Location of Subcutaneous Ruptures. J. Bone Joint Surg., **15:**705–722, 1933.

523. Preston, E. T.: Avulsion of both Quadriceps Tendons in Hyperparathyroidism. J.A.M.A., **221:**406–407, 1972.

524. Quenu, E., and Duval, P.: Traitement operatoire des ruptures sousrotuliennes du quadriceps. Rev. Chir., **31:**169–194, 1905.

525. Ramsey, R. H., and Müller, G. E.: Quadriceps Tendon Ruptures: A Diagnostic Trap. Clin. Orthop., **70:**161–164, 1970.

526. Rao, J. P., and Siwek, K. W.: Bilateral Spontaneous Rupture of the Patellar Tendons. A New Method of Treatment. Orthop. Rev., **7:**49–51, 1978.

527. Rascher, J. J.; Marcolin, L.; and James, P.: Bilateral Sequential Rupture of the Patellar Tendon in Systemic Lupus Erythematosis. J. ·Bone Joint Surg., **56A:**821–822, 1974.

528. Scuderi, C.: Ruptures of Quadriceps Tendon. Study of Twenty Tendon Ruptures. Am. J. Surg., **95:**626–635, 1958.

529. Scuderi, C., and Schrey, E. L.: Rupture of the Quadriceps Tendon. Arch. Surg., **61:**42–54, 1950.

530. Scuderi, C.: Ruptures of the Quadriceps Tendon. Am. J. Surg., **95:**626–635, 1958.

531. Siwek, K. W., and Rao, J. P.: Bilateral Simultaneous Rupture of the Quadriceps Tendons. Clin. Orthop., **131:**252–254, 1978.

532. Siwek, C. W., and Rao, J. P.: Ruptures of the Extensor Mechanism of the Knee Joint. J. Bone Joint Surg., **63A:**932–937, 1981.

533. Steiner, C. A., and Palmer, L. H.: Simultaneous Bilateral Rupture of the Quadriceps Tendon. Am. J. Surg., **78:**752–755, 1949.

534. Wagner, L. C.: Complete Rupture of Infrapatellar Tendon and Adjacent Capsular Ligaments. Ann. Surg., **86:**787–789, 1927.

535. Watson-Jones, R.: Fractures and Joint Injuries, 4th ed. Baltimore, Willliams, & Wilkins, 1956.

536. Wener, J. A., and Achein, A. J.: Simultaneous Bilateral Rupture of the Patellar Tendon and Quadriceps Expansions in Systemic Lupus Erythematosus. J. Bone Joint Surg., **56A:**823–824, 1974.

537. Wetzler, S. H., and Merkow, W.: Bilateral, Simultaneous and Spontaneous Rupture of the Quadriceps Tendon. J.A.M.A., **144:**615–617, 1950.

538. Unvesferth, L. J., and Olix, M. L.: The Effect of Local Steroid Injections on Tendon. J. Sports Med., **1:**31–37, 1973.

539. Zerricke, R. F.; Garhammer, J.; and Jobe, F.: Human Patellar-Tendon Rupture. J. Bone Joint Surg., **59A:**179–183, 1977.

Traumatic Dislocation of the Patella

540. Ahstrom, J. P.: Osteochondral Fracture in the Knee Joint Associated with Hypermobility and Dislocation of the Patella. J. Bone Joint Surg., **47A:**1491–1502, 1965.

541. Andersen, P. T.: Congenital Deformities of the Knee Joint in Dislocation of the Patella and Achondroplasia. Acta Orthop. Scand., **28:**27–50, 1958.

542. Arenberg, A. A., and Kalantarova, S. S.: Case of Unreduced Dislocation of the Knee Joint. Orthop. Travmatol. Protez, **35:**58–59, 1974.

543. Ashby, M. E.; Shields, C. L.; and Karmy, J. R.: Diagnosis of Osteochondral Fractures in Acute Traumatic Patellar Dislocations using Air Arthrography. J. Trauma, **15:**1032–1033, 1975.

544. Baker, R. H.; Carroll, N.; Dewer, P. P.; and Hall, J. E.: The Semitendinosus Tenodesis for Recurrent Dislocation of the Patella. J. Bone Joint Surg., **54B:**103–109, 1972.

545. Ballester, J.: Operative Treatment for Recurrent Dislocation of the Patella. Reconstr. Surg. Traumatol., **12:**46–52, 1971.

546. Baum, C., and Bensahel, H.: Recurrent Dislocation of the Patella in Children. Rev. Chir. Orthop., **59:**583–592, 1973.

547. Bassett, F. H. III: Acute Dislocation of the Patella, Osteochondral Fractures, and Injuries to the Extensor Mechanism of the Knee. A.A.O.S. Instructional Course Lectures, **25:**40–49, 1976.

548. Benoit, J.; Ruc, D. E.; and Bat, J. M.: Unbalanced Patella. 1. Introduction. Definitions. Classifications and Symptomatology. Rev. Chir. Orthop., **66:**205–208, 1980.

549. Blackburne, J. S., and Peel, T. E.: A New Method of Measuring Patellar Height. J. Bone Joint. Surg., **59B:**241–242, 1977.

550. Blazina, M. E.: Complications of the Hauser Procedure. Presented at A.A.O.S. Annual Meeting, San Francisco, 1975.

551. Blazina, M. E.; Fox, J. M.; Carlson, G. J.; and Jurgutis, J. J.: Patella Baja. A Technical Consideration in Evaluating Results of Tibial Tubercle Transplantation. J. Bone Joint Surg., **57A:**1027, 1975.

552. Bowker, J. H., and Thompson, E. B.: Surgical Treatment of Recurrent Dislocation of the Patella. J. Bone Joint Surg., **46A:**1451–1461, 1964.

553. Brady, T. A., and Russell, D.: Interarticular Horizontal

554. Brattstrom, H.: Shape of the Intercondylar Groove Normally and in Recurrent Dislocation of the Patella. Acta Orthop. Scand. (Suppl.) **68:**5–148, 1964.

555. Brattstrom, H.: Patella Alta in Non-dislocating Knee Joints. Acta Orthop. Scand., **41:**578–588, 1970.

556. Carter, C.: Recurrent Dislocation of the Patella and of the Shoulder. J. Bone Joint Surg., **42B:**721–727, 1960.

557. Cave, E. F., and Rowe, C. R.: The Patella, Its Importance in Derangement of the Knee. J. Bone Joint Surg., **32A:**542–553, 1950.

558. Chrisman, O. D.; Snook, G. A.; and Wilson, T. C.: A Long-term Prospective Study of the Hauser and Roux-Goldthwait Procedures for Recurrent Patellar Dislocation. Clin. Orthop., **144:**27–30, 1979.

559. Cofield, R. H., and Bryan, R. S.: Acute Dislocation of the Patella. Results of Conservative Treatment. J. Trauma, **17:**526–531, 1977.

560. Cox, J. S.: An Evaluation of the Elmslie-Trillat Procedure for Management of the Patellar Dislocations and Subluxations: A Preliminary Report. Am. J. Sports Med., **4:**72–77, 1976.

561. Crosby, E. B., and Insall, J.: Recurrent Dislocation of the Patella. Relation of Treatment to Osteoarthritis. J. Bone Joint Surg., **58A:**9–13, 1976.

562. Cross, M. J., and Waldrop, J.: The Patellar Index as a Guide to the Understanding and Diagnosis of Patellofemoral Instability. Clin. Orthop., **110:**174–176, 1973.

563. Dandy, D. J., and Poirier, H.: Chondromalacia and the Unstable Patella. Acta Orthop. Scand., **46:**695–699, 1976.

564. DaSilva, O. L., and Bratt, J. F.: Stress Trajectories in the Patella. Study by the Photoelastic Method. Acta Orthop. Scand., **41:**608–618, 1970.

565. DeCesare, W. F.: Late Results of Hauser Procedure for Recurrent Dislocation of the Patella. Clin. Orthop., **140:**137–144, 1979.

566. DeHaven, K. E.; Dolan, W. E.; and Mayer, P. J.: Chondromalacia in Athletes. Clinical Presentation and Conservative Management. Presented at the American Orthopaedic Society Sports Medicine Annual Meeting. San Diego, July 5–7, 1977.

567. DeHaven, K. E.; Dolan, W. A.; and Mayer, P. J.: Chondromalacia Patellae in Athletes. Clinical Presentation and Conservative Management. Am. J. Sports Med., **7:**12–14, 1979.

568. DeJour, H.; Goutallier, D.; and Furioli, J. Unbalanced Patella. X-Criticism of Therapeutic Methods and Indications. Rev. Chir. Orthop., **66:**238–244, 1980.

569. Delgado-Martins, H.: Treatment of the Patellar Syndrome in Nondislocated Patellae. Arch. Orthop. Trauma Surg., **97:**275–279, 1980.

570. Dexel, M., and Afifi, K.: Pathology of the Patella. Ten Year Results of Surgically Treated Patella Dislocations (author's transl.) Orthopaede, **8:**98–104, 1979.

571. Dickson, R. A.: Reversed Dynamic Slings. A New Concept in the Treatment of Post-traumatic Elbow Flexion Contractures. Injury, **8:**35–38, 1976.

572. Dougherty, J.; Wirth, C. R.; and Akbarnia, B. A.: Man-

agement of Patellar Subluxation. A Modification of Hauser's Technique. Clin. Orthop., **115:**204–208, 1976.

573. Duchenne, G. B. (transl. by Kaplan, E. B.): Physiology of Motion. W. B. Saunders, Philadelphia, 1959.

574. Ellis, J. S.: Primary Dislocation of the Patella. J. Bone Joint Surg., **36B:**145–146, 1954.

575. Feneley, R. C. L.: Intraarticular Dislocation of the Patella. J. Bone Joint Surg., **50B:**653–655, 1968.

576. Fielding, J. W.: The Extensor Mechanism of the Knee. Presented at A.A.O.S. Post-Graduate Course "The Injured Knee in Sports, Special Reference to the Surgical Knee." Eugene, Oregon, July 23, 25, 1973.

577. Fielding, J. W.; Liebler, W. A.; Urs, D.; Wilson, S. A.; and Puglisi, A.: Tibial Tubercle Transfer. A Long Range Follow up Study (Abstract). J. Bone Joint Surg., **56A:**1315–1316, 1974.

578. Fielding, J. W.; Liebler, W. A.; Krishne, Urs, N. D.; Wilson, S. W.; and Puglisi, A. S.: Tibial Tubercle Transfer. A Long Range Follow up Study. Clin. Orthop., **144:**43–44, 1979.

579. Floare, S. G., and Georgeson, N.: Traumatic Dislocations of the Patella. Rev. Med. Chir. Soc. Med. Nat. Iasi., **78:**359–364, 1974.

580. Fontaine, C.: Habitual Dislocations of the Patella in the Adult. Rev. Chir. Orthop., **66:**246–248, 1980.

581. Fox, T. A.: Dysplasia of the Quadriceps Mechanism. Hypoplasia of the Vastus Medialis Muscle as Related to the Hypermobile Patella Syndrome. Surg. Clin. North Am., **55:**199–226, 1975.

582. Frangakes, E. K.: Intraarticular Dislocation of the Patella. J. Bone Joint Surg., **56A:**423–426, 1974.

583. Gartland, J. J., and Benner, J. H.: Traumatic Dislocations in the Lower Extremities in Children. Orthop. Clin. North Am., **7:**687–700, 1976.

584. Geneste, R.: Unbalanced Patella. III. Physiological Bases of Nonsurgical Treatment. Kinesitherapy and its Results. Rev. Chir. Orthop., **66:**212–213, 1966.

585. Girgis, F. G.; Marshall, J. L.; and al Monajem, A. R. S.: The Cruciate Ligaments of the Knee Joint. Anatomical, Functional and Experimental Analysis. Clin. Orthop., **106:**216–231, 1975.

586. Gledhill, R. B., and McIntyre, J. M.: Interarticular Horizontal Dislocation of the Patella. Can. J. Surg., **11:**57–59, 1968.

587. Goodfellow, J.; Hungerford, D. S.; and Zindel, M.: Patellofemoral Joint Mechanics and Pathology. Functional Anatomy of the Patellofemoral Joint. J. Bone Joint Surg., **58B:**287–290, 1976.

588. Gore, D. R.: Horizontal Dislocation of the Patella. J.A.M.A., **214:**1119, 1970.

589. Goutallier, D.; Bernageau, J.; and Lecudonne, C. B.: The Measurement of the Tibial Tuberosity. Patella Groove Distanced Technique and Results. (author's transl.) Rev. Chir. Orthop., **64:**423–428, 1978.

590. Grana, W. A., and O'Donoghue, D. H.: Patellar Tendon Transfer by the Slot-block Method for Recurrent Subluxation and Dislocation of the Patella. J. Bone Joint Surg., **59A:**736–741, 1977.

591. Grimes, H. A.: Subluxating and Luxating Patellae. J. Arkansas Med. Soc., **72:**173–176, 1975.

592. Hall, J. E.; Micheli, L. J.; and McManama, G. B., Jr.: Semitendinosus Tenodesis for Recurrent Subluxation or Dislocation of the Patella. Clin. Orthop., **144:**31–35, 1979.

593. Handelsman, J. A.: Management of Subluxating Patella in Juveniles. J. Bone Joint Surg., **58B:**388, 1976.

594. Hampson, W. G., and Hill, P.: Late Results of Transfer of the Tibial Tubercle for Recurrent Dislocation of the Patella. J. Bone Joint Surg., **57B:**209–213, 1976.

595. Harrison, M. H. M.: The Results of a Realignment Operation for Recurrent Dislocation of the Patella. J. Bone Joint Surg., **37B:**559–567, 1955.

596. Hauser, E. D. W.: Total Tendon Transplant for Slipping Patella. Surg. Gynecol. Obstet., **66:**199–214, 1958.

597. Hejgaard, N.; Skive, L.; and Perrild, C.: Acute Traumatic Patellar Dislocation Treated by Simple Medical Capsulorrhaphy. Ugeskr. Laeger, **142:**238–240, 1980.

598. Hejgaard, N.; Skive, L.; and Perrild, C.: Recurrent Dislocation of the Patella. Treatment by a Modification of the Method of McCarroll and Schwartzmann. Acta Orthop. Scand., **51:**673–678, 1980.

599. Helfet, A. H.: Disorders of the Knee, pp. 13–14. Philadelphia, J. B. Lippincott Co., 1974.

600. Henry, J. H., and Craven, P. R.: Surgical Treatment of Patellar Instability: Indications and Results. J. Sports Med., **9:**82–85, 1981.

601. Henry, J. H., and Crosland, J. W.: Conservative Treatment of Patellofemoral Subluxation. Presented at the American Othopaedic Society Sports Medicine Annual Meeting. San Diego, July 5–9, 1977.

602. Heywood, A. W. B.: Recurrent Dislocations of the Patella. J. Bone Joint Surg., **43B:**508–517, 1961.

603. Houkom, S. S.: Recurrent Dislocation of the Patella. A Study of End Results in Twenty-Seven Cases. Arch. Surg., **44:**1025–1037, 1942.

604. Hoyt, W. A.; Davis, W. M.; and Schulze, K. W.: Reconstruction of the Quadriceps Mechanism by Vastus Medialis Transposition in Selected Cases of Patellar Luxation. A Preliminary Report. J. Bone Joint Surg., **51A:**1040, 1969.

605. Huang, T. L.; Fossier, C.; Ray, R. D.; and Ghosh, L.: Intra-articular Rheumatoid Nodule of the Knee Joint Associated with Recurrent Subluxation of the Patella. A Case Report. J. Bone Joint Surg., **61A:**438–440, 1979.

606. Huc, D. E.; Bat, J. M.; and Benoit, J.: Traumatic Dislocations of the Patella. Rev. Chir. Orthop. **66(4):**245–246, 1980.

607. Hughston, J. C.: Subluxation of the Patella. J. Bone Joint Surg., **50A:**1003–1026, 1968.

608. Hughston, J. C.: Subluxation of the Patella in Athletes. American Academy of Orthopaedic Surgeons Symposium on Sports Medicine, pp. 162–177. St. Louis, C. V. Mosby Co., 1969.

609. Hughston, J. C.: Reconstruction of the Extensor Mechanism for Subluxating Patella. J. Sports Med., **1:**6–13, 1972.

610. Hughston, J. C., and Walsh, W. M.: Proximal and Distal Reconstruction of the Extensor Mechanism for Patellar Subluxation. Clin. Orthop., **144:**36–42, 1979.

611. Insall, J.; Falvo, K. A.; and Wise, D. W.: Chondromalacia Patellae. J. Bone Joint Surg., **58A:**1–8, 1976.

612. Insall, J.; Goldberg, V.; and Salvati, E.: Recurrent Dislocation and the High-riding Patella. Clin. Orthop., **88:**67–69, 1972.

613. Insall, J., and Salvati, E.: Patella Position in the Normal Knee Joint. Radiology, **101:**101–104, 1971.

614. Jackson, R. W.: Examination of the Patella. A.A.O.S. Instructional Course Lectures, **25:**31–36, 1976.

615. Jacobsen, K., and Bertheussen, K.: The Vertical Location of the Patella. Fundamental Views on the Concept Patella Alta, Using a Normal Sample. Acta Orthop. Scand., **45:**436–445, 1974.

616. Jacobsen, K., and Metz, P.: Occult Traumatic Dislocation of the Patella. J. Trauma, **16:**829–835, 1976.

617. Jacobsen, K., and Rosenkilde, P.: A Clinical and Stress Radiographical Follow-up Investigation after Jones Operation for Replacing the Anterior Cruciate Ligament. Injury, **8:**221–226, 1977.

618. Jeffreys, T. E.: Recurrent Dislocation of the Patella due to Abnormal Attachment of the Ilio-tibial Tract. J. Bone Joint Surg., **45B:**740–743, 1963.

619. Jones, J. B.; Francis, K.; and Mahoney, J.: Recurrent Dislocating Patella. Clin. Orthop., **20:**230–239, 1961.

620. Jones, R. D.; Fisher, R. L.; and Curtis, B. H.: Congenital Dislocation of the Patella. Clin. Orthop. **119:**177–183, 1976.

621. Kaufman, I., and Habermann, E. T.: Intercondylar Vertical Dislocation of the Patella. A Case Report. Bull. Hosp. Joint. Dis., **34:**222–225, 1973.

622. Kennedy, J. C.; Weinberg, H. W.; and Wilson, A. S.: The Anatomy and Function of the Anterior Cruciate Ligament. As Determined by Clinical and Morphological Studies. J. Bone Joint Surg., **56:**223–235, 1974.

623. Kettlekamp, D. B., and DeRosa, G. P.: Biomechanics and Functional Role of the Patellofemoral Joint. A.A.O.S. Instructional Course Lectures, **25:**27–31, 1976.

624. Kummel, B. M.: The Treatment of Patellofemoral Problems. Primary Care, **7:**217–229, 1980.

625. Kummel, B. M., and Crutchlow, W. P.: Stabilization of the Subluxating Patella by Semitendinosus Transfer to the Third of the Infrapatellar Tendon. Am. J. Sports Med., **5:**194–203, 1977.

626. Labelle, H., and Laurin, C. A.: Radiological Investigation of Normal and Abnormal Patellae. J. Bone Joint Surg., **57B:**530, 1976.

627. Laing, P. G., Caulson, D. B., and Janeway, T.: Gracilis, Transplantation for Recurrent Dislocation of the Patella. J. Bone Joint Surg., **56A:**1540, 1974.

628. Languepin, A., and Aucoutorier, P.: Unbalanced Patella. IV. Operations on the Soft Portions. Rev. Chir. Orthop., **66:**214–215, 1980.

629. Lanier, B. E.: Stuck Medial Patella: Unusual Complication of a Hauser-Hughston Patellar Shaving Procedure. NY State J. Med., **77:**1955–1957, 1977.

630. Lanscourt, J. E., and Cristini, J. A.: Patella Alta and Patella Infera. J. Bone Joint Surg., **57A:**1112–1115, 1975.

631. Larson, R. L.: The Patella of the Female Athlete. Sub-

luxation, Chondromalacia and Patellar Compression Syndrome. Med. Aspects of Sports, **16:**12–18, 1974.

632. Larson, R. L.; Cabad, H. E.; Slocum, D. B.; James, S. L.; Keenan, T.; and Hutchinson, T.: The Patellar Compression Syndrome. Surgical Treatment by Lateral Retinacular Release. Clin. Orthop., **134:**158–167, 1978.

633. Laurin, C. A.; L'evesque, H. P.; Dussault, R.; Labelle, H.; and Peides, J. P.: The Abnormal Lateral Patellofemoral Angle. A Diagnosis, Roentgenographic Sign of Recurrent Patellar Subluxation. J. Bone Joint Surg., **60A:**55–60, 1978.

634. Lieb, F. J., and Perry, J.: Quadriceps Function. An Electromyographic Study under Isometric Conditions. J. Bone Joint Surg., **53A:**749–758, 1971.

635. Liebler, W. A.: Treatment of Patella Lesions for Instability, a Perplexing Problem. Orthop. Rev., **3:**25–37, 1974.

636. MacNab, I.: Recurrent Dislocation of the Patella. J. Bone Joint Surg., **34A:**957–967, 1952.

637. Madigan, R.; Wissinger, H. A.; and Donaldson, W. F.: Preliminary Experience with a Method of Quadriceps Plasty in Recurrent Subluxation of the Patella. J. Bone Joint Surg., **57A:**600–607, 1975.

638. Mansat, C.; Duboureau, L.; Cha, P.; and Dorbes, R.: Patellar Imbalance and External Rotary Instability of the Knee. Rev. Rhum. Mal. Osteoartic., **44:**115–123, 1977.

639. Mansat, C.: Unbalanced patella. VIII. Unbalanced Patella and Rotatory Instabilities. Therapeutic and Physiopathologic Concepts. Internal Dynamic Stabilization. Rev. Chir. Orthop., **66:**226–232, 1980.

640. Maquet, P.: Unbalanced patella. II. Biomechanical Back Motion. Rev. Chir. Orthop., **66:**209–211, 1980.

641. Masse, Y.: Trochleoplasty. Restoration of the Intertcondylar Groove in Subluxations and Dislocations of the Patella. Rev. Chir. Orthop., **64:**3–17, 1978.

642. McCarroll, H. R., and Schwartzmann, J. R.: Lateral Dislocation of the Patella. J. Bone Joint Surg., **27:**446–452, 1945.

643. McCarrol, J. R.: Acute Dislocation of the Patella Resulting in a Comminuted Patella Fracture. J. Sports Med., **9:**117–118, 1981.

644. McDougall, A., and Brown, D.: Radiological Signs of Recurrent Dislocation of the Patella. J. Bone Joint Surg., **50B:**841–843, 1968.

645. Merchant, A. C. and Mercer, R. L.: Lateral Release of the Patella. A Preliminary Report. Clin. Orthop., **103:**40–145, 1974.

646. Merchant, A. C.; Mercer, R. L.; Jacobsen, R. H.; and Cool, C. R.: Roentgenographic Analysis of Patellofemoral Congruence. J. Bone Joint Surg., **56A:**1391–1396, 1974.

647. Miller, G. F.: Familial Recurrent Dislocation of the Patella. J. Bone Joint Surg., **60B:**203–204, 1978.

648. Ober, F. R.: Recurrent Dislocation of the Patella. Am. J. Surg., **43:**497–500, 1939.

649. O'Donoghue, D. H.: Treatment of Injuries to Athletes, 2nd ed., p. 547. Philadelphia, W. B. Saunders, 1970.

650. Oki, T.; Terashima, Y.; Murachi, S.; and Nugami, H.: Clinical Features and Treatment of Joint Dislocations in Larsen's Syndrome. Report of Three Cases in One Family. Clin. Orthop., **119:**206–210, 1976.

651. Palumbo, P. M.: Dynamic Patellar Brace: A New Orthosis in the Management of Patellofemoral Disorders. Am. J. Sports Med., **9**:45–49, 1981.

652. Paulos, L.; Rusche, K.; Johnson, C.; and Noyes, F. R.: Patellar Malalignment; A Treatment Rationale. Phys. Ther., **60**:1624–1632, 1980.

653. Pendergrass, T. W., and Hayes, H. M., Jr.: Cryptorchism and Related Defects in Dogs: Epidemiologic Comparisons with Man. Teratology, **12**:51–55, 1975.

654. Percy, E. C.: Acute Dislocation of the Patella. Can. Med. Assoc. J., **105**:1176–1178, 1971.

655. Radin, E. L.: A Rational Approach to the Treatment of Patellofemoral Pain. Clin. Orthop. **144**:107–109, 1979.

656. Rengeval, J. P.: Recurrent Luxations of the Patella in Children. Rev. Chir. Orthop., **66**:216–218, 1980.

657. Robbins, H., and Ulin, R. I.: A Procedure for Recurrent Dislocation of the Patella. Bull. Hosp. Joint Dis., **34**:148–155, 1973.

658. Rorabeck, C. H., and Bobechko, W. P.: Acute Dislocation of the Patella with Osteochondral Fracture. J. Bone Joint Surg., **58B**:237–240, 1976.

659. Rosenberg, N. J.: Osteochondral Fractures of the Lateral Femoral Condyle. J. Bone Joint Surg., **45A**:1013–1026, 1964.

660. Roux, C.: The Classic. Recurrent Dislocation of the Patella: Operative Treatment. Clin. Orthop., **144**:4–8, 1979.

661. Ruder, B.; Marshall, J. L.; and Warren, R. F.: Clinical Characteristics of Patellar Disorders in Young Athletes. Am. J. Sports Med., **9**:270–273, 1981.

662. Sargent, J. R., and Teipner, W. A.: Medial Retinacular Repair for Acute and Recurrent Dislocation of the Patella. A Preliminary Report. J. Bone Joint Surg., **53A**:386, 1971.

663. Savastano, A. A., and Croni, R. J.: Recurrent Subluxation of the Patella. Int. Surg., **60**:25–29, 1975.

664. Saxena, P. S., and Sharma, K. K.: Compound Complicated Intra-articular Horizontal Dislocation of Patella. Indian J. Med. Sci., **29**:19–20, 1975.

665. Scheller, S., and Martenson, L.: Traumatic Dislocation of the Patella. A Radiographic Investigation. Acta Radiol., (Suppl.) **336**:6–160, 1974.

666. Shoji, H., and Granda, J. L.: Acid Hydrolaoes in the Articular Cartilage of the Patella. Normal Chondromalacia Patellae and Osteoarthritis. Clin. Orthop., **99**:293–297, 1974.

667. Slocum, D. B.; James, S. L.; and Larson, R. L: Surgical Treatment of the Dislocating Patella in Athletes. Presented at American Orthopaedic Association Annual Meeting, Hot Springs, Va., 1973.

668. Smillie, I. S.: Injuries of the Knee Joint, 4th ed., pp. 205–223, Baltimore, Williams & Willkins, 1971.

669. Smillie, I. S.: Diseases of the Knee Joint, pp. 82–97. London. Churchill Livingstone, 1974.

670. Southwick, W. O.; Becker, G. E.; and Albright, J. A.: Dovetail Patellar Tendon Transfer for Recurrent Dislocating Patella. J.A.M.A., **204**:665–669, 1968.

671. Stanisavljevic, S.; Zemenick, G.; and Miller, D.: Congenital Irreducible Permanent Lateral Dislocation of the Patella. Clin. Orthop., **116**:190–199, 1976.

672. Stewart, M.: Dislocations. *In* Crenshaw, A. H. (ed.). Campbell's Operative Orthopaedics, 5th ed. Vol. 1, pp. 448–454. St. Louis, C. V. Mosby., 1971.

673. Stover, C. N.: Interarticular Dislocation of the Patella. J.A.M.A., **200**:996, 1967.

674. Strong, T. E., and Bell, S.: The Campbell-Goldthwait Procedure for Recurrent Dislocation of the Patella. J. Bone Joint Surg., **56A**:1304–1305, 1974.

675. Sutro, C. J.: Hypermobility of Bones due to "Overlengthened" Capsular and Ligamentous Tissues. Surgery, **21**:67–76, 1947.

676. Trillat, A.; DeJour, J.; Couette, A.: Diagnostic et Traitement des 36 Subluxations Rescidiventes de la Rotule. Rev. Chir. Orthop., **50**:813–864, 1964.

677. Wall, J. J.: Compartment Syndrome as a Complication of the Hauser Procedure. J. Bone Joint Surg., **61**:185–191, 1979.

678. Watson-Jones, R.: Fractures and Joint Injuries. 4th ed., Vol. 2. Baltimore, Williams & Wilkins, 1956.

680. Wiberg, G.: Roentgenographic and Anatomic Studies on the Femoropatellar Joint. With Special Reference to Chondromalacia Patellae. Acta Orthop. Scand., **12**:319–409, 1941.

681. Wiggins, H. E.: The Anterior Compartment Syndrome. A Complication of the Hauser Procedure. Clin. Orthop., **113**:90–94, 1975.

682. Wilber, M. C.: Recurrent Lateral Dislocation of the Patella. Preliminary Results of Pes Anserinus Transfer. South. Med. J., **67**:531–533, 1974.

683. Williams, P. F.: Quadriceps Contracture. J. Bone Joint Surg., **50B**:278–284, 1968.

684. Willner, P.: Recurrent Dislocation of the Patella. Clin. Orthop., **69**:213–215, 1970.

685. Wimsalt, M. H., and Carey, R. J. J.: Superior Dislocation of the Patella. J. Trauma, **17**:77–80, 1977.

686. Wright, J. C.: The Cave-Rowe Patelloplasty: Report of a Series. Presented at Society of Military Orthopaedic Surgeons 14th Annual Meeting, San Antonio, Nov. 29, 1977.

687. Zeier, F. G., and Dissanayake, C.: Congenital Dislocation of the Patella. Clin Orthop., **148**:140–146, 1980.

Dislocation of the Knee

688. Aho, A. J.; Inberg, M. V.; and Wegelius, U.: Dislocation of the Knee with Total Rupture of the Popliteal Artery. A Case Report. Acta Chir. Scand., **137**:387–389, 1971.

689. Anderson, R. L.: Dislocation of the Knee. Report of Four Cases. Arch. Surg., **46**:598–603, 1943.

690. Apoil, A.; Langlais, F., and Vivier, J.: Fractures of the Tibial Margin in Serious Dislocations of the Knee. J. Chir. (Paris), **107**:611–616, 1974.

691. Arenberg, A. A., and Kalantarova, S. S.: Case of Unreduced Dislocation of the Knee Joint. Orthop. Travmatol. Protez., **35**:58–59, 1974.

692. Bruckner, H., and Bruckner, H.: Reconstruction Ligament Surgery in the Knee Area Following the "Building Block" Principle. Zentralbl. Chir., **97**:65–77, 1972.

693. Cole, W. G.: Fractures and Dislocations Complicated by Distal Ischaemia. Med. J. Aust., **1**:98–101, 1975.

694. Dart, C. H., Jr., and Braitman, H. E.: Popliteal Artery Injury following Fracture or Dislocation at the Knee. Diagnosis and Management. Arch. Surg., **112**:969–973, 1977.

695. DeBakey, M. E., and Simeone, F. A.: Battle Injuries in World War II. Ann. Surg., **123**:534–579, 1946.

696. Diatlov, M. M.: Vascular Disorders in Dislocations of the Knee. Vestn. Khir., **108**:57–61, 1972.

697. Doporto, J. M., and Rafique, M.: Vascular Insufficiency Complicating Trauma to the Lower Limb. J. Bone Joint Surg., **51B**:680–685, 1969.

698. Eger, M.; Huler, T.; and Hirsch, M.: Popliteal Artery Occlusion Associated with Dislocation of the Knee Joint. Br. J. Surg., **57**:315–317, 1970.

699. Fiala, O.; Dvo, R. A. L.; and Urb Anek, K.: Traumatic Dislocation of the Knee Joint (author's transl.). Acta Chir. Orthop. Traumatol. Cech., **40**:444–453, 1973.

700. Ficat, P.; Cuzacq, J. P.; and Ricci, A.: Surgical Repair of Chronic Instabilities of the Cruciate Ligaments of the Knee. Rev. Chir. Orthop., **61**:89–100, 1975.

701. Floare, S. G., and Georgescu, N.: On Irreducible Dislocation of the Knee. Rev. Med. Chir. Soc. Med. Nat. Iast., **77**:867–870, 1973.

702. Ford, G. L., and Goldner, J. L.: Dislocation of the Knee Joint. No. Carolina Med. J., **20**:463–468, 1959.

703. Gartland, J. J., and Benner, J. H.: Traumatic Dislocations in the Lower Extremity in Children. Orthop. Clin. North Am., **7**:687–700, 1976.

704. Geneste, R.; Senegas, J.; Gautier, D.; and Liorzoo, G.: Traumatic Dislocations of the Knee. Current Therapeutic Trend Apropos of a Series of 16 Cases. Bord. Med., **5**:2051–2058, 1972.

705. Green, N. E., and Allen, B. L.: Vascular Injuries Associated with Dislocation of the Knee. J. Bone Joint Surg., **59A**:236–239, 1977.

706. Goldman, H.: Complete Dislocation of the Knee with Rupture of the Popliteal Vessels. J. Int. Coll. Surgeons, **19**:237–242, 1953.

707. Hardy, E. G., and Tibbs, D. J.: Acute Ischemia in Limb Injuries. Br. Med. J., **4**:1001–1005, 1960.

708. Hill, J. A., and Rana, N. A.: Complications of Posterolateral Dislocation of the Knee: Case Report and Literature Review. Clin. Orthop., **154**:212–215, 1981.

709. Honton, J. L.; LeRebeller, A.; Legroux, P.; Kagni, R.; and Tramond, P.: Traumatic Dislocation of the Knee Treated by Early Surgical Repair (author's transl.). Rev. Chir. Orthop., **64**:213–219, 1978.

710. Hoover, N. W.: Injuries of the Popliteal Artery Associated with Fractures and Dislocations. Surg. Clin. North Am., **41**:1099–1112, 1961.

711. Houch, W. S., Jr.: Blunt Trauma to the Popliteal Artery: A Review and a Presentation of Four Cases. Am. Surg., **43**:434–437, 1977.

712. Hughes, C. W.: Arterial Repair during the Korean War. Am. Surg., **147**:555–561, 1958.

713. Jones, R. E., Smith, E. C., and Bone, G. E.: Vascular and Orthopedic Complications of Knee Dislocation. Surg. Gynecol. Obstet., **149**:554–558, 1979.

714. Kaczmarczyk, W., and Nowak, R.: Results of Surgical Treatment of 3 Cases of Traumatic Unreducible Subluxation of the Knee Joint. Chir. Narzadow Ruchu Ortop. Pol., **38**:535–539, 1973.

715. Kennedy, J. C.: Complete Dislocation of the Knee Joint. J. Bone Joint Surg., **45A**:889–904, 1963.

716. Lefrak, E. A.: Knee Dislocation. An Illusive Cause of Critical Arterial Occlusion. Arch. Surg., **111**:1021–1024, 1976.

717. Liebenberg, F.; Cloete, G. N. P.; Domisse, G. F.; and van Wyk, F. A. K.: Injuries of the Popliteal Artery Associated with Dislocation of the Knee. So. African Med. J., **44**:81–86, 1970.

718. MacGowan, W.: Acute Ischaemic Complicating Limb Trauma. J. Bone Joint Surg., **50B**:472–481, 1968.

719. Mayr, K.: Nursing Care of a Patient following Dislocation of the Knee Joint with Resulting Fistula and Empyema Formation. Osterr. Krankenpflegez, **25**:414–416, 1976.

720. Meyers, M. H.; Moore, T. M.; and Harvey, J. P., Jr.: Traumatic Dislocation of the Knee Joint. J. Bone Joint Surg., **57A**:430–433, 1975.

721. Miller, H. H.: Quantitative Studies on the Time Factor in Arterial Injuries. Ann. Surg., **130**:428–438, 1949.

722. Myles, J. W.: Seven Cases of Traumatic Dislocation of the Knee. Proc. R. Soc. Med., **60**:279–281, 1967.

723. O'Donnell, T. F., Jr.; Brewster, D. C.; Darling, R. C.; Veen, H.; and Waltman, A. A.: Arterial Injuries Associated with Fractures and/or Dislocations of the Knee. J. Trauma, **17**:775–784, 1977.

724. O'Donoghue, D. H.: An Analysis of End Results of Surgical Treatment of Major Injuries to the Ligaments of the Knee. J. Bone Joint Surg., **37A**:1–13, 1955.

725. Ottolenghi, C. E., and Traversa, C. H.: Vascular and Nervous Complications in Injuries of the Knee Joint. Reconstr. Surg. Traumatol., **14**:114–135, 1974.

726. Potter, A., and Chatelin, C. L.: Popliteal Artery Injury in an Open Dislocation of the Knee (author's transl.). Ann. Chir., **33**:109–112, 1979.

727. Quinlan, A. G., and Sharrard, W. J. W.: Posterolateral Dislocation of the Knee with Capsular Interposition. J. Bone Joint Surg., **40B**:660–663, 1958.

728. Reckling, F. W., and Peltier, L. F.: Acute Knee Dislocations and their Complications. J. Trauma, **9**:181–191, 1959.

729. Rich, N. M.; Bauch, J. H.; and Hughes, C. W.: Popliteal Artery Injuries in Viet Nam. Am. J. Surg., **118**:531–534, 1969.

730. Richard, D. R.: Unreduced Dislocations. Trop. Doct., **3**:119–122, 1973.

731. Richie, R. E.; Conkle, D. M.; Sawyers, J. L.; and Scott, H. W.: Proceedings: Surgical Management of Injuries of the Popliteal Artery and Associated Structures. J. Cardiovasc. Surg. (Torino), **17**:87, 1976.

732. Saggau, W., and Laubach, K.: Treatment of the Injured Popliteal Artery. Fortschr. Med., **92**:719–721, 1974.

733. St. Grabski, R., and Suchodolski, R.: Treatment of Traumatic Dislocation and Subluxation of the Knee Joint. Chir. Narzadow Ruchu Ortop. Pol., **43**:109–114, 1978.

734. Savage, R.: Popliteal Artery Injury Associated with Knee Dislocation: Improved Outlook? Am. Surg., **46**:627–632, 1980.

735. Schulze-Bergmann, G.: Injuries of the Popliteal Artery. Chirurg, **45:**391–394, 1974.

736. Schuster, G.: Dislocations of the Knee Joint. Fortschr. Med., **98:**415–418, 1980.

737. Shields, L.; Mital, M.; and Cave, E. F.: Complete Dislocation of the Knee: Experience at the Massachusetts General Hospital. J. Trauma, **9:**192–215, 1969.

738. Subbarao, K., and Jacobson, H. G.: Fractures and Dislocations around the Adult Knee. Semin. Roentgenol., **13:**135–143, 1978.

739. Taylor, A. R.; Arden, G. P.; and Rainey, M. A.: Traumatic Dislocation of the Knee. A Report of 43 Cases with Special Reference to Conservative Treatment. J. Bone Joint Surg., **54B:**96–102, 1972.

740. Vaccard, E.; Solitro, A.; Locantoni, A.; and Peverini, M.: Venous Gangrene due to Traumatic Dislocation of the Knee in a Patient with Ependymoblastoma of the Dorsispinal Medulla. Description of a Case. Minerva Med., **67:**1371–1376, 1976.

741. Zhelev, Z. H., and Minchev, M.: Treatment of Traumatic Crural Dislocation. Orthop. Travmatol. Protez., **33:**23–27, 1972.

742. Zhukov, P. P., and Bulatova, O. N.: Dislocations and Subluxations of the Knee Joint. Orthop. Travmatol. Protez., **2:**37–39, 1976.

Dislocation of the Proximal Tibiofibular Joint

743. Crothers, D. C., and Johnson, J. T. H.: Isolated Acute Dislocation of the Proximal Tibio-fibular Joint. J. Bone Joint Surg., **55A:**181–183, 1973.

744. Dennis, J. B., and Rutledge, B. A.: Bilateral Recurrent Dislocation of the Superior Tibio-fibular Joint with Peroneal Nerve Palsy. J. Bone Joint Surg., **40A:**1146–1148, 1958.

745. Harrison, R., and Hindenach, J. C. R.: Dislocations of the Upper End of the Fibula. J. Bone Joint Surg., **41B:**114–120, 1959.

746. Helfet, A. J.: The Management of Internal Derangement of the Knee. Philadelphia, J. B. Lippincott, 1963.

747. Lord, D. C., and Coutts, J. W.: A Study of Typical Parachute Injuries Occurring in 250,000 Jumps at the Parachute School. J. Bone Joint Surg., **26:**547–577, 1944.

748. Lyle, H. H. M.: Traumatic Luxation of the Head of the Fibula. Ann. Surg., **82:**635–639, 1925.

749. Ogden, J. A.: Subluxation and Dislocation of the Proximal Tibiofibular Joint. J. Bone Joint Surg., **56A:**145–154, 1974.

750. Owen, R.: Recurrent Dislocation of Superior Tibio-fibular Joint. J. Bone Joint Surg., **50B:**342–345, 1968.

751. Parkes, J. C. II, and Zelko, R. R.: Isolated Acute Dislocation of the Proximal Tibio-fibular Joint. J. Bone Joint Surg., **55A:**177–180, 1973.

752. Sijbeandij, S.: Instability of the Proximal Tibio-fibular Joint. Acta Orthop. Scand., **49:**621–626, 1978.

753. Vitt, R. J.: Dislocation of the Head of the Fibula. J. Bone Joint Surg., **30A:**1012–1013, 1948.

Chondral and Osteochondral Fractures

754. Ahstrom, J. P.: Osteochondral Fracture in the Knee Joint

755. Anderson, L. D.: Fractures. *In* Crenshaw, A. H. (ed.): Campbell's Operative Orthopaedics, 5th ed., St. Louis, C. V. Mosby, 1971.

756. Ashby, M. E.; Shields, C. L.; and Karmy, J. R.: Diagnosis of Osteochondral Fractures in Acute Traumatic Patellar Dislocations Using Air Arthrography. J. Trauma, **15:**1032–1033, 1975.

757. Blazina, M. E.: Classification of Injuries to the Articular Cartilage of the Knee in Athletes. *In* A.A.O.S. Symposium on Sports Medicine. St. Louis, C. V. Mosby, 1969.

758. Cavlak, Y., and Rucker, P.: Overlooked Osteochondral Fractures of the Knee Joint among Juveniles. Med. Klin., **73:**1555–1558, 1978.

759. Edwards, D. H., and Bentley, G.: Osteochondritis Dissecans Patellae. J. Bone Joint Surg., **59B:**58–63, 1977.

760. Frandsen, P. A., and Kristensen, H.: Osteochondral Fracture Associated with Dislocation of the Patella: Another Mechanism of Injury. J. Trauma, **19:**195–197, 1979.

761. Gilley, J. S.; Gelman, M. I.; Edson, D. M.; and Metcalf, R. W.: Chondral Fractures of the Knee. Arthrographic, Arthroscopic, and Clinical Manifestations. Radiology, **138:**51–54, 1981.

762. Glinz, W.: Diagnosis of Chondral Injury in Trauma of the Knee Joint (author's transl.). Langenbecks Arch. Chir., **345:**423–429, 1977.

763. Green, W. T., and Banks, H. H.: Osteochondritis Dissecans in Children. J. Bone Joint Surg., **35A:**26–79, 1953.

764. Hammerle, C. P., and Jacob, R. P.: Chondral and Osteochondral Fractures after Luxation of the Patella and their Treatment. Arch. Orthop. Trauma Surg., **97:**207–211, 1980.

765. Hughston, J. C.: Subluxation of the Patella. J. Bone Joint Surg., **50A:**1003–1026, 1968.

766. Kennedy, J. C.; Grainger, R. W.; and McGraw, R. W.: Osteochondral Fractures of the Femoral Condyles. J. Bone Joint Surg., **48B:**437–440, 1966.

767. Kondo, H.: Classification and Growth of Loose Bodies in Joints (author's transl.). Nippon Seikeigeka Gakkai Zasshi, **53:**1767–1789, 1979.

768. Landells, J. W.: The Reactions of Injured Human Articular Cartilage. J. Bone Joint Surg., **39B:**548–562, 1957.

769. Makin, M.: Osteochondral Fracture of the Lateral Femoral Condyle. J. Bone Joint Surg., **33A:**262–264, 1951.

770. Matthewson, M. H., and Dandy, D. J.: Osteochondral Fractures of the Lateral Femoral Condyle: A Result of Indirect Violence to the Knee. J. Bone Joint Surg., **60B:**199–202, 1978.

771. Milgram, J. E.: Tangential Osteochondral Fracture of the Patella. J. Bone Joint Surg., **25:**271–280, 1943.

772. Milgram, J. E.: Osteochondral Fractures of the Articular Surfaces of the Knee. *In* Helfet, A. J. (ed.): The Management of Internal Derangements of the Knee. Philadelphia, J. B. Lippincott, 1963.

773. Milgram, J. W.; Rogers, L. F.; and Miller, J. W.: Osteochondral Fractures: Mechanisms of Injury and Fate of Fragments. A.J.R., **130:**651–658, 1978.

774. Mollan, R. A.: Osteochondritis Dissecans of the Knee. Acta Orthop. Scand., **48:**517–519, 1977.

775. Newberg, A. H.: Osteochondral Fractures of the Dome of the Talus. Br. J. Radiol., **52**:105–109, 1979.

776. O'Donoghue, D. H.: Chondral and Osteochondral Fractures. J. Trauma, **6**:469–480, 1966.

777. O'Donoghue, D. H.: Treatment of Injuries to Athletes, 2nd. ed. Philadelphia, W. B. Saunders, 1970.

778. Orava, S.; Weitz, H.; and Holopainen, O.: Osteochondritis Dissecans of the Patella (author's transl.). Z. Orthop., **117**:906–910, 1979.

779. Puddu, G., and Mariani, P.: Osteochondral Fractures of the Knee. Ital. J. Orthop. Traumatol., (Suppl.)**3**:128–137, 1977.

780. Rorabeck, C. H., and Bobechko, W. P.: Acute Dislocation of the Patella with Osteochondral Fracture: A Review of Eighteen Cases. J. Bone Joint Surg., **58B**:237–240, 1976.

781. Rosenberg, N. J.: Osteochondral Fractures of the Lateral Femoral Condyle. J. Bone Joint Surg., **46A**:1013–1026, 1964.

782. Smillie, I. S.: Injuries of the Knee Joint, 4th ed. Baltimore, Williams & Wilkins, 1971.

783. Specchiulli, F., and Florio, O.: Osteochondral Fracture of the Patella. Chir. Organi Mov., **52**:75–79, 1975.

Injuries of the Ligaments of the Knee

784. Abbott, L. C.; Saunders, J. B.; Bost, F. C.; and Anderson, C. E.: Injuries to the Ligaments of the Knee Joint. J. Bone Joint Surg., **26**:503–521, 1944.

785. American Medical Association: Standard Nomenclature of Athletic Injuries. Chicago, American Medical Association, 1966.

786. Andrews, J. R.: Clinical Diagnosis of Acute Ligament Injury. Presented at the A.A.O.S. Postgraduate Course, The Injured Knee in Sports. Special Reference to the Surgical Knee. Eugene, Oregon, July 23–25, 1973.

787. Andrews, J. R.: Chronic Ligamentous Instability of the Knee. II. A.A.O.S. Instructional Course Lectures. New Orleans, 1982.

788. Aritomi, H., and Yamamoto, M.: A Method of Arthroscopic Surgery. Clinical Evaluation of Synovectomy with the Electric Resectoscope and Removal of Loose Bodies in the Knee Joint. Orthop. Clin. North Am., **10**:565–584, 1979.

789. Arnold, J. A.; Coker, T. P.; Heaton, L. M.; Park, J. P.; and Harris, W. D.: Natural History of Anterior Cruciate Tears. Am. J. Sports Med., **7**:305–313, 1974.

790. Augustine, R. W.: Technic. *In* Speed, J. S., and Knight, R. H. (eds.): Campbell's Operative Orthopaedics, 3rd ed., Vol. 1. St. Louis, C. V. Mosby, 1956.

791. Barfod, B.: Posterior Cruciate Ligament—Reconstruction by Transposition of the Popliteal Tendon. Acta Orthop. Scand., **42**:438–439, 1971.

792. Bots, R. A., and Slooff, T. J.: Arthroscopy in the Evaluation of Operative Treatment of Osteochondrosis Dissecans. Orthop. Clin. North Am., **10**:685–696, 1979.

793. Brennan, J. J.: Avulsion Injuries of the Posterior Cruciate Ligaments. Clin. Orthop., **18**:157–162, 1960.

794. Broukhim, B.; Fox, J. M.; Blazina, M. E.; Pizzo, W. D.; and Hirsh, L.: The Synovial Shelf Syndrome. Clin. Orthop., **142**:135–138, 1979.

795. Camerlain, M.: Arthroscopy and Its Rheumatologic Perspectives. Union Med. Can. **103**:1262–1265, 1974.

796. Campbell's Operative Orthopaedics. Crenshaw, A. H. (ed.), 5th ed., Vol. 1, pp. 79–82. St. Louis, C. V. Mosby, 1971.

797. Campbell's Operative Orthopaedics. Crenshaw, A. H. (ed.) 5th ed., Vol. 1, pp. 927–931. St. Louis, C. V. Mosby, 1971.

798. Carruthers, C. C., and Kennedy, M.: Knee Arthroscopy: A Follow-up of Patients Initially Not Recommended for Further Surgery. Clin. Orthop., **147**:275–277, 1980.

799. Carson, R. W.: Arthroscopic Meniscectomy. Orthop. Clin. North. Am., **10**:619–627, 1979.

800. Carter, C., and Wilkinson, J.: Persistent Joint Laxity and Congenital Dislocation of the Hip. J. Bone Joint Surg., **46B**:40–45, 1964.

801. Casscells, S. W.: Arthroscopy of the Knee Joint. A Review of 150 Cases. J. Bone Joint Surg., **53A**:287–298, 1971.

802. Casscells, S. W.: The Arthroscope in the Diagnosis of Disorders of the Patellofemoral Joint. Clin. Orthop., **144**:45–50, 1979.

803. Casscells, S. W.: The Place of Arthroscopy in the Diagnosis and Treatment of Internal Derangement of the Knee: An Analysis of 1000 Cases. Clin. Orthop., **151**:135–142, 1980.

804. Cassidy, R. E., and Shaffer, A. J.: Repair of Peripheral Meniscus Tears. Am. J. Sports Med., **9**:209–214, 1981.

805. Chassaing, V.: Palliative Ligamentoplasty (Lemaire technique) for Rupture of the Anterior Cruciate Ligament. A Study of Forty-Four Cases. Orthop. Transactions, **4**:136–137, 1980.

806. Clayton, M. L., and Weir, G. L., Jr.: Experimental Investigation of Ligamentous Healing. Am. J. Surg., **98**:373–378, 1959.

807. Cohen, S. H.; Ehrlich, G. E.; Kauffman, M. S.; and Cope, C.: Thrombophlebitis following Knee Surgery. J. Bone Joint Surg., **55A**:106–112, 1973.

808. Dashefsky, J. R.: Arthroscopy of the Knee. NY State J. Med., **74**:1049–1053, 1974.

809. DeHaven, K. E.: Diagnosis of Acute Knee Injuries with Hemarthrosis. Am. J. Sports Med., **8**:9–14, 1980.

810. DeHaven, K. E.: The "sprained" Knee: Diagnosis and Early Management. Contemp. Orthop., **2**:286–288, 1980.

811. DeHaven, K. E., and Collins, H. R.: Role of Arthroscopy in the Diagnosis of Internal Derangements of the Knee. Presented at the American Orthopaedic Society for Sports Medicine. Dallas, Jan. 22, 1974.

812. DeHaven, K. E. and Collins, H. R.: Diagnosis of Internal Derangements of the Knees. The Role of Arthroscopy. J. Bone Joint Surg., **57A**:802–810, 1975.

813. Dehne, E.: The Spinal Adaptation Syndrome: A Theory Based on the Study of Sprains. Clin. Orthop., **5**:211–220, 1955.

814. Dehne, E., and Torp, R. P.: Treatment of Joint Injuries by Immediate Immobilization. Clin. Orthop., **77**:218–232, 1971.

815. Dorfmann, H.; Figueroa, M.; and Eze, S. D. D.: Value of Arthroscopy in Isolated Monoarthritis of the Knee. Sem. Hop. Paris, **50**:179–188, 1974.

816. DuToit, G. T.: Knee Joint Cruciate Substitution. The

Lindemann (Heidelberg) Operation. S. Afr. J. Surg., **5:**25–30, 1967.

817. Edgar, M. A., and Lowy, M.: Arthroscopy of the Knee: A Preliminary Review of Fifty Cases. Proc. R. Soc. Med., **66:**512–515, 1973.

818. Eilert, R. E., and Hamilton, W.: Arthroscopy and Treatment of Osteochondritis Dissecans of the Knee. Presented at the Meeting of the American Orthopaedic Society for Sports Medicine. Dallas, February, 1978.

819. Ellison, A. E.: Distal Iliotibial Band Transfer for Anterolateral Rotatory Instability of the Knee. J. Bone Joint Surg., **61A:**330–337, 1979.

820. Ellison, A. E.: The Pathogenesis and Treatment of Anterolateral Rotatory Instability. Clin. Orthop., **147:**51–55, 1980.

821. Feagin, J. A.; Abbott, H. G.; and Rokous, J. R.: The Isolated Tear of the Anterior Cruciate Ligament. J. Bone Joint Surg., **54A:**1340–1341, 1972.

822. Ficat, R. P.; Philippe, J.; and Hungerford, D. S.: Chondromalacia Patellae: A System of Classification. Clin. Orthop., **144:**55–62, 1979.

823. Fisher, R. C., and Winkler, L. H.: Arthrography and Arthroscopy in the Small Hospital. Surg. Clin. North. Am., **59:**483–493, 1979.

824. Fowler, P. J.: The Classification and Early Diagnosis of Knee Joint Instability. Clin. Orthop., **147:**15–21, 1980.

825. Franken, T.; Frommhold, H.; and Klemmer, H. L.: Xeroradiographic Examination of the Capsule and Ligaments of the Knee Joint. II. Demonstration of injuries to the cruciate and lateral ligaments and menisci (English Abst.). Fortschr. Geb. Roentgenstr. Nuklearmed., **4:**381–386, 1977.

826. Fujisawa, Y.; Masuhara, K.; and Shiomi, S.: The Effect of High Tibial Osteotomy on Osteoarthritis of the Knee. An Arthroscopic Study of 54 Knee Joints. Orthop. Clin. North Am., **10:**585–608, 1979.

827. Fullerton, L. R.; Protzman, R. W.; and Wincheski, J.: Arthroscopy Training. Am. J. Sports Med., **9:**38–39, 1981.

828. Funk, F. J.: Color Atlas of Arthroscopy. J. Sports Med., **1:**24–26, 1972.

829. Gallannaugh, S.: Arthroscopy of the Knee Joint. Br. Med. J., **3:**285–286, 1973.

830. Galway, R. D.; Beaupre, A.; and Macintosh, D. L.: Pivot Shift: A Clinical Sign of Symptomatic Anterior Cruciate Instability. J. Bone Joint Surg., **54B:**763–764, 1972.

831. Gilley, J. S.; Gelman, M. I.; Edson, D. M.; and Metcalf, R. W.: Chondral Fractures of the Knee. Arthrographic Arthroscopic, Clinical Manifestations. Radiology, **138:**51–54, 1981.

832. Gillies, H., and Seligson, D.: Precision in the Diagnosis of Meniscal Lesions: A Comparison of Clinical Evaluation, Arthrography, and Arthroscopy. J. Bone Joint Surg., **61A:**343–346, 1979.

833. Girgis, F. G.; Marshall, J. L.; and al Monajem, A. R. S.: The Cruciate Ligaments of the Knee Joint. Anatomical, Functional and Experimental Analysis. Clin. Orthop., **106:**216–231, 1975.

834. Glick, J. M.; Chafetz, N.; Mark, A. S.; Helms, C.; Cann, C. E.; and Genant, H. K.: Computed Tomography (CT

of the Menisci and Cruciate Ligaments. Presented at A.A.O.S. Annual Meeting. New Orleans, Jan. 23, 1982.

835. Goldfuss, A. J.; Morehouse, C. A.; and le Veau, B. F.: Effect of Muscular Tension on Knee Stability. Med Sci. Sports, **5:**267–271, 1973.

836. Groves, E. W. Hey: Technique. In Crenshaw, A. H. (ed.). Campbell's Operative Orthopaedics, 5th ed., Vol. 1, pp. 937–938. St. Louis, C. V. Mosby, 1971.

837. Guhl, J. F.: Operative Arthroscopy. Am. J. Sports Med., **7:**328–335, 1979.

838. Guhl, J. F.: Arthroscopic Treatment of Osteochondritis Dissecans: Preliminary Report. Orthop. Clin. North Am., **10:**617–683, 1979.

839. Haage, H., and Watenabe, M.: Arthrography and Arthroscopy. An Assessment of the Value of These Techniques (author's transl.). Z. Orthop., **111:**178–183, 1973.

840. Hallen, L. G., and Lindahl, D.: Rotation in the Knee-joint in Experimental Injury to the Ligaments. Acta Orthop. Scand., **36:**400–407, 1965.

841. Halperin, N.; Axer, A.; Hirschberg, E.; and Agasi, M.: Arthroscopy of the Knee under Local Anesthesia and Controlled Pressure Irrigation. Clin. Orthop., **134:**176–179, 1978.

842. Hardaker, W. T.; Whipple, T. L.; and Bassett, F. J.: Diagnosis and Treatment of the Plica Syndrome of the Knee. J. Bone Joint Surg., **62A:**221–225, 1980.

843. Hauser, E. D. W.: Extra-articular Repair for Ruptured Collateral and Cruciate Ligaments. Surg. Gynecol. Obstet., **84:**339–345, 1947.

844. Hawkins, R. J., and Kennedy, J. C.: Tension Studies of Knee Ligaments. Presented at American Orthopaedic Society for Sports Medicine. Dallas, Jan. 22, 1974.

845. Henche, H. R.: Arthroscopy of the Knee Joint. Beitr. Orthop. Traumatol., **24:**217–220, 1977.

846. Henry, A.: Arthroscopy of the Knee Joint. Guys Hosp. Rep., **121:**25–30, 1972.

847. Henry, A.: Arthroscopy in Practice. Br. Med. J., **1:**87–88, 1977.

848. Hernandez, V., and O'Connor, M.: Case Study: Arthroscopy for Internal Knee Derangement. O.N.A. J., **5:**25–27, 1978.

849. Hertel, E.: Possibilities and Limits of Arthroscopy of Rheumatic Joints. Z. Orthop., **113:**798–801, 1975.

850. Hertel, P., and Schweiberer, L.: Arthroscopy of the Knee Joint as a Diagnostic and Therapeutic Operation (author's transl.). Unfallheilkunde, **83:**233–240, 1980.

851. Hesse, W., and Hesse, I.: Arthroscopy of the Knee Joint. Med. Klin., **74:**1257–1263, 1979.

852. Huang, T. L.; Rieger, R. W.; Barmada, R.; and Ray, R. D.: Correlation of Arthroscopy with Other Diagnostic Modalities. Orthop. Clin. North Am., **10:**523–534, 1979.

853. Hughston, J. C.: Acute Knee Injuries in Athletes. Clin. Orthop., **23:**114–133, 1962.

854. Hughston, J. C.: Surgical Repair of Acute Ligamentous Tears of the Knee. Presented at A.A.O.S. Postgraduate Course, The Injured Knee in Sports. Special Reference to the Surgical Knee. Eugene, Oregon, July 23–25, 1973.

855. Hughston, J. C.; Andrews, J. R.; Cross, M. J.; and Moschi, A.: Classification of Knee Ligament Instabilities.

Part I. The Medial Compartment and Cruciate Ligaments. J. Bone Joint Surg., **58A:**159–172, 1976.

856. Hughston, J. C.; Andrews, J. R.; Cross, M. J.; and Moschi, A.: Classification of Knee Ligament Instabilities. Part II. The Lateral Compartment. J. Bone Joint Surg., **58A:**173–179, 1976.

857. Hughston, J. C., and Eilers, A. F.: The Role of the Posterior Oblique Ligament in Repairs of Acute Medial (Collateral) Ligament Tears of the Knee. J. Bone Joint Surg., **55A:**923–940, 1973.

858. Hughston, J. C., and Norwood, L. A.: The Posterolateral Drawer Test and External Recurvatum Test for Postero-lateral Rotatory Instability of the Knee. Clin. Orthop., **147:**82–87, 1980.

859. Imbert, J. C.; Bolze, O.; and Mouilleseaux, B.: Value of Arthroscopy for the Diagnosis and Treatment of Intra-articular Disorders of the Knee. Rev. Chir. Orthop., **62:**137–141, 1976.

860. Ireland, J.; Trickey, E. L.; and Stocker, D. J.: Arthroscopy and Arthrography of the Knee: A Critical Reveiw. J. Bone Joint Surg., **62B:**3–6, 1980.

861. Ireuchi, H.: Meniscus Surgery Using the Watanabe Arthroscope. Orthop. Clin. North Am., **10:**629–642, 1979.

862. Ivey, F. M.; Blazina, M. E.; Fox, J. M.; and Del Pizzo, W.: Arthroscopy of the Knee under General Anesthesia: An aid to the Determination of Ligamentous Instability. Am. J. Sports Med., **8:**235–238, 1980.

863. Jackson, R. W.: Arthroscopy of the Knee. Presented at the A.A.O.S. Postgraduate Course, The Injured Knee in Sports. Special Reference to the Surgical Knee. Eugene, Oregon, July 23–25, 1973.

864. Jackson, R. W.: Rehabilitation of the Injured and Post-operative Knee. Presented at A.A.O.S. Postgraduate Course, The Injured Knee in Sports. Special Reference to the Surgical Knee. Eugene, Oregon, July 23–25, 1973.

865. Jackson, R. W.: The Role of Arthroscopy in the Management of the Arthritic Knee. Clin. Orthop., **101:**28–35, 1974.

866. Jackson, R. W., and Abe, L.: The Role of Arthroscopy in the Management of Disorders of the Knee. An Analysis of 200 Consecutive Examinations. J. Bone and Joint Surg., **54B:**310–322, 1972.

867. Jackson, R. W., and Dandy, S. J.: Arthroscopy of the Knee, pp. 87–91. New York, Grune & Stratton, 1976.

868. Jackson, R. W., and DeHaven, K. E.: Arthroscopy of the Knee. Clin. Orthop., **107:**87–92, 1975.

869. James, S. L., and Brubaker, C. E.: Biomechanics of Running. Orthop. Clin. North Am., **4:**605–615, 1973.

870. Janecki, C. J., Jr.; Hill, O. H.; and Eubanks, R. G.: Arthroscopy of the Knee. Am. Fam. Physician, **17:**109–116, 1978.

871. Johnson, L. L.: Arthroscopy of the Knee Using Local Anesthesia: A Review of 400 Patients. J. Bone Joint Surg., **58A:**736, 1976.

872. Jones, K. G.: Reconstruction of the Anterior Cruciate Ligament. J. Bone Joint Surg., **45A:**925–932, 1963.

873. Kay, J. J., and Himmelfarb, E.: Knee Arthrography. Orthop. Clin. North Am., **10:**51–60, 1979.

874. Kellam, J. F.; Larson, R. L.; and James, S. L.: The Use of Ligament Augmentation Surgery in the Treatment of Acute Injuries of the Anterior Cruciate Ligament. Presented at American Orthopaedics Society for Sports Medicine, New Orleans, Jan. 19–21, 1982.

875. Kennedy, J. C.: Complete Dislocation of the Knee Joint. J. Bone Joint Surg., **45A:**889–904, 1963.

876. Kennedy, J. C.: Ligamentous Injuries in the Adolescent. *In* The Injured Adolescent Knee. Baltimore, Williams & Wilkins, 1979.

877. Kennedy, J. C., and Fowler, P. J.: Medial and Anterior Instability of the Knee. An Anatomic and Clinical Study Using Stress Machines. J. Bone Joint Surg., **53A:**1257–1270, 1971.

878. Kennedy, J. C., and Grainger, R. W.: The Posterior Cruciate Ligament. J. Trauma, **7:**367–377, 1967.

879. Kennedy, J. C.; Weinberg, H. W.; and Wilson, A. S.: The Anatomy and Function of the Anterior Cruciate Ligament. J. Bone Joint Surg., **56A:**223–237, 1974.

880. Kieser, C. R., and Uttmann, A.: Arthroscopy of the Knee Joint. Schweiz Med. Wochenschr., **106:**1631–1637, 1976.

881. Klein, W.; Schulitz, K. P.; and Huth, F.: Plica Disease (Synovial Folds) of the Knee Joint: Arthroscopic and Histological Findings, with Suggestions for Treatment (author's transl.). Dtsch. Med. Wochenschr., **104:**1261–1264, 1979.

882. Korn, M. W.; Spitzer, R. M.; and Robinson, K. E.: Correlations of Arthrography with Arthroscopy. Orthop. Clin. North Am., **10:**535–543, 1979.

883. Koshino, T.; Okamoto, R.; Takamura, K.; and Tsuchiya, K.: Arthroscopy in Spontaneous Osteonecrosis of the Knee. Orthop. Clin. North Am., **10:**609–618, 1979.

884. Kovesdi, J. M., Jr.: Arthroscopy of the Knee: An 18-Month Review. J. Am. Osteopath Assoc., **76:**186–188, 1976.

885. Kraus, M., and Charuzi, I.: Arthroscopy of the Knee. Harefuah, **91:**94–96, 1976.

886. Kreft, E.: Arthroscopy: Its Place in the Diagnosis of Knee Lesions (Abstract). J. Bone Joint Surg., **57B:**258, 1975.

887. Krempen, J. F.; Silver, R. A.; and Hadley, J.: The Use of a Peritoneal Catheter for the Irrigating System in Arthroscopy: A Better System for Accurate Diagnosis. Clin. Orthop., **128:**214–215, 1977.

888. Krockow, K. G., and Vetter, W. L.: Knee Motion in a Long Leg Cast. Am. J. Sports Med., **9:**233–239, 1981.

889. Lam, J. S.: Reconstruction of the Anterior Cruciate Ligament using the Jones Procedure and its Guy Hospital Modification. J. Bone Joint Surg., **50A:**1213–1224, 1968.

891. Larson, R. L.: Acute Disruptions around the Knee. *In* Straub, L. R.; and Wilson, P. D. (eds.): Clinical Trends in Orthopaedics. New York. Thieme-Stratton, 1982.

892. Lee, H. G.: Avulsion Fracture of the Tibial Attachments of the Crucial Ligaments. J. Bone Joint Surg., **19:**460–468, 1937.

893. Leslie, I. J., and Bentley, G.: Arthroscopy in the Diagnosis of Chondromalacia Patellae. Ann. Rheum. Dis., **37:**540–547, 1978.

894. Levinsohn, E. M., and Baker, B. E.: Prearthrotomy Diagnostic Evaluation of the Knee: Review of 100 Cases Diagnosed by Arthrography and Arthroscopy. A.J.R., **134:**107–111, 1980.

895. Liljedahl, S. O.; Lindevall, N.; and Wetterfors, J.: Early

Diagnosis and Treatment of Acute Ruptures of the Anterior Cruciate Ligament. J. Bone Joint Surg., **47A:**1503–1513, 1965.

896. Liljedahl, S. O.; Lindevall, N.; and Wetterfors, J.: Roentgen Diagnosis of Rupture of Anterior Cruciate Ligament. Acta Radiol., **4:**225–239, 1966.

897. Lipscomb, A. B.; Johnston, R. K.; and Snyder, R. B.: The Technique of Cruciate Reconstruction. Am. J. Sports Med., **9:**77–81, 1981.

898. Losee, R. E.; Johnson, T. R.; and Southwick, W. O.: Anterior Subluxation of the Lateral Tibial Plateau. A Diagnostic Test and Operative Repair. J. Bone Joint Surg., **60A:**1015–1030, 1978.

899. McDaniel, W. J.: Insulated Partial Tear of the Anterior Cruciate Ligament. Clin. Orthop., **115:**209–212, 1976.

900. McGinty, J. B., and Freedman, P. A.: Arthroscopy of the Knee. Clin. Orthop., **121:**173–180, 1975.

901. McGinty, J. B., and Matza, R. A.: Arthroscopy of the Knee. Evaluation of an Out-patient Procedure under Local Anesthesia. J. Bone Joint Surg., **60A:**787–789, 1978.

902. MacIntosh, D. L., and Darby, T. A.: Lateral Substitution Reconstruction (abst.). J. Bone Joint Surg., **58B:**142, 1976.

903. Magill, C. D.: Value of Knee Arthroscopy. Rocky Mt. Med. J., **74:**203–205, 1977.

904. Marone, P. J., and Cohen, D. L.: Arthroscopy of the Knee Joint. Pa. Med., **82:**29–31, 1979.

905. Marshall, J. L.: Periarticular Osteophytes. Initiation and Formation in the Knee of the Dog. Clin. Orthop., **62:**37–47, 1969.

906. Marshall, J. L.: A Diagnostic Aid in the Treatment of Ligamentous Injuries of the Knee. Paper presented at A.A.O.S., Postgraduate Course on Skiing Injuries. Snowman Resort, Colorado, March 6, 1974.

907. Marshall, J. L., and Olsson, S.: Instability of the Knee. A Long-term Experimental Study in Dogs. J. Bone Joint Surg., **53A:**1561–1570, 1971.

908. Matsui, N., Moriya, H., and Kitahara, H.: The Use of Arthroscopy for Follow-up in Knee Joint Surgery. Orthop. Clin. North Am., **10:**697–709, 1979.

909. Mennet, P.: Potential and Limits of Knee Arthroscopy. Schweiz Med. Wochenschr., **101:**1591, 1971.

910. Miller, A. F.: Arthroscopy of the Knee. Ariz. Med., **34:**553–556, 1977.

911. Minkoff, J.: Arthroscopy: Its Value and Problems. Orthop. Clin. North Am., **8:**683–706, 1977.

912. Minkoff, J.: The Philosophy and Application of Arthroscopy in Nonmeniscal Problems of the Knee. Orthop. Clin. North Am., **10:**37–50, 1979.

913. Mital, M. A., and Hayden, J.: Pain in the Knee in Children: The Medial Plica Shelf Syndrome. Orthop. Clin. North Am., **10:**713–722, 1979.

914. Mockwitz, J.; Tamm, J.; and Contzen, H.: Extended Diagnosis for Lesions of the Capsule and the Ligament of the Knee Joint (author's trans.). Unfallchirurgie **6:**94–100, 1980.

915. Moore, H. A., and Larson, R. L.: Posterior Cruciate Ligament Injuries. Results of Early Surgical Repair. Am. J. Sports Med., **8:**68–78, 1980.

916. Moriya, H.: The Use of Arthroscopy and Biopsy in the Diagnosis of Monarticular Chronic Arthritis of the Knee Joint. Ryumachi, **16:**12–34, 1976.

917. Nakajima, H.; Rundo, M., Kurosawa, H., and Fukubayashi, I.: Insufficiency of the Anterior Cruciate Ligament. Review of Our 118 Cases. Arch. Orthop. Trauma. Surg., **95:**233–240, 1979.

918. Nicholas, J. A.: Injuries to the Knee Ligaments. Relationship to Looseness and Tightness in Football Players. J.A.M.A., **212:**2236–2239, 1970.

919. Nicholas, J. A.: Correction of Lateral Instability—"Nicholas Method." Presented at A.A.O.S. Postgraduate Course, The Injured Knee in Sports. Special Reference to the Surgical Knee. Eugene, Oregon, July 23–25, 1973.

920. Nicholas, J. A.: The Five-one Reconstruction for Anteromedial Instability of the Knee. J. Bone Joint Surg., **55:**899–922, 1973.

921. Nicholas, J. A.; Freiberger, R. H.; and Killoran, P. H.: Double Contrast Arthrography of the Knee. Its Value in the Management of 225 Knee Derangements. J. Bone Joint Surg., **52A:**203–220, 1970.

922. Norwood, L. A.; Shields, C. L.; and Russo, J.; Kerlan, R. K.; Jobe, F.W.; Carter, V. S.; Blazina, M. E.; Lombardo, S. J.; and Del Pizzo, W.: Arthroscopy of the Lateral Meniscus in Knees with Normal Arthrograms. Am. J. Sports Med., **5:**271–274, 1977.

923. Novich, M. M.: Adduction Injury of the Knee with Rupture of the Common Peroneal Nerve. J. Bone Joint Surg., **42A:**1372–1376, 1960.

924. Noyes, F. R.; Bassett, R. W.; Grood, E. S.; and Butler, D. L.: Arthroscopy in Acute Traumatic Hemarthrosis of the Knee. Incidence of Anterior Cruciate Tears and Other Injuries. J. Bone Joint Surg., **62A:**687–694, 1980.

925. Noyes, F. R., Butler, D. L., Grood, E. S., Basse, H, R. W., and Hosea, T.: Clinical parodoxes of anterior cruciate instability and a new test to detect its instability. Ortho Trans., **2:**36, 1978.

926. Noyes, F. R.; DeLucas, J. L.; and Torvik, P. J.: Biomechanics of Anterior Cruciate Failure: An Analysis of Strain-rate Sensitivity and Mechanism of Failure in Primates. J. Bone Joint Surg., **56A:**236–253, 1974.

927. Noyes, F. R., and Sonstegard, D. A.: Biomechanical Function of the Pes Anserinus at the Knee and the Effect of its Transplantation. J. Bone Joint Surg., **55A:**1225–1241, 1973.

928. O'Connor, R. L.: The Arthroscope in the Management of Crystal-induced Synovitis of the Knee. J. Bone Joint Surg., **55A:**1443–1449, 1973.

929. O'Connor, R. L.: Arthroscopy in the diagnosis and treatment of acute ligament injuries of the knee. J. Bone Joint Surg., **56A:**333–337, 1974.

930. O'Connor, R. L.: Arthroscopy of the knee. Surg. Annu., **9:**265–289, 1977.

931. O'Donoghue, D. H.: Surgical Treatment of Fresh Injuries to the Major Ligaments of the Knee. J. Bone Joint Surg., **32A:**721–738, 1950.

932. O'Donoghue, D. H.: An Analysis of End Results of Surgical Treatment of Major Injuries to the Ligaments of the Knee. J. Bone Joint Surg., **37A:**1–13, 1955.

933. O'Donoghue, D. H.: Surgical treatment of injuries to the knee. Clin. Orthop., **18**:11–36, 1960.

934. O'Donoghue, D. H.: A Method of Replacement of the Anterior Cruciate Ligament of the Knee. J. Bone Joint Surg., **45A**:905–924, 1963.

935. O'Donoghue, D. H.; Frank, G. R.; Jeter, G. L.; Johnson, W.; Zeiders, J. W.; and Kenyon, R.: Repair and Reconstruction of the Anterior Cruciate Ligaments in Dogs. J. Bone Joint Surg., **53A**:710–718, 1971.

936. Oretorp, N., and Gillquist, J.: Transcutaneous Meniscectomy under Arthroscopic Control. Int. Orthop., **3**:19–25, 1979.

937. Oster, A.; Kaj, O.; and Hulgaard, J.: Operative Treatment of Rupture in the Medial Collateral Ligament of the Knee. Acta Orthop. Scand., **42**:439, 1971.

938. Palmer, I.: On the Injuries to the Ligaments of the Knee Joint. Acta Chir., (Suppl.) **81**:3–282, 1938.

939. Palmer, I.: Injuries to the Crucial Ligaments of the Knee Joint as a Surgical Problem. Reconstruct. Surg. Traumatol, **4**:181–196, 1957.

940. Parks, V. J.: Arthroscopy. Natl. News, Dec., **12**:8, 1975.

941. Park, V. J.: Arthroscopy. Nurs. Times, **71**:2058–2059, 1975.

942. Patel, D.: Arthroscopy of the Plicae—Synovial Folds and Their Significance. Am. J. Sports Med., **6**:217–225, 1978.

943. Paulos, L.; Noyes, F. R.; Girod, E.; and Butler, D. L.: Knee Rehabilitation after Anterior Cruciate Reconstruction and Repair. Am. J. Sports Med., **9**:140–149, 1981.

944. Pavlov, H.; Warren, R. F.; Cayea, P. D.; and Ghelman, B.: The Accuracy of the Arthroscopic Evaluation of the Anterior Cruciate Ligament. Presented at A.A.O.S. Annual Meeting. New Orleans, Jan. 21, 1982.

945. Pevey, J. K.: Outpatient Arthroscopy of the Knee under Local Anesthesia. Am. J. Sports Med., **6**:122–126, 1978.

946. Pickett, J. C., and Altizer, T. J.: Injuries of the Ligaments of the Knee. A Study of Types of Injury and Treatment in 129 Patients. Clin. Orthop., **76**:27–32, 1971.

947. Platt, H.: On the Peripheral Nerve Complications of Certain Fractures. J. Bone Joint Surg., **10**:403, 1928.

948. Poehling, G. G.: Arthroscopic Teaching Technics. South. Med. J., **71**:1067–1069, 1978.

949. Poehling, G. G.; Bassett, F. H.; and Goldner, J. L.: Arthroscopy: Its Role in Treating Non-traumatic and Traumatic Lesions of the Knee. South. Med. J., **70**:465–469, 1977.

950. Pokorn, Y. V., Bur, Y.; and Sek, P.: Our Experiences with Arthroscopy in the Diagnosis of Injured Menisci of the Knee Joint. Rozhl. Chir., **54**:108–115, 1975.

951. Rasmussen, F.: Arthroscopy of the Knee Joint. Ugeskr. Laeger. **137**:501–502, 1976.

952. Scheuer, I., and Rehn, J.: The Technique of Arthroscopy with Nitrous Oxide Insufflation (author's transl.). Unfallheilkunde, **81**:661–663, 1978.

953. Schonholtz, G. J.: Arthroscopy of the Knee Joint. South. Med. J., **69**:1493–1495, 1976.

954. Schreiber, S. N.: Diagnostic and Operative Arthroscopy of the Knee: An Analysis of 400 Consecutive Cases. Ariz. Med., **37**:265–272, 1980.

955. Schweitzer, G.: The Value of Arthroscopy of the Knee

956. See-Toh, C. W.: Arthroscopy—A Diagnostic Aid to Knee Injury. Ann. Acad. Med. (Singapore), **8**:67–72, 1979.

957. Slocum, D. B., and Larson, R. L.: Pes Anserinus Transplant. A Simple Surgical Procedure for Control of Rotary Instability of the Knee. J. Bone Joint Surg., **50A**:226–242, 1968.

958. Slocum, D. B., and Larson, R. L.: Rotary Instability of the Knee. Its Pathogenesis and a Clinical Test to Demonstrate its Presence. J. Bone Joint Surg., **50A**:211–225, 1968.

959. Slocum, D. B.; Larson, R. L.; and James, S. L.: Late Reconstruction Procedures used to Stabilize the Knee. Orthop. Clin. North Am., **4**:679–689, 1973.

960. Slocum, D. B.; Larson, R. L., and James, S. L.: Late Reconstruction of the Medial Compartment of the Knee. Clin. Orthop., **100**:23–55, 1974.

961. Slocum, D. B., Larson, R. L., and James, S. L.: Pes Anserine Transplant: Impressions after the Experience of a Decade. Am. J. Sports Med., **2**:123–136, 1974.

962. Smillie, I. S.: Injuries of the Knee Joint, 4th ed. Baltimore, Williams & Wilkins, 1971.

963. Solares, R.: Radiodiagnosis of the Rupture of the Meniscus of the Knee. Auxiliary Maneuver without Contrast Medium. Preliminary Report (author's transl.). Prensa Med. Mex., **40**:331–335, 1975.

964. Solonen, K. A., and Rokkanen, P.: Operative Treatment of Torn Ligaments in Injuries of the Knee Joint. Acta Orthop. Scand., **38**:67–80, 1967.

965. Starr, D. E.: Repair of Old Ligamentous Injuries of the Knee. Clin. Orthop., **23**:162–170, 1962.

966. Sutro, C. J.: Hypermobility of Bones due to "Overlengthened" Capsular and Ligamentous Tissues. A Cause for Recurrent Intra-articular Effusions. Surgery, **21**:67–76, 1947.

967. Taylor, M. D.; Shields, C. L., Jr.; Kerlan, R. K.; Jobe, F. W.; Carter, V. S.; and Lombardo, S. J.: Pes Anserinus Transplantation without Medial Meniscectomy: A Review of Twenty-two cases. Presented at Annual Meeting of Am. Orthop. Soc. Sports Med., San Francisco, Feb. 21, 1979.

968. Thomas, R. H.; Resnick, D.; Alazraki, N. P.; Daniel, D.; and Greenfield, R.: Compartmental Evaluation of Osteoarthritis of the Knee. A Comparative Study of Available Diagnostic Modalities. Radiology, **116**:585–594, 1975.

969. Tongue, J. R., and Larson, R. L.: Limited Arthrography in Acute Knee Injuries. Am. J. Sports Med., **8**:19–23, 1980.

970. Torg, J. S.; Conrad, W.; and Kalen, V.: Clinical Diagnosis of Anterior Cruciate Instability in the Athlete. Am. J. Sports Med., **4**:84–93, 1976.

971. Towne, L. C.; Blazina, M. D.; Marmor, L.; and Lawrence, J. F: Lateral Compartment Syndrome of the Knee. Clin. Orthop., **76**:160–168, 1971.

972. Trickey, E. L.: Rupture of the Posterior Cruciate Ligament of the Knee. J. Bone Joint Surg., **50B**:334–341, 1968.

973. Van Linge, B.: Diagnostic Problems in the Knee: Arthrog-

in the Management of Sports Injuries. S. Afr. Med. J., **59**:66–68, 1981.

raphy, Arthroscopy, or Both? Ned Tijdschr Geneeskd, **124**:507–508, 1980.

974. Van Rens, J. G.: Knee Arthroscopy. Ned. Tijdschr. Geneeskd., **119**:1943–1944, 1975.

975. Vignon, E.: Combe, B.; and Patricot, L. M.: Arthroscopic Study after Failure of Synoviorthesis (author's transl.). Nouv. Presse Med., **8**:1409–1412, 1979.

976. Wall, J. J.: Isolated Tears of the Anterior Cruciate Ligament. Presented at A.A.O.S. Annual Meeting. New Orleans, Jan 21–26, 1982.

977. Walsh, J. J., Jr.: Reconstruction of the Anterior Cruciate Ligament. Clin. Orthop., **89**:171–177, 1972.

978. Warren, L. F.; Marshall, J. L.; and Girgis, F.: The Prime Static Stabilizer of the Medial Side of the Knee. J. Bone Joint Surg., **56A**:665–674, 1974.

979. Whipple, T. L., and Bassett, F. H.: Arthroscopic Examination of the Knee. Polypuncture Technique with Percutaneous Intra-articular Manipulation. J. Bone Joint Surg., **60A**:444–453, 1978.

980. Whipple, T. L.; Wolbarsht, M. L.; Hickingbotham, D. W.; and Fondren, F.: Arthroscopic Surgery: Simple Devices to Facilitate Multiple Entries and Manipulations of the Knee. Clin. Orthop., **154**:331–335, 1981.

981. White, J.: The Results of Traction Injuries to the Common Peroneal Nerve. J. Bone Joint Surg., **50B**:346–350, 1968.

982. Wirtz, P. D.: Knee Arthroscopy. J. Iowa Med. Soc., **68**:447–448, 1978.

983. Wruhs, O.: Arthroscopy and Endophotography of Diagnosis and Documentation of Knee Joint Injuries. Wien Med. Wochenschr., **120**:126–133, 1970.

984. Wruhs, O.: Arthroscopy of the Knee Joint. Z. Orthop., **111**:664–665, 1973.

985. Wruhs, O.: Arthroscopy of Tibial-head Fractures. Hefte Unfallheilkd., **126**:234–236, 1975.

986. Wruhs, O.: Arthroscopic findings in antepositioning of the tibial tuberosity. Hefte Unfallheilkd., **127**:187–194, 1975.

987. Yates, D. B.: Arthroscopy of the Knee after the Injection of 90Y. Ann. Rheum. Dis., (Suppl.) **32**:48–50, 1973.

Meniscus Injuries

988. Aarstand, T.: Treatment of Meniscal Rupture of the Knee Joint. Acta Chir. Scand., **107**:146, 1954.

989. Abbott, L. C., and Carpenter, W. F.: Surgical Approaches to the Knee. J. Bone Joint Surg., **27**:277–310, 1945.

990. Ahlers, J., and M. Uller, W.: Simultaneous Meniscus Injuries in Tibial Head Fractures. Hefte Unfallheilkd., **126**:266–267, 1975.

991. Aichroth, P. M.: Osteochondral Fractures and Osteochondritis Dissecans. J. Bone Joint Surg., **59B**:108, 1977.

992. Anderson, P. W., and Maslin, P.: Tomography Applied to Knee Arthrography. Radiology, **110**:271–275, 1974.

993. Andrews, J. R.; Norwood, L. A.; and Cross, M. J.: The double bucket-handle tear of the medial meniscus. Am. J. Sports Med., **3**:232–236, 1975.

993a. Arnoczky, S. P., and Warren, R. F.: Microvasculature of the Human Meniscus. Am. J. Sports Med., **10**:90–95, 1982.

994. Appel, H.: Late Results after Meniscectomy in the Knee Joint. Acta Orthop. Scand., (Suppl.) **133**:1–111, 1970.

995. Aufdermaur, M.: Histological Examination of the Knee Joint Meniscus. Schweiz Med. Wochenschr. **101**:1441–1445, 1971.

996. Bailey, W. H., and Blundell, G. E.: An Unusual Abnormality Affecting both Knee Joints in a Child. J. Bone Joint Surg., **56A**:814–816, 1974.

997. Baird, M.: Double Contrast Arthrography of the Knee. Radiography, **46**:206–208, 1980.

998. Baryluk, M.; Oblonczek, G.; and Zolmowski, J.: Injury of the Semilunar Cartilages of the Knee Joint in Childhood (author's transl.). Arch. Orthop. Unfallchir., **87**:65–71, 1977.

999. Bednarski, W.; Krawczyk, E.; and Pilarek, M.: Levels of Various Blood Serum Glycoproteins in Coal Miners Operated on for Injuries of the Knee Meniscus. Chir. Narzadow Ruchu Ortop. Pol., **421**:377–381, 1977.

1000. Bir, O. T.; and Bihari-Varga, M.: Biochemical Investigation of the Knee Joint after Meniscus Injuries. Acta Chir. Acad. Sci. Hung., **14**:59–67, 1973.

1001. Bonnin, J. G.: *In* Platt, H. (ed.): Modern Trends in Orthopedics, Second Series. London, Butterworth's, 1956.

1002. Bramson, R. T., and Staple, T. W.: Double Contrast Knee Arthrography in Children. Am. J. Roentgenol. Rad. Ther. Nucl. Med., **123**:838–844, 1975.

1003. Brantigan, O. C., and Voshell, A. F.: The Mechanics of the Ligaments and Menisci of the Knee Joint. J. Bone Joint Surg., **23**:43–66, 1941.

1004. Brown, C. W.; Odom, J. A.; Messner, D. G.; and Mitchelfree, R. G.: A Simplified Operative Approach for the Lateral Meniscus. Am. J. Sports Med., **3**:265–269, 1975.

1005. Bruser, D. M.: A Direct Lateral Approach to the Lateral Compartment of the Knee Joint. J. Bone Joint Surg., **42B**:348–352, 1960.

1006. Brunner, C.: Meniscus Injuries in Child and Adolescent. Z. Unfallmed. Berufskr., **63**:96–100, 1970.

1007. Bryan, R. S.; Dickson, J. H.; and Taylor, W. F.: Recovery of the Knee following Meniscectomy. An Evaluation of Suction Drainage and Cast Immobilization. J. Bone Joint Surg., **51A**:973–978, 1969.

1008. Bullough, P. G.; Munuera, L.; Murphy, J.; and Weinstein, A. M.: The Strength of the Menisci of the Knee as it Relates to their Fine Structure. J. Bone Joint Surg., **52B**:564–570, 1970.

1009. Burgan, D. W.: Arthrographic Findings in the Meniscal Cysts. Radiology, **101**:579–581, 1971.

1010. Burri, C.: Meniscus Lesions. Z.F.A. (Stuttgart), **56**:2090–2100, 1980.

1011. Cabaud, H. E.; Rodkey, W. G.; and Fitzwater, J. E.: Medial Meniscus Repairs: An Experiment and Morphologic Study. Am. J. Sports Med., **9**:129–133, 1981.

1012. Cameron, H. U., and Macnab, I.: The Structure of the Meniscus of the Human Knee Joint. Clin. Orthop., **89**:215–220, 1972.

1013. Cargill, A. O'R., and Jackson, J. P.: Bucket-handle Tear of the Medial Meniscus. A Case for Conservative Surgery. J. Bone Joint Surg., **58A**:248–251, 1976.

1014. Casscells, S. W.: Torn or Degenerated Meniscus and its Relationship to Degeneration of the Weight-bearing Areas of the Femur and Tibia. Clin. Orthop., **132**:196–205, 1978.

1015. Cassidy, R. E., and Shaffer, A. J.: Repair of Peripheral Meniscus Tears. Am. J. Sports Med., **9**:209–214, 1981.

1016. Chandler, F. A.: Closed Drainage of the Knee Joint following Arthrotomy. J. Bone Joint Surg., **31A**:580–581, 1949.

1017. Claessens, S.; Stuyck, J.; and Martens, M.: Repeat Exploratory Arthrotomy of the Knee. Acta Orthop. Belg., **42**:183–186, 1976.

1018. Contzen, H.: Expert Testimony on Meniscus Lesions. Hefte Unfallheilkd., **128**:66–72, 1976.

1019. Cotta, H.: Childhood Lesions of the Meniscus. Hefte Unfallheilkd., **128**:59–65, 1976.

1020. Cotta, H.: Acute Traumatic Cartilage Damage. Experimental Studies and their Practical Consequences. Langenbecks Arch. Chir., **345**:415–422, 1977.

1021. Cox, J. S., and Cordell, L. D.: The Degenerative Effects of Medial Meniscus Tears in Dogs' Knees. Clin. Orthop., **125**:236–242, 1977.

1022. Cox, J. S.; Nye, C. E.; Schaefer, W. W.; and Woodstein, I. J.: The Degenerative Effects of Partial and Total Resection of the Medial Meniscus in Dogs' Knees. Clin. Orthop., **109**:178–183, 1975.

1023. Cullen, J. C.: Meniscectomy. NZ Med. J., **89**:138–140, 1979.

1024. Czipott, Z.: Pathogenesis of arthroses following meniscus surgery. Z. Orthop., **109**:82–94, 1971.

1025. Czipott, Z., and Herpai, S.: Electromyographic Studies in Meniscus, Knee and Ligament Injuries. Z. Orthop., **109**:758–778, 1971.

1026. Dalinka, M. K.: Lally, J. F.; and Gohel, V. K.: Arthrography of the Lateral Meniscus. Am. J. Roentgenol. Rad. Ther. Nucl. Med., **121**:79–85, 1974.

1027. Dandy, D. J.: Early Results of Closed Partial Meniscectomy. Br. Med. J., **1**:1099–1101, 1978.

1028. Dandy, D. J., and Jackson, R. W.: Meniscectomy and Chondromalacia of the Femoral Condyle. J. Bone Joint Surg., **57A**:1116–1119, 1975.

1029. Dashefsky, J. H.: Discoid Lateral Meniscus in Three Members of a Family. J. Bone Joint Surg., **53A**:1209–1210, 1971.

1030. DeHaven, K.: A Selective Approach to Meniscal Surgery. Presented to Annual Meeting of the Herodicus Society, Basin Harbor, Vermont, 1978.

1031. DeHaven, K. E., and Collins, H. R.: Diagnosis of Internal Derangements of the Knee. The Role of Arthroscopy. J. Bone Joint Surg., **57A**:802–810, 1975.

1032. Dem'lanov, V. M.; Ovchinnikov, I. U. I.; and Ior'Ev Ion.: Injury and Cyst of a Discoid Lateral Meniscus in the Knee Joint. Orthop. Travmatol. Protez., **33**:42–46, 1972.

1033. Despontin, J.: Treatment of Meniscal Lesions. Acta. Orthop. Belg., **42**:174–182, 1976.

1034. DiStefano, V. J.: Function, Post-traumatic Sequelae and Current Concepts of Management of Knee Meniscus Injuries. A Review Article. Clin. Orthop., **151**:143–146, 1980.

1035. Drugov, A. B.: Arthrography of the Knee. Possibilities—limits—perspectives. S. Lek., **74**:15–19, 1972.

1036. Duffin, D. A.: Knee Strength and Function following Meniscectomy. Physiotherapy, **63**:362–363, 1977.

1037. Durrschmidt, V. V., and Crasselt, C.: Role of Sport in the Pathogenesis of Meniscus Injuries. Beitr. Orthop. Traumatol., **20**:270–276, 1973.

1038. DuToit, G. T., and Enslin, T. B.: Analysis of 100 Consecutive Arthrotomies for Traumatic Internal Derangement of the Knee Joint. J. Bone Joint Surg., **27**:412–425, 1945.

1039. Dwight, R. D., and Loniewski, E. A.: Arthroscopy of the Knee: A Needed Adjunct to the Management of Meniscus Disease. J.A.O.A., **79**:179–185, 1979.

1040. Eckel, H.; Lindner, J.; Petzold, M. V.; Meyne, K.; and D. Orges, J.: The Significance of Arthrography and Arthroscopy in the Diagnosis of Meniscus Injury: A Comparative Study (author's transl.). Roentgenblaeter, **34**:43–50, 1981.

1041. Fairbank, H. A. T.: Internal Derangement of the Knee in Children and Adolescents. Proc. R. Soc. Med., **30**:427–432, 1936.

1042. Fairbank, T. J.: Knee Joint Changes after Meniscectomy. J. Bone Joint Surg., **30B**:664–670, 1948.

1043. Fisher, V.; Matzen, K.; and Bruns, H.: Arthroseauslosende Faktoren der Meniskektomie. Z. Orthop., **114**:735–737, 1976.

1044. Fowler, P. J., and Brock, R. M.: Meniscal Lesions in the Adolescent. Presented at the Annual Meeting of the American Academy of Orthopaedic Surgeons. Las Vegas, Nevada, February 1977.

1045. Fox, J. M.; Blazina, M. E.; and Carlson, G. J.: Multiphasic View of Medial Meniscectomy. Am. J. Sports Med., **7**:161–164, 1979.

1046. Frahm, W., and Rinke, W.: Value of Positive Contrast-media Arthrography in the Diagnosis of Meniscus Injuries. Zentralbl. Chir., **981**:1463–1467, 1973.

1047. Franchin, F.: Late Results of Meniscectomy Using Smillie's Technic. Chir. Organi Mov., **64**:51–57, 1978.

1048. Frankel, U. H.; Burstein, A. H.; and Brooks, D. B.: Biomechanics of Internal Derangement of the Knee. J. Bone Joint Surg., **53A**:946–962, 1971.

1049. Gear, M. W.: The Late Results of Meniscectomy. Br. J. Surg., **54**:270–272, 1967.

1050. Gillquist, J., and Hagberg, G.: Findings at Arthroscopy and Arthrography in Knee Injuries. Acta Orthop. Scand., **491**:398–402, 1978.

1051. Glinz, W.: Arthroscopy in Injuries Meniscus. Z. Unfallmed. Berufskr., **69**:106–115, 1976.

1052. Glinz, W.: Diagnostic Arthroscopy and Arthroscopic Surgery: Experiences with 500 Knee Arthroscopies. Helv. Chir. Acta, **46**:25–32, 1979.

1053. Grepl, J.: Suggestion for the New Method of Aimed Picturing of Knee Joint Arthrography (author's transl.). Cesk. Radiol., **28**:233–237, 1974.

1054. Gronert, H. J., and Stewin, J.: Potentials and Limits of Arthroscopy in the Diagnosis of Fresh Injuries of the Knee Joint (author's transl.). Unfallheilkunde, **83**:108–114, 1980.

1055. Grossman, R. B., and Nicholas, J. A.: Common Disorders of the Knee. Orthop. Clin. North Am., **8**:619–639, 1972.

1056. Gudushauri, O. N.; Gogoadze, D.; and Bukhaidze, Z. A.: Diagnosis and Surgical Treatment of Meniscus Injuries of the Knee Joint. Orthop. Travmatol. Protez., **7**:13–15, 1980.

1057. Guhl, J. F.: Operative Arthroscopy. Am. J. Sports Med., **7**:328–335, 1979.

1058. Gurin, J.: Evaluation of Operations on Discoid Meniscus. Magy. Traumatol. Orthop., **21**:44–46, 1978.

1059. Hall, F. M.: Arthrography of the Discoid Lateral Meniscus. Am. J. Roentgenol., **128**:993, 1977.

1060. Hall, F. M.: Further Pitfalls in Knee Arthrography. J. Can. Assoc. Radiol., **29**:179–184, 1978.

1061. Hanse, F. W.: Underside Lesions of the Meniscus. Acta Orthop. Scand., **49**:610–614, 1978.

1063. Heatley, F. W.: The meniscus—Can It Be Repaired? J. Bone Joint Surg., **62B**:397–402, 1980.

1064. Helfet, A. J.: Mechanism of Derangements of the Medial Semilunar Cartilage and their Management. J. Bone Joint Surg., **41B**:319–336, 1959.

1065. Helfet, A. J.: The Management of Internal Derangements of the Knee. Philadelphia, J. B. Lippincott, 1963.

1066. Hertel, P., and Schweiberer, L.: Diagnosis of Meniscus Lesions. Hefte Unfallheilkd., **128**:14–20, 1976.

1067. Hess, H.: Degenerative Meniscus Lesions in Occupational Soccer Players—An Occupational Disease? Z. Orthop., **113**:669–672, 1975.

1068. Hierholzer, G.: Therapy of Meniscus Injuries. Hefte Unfallheilkd., **128**:21–31, 1976.

1069. Hierholzer, G., and Ludolph, E.: Diagnosis of Ligamentous Injuries of the Knee Joint (author's transl.). Langenbecks Arch. Chir., **345**:445–449, 1977.

1070. Huckell, J. R.: Is Meniscectomy a Benign Procedure? A Long-term Follow-up Study. Can J. Surg., **8**:254–260, 1965.

1071. Hughston, J. C.: Acute Knee Injuries in Athletes. Clin. Orthop., **23**:114–133, 1962.

1072. Hughston, J. C.: Editorial comment. Am. J. Sports Med., **3**:269–270, 1975.

1073. Hughston, J. C.: A Simple Meniscectomy. Am. J. Sports Med., **3**:179–187, 1975.

1074. Iakovets, V. V.: Symptoms of Injuries of the Knee Joint Menisci in Contrast Arthrography. Orthop. Travmatol. Protez., **34**:25–29, 1973.

1075. Iseki, F., and Imai, N.: The Regenerated Meniscus with Special Reference to Functional Anatomy. In. Rev. Rheum., **33**:75–80, 1976.

1076. Iselin, M.: Is It Possible To Trust an X-ray Diagnosis: Meniscus Injury? Z. Unfallmed. Berufskr., **63**:90–95, 1970.

1077. Jackson, J. P.: Degenerative Changes in the Knee after Meniscectomy. Br. Med. J., **2**:525–527, 1968.

1078. Jackson, R. W.: Arthroscopy of the Knee. Presented at the A.A.O.S. Postgraduate Course, The Injured Knee in Sports. Special reference to the surgical knee. Eugene, Oregon, July 23–25, 1973.

1079. Jackson, R. W., and Dandy, D. J.: Partial Meniscectomy. J. Bone Joint Surg., **58B**:142, 1976.

1080. Jackson, R. W., and Rouse, D. W.: The Results of Partial Meniscectomy in Patients Over Forty. Presented at the American Association of Orthopaedic Surgeons Annual Meeting. New Orleans, Jan. 21–26, 1982.

1081. Johnson, L. L.: Diagnostic and Surgical Arthroscopy. St. Louis, C. V. Mosby, 1981.

1082. Johnson, R. J.; Kettlekamp, D. B.; Clark, W.; and Leaverton, P.: Factors Affecting Late Results after Meniscectomy. J. Bone Joint Surg., **56A**:719–728, 1974.

1083. Johnson, R. J., and Pop, M. H.: Functional Anatomy of the Meniscus, In A.A.O.S. Symposium on Reconstructive Surgery of the Knee, Rochester, N.Y., 1976. St. Louis, C. V. Mosby, 1978, p. 3.

1084. Jones, R. E., Smith, E. C., and Reisch, J. S.: Effects of Medial Meniscectomy in Patients Older than Forty Years. J. Bone Joint Surg., **60A**:783–786, 1978.

1085. Kaplan, E. B.: The Embryology of the Menisci of the Knee Joint. Bull. Hosp. Joint Dis., **16**:111, 1955.

1086. Karoyi, M.: Diagnosis of Meniscus Injuries by Arthrography in Acute Knee Joint Trauma. Ortop. Travmatol. Protez., **7**:20–23, 1980.

1087. Karpf, P. M., and Rupp, N.: The Clinical Importance of Arthrography after Lesions of the Meniscus and Capsular Ligament (author's transl.). Z. Orthop., **118**:73–84, 1980.

1088. Karumo, I.: Intensive Physical Therapy after Meniscectomy. Ann. Chir. Gynaecol., **66**:41–46, 1977.

1089. Karumo I.; Rehunen, S.; N. Averi, H.; and Alho, A.: Red and White Muscle Fibers in Meniscectomy Patients. Effects of Postoperative Physiotherapy. Ann. Chir. Gynaecol., **66**:164–169, 1977.

1090. Kasperek, M. G., and Kienzler, G.: The Treatment of Degeneration of Cartilage in Research and Practice (author's transl.). Z. Orthop., **112**:1256–1259, 1974.

1091. Kaye, J. J., and Friegerger, R. H.: Arthrography of the Knee. Clin. Orthop., **107**:73–80, 1976.

1092. Kempf, F. K.: Treatment of Meniscus Defects with Reference to Our Operative Method. Subtotal Meniscectomy, Resection of Hoffa's Corpus Adiposum, Inner Drainage. Arch. Orthop. Trauma. Surg., **96**:95–194, 1980.

1093. King, D.: The Function of the Semilunar Cartilages. J. Bone Joint Surg., **18**:1069–1076, 1936.

1094. Kingertz, H. G.: Arthrography of the Knee. I. Localization of Lesions. Acta Radiol. [Diagn.] (Stockh), **141**:138–144, 1973.

1095. Klimov, G. I.: Roentgen Diagnosis of Injuries to the Meniscus of the Knee Joint. Voen. Med. ZH., **12**:62–64, 1971.

1096. Klimov, G. I.: Diagnosis of Injuries of the Knee Joint Menisci with the Aid of Arthrography with Double Contrasting. Ortop. Travmatol. Protez., **35**:40–43, 1974.

1097. Klimov, G. I., and Dasaev, R. A.: Possibilities of the Roentgen Diagnosis in Experimental Injuries. Vestn. Khir., **111**:112–115, 1973.

1098. Kobayashi, A.: Diagnosis and Management of Knee Joint Meniscus Injuries. Nippon Seikeigeka Gakkai Zasshi, **53**:253–265, 1979.

1099. K. Onn, G., and R. Uther, M.: Pathological Anatomy and Assessment of Tibial Meniscus Lesion. Hefte Unfallheilkd., **128**:7–13, 1976.

1100. Krause, W.: Indications for Meniscectomy—Results of Surgery. Z. Allgemeinmed., **49**:1641–1643, 1973.

1101. Krause, W. R.; Pope, M. H.; Johnson, R. J.; and Wilder, D. G.: Mechanical Changes in the Knee after Meniscectomy. J. Bone Joint Surg., **58A:**599–604, 1976.

1102. Krawczyk, E.; Pilarek, M.; Bednarski, W.; Kochman, F.; and St. Epniewski: Blood serum proteins in patients with lesions of the knee joint meniscus. Chir. Narzadow Ruchu Ortop. Pol., **44:**537–541, 1979.

1103. Kunitsch, G.; Muhr, G.; and Oestern, J. H.: Significance of Arthrography in the Diagnosis of Meniscus Lesions (author's transl.). Arch. Orthop. Unfallchir., **79:**335–340, 1974.

1104. Kunitsch, G.; Oestern, H. J.; and Meyer, G.: Significance of Arthrography of the Knee Joint (author's transl.). Roentgenblaettier, **33:**48–56, 1980.

1105. Kurosawa, A; Fukubayashi, T.; and Nakajima, H.: Load-bearing Mode of the Knee Joint With or Without Menisci. Clin. Orthop., **149:**283–290, 1980.

1106. Kvist, E., and Kjaergaard, E.: Vascular Injury Complicating Meniscectomy. Report of a Case. Acta Chir. Scand., **145:**191–193, 1979.

1107. Laarmann, A.: Ganglia of the Meniscus of the Knee Joint and the Adjoining Tissue. Their Significance in the Evaluation of Occupational Meniscus Injuries. Arch. Orthop. Unfallchir., **67:**187–198, 1970.

1108. Laasonen, E. M., and Wilppula, E.: Why a Meniscectomy Fails. Acta Orthop. Scand., **47:**672–675, 1976.

1109. Laczay, A., and Csap, O. K.: The Vacuum Phenomenon in the Knee Joint (author's transl.). Roentgenblaetter, **27:**315–320, 1974.

1110. Lauttamus, L.; Haikara, J.; and Korkala, O.: Late Results of Meniscectomy of the Knee. A Follow-up Study of Patients. Ann. Chir. Gynaecol., **68:**169–171, 1979.

1111. Leach, R. E.; Stryker, W. S.; and Zohn, D. A.: A Comparative Study of Isometric and Isotonic Quadriceps Exercise Programs. J. Bone Joint Surg., **47A:**1421–1426, 1965.

1112. Lev, En H.: Evaluation of a Modified Method for Arthrography of the Knee. Acta Radiol. [Diagn.] (Stockh), **18:**351–356, 1977.

1113. Lewin, P.: The Knee and Related Structures. Philadelphia, Lea & Febiger, 1952.

1114. Lipscomb, P. R., and Henderson, M. S.: Internal Derangement of the Knee. J.A.M.A., **135:**827–830, 1947.

1115. Lotke, P. A.; Lefkoe, R. T.; and Ecker, M. L.: Late Results following Medial Meniscectomy in an Older Population. J. Bone Joint Surg., **63A:**115–119, 1981.

1116. Lutfi, A. M.: Morphological Changes in the Articular Cartilage after Meniscectomy. J. Bone Joint Surg., **57B:**525–528, 1975.

1117. Lysholm, J.; Gillquist, J.; and Lilhedahl, S. O.: Arthroscopy in the Early Diagnosis of Injuries to the Knee Joints. Acta Orthop. Scand., **52:**111–118, 1981.

1118. McGinty, J. B.: Arthroscopic Surgery in Sports Injuries. Orthop. Clin. North Am., **11:**787–799, 1980.

1119. McGinty, J. B.; Geuss, L. E.; and Marvin, R. A.: Partial or Total Meniscectomy: A Comparative Analysis. Orthop. Trans., **1:**81, 1977.

1120. McIntyre, J. L.: Arthrography of the Lateral Meniscus. Radiology, **105:**531–536, 1972.

1121. McMurty, R.: The Meniscus in Childhood. *In* Rang, M. (ed.): Children's Fractures, p. 186. Philadelphia, J. B. Lippincott, 1974.

1122. Man, W.; Birk, M.; and Bl. Umel, G.: Practical Application of Phonoarthrography in the Diagnosis of Knee Joint Disease (author's transl.). Z. Orthop., **118:**85–90, 1980.

1123. Masshoff, W., and Schultz-Ehrenburg, U.: Studies in the Nature of Meniscal Ganglia (author's transl.). Z. Orthop., **112:**369–382, 1974.

1124. Mayer, G.: Importance of Double-contrast Arthrography for the Diagnosis of Injuries of the Meniscus. Beitr. Orthop. Traumatol., **22:**394–397, 1975.

1125. Mazzarri, N. F., and Luiti, A.: Internal Knee Lesions and Medial Discoid Meniscus. Ital. J. Orthop. Traumatol., **1:**119–131, 1977.

1126. Medlar, R. C.; Mandiberg, J. J.; and Lyne, E. D.: Meniscectomies in Children. Am. J. Sports Med., **8:**87–92, 1980.

1127. Meier, W.: The Saphenous Nerve Syndrome in Differential Diagnosis of Tibia Meniscus Injury. Z. Unfallmed. Berufskr., **63:**129–132, 1970.

1129. Meittelmeier, H.: Meniscus Injuries. Z. Orthop., **111:**386–394, 1973.

1130. Mironova, Z. S.: Injuries of the Knee Joint Menisci. Khirurgiia (Mosk), **11:**124–128, 1975.

1131. Montgomery, C. E.: Synovial Recesses in Knee Arthrography. Am. J. Roentgenol. Rad. Ther. Nucl. Med., **121:**86–88, 1974.

1132. Muller, W.: Various Types of Meniscus Lesions and their Etiology. Hefte Unfallheilkd., **128:**39–50, 1976.

1133. Murdoch, G.: Errors of Diagnosis Revealed at Meniscectomy. J. Bone Joint Surg., **39B:**502–507, 1957.

1134. Murdoch, G.: Meniscus Removed in Error. Clin. Orthop., **18:**123–130, 1960.

1135. Navarre, L.: Cystic Degeneration of the External Meniscus. Acta Orthop. Belg., **42:**187–192, 1976.

1136. Neilsen, N. S.; Kristensen, O. K.; and Hansen, N. R.: Value of Arthrography of the Knee in the Diagnosis of Meniscal Lesions. Ugeskr. Laeger, **142:**2759–2760, 1980.

1137. Nemchak, A. L.: Instruments for Meniscectomy. Orthop. Travmatol. Protez., **11:**61–63, 1979.

1138. Nicholas, J. A.: Internal Derangement of the Knee: Diagnosis and Management. *In* A.A.O.S. Symposium on Sports Medicine, pp. 152–161. St. Louis, C. V. Mosby, 1969.

1139. Nicholas, J. A.: Injuries to the Menisci of the Knee. Orthop. Clin. North Am., **4:**647–664, 1973.

1140. Nicholas, J. A.; Frieberger, R. H.; and Killoran, P. J.: Double-contrast Arthrography of the Knee. Its Value in the Management of 225 Knee Derangements. J. Bone Joint Surg., **52A:**203–220, 1970.

1141. Niinikoski, J., and Einola, S.: Postoperative Synovial Fluid. Metabolic Response to Meniscectomy or Synovectomy. Acta Orthop. Scand., **48:**129–137, 1977.

1142. Norman, A., and Baker, N. D.: Spontaneous Osteonecrosis of the Knee and Medial Meniscal Tears. Radiology, **129:**653–656, 1978.

1143. Novikov, N. V.: Treatment Tactics in Fractures of the

Tibial Condyle Associated with Injuries to the Menisci. Orthop. Travmatol. Protez., **33**:17–21, 1972.

1144. O'Donoghue, D. H.: Discussion (of Tapper and Hoover [Ref. #1195]). J. Bone Joint Surg., **51A**:600, 1969.

1145. Oestern, H. J.; Murh, G.; and Kunitsch, G.: Significance of Roentgenological Studies in Post-traumatic Cartilage Injuries of the Knee Joint. Hefte Unfallheilkd., **126**:407–410, 1975.

1146. Olson, R. W.: Arthrography of the Knee. Presented at the A.A.O.S. Postgraduate Course, The Injured Knee in Sports. Special Reference to the Surgical Knee. Eugene, Oregon, July 23–25, 1973.

1147. O'Malley, B. P.: Value of Delayed Films in Knee Arthrography. J. Can. Assoc. Radiol., **25**:144–146, 1974.

1148. Oretorp, N.; Gillquist, J.; and Liljedahl, S.O.: Long-term Results of Surgery for Non-acute Anteromedial Rotary Instability of the Knee. Acta Orthop. Scand., **50**:329–336, 1979.

1149. Pallesen, J.: Results following Meniscus Lesions. Hefte Unfallheilkd., **128**:32–39, 1976.

1150. Parry, B. W.; Nichols, P. J.; and Lewis, N. R.: Meniscectomy, A Review of 1,723 Cases. Ann. Phys. Med., **4**:201–215, 1958.

1151. Pe Cina, M.; Kova, Cevi, C. D.; and Anti Cevi, C. D.: Diagnostic Possibilities of the Arthrography of the Knee in Meniscus Injuries (author's transl.). Lijec. Vjesn., **99**:678–682, 1977.

1152. Pizio, Z.; Chromik, D.; and Geiger, L.: Knee Joint Cartilage Injuries after Traumatic Rupture of the Semilunar Cartilage. Chir. Narzadow Ruchu Orthop. Pol., **45**:431–435, 1980.

1153. Podkuzhko, A. S.: Operative Treatment of Meniscus Injuries to the Knee Joint. Vestn. Khir. **117**:87–89, 1976.

1154. Pokorn, Y. V; Bur, Y.; and Sek, P.: Our Experiences with Arthroscopy in the Diagnosis of Injured Menisci of the Knee Joint. Rozhl. Chir., **54**:108–115, 1976.

1155. Powers, J. A.: Meniscectomies in Women. J.A.M.A., **208**:663–665, 1969.

1156. Price, C. T., and Allen, W. C.: Ligament Repair in the Knee with Preservation of the Meniscus. J. Bone Joint Surg., **60A**:61, 1978.

1157. Reichelt, A.: Clinical and Radiological Results after Cruciate Ligament Repairs Using the Meniscus (author's transl.). Arch. Orthop. Unfallchir., **88**:37–48, 1977.

1158. Ricklin, P.: Spatergebnisse Nach Meniskektomi. Hefte Unfallheilkd., **128**:51–58, 1976.

1159. Ricklin, P., and Fornaro, E.: Resultats Tardifs des Meniscectomies. Z. Unfallmed. Berufskr., **69**:121–216, 1976.

1160. Ricklin, P.; Ruttiman, A.; and del Buono, M. S.: Meniscus Lesions, Practical Problems of Clinical Diagnosis, Arthrography, and Therapy. New York, Grune & Stratton, 1971.

1161. Ringertz, H. G.: Arthrography of the Knee. II. Isolated and Combined Lesions. Acta Radiol. [Diagn.] (Stockh), **17**:235–248, 1976.

1162. Rondi, L., and Marty, A.: Zur Problematik der Spatfolgen nach Meniskektomie. Helv. Chir. Acta, **42**:489–492, 1975.

1163. Scheidegger, A.; K. Upfer, K.; and Stirnemann, H.: Late

Results in Nonoperated Patients with Suspected Meniscus Lesions. Helv. Chir. Acta, **42**:485–488, 1975.

1164. Schettler, G., and Ziai, A.: Injury to the Semilunar Cartilages of the Knee Joint in Childhood. Z. Orthop., **110**:443–449, 1972.

1165. Schilling, H.: Retrospective and Prospective Studies on Meniscus Surgery. Monatsschr. Unfallheilkd. **76**:549–554, 1973.

1166. Schilling, H.: The Meniscus from Embryonal and Functional Points of View (author's transl.). Munch. Med. Wochenschr., **117**:977–980, 1975.

1167. Schilling, H.: Is There a Relationship between the "Miner's Meniscus" and Patellar Chondropathy? Hefte Unfallheilkd., **129**:324–327, 1977.

1168. Schlonsky, J., and Eyring, E. J.: Lateral Meniscus Tears in Young Children. Clin. Orthop., **97**:117–118, 1973.

1169. Schneider, P. G.: Damage to the Meniscus in Professional Footballers. Munch. Med. Wochenschr., **117**:153–156, 1975.

1170. Schneider, P. G.: Meniscus Lesions in Occupational Soccer Players. Z. Orthop., **113**:666–668, 1975.

1171. Scholz, O., and Tauchmann, R.: Results and Experiences with Double-contrast Arthrography in the Diagnosis of Meniscus Damage. Zentralbl. Chir., **96**:1049–1053, 1971.

1172. Schramm, W.: Problems in Evaluation of Meniscus Injuries in Miners. Hefte Unfallheilkd., **121**:266–267, 1975.

1173. Schreiber, A.; Dexel, M.; and Dietschi, C.: Spatresultate nach Meniskektomie. Z. Unfallmed. Berufskr., **70**:63–70, 1977.

1174. Schulitz, K. P.: Meniscus Lesion in Childhood (author's transl.). Arch. Orthop. Unfallchir., **76**:195–204, 1973.

1175. Schulitz, K. P.; Geldh, and Auser, H.: Degenerative Changes in the Knee Joint following Removal of Discoid Semilunar Cartilages (author's transl.). Z. Orthop., **111**:127–134, 1973.

1176. Seedom, B. B.; Dowson, D.; and Wright, V.: Functions of Menisci. A Preliminary Study. J. Bone Joint Surg., **56B**:381–382, 1974.

1177. Shelukhin, N. I.: Causes of Unfavorable Outcome of Surgical Treatment of Injuries of the Menisci of the Knee Joint. Vestn. Khir., **115**:130–132, 1975.

1178. Shelukhin, N. I.: Diagnosis of Injuries of the Knee Joint Menisci. Vestn. Khir., **115**:104, 1975.

1179. Sichkaruk, I. A.; Gubenko, V. P.; Skrobonski, I. and Tikhumirov, D. N.: Military Medicine Expertise in Meniscus Injuries of the Knee Joints. Voen. Med. Zh., **1**:32–34, 1976.

1180. Simenach, B. I.: Pathology of the Menisci of the Knee Joint in Children and Adolescents. Ortop. Travmatol. Protez, **3**:55–60, 1976.

1181. Slocum, D. B.: Early Degenerative Arthritis following Meniscal or Ligamentous Injury. Presented as part of symposium, Early Degenerative Arthritis of the Knee, at A.A.O.S. Annual Meeting. New York, January 19, 1969.

1182. Slocum, D. B., and Larson, R. L.: Rotatory Instability of the Knee: Its Pathogenesis and a Clinical Test to Demonstrate its Presence. J. Bone Joint Surg., **50A**:211–225, 1968.

1183. Smillie, I. S.: Injuries of the Knee Joint, 1st ed. Edinburgh, London, E & S Livingston, 1946.

1184. Smillie, I. S.: The Congenital Discoid Meniscus. J. Bone Joint Surg., 30B:671–682, 1948.

1185. Smillie, I. S.: Injuries of the Knee Joint, 4th ed. Baltimore, Williams & Wilkins, 1971.

1186. Solares, R.: Radiodiagnosis of the Rupture of the Meniscus of the Knee, Auxiliary Maneuver without Contrast Medium. Preliminary Report (author's transl.). Prensa Med. Mex., 40:331–335, 1975.

1187. Sonne-Holm, S.; Fleelius, I.; and Ahn, N. C.: Results after Meniscectomy in 147 Athletes. Acta Orthop Scand., 51:303–309, 1980.

1188. Soustre, L.; Larroud, E. C.; Diard, F.; and Delurme, G.: Radiological Study of the Menisci in Injuries of the Knee. Bord. Med., 5:1411–1417, 1972.

1189. Stensir, O. M. A.; Hagstedt, B.; Hansson, L. I.; and Ljung, P.: Meniscectomy: A Comparison of Two Series Treated as Outpatients and Inpatients. Acta Orthop. Scand., 49:403–406, 1978.

1190. Stewart, J. P., and Erskine, C. A.: An Experimental Analysis of Injuries to the Menisci of the Knee Joint. Int. Orthop., 3:9–12, 1979.

1191. Stewart, M.: Traumatic Affections of Joints. In Crenshaw, A. H. (ed.): Campbell's Operative Orthopaedics, 5th ed., Vol. 1, pp. 907–908. St. Louis, C. V. Mosby, 1971.

1192. Stone, R. G.: Peripheral Detachment of the Menisci of the Knee. A Preliminary Report. Orthop. Clin. North Am., 10:643–658, 1979.

1193. Swito, N.: Contribution to the Theory on the Etiology and Treatment of Lesions of the Knee Joint Meniscus. Chir. Narzadow Ruchu Ortop. Pol., 44:543–546, 1979.

1194. Tagadiur, M. I., and Shalin, K. V.: Expertise in the Disability Evaluation of Military Construction Workers with Injuries of the Knee Joint Meniscus. Voen. Med. Zh., 4:63–64, 1972.

1195. Tapper, E. M., and Hoover, N. W.: Late Results after Meniscectomy. J. Bone Joint Surg., 51A:517–526, 1969.

1196. Tauber, C.; Heim, M.; Horoszowki, H.; and Farine, I.: Tear of the Anterior Cruciate Ligament as a Late Complication of Meniscectomy. Injury, 10:223–224, 1979.

1197. Thomsen, W.: Basic Principles for the Diagnosis of Meniscus Injuries. Z. Orthop., 111:394–396, 1973.

1198. Tokarowski, A.; and Bujarski, L.: Value of Electromyographic Examination of the Quadriceps Muscle in the Diagnosis of Lesions of the Medial Meniscus of the Knee Joint. Chir. Narzadow Ruchu Orthop. Pol., 40:309–314, 1975.

1199. T. Onnis, D.: Treatment of Semilunar Cartilage Injuries in the Aged. Hefte Unfallheilkd., 121:49–51, 1975.

1200. Vahvanen, V., and Aalto, K.: Meniscectomy in Children. Acta Orthop. Scand., 50:791–795, 1979.

1201. Van Gaver, P.; Delmotte, S.; and Mettewie: 236 Meniscectomies Performed at Discca, Brussels. Acta Orthop. Belg., 42:166–173, 1976.

1202. Veber, K. H.: Results of the Clinical Examination of Meniscus Injuries. Orthop. Travmatol. Protez., 7:12–13, 1979.

1203. Walker, P. S., and Erkman, M. J.: The Function of the Menisci of the Knee. J. Bone Joint Surg., 57A:1028, 1975.

1204. Watson-Jones, R.: Fractures and Joint Injuries, 4th ed. Baltimore, Williams & Wilkins, 1956.

1205. Weigand, H.; Rahmanzadeh, K.; and Sarvestani, M.: Late X-ray Observations on the Knee Joint following Meniscectomy. Hefte Unfallheilkd., 126:404–407, 1975.

1206. Wickstrom, K. T.; Spitzer, R. M.; and Olsson, H. E.: Roentgen Anatomy of the Posterior Horn of the Lateral Meniscus. Radiology, 116:617–619, 1975.

1207. Woxholi, G., and Westgaard, T.: Lateral Discoid Meniscus. Presentation of Roentgenologic Findings in 2 Patients. Tidsskr. Nor. Laegeforen., 93:1745–1747, 1973.

1208. Wrohs, O.: Arthroscopy and Endophotography for Diagnosis and Documentation of the Knee Joint Injuries. Wien Med. Wochenschr., 120:126–133, 1970.

1209. Yocum, L. A.; Kerlan, R. K.; Job, F. W.; Carter, V. S.; Shields, C. L.; Lombardo, S. J.; and Collins, H. R.: Isolated Lateral Meniscectomy: A Study of Twenty-six Patients with Isolated Tear. J. Bone Joint Surg., 61A:338, 1979.

1210. Zaman, M., Leonard, M. A.: Meniscectomy in Children. Injury, 12:425–428, 1980.

1211. Zejer, B., and Drozd, L.: Treatment of Injuries to the Shock-absorbing Mechanism of the Knee Joint. Pol. Przegl. Chir., 46:515–518, 1974.

17

Fractures of the Tibia and Fibula *Robert E. Leach*

The tibia is the most commonly fractured of all the long bones. Because a fracture of this bone usually appears uncomplicated and is generally inclined to do well, it is often relegated to the care of the junior physician on a fracture service. Yet, with the exception of intracapsular fractures of the femoral neck, no fracture arouses more controversy in regard to method of treatment than a tibial fracture. Although all treatment modes attempt to encourage early bony union and complete functional return, tibial fractures, because of their frequency and the number of postfracture complications, have become a major source of both temporary and permanent disability. This is particularly true of tibial fractures that are secondary to high-energy impact such as occurs in vehicular accidents.

The expected result after a tibial shaft fracture has changed radically in the past 40 years. Speed's *Textbook of Fractures and Dislocations,*[228] published in 1928, refers to a series of cases from St. Michael's Hospital in Toronto[228] in which 54 consecutive leg fractures resulted in four deaths, two amputations, six infections, seven delayed unions, and one non-union. Contrast these statistics with those reported by Weissman in a 1966 article.[250] In 140 consecutive adult tibial shaft fractures, there were no deaths, no amputations, no infections, 24 delayed unions, and one nonunion. The definition of *delayed* union, however, was based on the arbitrary time of 6 months. Only one of these delayed unions went on to nonunion. Of the 140 patients, 90% ultimately had normally functioning legs after their tibial shaft fractures.

Also in Speed's textbook, Singer and Norman reported on 231 open fractures of the tibia of which 21 became infected, 31 failed to unite, and 11 required amputation. In 1969, Brown and his colleagues[37] reported 63 open fractures of which only 4 had chronic drainage, all united, and none required amputation. Normal function resulted in 57 of the 63.

Wilson,[255] in his textbook published in 1938, referred to a nonunion rate of 20% in tibial fractures treated by skeletal traction, which was the treatment method of choice at Massachusetts General Hospital in that era. The contrast between the figures in older texts and those in more recent articles by Brown,[37] Sarmiento,[212] and Nicoll[187] is striking. In the past four decades movement has been away from the position of accepting a definite percentage of delayed unions and nonunions plus a number of infections and joint disabilities toward the position of demanding no nonunions or chronic infections and more than 90% functionally and cosmetically excellent results.

Because of the frequency of tibial and fibular shaft fractures, the literature in all languages is voluminous. The bibliography at the end of this chapter is almost exclusively limited to English-language publications on the theory that most significant advances or series on the subject will eventually make their way into the English-language literature or at least have been abstracted into English.

The methods of treatment advocated in the literature are as diverse as the literature itself. This chapter includes discussions of all generally accepted methods of treatment but not those that have become obviously archaic. During the past 20 years movement has been away from the operative methods of treatment that were popular in the 1940s and 1950s toward the nonoperative methods. This chapter places emphasis on the nonoperative methods of treatment, realizing that there is a definite role for operative treatment and internal fixation in certain tibial fractures. It also discusses the role of closed intramedullary nailing with Lottes[154] nails and Ender's nails.[191]

As with many operative procedures, the results are often better in the hands of the major proponents and practitioners of that particular operation. Although many publications attest to the value of rigid internal fixation in tibial fractures, there has been a definite rejection of many previous methods of fixation that now seem to provide only internal splinting and not the rigid fixation advocated by Müller and his co-workers,[183] Lottes,[153] and others.

Although this chapter deals with fractures of both the tibial and fibular shafts, virtually all the material is devoted to the tibia. Most fibular shaft fractures occur as the result of violence incurred with a tibial shaft injury. Fibular fractures that occur alone are relatively simple to treat. This is discussed at the end of the chapter, on page 1652. Fractures of the tibial plafond at the ankle will be discussed, but fractures around the knee (although technically they involve the upper tibial shaft) are included in Chapter 16 and are not discussed here.

SURGICAL ANATOMY

The anatomical position of the tibia, which makes it so vulnerable to injury, particularly by direct impact, also makes it relatively easy to approach surgically. The anterior medial surface and the anterior crest are covered only by skin and thin subcutaneous tissue. Any incision made to approach the tibia should be placed so as to have the majority of the incision over the muscles, which usually requires a long curved incision, starting anteriorly and then going posterolaterally and coming back to the anterior aspect. Less commonly, the tibia may be approached from the posteromedial aspect.

ANTERIOR COMPARTMENT

The anterior compartment of the leg contains the tibialis anterior, extensor digitorum longus, exten-

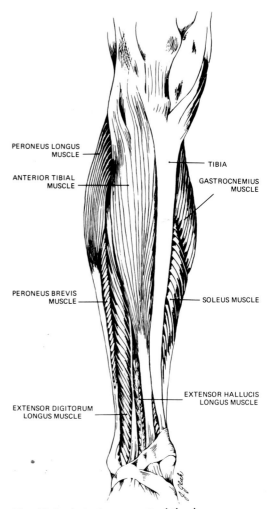

Fig. 17-1. Anterior aspect of the leg.

sor hallucis longus, and the peroneus tertius muscles (Fig. 17-1). They are enclosed in a relatively unyielding compartment made up of the tibia medially and the fibula laterally, the interosseous membrane posteriorly, and the tough anterior investing fascia, which goes from the tibia to the fibula anteriorly. This anterior compartment also contains the anterior tibial artery plus the deep peroneal nerve. Both the artery and the nerve run deep to the muscles, being normally protected from injury by them (Fig. 17-2). Near the ankle, the tendons of the tibialis anterior, extensor hallucis longus, and extensor digitorum longus are close to the tibia, and fractures in this area may cause callus formation that can partially restrict gliding of these tendons.

Because of the unyielding walls of the anterior

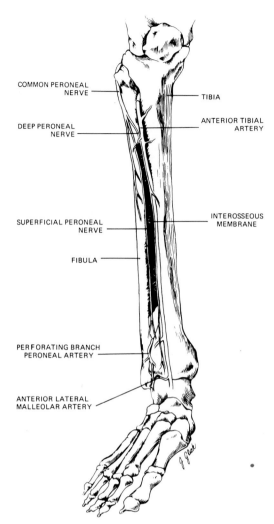

COMMON PERONEAL NERVE

TIBIA

DEEP PERONEAL NERVE

ANTERIOR TIBIAL ARTERY

SUPERFICIAL PERONEAL NERVE

INTEROSSEOUS MEMBRANE

FIBULA

PERFORATING BRANCH PERONEAL ARTERY

ANTERIOR LATERAL MALLEOLAR ARTERY

Fig. 17-2. The peroneal nerve and the anterior tibial artery lie deep to muscles.

compartment, increased tissue pressure there may give rise to the ischemic process called the anterior tibial compartment syndrome. This may occur secondary to tibial fractures or even as the result of prolonged exercise without a fracture. Decreased arterial oxygen supply causes muscle ischemia and, eventually, muscle necrosis. The peroneal nerve may be damaged directly by the intracompartmental pressure or by decreased blood supply to the nerve.

LATERAL COMPARTMENT

The peroneus brevis and peroneus longus muscles fill the lateral compartment. They protect the fibular shaft, except near the ankle, so isolated fractures

of the fibula owing to direct trauma are uncommon. The superficial peroneal nerve runs in the intermuscular septum between the peronei and the extensor digitorum longus. Thus the nerve is rarely involved in fractures of the fibular shaft, although it is at risk in a fracture of the fibular neck. Ischemic changes in the lateral compartment are uncommon and are more likely to be caused by a rigid compression dressing, such as a cast, than by external physical trauma.

POSTERIOR COMPARTMENT

The posterior compartment muscles include the soleus, gastrocnemius, tibialis posterior, flexor hallucis longus, and flexor digitorum longus. The posterior tibial nerve is isolated from the shaft of the tibia by the tibialis posterior and flexor digitorum longus. It is not likely to be injured directly in fractures of the tibia. The posterior tibial artery and its large branch, the peroneal artery, also run in the posterior compartment and are also protected by the same muscles, so that direct damage to them from a tibial fracture is uncommon (Fig. 17-3). The posterior tibial artery and nerve and the peroneal artery plus the deep muscles of the calf lie within a posterior compartment that is larger and more elastic than the anterior compartment. However, posterior muscle ischemia owing to increased pressure within the posterior compartment can result from a tibial fracture. The symptoms are usually less striking than those of the anterior compartment but may cause some clawing of the toes, which would be a late manifestation of a transient or partial ischemia of the posterior compartment muscles.[58]

BLOOD SUPPLY

The blood supply of the tibial shaft comes from the nutrient artery and the periosteal vessels. The nutrient artery of the tibia arises from the posterior tibial artery and enters the posterior lateral cortex of the bone at the origin of the soleus muscle, just below the oblique line of the tibia posteriorly. This artery divides into three ascending branches and only one main descending branch, which gives off smaller branches to the endosteal surface. The periosteum has an abundant blood supply from branches of the anterior tibial artery as it courses down the interosseous membrane. There is controversy as to which blood supply plays the larger role in fracture healing in the tibia.[160] Nelson[186] and others feel that the periosteal blood supply plays a relatively minor role in supplying the normal adult tibial cortex. They state that the intramedullary vascular supply is the most important. However, after injury that disrupts the intramedullary vascular pattern, the periosteal blood vessels increase their contribution and are prominent in the formation of new bone.

The anterior tibial artery may be subject to injury shortly after it takes off from the popliteal artery. At that point, it passes through a small hiatus in the upper portion of the interosseous membrane, toward the front of the leg on the anterior portion of the interosseous membrane. Physicians must realize that the peroneal artery in the posterior compartment has an anterior communicating branch to the dorsalis pedis and that the anterior tibial artery may be occluded even though there is still a palpable dorsalis pedis pulse from this communication.

ANTERIOR APPROACH

The most common approach to the tibia is anterolateral, because it is easily accessible, and the anterior compartment muscles can cover any internal fixation device or bone graft. Unfortunately, as a result of an open wound or secondary to previous operative procedures, skin and subcutaneous tissue in this area is often of poor quality or infected. Thus another incision may have to be employed. The anteromedial approach to the tibia is less popular than the anterolateral. The incision is made along the anteromedial aspect of the tibia, and dissection is carried between the soleus and the flexor digitorum longus and the posterior border of the tibia. This gives somewhat limited access to the tibia for open reduction, but it is satisfactory in cases of simple bone grafting.

POSTEROLATERAL APPROACH

A most useful approach to the tibia is the posterolateral one described by Harmon[120] and used effectively by both Jones,[135] and Hanson and Eppright.[117] Because the skin and subcutaneous tissue over the tibia are often involved by trauma, infection, or operative incisions, anterior incisions may prove risky or impossible. The posterolateral approach goes behind the fibula and the peroneal compartment muscles but in front of the posterior compartment muscles (Fig. 17-4). The patient must be positioned either on his side or at a 45° angle, so that the posterior aspect of the fibula is accessible. The incision is made along the posterior border of

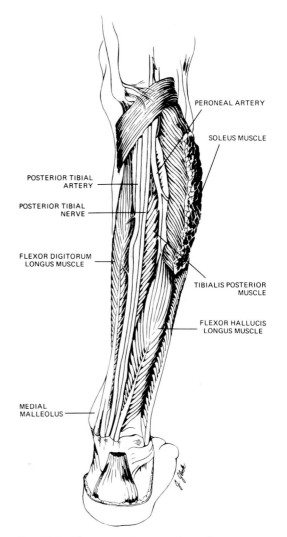

Fig. 17-3. The posterior vessels and nerve are protected by deep muscles.

PERONEAL ARTERY

SOLEUS MUSCLE

POSTERIOR TIBIAL ARTERY

POSTERIOR TIBIAL NERVE

FLEXOR DIGITORUM LONGUS MUSCLE

TIBIALIS POSTERIOR MUSCLE

FLEXOR HALLUCIS LONGUS MUSCLE

MEDIAL MALLEOLUS

the fibula and must be quite long, because the tissues tend to be tight. The surgeon needs superficial relaxation to be able to see deep into the leg, or else he finds himself working in a small, deep, V-shaped wound. After going through the superficial fascia, he must locate the plane between the peroneal muscles anteriorly and the flexor hallucis longus taking origin from the fibula posteriorly. There is a tendency to go between the flexor hallucis longus and the soleus muscle. This mistake can be easily recognized, because as the surgeon goes deeper into the leg he will find that the interosseous membrane and the tibia are covered by muscle. If the surgeon stays subperiosteally directly on the fibula, he dissects the flexor hallucis off the posterior

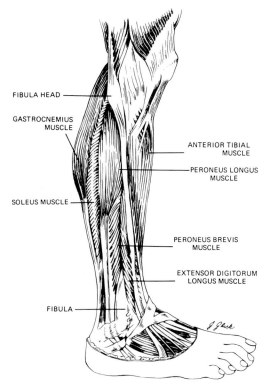

FIBULA HEAD

GASTROCNEMIUS
MUSCLE

ANTERIOR TIBIAL
MUSCLE

PERONEUS LONGUS
MUSCLE

SOLEUS MUSCLE

PERONEUS BREVIS
MUSCLE

EXTENSOR DIGITORUM
LONGUS MUSCLE

FIBULA

Fig. 17-4. A lateral view of the leg shows the plane between the lateral and posterior compartment muscles.

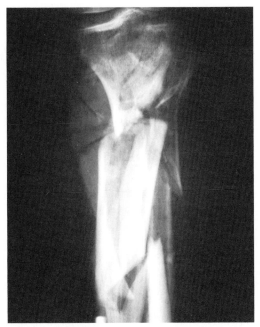

Fig. 17-5. This high-energy fracture was caused by a car accident. The anteroposterior view shows marked comminution.

surface of the fibula and the interosseous membrane. Dissection is then continued across the interosseous membrane onto the posterior surface of the tibia, where both the tibialis posterior and the flexor digitorum longus are taken off the tibia subperiosteally. The posterior tibial artery and nerve and the peroneal artery are all protected by the muscles so long as dissection is continued along the plane of the fibula, the interosseous membrane, and the posterior tibia.

Approaches to the fibula are simple. The incision is made over the subcutaneous lateral border. Either the anterior or posterior part of the fibula can be cleared by subperiosteal dissection. If need be, the middle segment of the fibula can be resected for bone graft or any other reason, because it functions only as a muscle attachment.

MECHANISMS OF INJURY

Tibial shaft fractures are caused by direct violence to the tibia, such as occurs in auto accidents and

gunshot wounds, or by indirect stress, such as ski injuries and falls with the foot fixed.

Direct violence accounts for an increasing number of tibial fractures. The exposed subcutaneous location of the tibia offers little protection against any direct blow, and the incidence of tibial fractures has increased with the use of automobiles and motorcycles and the frequency of criminal violence. Riding or walking, people are at great risk from motor vehicles. Hoaglund and States[127] found that these high-energy fractures had a worse prognosis than the low-energy group. High-energy and direct violence injuries cause more open wounds, more loss of skin, more soft tissue damage, and more bone displacement and comminution (Fig. 17-5). The fracture line is more likely transverse or comminuted, in contrast to the usual oblique or spiral fractures caused by indirect violence. Missile wounds from both war and civil strife cause tibial fractures. The higher-velocity missiles from military weapons and hunting rifles cause more soft tissue damage with the attendant poorer prognosis for that tibial fracture. The relatively low-velocity, lighter bullets of civilian life cause fewer problems.

Most indirect injuries result from recreational activities or falls within the normal course of life. The foot may be anchored while the person falls, and torque is applied to the leg. The foot itself may

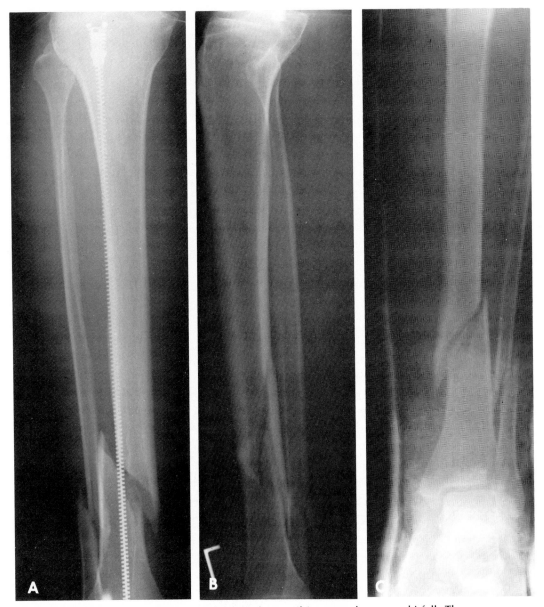

Fig. 17-6. (*A, B*) A low-energy fracture of the lower tibia secondary to a ski fall. The fracture line was oblique and there was no soft tissue wound. (*C*) Closed reduction produced adequate position with mild valgus deformity.

be twisted and force transmitted to the tibia in that fashion. This type of injury usually results in a longitudinal fracture line, either spiral or oblique, and the injuries are less severe than those caused by direct violence (Fig. 17-6).

Virtually all fibular shaft fractures result from the same injury that caused the tibial fracture. In those few cases in which only the fibula is fractured, it usually results from violence applied directly to the

fibula. A fibular shaft fracture concurrent with a tibial shaft injury implies that the tibial fracture is relatively severe. The less violence applied to the tibia, the less likely the fibula is to be fractured. The greater the force applied to the tibia, the greater will be the angulation and displacement, and the more likely the fibula is to be fractured.

Fractures involving the tibial shaft and tibial plafond are much less common than fractures of the shaft alone. They generally result from a fall from a height or, less commonly, from a blow on the anchored foot that drives the talus up into the tibial plafond. These fractures are associated with varying combinations of ankle fractures and tend to be comminuted.

CLASSIFICATION

Any classification of tibial fractures is useless unless it helps the surgeon choose a treatment method or helps to predict the prognosis. Many previous classifications have been of little use in achieving either of these aims. For instance, tibial fractures are often termed stable or unstable. This implies that certain fractures are difficult to reduce and to hold. Some surgeons seize on this classification as an excuse to open and fix internally a fracture that looks unstable to them. Yet, fractures that may be classified as unstable (such as a short, oblique, midshaft fracture) once reduced, usually maintain a functional, although not anatomical, position.

When classifying a fracture one should describe the precise anatomical location in the tibia, the pattern of the fracture line, and the position of the fragments and should note whether there is comminution and whether the wound is open or closed. These descriptive terms help the surgeon evaluate the injury and the prognosis, and this information is used to formulate a classification.

In the literature of the past 25 years, there have been many attempts to classify tibial fractures. Ellis[92,93,94] classified fractures into three basic groups: minor severity, moderate severity, and major severity. A minor severity fracture is a fracture that is undisplaced, not angulated, and has only a minor degree of comminution or a minor open wound (Fig. 17-7). Moderate severity is total displacement or angulation with a small degree of comminution or a minor open wound (Fig. 17-8). Finally, in an injury of major severity there is complete displacement of the fracture fragments with major comminution or a major open wound (Fig. 17-9). In the minor group, Ellis found that bony union took roughly 10 weeks, with a delayed union rate of only 2%. In fractures of moderate severity, union took approximately 15 weeks, with an 11% rate of delayed union. However, in the major fractures, healing took 23 weeks with a 60% rate of delayed union.

Weissman[250] based his classification of tibial fractures largely on the initial displacement of the fragments. He felt that this was an accurate indi-cation of the severity of the initial trauma and that the degree of initial angulation was of less importance. Although he agreed that both comminution and open wounds were important, he did not use them in his classification. In his system, minimal displacement was defined as being one fifth the width of the tibial shaft in the horizontal plane and was usually associated with slight angulation (10° or less). Mild displacement was one fifth to two fifths the width of the tibia with angulation of approximately 10° to 30°. Marked displacement occurred when there was more than 50° horizontal shift of the shaft of the tibia, and severe cases had total displacement with total loss of contact between the fragments.

Nicoll,[187] in a large study of tibial fractures, defined those characteristics of a fracture that seemed to have the most effect on the prognosis. These were degree of initial displacement, comminution, and soft tissue wounds. He then created an arbitrary range of three grades for each factor: nil or slight, moderate, and severe. Combining the three groups, he came up with a classification that made the outcome of any given fracture reasonably predictable.

Those fractures that had little or no displacement, no comminution, and no soft tissue wound had accelerated or normal union in over 90% of cases, and the delayed union or nonunion rate was about 9%. For fractures with severe displacement, severe comminution, and severe wounds, the incidence of accelerated and normal union fell below 70%, and the incidence of delayed and nonunion rose to the 30% to 55% range.

Although I believe that each of these classifications has something to recommend it, Ellis' classification is the easiest to work with. However, I believe that his minor and moderate severity groups could be modified. I would suggest that fractures with horizontal displacement of 0% to 50% be called minor fractures and those with more than 50% displacement be called moderate. In both instances for a fracture to be called minor or moderate, it would mean that there was only minor comminution or a minor open wound. Displaced fractures with a major open wound or comminution would go into the major severity group.

SIGNS AND SYMPTOMS

The signs and symptoms of a tibial or fibular shaft fracture depend primarily on the severity of the injury and the mechanism whereby it was pro-

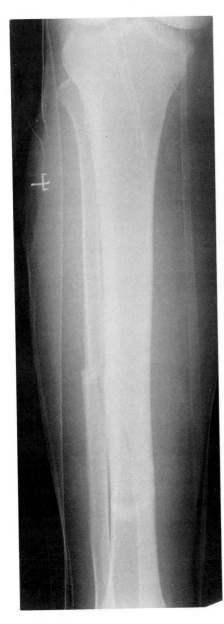

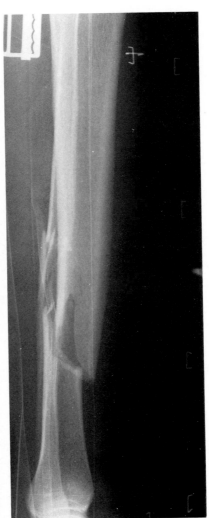

Fig. 17-7. This closed fracture of the lower third of the tibia shows minimal displacement and would be classified in the mild or minor category.

duced. The location of the fracture may also determine certain signs and symptoms. Obviously, an open, comminuted, displaced fracture of the lower tibia produced by a motorcycle accident will cause more pain and more signs than a closed, short oblique fracture of the midshaft produced by a skiing injury.

SYMPTOMS

The major symptom produced by either a tibial or fibular shaft fracture is pain. Pain associated with an isolated fibular shaft fracture produced by direct impact is relatively minor and might be thought by a spartan patient to be simply the result of a muscle contusion. On the contrary, the immediate pain produced by a tibial fracture, in almost all instances, will be severe and well localized to the site of the fracture. When the fracture is relatively stable with little displacement or soft tissue injury, pain may quickly subside after the initial onset, provided the fracture remains immobile. However, motion of the fracture fragments causes a marked increase in pain. Although the isolated fibular shaft fracture

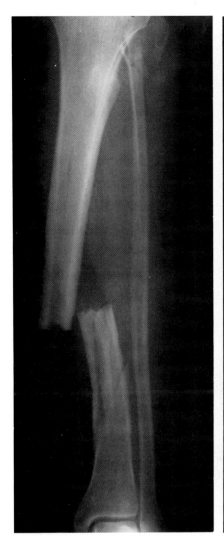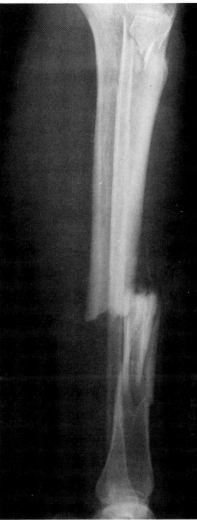

Fig. 17-8. This closed fracture had mild comminution but the fracture was totally displaced and would therefore be classified as moderate.

may not prevent walking, in almost all instances of a tibial shaft fracture, walking without adequate casting or splinting would be most difficult because of pain and lack of stability.

SIGNS

The most obvious sign in the usual tibial shaft fracture is deformity, which takes the form of angulation or rotation. With injuries produced by direct impact, particularly high-energy force, deformity is significant, and there can be any combination of angulation, displacement, rotation, or shortening, depending on the force and direction of the impact. In the common injuries produced by simple falls and twists, there is less deformity, commonly taking the form of external rotation and valgus angulation. Local swelling occurs quickly as

the result of bleeding and soft tissue reaction. An open fracture or soft tissue wound would be obvious; they usually result from direct vehicular violence to car passengers or pedestrians. A puncture wound produced by the fractured tibia penetrating the skin from the inside to the outside is common, and although technically an open wound, it usually does not have the poor prognosis of more severe open wounds. However, such a puncture wound does have the potential for secondary infection and must not be completely disregarded in the treatment of the fracture.

Tenderness, always present in tibial or fibular shaft fractures, is maximal over the anatomical site. Although mobility may be demonstrated in a tibial fracture, it is senseless to test this, because it causes the patient pain and may damage the soft tissues and increase deformity.

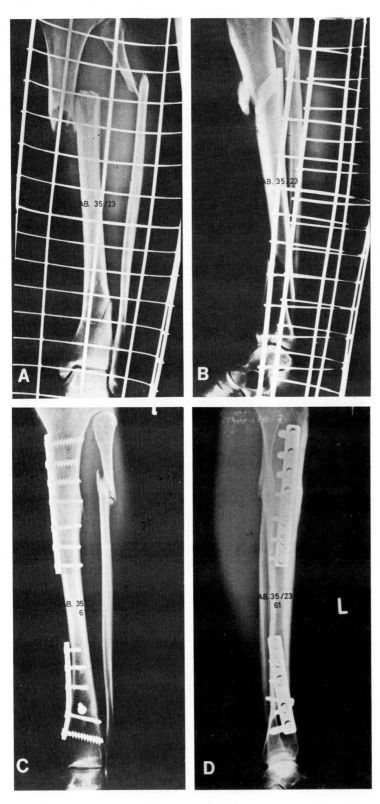

Fig. 17-9. (*A, B*) This markedly comminuted open fracture was totally displaced. The classification was severe. (*C, D*) It was treated by two compression plates and early immobilization. Solid bone union and excellent function occurred 6 months later. (Courtesy of Professor M. Allgöwer.)

Direct nerve damage is uncommon in tibial and fibular shaft fractures. A fibular neck fracture produced by direct impact or a fracture of the upper tibia and fibula, such as might occur from being hit by a car, can stretch or contuse the peroneal nerve. In all lower leg fractures, the examiner should check for dorsiflexion and plantar flexion of the toes and foot and sensation of the foot and leg. This picks up any early damage and establishes a baseline in case there are any future problems such as might occur from a tight cast compromising the peroneal nerve or producing an anterior or posterior tibial compartment syndrome. A compartment syndrome may result just from the fracture with the resultant soft tissue swelling.[78]

Damage to major blood vessels is unlikely to occur in the common shaft fracture. However, in a fracture of the upper tibia, where the anterior tibial artery passes through the interosseous membrane, there may be a laceration of the artery or pressure from an adjacent bony fragment. Another fracture that can damage vessels is that which involves the lower tibia. In all shaft fractures, one should check for both the dorsalis pedis and posterior tibial pulses. Other signs of circulation must be observed, such as capillary filling, muscle contractility, and sensation, and the pain pattern must be monitored carefully.

Soft tissue damage must be assessed carefully. The presence or absence of an open wound or potential areas of skin necrosis has important prognostic significance. Crush injuries have potentially severe effects on both the skin and soft tissue, and it may take several days to evaluate the extent of such damage. Injury to underlying muscles or tendons is uncommon except in open wounds, particularly those that involve the lower quarter of the tibia.

RADIOGRAPHIC FINDINGS

With any suspected tibial or fibular fracture, proper x-rays must be taken at two or more planes. Generally, in the acute stage the only films needed are anteroposterior and lateral views. Films must be of good quality, not only to see any obvious fracture line, but to see small linear cracks that could cause complications, particularly if open reduction is being considered. In later weeks, when healing is being evaluated and particularly when there is any question of delayed union or nonunion, oblique views must be taken as well as the obligatory anteroposterior and lateral films. Sometimes when a nonunion is being considered, tomograms may help.

Postreduction films should include both the knee and ankle joints on the same large plate, so that the treating physician can see that there is proper parallel alignment of these two joint surfaces. Obviously, x-rays must include the entire tibia and fibula to be sure there is not a low tibial fracture with a high fibular fracture.

FRACTURE DESCRIPTION

When describing the x-ray of a tibial or fibular shaft fracture, start with the location of the fracture: in the proximal, middle, or lower third. Then the fracture is classified as to the nature of the fracture line: transverse, oblique, or spiral. The presence or absence of comminution must be mentioned, and if it is a segmental fracture, this is noted. Angulation is measured on both the lateral and anteroposterior views. In the lateral view, angulation is measured in the direction of the apex of the fracture fragments; thus it is either posterior or anterior angulation. In the anteroposterior view, angulation is described by stating that the distal fragment is either in varus or valgus. Another way of describing valgus angulation is to say that the distal fragment is angulated with the apex medially. If the distal fragment were in varus position, it would indicate that the fragment is angulated with the apex pointing laterally. Angulation is always measured in degrees. Perhaps the most important measurement is the displacement of the fracture fragments. The displacement of the distal fragment is described in its relationship to the proximal fragment. For instance, the distal fragment may be displaced laterally 50% of the width of the shaft; this would mean that the two fragments have half their shafts in apposition. In another case, the distal fragment could be displaced laterally 100% of the width of the shaft. In that instance the fracture surfaces would not be in apposition. Displacement assumes a most important prognostic significance, because fractures that are displaced the total width of the shaft have a much poorer healing prognosis than those with less displacement. Shortening is noted on the x-ray, and the amount of overlap or distraction should be measured. Ellis[93] reported that distraction of as much as $\frac{1}{16}$ inch had to be noted and was important for the length of time for fracture healing. Rotation is difficult to judge on x-rays and must be measured clinically.

DIFFERENTIAL DIAGNOSIS

There are few entities likely to be confused with a routine traumatic fracture of either the tibia or the fibula. Nutrient foramina are not large enough to cause confusion, but a stress fracture of either bone may present difficulty. A stress fracture simply shows some periosteal reaction with perhaps a small radiolucent line at the site of the fracture. In young adults, this periosteal reaction may be quite marked, but in adults it may be insignificant. A stress fracture could be confused with a chronic, indolent infection or, in an adolescent, even with a bone sarcoma. However, the localized tenderness and the clinical course plus the findings on repeat x-rays should make the differentiation easy.

In evaluating any bone for a fracture, one looks carefully for an underlying lesion that might have been the cause of the break. Obviously, both benign and malignant bone lesions can be the cause of pathologic fractures. Osteoporosis, even in the younger person, may be a potential cause of fracture.

EPONYMS

Appellations that describe the location and characteristics of the fracture have taken the place of eponyms in tibial and fibular shaft fractures, and for this students and practitioners of orthopaedic surgery may be thankful.

METHODS OF TREATMENT

The basic principles of fracture treatment change little over the years, but application of these principles undergoes radical changes from generation to generation. Nowhere is this more evident than in the treatment of tibial shaft fractures. The primary aims of any orthopaedic surgeon treating this fracture are to place the fracture fragments into a functional and as near anatomical position as possible and then to maintain these fragments in that position until the natural body processes attain bony union. The methods by which the fracture fragments are reduced and held have changed almost from decade to decade. With regard to tibial fractures, there have been wide swings of opinion from the closed methods of the 1930s and 1940s to the use of open reduction more popular in the 1950s and early 1960s. This latter swing seems to have been replaced by a return to the nonoperative methods of treatment with occasional judicial use of open reduction in selected instances by experienced surgeons. Although not as popular as closed intramedullary rodding of the femur, closed nailing continues to be useful for certain acute fractures and in selected instances of nonunions of the tibia. Compression plates give excellent results in selected cases.

In fractures of both bones of the leg, the treatment of the fibular shaft fracture is the same as for the associated tibial shaft injury. The importance of the fibular fracture is that it is an indication of the potential stability or lack of it in the tibial fracture. With the fibula intact, there is generally less initial displacement of the tibia, and the prognosis is better. In instances in which both the tibia and the fibula are fractured and the fibula heals quickly, there is the possibility that the healed fibula may hold apart the tibial fracture and thus delay union of the tibia. Varus angulation may result with an intact fibula.[234]

ACCEPTABLE REDUCTION

Acceptable position implies that there is functional position of the tibial fracture, virtually normal rotation, minimal shortening, and minor angulation in both the anteroposterior and lateral planes. Although no displacement obviously offers the best chance for rapid osseous union plus perfect function and cosmesis, some degree of displacement can be tolerated. It is difficult to be precise in stating how much short of a perfect anatomical reduction may be accepted. Most authorities agree that rotation should be nearly perfect. If the other tibia is intact, the surgeon should check the healthy leg to see the precise amount of rotation present on that side. A line drawn from the anterosuperior iliac spine to the middle of the patella down to the foot shows the amount of rotation present on the normal side, and this should be attained on the fractured side. Generally, that line will fall between the first and second toes.

The ankle and knee joint surfaces should be parallel to each other to prevent maldistribution of weight-bearing stresses. Nicoll[188] stated that more than 10° of angulation in any plane was unacceptable. However, I believe the goal should be 5° of varus or valgus on the anteroposterior film and 10° of anterior or posterior angulation on the lateral film. Having stated that this is what the goal should be, more angulation in either plane may still give a functionally excellent result with only a minor cosmetic deformity. Some varus is cosmetically better than some valgus. The surgeon must always view the opposite extremity during reduction and casting to be sure he is matching the normal configuration of the uninjured side. Either anterior or posterior angulation will cause some shortening of the tibia, but anterior angulation is cosmetically more noticeable, and the patient may have to walk with the foot in slight equinus. The more precise the anatomical reduction, the better, but an allowable leeway must be taken into account, particularly when one is dealing with difficult tibial fractures having open wounds, loss of bony substance, or marked comminution.

How much displacement is acceptable? Tibial fractures may heal with the shaft 100% displaced and yet function well; cosmetically, there is often less noticeable deformity than one might anticipate. However, healing is obviously more rapid and delayed union or nonunion is much less of a possibility when there is little or no displacement of the shaft fragments. The surgeon should try to reduce the fragments to 100% apposition; yet 50% apposition in some severe fractures may be reasonable, provided that rotation, alignment, and angulation are acceptable. Some physiologic shortening of the tibia can be expected and is felt by most authorities to contribute to rapid healing of the fracture. In most instances this shortening should be no more than 5 mm to 7.5 mm. An attempt should be made to correct shortening of as much as 1 cm, but in some instances it may not be practical. In certain comminuted or open fractures or when there is a loss of bony substance, shortening may have to be allowed, and this may be advisable to obtain union. In routine tibial fractures an attempt should be made to limit shortening to 5 mm to 7.5 mm. No distraction of the fracture fragments should be allowed, because as little as 5 mm may increase the healing time of a tibial fracture to 8 to 12 months,[241] as opposed to the usual mean healing time of 4 months. Function and union must be the first consideration in determining what is an acceptable reduction. Guidelines can be given in textbooks such as this, but the final decision as to what is acceptable depends on the fracture that one is dealing with and, in some instances, other patient considerations.

CLOSED TREATMENT

Most tibial fractures can be handled by a closed reduction and application of a long leg cast. If the fracture is relatively undisplaced, classified as minor or moderate, the patient may need only sedation

and pain medication (given either intramuscularly or intravenously). The leg is then hung over the end of the table so that the weight of the leg provides traction.[202] Also by hanging the leg over the end of the table one can compare the involved leg to the normal leg for control of rotation and angulation. If needed, the operator can apply further traction and manually reduce the fracture. Once a satisfactory reduction is confirmed by visual inspection of the leg, a long-leg cast is applied. After careful padding with Webril or similar material, a well-molded cast is applied from the toes to the tibial tubercle as the leg is held in the reduced position. The rest of the cast is then applied across the knee to the high thigh region after the lower cast is hard. The foot should be in neutral position, except in some fractures of the lower tibia, when putting the foot in neutral may cause posterior angulation at the fracture site. In these fractures some equinus is acceptable for a period of 4 to 6 weeks. The cast is changed when the fracture is sticky, and the foot is brought back to neutral position.

Most of the older texts emphasize that the knee should be flexed anywhere from 20° to 45° to control rotation of the leg and maintain reduction. This flexion also helps to clear the foot for crutch walking. However, Böhler,[26] Dehne,[73] and others have shown that early weight bearing in a cast applied with the knee straight does not cause a reduction to be lost and does not increase the incidence of nonunion due to rotatory stress on the tibia. Flexing the knee does contribute to the patient's initial comfort by relaxing the pull of the gastrocnemius and preventing some rotatory stress, which may cause pain.

EARLY WEIGHT BEARING

Thirty years ago the routine treatment for an uncomplicated tibial fracture was a closed reduction followed by a long leg cast with the knee flexed, worn for approximately 10 weeks. During that time the patient would be on crutches, bearing no weight on the injured leg. If it were then felt that clinical union was progressing, a new long leg cast might have been applied with the knee in somewhat less flexion; the patient would be allowed partial weight bearing with crutches until the fracture was clinically and radiographically healed. Böhler,[26] and particularly Dehne[73] in the United States, popularized the early weight-bearing treatment method. For early weight bearing, the cast is applied with the knee straight, and the patient is encouraged to bear as much weight on the leg as desired. Usually from 10 to 16 days are required to bear a great deal of weight, but between the second and fourth weeks after fracture, many patients are bearing full weight. Position of the fracture is checked immediately after reduction and after 7 to 10 days. If the reduction is maintained, increased weight bearing is gradually encouraged. X-rays are taken at the end of the second week, when the cast is checked and the clinical position of the leg is noted. The cast must remain snug and must be changed if it loosens. Weight bearing continues until osseous union is clinically and radiographically present. Building up the opposite shoe helps the fractured leg to clear the ground, and a fracture boot provides a more effective means of bearing weight than a walking heel. The boot allows greater surface area to come into contact with the ground and prevents the pivoting action that may apply rotatory stress.

Early weight bearing seems to allow less muscle atrophy of the leg, and the pumping action of the muscles helps to reduce tissue edema. After cast removal the patient regains joint motion quickly and has a shorter postcast rehabilitation period. Bony union may be enhanced, because the incidence of nonunion with early weight bearing is low, as reported by Brown,[37] but the major effect of early weight bearing is on the soft tissues by helping to prevent the usual sequelae from trauma and immobilization.[75]

BELOW-KNEE CAST

Even more innovative has been the approach of Sarmiento,[209,212] who has pioneered the use of a total contact below-knee cast in tibial fractures. The cast is carefully molded around the tibial condyles and patella in the fashion of the patellar tendon–bearing prosthesis (Fig. 17-10). Sarmiento believes that careful molding decreases rotation of the tibia and may allow some body weight to be borne on the tibial condyles, but the majority of weight is borne by the compressed soft tissues in accordance with hydrostatic principles, because weight is borne on the heel and passed to the cast and compressed soft tissues. Sarmiento[211] generally reduces the fracture and applies a long leg cast for several weeks. Then, when the fracture is stable and the pain is decreased, he applies the total contact below-knee cast. Graduated weight bearing is allowed with crutches and finally full weight bearing with either a cane or no support.

In his first published series of patients with total contact below-knee casts, Sarmiento found that several ended with a centimeter or so of shortening,

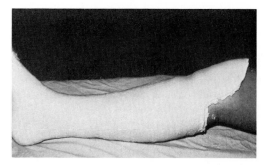

Fig. 17-10. Below-knee PTB cast. It is higher over the patella than Sarmiento recommends.

but angulation presented no problems. He had no nonunions, and if one accepts the definition of delayed union as union occurring at least 20 weeks after fracture, he had only 1 case in 100, which took 21 weeks to heal. His latest series[211] with an initial long leg cast followed by a below-knee cast has shown even less shortening and no loss of position. The major problem with this particular cast is that it must be meticulously applied— carefully molded over the tibial condyle, patellar tendon, and patella—and that no pressure is allowed in the popliteal area. It is not a cast for the casual bone setter. It has the advantage of allowing knee motion, which is particularly good for older patients. It also allows sitting more easily and provides ease of ambulation for patients with bilateral fractures. Early weight bearing in the short leg cast seems to decrease the rate of delayed union and nonunion, although no more effectively than early weight bearing in the long leg cast.

SHORT LEG BRACE

Sarmiento[210,211] has devised a short leg brace with a free ankle, which he applies after the tibial fracture appears on its way to clinical union, 4 to 8 weeks after the initial fracture. The fracture brace for tibial shaft fractures has not been as well accepted as a cast brace for femoral shaft fractures. Perhaps this is because patients do not seem to have as much trouble regaining ankle motion, or it may be that the techniques and materials to make the fracture brace cause more problems for the surgeon. With the use of early bracing in certain ankle fractures, there may be more use for the free ankle fracture brace in tibial fractures. Its best use appears to be for older patients, particularly those who have bilateral fractures and need mobility of both the knee and the ankle to ambulate.

DELBET GAITER CAST

Another protective device applied later in fracture healing is the Delbet[76] gaiter cast, which Weissman[250] stated he used routinely (Fig. 17-11). It allows knee and ankle motion while giving some protection to the fracture site. Its principal use is for the fracture that is clinically united but thought not strong enough to allow completely unprotected weight bearing.

CAST WEDGING

Wedging of casts seems to be a gradually diminishing art. Charnley,[52] Böhler,[26] and Watson-Jones[246] all have discussed wedging and have encouraged the practice. It seems that most doctors prefer to re-reduce the fracture and apply a new cast or to operate rather than to wedge a cast. If position of a tibial fracture proves unsatisfactory, the surgeon has the choice of wedging the cast, doing a new reduction and casting, employing another reduction technique, or performing open reduction. Anderson and Hutchins,[8] Dehne and his associates,[73] Brown and Urban,[37] and others use wedging to improve position. The technique must be done carefully, but in selected instances it is most helpful. Sometimes a reduction is difficult to hold, and when one sees that there is still angulation, particularly in one plane, an attempt at wedging may be performed more easily than a whole new reduction and cast.

How does one determine where to wedge the cast? Böhler[26] and Charnley[52] wedged at the intersection of the long axes of the two fragments. Watson-Jones wedged over the fracture itself. If the intersection of the long axes occurs at quite a distance from the fracture site, it may be best to wedge somewhat closer to the fracture. To determine the point of the fracture, x-rays are taken with several metal markers on the cast as reference points.

Böhler[26] advised using an opening wedge. The cast is cut on the concave side with the fulcrum on the convex side. The cast is wedged open and a small piece of wood or plaster is put in the opening on the concave side; then plaster is re-applied (Fig. 17-12). This technique is safer than a closing wedge, because the skin cannot be pinched, but it has the theoretical disadvantage of possible distraction at the fracture site. I prefer an opening wedge despite this theoretical disadvantage. With a closing wedge, an ellipse is cut out on the convex side and the two edges are brought together to close the wedge. This will not lead to distraction but may cause pressure on the skin and even some

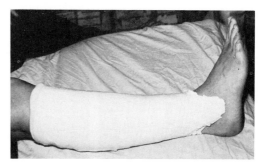

Fig. 17-11. The Delbet gaiter allows knee and ankle motion in patients with clinical union.

increased soft tissue pressure; consequently, it is more dangerous.

PINS ABOVE AND BELOW THE FRACTURE

With an unsatisfactory closed reduction, the surgeon must consider rereduction, wedging, or another method of treatment. Some fractures classified as moderate or severe may respond well to the use of Steinmann pins placed above and below the fracture and a below-knee plaster incorporating these pins.[8,9,26,132] I do not know to whom credit should be given for first using this technique. Böhler[26] described it years ago, and an external fixation apparatus using pins above and below was popularized by both Roger Anderson[10] and Stader.[219] Lewis Anderson and his colleagues[9] and Hughston[132] have reported separate series of patients and have outlined the technique of using pins above and below plus plaster.

Under spinal or general anesthetic in sterile conditions, two smooth Steinmann pins $\frac{3}{32}$ inch to $\frac{1}{8}$ inch in diameter are drilled across the proximal tibia, well above the fracture site. One is directly below the level of the tibial tubercle and the other, 25 mm to 40 mm more distal, avoiding the fracture site. Two other pins are placed in the lower third of the tibia, below the fracture, being careful not to impale any of the structures in the anterior tibial compartment that run close to the tibia in its distal third (Fig. 17-13). With the pins in place, the fracture fragments can be manipulated by an operator with the patient's leg hanging over the table. The complete relaxation provided by anesthetic plus the ability to grip the lower pin firmly provides adequate traction to align the fracture fragments. A traction bow may be put on the lower pin to apply traction. After reduction, the cast is applied from the toes to the tibial tubercle in the usual

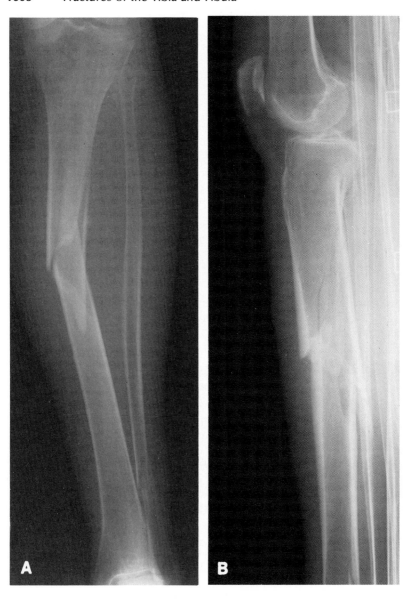

Fig. 17-12. (A, B) A midshift tibial fracture. The classification was mild.

fashion, with the pins firmly incorporated in plaster (Fig. 17-14). After the lower cast hardens, a long leg cast may be continued onto the thigh if needed, but a short leg cast is usually sufficient. Two pins are used, because a single pin would allow rotation of the fragment, particularly the proximal, which could cause pressure necrosis of the anterior skin and possible loss of position. The pins are left in place for 4 to 6 weeks, usually until the fracture has become sticky. Pin tract infections have been only a minor problem. The aftercare with pins above and below varies. Anderson[9] states that he removes the pins at approximately 6 weeks, and

his patients then start weight bearing in a long leg plaster cast. In his first article the pins were left in longer and weight bearing was subsequently more delayed.[8] Other authors have advocated the use of weight bearing with pins in place and have started patients walking several weeks after the initial fracture. Because it is not the mild type of fractures that are handled in this manner but usually those with significant displacement and often with extensive soft tissue wounds, the patients are probably served best by not walking immediately but allowing some time for soft tissue healing (Fig. 17-15). Perhaps at the end of the fourth week partial weight

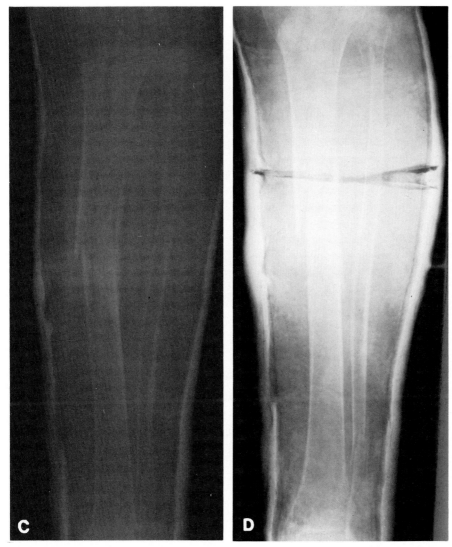

Fig. 17-12 (*Continued*). (*C*) After casting there was 14° of valgus angulation. (*D*) An opening wedge on the lateral side corrected angulation.

bearing would not be harmful, even with the pins in place, although I now usually remove them by that time.

EXTERNAL FIXATION TECHNIQUE

The use of pins-in-plaster has become less common as the use of external fixation devices has increased.[85,86,98,138] Despite the early popularity of the Roger Anderson apparatus and the Stader splint, both of these fell out of favor by the 1950s. However, there has been a return to the use of external fixation devices with excellent results in certain types of fractures and wounds. The fixation devices presently available give more rigid bone fixation, and with good skin care, pin tract infections have not been a major problem (Fig. 17-16). One must be careful drilling the pins into the bone. The use of high-speed drills is condemned, because they may cause segmental necrosis of a portion of the tibial cortex, with subsequent sequestration and infection. Bonnel pins, which are threaded in the middle, help to hold the bone securely and prevent loosening.

An external fixation device seems to be most useful in instances involving severe soft tissue

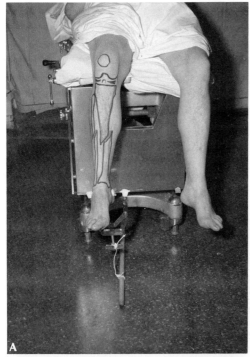

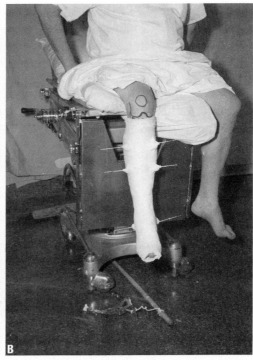

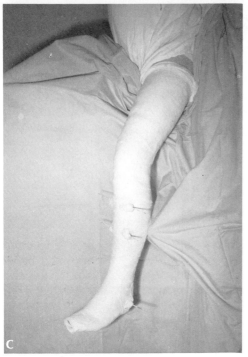

Fig. 17-13. (*A*) A patient's leg over the end of a table with an os calcis pin in place. A lower tibia pin gives better control. (*B*) Two pins were placed above the fracture and one below with the below-knee portion of the cast applied. (*C*) The finished long leg cast with pins in place. (Courtesy of T. B. Quigley, Jr.)

wounds. The external fixator gives bony stabilization while allowing for the easy access and care of the soft tissues. This method is particularly applicable in instances that involve circumferential wounds, such as degloving injuries or burns. The apparatus is also useful when there has been loss of bone substance. With the application of rigid fixation, length may be gained and maintained

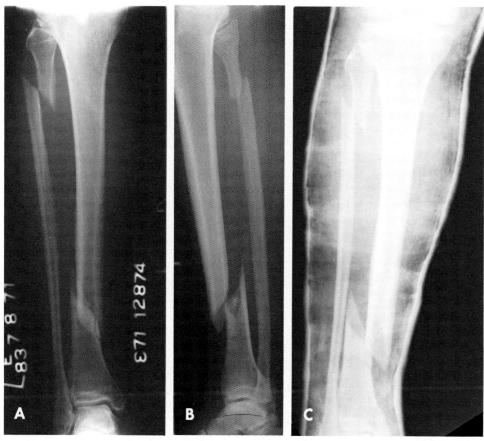

Fig. 17-14. (*A, B*) This fracture of the lower tibia was moderately displaced. (*C, D*) Attempted closed reduction resulted in poor position. (*continued on next page*)

while allowing soft tissue healing. A later bone graft may allow bony union without the loss of tibial length. Other advantages of the external fixation device include knee and ankle motion. The patient may even be ambulatory with the fixation apparatus in place. I do not usually allow patients to be weight bearing in the apparatus.

A variety of external fixation devices are available, and each surgeon should learn how to use one. Some refinements of the newer fixation devices include more pins for fixation and the possibility of reducing the fracture by manipulation of the external fixation apparatus. A major worry with pins-in-plaster or the external fixation devices is that if distraction is produced, delayed union or nonunion may ensue. One must be careful with the use of these devices not to allow distraction. The external fixation device is used long enough to allow soft tissue care or until early bony union has been achieved. When there is loss of bony substance, one may have a major problem in

determining when the fixation apparatus should be taken out to prevent bony collapse.

For more details about the use of external fixators, see Chapter 1.

TRACTION

The use of external fixation devices has almost replaced the low tibial or os calcis traction to treat tibial fractures. It is, however, still a method that can be used in particular instances, such as in massive soft tissue injuries, where the surgeon prefers not to use an external fixation apparatus. Patients with tibial fractures may be treated in traction with the leg in a Thomas splint or Böhler frame. A posterior plaster slab going from the toes up past the knee makes the patient more comfortable. Usually 7 to 10 pounds of weight are required to align the fracture. X-rays are taken after 24 hours and necessary adjustments are made then. When the fracture is reduced, traction weight is decreased to 5 or 6 pounds to prevent distraction

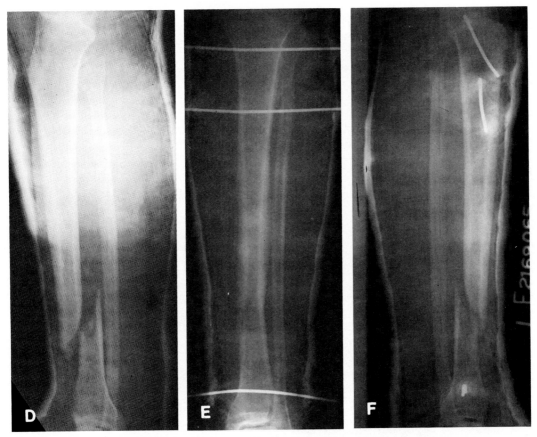

Fig. 17-14. *(Continued).* *(E, F)* Pins above and below secured and held adequate reduction.

at the fracture site. At 3 weeks, with the fracture more stable, the leg can be placed in a long leg cast.

Traction could be used temporarily in a patient who has an anterior compartment syndrome resulting from a tibial shaft fracture (Fig. 17-17). It may also be used in tibial plafond fractures where fixation is not secure but early motion is desired.

IPSILATERAL FEMORAL AND TIBIAL FRACTURES

A particularly difficult problem is the combination of ipsilateral femoral and tibial fractures.[103] The femoral fracture can usually be treated either by intramedullary fixation or by traction followed by a cast brace. In most instances it is preferable to use intramedullary fixation, particularly closed intramedullary nailing. The reason for internally fixing the femur is to allow the option of getting the patient out of bed as soon as possible. Then

the only worry is his tibial injury plus the other bodily injuries suffered by patients with such fractures who are often the victims of multiple trauma.

A number of options are available for treating the tibial fracture. The aim is to make the patient ambulatory as quickly as possible, and therapy should be directed toward this aim while doing nothing to retard fracture healing. If the tibial fracture is amenable to closed intramedullary nailing, this is one possibility that allows the patient to start early weight bearing. Frequently, the tibial fracture can be treated with a long leg cast, later progressing to a total contact below-knee cast, which will allow early ambulation, particularly if the femur has already been fixed.

If, for some reason, internal fixation of the femur is not feasible, an alternate method of treatment is to apply an external fixation device with Steinmann pins to the tibia and apply traction to the uppermost tibial pin for the femur. This method is particularly attractive when there are major soft tissue wounds

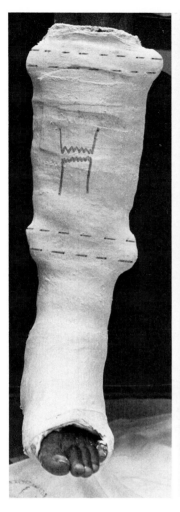
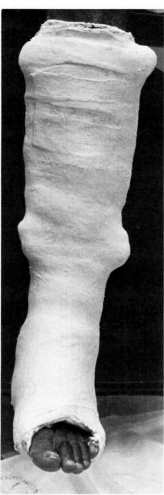

Fig. 17-15. (*Left*) The dotted lines indicate the paths of the Steinmann pins above and below the fracture. (*Right*) Below-knee cast with pins encased in plaster.

of the leg. Once the femur has become sticky, if the tibial fracture and the soft tissue wounds are coming along well, a cast brace can be applied for the femur, and pins-in-plaster will hold the tibia, which will allow the patient to be up and around. The use of traction followed by a cast brace for the femoral fracture and an external fixation device followed by pins-in-plaster for the tibial fracture is best in those patients who have other severe bodily injuries that may keep them in bed. In such cases, however, particularly if there is a head injury, internal fixation of both the femur and the tibia may make it a great deal easier for nursing care, provided there are not extensive soft tissue wounds.

For this difficult combination—the ipsilateral femoral and tibial fracture—a number of treatments are possible and the one that is best for the individual patient must be chosen.

OPEN REDUCTION

The first part of this section has been devoted to closed treatment of tibial fractures, which is my primary method of choice. However, many tibial fractures can be handled well by operative methods, and some may be treated best by open reduction. I do not plan to discuss various methods using internal suture devices, such as Parham bands[178] or isolated screws.[251] Although they were once popular, enthusiasm for this type of operative procedure seems to be waning rapidly. Neither of these methods achieves rigid fixation, and although a better x-ray is often produced, it is at the usual risk inherent in any open reduction without the benefit of firm fixation, which allows earlier joint motion, earlier weight bearing, and a subsequent shorter rehabilitation period. I shall discuss only

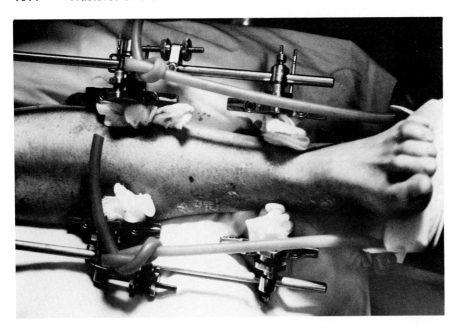

Fig. 17-16. The Hoffmann-type external fixation apparatus used in comminuted, open tibial fractures.

intramedullary nails and compression plates, both of which may give firm fixation of tibial fractures. I shall also comment on the use of closed Ender's nails as a means of aligning tibial fractures and providing internal suture.

COMPRESSION PLATING

Plating of tibial fractures has been popular for years. Noncompression plates have almost universally been replaced by compression plates. With the risks of open surgery, the only logical reason to do an open reduction of a fractured tibia is to obtain an anatomical reduction, which should be held by firm fixation. The compression plating system of Müller, Allgöwer, and their associates[182,183,184] makes this possible. The procedure, popular in Switzerland and France, has ardent advocates in England,[18] the United States, and throughout the world. This technique, as practiced by the AO group,[183] is meticulous and demanding, which may be the secret of its success. Fracture fragments are reassembled with the soft tissues attached, and the periosteum is left undisturbed. Then the fragments are bound together firmly by a well-engineered rigid plate, using bone-holding screws and the compression system.

The advantages of compression plating are several.[243] An anatomical reduction is obtained. Firm fixation should result, which allows the patient to be out of plaster the first few weeks postoperatively, and during that time, motion of the knee, ankle, and foot is allowed. Most surgeons will then apply a cast and allow early weight bearing. The question remains as to whether or not compression plating has any great advantage over nonoperative treatment of tibial fractures, particularly if the treating physician advocates an early-weight-bearing technique. In both compression plating and nonoperative early-weight-bearing techniques, union seems enhanced, and severe soft tissue problems decreased. Does compression plating further increase joint motion and soft tissue healing and allow for earlier functional return?

The argument has been made that the best results of compression plating occur in those fractures that could also be well handled by closed methods. This may be true, but certain tibial fractures are well handled by compression techniques[213,236] and some are best handled by open reduction and internal fixation. Intra-articular fractures involving the tibial shaft and knee joint or tibial shaft and ankle joint need anatomical reconstitution of the joint surface plus firm fixation and are best handled with the use of compression plates and intrafragmentary screws.[204–206] Patients with an arterial injury often require stabilization of fracture fragments, and compression plates do this well.[196,197,198] A difficult segmental fracture may sometimes be managed by one large or two small compression plates, provided that soft tissue dissection is performed so as to not devitalize the fracture fragments (Fig. 17-18).[140] The segmental fracture may also be stabilized by an intramedullary Lottes nail or aligned by Ender's nails, which will need external plaster fixation.

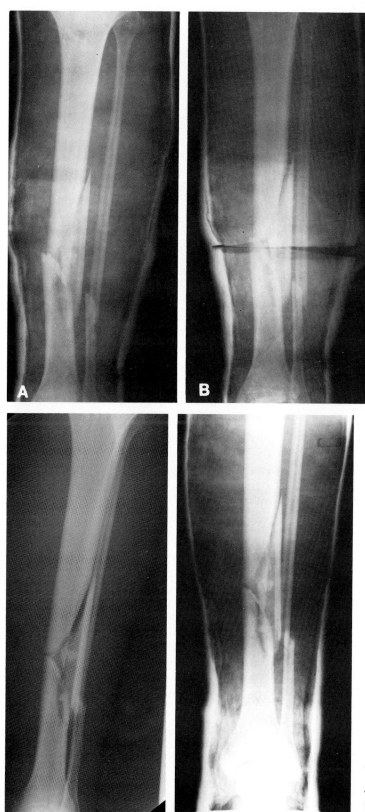

Fig. 17-17. (*A*) Ski fracture. The first reduction showed some valgus deformity. (*B*) The deformity was lessened by open wedging. (*C*) Os calcis traction was used because of anterior tibial compartment syndrome. (*D*) Later casting with pin in place.

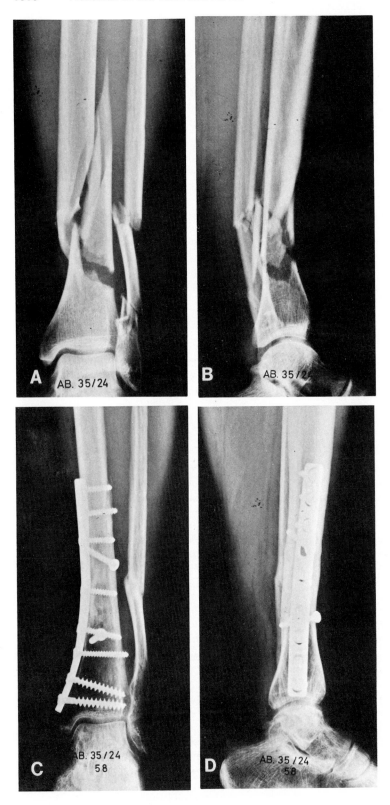

Fig. 17-18. (*A, B*) A comminuted, segmental fracture of the lower tibia. (*C, D*) A compression plate was used. There was solid union and excellent anatomical and functional results 6 months later. (Courtesy of Professor M. Allgöwer.)

In certain severe tibial injuries with major soft tissue wounds, it is advantageous to stabilize the tibia as a means of maintaining limb length and soft tissue integrity. This may be done with an external fixation device but, in some instances, may be best accomplished by a compression plate. In such instances the wound is left open and the soft tissues may heal right over the plate. Sometimes a secondary closure is done. This treatment has been well described by Chapman[50,51] and often may be a means of saving a severely damaged leg (see Part II of Chapter 3, p. 199).

Sometimes a short, oblique fracture of the lower third of the tibia cannot be reduced and held by closed means, and after several reductions the surgeon needs an alternative treatment method. An external fixator or pins above and below in plaster can be used. But the short, oblique fracture can be managed by open reduction and internal fixation with a compression plate. A major concern with the use of compression plates is the problem of devitalization of tissue and subsequent skin breakdown and wound sepsis. The use of intra-operative and postoperative antibiotics has decreased the incidence of wound infections in clean wounds, and with meticulous soft tissue surgery, the point has been reached where the incidence of sepsis after plating should be minimal. The use of multiple screws in the long, oblique tibial fracture is still rarely indicated, because this type of fracture can usually be managed with closed reduction and a long leg cast.

The operative techniques and postoperative care are covered thoroughly in the AO manual.[184] The results in the hands of many surgeons using compression techniques appear impressive. Although certainly not the procedure of choice in most fractures, one must consider each tibial fracture individually and see if it is best handled by closed or operative means. Most tibial fractures can be handled by closed techniques. With fractures produced by high-energy violence the incidence of complications after open plating may be high,[96] and the causative agent, along with skin wounds, must be considered in the treatment of tibial fractures.

Much clinical success has been gained using rigid compression plates, but recently Taylor and his co-workers[233] have started using a semirigid, non-compression plate for tibial fractures. This carbon fiber-reinforced plastic plate is load sharing and may result in a lesser incidence of osteopenia under the plate, which in turn may lead to fewer refractures after removal of tibial plates and fewer stress

fractures at the junction of the plate and normal bone. The semirigid plates appear to give enough support to allow bony union. Presently, experimental work is going on using biodegradable materials for plates, which may have a use in the future.

INTRAMEDULLARY NAILING

Intramedullary nails, although popular for the femur, have never reached the same status in tibial shaft fractures. This may be because (1) tibial shaft fractures are handled so well by nonoperative means; (2) the technique is not as successful; or (3) a surgeon is not so willing to operate on a tibial fracture, which will keep the patient in bed for a shorter period than would a femoral fracture. Nonetheless, the intramedullary nail plays a role in the treatment of tibial shaft fractures. Dr. Otto Lottes has been the principal proponent of intramedullary nailing of the tibia in the United States, and the Lottes[152–154] nail has been the most popular of these devices in this country. Other nails and several men in various countries[16,225] have proved the concept to be successful. Among others, Alms[5] and Zucman[257] have published highly successful reports of intramedullary nailings of the tibial shaft. Küntscher helped to lead the way in this field, and the AO group has devised a total system for intramedullary fixation of long bones.

Intramedullary nailing of the tibia appears most useful in two types of fractures: the noncomminuted transverse or short oblique fracture of the middle third of the tibial shaft, in which there has been major displacement or angulation, and the segmental fracture (Fig. 17-19). The method is not applicable for fractures in the lower third or upper fourth of the tibia. Lottes has at times used it for fractures both higher and lower than the usual cases, but he has extensive experience in the technique. Comminution is generally a contraindication for its use, although in mildly comminuted fractures and in particular with segmental fractures that have an intact middle fragment, it may be successful.

The procedure works best when carried out as a blind nailing, so that the fracture site is not opened. This decreases the potential for infection while not denuding the blood supply of the periosteum and adjacent muscle. With the intramedullary blood supply being cut off by the nail, the soft tissue vascularity must not be impaired. The use of an image intensifier in the operating room cuts down both operating time and difficulty. Lottes's[154] technique of positioning and applying traction should be followed carefully to avoid opening the fracture

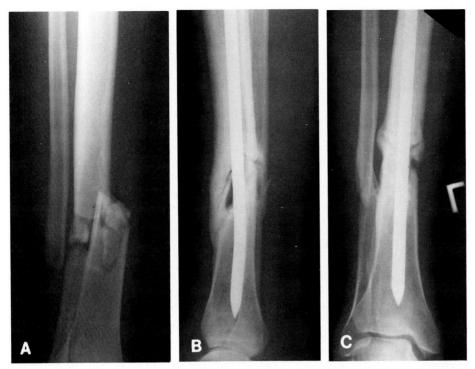

Fig. 17-19. (*A*) A transverse, slightly comminuted fracture of the lower third of the tibia. (*B, C*) Bony union 6 months later with Lottes nail. This fracture was more distal than is usual for the Lottes nail. (Courtesy of Otto Lottes, M.D.)

site, because the procedure loses some of its advantages otherwise. As with compression plating, the procedure's major advantage is that it usually stabilizes the tibial fracture so that the patient does not have to be in a cast in the immediate postoperative period. He is free to move the knee, ankle, and foot while soft tissue healing progresses. Most people who use intramedullary nails do apply a cast after soft tissue healing and then allow the patient to commence bearing weight early. The narrow area of the tibia must be reamed to allow use of a nail large enough to control rotation, but even then the wide medullary canal of the distal tibia causes most surgeons to use some type of external support. However, weight bearing is usually allowed after cast application, and the stability of the nail may allow the cast to be removed when early clinical union is thought to be present.

Ender's Nails

Most orthopaedic surgeons have had problems with tibial fractures that can be reduced by closed means but slip after reduction has been achieved. This development may lead to the use of an external fixation device or even open reduction and internal fixation. One tibial fracture with this well-recognized propensity to slip is the short, oblique fracture of the distal third of the tibia. Pankovich and his associates[191] have used Ender's nails in a series of tibial fractures with reported good results. It must be remembered that Ender's nails do not give firm fixation and, in most instances, are going to be supplemented with external plaster support (Fig. 17-20). Also, one must be careful in inserting the Ender's nails that their introduction does not cause further comminution.

One worry I have is that the use of Ender's nails could be popular at the expense of obtaining closed reductions, which have proved to be exceedingly effective in tibial fractures. It is, however, another method of handling certain difficult fractures.

SEGMENTAL FRACTURES

Segmental fractures of the tibia are notorious for developing nonunion at one fracture site and are difficult to reduce and hold.[140] The intramedullary nail may give excellent control of the intermediate fragment and may allow earlier weight bearing and enhance union. Again, it is preferable if this can

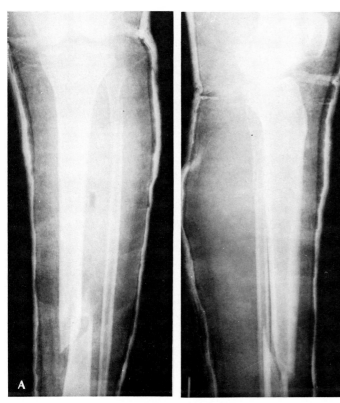

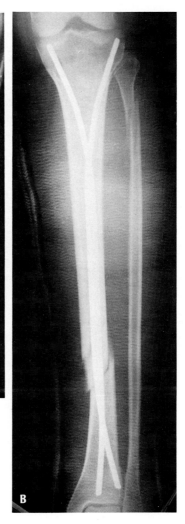

Fig. 17-20. (*A*) Oblique tibial fracture that has slipped twice. (*B*) Reduction after Ender's nails have been inserted.

be performed in a blind nailing fashion, but at times a small incision has to be made to accomplish reduction. Its usefulness in segmental fractures has been well proved and can be considered even if the fracture is open. This may increase the risk of infection, but it also increases the possibility of union, which must be considered, particularly in severe segmental fractures.

SOFT TISSUE WOUNDS

The prognosis for bony union is much worse in open fractures of the tibia than in closed fractures. The incidence for delayed union or nonunion and for infection is higher in open fractures,[109,111] and the more severe the open wound, the worse the prognosis. Gustilo[110,112,113] and others have classi-

fied wounds as mild, moderate, and severe, and by doing this allow a prognosis to be made for the tibial fracture. All would agree that all open wounds should be cleaned, irrigated, and debrided of necrotic or contaminated tissue. If the wound is a small one and can be easily closed without any tissue tension, primary closure *may* be done. However, if there is any question as to whether or not the closure will put tension on the skin edges, or if it is believed that the wound could not be adequately debrided, the wound should be left open and either a secondary closure done or the wound allowed to granulate in. Puncture wounds caused by fractured bones that penetrate from the inside to the outside are not as serious but still need debridement and are the least likely to cause long-term problems.

Modern techniques of fracture fixation have permitted a different approach to stabilizing open tibial fractures. The biggest problems are those that involve major soft tissue wounds, and these fractures can be well handled by the use of an external fixation device.[138] The external fixators are probably preferable to the use of pins above and below in plaster, because they allow adequate wound debridement, and when bony union is progressing the next step could be the conversion to pins above and below in plaster or even removing the pins and using a long leg weight-bearing cast.

There is controversy as to the use of internal fixation devices in open fractures. Chapman[51] and Gustilo's[109,111] figures have shown the dangers of internal fixation with open wounds. In their two different series there was a marked increase in the infection rate of open wounds treated with internal fixation as opposed to those that were not treated with internal fixation. However, not all authorities agree that open reduction and internal fixation in the face of an open wound has a greater risk of infection. McNeur[166] reported on severely damaged arms and legs in the Vietnam War and believed that in many instances the judicious use of open reduction and internal fixation may save arms and legs that have been severely damaged. Closure of contaminated wounds is contraindicated, and although secondary closure and healing by secondary intention goes on, the bone is stabilized in the interim. Either an intramedullary nail or compression plate may be the stabilizing device. Chapman[51] and others have reported on the same type of patients and have used rigid internal fixation as a means of saving severely damaged arms and legs. It is axiomatic that the wounds are not closed in these cases and that they will heal by secondary intention or by late secondary closure.

Of importance is the experience of Brown and Urban[37] who treated 63 consecutive open fractures by early weight bearing. All these fractures went on to bony union, which demonstrates the efficacy of this method of treatment. If there is an open wound and a cast is applied, the cast may be windowed over the wound so the dressings can be changed daily. As soon as clean granulation tissues appear, a well-fitting long leg cast is applied and early weight bearing performed in the usual manner.

When operating on open fractures, antibiotics should be used preoperatively, intra-operatively, and postoperatively.[193] The question always has to be considered as to how long antibiotics should be used postoperatively and has not been resolved at this point. Adequate soft tissue debridement and bony stabilization and leaving the wound open appear to be the key factors for obtaining bony union and preventing long-term effects.

Gustilo's[111] most recent series shows a marked increase in infections caused by gram-negative organisms. He recommends the routine use of cephalosporin plus an aminoglycoside for 72 hours in type III open fractures. Even with this regimen, those fractures that were internally fixed had an increased incidence of wound infection, with intramedullary nailing having the highest rate of infection.

OPEN VERSUS CLOSED REDUCTION

Throughout this chapter, there is a bias toward the nonoperative treatment of tibial fractures. This bias has been influenced by personal experience plus the large number of cases in series published by such authors as Dehne,[73] Sarmiento,[212] Brown,[37] Weissman,[250] Nicoll,[187] and Anderson.[8] All these authors have demonstrated the efficacy of the nonoperative treatment of tibial fractures. With the excellent results obtainable by the nonoperative treatment, we may question whether there is any indication for open reduction of a fractured tibia.

Advocates of open reduction include Lottes,[156] Alms,[5] Burwell,[39,40] Hicks,[125] Müller,[183] and Ruedi.[207] It is hoped that even these advocates would not routinely use open reduction for all tibial fractures, but there are many instances in which an open reduction of the tibia is a procedure of choice in their hands. Whether the operative procedure would always work as well in the hands of most orthopaedic surgeons is open to question. However, this holds true for the nonoperative methods too, because practice and skill are required to reduce and hold tibial fractures by closed methods. Unfortunately, many surgeons feel the easier course is to open the fracture and fix it with a plate or screws, so that they can know it is together rather than having to worry about a closed reduction holding the fracture. This Pavlovian thinking leads to nonunions, infections, and even amputations. The advantages and disadvantages of both methods must be examined in preparation for treating correctly any tibial fracture, no matter what the circumstances.

ADVANTAGES OF OPEN REDUCTION

What are the advantages[137] of open reduction? It is a definitive form of treatment, and one does not have to worry about later loss of position or shortening. There should be no postfracture deformity, because an open reduction should obtain a precise anatomical position and hold it. Certain fractures are exceedingly difficult to reduce by closed means, and open reduction may be the easiest method to achieve an acceptable reduction. With rigid internal fixation, the leg is not put into a cast initially, and adjacent joints are allowed to move, so there may be less stiffness in the joints after the fracture heals and less muscle wasting. Advocates state that less time is spent in the cast and weight bearing is allowed sooner. Lucas[157] reported an earlier return to work.

DISADVANTAGES OF OPEN REDUCTION

The major disadvantages of open reduction of tibial fractures are the complications that may follow any open reduction. Boyd, Lipinski, and Wiley[33] reported on a large series of nonunions seen at the Campbell Clinic up to 1959. Of that total series, 35% of the nonunions were tibial fractures. One third of these nonunions had been treated primarily by open reduction of the tibial fracture. In a later series by Boyd and his co-workers,[31] covering the period from 1959 to 1964, nonunions of the tibia comprised only 20% of that total series. The authors felt that this lower incidence of nonunion of the tibia was due to the fact that fewer primary operative reductions were performed during that period. Primary open reduction has long been cited as one of the principal causes of both delayed union and nonunion in tibial fractures.[208] However, the open reduction generally referred to has used such internal devices as Parham bands, screws, and noncompression plates. The incidence of both delayed union and nonunion after open reduction with intramedullary nails or compression plates seems substantially lower than the incidence of these complications after the use of these other devices.

Yet, even intramedullary nails and compression plates have certain undesirable qualities. An intramedullary nail destroys the intramedullary blood supply to the tibia, and thus union on the endosteal side has to be slowed and healing must come from the periosteal blood supply. The nail may give enough stability to allow for eventual healing in most instances, but it does not speed bony union. With the meticulous technique advised by the advocates of compression plating, the bone is not denuded of the periosteum and its soft tissues, and the blood supply for the bone is only partially lost in a compression plating properly performed. This assumes, of course, that all surgeons will follow the meticulous soft tissue technique advocated.

Compression plates have a certain bulk to them, which, in a subcutaneous bone such as the tibia, can be a problem. Lucas and Todd[157] reported imperfect wound healing in 15% of his series, and the bulk of the plate in this relatively exposed area was thought to play a role. One other disadvantage is that internal fixation devices must generally be removed. An intramedullary nail can penetrate the ankle or, more likely, back out into the knee. Compression plates, screws, and other devices should be removed, because if they are left in place, they form focal points of weakness for fracture if the tibia is subjected to unusual stress.

Technique is important in open reduction but particularly when using an intramedullary nail or a compression plate. The closed method of intramedullary nailing is far superior to open reduction, but it may require special equipment, such as an image intensifier, in the operating room. As with many surgical procedures, the surgeon sometimes has casual acceptance of the concept of open reduction without a skillful application of the principles and technique.

INFECTION

Open reduction does have other disadvantages inherent in any operation (*i.e.,* the necessity for hospitalization, the requirement of an anesthetic with all its attendant risks, and of course, the possibility of sepsis). The possibility of sepsis is a major worry, because all authorities on tibial fractures agree that sepsis increases dramatically the possibility of delayed union and nonunion of the tibia and may even necessitate secondary amputation. Veliskakis[243] reported a series of 80 open tibial fractures treated by open reduction in which there was a 10% sepsis rate. Of these fractures, 61 were fixed by plates and the other 19, by screws. In the same hospital, at the same time, a series of open reductions were done on 95 closed tibial fractures in which there was a 2.1% infection rate. Burwell,[39] advocating open reduction of the tibia, reported a corrected infection rate of 3.9%, whereas Blockey[24] had four deep infections out of 33 operative reductions of the tibia (12%). Fisher and Hamblen[100] reported a 10.5% infection rate and a 10.6% fixation failure rate in a series of patients treated from 1973 to 1976. Kristensen's[141] series of tibial shaft fractures treated by internal fixation showed an infection rate of only 1.3%. However, this percentage may represent an irreducible incidence of infection after open reduction. Lottes[156] reported a lower incidence of infection in intra-medullary nailing of the tibia, particularly in those reductions done by the closed method, and compression plates in many hands have an admirably low infection rate. However, there may be an irreducible incidence of infection following open reduction. Even if we grant that this may be admirably low, say less than 1% in clean, closed cases, that is still greater than the theoretical 0% that we should expect in clean, closed cases in which no surgery is performed. Considering the number of tibial fractures seen in any one year throughout the world, even an infection rate of 0.5% could be quite significant in terms of the total number of patients and hospital days.

In open wounds the incidence of infection is much higher with both closed and operative methods of treatment, but it is particularly high in cases managed by internal fixation. In one series of patients, Gustilo's[110] statistics showed an incidence of six deep infections in 29 open cases in which primary metallic fixation was performed, whereas in 144 cases of open fractures of the tibia treated by either a cast or the pins above and below technique, only six deep infections developed. Most recently, in a series of patients with type III open fractures of the tibia,[111] he found a 33% incidence of wound infection with patients treated with intramedullary nailing of the tibia and two of nine patients treated by early plating had wound infections. However, these were all severe fractures with extensive soft tissue damage. He points out that those patients who have either arterial injury or severe soft tissue injury with loss of substance and periosteal stripping or bare bone have the worst prognosis.

Some authors[39,51,130,166,169] have stated that, in some instances, open reduction with rigid fixation may be needed in open fractures of the tibia to stabilize the bone, which will aid soft tissue healing. The rationale is that rigid internal fixation maintains position and length and decreases tissue reaction caused by motion. However, there are alternative methods of treatment for this type of wound, including in particular the use of external fixators. Open reduction in the face of an open tibial fracture clearly has a high incidence of subsequent infection.

The use of external fixators, as shown by Edwards and his associates[89] and Widenfolk and his co-workers[253] demonstrates that rigid fixation of an open tibial fracture can be obtained without the risk of introducing plates and screws. If one chooses to use plate fixation in open fractures, the principles advocated by Chapman[51] and others must be fol-lowed closely or long-term wound sepsis is likely and, in some instances, may lead to chronic osteo-myelitis.

The question, then, to be considered is whether by operating and risking some infections the surgeon avoids later operations for nonunion or malunion, which carries its own risk of infection plus the disability caused by the nonunion. Does open reduction decrease the rate of delayed union, non-union, and other complications so that its risks are outweighed by its advantages?

Even accepting the now lower incidence of infection after open reduction of closed tibial fractures, my major reason for playing down the role of operative over nonoperative treatment in the care of tibial fractures is that nonoperative treatment does so well. In the recent literature, there seem to be few cases of tibial fracture that cannot be adequately reduced, with sound functional and cosmetic results, without operative intervention. Using function rather than radiographic results as the index of success, nonoperative treatment seems to be applicable in most cases. The incidence of delayed union and nonunion is so low in the nonoperative series of Dehne and his associates,[73] Sarmiento,[212] and Anderson,[8] that I do not feel open reduction could lessen this incidence.

How about the postfracture complications of joint stiffness and soft tissue edema? There is little question that the use of intramedullary nails and compression plates minimizes these problems, because rigid fixation allows early motion. Nonetheless, the early-weight-bearing technique in a plaster cast also handles the problem well. In my mind, any comparisons of soft tissue injuries and their complications should be between rigid internal fixation and the early-weight-bearing technique. It may be that the important factor is the initial amount of soft tissue injury and that this, rather than treatment, determines the amount of joint stiffness and soft tissue disability.

VASCULAR PROBLEMS

Are there any absolute indications for open reduction? In a tibial fracture with an associated vascular or neural injury that must be repaired, should there be rigid fixation of the tibial fracture? How is this best accomplished? In many but not all instances an intramedullary nail or compression plate will be indicated. However, according to Connolly and his colleagues,[63] internal fixation may not always be needed, and the use of an external fixator or even traction alone may be enough. The personality of the fracture indicates the best method of treatment. With large open wounds and soft tissue loss in a comminuted fracture, the surgeon has to decide whether an external fixator, plate fixation, or an intramedullary nail is going to give the best fixation, allowing access to the wound, and yet do the least damage to the soft tissues. However, in many vascular repairs, particularly if the ends of the fractured tibia are immediately adjacent to the arterial repair, it may be mandatory to have the fracture stabilized before performing the vascular anastomosis; an intramedullary nail or compression plate gives stable fixation and allows the surgeon easy access to the wound. The method that gives best fixation with minimal soft tissue dissection should be used. Pins above and below generally have to be inserted after the anastomosis is performed, and the surgeon may worry about the injury to the vascular repair during this procedure.

SEGMENTAL FRACTURES

Segmental fractures are comminuted and usually markedly displaced; they have a poor prognosis.[146] Certain ones are amenable to open reduction and internal fixation. They are usually caused by major direct violence and may have associated soft tissue wounds. Some still in reasonable anatomical position and without significant shortening can be handled by the usual methods of casting. If the fracture does not lose position in the first few days, even early weight bearing may be reasonable with such a fracture. Still others are best handled by either an external fixator or pins above and below. Because anatomical restoration in the middle fragment need not be exact, as long as the fragments allow bony contact, they can go on to union.

The flexible nails of the Ender's type can also be used in segmental fractures as a means of aligning the fracture. They do not give stability, but when combined with external casting, they may allow a good reduction with a relatively minor procedure.

Some segmental fractures, despite assiduous nonoperative attempts, simply cannot be reduced to allow bony contact. The incidence of nonunion of such fractures is substantial. Charnley[52] felt that most segmental fractures would go on to nonunion at one site or the other and advised early grafting. Another danger from segmental fractures is that one fragment, particularly the upper, may be tilted forward so that there is pressure on the skin, which causes necrosis (Fig. 17-21). Such fractures are handled well by intramedullary nailing. If the procedure can be done without opening the fracture

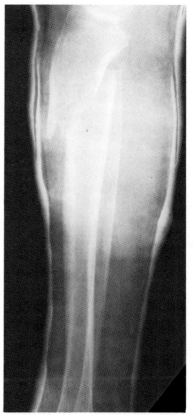

Fig. 17-21. The upper tibial fragment was tilted forward causing skin necrosis. The cast was poorly laminated.

site, that is preferable, because the intramedullary blood supply is destroyed by the nailing. With a blind nailing, such as Lottes[152] and others[5] advocate, soft tissue attachments are preserved. It may be difficult to drive the nail from the proximal fragment into the middle one, and a limited open reduction may have to be done for that fragment. After that, it is usually possible to drive the nail from the middle to the distal fragment without opening the fracture site (Fig. 17-22). Treatment after this would be the same as for any intramedullary nailing and depends on the stability. One must not assume that fixation is always rigid, because the middle fragment cannot be reamed. A smaller nail may have to be used to align the fracture, and rigid fixation may not be possible. Postoperative casting is usually needed.

Müller and Allgöwer,[182] and their AO associates use compression plates for such fractures. Again, limited dissection is needed to keep from denuding the middle fragment of its blood supply. Because

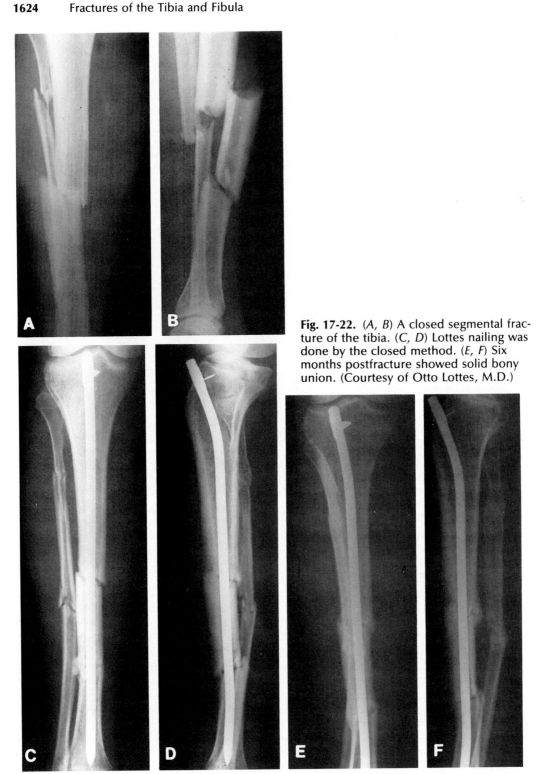

Fig. 17-22. (*A, B*) A closed segmental fracture of the tibia. (*C, D*) Lottes nailing was done by the closed method. (*E, F*) Six months postfracture showed solid bony union. (Courtesy of Otto Lottes, M.D.)

most segmental fractures require a large plate to go from the proximal across the middle to the distal fragment, or two plates, this implies a great deal of dissection. The dangers of a large wound with much dissection in a segmental fracture are obvious, but the advantages of rigid fixation cannot be denied.

INADEQUATE REDUCTION

Soft tissue interposition is not a common cause of inadequate reductions but can occur, particularly in the lower quarter of the tibia. Here, the distal muscle bellies and tendons can intervene, particularly in the short, oblique fractures, and open reduction and internal fixation may be necessary (Fig. 17-23).

Poor reduction usually results from insufficient traction of the distal fragment, which will not allow the distal fragment to engage the proximal fragment. If, with several tries at a closed reduction, suitable reduction cannot be obtained, internal fixation may be justified. Internal fixation is not justified simply to secure anatomical reduction. Most tibial fractures can easily accept some displacement and angulation with no functional impairment or major cosmetic effect.

ASSOCIATED KNEE PROBLEMS

Open reduction of the tibia might be considered when there is an associated knee problem that requires operation and the surgeon would like to have the knee moved before the tibial fracture would ordinarily be healed. In this instance an open reduction and rigid internal fixation, as with a compression plate, would allow earlier motion of the knee. Other tibial fractures can be adequately handled with an external fixator or pins above and below that will allow knee motion, although this is less secure than compression plating and the external apparatus may make it difficult to get good knee motion.

TREATMENT OF TIBIAL PLAFOND FRACTURES

Open reduction may be preferable in certain fractures involving the tibial plafond. For best long-term results, intra-articular fractures should be anatomically reduced. If fracture fragments have been driven up into the tibial shaft, neither closed reduction nor traction is going to bring these fragments into position, and anatomical restoration

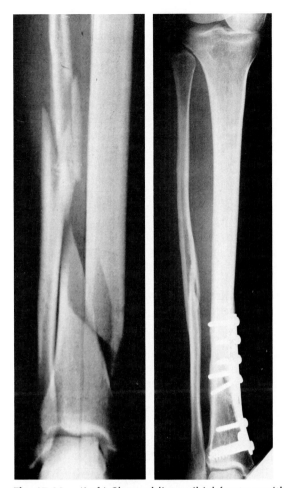

Fig. 17-23. (*Left*) Short oblique tibial fracture with soft tissue interposition. (*Right*) Healing after compression plate was applied medially because of an open wound.

with compression plates and cancellous bone screws would be best. This allows reposition of the fragments, and early joint motion is possible because of the rigid fixation. The surgeon must ascertain that the fragments are not so comminuted that he cannot obtain an anatomical reduction at the time of operative intervention.

I believe that open reduction and rigid internal fixation can be successful and that it is preferable in some instances. The surgical techniques must be performed meticulously. Most important, the physician must recognize that the vast majority of tibial fractures can be adequately handled by nonoperative means and there must be a compelling reason to use internal fixation, as opposed to the closed treatment methods, on tibial fractures.

AUTHOR'S PREFERRED METHOD OF TREATMENT

My basic approach is to assume that virtually all tibial fractures can be treated by nonoperative methods but that certain fractures and soft tissue problems will require variations of the nonoperative method. Furthermore, some selected fractures may do better with open reduction and internal fixation, but this number is few in my hands.

EXAMINATION

When seeing a patient with a suspected tibial fracture for the first time, I start by doing a quick general physical examination. After being sure there is no major respiratory, cardiovascular, abdominal, or neurologic problem, I examine the leg for deformity, open wounds, and any associated skin necrosis or soft tissue injury. Both the dorsalis pedis and posterior tibial pulses are checked, as well as function of the posterior tibial and peroneal nerves. The examination may be difficult because of pain, but with proper splinting the patient should be able to move his toes up and down to give baseline function. Sensation is easier to ascertain. With adequate splinting the patient is taken to x-ray for necessary films.

After radiography, an assessment is made of the type of fracture being dealt with. It is classified as minor, moderate, or severe, and plans for treatment are based on this classification and the soft tissue injuries. With questionable damage to the arterial circulation of the leg, all the above steps are speeded up. In such an instance an obvious deformity might be partially reduced, and routine x-rays might include an arteriogram.

TECHNIQUE OF CLOSED REDUCTION

With a closed tibial shaft fracture with minor or moderate displacement, I would intend to perform a closed reduction and apply a long leg cast with the knee straight. If pain is mild and little or no reduction is required, intramuscular or intravenous sedation or analgesia may be enough to allow accurate reduction and casting of the fracture. In instances where attempted reduction has already failed or if it may prove difficult, spinal anesthesia allows not only complete pain relief, but also excellent relaxation of the leg muscles.

The patient lies supine on a stable plinth or table with the leg hanging over the end of the table, allowing the weight of the leg to apply traction.

This may be sufficient to allow the surgeon to manipulate the fracture into proper position. If more traction is needed, the distal leg and foot are firmly gripped, applying longitudinal traction. The fracture fragments are brought into proper position, alignment, and especially rotation by manual manipulation. It is easier to check rotation with the leg over the end of the table rather than over the side, where external rotation may result. If the reduction appears reasonable, the surgeon maintains position, and his assistant applies Webril or some other form of soft tissue padding, starting at the toes and padding the heel, both malleoli, and the fibular neck where the peroneal nerve crosses. This first soft tissue padding should go across the knee and should not stop at the fibular neck, where pressure might be applied to the nerve. The surgeon continues to hold the reduction, and plaster is applied from the toes to the tibial tubercle area by the assistant. With only one assistant, it is easiest to have the leg over the bottom of the table while the surgeon maintains reduction and traction. After the lower leg plaster is dried, the padding is continued to the high thigh region, to approximately 2 fingerbreadths below the greater trochanter of the femur. With the leg now up on the table and the knee between 0° and 5° of flexion, the alignment, position, and rotation are carefully noted. Again the surgeon maintains position while the assistant wraps the plaster, going from the lower leg cast up to the high thigh. The cast must be molded well over both the tibial condyles and the lower femur to help prevent rotation, because the cast is applied with the knee in almost full extension. The junction of the lower leg cast and the upper leg cast must be strong to prevent breakage and well padded where the peroneal nerve crosses the fibula.

With the cast dry, x-rays in two planes are taken, and the reduction is checked. Provided the reduction is adequate, the patient may be admitted to the hospital or, in some instances, sent home. If the fracture has been of minor displacement with no open wounds and the patient has little pain, is trustworthy, and has someone to take care of him, it is reasonable to allow the patient to go home. He is shown how to use crutches with a non-weight-bearing gait, and his walking is tested before he leaves. He must be given explicit instructions on what he is to do after arriving home. He is told to keep the leg elevated and to move his toes up and down. He is given an appointment for the next day for circulation and cast checks and further instructions. (If pain increases or if the patient cannot perceive feeling in toes or move them either up or down, he must call his physician immediately and return to the hospital.) If the fracture is open, severely displaced, or, in some instances, moderately displaced but the patient does not have anyone to take care of him, it is better to admit him to the hospital. With any patient, check x-rays are always taken the next day to be sure that the reduction is maintained and that the leg and cast are fine.

WEDGING

If, after a reduction, the check x-rays show that the position is not good enough or that the fracture has slipped, the cast may be wedged. This procedure must be planned as carefully as the initial reduction of the fracture was. If, for instance, there is 16° of valgus angulation in a midshaft fracture of the tibia, the long axes of the proximal and distal fragments are drawn and at that point where these lines intersect, the wedging of the plaster should be carried out. I prefer to use an opening wedge so that with a valgus angulation of the tibia, the apex of the wedge will be based on the medial aspect of the tibia. The plaster is opened anteriorly, posteriorly, and laterally but left intact on the medial side, which acts as a fulcrum. The lower leg fragment is then angled into a more neutral position, thus opening the lateral side of the cast and taking the leg out of valgus. Some plaster or a small piece of wood is inserted in the opening on the lateral aspect, and then the whole area is wrapped in plaster and a check x-ray is taken.

Closing wedges may be used, but one has to be exceedingly careful not to cause pressure against the skin. Wedging is usually performed the day after casting to allow the plaster to dry.

EARLY WEIGHT BEARING

I intend to treat all minor and moderate fractures of the tibia with the early-weight-bearing technique. Patients do quadriceps sets and straight-leg raisings during the first 48 hours. Two days after the cast application, the patient is taught how to walk with crutches by the physical therapist. He will take virtually all his weight on the hands but go through the normal walking motion with a heel-toe gait. A walking boot or cast and shoe is preferred to a rubber walking heel, because it seems more stable and there is less tendency to rotate externally. Walking is easier if the shoe on the opposite leg is built up about 1 inch. The patient is told that he may increase weight on the leg

gradually as pain decreases, taking as much weight as he cares to. In most instances he bears little or no weight during the first 7 to 10 days and then gradually increases weight bearing. Check x-rays are taken between the seventh and tenth postreduction days. It has been my experience that if a fracture has not slipped at that point, it is unlikely to move.

Young people seem to bear much weight even by the sixth to the tenth postfracture days, and the problem is to make sure that the cast holds up under the stress of this weight bearing. The cast must be changed if any part breaks down or becomes loose. For walking casts, I use some of the lightweight, but durable synthetic materials. If the reduction is difficult to hold, I use plaster of paris for the first cast and then apply another material for a second cast. Patients can walk on these, and the light weight, coolness, and easy ventilation are appreciated. *Sometimes* I even allow the cast to be immersed in water because it can usually be dried with a hand-held hair dryer. However, the material underneath, even though non-water-absorbable material is available, does not always dry well, so patients should be cautioned about getting the cast wet.

I believe that early weight bearing enhances bony union, although hard data to support this are lacking. Both delayed union and nonunion appear less common with early weight bearing. However, its greatest attribute for me is that it keeps the muscles in a more physiologic state and that after the cast is removed, knee, ankle, and foot motion are regained more quickly. There is also less muscle atrophy and tissue edema. Because my patients have had no great difficulty regaining knee motion after the use of early-weight-bearing long leg casts with the knee straight, I have not been inclined to regularly use the below-knee walking cast described by Sarmiento. However, in some older patients who may have trouble regaining knee motion and in some bilateral tibial fractures and certain others, the long leg plaster is changed at 6 to 8 weeks to a Sarmiento patellar tendon-bearing cast (see Fig. 17-10). This cast is then worn until osseous union occurs.

Certain patients are put in the Delbet gaiter cast (see Fig. 17-11). These are usually younger patients who will literally beat a cast to death and in whom I believe clinical union has occurred but I would like to have a bit more protection for the fracture site. The Delbet gaiter cast is applied for another 4 to 6 weeks to restrict activity, to protect the leg, and to allow the surgeon to sleep more easily.

Although it allows knee and ankle motion, it may be problematical with swelling below the cast in the foot. This may be handled with a Gelocast or some other type of compression bandaging under the Delbet gaiter.

EXTERNAL FIXATION DEVICES

If x-rays show an unacceptable reduction that will not respond to wedging, despite having had adequate anesthesia, I used to use pins above and below the fracture site. At this stage I still use pins above and below in some patients, particularly if I believe a reduction can be obtained relatively easily. If the fracture is more comminuted and I think it may be more difficult to get a reduction, I use one of the external fixation devices, such as the modifications of the Hoffmann frame.[132]

To use pins above and below, the patient is anesthetized and the skin prepped and draped in the usual fashion. The surgeon should scrub and use gloves and a smooth mask. Steinmann pins $3/32$ inch or $1/8$ inch are used, with two above the fracture site and two below. Bonnel pins, which are strong and threaded in the middle, have secure fixation in the cortex and are not as likely to break as ordinary Steinmann pins. Pins in the lower tibia give better control than they do in the os calcis. The pins must not traverse the fracture site and should be inserted from the lateral side to avoid the peroneal nerve. One must also be careful about impaling any of the muscle or tendon or neurovascular structures in the lower part of the leg.

Once pins are in place, traction can be applied to the lower tibia by holding on to the lower Steinmann pin or even by using a traction bow applied to the pin. Reduction is accomplished and maintained while soft tissue padding for the cast is applied. The cast is applied in the same fashion as for routine tibial fractures, with the pins being incorporated. It is unnecessary to go above the knee once the pins above and below the fracture site have been incorporated in the plaster. X-rays are taken, and if the reduction is adequate, the patient is admitted to the hospital. If proper reduction has not been obtained, a second try is made. If a second attempt is unsuccessful, there are two alternatives: One is to leave the cast intact and wedge it 1 or 2 days later, and the other is to abandon this method and do an open reduction and internal fixation.

External fixation devices are more expensive and more difficult to apply. However, without question,

once one is accomplished in the technique of using such devices, they can be helpful in obtaining reductions and in maintaining adequate tibial position. I advise surgeons to become competent in the use of one of these external fixation devices. I tend to use the external fixation devices in the more severe fractures and particularly in those in which there are soft tissue wounds that must be considered or other injuries that may necessitate the patient being in the hospital.

TRACTION

Traction as a means of holding tibial fractures is slowly disappearing from the armamentarium. It still can be used in selected instances in which the use of other techniques is undesirable. Traction can be applied either to the lower tibia or to a pin in the os calcis and the leg placed in a Thomas splint with the knee partly flexed. Approximately 7 to 10 pounds needs to be applied and, generally speaking, within 48 hours a satisfactory reduction can be obtained. Check x-rays must be taken during the first several days to be sure the fracture fragments are in proper position and that there has been no distraction. Traction weight is quickly reduced to 5 or 6 pounds as soon as reduction is obtained, and within several weeks it is desirable to apply a long leg cast, to allow early weight bearing.

There are fewer instances now in which traction is needed, because other methods of treatment, particularly the use of external fixation devices and even internal fixation, seem to be more helpful.

SEGMENTAL FRACTURES

A difficult fracture for me to handle is the segmental fracture of the tibia. A simple, closed reduction is unlikely to suffice unless the fracture remains in good position at the time it is originally seen. Such an injury is treated as a routine fracture with a long leg cast and even early weight bearing. In my experience if the fracture, although it is segmental, is in relatively good overall alignment, it does not displace further with early weight bearing. However, when there has been displacement of the fracture fragments, the use of an external fixation device or pins above and below has been a successful method of treatment. It is usually possible to obtain an adequate reduction with either of these methods (Fig. 17-24). A disadvantage in using pins across the tibia is that if the method does not work, the pins must be removed and the wounds allowed

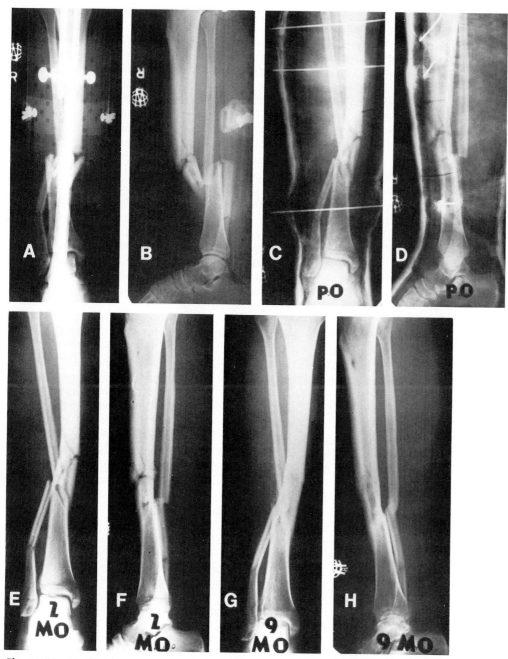

Fig. 17-24. (*A, B*) A severe segmental tibial fracture. (*C, D*) Pins above and below secured satisfactory reduction. (*E, F*) Two months following fracture the position was maintained. (*G, H*) Nine months after fracture solid union in good position. (Anderson, L. D., and Hutchins, W. C.: Fractures of the Tibia and Fibula Treated with Casts and Transfixing Pins. South. Med. J., **59**:1026, 1966.)

to heal before any operative internal fixation method of treatment can be applied. The healing of pin tracts may take 7 to 14 days and thus delay open reduction. However, because some authors believe that all open reductions of long bones should be delayed from 7 to 14 days for quicker fracture healing, the delay may not be catastrophic.

If pins either in plaster or in an external fixation device cannot handle the segmental fracture, and in particular if there is a problem with the proximal or middle fragment tenting against the anterior skin, which will cause necrosis of the skin, internal fixation of the fracture may be best. With a non-comminuted fracture, I prefer to use an intramedullary nail. I follow Lottes' technique and pass the nail through both fragments in the closed manner. An image intensifier in the operating room is a necessity for this procedure. In some instances it is impossible to manipulate the fracture fragments into position without opening the fracture site through a limited incision. With comminution of the fracture fragments, I would not use an intramedullary nail but would try to treat it with an external fixation device. Occasionally, this is unsuccessful, and compression plating may be applicable even in the face of some comminution. As previously stated, another possibility is the use of Ender's nails to obtain alignment, which can be combined with external plaster fixation and may be successful in certain of these segmental fractures.

Those fractures that involve the lower tibia and tibial plafond are covered later in the chapter. In most instances if it is impossible to obtain a good reduction by closed means, I use compression plates and intrafragmentary bone screws to reconstitute the lower tibia and tibial plafond. The basic concept is to restore anatomical continuity as early as possible with rigid fixation, which will allow early motion.

OPEN FRACTURES

Open fractures have a worse prognosis than closed fractures.[193] An open wound is irrigated and necessary debridement is performed in the usual fashion.[121] If the soft tissue wound is relatively minor, the skin may be closed primarily. In any instance in which it is felt that the wound is contaminated or the skin closure would be too tight, the wound is left open and a secondary closure is planned. Relaxing incisions may be used, but if there is any question about the viability of the skin or a tight closure, I prefer to leave it open and do a secondary closure. If the fracture can be handled by closed

reduction and a long leg cast, that is the method used. If the fracture cannot be handled by this method, an external fixation device or pins above and below in plaster will stabilize the fracture. If the wound is relatively minor, the pins in plaster technique can be adequate and the wound allowed to granulate in. If the wound is more major, the external fixation device allows care of the wound until the fracture fragments become sticky. At that point the apparatus may be removed and a long leg cast applied. It is not always necessary to do a secondary closure or even a skin graft, because many of these wounds granulate in nicely.[37] I do try to get the patient into a long leg cast and allow weight bearing as quickly as possible.

Certain severe, open fractures with large soft tissue wounds and bony loss or lack of continuity may sometimes be best handled by internal fixation with plates and leaving the wounds open. In more instances, however, with such a wound, I tend to use an external fixation device.

FRACTURE HEALING

Determination of fracture healing is partially based on prior knowledge of how most fractures will heal in any particular area. Patients should be checked at roughly 6- to 8-week intervals, and any cast change must be followed by x-rays to be sure that no change in position has occurred. Most uncomplicated tibial fractures will heal between the 14th and 18th weeks. To check healing, the cast must be removed to allow a clinical determination based primarily on the lack of both tenderness and pain under stress at the fracture site. Anteroposterior, lateral, and oblique x-rays determine if union is radiographically evident. When there is evidence of both clinical and radiographic union, the cast is removed. If the fracture is clinically sound but on x-rays does not appear to be completely united, I prefer to be on the safe side and apply a new weight-bearing cast, perhaps a patellar tendon-bearing cast or occasionally, the Delbet gaiter cast.

If at 16 to 20 weeks the fracture is not healed but x-rays appear to show progression of the healing, and if this fracture is known by its "personality" to require a longer period of healing, I wait for the fracture to declare its intent. As long as the patient is bearing weight and there is no radiographic sign of nonunion, it appears to me that most fractures go on to union. If, however, at the end of 20 weeks the fracture shows no obvious sign of healing as well as an expected poor prognosis, I give consideration to some type of procedure. In some instances, partial resection of 1 inch of the fibula,[77] if previously healed, allows closer approximation of the tibial fracture and may help union. In other instances I consider cancellous bone grafting. At 6 months any unhealed fracture of the tibia must be carefully studied to see if something should be done to increase the possibilities of bony union. These problems are discussed in the section on complications of tibial fractures.

CARE AND REHABILITATION AFTER TREATMENT

The rehabilitation of tibial fractures starts with selection of the treatment method. The objective is to have the fracture heal as quickly as possible so as to minimize the time spent in a cast. While awaiting fracture healing, the aim is to minimize the harmful effects of immobilization: muscle atrophy, soft tissue and joint contracture, and bony osteoporosis. Thus treatment methods are chosen with both fracture healing and leg rehabilitation in mind.

The majority of tibial fractures require a cast during the healing period. The type of cast, to some extent, determines the care. However, the casting procedure is different for those fractures that had open reduction with rigid fixation. The following section discusses the details of fracture care after nonoperative treatment and after operative intervention.

Fracture rehabilitation requires careful cast application. An appropriately padded and nicely molded cast with the foot in neutral position prevents cast sores and heel cord contractures. For fractures of the lower third of the tibia, the foot may have to be in some equinus to prevent posterior angulation at the fracture site, but the cast should be changed at 4 to 6 weeks so the foot may be brought to neutral position. Elevation of the leg during the first few days helps to reduce the immediate edema of the fracture. Whenever the patient is not up and actually walking in the first week, the leg should be elevated.

CARE AFTER CASTING

Most important in the immediate postreduction and casting phase are the instructions to a patient concerning his aftercare and the possible consequences of the fracture and treatment. Not all pain will disappear immediately after reduction and casting, but it should be considerably reduced. An increase of pain after casting or operative reduction is a danger signal that requires the physician to examine the patient carefully. For this the patient must be seen in the hospital, or he must return to the emergency department or office. The patient must be made aware that any decrease of sensation in the toes or foot, any loss of toe motion, any muscle weakness, or any increase in pain is crucial. Toes will swell somewhat and may feel cool after a cast is applied, but if pain increases and swelling becomes tight, the patient must be checked. The color of the toes is less important. One must remember that an anterior tibial compartment syndrome may occur although the toes are pink and show good capillary return. A posterior compartment syndrome is more difficult to diagnose, and pain in the calf and pain with forced extension of the toes may be the only clinical signs on which to base this diagnosis.[58] Obviously, blue or black toes indicate a major problem. The patient must be told where to seek aid in the first 48 hours after fracture, whether he is going to a hospital, to his home, or to a ski lodge.

Patients must be taught the proper use of crutches before being discharged from the emergency department or hospital. To simply throw a pair of crutches at a patient and tell him to use them is to endanger him and his tibial reduction. Crutches should be measured properly to put the handpiece at proper height and take pressure off the axillary structures. The patient is instructed to take the weight on his hands and not in the axillae. He should be given practice on both flat surfaces and stairs if he has to navigate them. The patient is not started on weight bearing on the first day, but after this, the care of the patient depends on the fracture and the philosophy of the treating physician.

On the day after fracture the patient should be started on quadriceps sets in the cast. He is given a regular program to follow daily, which will minimize, to some extent, quadriceps atrophy and will help regain knee motion after cast removal. Both quadriceps sets and straight-leg raising, which cause the patella to move, appear to minimize knee stiffness. Routine toe exercises include both plantar flexion and dorsiflexion. Although this may be painful at first, pain gradually disappears.

Advocates of no weight bearing feel that the knee should be flexed 25° to 40° to help control rotation of the tibia and to help the foot clear the ground. In my opinion, the success of early weight bearing shows that rotation can be controlled even when the knee is straight, provided the cast is applied properly. Knee flexion may be of some help in controlling initial pain. If early weight bearing is advocated, this must be explained clearly to the patient. He should repeat the instructions and practice under a physician's or therapist's eye during the first week. Either a walking boot or a heel can be used; I prefer the boot, because ambulation seems easier with it. The opposite shoe needs a lift of ¾ to 1 inch to compensate for the straight knee and the thickness of the plaster on the volar aspect of the fractured leg. Initially, the patient bears most of his weight on his hands and gradually takes weight on the leg as he feels able. He must use a heel-toe gait and must not throw the leg out to the side. As pain in the leg subsides and strength increases, weight bearing on the fractured leg is increased. The patient may then go from two crutches to one, and finally to a cane in the opposite hand (or he may elect to use no walking aid).

CARE AFTER CAST REMOVAL

A cast should be removed when the fracture has healed. What constitutes healing of a fracture? For a fracture to be totally healed, there must be radiographic evidence of union, with no tenderness at the fracture site, and the patient must be able to bear weight unassisted and without pain. Radiographic union sometimes is later than clinical union. If there is any doubt as to whether the anteroposterior, lateral, and oblique films demonstrate union, I prefer to put the patient back in another cast and allow weight bearing for another 6 weeks. It would appear senseless to try to save a few weeks at the risk of refracture or nonunion.

To some extent, postcast rehabilitation depends on what happened while the leg was in the cast. If, for instance, a below-knee patella tendon-bearing cast was applied, the patient will have little work to do for knee rehabilitation. Even for those patients who have long leg casts with early weight bearing, knee rehabilitation has not been a major problem.

With the early-weight-bearing technique, Dehne[72] chooses to admit his patients to the hospital after cast removal. He keeps them in bed until knee and ankle motion are regained. In civilian practice this is not always practical, and exercises can usually be supervised on an outpatient basis.

Attention is given initially to range of motion of the knee, ankle, subtalar joints, and even the toes. For the knee and ankle, simple flexion and extension exercises usually suffice if done under the direction of a competent physical therapist. Dorsi-

flexion of the foot may be difficult to restore, but with active exercise and such tricks as walking upstairs backwards, this can be solved. Inversion and eversion require active motion and, occasionally, active assistive exercises by a therapist or family member. Clawing of the toes may sometimes be corrected by manual stretching.

After the cast is removed, walking at first may be difficult, because the patient has been depending on the cast. The patient is started with crutches and partial weight bearing, which goes on quickly to full weight bearing. In other instances only a cane is needed.

Swelling of the extremity may be a problem, particularly if there has been no early weight bearing. The patient is told that he must elevate the extremity whenever he is not actually walking. When he stands the muscles must be constantly contracted. In most instances it is wise to use an elastic compression type of stocking, which must be applied in the early morning.

As range of motion starts to return, more attention is paid to strengthening the muscle groups of the lower extremity. This includes the hip abductors, the knee flexors and extensors, and the dorsiflexors and plantar flexors of the foot. Walking does not increase muscle strength greatly, and resistance exercises must be done to strengthen muscle groups. In young people, returning to such activities as walking, bicycling, and swimming helps rehabilitation and increases endurance. As range of motion and strength increase, the patients progress to jogging and finally more active sports. (The latter should not be done until strength and range of motion of the extremity are near normal.) Any type of contact sports and risk sports, such as skiing or soccer, should not be done until the internal architecture of the bone has been restored and muscle strength is normal.

CARE AFTER INTERNAL FIXATION

Most but not all tibial fractures treated by intramedullary nailing will be casted eventually. However, the immediate postoperative regimen for an intramedullary nailing of the tibia depends on the stability of the fracture and the wishes of the surgeon. The nail usually gives excellent fixation, except for rotatory stability, which ranges from excellent to only fair. Most authors prefer to leave the leg out of plaster during the initial 10 to 14 postoperative days, a practice that allows free knee, ankle, and foot motion. After this, the leg is casted and weight bearing with crutches is allowed. Healing does not occur more quickly with an intramedullary nail than with nonoperative treatment. Ascertaining fracture union may be a bit difficult with an intramedullary nail, but the stability provided by the nail provides protection with weight bearing.

A regimen similar to this is followed with compression plates. After surgery, the leg is placed on a posterior padded splint or a Thomas splint, which allows comfort and soft tissue healing. Knee, ankle, and foot are put through a gentle range of motion several times daily. After the wound is healed and swelling is gone, a snug, total-contact cast is applied, and graduated weight bearing is allowed. Most advocates of internal fixation by compression plating believe that the period of 10 to 14 days without a cast after operation restores motion to the joints of the lower extremity and that this is one of the beneficial results of compression plating. Applying the cast 2 weeks after the open reduction permits a better fitting cast that does not have to be changed.

In many instances, members of the AO group do not use a cast at all after fracture fixation. Weight bearing with crutches increases gradually as bony union progresses. The decision as to whether or not to use a cast after internal fixation must be based on the surgeon's own estimate of the rigidity of fixation and an understanding of the possible complications if the fracture is not protected further with a cast.

After the cast is removed the routine is similar to that used for a nonoperative treatment of the tibial fracture. Some authors[157] believe that during the initial 8 months after fracture the patient with a compression plate does functionally better than one with a simple closed reduction. However, by a year the results seem to be roughly equal.

PROGNOSIS

The prognosis of tibial shaft fractures depends largely on the fracture itself and the mechanism that produced the injury. The treatment method undoubtedly contributes to the prognosis, but often the method of treatment depends not only on the surgeon and his prejudices, but also on the fracture's characteristics. Thus what Nicoll[187] describes as the "personality of the fracture" seems to be the major determinant for prognosis. By this he means that there are factors inherent in all fractures that will adversely affect the prognosis, no matter what the treatment. Nicoll identifies the major adverse factors

as these: initial displacement of the fracture, soft tissue damage that includes open wounds, comminution of the fracture, and intervening infection. Each factor adversely affects healing and thus the prognosis. Many authors, including Ellis,[92] Weissman,[250] and Clancey,[55] agree that these appear to be the major determinants in the prognosis of any particular fracture. Also of importance is the violence causing the fracture, with high-energy forces causing a poorer prognosis.

HEALING TIME

The average time required for osseous union has been described for various tibial fractures by numerous authors. It is sometimes difficult to define bony union, but most authorities agree that this means radiographic evidence of trabeculae crossing the fracture line, plus the patient's ability to bear full weight on the limb without support and without pain. In adults the average time for osseous union for a closed undisplaced, uncomplicated fracture of the tibia might be 10 to 13 weeks; whereas it could be 13 to 16 weeks for a displaced fracture of the tibia and 16 to 26 weeks for an open or comminuted fracture. These are "ballpark figures." Several authors[94,187] have suggested that a mean healing time for tibial fractures should be 16 weeks, with a standard deviation of ±4 weeks. They would then arbitrarily define lack of bony union after 20 weeks as delayed union. Other authors[208,250] have stated that 26 weeks without osseous union should be the criterion for delayed union. I consider 20 weeks to be the point at which I identify delayed union.

It is also difficult to define the precise moment when delayed union becomes nonunion. Nonunion is a clinical diagnosis made by the surgeon on the basis of radiographic and clinical findings. The surgeon must see that there is obvious lack of bony union as evidenced by sclerosis of the fractured bone ends, flaring of these ends, or clinical motion in the area. When this occurs and the surgeon believes that there is no longer any potential for bony union and that the fracture must be treated by some means to obtain union, nonunion has occurred.

PROGNOSTIC SIGNS

Of the immediate prognostic signs for bony healing, probably the single best is the amount of initial displacement of the fracture. The more displaced the fracture is, the greater the likelihood of a longer healing time. Comminuted fractures take longer to heal than noncomminuted fractures. Severe initial displacement is often associated with comminution, and this combination further increases healing time. Open injuries and soft tissue wounds are other poor prognostic signs that increase the expected healing time.[4] Hoaglund and States[127] found that it was high-energy forces that caused the most severe fractures and soft tissue damage and thus fractures that took longer healing. If infection intervenes, healing time is again increased; infection is the most potent factor in producing a poor prognosis.

In summary, a high-energy force that causes an open tibial fracture with severe initial displacement, obvious comminution, and soft tissue injury with a subsequent infection has the worst prognosis.

The direction of the fracture line—oblique, transverse, spiral, or whatever—seems to have little to do with the healing time of the fracture, provided that displacement is not present and that there is no open wound or comminution. For example, an undisplaced transverse fracture seems to heal in approximately the same time as an oblique or spiral fracture in comparable position. However, transverse fractures tend to occur more often as a result of direct violence and from high-energy forces. Fractures produced this way are more likely to be initially displaced and have comminution and possibly open wounds. Oblique or spiral fractures are more likely to occur as the result of indirect violence and tend not to have as much displacement. This may indicate why some people feel that the spiral fracture inherently has a better outcome than the transverse fracture. It is the displacement that is the prognostic sign. A transverse fracture totally displaced initially has a poorer healing time than an undisplaced transverse fracture in the same area.

Segmental fractures are by definition comminuted. These have a notoriously poor prognosis. Healing time is usually longer than 6 months, and because of this poor prognosis, special treatment is recommended by many authors. This is one of the few fractures of the tibia that I believe may deserve an internal fixation device to decrease the healing time and disability. Segmental and comminuted fractures may have actual loss of bony substance, which also increases healing time. Bone loss generally results from high-energy forces that produce the other poor prognostic signs in tibial fractures.

Location of the Fracture. It has long been part of the tibial fracture folklore that fractures in the lower third heal less quickly than those in other sites. However Nicoll,[187] Ellis,[93] Weissman,[249] and Sarmiento[209] all agree that fracture healing time appears to be roughly equal in the upper, middle, and lower thirds of the tibia. Sarmiento[209] found somewhat quicker union in the upper third, but this difference of healing rate was insignificant.

Concomitant Fibular Fracture. Another factor many times thought to be significant has been the presence or absence of an associated fibular fracture.[234] Nicoll[187] and Weissman[250] found that an intact fibula may in fact indicate a better prognosis. This is because the intact fibula gives some stability and shows that, because the original force was not severe enough to cause a fracture of the fibula, displacement of the tibia is probably less severe. Sarmiento found a prolonged healing time in those patients with an intact fibula, and Teitz[234] recently reported that in patients older than age 20 the intact fibula caused delayed union in 26%. However, other evidence seems to favor a good prognosis with an intact fibula, primarily because it indicates that there was less initial displacement and damage. Although an intact fibula may at times contribute to angular deformities, particularly varus, and may make it somewhat more difficult to reduce certain tibial fractures, the intact fibula should now be thought of as a good prognostic sign rather than a poor one. However, once delayed union or nonunion has been established, resection of 1 inch (2.5 cm) of an intact or healed fibula may aid in the healing of that fracture by allowing physiologic[77] impaction of the tibia with weight bearing.

Patient's Age. The age of the patient, provided he is older than age 16, seems to have little to do with the healing of tibial fractures. All fractures of the tibia and fibula appear to heal more quickly in children under 16 than in older patients. In patients older than age 65 there may be some delay in union of shaft fractures, but it is probably insignificant and more likely is related to poor soft tissue nutrition and the incidence of soft tissue injury in that group rather than to other age factors.

Distraction. Distraction at the fracture site materially increases the chances of delayed union or nonunion. Urist[241] has estimated that a gap of 0.5 cm would take 12 months to fill in. Ellis[94] believes that as little as 1.5 mm is detrimental. However, in the absence of distraction the use of traction as a means of treatment does not delay union. It is the distraction that delays union. Many patients treated in traction are initially thought to be unsuitable for other methods of treatment (owing to severe comminution, an open wound, or other factors), and thus it appears it is the characteristics of the fracture itself rather than the treatment that implies a longer healing time.

Soft Tissue Injury. The prognosis for either residual bony deformity or residual joint stiffness and other soft tissue problems to a large degree parallels the prognosis for healing time of the fracture. Nicoll[187] in his large series found that 8.6% of the patients had significant residual deformity and 8% had disabling joint stiffness. It is assumed that a number of these patients had both residual deformity and joint stiffness. He found that the incidence of joint stiffness was nearly three times higher in moderate or severe soft tissue wounds. The time of immobilization *per se* did not significantly increase joint stiffness, but the amount of soft tissue damage seems to be the major determinant. Müller,[181] Ruedi,[207] Kristensen,[141] and other advocates of rigid internal fixation believe that they can significantly decrease the number of patients who have residual joint stiffness after tibial shaft fractures. They state that the early motion before casting (or not casting) decreases joint stiffness even in fractures with poor prognosis. They also note that compression fixation decreases the likelihood of residual bony deformity. Dehne[72,73] advocates early weight bearing, saying that it may increase the rate of bony union and does decrease the risk of residual joint stiffness. He believes that one not need risk the dangers of internal fixation to minimize joint stiffness.

Ellis,[92] in his important study of tibial shaft fractures, agreed that the severity of the initial bone and soft tissue trauma is the most important determinant of eventual function and that soft tissue loss or damage accounts for most of the residual problems. He found that 86% of 343 people with fractured tibias had excellent functional and anatomical results. Knee flexion was somewhat limited in 2.5%, and 6% had some limitation of ankle or foot motion. There were virtually no angular deformities, but 5.5% had 13 mm to 19 mm of shortening. Like others, Ellis[92] asked whether it was the immobilization in a cast that allowed organization of traumatic exudate and thus formation of fibrous adhesions with resulting stiffness, or whether the initial severity of the injury caused this reaction. The results of early weight bearing seem to indicate that mere immobilization in the cast is not the major factor.

To one reviewing the literature from 1960 to 1980, it becomes obvious that there are fewer and fewer poor results of tibial fractures. Weissman's study[250] of 140 consecutive adult tibial fractures showed only one nonunion after fracture, and 90% of his patients had normally functioning legs. The other 10% had generally minor degrees of disability. Anderson and Hutchins[9] presented 128 fractures, which were not consecutive but thought to be severe and which were selected for treatment by pins above and below the fracture site. They reported three deaths and five patients who had to undergo primary amputation of the fractured leg because of circulatory complications or massive soft tissue loss associated with severe infection. Of a total of 107 patients who had adequate follow-up, 2 developed nonunion and 3 had delayed union. All 5 of these patients were treated with cancellous bone grafts and united. Of these 107 fractures, 48 were open, 22 had major comminution, and 8 were segmental fractures. Of their 91 patients for whom final results are known, only 4 were rated as having a fair functional or anatomical result and 1 as poor. All the rest were good to excellent. Two patients had shortening of greater than 13 mm and only three had angulation of more than 10 degrees. Brown and Urban[37] reported on a series of 63 open fractures of the tibia treated with early weight bearing. All went on to union, and only 4 of the 63 had continued drainage after the fracture was healed. Although they had open comminuted wounds from missiles, 40 of these patients had no shortening, whereas 10 had shortening of 20 mm or more. Finally, in a series of segmental fractures of the tibia treated by closed intramedullary nailing, Zucman and Maurer[257] reported that of 17 segmental closed fractures, 2 nonunions developed and 15 healed primarily. In 19 open segmental fractures, 15 healed primarily, 3 developed sepsis but went on to healing, and 1 developed sepsis and nonunion.

By all accounts it would appear that the prognosis in tibial shaft fractures is improving. This is based on the recognition of the factors that adversely affect union and function and on treatment that is now based on the ability to deal with these adverse factors.

COMPLICATIONS

Many complications are possible after tibial and fibular shaft fractures. These complications may be grossly divided into those resulting from the fracture itself, perhaps because of the "personality of the fracture,'' and those complications that result from the management. Those resulting from the fracture's characteristic are more numerous and usually more severe. Much of the diversity of treatment of leg fractures has occurred in an effort to avoid complications. This section discusses not only the complications, but also their prevention and treatment.

DELAYED UNION

Delayed union is a common complication of tibial fractures. Because of statistics cited earlier in this chapter, I have chosen to call a delayed union a fracture of the tibia that does not show osseous union after 20 weeks. By this measure a certain percentage of patients do show delayed union of tibial fractures. Even in those series that have excellent results in the treatment of tibial fractures, the delayed union rate may be from 1% to 17%.[187,212] The more important figure, however, is the proportion of these delayed unions that go on to nonunion. Seemingly, the vast majority of delayed unions heal without operative intervention. Yet, delayed union is important, because it increases the patient's disability time, and the extra weeks spent in a cast increase the potential for muscle atrophy and joint stiffness.

Souter[227] has suggested that a fracture that is mobile and not united at 12 to 16 weeks should be subjected routinely to cancellous bone grafting. This does not seem reasonable to me, because many patients with delayed union at that point still have healing potential and go on to bony union. Even at 20 weeks few, if any, ununited tibias show obvious radiographic signs of nonunion. At 12 weeks, if they have not done so before, these patients should be started on full weight bearing in a long leg cast (preferable in my hands) or a patellar tendon-bearing below-knee cast. With weight bearing, most of these patients go on to union (Fig. 17-25). Resection of 1 inch (2.5 cm) of the fibula may be considered in such instances, as it has been shown to be beneficial in either delayed union or early nonunion.[77] If there is a gap between the bone ends at 20 weeks, one should consider cancellous bone grafting. At what point after 20 weeks the surgeon decides the fracture will not heal and grafting should be done is an individual decision based on clinical and radiographic signs that there is no further healing potential in the bone. With obvious radiographic signs of nonunion, ununited fractures should be treated in some way, either by grafting, by rigid internal fixation, or

perhaps by electrical stimulation.[17,36,221] If 26 weeks after a fracture, union has not occurred with an atrophic nonunion, again something must be done to increase healing potential of the fracture.

NONUNION

Nonunion of a tibia can be identified as that point in time at which the surgeon believes that radiographic and clinical signs show that the fracture no longer has potential for union and that something further must be done to enhance bony union. The usual radiographic signs of nonunion are well known and include sclerosis and flaring of the fractured ends plus lack of bone continuity (Fig. 17-26). In some instances an atrophic nonunion is seen without the usual sclerosis and flaring of the fracture ends. Clinical signs and symptoms include angulation, pain with weight bearing, and local stress tenderness. Most causes of nonunion are probably inherent in the fracture itself. Fractures that are severely displaced, have open wounds[203] or skin loss, and are severely comminuted are more likely to go on to nonunion than other fractures. There is an increased incidence in those fractures that have infection following from either an open reduction or an open wound. Other causes often cited include distraction or improper use of pins above and below the fracture, which literally hold the fracture apart instead of allowing physiologic impaction. Inadequate external immobilization and inadequate internal fixation are obvious causes of nonunion (Fig. 17-27). The present methods of compression plating and intramedullary nailing are less likely to cause nonunion than older fixation devices.[224]

Sometimes there is a fine line between delayed union and nonunion. If the surgeon thinks there is still some potential for bony union, the stimulation of weight bearing alone may induce osteogenesis. It would not be effective alone in those cases in which there is an actual pseudarthrosis.

METHODS OF TREATMENT

The easiest way to induce bony union in an ununited fracture that has firm fibrous union and reasonably good position is to add cancellous bone strips without taking down the fracture site. An ample supply of good cancellous bone must be packed around the fracture with good, vascular soft tissue adjacent. In many instances nonunion of the tibia occurs secondary to an open wound or open reduction that becomes infected. The skin anteriorly

(*Text continues on p. 1640.*)

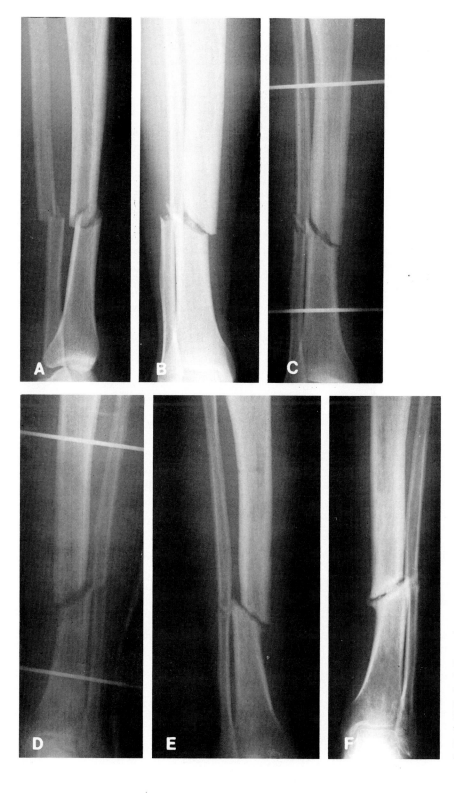

Fig. 17-25. (*A, B*) A midshaft tibial fracture. (*C*) Pins were placed above and below and an external splint was used. (*D*) Plaster was applied including the pins. The fracture was distracted. (*E*) After 6 months, avoidance of weight bearing plus the initial distraction had delayed union. (*F*) After 5 months of full weight bearing in a fiberglass cast there was clinically solid union and evidence on x-ray of early union.

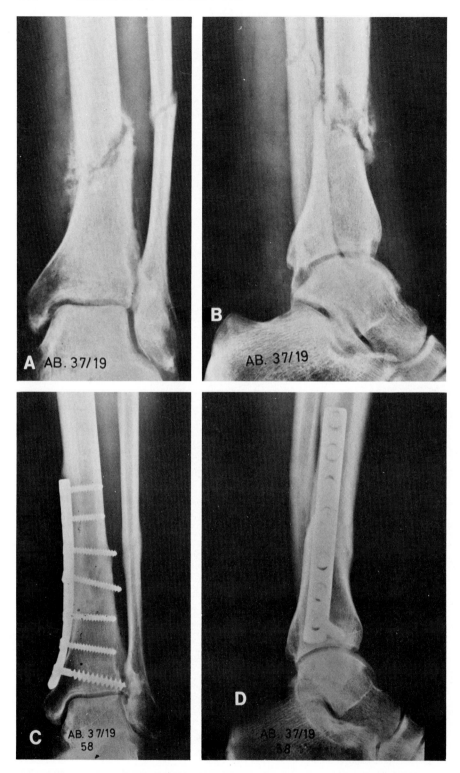

Fig. 17-26. (*A, B*) Eight-month-old nonunion of the lower tibia. (*C, D*) Eight months after application of a compression plate and weight bearing the tibia had healed. (Courtesy of Professor M. Allgöwer.)

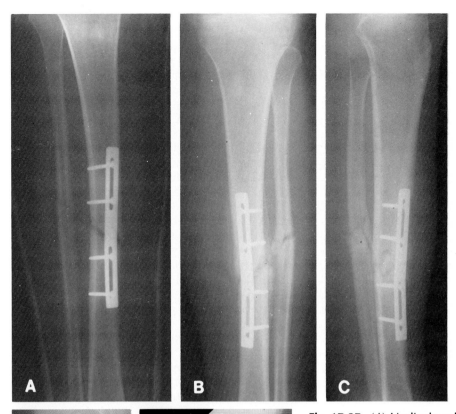

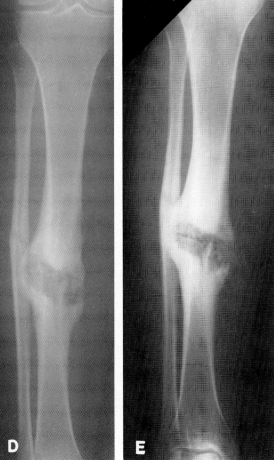

Fig. 17-27. (A) Undisplaced open tibial fracture treated with noncompression plate. (B, C) Six months later there was infection and delayed union. (D) Eleven months after fracture the drainage had stopped, but the fracture had not united. (E) Nineteen months after fracture nonunion persisted despite weight bearing in a caliper.

and medially may be poor. In such cases the posterolateral or posteromedial bone grafting approach is necessary.[117,120] Although the fracture site with its fibrous tissue is usually left intact, "fish scaling" or "shingling" of the cortical bone on either side of the fracture may be useful.

One other operation used in some instances of early nonunion is osteotomy of the fibula.[77] Lottes[155] uses this with his intramedullary nail, believing that this allows some physiologic impaction at the fracture site. This procedure has been successful in the hands of other authors, such as Brown,[37] Sorenson,[226] and Fernandez-Palazzi,[99] but it seems best for those nonunions that are either very early or in fact are delayed unions. The procedure is not indicated when there is a true pseudarthrosis, although it may be combined with grafting and internal fixation. If the fibula is healed and holding the tibia apart, one must consider osteotomy as a part of combined procedure.

Müller,[182] Ruedi,[207] and others report that rigid compression plating and early weight bearing successfully manage many nonunions. They do not advise bone grafting, which they reserve for those instances in which there is no potential left for bone healing. If the nonunion is in malposition or without a firm fibrous union, it would be wise to use internal fixation to place the fragment in proper position and maintain it firmly. In such cases, cancellous bone grafts should be added.

Intramedullary nails are also used for nonunion. Lottes[155] and others use an intramedullary nail after widely reaming out the medullary canal. They recommend fibular osteotomy plus weight bearing. Bone grafting has not always been necessary, depending to some extent on how much healing potential is present. In most instances I deem it prudent to add bone grafting to the rigid fixation.

Previously, tibial nonunions have been treated with only bone grafts, but this method of treatment is less popular and successful than the use of grafting plus compression plates. With marked loss of bony substance, dual onlay bone grafts with firm fixation can be used. There should be good vascular tissue in the area, and cancellous bone is laid in the defect between the onlay grafts.

The role of electrical stimulation as a means of combating tibial nonunions is still being delineated. There seems no doubt that it is a valuable nonoperative addition to the treatment of bony nonunion. Both pulsating electromagnetic fields and direct current have been used with success. Bassett[17] is convinced of its efficacy and has reported an 87% healing rate in 127 unhealed tibial fractures.

He did not think the presence of previous metallic implants or infection was a deterrent to its use or success. A cast must be worn throughout the treatment period and non-weight bearing is the rule during this phase.

Most advocates of electrical stimulation agree that in the presence of a true pseudarthrosis, the method is of no value. Brighton's[36] series of 178 patients with tibial nonunions had a success rate of 84%. He found that the presence of infection decreased the success rate to 74% and cautioned against electrical stimulation in a case of pseudarthrosis or when there was a gap of more than 1 cm in the bone. Other workers[221] have had similar success, and electrical stimulation presents an interesting alternative to surgery and bone grafting in the treatment of tibial nonunions.

INFECTED NONUNION

The most severe tibial problem is infected nonunion. Then the surgeon must use all modalities at his disposal. It may be difficult or impossible to eradicate the infection before attempting to obtain union. Like many authors, including Jones,[135,136] Hanson and Eppright,[117] and Reckling,[200] I believe that there is no need to clear the infection completely before trying to obtain bony union. If debridement or other procedures on the anterior aspect of the tibia have failed to eradicate the infection, but it is localized anteriorly, I believe that a posterolateral cancellous bone graft is a logical next step.[117,120] The soft tissues in this area are left intact, and no attempt is made to take down the fracture site. The object is to create a synostosis from the tibia across the interosseous membrane to the fibula, by a solid mass of bone posteriorly (Fig. 17-28). Eventually, as this area unites and weight bearing is permitted, the tibia unites. In many instances the infection previously present gradually clears after union is obtained. I do not use internal fixation if there is firm fibrous union, and one must be careful not to violate the infected anterior compartment of the leg. I allow early weight bearing in such instances after soft tissue healing. One may use the posteromedial approach if the skin is intact on that side.

With gross mobility at the fracture site, a fixation device must be considered, but there is obvious risk if there is an open anterior wound. Intramedullary nails have been used. Pins above and below, fixed either in plaster or an external device, is safer. External fixation devices can help in securing firm fixation while allowing various methods of osteogenesis to work. It is particularly helpful when there are open wounds in the presence of infection and when there is bone loss. Bone grafting can be accomplished and an external fixation device used to hold the limb out to length while waiting for healing. At the same time, infected or open wounds can be treated without difficulty.

A number of procedures have been described to establish union when there has been a loss of substance of the tibia.[49] The primary objective has been to use the fibula as a stable strut and to gradually induce union through the fibula and interosseous membrane, hoping that the tibia either will eventually bridge or that the fibula will hypertrophy enough to allow weight bearing. Initially, procedures were described by Huntington[132a] and Codivilla[59] and later by Wilson.[255] The principle is to bypass the area of bone loss in the tibia. In more recent years the use of peg grafting from fibula to tibia, as described by McMaster and Hohl,[164] has been successful, as has the procedure described by Companacci and his co-workers,[62] in which the fibula is united to the tibia proximally and distally. The latter has been exceedingly effective in their hands. These wounds with loss of bony substance, often associated with anterior infection, are the most difficult problems in the tibia, and the operative procedure must be carefully planned or disaster will ensue. A new approach to treating a bony gap in the tibia is by use of a vascularized fibular graft transferred into the tibial gap. Chacha and his associates[49] have reported good success in some patients who have had large gaps in the tibia. The procedure appears technically difficult but may help to solve this problem. It is definitely a salvage procedure and requires the use of some type of fixation device while awaiting healing.

MALUNION

What constitutes malunion of a tibial shaft fracture? Many fractures not anatomically reduced are functionally and cosmetically acceptable. How much deviation from the normal anatomical configuration constitutes a malunion? Is a fracture displaced laterally 100% the width of the shaft but solidly healed, in excellent alignment, with no angulation, and a functionally excellent result, a malunion? It might constitute some cosmetic deformity, but it would not be reasonable to take this fracture down, perform an osteotomy, and reduce it to anatomical position.

Displacement is less likely to constitute malunion than rotational or angular deformity (Fig. 17-29).

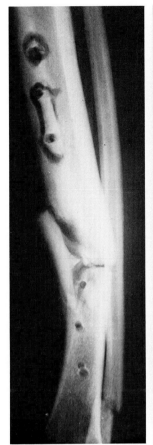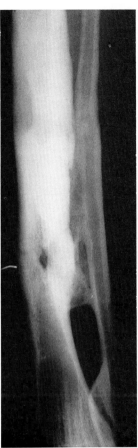

Fig. 17-28. (*Left*) Infected nonunion with bony sequestra after use of external fixation apparatus. (*Right*) Union following posterolateral bone grafting and removal of sequestra.

When reducing a fracture, I would not usually accept varus or valgus angulation of greater than 5° or an anterior or posterior angulation of the same margin. I would try to reduce such deformity by a cast change or wedging. However, if a fracture is already clinically solid with that degree of angulation, whether or not something more should be done depends on the functional and cosmetic results. More external rotation than internal may be accepted. Internal rotation of more than 5° may make for an unsightly gait, whereas external rotation of as much as 20° could be tolerated without causing a significant gait disorder.

Significant malunion appears uncommon in tibial fractures. Mild rotational disorders and angulation may occur in severe fractures with soft tissue loss, comminution, and marked initial displacement. Because most of these occur as a result of

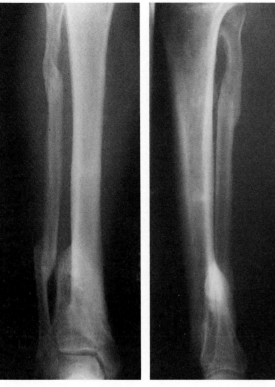

Fig. 17-29. A healed tibial fracture with the shaft offset 50%. There was an excellent cosmetic and functional result.

difficult fractures that may have had trouble with initial healing, function must be considered primarily and cosmesis, secondarily. If a malunion requires correction, a controlled osteotomy with internal fixation and cancellous bone grafting should be done. Compression plates are the most effective way to hold this osteotomy (Fig. 17-30).

Significant malunion is an avoidable complication and, fortunately, a comparatively rare occurrence in fractures of the tibia.

SHORTENING OF THE EXTREMITY

Shortening occurs frequently in tibial fractures, but it is usually minor. Early weight-bearing advocates such as Dehne,[73] Brown,[37] and Sarmiento,[212] believe that physiologic shortening allows impaction of the fracture site and promotes union. The early-weight-bearing technique may be the treatment method that causes the most shortening of tibial fractures, but even Sarmiento,[212] using the below-knee cast or brace, had a maximum shortening of 22 mm and an average of only 6.5 mm. Brown's[37]

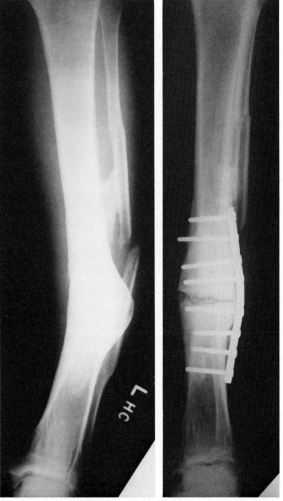

Fig. 17-30. (*Left*) Malunion of the tibia with 25° of varus. (*Right*) Normal alignment following osteotomy and plate fixation.

study of 63 patients with severe open fractures had only 10 cases with 20 mm or more of shortening. Nicoll,[187] studying many fractures treated with various closed methods, found 2.5% of his patients with 2 cm or more of shortening, while Ellis had 5.5% with 13 mm to 19 mm of shortening. Shortening does occur in tibial fractures, but in most instances it is not significant. I would agree with Sarmiento that shortening of 8 mm or less is cosmetically and functionally insignificant.

Distraction must be avoided at all costs, as even a small gap can cause a severe delay in union. Shortening of 5 mm to 8 mm seems a minor price to pay for early union of a tibial fracture, and overzealous attempts to regain complete length of the tibia as a result of repeated manipulations and traction should be discouraged.

The worst shortening problems result from either bone loss from the initial trauma or infection, primary or secondary. In such instances some shortening of the tibia may have to be accepted to allow bone union.

INFECTION

Aside from an initial major soft tissue or vascular injury that necessitates primary amputation, infection is the most significant problem in the tibia. Of all the fracture characteristics described by Nicoll,[187] the factor that implied the worst prognosis was infection. Infection, when combined with nonunion, is disastrous and always results in long-term disability and, in some instances, amputation. Infection may result from an initial open wound, usually the high-energy type associated with skin necrosis or skin loss. The other major cause of tibial infection is surgery for internal fixation and open reduction of a fracture.

A strong bias exists against the use of internal fixation in open tibial fractures. Adequate statistical evidence shows that the infection rate is higher in these instances than if no internal fixation is used, and most open tibial fractures should be treated without internal fixation. External fixation devices and pins above and below the fracture site offer other possible treatment modes. In these cases the wounds should either be closed secondarily or allowed to granulate in.

The surgeon must use every modality at his control to prevent infection. There is little controversy now regarding the use of preoperative, intraoperative, and postoperative antibiotics in open wounds[193] of the extremities, because they are effective in lowering the rate of deep wound infection. Antibiotics are never a substitute for good surgical technique, but given judiciously and combined with adequate irrigation, debridement, and proper handling of the tissues, they may be another factor in preventing wound infection.

Once infection of the tibia is established, attention must be directed not only to eradicating the infection, but also primarily to obtaining bony union. A patient may tolerate a leg with a united tibia and a draining sinus, but he cannot get by with an ununited tibia with a draining sinus.

An infected wound must be opened and adequate drainage established. The extent of the infection is delineated by x-rays, which may have to include tomograms to identify possible bony sequestra, and a sinogram to see where the infection leads. Obviously necrotic and contaminated tissue is debrided. After this, the wound may be packed open to allow secondary healing or later skin grafting, or local flap closure may be done. If the wound becomes clean, the surgeon may proceed with posterolateral bone grafting. Sometimes this has to be done even in the face of anterior infection, if this is adequately drained.

The principle of leaving an internal fixation device in place in the presence of infection if the device does stabilize the fracture is established.[159] If there is no fibrous union of a fracture that is mobile, one must consider some type of fixation device, possibly an external fixation apparatus. An intramedullary nail is risky in the face of infection, but it has been used by some authors in desperate situations.

Again, the most serious problem is the nonunion associated with infection. I have already discussed how I would deal with that in the previous section on nonunion (see p. 1640). The basic concept is to secure union first, because drainage often will cease after that. There may be some minor potential danger in a long-term draining sinus, but this is infinitely preferable to an infected nonunion, which may lead to amputation.

SKIN LOSS

The subcutaneous position of the tibia makes the leg vulnerable to skin damage or loss at the time of fracture. Open tibial fractures are common but do not always entail actual loss of skin, which usually results from massive trauma to the leg. Damaged or necrotic skin should be judiciously excised at the time of wound debridement. If, after excision of the necrotic edges, the skin may be closed without tension, this should be done. However, if there is any question of a tight closure or the skin's viability, the wound should be left open. Grafting or secondary closure may be done at a later time. Occasionally, it may be possible to make a relaxing incision over the muscle, away from the wound, and thus allow primary skin closure over the bone.

The second most common cause of skin loss in tibial fractures is secondary to an open reduction. If performed through skin previously damaged, the consequences can be a necrotic area immediately over the bone. Also, infection secondary to an open reduction may cause skin loss directly over the fracture. Skin loss may occur as the result of pressure of underlying bone fragments on the anterior skin, most common in fractures of the proximal third when the proximal fragment is anteriorly angulated. This danger is noted on a lateral x-ray and can be avoided.

An open wound, and particularly skin loss, implies a poor prognosis for the fracture. Healing time is longer and the incidence of infection, delayed union, and nonunion is increased. Yet, the principles of Winnett Orr embodied in a series by Paul Brown and Urban[37] have shown us that tibial fractures can heal despite open wounds. With this method of treatment (popularized as a result of its use in severe tibial fractures from war missile wounds), wounds are packed open and casted in plaster. The wound is allowed to heal by secondary intention. Although it has been thought that these atrophic scars may break down, many are perfectly serviceable.

Many such wounds will heal by secondary intention, but others require some type of coverage. Split-thickness skin grafts take poorly over bare bone and the process of decorticating or drilling the medullary cavity is relatively ineffective and damages the bone itself. Coverage may be gained by a vascularized flap or a flap from adjacent tissues. Pedicle flaps from the other leg are generally inadvisable. These cross-leg flaps have been replaced by the use of the vascularized free flaps[169a,218a,248a] or transposition of muscle tissue from the same leg.[105a] Split-thickness skin is then grafted on top of the vascularized muscle bed. Recent studies[55a] suggest that the earlier these free flaps are done, the better the prognosis. However, these procedures require much planning and knowledge and are best done in conjunction with someone who has had special training in these techniques, whether an orthopaedic, general, or plastic surgeon.

If there is chronic infection in the area, the infection must be cleared before an attempt is made to close the skin. Closure by secondary granulation, although slow for the patient, is sometimes the safest and most effective means of allowing these wounds to close.

AMPUTATION

Below-knee amputations may result directly from the trauma that causes a tibial fracture. The majority of such amputations are secondary to an open wound with severe soft tissue and associated vascular injuries. Vehicular accidents and crush injuries are the major causes. In any published series the rate of occurrence of primary amputations seems to depend on the type of fracture that any individual author or hospital treats. A primary accident hospital would obviously have a larger series of severely injured legs than a hospital that treats skiing injuries. The exact statistics for primary amputations resulting from tibial shaft fractures is difficult to estimate, because most authors, in discussing the treatment of tibial shaft fractures, do not include those that resulted in primary amputation.

Secondary amputations may result from secondary vascular problems or from open wounds and infection. There is probably little that can be done operatively to decrease the number of primary amputations secondary to soft tissue or bone loss or vascular injury. Many limbs are saved by arterial reconstruction, but there will still be some in which the initial injury is too great for the limb to survive. It appears that a number of tibial fractures result in secondary amputations as sequelae to infection and nonunion. Orthopaedic surgeons should be able to improve these results. Hicks[125] reported from a large accident hospital on a 12-year study of amputations due to fractures or their complications (including treatment). He stated that primary amputations occurred in 1.7% to 3.5% of the total number of fractured tibias seen at his hospital, which treats many severe automobile injuries. He felt that the single most important cause of secondary amputation was the occurrence of skin necrosis from the accident or subsequent surgery. He stated that some cases fall into the "inevitable amputation" category, and certain iatrogenic amputations are the ones that should be decreased significantly. It was his opinion that rigid internal fixation did not necessarily increase iatrogenic amputations but could decrease them. This would be difficult to prove at present, but in those severe soft tissue injuries with tibial fractures, perhaps one should look longer at rigid stabilization procedures, whether by internal fixation with plates or intramedullary nail or by the use of pins above and below and a rigid external stabilization apparatus.

VASCULAR INJURIES

Vascular injury as a direct result of tibial shaft fractures is relatively rare, except after extreme violence of the high-energy type, which causes comminuted, markedly displaced, and often open fractures of the tibia. The most common area for vascular injury is the upper quarter of the tibia, where the anterior tibial artery passes from behind through the interosseous membrane. The fracture fragment may lacerate the artery or occlude it by direct bone pressure or by soft tissue swelling (Fig.

17-31). With such injuries and irreparable vascular damage, treatment may have to be primary amputation at the level of injury.

With any lower leg fracture, the possibility of vascular injury must be considered. An obvious deformity or open wound may draw attention away from vascular injury. The examiner must feel for both the dorsalis pedis and posterior tibial pulses. If either is absent, immediate diagnostic measures are taken to ascertain the cause and correct it. With the advance of vascular surgery, microvascular repairs of even the anterior and posterior tibial arteries are seen. The decision as to whether or not a repair of this sort should be attempted depends on the vascular status of the leg, because the lower leg can usually well survive the loss of either one of these major arteries. One must remember that there can be a dorsalis pedis pulse despite occlusion of the anterior tibial artery high in the leg, if blood is shunted from the posterior tibial to the peroneal artery and then to the dorsalis pedis. Thus, even with peripheral pulses, if there is clinical concern about the arterial blood supply to a leg because or poor color, slow capillary filling, or signs of muscle ischemia, an arteriogram should be obtained to demonstrate the patency or lack thereof of the arterial tree.

One other fracture that may involve the anterior tibial artery occurs in the lower tibia when the foot and lower tibia are displaced posteriorly. This causes the anterior tibial artery to go over a sharp proximal fragment and course backward, which may cause pressure on the artery. With such a deformity, the surgeon should immediately try to reduce the fracture at least partially by bringing the distal fragment forward. Again, without immediate return of normal circulation, an arteriogram is needed. The anterior tibial artery is more likely to be involved in tibial fractures, and with the posterior tibial artery completely patent, it is probable that a limb would survive, even with complete occlusion of the anterior tibial artery. However, the anterior compartment muscles would not survive. Exploration of either anterior or posterior tibial artery is imperative if a block is suspected. Sometimes pressure may be relieved by reducing the bony fragments. Other times the artery will be decompressed, stripped, and injected with papaverine to decrease spasm. In many instances repair of the artery may be needed. I believe that a vascular surgeon should do the arterial repair, but there can be a problem of availability. In such an instance one would try to call a vascular surgeon and then have the most experienced member of the team be prepared to

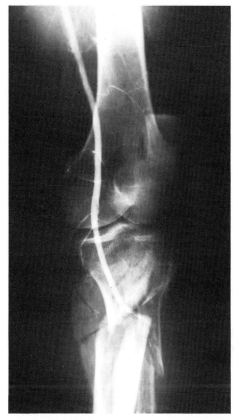

Fig. 17-31. Severe comminuted fracture of the upper tibia. The arteriogram showed blockage of the anterior tibial artery.

go ahead with the vascular repair in emergency cases. The orthopaedic surgeon must be prepared to stabilize the fracture in some manner so as to not jeopardize this arterial repair. This may be done with an intramedullary rod, a compression plate, pins above and below in plaster, or an external fixation apparatus. Internal fixation may not always be necessary, but stability is needed for the arterial repair to survive. If internal fixation is to be performed before the arterial repair, it must be done quickly. Ideally, rigid fixation of the fracture before arterial repair would be best. However, the viability of the limb is of primary concern, and if some hours have elapsed since injury, it may be necessary to do the arterial repair first and then stabilize the fracture, either by internal or external fixation.

The posterior tibial artery is less likely to be involved in fractures of the tibia than the anterior tibial artery. Cases have been reported with posterior intracompartmental pressure rises in which the posterior tibial artery has been partially occluded. Jefferys[134] recorded three cases that responded well to exploration and stripping of the arteries plus papaverine injection. Both Owen[190] and Seddon[217] have reported on ischemic changes in the posterior compartment that led to claw toes in the postfracture period. This may be difficult to recognize and to treat, because the symptoms are certainly not as dramatic as those of an elevated pressure in the anterior compartment.

Several instances of aneurysms[68] of the upper portion of the anterior tibial artery have been reported after tibial fracture. In such an instance, with the fracture healed, the arterial supply to the foot appeared to be intact initially, but severe local swelling plus a bruit in the area of the aneurysm led to the discovery of this vascular complication. It is a rare finding.

ANTERIOR COMPARTMENT SYNDROME

One treatable complication of tibial fractures is the anterior tibial compartment syndrome. It tends to follow minor closed fractures[142,151,222] rather than the severer ones in which the interosseous membrane is disruptured, or open fractures, because in those instances the anterior compartment decompresses itself. However, it has been reported in open fractures of the tibia; thus an open fracture does not rule out the possibility of a compartment syndrome occurring. A compartment syndrome can occur with an undisplaced fracture. I have seen several patients with compartment syndromes occurring 48 hours after fracture, apparently secondary to repeated manipulations.

Although the anterior tibial compartment syndrome was the first to be well recognized, it is now understood that both the posterior and lateral compartments can be involved secondary to tibial fractures. These are discussed in the next section.

The anterior compartment syndrome comes about because of increased pressure in the closed confines of the anterior tibial compartment, which is bounded by the tibia, the fascia of the anterior compartment, the fibula, and the interosseous membrane. After a tibial fracture with the resultant hemorrhage and soft tissue edema secondary to trauma, there is increased pressure within the compartment. This pressure impedes venous outflow and gradually occludes the small arterioles and capillaries carrying blood to the muscles. Ischemia of the anterior compartment muscles soon follows, and eventually pressure occludes the anterior tibial artery. Symptoms may not appear for 24 hours after injury, at which point a cast has been in place. This cast may cause further embarrassment and increased pressure.

Clinically, pain in the leg becomes more severe despite the fact that the fracture has been reduced and casted. If pain increases, the cast should be bivalved immediately and the leg should be inspected. If the most severe tenderness is not over the fracture site but over the muscles of the anterior compartment, this is highly suspicious. Usually, the anterior compartment muscles are hard on palpation. The dorsalis pedis pulse may be intact, although late in the course of the syndrome it may disappear. However, a full-blown anterior tibial compartment syndrome is possible with a booming dorsalis pedis pulse and normal sensation. After muscle pain the most common signs relate to the common peroneal nerve. One may find lack of sensation, particularly in the first dorsal cleft between the great and second toes. First weakness and, eventually, paralysis occur in the extensor hallucis longus, extensor digitorum longus, and anterior tibial muscles.

Once the diagnosis of the anterior compartment syndrome is suspected, one should proceed immediately, with either studies to document the anterior compartment pressure or a complete fasciotomy of the anterior compartment. In some instances the diagnosis is so obvious that compartmental pressures do not have to be taken, and one should go ahead with the fasciotomy rather than procrastinate. However, the compartmental syndromes can be accurately measured by a variety of the techniques that have been recently reported by Mubarak and his associates,[180] Matsen,[170] and Whitesides.[252] To acquaint himself thoroughly with the findings in the compartment syndromes, the reader should refer to these articles[180,252] and, in particular, to the complete text by Matsen.[170]

Ischemic muscle will not survive longer than 6 to 8 hours. The diagnosis is made on an index of clinical suspicion, acute tenderness over the anterior compartment, weakness or paralysis of these same muscles, and often sensation loss in the first dorsal cleft region of the toes. In the late stages there is no dorsalis pedis pulse. Fasciotomy of the anterior compartment must be total, but the surgeon should try to keep away from the fracture site itself. A longitudinal fasciotomy is performed, plus several horizontal fascial incisions. The skin may sometimes be closed, but if it is tense, it is best left open and closed secondarily.

After fasciotomy the patient may be treated with an external fixation device or even with traction from a pin in the lower tibia or os calcis for a short period. The foot must be kept in neutral position, in case there is subsequent paralysis of the anterior compartment muscles. This prevents the foot from going into equinus, and the patient even with paralyzed compartment muscles may have a tenodesis of the anterior tibial muscle and no resulting foot drop.

POSTERIOR AND LATERAL COMPARTMENT SYNDROMES

Involvement of both the posterior and the lateral compartments is less common than the involvement of the anterior compartment. Nonetheless, the consequences of posterior or lateral compartment syndromes, particularly involving the posterior deep compartment, can be as disastrous as that of the anterior compartment. Owen and his associates[190] and Matsen and Clawson[171] have called attention to the posterior compartment syndrome. This is characterized by severe pain in the posterior compartment, plantar hypesthesia, and weakness of toe flexion. Pain is intensified by passive toe extension. The examiner will see tenseness of the fascia between the tibia and the triceps surae in the distal medial aspect of the leg.

If this condition is left untreated, it will lead to claw toes and a possible posterior tibial neuropathy. Some of the claw toes seen in previous years that were thought to be caused by poor casting, were undoubtedly caused by a mild posterior compartment syndrome.

The compartment pressures can be studied in the manner referenced under the anterior compartment syndrome.[180,252] If the pressure is up or if the diagnosis is thought to be obvious, a medial approach is used to incise the transverse crural septum and the crural fascia. The tibial origin of the soleus has to be released and, in some instances, individual muscle epimysium has to be released.

The lateral compartment includes the peroneal muscles and is characterized by severe pain in this area plus weakness of those two muscle groups. It is less likely to be involved in either the anterior or posterior compartment but may be involved in a tricompartmental syndrome. In some cases in which there has been severe trauma to the lower extremity and a compartment syndrome is either recognized or worried about in all three compartments, Ernst[96] has advised doing a fibulectomy as a means of decompressing all three compartments. This would be an unusual circumstance, but it is a possible way of decompressing the compartments.

The basic therapeutic concept with all the compartment syndromes is to recognize the possibility of occurrence. Accurate muscle and nerve testing must be done, and if a compartment syndrome is suspected, pressures should be taken. Once the diagnosis is considered and then confirmed, either clinically or by studies, a release of the involved compartment must be done immediately.

NERVE INJURY

Primary nerve injury as a direct result of the trauma causing a fracture of the tibial or fibular shaft is uncommon. The combination of high-energy upper tibial and fibular fractures with gross displacement of the distal fragment into a varus position could produce immediate injury to the peroneal nerve as could direct trauma to the fibular neck area. Both injuries are rare, but in any fracture of the lower leg, function of the posterior tibial, deep peroneal, and superficial peroneal nerves must be checked immediately, because secondary nerve dysfunction is not uncommon. Dorsiflexion and plantar flexion of both the foot and toes can usually be accomplished if the fracture is stabilized and if the patient can be cajoled into moving his toes. Sensation is checked over the leg and foot and particularly in the first dorsal cleft region.

Nerve injury in the lower leg as a result of fracture is more likely to be secondary to swelling in the soft tissues of the leg or to cast pressure over the fibular neck where the peroneal nerve crosses into the anterior compartment of the leg. Function of the nerve is checked before fracture reduction and then immediately after the reduction and cast application. When applying a cast, carefully pad the area around the fibular head and neck. Do not pull the padding tight, and be sure that the free edge of the lower leg cast does not impinge where the peroneal nerve crosses. During the first 48 hours, dorsiflexion and plantar flexion of the toes should be checked at 4-hour intervals, to be sure there is no cast pressure. A physician or nurse, the patient, or his family should be able to note this. Secondary nerve paralysis is an avoidable complication. Pressure on a nerve for even an hour may cause neurapraxia. If the cast and soft padding are quickly split and pressure is completely relieved, the nerve should recover. Pressure for 6 to 12 hours may result in permanent nerve damage. If at any time the physician is suspicious of a peroneal nerve palsy, this dictates bivalving the cast and cutting the Webril. Once a palsy has occurred, the patient's foot must be splinted in neutral position while waiting to see if function will return. Serial electromyograms may be done after 3 weeks to follow the progress of the nerve. If after 10 to 12 weeks there is no sign of return of sensory or motor function, no advancing Tinel's sign, and no progress on an electromyogram, it may be wise to explore the nerve at the fibular neck and do a neurolysis and possibly resection of the fibular head. With no late return and total paralysis of the dorsiflexors of the foot, a transfer of the posterior tibial muscle through the interosseous membrane onto the dorsum of the foot usually provides satisfactory function.

JOINT STIFFNESS AND ANKYLOSIS

Bony or fibrous ankylosis of any lower leg joint after tibial fracture is uncommon. However, joint stiffness involving the knee, ankle, or subtalar joints occurs. There are two schools of thought relating to joint stiffness after fracture. One believes that it is a result of prolonged immobilization; the other, that it is the result of the initial soft tissue injury or secondary infection consequent to the injury or fracture treatment. The dispute is difficult to resolve, because those fractures that have the most severe soft tissue injury or infection are precisely those that are immobilized the longest.

Any loss of knee extension would be significant but fortunately this is rare in lower leg fractures. Some loss of knee flexion is common, but it is generally relatively insignificant. Ankle and foot stiffness are more common. Nicoll found in his study of 241 patients that severe ankle stiffness, defined as 50% loss of extension or flexion, occurred in 5 cases and severe foot stiffness, defined as 50% loss of inversion or eversion, in 11 cases.

Many of the treatment methods of the past two decades have been predicated on the possibility of getting joints to move more quickly. The proponents of rigid internal fixation cite joint stiffness as a major reason for using compression plates. After compression plating the patient is left out of plaster and all joints are moved for 10 to 14 days. This has definite advantages. However, in a series reported by Lucas,[157] it was found that although these patients seemed to be doing better 8 months after fracture, by a year after fracture, patients treated in a cast and those treated by compression plating had essentially the same functional result. One problem is that certain fractures that have a poor prognosis (*i.e.*, those with open wounds or soft tissue loss) may not be amenable to treatment by a compression plate and would have to be treated by casting. Thus those poor results attributed to cast treatment may actually be the result of the severity of the soft tissue wound.

Sarmiento,[212] with his use of a patellar tendon-bearing cast and the short leg brace, has tried to mobilize the knee and the ankle as soon as possible. Early weight bearing in tibial fractures also seems

to decrease stiffness of the joints of the lower extremity.

Once the patient is out of plaster, it is relatively easy, by active exercises, to mobilize the knee and the ankle. Normal walking helps both, and going up and down stairs increases knee motion and ankle motion. It is more diffcult to regain inversion and eversion of the foot, and this often requires the assistance of a therapist with active assistive exercises.

Joint stiffness has remained a significant problem with tibial shaft fractures. The use of rigid internal fixation, early weight bearing, and various casts and appliances to allow free motion of lower extremity joints is helpful but has not solved the problem.

TRAUMATIC ARTHRITIS

Traumatic arthritis may occur in tibial shaft fractures that involve the tibial plafond. The key to reducing the incidence is to reconstruct the joint accurately. A poorly reduced tibial plafond fracture eventually deteriorates, causing traumatic arthritis and necessitating a future ankle arthrodesis if pain increases.

POST-TRAUMATIC DYSTROPHY

Post-traumatic dystrophy follows tibial fractures more commonly in patients who cannot bear weight early and in those who are in a cast for a long time. Consequently, it is more common in severe fractures, particularly those with soft tissue damage. The condition occurring in the leg and foot is a massive sympathetic response resulting initially in swelling and pain in the extremity and going on to a late atrophic stage.

Post-traumatic dystrophy can always be treated, provided the patient can be convinced that graduated weight bearing is the answer. The swelling causes pain, and this must be decreased. Elastic stockings, intermittent elevation, and active muscle exercises all help to decrease swelling. I have occasionally tried to decrease swelling swiftly by hospitalizing the patient, putting a cast on the lower leg and foot, and suspending it from a Balkan frame for constant elevation. Usually, after 2 to 3 days all the soft tissue swelling is gone. With a well-fitted support stocking the patient ambulates briefly several times a day and elevates the leg the rest of the time. If such a regimen is followed, the swelling decreases gradually. The key is to have the patient bear weight gradually. This may be a long and tedious process for both physician and patient. Initially, crutches are used, but weight bearing is increased gradually to the point where no support is used. Some pain must be accepted by the patient so that weight bearing can continue.

The radiographic finding is marked demineralization, spotty in nature and involving the bones of the foot and the lower tibia (Fig. 17-32). Gradual remineralization occurs as the patient bears weight. There is probably no sure way to avoid posttraumatic dystrophy, but prompt mobilization of the leg and early weight bearing appears most likely to help. This condition has often been called Sudeck's atrophy, but the better term is post-traumatic dystrophy.

CAUSES AND MANAGEMENT OF REFRACTURE

An inadequately healed fracture may refracture if the cast is removed too soon or if unusually great stress is applied to a healed but still weaker-than-normal tibia. This is particularly likely in young patients who are engaged in athletic activities. Athletically inclined people should not be allowed to participate in contact or stress sports until the musculature of the involved leg regains normal strength and until the intramedullary canal of the tibia has remodelled. This remodelling may take 9 to 24 months.

One major problem with the use of rigid compression plates has been the occurrence of bone osteopenia underneath the compression plate. This may lead to a fracture through this weakened bone after the removal of the plate and this can occur up to 9 months after plate removal. A better known cause of pathologic fractures are the screws and screw holes used for various reductions. A screw hole takes about 6 months to fill in with normal bone and even a screw in intact bone acts as a stress point. If the bone is subjected to unusual forces, this may cause a fracture going through the old screw hole or, in more rare instances, through the area where the screw is still present.

In most instances refracture can be treated simply by casting and treating as if it were a primary fracture. If possible, the patient should attempt weight bearing early to prevent gross bone demineralization. If the initial fracture showed delayed union, and if it appears that the patient is in for another long-term treatment, the surgeon should consider cancellous bone grafts early.

Some refractures are seen in healthy young adults who had a skiing fracture of the lower quarter of

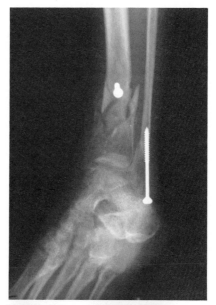

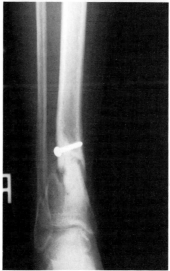

Fig. 17-32. (*Top*) Painful post-traumatic dystrophy followed open reduction, delayed union, and non-weight bearing. (*Bottom*) One year later, after 4 months of full weight bearing in a cast, there was solid union and no pain.

the tibia, commonly called a boot-top fracture.[54] After such a fracture there may be poor remineralization of the lower part of the bone, which appears weaker than normal and can be subject to fracture with athletic activities. Such a patient must be protected and not allowed to engage in skiing or other active sports until remineralization of the lower part of the tibia has occurred.

Refracture would be most severe in a tibia that had poor bone substance because of previous bone loss or infection. In such a case, with no active infection, it might be wise to add bone graft to this area.

PATHOLOGIC FRACTURES

Pathologic fractures of the tibia may occur secondary to a variety of benign or malignant bone tumors and to a number of other conditions. It is, however, not a common cause of fractures of the tibia. Possibly the most common benign lesion that causes pathologic fractures is a nonosteogenic fibroma. Treatment for the fracture is as for any tibial fracture, although occasionally, after the fracture has healed, the benign tissue may be removed and bone grafting accomplished.

One other bone lesion that can lead to pathologic fractures of the tibia is Paget's disease. In some instance the fracture is secondary to a malignant degeneration of the pagetoid tissue. In other cases it occurs simply because the bone is weaker than normal. These fractures will heal. Closed treatment is generally applicable, but the patient should be started on weight bearing early to possibly decrease calcium loss, which further weakens the bone. Intramedullary nails seem contraindicated because of the difficulty of reaming. If internal fixation were to be used, compression plates would seem most reasonable. As in all pagetoid bone, bleeding may be unusually profuse. It seems essential that the patient bear weight on the limb and that protection continue longer than usual.

CLAW TOES

Claw toes are an uncommon cause of significant disability at the conclusion of fracture healing. They can be severe, particularly if they occur as a result of ischemia of the posterior compartment muscles.[58] They are rarely caused by tethering of the long extensor tendons by callus on the anterior aspect of the tibia. While in a cast the patient should be encouraged to flex and extend his toes frequently during the day. Passive stretching should be done at least once a day.

FAT EMBOLISM

Fat embolism may occur secondary to a tibial fracture. The systemic signs and symptoms are the same as for other instances of fat embolism. The subject is covered thoroughly in Chapter 4.

STRESS FRACTURES

Stress fractures of the tibia or fibula occur in special groups of young people: athletes, particularly runners, ballet dancers, military recruits. Morris and Blickenstaff[179] found in their study of 700 military recruits with stress fractures that 17% of these fractures occurred in the tibia and 1% in the fibula. In military recruits the majority of stress fractures of the tibia occur in the upper third and involve both cortices with the reaction being most marked at the posterior medial aspect of the tibia. In young athletes there seems to be more involvement of the metaphyseal area at the junction of the middle and lower third,[80] whereas in ballet dancers reported by Burrows,[38] most of the fractures were found in the middle third of the tibia. Stress fractures of the fibula are inclined to occur just above the ankle, particularly in runners.

CLINICAL COURSE

The common clinical course is that of an onset of insidious soreness in the leg that occurs during and increases with activity. This prodromal period gradually moves into another stage in which pain occurs both during and after activity and even at night. Rarely, there is a significant fall or some trauma that causes displacement of what was apparently a preexisting stress fracture. This displaced fracture may then require reduction and casting, like that for any routine fracture. The ordinary stress fracture has direct tenderness over the site of the fracture plus swelling and thickening of the soft tissues in the area. Persistence of pain even in the face of an initial negative x-ray makes follow-up examination mandatory.

The diagnosis may be difficult to distinguish from the acute anterior compartment syndrome, the chronic anterior compartment syndrome, or "shin splints." The pain in either compartment syndrome is directly over the muscles of the anterior compartment. In the acute form, pain becomes severe even with rest and goes on to cause muscle ischemia, weakness, and loss of sensation in the foot and leg. In the chronic form, pain lessens quickly after activity and there is no bone tenderness. Shin splints characteristically cause pain where the muscles attach to the tibia, particularly at the posteromedial border of the tibia. The rest of the bone is not tender. Only stress fractures have radiographic findings, even though they may take 2 to 4 weeks to develop.

X-rays taken within the first 2 to 4 weeks of the

onset of pain may show nothing. After that, there will be a soft periosteal reaction and a narrow transverse radiolucent line that may involve only one cortex or both. Some bony sclerosis, particularly around the cortex, surrounds this fracture line (Fig. 17-33). In some instances in which a stress fracture is suspected, it may be efficacious to do a bone scan to pick up the stress fracture.[106,197] Evidence shows that the bone scan will show a stress fracture several weeks before evidence is seen on the plain films and, in some instances, may show the best evidence of a stress fracture.

Fibular stress fractures generally occur in the lower portion of the fibula, particularly in the

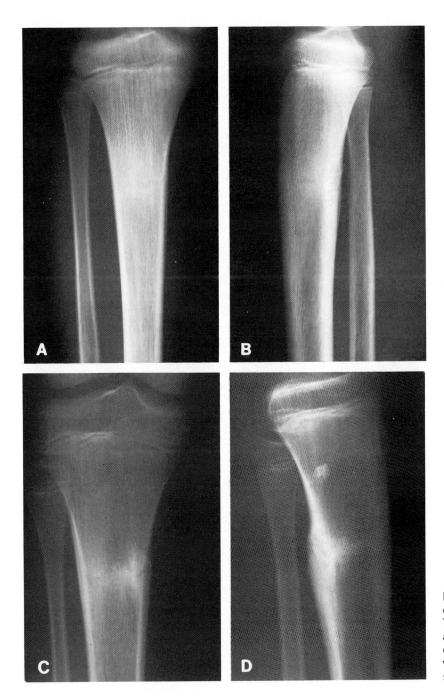

Fig. 17-33. (*A, B*) A military recruit had leg pain for 2 weeks. There was a faint periosteal reaction and the radiolucent line of a stress fracture. (*C, D*) Nine weeks after onset of pain the stress fracture had healed.

posterolateral aspect. The onset, although usually insidious, occasionally may be more acute, as reported by Devas.[82] The symptoms, signs, and radiographic findings are the same as for the tibia.

TREATMENT

Treatment is variable. In all instances activity must be markedly decreased or the patient will continue to have pain. Crutch walking without a cast may be enough in some instances. Some of these fractures may apparently heal in 2 to 3 months, but if the patient returns to full activity, symptoms may recur. Burrows reported a case in which, 3 months after apparent healing, symptoms recurred. Most patients will not require casting with stress fractures. They must be taken off the athletic activity or unusual activity that caused the stress fracture. In rare instances casting will be required. The time required for healing can be from 6 to 10 weeks, and weight bearing should be allowed during that time.

FRACTURES OF THE FIBULAR SHAFT

In contrast to fractures of the fibula near the ankle, isolated fibular shaft fractures are uncommon. Nearly all fibular shaft fractures occur as the result of the same violence that caused a tibial shaft fracture. In such cases the treatment of the fibular fracture is the same as that for the tibial fracture. Complications from a fibular fracture are most unlikely, and no real consequence would ensue, even should there be nonunion.

A simple fracture of the fibular shaft without associated tibial or ankle injury generally results from direct violence to the fibula. Local tenderness, swelling, and pain, plus difficulty walking are virtually the only signs and symptoms. One would expect no nerve or vascular damage, and the fracture generally is in excellent alignment and position.

For relief from pain, a cast should be applied, although healing of a fibular shaft fracture would probably occur even if there were no treatment. A long leg cast is most comfortable, but after 2 weeks it may be cut down to a short leg cast. Immediate weight bearing may be allowed, and the cast is removed by 6 weeks, when healing should be completed. The immediate use of a weight-bearing cast makes the postplaster rehabilitation period simple and short.

Ordinarily, the fibular shaft participates mini-mally in weight bearing[218] and serves primarily as a place of origin for some muscles of the leg and as an attachment for the interosseous membrane. Thus if pain is not severe (as is indeed the case with most undisplaced fibular shaft fractures), a cast may not be needed. The patient can be put on crutches, with the leg supported by an elastic bandage starting from the toes and going up to the knee. This may be all that is needed for a patient with good pain tolerance. Fibular nonunions are uncommon but can occur. If the nonunion is painful with weight bearing, it could be treated with a graft and internal fixation or by electrical stimulation.

FRACTURES OF THE TIBIAL PLAFOND

One of the least common but most difficult fractures to handle is that involving the lower tibia extending through the tibial plafond into the ankle joint[65,150] (Fig. 17-34). This usually results from a fall from a height as the talus is forced into the tibial plafond at the time of impact, initiating a fracture that may extend in a spiral or longitudinal fashion up the tibial shaft itself. The fracture may also occur as the result of an auto accident in which the foot is trapped and pressure is applied to the plantar surface, again forcing the talus against the tibial plafond.

The most important aspect of the injury is that it involves the articular surface of the ankle. However, there may also be extensive soft tissue injury with severe swelling. Provided there is no actual dislocation of the ankle, the dorsalis pedis and posterior tibial pulses are likely to be intact, but circulation should be checked carefully in lower tibial fractures. This injury may involve simply the tibial plafond and adjacent tibia or other parts of the ankle itself.

In instances in which the fracture is less severe with a simple crack through the plafond and lower tibia, it may be possible to manipulate and cast it in the usual fashion as a routine tibial shaft fracture. The foot may have to be in some equinus to avoid posterior angulation at the fracture site. The treatment of this particular fracture is the same as that for any other tibial fracture, except that bearing weight is inadvisable until solid bony union occurs.

In instances with comminution of the tibia plafond and perhaps of the talar dome itself, the surgeon has to decide whether the ankle joint surface can be reconstituted surgically or if this is

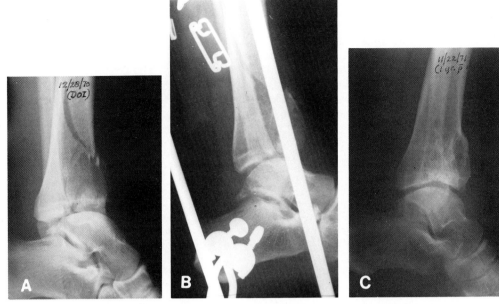

Fig. 17-34. (*A*) A comminuted fracture involving the lower tibia and plafond. (*B*) Ten days after traction was applied through a calcaneal pin, the patient could move the ankle. (*C*) One year after injury there was good joint space and excellent function. (Courtesy of Frank Wilson, M.D.)

impossible and the patient might best be treated by traction and early motion.[196] Primary arthrodesis does not seem a good choice, because an arthrodesis of the ankle can be done anytime with a good result. The ankle seems to react better to trauma than most joints, and every attempt should be made to preserve the ankle joint. Thus even if it is decided that the ankle joint cannot be reconstituted surgically, arthrodesis constitutes no emergency. It would be best to apply a cast for several weeks and reduce swelling by elevation, and after that any surgical procedure can be done with greater safety.

In many tibial plafond fractures with an intact talus a common method of treatment is to put a pin through the os calcis and apply traction on a Böhler–Braun frame or a Thomas splint. The traction allows reduction of pain and early motion and will help pull the fragments that are attached to ligaments into place (see Fig. 17-34). However, any articular fragments that have been driven up into the tibia in the middle will not be brought into position by this method. Traction may give excellent functional results in many instances, even when x-rays may not look perfect. Over a period of years a certain number of these patients may be

expected to develop traumatic arthritis, but x-rays do not necessarily parallel clinical symptoms.

Advocates of compression plating, particularly Rüedi[204–206] and Leach[150] believe that this fracture involving the lower tibia and tibial plafond is an excellent one for open reduction and internal fixation with compression plates and intrafragmentary screws. If the comminuted fragments are so small that they cannot be re-assembled, this may not be possible. However, most of the time a reasonable, if not perfect, reconstitution of the joint surface can be made (Fig. 17-35). Properly contoured compression plates plus cancellous bone screws will allow stability ranging from very firm to less firm fixation (Fig. 17-36). With less firm fixation, compression plating can be combined with os calcis traction to allow early motion. Autogenous bone grafting to fill in the defects above the plafond is usually necessary when open reduction is performed. The operation must be performed meticulously to avoid denuding bone fragments and thus increasing the risk of infection to delayed union. Fixation should be as rigid as possible to allow early motion, because there is less benefit from open reduction without early motion. Scheck[214] has advised the use of

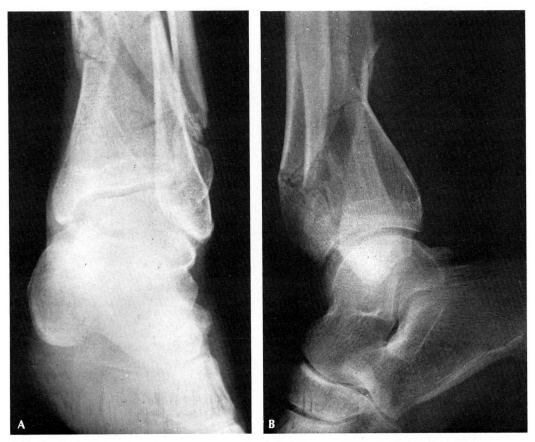

Fig. 17-35. (*A, B*) Comminuted tibial and tibial plafond fracture. (*C, D*) Restoration of length and articular surface after open reduction and internal fixation.

limited open reduction plus traction to stabilize these fractures. This may be reasonable in certain instances. However, if one is going to operate, one should try to do the complete job and reconstitute and hold the fragments firmly.

An alternative method of treatment with fractures of the tibial plafond and shaft and the fibular shaft is to stabilize only the fibular shaft (Fig. 17-37). This may aid in reduction of the other fracture fragments and restore the ankle joint anatomy without an operation over the major fracture area. This has limited use and might be used when there are open wounds or perhaps when it has been decided that there is no way of reconstituting the articular surface of the talus and plafond. It can be combined with os calcis pin traction.

As in all fractures involving the articular surface, the key is accurate repositioning of the joint fragments and firm fixation with early motion. If rigid fixation is impossible, traction may be a good alternative.

REFERENCES

1. Abbott, L. C.: The use of Iliac Bone in the Treatment of Ununited Fractures. A.A.O.S. Instructional Course Lectures, Vol. 2. Ann Arbor, J. W. Edwards, 1944.
2. Adler, J. B.; Shaftan, G. W.; Rabinowitz, J. G.; and Herbsman, H.: Treatment of Tibial Fractures. J. Trauma, **2:**59–75, 1962.
3. Albert, M.: Delayed Union in Fractures of the Tibia and Fibula. J. Bone Joint Surg., **26:**566–578, 1944.
4. Allum, R. L., and Mowbray, M. A. S.: A Retrospective Review of the Healing of Fractures of the Shaft of the Tibia with Special Reference to the Mechanism of Injury. Injury, **11:**304–308, 1980.
5. Alms, M.: Medullary Nailing for Fractures of the Shaft of the Tibia. J. Bone Joint Surg., **44B:**328–339, 1962.
6. Andersen, M. K.; McDonald, K.; and Stephens, J. G.: A

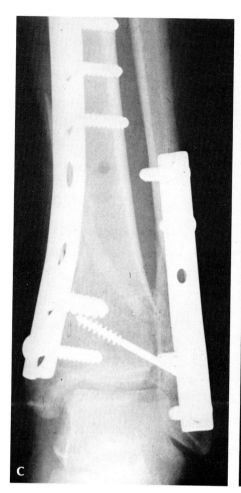

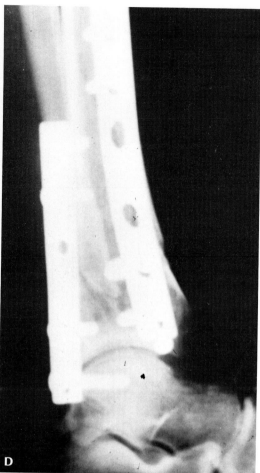

Study of the Effect of Open and Closed Treatment on Rate of Healing and Complications in Fractures of the Tibial Shaft. J. Trauma, **1:**290–297, 1961.

7. Anderson, L. D.: Compression Plate Fixation and the Effect of Different Types of Internal Fixation on Fracture Healing. J. Bone Joint Surg., **47A:**191–208, 1965.

8. Anderson, L. D., and Hutchins, W. C.: Fractures of the Tibia and Fibula Treated with Casts and Transfixing Pins. South. Med. J., **59:**1026–1032, 1966.

9. Anderson, L. D.; Hutchins, W. C.; Wright, P. E.; and Disney, J. M.: Fractures of the Tibia and Fibula Treated by Casts and Transfixing Pins. Clin. Orthop., **105:**179–191, 1974.

10. Anderson, R.: An Automatic Method of Treatment for Fractures of the Tibia and Fibula. Surg. Gynecol., Obstet., **58:**639–646, 1934.

11. Anson, B. J.: Morris' Human Anatomy. 12th ed. New York, McGraw-Hill, 1966.

12. Ashbaugh, D. G., and Petty, T. L.: The use of Corticosteroids in the Treatment of Respiratory Failure Associated with Fat Embolism. Surg. Gynecol., Obstet., **123:**493–500, 1966.

13. d'Aubigne, R. M.: Infection in the Treatment of Ununited Fractures. Clin. Orthop., **43:**77–82, 1965.

14. d'Aubigne, R. M.: Surgical Treatment of Non-union of Long Bones. J. Bone Joint Surg., **31A:**256–266, 1949.

15. d'Aubigne, R. M., and Maurer, P.: Traitment des Pseud-arthroses graves de Jambe. Mem. Acad. Chir., **85:**673–677, 1959.

16. d'Aubigne, R. M.; Maurer, P.; Zucman, J.; and Masse, Y.: Blind Intramedullary Nailing for Tibial Fractures. Clin. Orthop., **105:**267, 1974.

17. Bassett, C. A.; Mitchell, S. N.; and Gaston, S. R.: Treatment of Ununited Tibial Diaphyseal Fractures with Pulsing Electromagnetic Fields. J. Bone Joint Surg., **63A:**511–523, 1981.

18. Batten, R. L.; Donaldson, L. J.; and Aldridge, M. J.: Experience with the A-O Method in the Treatment of 142 Cases of Fresh Fracture of the Tibial Shaft Treated in the U.K. Injury. **10:**108–114, 1978.

19. Bauer, G., and Edwards, P. O.: Fracture of the Shaft of the Tibia. Incidence of Complications as a Function of Age and Sex. Acta Orthop. Scand., **36:**95–103, 1965–1966.

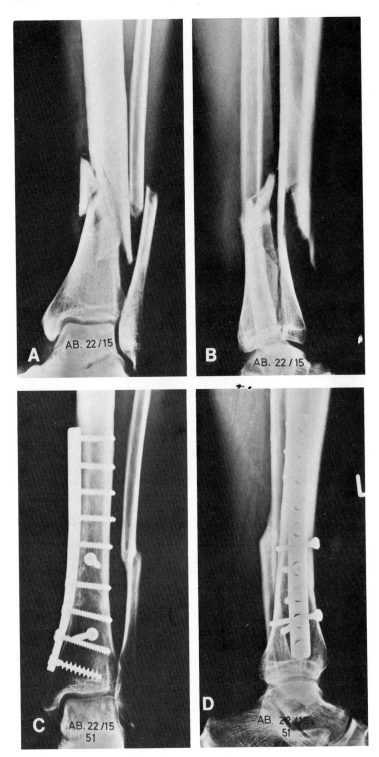

Fig. 17-36. (A, B) This comminuted distal tibial fracture extended into the tibial plafond. (C, D) Six months later there was solid union with a normal ankle joint. (Courtesy of Professor M. Allgöwer.)

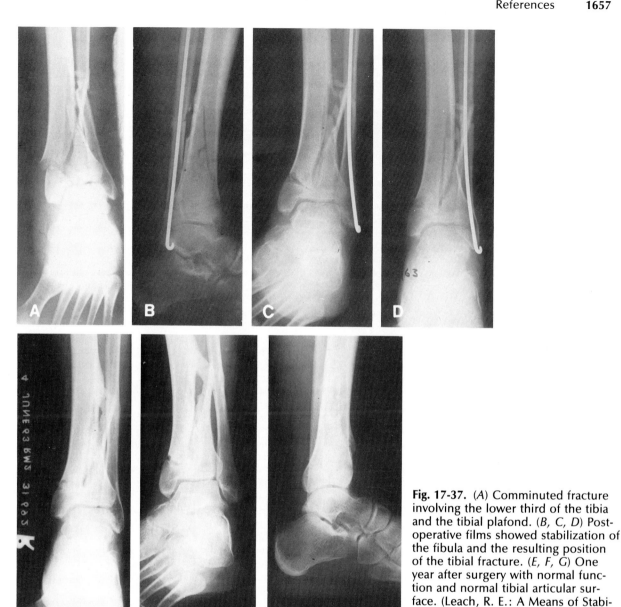

Fig. 17-37. (*A*) Comminuted fracture involving the lower third of the tibia and the tibial plafond. (*B, C, D*) Postoperative films showed stabilization of the fibula and the resulting position of the tibial fracture. (*E, F, G*) One year after surgery with normal function and normal tibial articular surface. (Leach, R. E.: A Means of Stabilizing Comminuted Distal Tibial Fractures. J. Trauma, **4**:722–725, 1964.)

20. Bauer, G.; Edwards, P. O.; and Widmark, P. H.: Shaft Fractures of the Tibia. Acta Chir. Scand., **124**:386–395, 1962.

21. Bauer, G.; Edwards, P. O.; and Widmark, P. H.: Shaft Fractures of the Tibia. Etiology of Poor Results in a Consecutive Series of 173 Fractures. Acta Chir. Scand., **124**:386–395, 1962.

22. Bayne, L. G.; Morris, H.; and Wickstrom, J.: Evaluation of Intermedullary Fixation of the Tibia with the Lottes Nail. South. Med. J., **53**:1429–1440, 1960.

23. Bergentz, S. E., and Thureborn, E.: Shaft Fractures of the Lower Leg; Open Versus Closed Reduction. Analysis of a Twenty-year Series. Acta Chir. Scand., **114**:235–241, 1957.

24. Blockey, N. J.: The Value of Rigid Fixation in the Treatment of Fractures of the Adult Tibial Shaft. J. Bone Joint Surg., **38B**:518–527, 1956.

25. Böhler, J.: Treatment of Non-union of the Tibia with Closed and Semiclosed Intramedullary Nailing. Clin. Orthop., **43**:92–102, 1965.

26. Böhler, L.: The Treatment of Fractures. English 5th ed., 3 Vols. New York, Grune & Stratton, 1956–1958.

27. Bonnin, J. G.: Injuries to the Ankle. London, William Heinemann, 1950.

28. Boutin, P.: 25 Cas de Fractures bifocales de Jambe. Rev. Chir. Orthop., **42**:647–663, 1956.

29. Boyd, H. B.: Non-union of the Shafts of Long Bones. Postgrad. Med., **36**:315–320, 1964.

30. Boyd, H. B.: The Treatment of Difficult and Unusual Non-unions. With Special Reference to the Bridging of Defects. J. Bone Joint Surg., **25**:535–552, 1943.

31. Boyd, H. B.; Anderson, L. D.; and Johnston, D. S.: Changing Concepts in the Treatment of Non-union. Clin. Orthop., **43**:37–54, 1965.

32. Boyd, H. B., and Lipinski, S. W.: Causes and Treatment of Non-union of the Shafts of the Long Bones, with a Review of 741 Patients. A.A.O.S. Instructional Course Lectures, Vol. 17. St. Louis, C. V. Mosby, 1960.

33. Boyd, H. B.; Lipinski, S. W.; and Wiley, J. H.: Observations of Non-union of the Shafts of the Long Bones with a Statistical Analysis of 842 Patients. J. Bone Joint Surg., **43A**:159–168, 1961.

34. Boylston, B. F., and Milam, R.: Segmental Fractures of the Tibia: An Analysis of Thirty Cases. South. Med. J., **50**:969–975, 1957.

35. Brighton, C. T.: Treatment of Non-union of the Tibia with Constant Direct Current. (1980 Fitts Lecture, A.A.S.T.) J. Trauma, **3**:189–195, 1981.

36. Brighton, C. T.; Black, J.; Friedenberg, C. B.; Esterhai, J. L.; Day, L. J.; and Connolly, J. F.: A Multi-center Study of the Treatment of Non-union with Constant Direct Current. J. Bone Joint Surg., **63A**:2–13, 1981.

37. Brown, P. W., and Urban, J. G.: Early Weight-bearing Treatment of Open Fractures of the Tibia. J. Bone Joint Surg., **51A**:59–75, 1969.

38. Burrows, H. J.: Fatigue Infraction of the Middle of the Tibia in Ballet Dancers, J. Bone Joint Surg., **38B**:83–94, 1956.

39. Burwell, H. N.: Plate Fixation of Tibial Shaft Fractures—A Survery of 181 Injuries. J. Bone Joint Surg., **53B**:258–271, 1971.

40. Burwell, H. N., and Charnley, A. D.: The Treatment of Displaced Fractures at the Ankle by Rigid Internal Fixation and Early Joint Movement. J. Bone Joint Surg., **47B**:634–660, 1965.

41. Campbell, W. C.: Transference of the Fibula as an Adjunct to Free Bone Graft in Tibial Deficiency. Report of Three Cases. Am. J. Orthop. Surg., **1**:625–631, 1919.

42. Carnesale, P. L., and Guerrieri, A. G.: Fibular Transplant for Loss of Substance of Tibia; Report of a Case. J. Bone Joint Surg., **37A**:204–206, 1955.

43. Carpenter, E. B.: Management of Fractures of the Shaft of the Tibia and Fibula. J. Bone Joint Surg., **48A**:1640–1646, 1966.

44. Carpenter, E. B., and Butterworth, J. F., III: The Conservative Treatment of Shaft Fractures of the Tibia and Fibula. South. Med. J., **50**:1209–1214, 1957.

45. Carpenter, E. B.; Dobbie, J. J.; and Sewers, C. F.: Fractures of the Shaft of the Tibia and Fibula. Comparative End-results from Various Types of Treatment in a Teaching Hospital. Arch. Surg., **64**:433–456, 1952.

46. Carrell, W. B.: Transplantation of Fibula in the Same Leg. J. Bone Joint Surg., **20**:627, 1938.

47. Cavadias, A. X., and Trueta, J.: An Experimental Study of the Vascular Contribution to the Callus of Fracture. Surg. Gynecol., Obstet., **120**:731–747, 1965.

48. Cave, E. F. (ed.): Fractures and Other Injuries. Chicago, Year Book Publishers, 1958.

49. Chacha, P. B.; Ahmed, M.; and Daruwalla, J. S.: Vascular Pedicle Graft of the Ipsilateral Fibula for Non-union of the Tibia with a Large Defect. An Experimental and Clinical Study. J. Bone Joint Surg., **63B**:244–253, 1981.

50. Chapman, M. W.: Immediate Internal Fixation in Open Fractures. Orthop. Clin. North Am., **11**:579–591, 1980.

51. Chapman, M. W., and Mahoney, M.: The Role of Internal Fixation in the Management of Open Fractures. Clin. Orthop., **138**:120–231, 1979.

52. Charnley, J.: The Closed Treatment of Common Fractures, 3rd ed. Edinburgh, E. & S. Livingstone, 1961.

53. Childress, H. M.: Vertical Transarticular-pin Fixation for Unstable Ankle Fractures. J. Bone Joint Surg., **47A**:1323–1334, 1965.

54. Chrisman, O. D., and Snook, G. A.: The Problem of Refracture of the Tibia. Clin. Orthop., **60**:217–219, 1968.

55a. Cierny, G.; Byrd, H. S.; and Jones, R. E.: Primary Versus Delayed Soft Tissue Coverage for Severe Open Tibial Fractures. A Comparison of Results. Clin. Orthop., **178**:54–63, 1983.

55. Clancey, G. J., and Hansen, S. T., Jr.: Open Fractures of the Tibia. J. Bone Joint Surg., **60A**:118–122, 1978.

56. Clark, J. M.: Modern Trends in Orthopaedic Treatment. London, Butterworth, 1962.

57. Clark, W. E. Vascularization of Muscles. Lancet, **1**:17, 1945.

58. Clawson, D. K.: Claw Toes Following Tibial Fracture. Clin. Orthop., **103**:47, 1974.

59. Codivilla, A.: On the Care of Congenital Pseudoarthrosis of the Tibia by Means of Periosteal Transplantation. Am. J. Orthop. Surg., **4**:163–169, 1906.

60. Codivilla, A.: Sur le Traitement des Pseudarthroses des Os longs. In Computes Rendu, XVI. Congres International de Medecine, Budapest, 1909, **8A**:266–343, 1910.

61. Cohen, S. M.: Traumatic Arterial Spasm. Lancet, **1**:1–6, 1944.

62. Companacci, M., and Zanoli, S.: Double Tibiofibular Synostosis for Non-union and Delayed Union of the Tibia. J. Bone Joint Surg., **48A**:44–56, 1966.

63. Connolly, J. F.; Whittaker, D.; and Williams, E.: Femoral and Tibial Fractures Combined with Injuries to the Femoral or Popliteal Artery. J. Bone Joint Surg., **53A**:56–67, 1971.

64. Conwell, H. E., and Reynolds, F. C.: Management of Fractures, Dislocations, and Sprains, 7th ed. St. Louis, C. V. Mosby, 1961.

65. Coonrad, R. W.: Fracture Dislocations of the Ankle Joint with Impaction Injury. J. Bone Joint Surgery, **52A**:1337–1347, 1970.

66. Cooper, A. P.: A Treatise on Dislocation and on Fractures of the Joints. London, Longman, Hurst, Rees, Orme & Brown, 1822.

67. Copeland, C. X., Jr., and Enneking, W. F.: Incidence of

Osteomyelitis in Compound Fractures. Am. Surgeon, **31:**156–158, 1965.

68. Crellin, R. Q., and Tsapogas, M. J. C.: Traumatic Aneurysm of the Anterior Tibial Artery. Report of a Case. J. Bone Joint Surg., **45B:**142–144, 1963.

69. Crenshaw, A. H.: Campbell's Operative Orthopedics, 5th ed. St. Louis, C. V. Mosby, 1971.

70. Davis, A. G.: Fibular Substitution for Tibial Defects. J. Bone Joint Surg., **26:**229–237, 1944.

71. DeHaas, W. G.; Watson, J.; and Morrison, D. M.: Non-invasive Treatment of Ununited Fractures of the Tibia using Electrical Stimulation. J. Bone Joint Surg., **62B:**465–470, 1980.

72. Dehne, E.: Treatment of Fractures of the Tibial Shaft. Clin. Orthop., **66:**159–173, 1969.

73. Dehne, E.; Metz, C. W.; and Deffer, P. A.: Nonoperative Treatment of the Fractured Tibia by Immediate Weight Bearing. J. Trauma, **1:**514–533, 1961.

74. Dehne, E.; Deffer, P. A.; Hall, R. M.; Brown, P. W.; and Johnson, E. V.: The Natural History of the Fractured Tibia. Surg. Clin. North Am., **41:**1495–1513, 1961.

75. Dehne, E.: Ambulatory Treatment of the Fractured Tibia. Clin. Orthop., **105:**192–201, 1974.

76. Delbet, P.: Methode de Traitement des Fractures de Jambes. Ann. Clin. Chev., (Paris), **5,** 1916.

77. DeLee, J. C.; Heckman, J. D.; and Lewis, A. G.: Partial Fibulectomy for Ununited Fractures of the Tibia. J. Bone Joint Surg., **63A:**1390–1395, 1981.

78. DeLee, J. C., and Stiehl, J. B.: Open Tibia Fracture with Compartment Syndrome. Clin. Orthop., **160:**175–184, 1981.

79. DePalma, A.: The Management of Fractures and Dislocations, 2nd ed. Philadelphia, W. B. Saunders, 1970.

80. Devas, M. B.: Stress Fractures of the Tibia in Athletes or ''Shin Soreness.'' J. Bone Joint Surg., **40B:**227–239, 1958.

81. Devas, M. B.: Shin Splints or Stress Fractures of the Metacarpal Bone in Horses and Shin Soreness or Stress Fractures of the Tibia in Man. J. Bone Joint Surg., **49B:**310–313, 1967.

82. Devas, M. B., and Sweetman, R.: Stress Fractures of the Fibula—A Review of Fifty Cases in Athletes. J. Bone Joint Surg., **38B:**818–829, 1956.

83. Dickerson, R. C.: Recent Developments in the Study and Treatment of Fractures. Surg. Gynecol., Obstet., **131:**537–554, 1970.

84. Dunlop, K., and Wirzalis, E. F.: Two-stage Transplant for Persistent Non-union with Gross Loss of Tibia—A Report of Five Cases. Milit. Surg., **107:**356–373, 1950.

85. Edge, A. J., and Denham, R. A.: The Portsmouth Method of External Fixation of Complicated Tibial Fractures. Injury, **11:**13–18, 1979.

86. Edge, A. J., and Denham, R. A.: External Fixation for Complication Tibial Fractures. J. Bone Joint Surg., **63B:**92–97, 1981.

87. Edwards, P.: Fracture of the Shaft of the Tibia: 492 Consecutive Cases in Adults. Importance of Soft Tissue Injury. Acta Orthop. Scand., (Suppl.) 76, 1965.

88. Edwards, P.; Baver, G.; and Widmark, P. H.: The Time of

Disability Following Fracture of the Shaft of the Tibia. Acta Orthop. Scand., **40:**501–506, 1969.

89. Edwards, C. C.; Jaworski, M. F.; Solana, J.; and Aronson, B. S.: Management of Compound Tibial Fractures using External Fixation. Am. Surg., **45:**190–203, 1979.

90. Eggers, G. W. N.: Indications and Operative Technique for Open Reduction and Internal Fixation of Fractures of the Shafts of the Tibia and Fibula. Surg. Clin. North Am., **41:**1515–1530, 1961.

91. Eggers, G. W. N.; Shindler, T. O.; and Pomerat, C. M.: The Influence of the Contact-Compression Factor on Osteogenesis in Surgical Fractures. J. Bone Joint Surg., **31A:**693–716, 1949.

92. Ellis, H.: Disabilities after Tibial Shaft Fractures. J. Bone Joint Surg., **40B:**190–197, 1958.

93. Ellis, H.: The Speed of Healing after Fracture of the Tibial Shaft. J. Bone Joint Surg., **40B:**42–46, 1958.

94. Ellis, H.: A Study of Some Factors Affecting Prognosis Following Tibial Shaft Fractures. Oxford, Bodleian Library, 1956.

95. Ellis, J.: Treatment of Fractures of the Tibial Shaft. J. Bone Joint Surg., **46B:**371–372, 1954.

96. Ernst, C. B., and Kaufer, H.: Fibulectomy and Fasciotomy: An Important Adjunct in the Management of Lower Extremity Arterial Trauma. J. Trauma, **2:**365–380, 1971.

97. Evans, E. B., and Eggers, G. W. N.: Internal Fixation of the Fibula in Fractures of both Bones of the Leg. J.A.M.A., **169:**321–326, 1959.

98. Evans, G. A.; Bang, R. L.; Cornah, M. S.; and Corps, B. V. M.: The Value of the Hoffmann Skeletal Fixation in the Management of Cross Leg Flaps, Particularly Those Injuries Complicated by Open Fractures of the Tibia. Injury, **11:**110–114, 1979.

99. Fernandez-Palazzi, F.: Fibular Resection in Delayed Union of Tibial Fractures. Acta Orthop. Scand., **40:**105–118, 1969.

100. Fisher, W. D., and Hamblen, D. L.: Problems and Pitfalls of Compression Fixation of Long Bone Fractures: A Review of Results and Complications. Injury, **10:**99–107, 1978.

101. Flanagan, J. J., and Burem, H. S.: Reconstruction of Defects of the Tibia and Femur with Apposing Massive Grafts from the Affected Bone. J. Bone Joint Surg., **29:**587–597, 1947.

102. Forbes, D. B.: Subcortical Iliac Bone Grafts in Fracture of the Tibia. J. Bone Joint Surg., **43B:**672–679, 1961.

103. Fraser, R. D.; Hunter, G. A.; and Waddell, J. P.: Ipsilateral Fracture of the Femur and Tibia. J. Bone Joint Surg., **60B:**510–551, 1978.

104. Furste, W.: Prophylaxis Against Tetanus and Gas Gangrene. In Blakemore, W. S. and Fitts, W. T.: Management of the Injured Patient, New York, Hoeber Medical Division, 1969.

105. Ganosa, A. C. L.; Carruiterro, J.; and Rogers, S.: Straight Nails in Tibial Fractures. Techniques and Reports of Thirty Cases. J. Bone Joint Surg., **49A:**280–284, 1967.

105a. Ger, R.: Muscle Transposition for Treatment and Prevention of Chronic Post-traumatic Osteomyelitis of the Tibia. J. Bone Joint Surg., **59A:**784–791, 1977.

106. Geslien, G. E.; Thrall, J. H.; and Espinosa, J. L.: Early

Detection of Stress Fractures Using 99m Tc-Polyphosphate. Radiology, **121**:683–687, 1976.

107. Gosselin, L.: Sur les Fractures en V du Tibia. Gazette des Hospitaux Civils et Militaires, (Paris), **28**:218, 1855.

108. Greenbaum, E., and O'Loughlen, B. J.: Value of Delayed Filming in the Anterior Tibial Compartment Syndrome Secondary to Trauma. Radiology, **93**:373–376, 1969.

109. Gustilo, R. B.: Management of Open Fractures and Their Complications. Philadelphia, W. B. Saunders, 1982.

110. Gustilo, R. B., and Anderson, J. T.: Prevention of Infection in the Treatment of 1025 Open Fractures of Long Bones. J. Bone Joint Surg., **58A**:453–458, 1976.

111. Gustilo, R. B., Mendoza, R. M.; and Williams D.: Problems in the Management of Type III (Severe) Open Fractures. Submitted to J. Bone Joint Surg., 1982.

112. Gustilo, R. B.; Simpson, L.; Nixon, R.; Ruiz, A.; and Indeck, W.: An Analysis of 511 Open Fractures at Hennepin County General Hospital. J. Bone Joint Surg., **50A**:830–831, 1968.

113. Gustilo, R. B.; Simpson, L.; Nixon, R.; Ruiz, A.; and Indeck, W.: Analysis of 511 Open Fractures. Clin. Orthop., **66**:148–154, 1969.

114. Hahn, E.: Eine Methode, pseudarthrosen der Tibia mit grossen Knochendefekt zur Heilung zubringen. Centralbl. f. Chir., **21**:337–341, 1884.

115. Hampton, O. P., Jr., and Holt, E. P., Jr.: The Present Status of Intramedullary Nailing of Fractures of the Tibia. Am. J. Surg., **93**:597–603, 1957.

116. Hand, F. M.: Crisscross Tibiofibular Graft for Nonunion of the Tibia. Clin. Orthop., **1**:154–160, 1953.

117. Hanson, L. W., and Eppright, R. H.: Posterior Bone Grafting of the Tibia for Nonunion. A Review of Twenty-four Cases. J. Bone Joint Surg., **48A**:27–43, 1966.

118. Harkins, H. N., and Phemister, D. B.: Simplified Technique of Onlay Grafts. For all Ununited Fractures in Acceptable Position. J.A.M.A., **109**:1501–1506, 1937.

119. Harmon, J. W.: A Historical Study of Skeletal Muscle in Acute Ischemia. Am. J. Pathol., **23**:551–565, 1947.

120. Harmon, P. H.: A Simplified Approach to the Posterotibia for Bone Grafting and Fibular Transferral. J. Bone Joint Surg., **27**:496–498, 1945

121. Harvey, J. P. Jr.: Management of Open Tibial Fractures. Clin. Orthop., **105**:154–166, 1974.

122. Hedenberg, I., and Pompeius, R.: Shaft Fractures of the Lower Leg. Comparing the Early Results of Open and Closed Treatment in 120 Cases. Acta Chir. Scand., **118**:339–348, 1960.

123. Hedrick, D. W.; Hawkins, F. B.; and Townley, C. O.: Primary Arterial Injury Complicating Extremity Fractures. J. Bone Joint Surg., **29**:738–744, 1947.

124. Hicks, J. H.: Amputation in Fractures of the Tibia. J. Bone Joint Surg., **46B**:388–392, 1964.

125. Hicks, J.H.: The Relationship Between Metal and Infection. Proc. Roy. Soc. Med., **50**:842–844, 1957.

126. Hjelmsted, A.: Fractures of the Tibial Shaft. A Study of Primary and Late Results in 105 Cases. Acta Chir. Scand, **121**:511–516, 1961.

127. Hoaglund, F. T., and States, J. D.: Factors Influencing the Rate of Healing in Tibial Shaft Fractures. Surg. Gynecol. Obstet., **124**:71–76, 1967.

128. Holden, C. E. A.: Bone Grafts in the Treatment of Delayed Union of Tibial Shaft Fractures. Injury, **4**:175–179, 1972.

129. Holderman, W. D.: Results Following Conservative Treatment of Fractures of the Tibial Shaft. Am. J. Surg., **98**:593–597, 1959.

130. Holstad, H. A.: Primary Osteosynthesis Versus Conservative Treatment of Compound Fractures of Long Tubular Bones. J. Oslo City Hosp., **12**:225–237, 1962.

131. Howe, J. J., Jr., and Sutherland, R.: Fracture Fixation by Transarticular Pin; A Technic for Control of Severe Ankle Fractures. Am. J. Surg., **74**:24–26, 1947.

132. Hughston, J. C., et al: Tibia Fractures. South. Med. J., **62**:931–940, 1969.

132a. Huntington, T. W.: Case of Bone Transference. Use of a Segment of Fibula to Supply a Defect in the Tibia. Ann. Surg., **41**:249–251, 1905.

133. Jackson, R. W., and Macnab, I.: Fractures of the Shaft of the Tibia. A Clinical and Experimental Study. Am. J. Surg., **97**:543–557, 1959.

134. Jefferys, C. C.: Spasm of the Posterior Tibial Artery after Injury. J. Bone Joint Surg., **45B**:223, 1963.

135. Jones, K. G.: Treatment of Infected Non-union of the Tibia Through the Posterolateral Approach. Clin. Orthop., **43**:103–109, 1965.

136. Jones, K. G., and Barnett, H. C.: Cancellous-Bone Grafting for Non-union of the Tibia Through the Posterolateral Approach. J. Bone Joint Surg., **37A**:1250–1260, 1955.

137. Karlstrom, G., and Olerud, S.: Fractures of the Tibial Shaft: A Critical Evaluation of Treatment Alternatives. Clin. Orthop., **105**:82–115, 1974.

138. Karlstrom. G., and Olerud, S.: Percutaneous Pin Fixation of Open Tibial Fractures: Double-Frame Anchorage Using the Vidal–Adrey Method. J. Bone Joint Surg., **57A**:915–924, 1975.

139. Kelly, R. P., and Murphy, F. E.: Fatigue Fractures of the Tibia. South. Med. J., **44**:290–297, 1951.

140. Kratochvil, B. L., and Premer, R. F.: The Delbet Splint: A Report of Three Cases. Clin. Orthop., **36**:151–155, 1964.

141. Kristensen, K. D.: Tibial Shaft Fractures: The Frequency of Local Complications in Tibial Shaft Fractures Treated by Internal Compression Osteosynthesis. Acta Orthop. Scand., **50**:593–598, 1979.

142. Kunkel, W. G., and Lynn, R. B.: The Anterior Tibial Compartment Syndrome. Canad. J. Surg., **1**:212–217, 1958.

143. Lam, S. J.: The Place of Delayed Internal Fixation in the Treatment of Fractures of the Long Bones. J. Bone Joint Surg., **46B**:393–397, 1964.

144. Lamb, R. H.: Posterolateral Bone Graft for Nonunion of the Tibia. Clin. Orthop., **64**:114–120, 1969.

145. Landoff, G. A.: A Comparative Study of Methods of Treatment of Diaphyseal Fractures of the Leg. Acta Orthop. Scand., **18**:37–60, 1948.

146. Langard, O., and Bo, O.: Segmental Tibial Shaft Fractures. Acta Orthop. Scand. **47**:354–357, 1976.

147. Laurence, M.; Freeman, M. A. R.; and Swanson, S. A. V.: Engineering Considerations in the Internal Fixation of Fractures of the Tibial Shaft. J. Bone Joint Surg. **51(B)**:754–768, 1969.

148. Laurent, L. E., and Langenskiold, A.: Osteosynthesis with

a Thick Medullary Nail in Non-union of Long Bones. Acta Orthop. Scand., **38**:341–358, 1967.

149. Leach, R. E.: A Means of Stabilizing Comminuted Distal Tibial Fractures. J. Trauma, **4**:722–725, 1964.

150. Leach, R. E.: Fractures of the Tibial Plafond. A.A.O.S. Instructional Course Lectures, **28**:88–93, 1979.

151. Leach, R. E.; Hammond, G.; and Stryker, W. S.: Anterior Tibial Compartment Syndrome—Acute and Chronic. J. Bone Joint Surg., **49A**:451–462, 1967.

152. Lottes, J. O.: Blind Nailing Technique for Insertion of the Triflange Medullary Nail. J.A.M.A., **155**:1039–1042, 1954.

153. Lottes, J. O.: Intramedullary Fixation for Fracture of Shaft of Tibia. South. Med. J., **45**:407–414, 1952.

154. Lottes, J. O.: Intramedullary Nailing of the Tibia. A.A.O.S. Instructional Course Lectures, **15.** Ann Arbor, J. W. Edwards, 1958.

155. Lottes, J.O.: Treatment of Delayed or Non-union Fractures of the Tibia by Medullary Nail. Clin. Orthop., **43**:111–128, 1965.

156. Lottes, J. O.; Hill, L. J.; and Key, J. A.: Closed Reduction, Plate Fixation and Medullary Nailing of Fractures of both Bones of the Leg. J. Bone Joint Surg., **34A**:861–877, 1952.

157. Lucas, K., and Todd, C.: Closed Adult Tibial Shaft Fractures. J. Bone Joint Surg., **55B**:878, 1973.

158. MacAusland, W. R., Jr.: Treatment of Sepsis after Intramedullary Nailing of Fractures of the Femur. Clin. Orthop., **60**:87–94, 1968.

159. MacAusland, W. R., Jr., and Eaton, R. G.: The Management of Sepsis Following Intramedullary Fixation for Fractures of the Femur. J. Bone Joint Surg., **45A**:1643–1653, 1963.

160. McCarroll, H. R.: The Surgical Management of Ununited Fractures of the Tibia. J.A.M.A., **175**:578–583, 1961.

161. McCormack, M. P., and Carr, M.: Alms Technique of Kuntscher Nailing for Fractures of the Tibia. J. Bone Joint Surg., **47B**:586, 1965.

162. McLaughlin, H. L.: On the Operative Treatment of Tibial Fractures. Surg. Clin. North Am., **41**:1489–1494, 1961.

163. McLaughlin, H. L.; Gaston, S. R.; Neer, C. S.; and Craig, F. S.: Open Reduction and Internal Fixation of Fractures of the Long Bones. J. Bone Joint Surg., **31A**:94–114, 1949.

164. McMaster, P. E., and Hohl, M.: Tibiofibular Cross-Peg Grafting. J. Bone Joint Surg., **47A**:1146–1158, 1965.

165. MacNab, I.: Blood Supply of the Tibia. J. Bone Joint Surg., **39B**:799, 1957.

166. McNeur, J. C.: The Management of Open Skeletal Trauma with Particular Reference to Internal Fixation. J. Bone Joint Surg., **52B**:54–60, 1970.

167. Maisonneuve, M. J. G.: Recherches sur la Fracture du Perone. Arch Gen. Med., **7**:165–187; 433–473, 1840.

168. Marmor, L.: How to Treat the Infected United Fracture of the Tibia. Am. J. Surg., **113**:475–478, 1967.

169. Marshall, D. V.: Three-side Plate Fixation for Fractures of the Femoral and Tibial Shafts. J. Bone Joint Surg., **40A**:323–345, 1958.

169a. Mathes, S. J., and Nahai, F.: Clinical Atlas of Muscle and Musculocutaneous Flaps. St. Louis, C. V. Mosby, 1979.

170. Matsen, F. A. III: Compartmental Syndromes. New York, Grune & Stratton, 1980.

171. Matsen, F. A., and Clawson, K.: The Deep Posterior Compartment Syndrome of the Leg. J. Bone Joint Surg., **57A**:34–41, 1975.

172. Milch, H.: Tibiofibular Synostosis for Nonunion of the Tibia. Surgery, **27**:770–779, 1950.

173. Miller, D. S.: Marken L.; and Grossman, E.: Ischemic Fibrosis of the Lower Extremity in Children. Am. J. Surg., **84**:317–322, 1952.

174. Miller, W.; Grady, L. J.; and Frank, G. R.: Posterior Bone Grafts in Non-union of Fractures of the Shafts of the Tibia: A Review of 27 Cases. South. Med. J., **62**:1254–1258, 1969.

175. Mooney, V.; Nickel, V. L.; Harvey, J. P.; and Snelson, R.: Cast Brace Treatment for Fractures of the Distal Part of the Femur. J. Bone Joint Surg., **52A**:1563–1578, 1970.

176. Moore, J. R.: The Closed Fracture of the Long Bones. J. Bone Joint Surg., **42A**:869–874, 1960.

177. Moore, S. T.; Storts, R. A.; and Spencer, J. D.: Fractures of the Tibial Shaft in Adults: A Ten Year Survey of such Fractures. South. Med. J., **55**:1178–1183, 1962.

178. Moritz, J. R., et al.: Spiral Fractures of the Tibia: Long Term Results of Parham Band Fixation. J. Trauma, **2**:147–161, 1962.

179. Morris, J. M., and Blickenstaff, L. D.: Fatigue Fractures—A Clinical Study. Springfield, Ill., Charles C. Thomas, 1967.

180. Mubarak, S. J.; Hargens, A. R.; Owen, C. A.; Garetto, L. P.; and Akeson, W. H.: The Wick Catheter Technique for Measurement of Intramuscular Pressure. J. Bone Joint Surg., **58A**:1016–1020, 1976.

181. Müller, M. E.: Internal Fixation for Fresh Fractures and for Non-union. Proc. Roy. Soc. Med., **56**:455–460, 1963.

182. Müller, M. E.; Allgöwer, M.; Schneider, R.; and Willenegger, H.: Treatment of Nonunions by Compression. Clin. Orthop., **43**:83–88, 1965.

183. Müller, M. E.; Allgöwer, M.; Schneider, R.; and Willenegger, H.: Manual of Internal Fixation, 2nd ed. New York, Springer-Verlag, 1979.

184. Müller, M. E.; Allgöwer, M.; and Willenegger, H.: Technique of Internal Fixation of Fractures. New York, Springer-Verlag, 1965.

185. Murray, W. R.; Lucas, D. B.; and Inman, V. T.: Treatment of Non-union of Fractures of the Long Bones by the Two-plate Method. J. Bone Joint Surg., **46A**:1027–1048, 1964.

186. Nelson, G.; Kelly, P.; Paterson, L.; and Janes, J.: Blood Supply of the Human Tibia. J. Bone Joint Surg., **42A**:625–635, 1960.

187. Nicoll, E. A.: Fractures of the Tibial Shaft. A Survey of 705 Cases. J. Bone Joint Surg., **46B**:373–387, 1964.

188. Nicoll, E. A.: Closed and Open Management of Tibial Fractures. Clin. Orthop., **105**:144–153, 1974.

189. Onnerfalt, R.: Fracture of the Tibial Shaft Treated by Primary Operation and Early Weight Bearing. Acta Orthop. Scand., (Suppl.), **171**:1–63, 1978.

190. Owen, R., and Tsimboukis, B.: Incidence of Ischemic Contracture Following Closed Injuries to the Calf. J. Bone Joint Surg., **49B**:268–275, 1967.

191. Pankovich, A. M.; Tarabisky, I. E.; and Yelda, S.: Flexible

Intramedullary Nailing of Tibial Shaft Fractures. Clin. Orthop., **160**:185–195, 1981.

192. Paradies, L. H., and Gregory, C. F.: The Early Treatment of Close-range Shotgun Wounds to the Extremities. J. Bone Joint Surg., **48A**:425–435, 1966.

193. Patzakis, M. J.; Harvey, J. P.; and Ivler, D.: The Role of Antibiotics in the Management of Open Fractures. J. Bone Joint Surg., **56A**:532, 1974.

194. Phemister, D. B.: Splint Grafts in the Treatment of Delayed and Non-union of Fractures. Surg., Gynecol., Obstet., **52**:376–381, 1931.

195. Phemister, D. B.: Treatment of Ununited Fractures by Onlay Bone Grafts without Screw or Tie Fixation and Without Breaking Down of the Fibrous Union. J. Bone Joint Surg., **29**:946–960, 1947.

196. Pierce, R. O., Jr., and Heinrick, J. H.: Comminuted Intra-articular Fractures of the Distal Tibia. J. Trauma, **19**:828–832, 1979.

197. Prather, J. L.; Nusynowitz, M. L.; and Snowdy, H. A.: Scintigraphic Findings in Stress Fractures. J. Bone Joint Surg., **59A**:869–874, 1977.

198. Ralston, E. L.: Handbook of Fractures. St. Louis, C. V. Mosby, 1967.

199. Ratliff, A. H. C.: Fractures of Femur and Tibia in same Limb. J. Bone Joint Surg., **47B**:586, 1965.

200. Reckling, F. W., and Waters, C. H.: Treatment of Non-unions of Fractures of the Tibial Diaphysis by Postero-lateral Cortical Cancellous Bone Grafting. J. Bone Joint Surg., **62A**:936–941, 1980.

201. Rittman, W. W.; Schibli, M.; Matter, P.; and Allgöwer, M.: Open Fractures: Long Term Results in 200 Consecutive Cases. Clin. Orthop., **138**:132–140, 1979.

202. Rix, R. R.: A Method of Treatment for Tibial Shaft Fractures. Surg., Gynecol, Obstet., **117**:647–650, 1963.

203. Rosenthal, R. E.; MacPhail, J. A.; and Ortiz, J. E.: Non-union in Open Tibial Fractures. J. Bone Joint Surg., **59A**:244–248, 1977.

204. Rüedi, T. P., and Allgöwer, M.: Fractures of the Lower End of the Tibia into the Ankle Joint. Injury, **1**:92–99, 1969.

205. Rüedi, T. P., and Allgöwer, M.: Fractures of the Lower End of the Tibia into the Ankle Joint: Results Nine Years After Open Reduction and Internal Fixation. Injury, **5**:130–134, 1973.

206. Rüedi, T. P., and Allgöwer, M.: The Operative Treatment of Intra-articular Fractures of the Lower End of the Tibia. Clin. Orthop., **139**:105–110, 1979.

207. Rüedi, T.; Webb, J. K.; and Allgöwer, M.: Experience with the Dynamic Compression Plate (DCP) in 418 Recent Fractures of the Tibial Shaft. Injury, **7**:252–265, 1976.

208. Sakellarides, H. T.; Freeman, P. A.; and Grant, B. D.: Delayed Union and Non-union of Tibial-Shaft Fractures. A Review of 100 Cases. J. Bone Joint Surg., **46A**:557–569, 1964.

209. Sarmiento, A.: A Functional Below-the-Knee Brace for Tibial Fractures. J. Bone Joint Surg., **52A**:295–311, 1970.

210. Sarmiento, A.: Functional Bracing of Tibial and Femoral Shaft Fractures. Clin. Orthop., **82**:2–13, 1972.

211. Sarmiento, A.: Functional Bracing of Tibial Fractures. Clin. Orthop., **105**:202–219, 1974.

212. Sarmiento, A.: A Functional Below-the-knee Cast for Tibial Fractures. J. Bone Joint Surg., **49A**:855–875, 1967.

213. Schatzker, J.: Compression in the Surgical Treatment of Fractures of the Tibia. Clin. Orthop. **105**:220–239, 1974.

214. Scheck, M.: Tratment of Comminuted Distal Tibial Fractures by Combined Dual-pin Fixation and Limited Open Reduction. J. Bone Joint Surg., **47A**:1537–1553, 1965.

215. Scott, J. C.: Fractures of the Tibia and Fibula. In Clark, J. M. P. (ed.): Modern Trends in Orthopedics. Fracture Treatment. London, Butterworth & Co., 1962.

216. Scudese, V. A.; Birotte, A.; and Gialenella, J.: Tibial Shaft Fractures: Percutaneous Multiple Pin Fixation, Short Leg Cast and Immediate Weight Bearing. Clin. Orthop., **72**:271–282, 1970.

217. Seddon, H. J.: Volkmann's Ischaemia in the Lower Limb. J. Bone Joint Surg., **48B**:627–636, 1966.

218. Segal, D.; Pick, R., Klein, H.; and Heskioff, D.: The Role of the Lateral Malleolus as a Stabilizing Factor of the Ankle Joint: Preliminary Report. Foot Ankle, **2**:25–29, 1981.

218a. Serafin, D.: Georgiade, N. G.; and Smith, D. H.: Comparison of Free Flaps with Pedicled Flaps for Coverage of Defects of the Leg or Foot. Plast. Reconstr. Surg., **59**:492–499, 1977.

219. Shaar, C. M.; Krenz, F. P., Jr.; and Jones, D. T.: Fractures of the Tibia and Fibula—Treatment with the Stader Reduction and Fixation Splint. Surg. Clin. North Am., **23**:599–630, 1943.

220. Shands, A. R., and Raney, R. B.: Handbook of Orthopaedic Surgery. St. Louis, C. V. Mosby, 1967.

221. Sharrard, W. J. W.; Sutcliff, M. L.; Robson, M. J.; and MacEachern, A. G.: The Treatment of Fibrous Non-union of Fractures by Pulsing Electromagnetic Stimulation. J. Bone Joint Surg., **64B**:189–193, 1982.

222. Sirbu, A. B.; Murphy, M. J.; and White, A. S.: Soft Tissue Complications of Fractures of the Leg. Calif. West. Med., **60**:53–56, 1944.

223. Slatis, P., and Rokkanen, P.: Closed Intramedullary Nailing of Tibial Shaft Fractures. Acta Orthop. Scand., **38**:88–100, 1967.

224. Smith, J. E. M.: Results of Early and Delayed Internal Fixation for Tibial Shaft Fractures. A Review of 470 Fractures. J. Bone Joint Surg., **56B**:469–477, 1974.

225. Solheim, K.; Bo, O., and Langard, O.: Tibial Shaft Fractures Treated with Intramedullary Nailing. J. Trauma, **17**:223–230, 1977.

226. Sorenson, K. H.: Treatment of Delayed Union and Non-union of the Tibia by Fibular Resection. Acta Orthop. Scand., **40**:92–104, 1969.

227. Souter, W. A.: Autogenous Cancellous Strip Grafts in the Treatment of Delayed Union of Long Bone Fractures. J. Bone Joint Surg., **51B**:63–75, 1969.

228. Speed, K.: A Textbook of Fractures and Dislocations. Philadelphia, Lea & Febiger, 1928.

229. Stein, A. H., Jr.: Arterial Injury in Orthopaedic Surgery. J. Bone Joint Surg., **38A**:669–676, 1956.

230. Stephens, J. G., and Andersen, M. N.: An Analysis of Open and Closed Treatment of Fractures of the Tibial Shaft. Canad. J. Surg., **4**:65–68, 1960.

231. Straub, L. R.: Brace Management in Complicated Fractures

of the Tibia. Surg. Clin. North Am., **41:**1579–1585, 1961.

232. Strobel, C. J., and Indeck, W.: Fractures of the Tibia. An Analysis of Treatment at Minneapolis General Hospital. Minn. Med., **43:**469–472, 1960.

233. Taylor, K.; Johnson–Nurse, C.; McKibbin, B.; Bradley, J.; and Hastings, G.: The Use of Semi-rigid Carbon-Fibre Reinforced Plastic Plates for Fixation of Human Fractures. J Bone Joint Surg., **64B:**105–111, 1982.

234. Teitz, C C.; Carter, D. R.; and Frankel, V. H.: Problems Associated with Tibial Fractures with Intact Fibulae. J. Bone Joint Surg., **62A:**770–776, 1980.

235. Thompson, J. E. M.: Nonunion and Malunion of Fractures of the Lower Extremity Treated by Medullary Fixation. In DePalma, A. F., (ed.): Clinical Orthopaedics, 2nd ed. Philadelphia, J. B. Lippincott, 1953.

236. Thunold, J.; Varhaug, J. E.; and Bjerkeset, T.: Tibial Shaft Fractures Treated by Rigid Internal Fixation: The Early Results in a 4-Year Series, Injury **7:**125–133, 1975.

237. Torok, G., and Serfati, A: Treatment of Fractures of the Tibial Shaft. Harefuah, **63:**467–470, 1962.

238. Trueta, J., and Cavadias, A. X.: Vascular Change Caused by the Kuntscher Type of Nailing. J. Bone Joint Surg., **37B:**492–505, 1955.

239. Tucker, J. T.; Watkins, F. P.; and Carpenter, E. B.: Conservative Treatment of Fractures of the Shaft of the Tibia. J.A.M.A., **178:**802–805, 1961.

240. Urist, M. R.: End Result Observations Influencing Treatment of Fractures of Shaft of Tibia. J.A.M.A., **159:**1088–1093, 1955.

241. Urist, M. R.; Mazet, R., Jr., and McLean, F. C.: The Pathogenesis and Treatment of Delayed Union and Non-Union. A Survey of Eighty-five Ununited Fractures of the Shaft of the Tibia and One Hundred Control Cases with Similar Injuries. J. Bone Joint Surg., **36A:**931–967, 1954.

242. Van Der Linden, W. Larsson, L.: Plate Fixation Versus Conservative Treatment of Tibia Shaft Fractures. J. Bone Joint Surg., **61A:**873–878, 1979.

243. Veliskakis, K. P.: Primary Internal Fixation in Open Fractures of the Tibial Shaft. The Problem of Wound Healing. J. Bone Joint Surg., **41B:**342–354, 1959.

244. Wade, P. A., and Campbell, R. D., Jr.: Open Versus Closed Methods in Treating Fractures of the Leg. Am. J. Surg., **95:**599–616, 1958.

245. Wagner, J. H.: Anterolateral Approach in Bone Grafting for Ununited Fractures of Tibia. Am. J. Surg., **73:**282–299, 1947.

246. Watson–Jones, R.: Fractures and Joint Injuries, 4th ed. Baltimore, Williams & Wilkins, Vol. 1, 1952; Vol. 2, 1955.

247. Watson–Jones, R.: Styloid Process of the Fibula in the Knee Joint with Peroneal Palsy. J. Bone Joint Surg., **13:**258–260, 1931.

248. Watson–Jones, R., and Coltart, W. D.: Slow Union of Fractures. With a Study of 804 Fractures of the Shafts of the Tibia and Femur. Br. J. Surg., **30:**260–276, 1942.

248a. Weiland, A. J.; Moore, J. R.; and Hotchkiss, R. N.: Soft Tissue Procedures for Reconstruction of Tibial Shaft Fractures. Clin. Orthop., **178:**42–53, 1983.

249. Weissman, S. L., and Herold, H. Z.: Treatment of Tibial Shaft Fractures. A Review of 103 Cases. Harefuah, **63:**462–466, 1962.

250. Weissman, S. L.; Herold, H. Z.; and Engelberg, M.: Fractures of the Middle Two-thirds of the Tibial Shaft. Results of Treatment without Internal Fixation in 140 Consecutive Cases. J. Bone Joint Surg., **48A:**257–267, 1966.

251. White, E. H.; Radley, T. J.; and Earley, N. N.: Screw Stabilization in Fractures of the Tibial Shaft. J. Bone Joint Surg., **35A:**749–755, 1953.

252. Whitesides, T. E., Jr.; Harada, H.; and Morimoto, K.: Compartment Syndromes and the Role of Fasciotomy, Its Parameters and Techniques. AAOS, Instructional Course Lectures, **26:**179, St. Louis, C. V. Mosby, 1977.

253. Widenfolk, B.; Ponten, B.; and Karlstrom, G.: Open Fractures of the Shaft of the Tibia: Analysis of Wound and Fracture Treatment. Injury, **11:**136–143, 1979.

254. Wiggins, H.; Bundens, W.; and Park, B.: Complications Following Open Reduction and Plating of Fractures of the Tibia. Am. J. Surg., **86:**273–281, 1953.

255. Wilson, P. D.: Management of Fractures and Dislocations. Philadelphia, J. B. Lippincott, 1938.

256. Wilson, P. D.: A Simple Method of Two-stage Transplantation of the Fibula for use in Cases of Complicated and Congenital Pseudarthrosis of the Tibia. J. Bone Joint Surg., **29:**639–675, 1941.

257. Zucman, J., and Maurer, P.: Two-level Fractures of the Tibia. J. Bone Joint Surg., **51B:**686–693, 1969.

18

Fractures and Dislocations of the Ankle *Frank C. Wilson*

The purpose of this chapter is to present the biomechanical and biologic concepts of ankle injuries so that therapy may be based on a reconciliation of these fundamentals with the characteristic features of specific injuries. An attempt has been made to avoid a "cookbook" approach to treatment on the premise that if principles are understood, methods will usually be self-evident.

HISTORICAL REVIEW

Knowledge of the forces involved in the production of ankle injuries is founded largely on the work of authors whose contributions were made over two centuries ago. One of the first investigators to consider these mechanisms was Sir Percivall Pott,[66] who in 1768 described a fracture of the fibula "within 2 or 3 inches of its lower extremity" associated with a tear of the deltoid ligament and lateral subluxation of the talus (Fig. 18-1). He ascribed the injury to "leaping or jumping." Since neither malleolus was fractured, use of the term "Pott's fracture" to indicate bimalleolar fracture should be avoided; and, as Pott failed to appreciate the syndesmotic damage associated with this injury, he did in fact describe a fracture that does not occur. He did, however, emphasize the importance of accurate reduction, which he achieved more easily than his predecessors by flexing the knee to relax the calf muscles.

After this early English contribution, the French dominated the field of ankle injuries until the work of Ashhurst and Bromer in 1922. In his 1771 prize essay for the Royal Academy of Surgery in Paris, Jean-Pierre David,[18] writing under the pseudonym of "Basylle," was the first to explain the role of indirect or "contre-coups" forces in the production of ankle fractures.

The contributions of Dupuytren[21] are difficult to assess because of internal inconsistencies in his writings, a tendency to mix opinion with observation, and clinical with autopsy findings. He emphasized the role of "inward and outward" movement of the foot in the production of ankle injuries, distinguishing fractures caused by ligamentous avulsion, which he believed to be the primary injury, and those caused by talar impact, which he thought to be the secondary one. By outward (abduction) movement of the foot, Dupuytren reproduced the fibular fracture observed by Pott; however, he also noted the rupture of the tibiofibular ligaments that is a necessary accompaniment of this fracture (Fig. 18-2) and was the first to describe the proximal intercrural dislocation of the talus that might follow diastasis. It is this lesion perhaps that most justifiably deserves to be called the Dupuytren fracture, although the eponym is a source of more confusion than clarification.

In 1840 Maisonneuve[48] emphasized the role of external rotation in the production of ankle injuries. Unfortunately, his work was neglected at the time in favor of the theories of Dupuytren and other contemporaries, a fact that does not diminish the value of his contributions. In cadaver experiments, he showed how the effects of external rotation

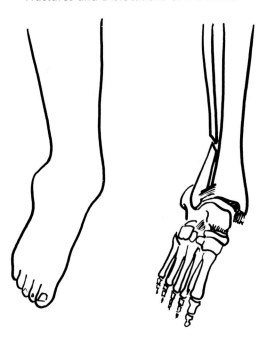

Fig. 18-1. Pott's fracture. (Redrawn from the original illustration by Sir Percivall Pott, 1768.)

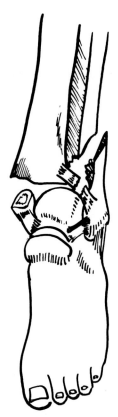

Fig. 18-2. Dupuytren-type fracture. Note "outward" movement of the foot and diastasis. Occasionally the talus dislocates proximally between the tibia and fibula.

forces applied to the foot were determined by the strength of the syndesmosis. If the forces developed were resisted by the anterior tibiofibular ligament (the most common occurrence), an oblique fracture of the fibula occurred beginning anteriorly just below the ligament and extending posterosuperiorly to just above the attachment of the posterior tibiofibular ligament. If the force continued, there was an associated fracture of the medial malleolus or a tear of the deltoid ligament. He then demonstrated that if the tibiofibular ligament yielded first, the fibular fracture might occur as high as the proximal third of the fibula, producing the fracture that bears his name (Fig. 18-3).

Huguier[36] confirmed the importance of external rotation by demonstrating that this force could produce a distal one-third or proximal one-third fibular fracture after rupture of the anterior tibiofibular and deltoid ligaments. He did not specify the position of the foot when the external rotation force was applied to the ankle.

Tillaux[78] described the lesions resulting from a combination of abduction and external rotation in 1872, suggesting that these forces usually occur together in the clinical situation. His experiments did not refute, as he had intended, the findings of Maisonneuve, but he observed, as a secondary lesion, a small bone fragment from the tibia (*frag-*

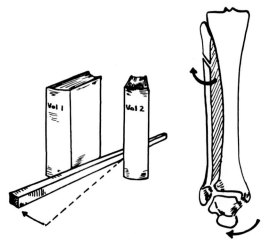

Fig. 18-3. Maisonneuve's fracture. Maisonneuve showed (*left*) how external rotation of the talus could produce a high fibular fracture (*right*). Although not depicted, these injuries usually include tearing of the interosseous membrane as far proximally as the fibular fracture.

ment troisième). Although he did not state whether its origin was anterolateral or posterolateral, his drawings show both fragments, so it must be presumed that either the anterior or posterior tibial tubercles could represent the source of the third fragment.

LeFort,[44] in 1886, described three patients with isolated fractures of the lateral malleolus corresponding to the fibular attachment of the anterior inferior tibiofibular ligament. These findings were confirmed experimentally by his pupil LeRoy[46] in 1887, although both interpreted the mechanism as supination and adduction rather than the more probable external rotation (Fig. 18-4).

With the 20th century came the x-ray, which added an important dimension to the study of ankle fractures by providing, when correlated with biomechanical principles, a means to assess more precisely the nature and mechanism of injury.

Marginal fractures of the distal tibia were probably first recorded by Sir Astley Cooper,[16] who in 1822 described a fracture of the posterior tibial margin that had healed with posterior talar subluxation. In the 1829 *Lancet*, Earle[23] presented the autopsy findings of a fresh posterior lip fracture, which he considered "perfectly novel." Lucas-Championnière[4] theorized in 1870 that vertical compression was necessary to produce this fracture, but it remained for Rochet[71] to document the mechanism 20 years later. He produced a fracture of the posterior articular lip of the tibia by dropping a weight on the upper end of the tibia while the ankle was held in plantar flexion. Destot[20] named the posterior lip of the tibia the third malleolus in 1912, the same year in which Cotton[17] presented a paper to the American Medical Association entitled "A New Type of Ankle Fracture," in which he called attention to fracture of the posterior articular margin of the tibia as a previously undescribed lesion. Many authors have responded by labeling the trimalleolar lesion "Cotton's fracture," an eponym that is clearly inappropriate. The term trimalleolar fracture was coined by Henderson[34] in 1932.

Fracture of the anterior articular margin of the distal tibia was recorded by Nélaton[60] in 1874 in a young patient who fell from the fourth story, a finding that was reported often after introduction of the roentgenogram.

The operative treatment of ankle fractures was pioneered by Lane[41] at the beginning of this century. He preferred screw to wire fixation and employed a "no touch" surgical technique, stating that the absence of "rarefying osteitis" in his cases could be accounted for by more careful precautions and better fixation.

ANATOMY

The ankle is a modified hinge joint consisting of three bones and the ligaments that bind them into a functional unit, upon which the muscles that cross the joint act to produce dorsiflexion or plantar flexion. It has been likened to a mortise and tenon joint in which the talar tenon fits into a mortise formed by the lower end of the tibia and the medial and lateral malleoli.

The lower end of the tibia usually ossifies from a single center that appears in the second year and unites with the shaft of the tibia about the 18th year. Its inferior surface is articular and is often referred to as the tibial plafond (ceiling). This articular surface is concave anteroposteriorly and mediolaterally, broader anteriorly than posteriorly, and longer on its lateral than medial side. The plafond is continuous medially with the medial malleolus, which projects below the plafond and articulates with the medial surface of the talus. The medial malleolus is grooved posteriorly by a shallow sulcus that transmits the tendons of the posterior tibial and flexor digitorum longus muscles. Its distal extremity is divided into two prominences, the anterior and posterior colliculi.

The lower end of the fibula, or lateral malleolus, also ossifies from a separate center; it appears about the second year and unites with the fibular shaft in the 20th year. The lateral malleolus projects about 1 cm distal and posterior to the medial malleolus and has a medial facet for articulation

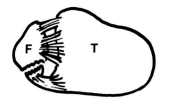 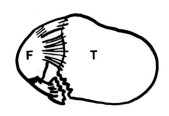

Fig. 18-4. (*Left*) Avulsion fracture of the anterior lip of the fibula by the anterior inferior tibiofibular ligament. (*Right*) Avulsion fracture of the anterolateral margin of the tibia. Either lesion may be produced by external rotation.

with the talus. The broad posterior surface is marked by a sulcus for passage of the peroneus longus and brevis tendons.

The talus, interposed between tibia and calcaneus, articulates distally with the navicular and laterally with the fibula and is covered largely by cartilage. Its body presents a superior trochlea, some 25° wider anteriorly than posteriorly, which is matched for articulation with the tibia. The superior articular surface is continuous with a comma-shaped medial facet and a triangular lateral facet that articulate respectively with the medial and lateral malleoli. The malleoli embrace the talus at an angle opening anteriorly. (Fig. 18-5). Uniting these osseous structures are the medial and lateral collateral ligaments and the ligaments of the tibiofibular syndesmosis.

For practical purposes, motion of the ankle joint may be said to occur about a single axis that is oriented obliquely to the long axis of the leg, passes between the tips of the malleoli, and is directed 20° to 25° laterally, posteriorly, and downward.[38]

The medial collateral or deltoid ligament is a thick triangular band consisting of two sets of fibers, superficial and deep. The superficial fibers arise largely from the anterior colliculus of the medial malleolus and run as a continuous sheet in the sagittal plane to attach to the navicular, the sustenaculum tali, and the talus. The important deep portion of this ligament is intra-articular and more horizontally directed, running from the intercollicular notch and posterior colliculus to the medial surface of the talus (Fig. 18-6 *top*). The deltoid ligament is crossed superficially by the tendons of the posterior tibial and flexor digitorum longus muscles (Fig. 18-6 *bottom*).

The ligamentous support on the lateral side of the ankle is derived from three separate liagments that have less bulk, and therefore provide less support, than the medial ligament. The anterior talofibular ligament runs anteriorly and medially from the anterior margin of the lateral malleolus to the talus anterior to its lateral articular facet. The posterior talofibular ligament runs horizontally from the sulcus on the back of the lateral malleolus to the posterior aspect of the talus lateral to the groove for the flexor hallucis longus tendon. The middle band, named the calcaneofibular ligament, extends downward and posteriorly from the tip of the fibular malleolus to a tubercle on the lateral aspect of the calcaneus (Fig. 18-7), spanning both the ankle and talocalcaneal joints. The ligament is positioned in relation to the axis of motion in these joints so that it causes no undue restriction of motion in either. (Failure to appreciate these unique relationships during reconstruction of the lateral ligaments may lead to unnecessary restriction of

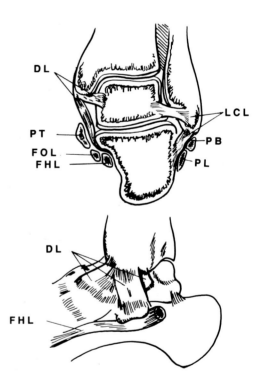

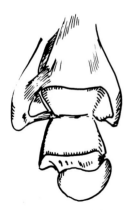

Fig. 18-5. The ankle mortise. The talus and tibial plafond are wider anteriorly than posteriorly.

Fig. 18-6. Deltoid ligament. (*Top*) Cross section showing the relationship of the collateral ligaments to nearby tendons. (*Bottom*) Medial view. (DL, deltoid ligament; PT, posterior tibial tendon; FDL, flexor digitorum longus; FHL, flexor hallucis longus; LCL, lateral collateral ligament; PB, peroneus brevis; PL, peroneus longus).

subtalar motion.) It is crossed by the peroneal tendons and often blends intimately with their sheath (see Fig. 18-6B). When the angle between the anterior talofibular and the calcaneofibular ligaments approximates 90°, the anterior talofibular ligament is tightened during plantar flexion to provide inversion stability, and the calcaneofibular ligament becomes the stabilizer in dorsiflexion. However, when this angle is more obtuse, as is usually the case, inversion stability, especially in plantar flexion, is weakened.[38]

The lower adjacent surfaces of the tibia and fibula are bound together by four ligaments and the interosseous membrane. This syndesmosis is formed by the convex medial surface of the fibula and a corresponding depression of variable depth on the lateral aspect of the tibia known as the peroneal groove. Above, these adjacent surfaces are rough; below, they are covered by articular cartilage separated by a projection of the synovial membrane

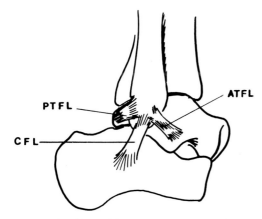

Fig. 18-7. Lateral collateral ligament. (ATFL, anterior talofibular ligament; PTFL, posterior talofibular ligament; CFL, calcaneofibular ligament)

from the ankle joint. The ligaments of the syndesmosis are the anterior and posterior inferior tibiofibular ligaments, the interosseous ligament, and the inferior transverse ligament. The anterior tibiofibular ligament is a quadrilateral band of fibers running downward between the anterior margins of the tibia and fibula. The posterior tibiofibular ligament is smaller and occupies a similar position on the posterior aspect of the tibia and fibula. The inferior transverse ligament is a strong band of fibers, almost continuous with the lower border of the posterior inferior tibiofibular ligament. It extends from the lateral malleolus across the back of the joint to the posterior articular margin of the tibia. The interosseous ligament is the name given to the lower portion of the interosseous membrane. Its fibers are directed obliquely downward from the tibia to the fibula and constitute the strongest bond between these bones (Fig. 18-8).

The arrangement of the syndesmotic ligaments permits slight fibular movement in the craniocaudal, anteroposterior, rotary, and mediolateral planes during normal movement of the ankle joint. These motions have considerable individual variation and provide additional "give" or flexibility to the ankle.[38] McCullough and Burge have shown that in the normal unloaded ankle there is 12° of rotary motion of the distal tibiofibular joint.[52]

The muscles that dorsiflex the ankle joint are the anterior tibial, peroneus tertius, and toe extensors; the triceps surae, posterior tibial, peroneus longus and brevis, and toe flexors provide plantar flexion.

The stability of the ankle joint depends on gravitational effects, positioning, and the arrangement of the bones, ligaments, and muscles. Gravity and muscle contraction tend to produce posterior displacement of the talus on the tibia; these forces are resisted by the bony architecture and ligaments. The shape of the talar dome and the intermalleolar

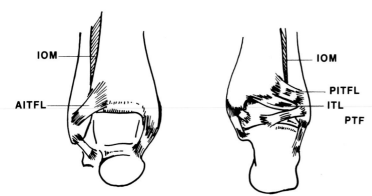

Fig. 18-8. Ligaments of the syndesmosis. (*Left*) Anterior view. (*Right*) Posterior view. (IOM, interosseous membrane; AITFL, anterior inferior tibiofibular ligament; PITFL, posterior inferior tibiofibular ligament; ITL, inferior transverse ligament; PTF, posterior talofibular ligament)

distance, both of which are wider anteriorly than posteriorly, confer greater stability in dorsiflexion. In addition, the posterior tibial margin projects further inferiorly than the anterior; this posterior talar "socket" is deepened by the fibers of the inferior transverse ligament (Fig. 18-9). Additional ligamentous stability is afforded by the medial and lateral collateral and syndesmotic ligaments.

RADIOGRAPHY

Routine radiographic examination of the ankle includes anteroposterior, lateral, and mortise views (Fig. 18-10). The special techniques of stress films and arthrography are discussed in the section on injuries of the ligaments.

The anteroposterior x-ray is taken in the long axis of the foot and is particularly useful for evaluation of medial or lateral shift of the talus, adduction fractures of the medial malleolus, or abduction fractures of the lateral malleolus.

In the lateral x-ray the fibula overlaps the posterior portion of the tibia, except for the posterior tibial tubercle. This view is especially useful to demonstrate external rotation fractures of the fibula and fractures of the anterior or posterior tibial articular margins. Superimposition of the talus and fibula makes visualization of the medial malleolus difficult in the lateral view.

The mortise view is an anteroposterior projection taken with the medial and lateral malleoli on a plane horizontal to the table. Since localization of the malleoli may be difficult in the presence of soft tissue swelling, this view may be more reliably obtained by positioning the foot on the table with the fifth metatarsal in 10 to 15° of internal rotation.[31] Since the anterior tubercle of the peroneal groove projects further laterally than the posterior, this view places the tubercles in approximately the same plane and thus provides the least obstruction to visualization of the inferior tibiofibular joint. Even so, the depth of the peroneal groove usually impairs visualization of this area. If a clear zone is visualized it is difficult to know whether it indicates a shallow peroneal groove or diastasis unless its width exceeds 3 mm in the mortise view, in which case one may be reasonably certain of diastasis.[4] The clear zone between the medial malleolus and the talus is also seen best in this view, although its width varies somewhat with the tube-to-target distance and the degree of plantar flexion of the talus.

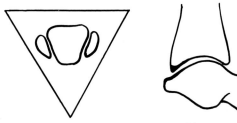

Fig. 18-9. Bony stability of the ankle joint. Posterior displacement of the foot is prevented by (*left*) greater anterior width of the talus and (*Right*) distal projection of the posterior tibia, which is further deepened by the inferior transverse ligament.

CLASSIFICATION OF ANKLE INJURIES

Destot,[4] in 1911, correlated radiographic findings with previous anatomical experiments, providing the basis for determining the mechanism of injury from the appearance of the x-rays.

In 1922 Ashhurst and Bromer[2] provided the first comprehensive classification of ankle fractures according to mechanism of injury. In their series of 300 cases, approximately 95% were caused by external rotation (60%), abduction (20%), or adduction (15%) of the foot relative to the leg. Within each major group they distinguished three degrees of injury that they attributed to progressively severe injuring force: first degree injuries involved only one malleolus; second degree injuries were bimalleolar or (malleolar fracture and contralateral ligament rupture); and third degree injuries involved a fracture of the entire lower end of the tibia as well as the fibular malleolus. Three per cent of these injuries were attributed to compression, which the authors felt could produce isolated anterior or posterior marginal lip fractures or comminution of the tibial plafond.

This classification has the following limitations: (1) it fails to emphasize ligamentous damage sufficiently, especially in relation to diastasis; (2) the third degree of injury in each group probably represents a different mechanism of injury rather than a progression in the severity of the injuring force; (3) it suggests that ankle fractures are produced by a unidirectional force rather than a combination of forces, which is more often the case.

A more detailed classification of ankle fractures was provided by Lauge-Hansen,[42] who, from ca-

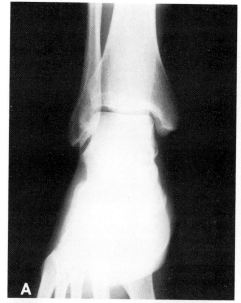

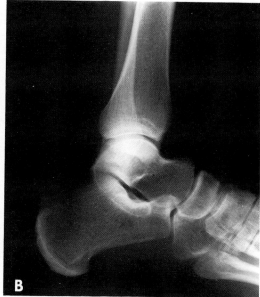

Fig. 18-10. (*A*) Anteroposterior, (*B*) lateral, and (*C*) mortise x-rays of a normal ankle.

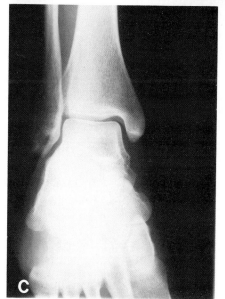

daver experiments, distinguished four major types of injury with several stages in each group. In this classification the first word refers to the position of the foot at the time of injury and the second to the direction of the injuring force; one must also understand that eversion refers to lateral or external rotation and inversion to medial or internal rotation:

SUPINATION–ADDUCTION

Stage 1. Transverse fracture of the lateral malleo-

lus at varying heights or tear of the lateral collateral ligaments

Stage 2. Stage 1 plus fracture of the medial malleolus

SUPINATION–EVERSION

Stage 1. Rupture of the anterior inferior tibiofibular ligament, sometimes by avulsion of a bone fragment from the tibia or fibula (Whether rupture of this ligament always precedes Stage 2 is a much debated point.)

Stage 2. Stage 1 plus a spiral oblique fracture of the lateral malleolus

Stage 3. Stage 2 plus a fracture of the posterior lip of the tibia

Stage 4. Stage 3 plus a fracture of the medial malleolus or tear of the deltoid ligament

PRONATION–ABDUCTION

Stage 1. Fracture of the medial malleolus or tear of the deltoid ligament

Stage 2. Stage 1 plus rupture of the anterior inferior tibiofibular and posterior inferior tibiofibular ligament, and transverse ligament, with fracture of the posterior lip of the tibia

Stage 3. Stage 2 plus an oblique supramalleolar fracture of the fibula, *i.e.,* the anterior and posterior tibiofibular ligaments tear but the interosseous does not

PRONATION–EVERSION

Stage 1. Same as Stage 1 of pronation–abduction injuries

Stage 2. Stage 1 plus a tear of the anterior inferior tibiofibular and interosseous ligaments

Stage 3. Stage 2 plus an interosseous membrane tear and spiral fracture of the fibula 7 to 8 cm proximal to the tip of the lateral malleolus

Stage 4. Stage 3 plus a fracture of the posterior lip of the tibia secondary to ligamentous avulsion by the posterior inferior and inferior transverse tibiofibular ligaments

About three fourths of Lauge-Hansen's cases fell into the first two groups (*i.e.,* occur with the foot inverted, which reflects the inclusion of sprains of the lateral collateral ligament).

It is of interest that the lesion produced by external rotation varied with the position of the foot: with external rotation of the supinated foot the first injury was on the lateral side of the ankle (as Maisonneuve suggested), whereas with external rotation of the pronated foot, the first injury was to the medial structures. External rotation produced extensive damage to the syndesmotic ligaments only when the foot was pronated, a concept that has been challenged by Pankovich,[65] who found syndesmotic injury also following external rotation of the supinated foot. Also, fracture of the posterior lip of the tibia involving more than a small portion of the articular surface of the tibia required vertical compression in addition to external rotational forces, whereas small posterior lip fractures were avulsed

by the posterior tibiofibular ligament as a result of talar rotation in the mortise.

Lauge-Hansen's experimentally based classification advanced pathogenetic understanding of ankle injuries by indicating the relationship of ligamentous damage to fracture patterns and the sequences in which different structures are damaged when specified forces are applied; however, it is unnecessarily detailed and cumbersome for routine use in manipulative reductions.

The Danis-Weber (AO) classification[58] emphasizes the fibular fracture, pointing out that the higher the fibular break the greater the syndesmotic injury and displacement of the mortise. Three types of fibular fracture are recognized: type A, caused by internal rotation and adduction, is a transverse fracture at or below the joint line, with a possible shear fracture of the medial malleolus; type B results from external rotation, which produces a fracture rising obliquely from the joint line in an anteroposterior plane (with or without rupture of the inferior tibiofibular ligament) and associated medial injury; type C fractures are divided into those resulting from abduction alone (C1), which causes an oblique medial to lateral fibular break above a ruptured tibiofibular ligament, and those resulting from a combination of abduction and external rotation (C2), wherein more extensive syndesmotic rupture leads to a similar but higher fracture that is often comminuted laterally. Both type C injuries may be associated with deltoid ligament ruptures or transverse medial malleolar fractures, and all types may occur with posterior malleolar fragments, either large or small. It is suggested by Hughes[35] that type A fractures may be managed successfully by nonoperative methods, whereas types B and C, because of associated ligamentous injury, usually cannot be reduced and held without internal fixation. Although pointing out that more extensive injury may require more complex treatment, this classification adds little to our understanding of the pathogenesis of ankle injuries.

Since fracture reduction involves reversal of the force causing the injury, the practical value of any pathogenetic classification lies in its applicability to treatment. By careful analysis of the x-rays, it is possible to identify the primary movement of the foot (in relation to the leg) that produced the fracture. These primary movements are external rotation, abduction, adduction, and vertical compression (Fig. 18-11). The common occurrence of these movements in combination produces subtle radiographic differences and therapeutic implica-

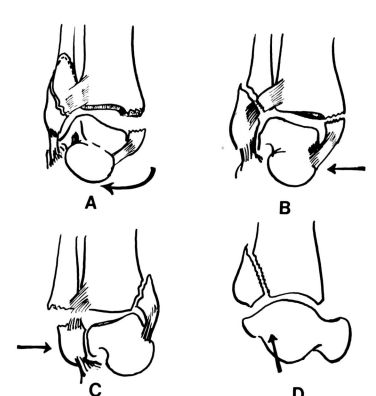

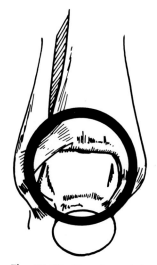

Fig. 18-11. Basic mechanisms of ankle injury with the characteristic fractures produced by each. (*A*) External rotation, (*B*) abduction, (*C*) adduction, (*D*) vertical compression.

tions that will be described in the sections that follow.

FRACTURES OF THE ANKLE

As Neer[59] has pointed out, the ankle mortise actually constitutes a ring of three bones and their uniting ligaments (Fig. 18-12). Since most ankle injuries are produced by abnormal motion of the talus, in which a malleolus is either pushed off or pulled off by means of its ligamentous attachments, the talus may be said to be the ringleader. Because these ligaments do not stretch, a single break in the ring permits no anteroposterior or lateral shift of the talus in the mortise. For talar shift to occur, there must be at least two breaks—either a fracture of both malleoli or a fracture of one malleolus and rupture of one ligament (Fig. 18-13). This fact is important in assessing the stability or potential for displacement of any ankle injury. In general, fractures produced by ligamentous avulsion are transverse; those produced by talar impact are oblique, often with comminution on the side of the bone subject to compression forces. The plane of obliquity of the fracture is determined by the direction of the forces involved in its production. Thus, in a fracture

Fig. 18-12. The ring of the ankle mortise.

of the fibula produced by abduction, tension forces are developed in the medial cortex at the point of talar impact, and compression occurs laterally, producing a fracture line directed from inferomedial to superolateral and lateral comminution (Fig. 18-14). In pure external rotation injuries, talar

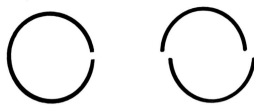

Fig. 18-13. The potential for talar shift is determined by the number of breaks in the mortise ring; (*left*) stable, (*right*) unstable.

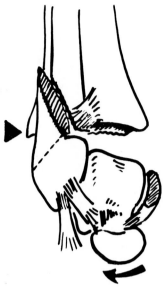

Fig. 18-15. External rotation of the foot produces an oblique fibular fracture in the anteroposterior plane, often with posterior comminution.

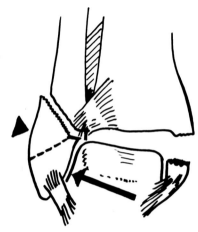

Fig. 18-14. Abduction of the foot produces a short oblique fracture of the fibula in the mediolateral plane, often with lateral comminution.

impact is directed posteriorly so that the fracture line usually runs from anteroinferior to posterosuperior. Since the compression forces develop posteriorly under these circumstances, fragmentation tends to occur in the posterior cortex (Fig. 18-15).

Whether ligament or bone fails when a ligamentous-osseous complex is stressed depends on the relative ability of each to withstand the type of stress applied. Frequently a malleolar fracture occurs on one side of the ankle and a ligamentous disruption on the other. When fractures and ligamentous lesions coexist, the soft-tissue lesion is often ignored in favor of the more visible bone lesion. Because ligamentous injury frequently has more serious implications than fracture, it is important that it be recognized and included in the plan of treatment. The diagnosis of ligamentous injury may be inferred if the x-ray shows a *displaced* malleolar fracture, since there must be another injury in the ring to permit such displacement (Fig. 18-16).

FRACTURES RESULTING PRIMARILY FROM EXTERNAL ROTATION

MECHANISM OF INJURY

In the clinical situation, external rotation of the talus and the ankle mortise usually results from internal rotation of the body on the fixed foot. The first pathologic event is tearing of the deltoid ligament, which begins with its anterior fibers and may extend through the entire ligament. Alternatively, the anterior colliculus or entire medial malleolus is avulsed. The fibula is then compressed in a predominantly anteroposterior direction by the rotating talus, producing a spiral or oblique fracture line directed from anteroinferior to posterosuperior that begins below an intact anterior tibiofibular ligament, or above a torn one. In general, the more proximal the fibular fracture, the greater the damage to the tibiofibular ligaments. The most extensive tearing is found with fractures of the proximal third of the fibula (Maisonneuve fracture), in which the interosseous membrane is usually torn as far proximally as the fibular fracture (Fig. 18-17).

External rotation of the supinated or adducted foot occurs less frequently and is radiographically similar to external rotation fracture of the pronated foot, except that the interosseous ligaments are less likely to be injured, and the fibular fracture therefore rarely begins above the tibial plafond.

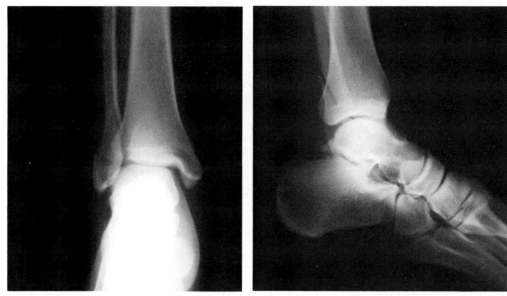

Fig. 18-16. External rotation injury. Tear of the deltoid ligament may be inferred from the displacement of the fibular fracture and widening of the medial clear space.

CLINICAL FINDINGS

The clinical findings vary with the degree of injury. Examination should include all structures about the ankle, the interosseous area and the proximal fibula. Once the neurovascular status of the foot has been assessed, each of the bones and ligaments should be carefully examined. Tenderness, swelling, and ecchymosis occur with either fracture or ligament injury, but their location and the presence of crepitus will usually distinguish osseous injuries. With stable injuries (*i.e.* no more than one break in the ring) the patient may be able to bear weight on the injured limb; walking is rarely possible with unstable lesions. If the lesion is unstable, and the talus has shifted, there will also be a valgus deformity of the ankle.

RADIOGRAPHIC FINDINGS

The spectrum of radiographic findings following external rotation injury ranges from soft-tissue swelling to trimalleolar fracture with dislocation of the talus. Three different types of fibular fracture occur: long oblique, short oblique, or a combined transverse and oblique. Comminution, if present, is posterior. Although it is usually in the distal third, the exact level of the fibular fracture varies with the degree of syndesmotic disruption and is best seen in the lateral x-ray; in fact, if undis-

placed, it may be seen *only* in the lateral view (Fig. 18-18). The distal fibular fragment is usually externally rotated and may be displaced superiorly and posteriorly. Medial malleolar fractures are usually slightly oblique in the anteroposterior plane, usually at or below the tibial plafond, and may be displaced inferiorly by the attached deltoid ligament. If the fibular fracture is displaced and no other fracture exists, either the syndesmotic or the deltoid ligaments or both are torn. Incomplete (anterior) rupture of the syndesmosis is often difficult to infer without an avulsed bone fragment, but at least partial rupture of the deltoid ligament must be suspected if the medial clear space is widened. Posterior lip fractures are usually small, unless vertical compression has been a component of the injury. If only the tubercle is involved, the fracture may be invisible. When displaced, the posterior fragment is usually shifted upward and posteriorly. If the anteroposterior x-ray shows the proximal fibular fragment superimposed behind the tibia, this fragment may be locked behind the lateral edge of the tibia, a complication that often, but not invariably, requires open reduction.[5,50]

When abduction is associated with external rotation, the obliquity of the fracture line is shorter, its direction shifted from the anteroposterior toward the mediolateral plane, and its location is some 2½ inches above the tip of the lateral malleolus.

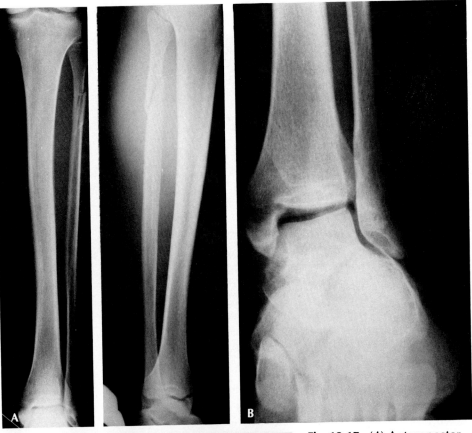

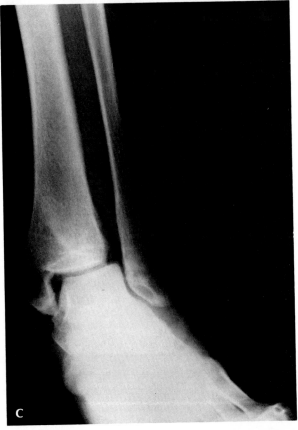

Fig. 18-17. (*A*) Anteroposterior and lateral views of the Maisonneuve fracture. There is a small undisplaced fracture of the posterior lip of the tibia. With abduction stress (*B*), the extent of the syndesmotic injury cannot be appreciated, but with external rotation stress (*C*) complete diastasis is apparent. (Courtesy of Charles A. Rockwood, Jr., M.D.)

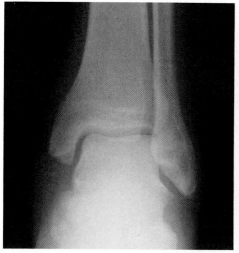

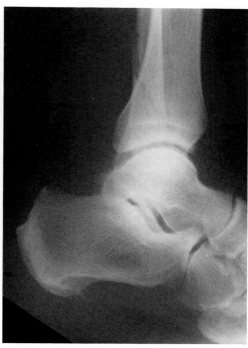

Fig. 18-18. An undisplaced external rotation fracture of the fibula. These injuries are frequently invisible on the anteroposterior view.

TREATMENT

The goals of treatment are the same for all ankle injuries: anatomical positioning of the talus in the mortise, a joint line that is parallel to the ground, and a smooth articular surface. Unless these requisites are achieved by treatment, post-traumatic arthritis is likely to occur.[69]

Stable injuries requiring no reduction are immobilized only for comfort and protection. I use a posterior molded splint from toe to knee, held in place with an elastic bandage until swelling has subsided. No weight bearing is permited during this period, and elevation is encouraged. A below-knee walking cast is then applied with the foot and ankle in a neutral position and weight bearing progressed as tolerated. After 3 to 4 weeks, healing is sufficiently advanced to terminate immobilization.

Unstable injuries, such as bimalleolar fractures or fracture of one malleolus with contralateral ligament rupture, require reduction. Most surgeons would probably agree that if a satisfactory reduction cannot be achieved by closed methods, the fracture should be treated operatively. Difficulty arises in the definition of a satisfactory reduction. How much displacement of the talus or malleoli may be accepted with the expectation of a satisfactory result? For the talus the answer is clear: it must be positioned anatomically under the tibial plafond. Even slight talar shift may cause sufficient joint

incongruity to result in degenerative changes.[40,81] Ramsey and Hamilton have shown that a lateral shift of the talus of just 1 mm can lead to abnormal wear on the tibiotalar joint.[69] The sequelae of isolated malleolar displacement are less predictable. Failure to reposition a malleolus anatomically is less likely to be associated with a poor end result than is talar displacement, although symptomatic nonunions and malunions do occur.[81] Occasionally, persistent malleolar displacement prevents stable talar reduction, as in medial malleolar fractures at the level of the plafond, where interposed periosteum and retinacular ligament may prevent bone union, allowing sufficient mediolateral talar instability to cause degenerative changes in the ankle joint.

The primary indication for operative treatment, therefore, is the inability to obtain or maintain *anatomical* position of the talus in relation to the tibia. The major contraindication is the presence of extensive comminution, which precludes anatomical reduction or rigid fixation, leaving the patient subject to the risks of operative intervention without its benefits.

Technique of Closed Reduction

Knowledge of the mechanism of injury is necessary to carry out manipulative reduction. What-

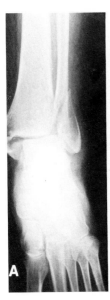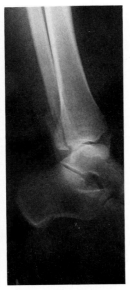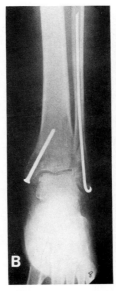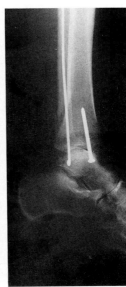

Fig. 18-19. (A) Anteroposterior and lateral x-rays of an abduction-external rotation fracture treated by (B) internal fixation. Stabilization of both malleoli reduces the need for external immobilization.

ever the method employed, the principle is the same: reversal of the injuring forces. For example, fractures produced by external rotation and abduction are reduced by internal rotation and adduction of the foot. Plaster immobilization should extend above the flexed knee to control rotation of the tibia. That portion of the cast from the supramalleolar area to the groin is applied first so that only the foot and ankle require manual control during manipulation. If posterior subluxation of the talus is present, the foot should be held forward during application of the cast. Care must be taken to avoid plantar flexion of the ankle, since in this position, the taut anterior fibers of the deltoid ligament are tightened and prevent replacement of the medial malleolus. Interposition of periosteum at the fracture site or impingement of the lateral malleolus on the proximal fibular fragment may also prevent its reduction.[82] Union of the fracture is usually sufficiently advanced within a month to permit application of a walking cast with the foot and ankle returned to a neutral position. All immobilization may normally be discontinued after an additional month. It is not necessary or desirable to await radiographic evidence of fibular union, since union occurs clinically long before it becomes visible on the x-ray. If there is damage to the syndesmotic ligaments, weight bearing should be deferred until 3 months or more after injury, since solid ligamentous healing is necessary to prevent late spread of the syndesmosis.[40]

Open Reduction

Primary operative treatment for ankle fractures has been recommended with increasing frequency in recent years, in spite of tenuous data to support this position and infection rates as high as 18%.[26,35,49,56,57] Many authors have advocated the AO technique, which emphasizes rigid anatomical reconstruction of the mortise. However, the admonition of the AO group that "internal fixation of the lower end of the fibula should be done with a minimum amount of internal fixation"[58] is often overlooked or sacrificed to achieve more rigid stabilization than is necessary for early movement. In general, the application of heavy plates on a subcutaneous bone surface should be avoided. Except for the occasional comminuted fracture, plating of the fibula is unwarranted for either reduction or fixation.

Should open reduction be necessary, several principles should be observed: (1) the need for anatomical reduction of the mortise, always important, is even more critical after internal fixation, since no further spontaneous or manipulative adjustments are possible; (2) fixation should be rigid enough to permit early motion; and (3) all bone or cartilage debris must be removed from the joint. If surgery is planned, it should be done promptly, since operative delay, especially after repeated manipulations, has been correlated with less satisfactory end results.[26]

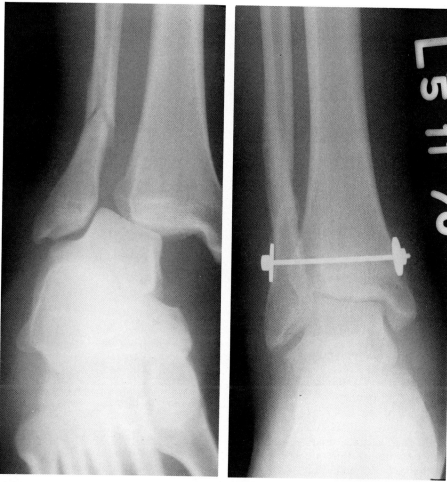

Fig. 18-20. A Dupuytren-type fracture with rupture of the distal tibiofibular ligaments and the interosseous ligament up to the level of the fractured fibula, along with a rupture of the deltoid ligament. (*Left*) Note the complete tibiofibular diastasis. (*Right*) Closed reduction was unsuccessful and transsyndesmotic bolting and deltoid ligament repair were necessary.

I prefer to fix both malleoli, beginning with the lateral malleolus, which may be stabilized with an intramedullary screw or Rush pin. A single screw, directed perpendicular to the fracture line, is sufficient for most medial malleolar fractures,[81] (Fig. 18-19). If both malleoli are fixed securely, the only external immobilization needed is a below-knee posterior molded splint, which should be removed several times daily for active range of motion exercises of the foot and ankle. After suture removal, a below-knee walking cast is applied, and full weight bearing permitted. Immobilization is maintained for about 2 months following injury. Direct suture of a fresh rupture of the syndesmotic ligaments is usually unnecessary, since anatomical replacement of the malleoli compels reduction of

the syndesmosis; however, in injuries over a week old consolidation of the hematoma in the syndesmosis makes reduction difficult and transsyndesmotic bolting is preferred to insure anatomical reduction (Fig. 18-20). Since it prevents normal motion of the syndesmosis, rigid tibiofibular fixation should be removed before unprotected ambulation is begun.

If swelling precludes definitive treatment of external rotation-abduction injuries by either open or closed methods, the foot may be suspended in stockinette as recommended by Quigley.[68] After application of stockinette from toe to groin, the limb is suspended at the knee and foot by means of weights (Fig. 18-21). Thus balanced, the foot will assume a position of internal rotation and

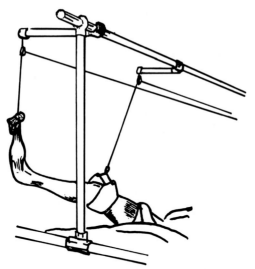

Fig. 18-21. Suspension treatment of external rotation injuries. (Redrawn from Quigley, T. B.: Management of Ankle Injuries in Sports. J.A.M.A., **169**:1434, 1959).

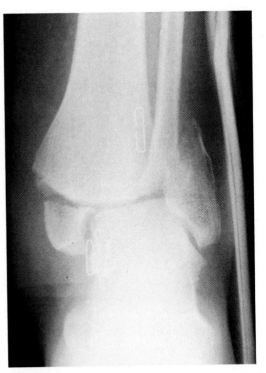

Fig. 18-22. Low abduction fracture of the fibula. Note the short oblique fibular fracture and transverse medial malleolar fracture.

adduction, which often accomplishes the reduction by the time the swelling has subsided. A further convenience of this method is that the cast may be easily applied to the leg while it is suspended.

When the medial component of an external rotation injury is a tear of the deltoid ligament (usually at its attachment to the medial malleolus), the indications for open reduction are no different from those in bimalleolar fractures, *i.e.,* inability to obtain or maintain satisfactory position by closed reduction and casting. In about 10% of the cases, anatomical reduction of the talus will be prevented by infolding of the ligament or displacement of the posterior tibial tendon into the joint.[28] After the interposed soft tissue is removed from the joint and the ligament is repaired, additional stability is obtained by internal fixation of the fibula. Above-knee casting is used for about 1 month, followed by a similar period in a below-knee cast. Early motion is not permitted. (See also section on injuries of the deltoid ligament.)

External rotation injuries associated with large posterior lip fractures are discussed under vertical compression fractures.

FRACTURES RESULTING PRIMARILY FROM ABDUCTION

MECHANISM OF INJURY

Injuries of the ankle from abduction forces alone are less common than those caused by external rotation. When pure abduction of the foot does occur, the first injury is to either the medial malleolus or, more rarely, the deltoid ligament. Medial injury is followed by fracture of the fibula below the syndesmotic ligaments or rupture of these ligaments (Fig. 18-22). If the ligaments yield first, fracture of the fibula occurs between the supramalleolar level and the junction of the middle and distal thirds of the fibula (Fig. 18-23). The most proximal level of the interosseous tear corresponds to the level of the fibular fracture. Small anterior or posterior marginal fractures of the tibia or fibula may be produced if rupture of the syndesmotic ligaments occurs through their attachments to bone. If external rotation accompanies abduction, the fibular fracture is likely to be higher and more helical than with abduction injuries alone, since ligaments have less resistance to shear than to tension. The association of vertical compression with abduction often produces an impacted fracture of the lateral plafond with tilting of the joint and late degenerative changes[15] (Fig. 18-24).

CLINICAL FINDINGS

The clinical findings depend on the severity of the injury. If both sides of the mortise are disrupted, the foot is abducted in proportion to the amount

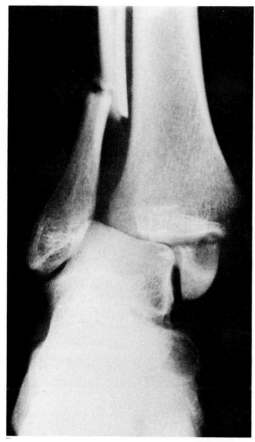

Fig. 18-23. High abduction fracture (Dupuytren-type) of the fibula. This injury must be accompanied by tearing of the tibiofibular ligaments and the interosseus membrane as far proximally as the fibular fracture.

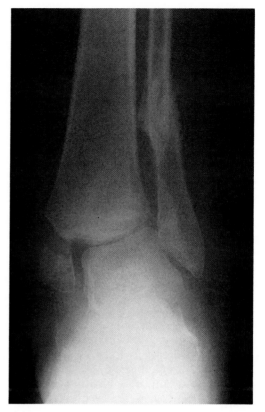

Fig. 18-24. Compression fracture of the lateral plafond. These injuries are usually the result of abduction and vertical compression forces.

of talar displacement, producing increased prominence of the lower medial tibia. If sufficient lateral displacement of the foot occurs, the medial malleolus may protrude through the skin, allowing bacterial contamination of both the fracture and the joint. Tenderness, swelling, ecchymosis, and crepitus are present at the fracture sites.

RADIOGRAPHIC FINDINGS

The typical fibular lesion is seen on the anteroposterior x-ray as a short oblique fracture directed from inferomedial to superolateral. The lateral cortex is frequently comminuted. Fractures of the medial malleolus are transverse and usually occur below the level of the plafond. Absence of a medial malleolar fracture in the presence of a displaced fibular fracture and lateral talar shift is evidence of a tear of the deltoid ligament. Since all syndesmotic ligaments are frequently torn with this injury,

diastasis is more apparent than in external rotation injuries, which usually spare the posterior ligaments. Variation in the depth of the peroneal groove and in radiographic projection make it difficult to determine the status of the syndesmotic ligaments from the x-ray unless gross separation of the tibia and fibula has occurred. Small fracture fragments avulsed from the anterior or posterior margins of the tibia or fibula are occasionally seen, as is compression of the lateral plafond.

TREATMENT

The principles of treatment are no different from those for external rotation fractures, except that adduction is required for reduction. Open reduction is necessary if anatomical replacement of the talus cannot be achieved and maintained by closed methods. Since loss of position in unstable ankle fractures may occur as late as 18 days following fracture, x-rays should be taken at regular intervals during this period to insure that the talus has not become displaced. If open reduction is required, both malleoli are internally fixed in order to insure reduction of the syndesmosis. A below-knee cast is required for about 2 months, and weight bearing is deferred for an additional month. When treatment has been delayed for a week or more after injury, it is probably advisable to fix the tibiofibular joint with a bolt, which should be inserted with the talus in neutral position or slight dorsiflexion; if it is inserted with the talus in plantar flexion, the malleoli will be drawn together to grip the narrower posterior portion of the talus, and dorsiflexion will be restricted.

Compression fractures of the lateral plafond that allow tilting of the talus should be managed by elevation of the fragments and packing of the subchondral area with bone;[55] otherwise obliquity of the joint line causes abnormal concentration of weight-bearing forces medially, which may result in painful degenerative changes.

FRACTURES RESULTING PRIMARILY FROM ADDUCTION

MECHANISM OF INJURY

In contrast to external rotation and abduction forces, adduction violence is more frequently an isolated event. Injuries produced by pure adduction are never associated with diastasis, and posterior marginal fractures are uncommon. Adduction commonly results in a tear of the lateral collateral ligament; however, if the collateral ligaments prove stronger than the fibula, fracture of the lateral malleolus occurs and, with continuation of the force, the medial malleolus is fractured by talar impact.

If vertical compression is associated with adduction forces, the type of fracture produced depends on the position of the ankle. If the talus is dorsiflexed at the time of injury, the medial malleolar fragment may contain a portion of the anterior articular margin of the tibia; if the talus is plantar flexed, the posteromedial margin of the tibia may be included with the medial malleolar fracture.

The combination of adduction and external rotation is discussed in the section on external rotation injuries.

CLINICAL FINDINGS

The findings on examination range from those of a sprain of the lateral collateral ligament to those of bimalleolar fracture. If the talus is displaced medially, there will be a varus deformity of the foot.

RADIOGRAPHIC FINDINGS

The fibula is fractured transversely, usually at or below the level of the plafond; the medial malleolus

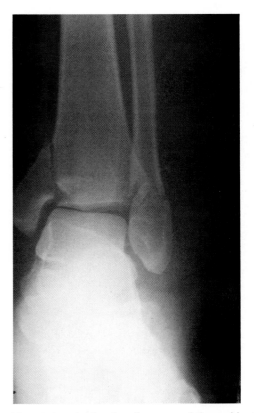

Fig. 18-25. Adduction fracture of the ankle. Note the transverse fracture of the avulsed lateral malleolus and the vertical oblique fracture of the compressed medial malleolus.

is fractured more vertically, the fracture line extending upward and medially from the junction of the medial malleolus with the plafond (Fig. 18-25). Careful inspection of the x-ray will frequently reveal comminution of the medial corner of the plafond. Medial displacement of the malleoli accompanies medial shift of the talus.

TREATMENT

Wedging of small comminuted fragments into the fracture line often prevents closed reduction, so that open reduction with internal fixation may be required to restore a smooth joint surface. Open reduction also provides the opportunity to remove detached pieces of bone and cartilage from the joint. The medial malleolus is approached first, since the compressed side of the joint is more likely to contain comminuted fragments that may block reduction. Adduction produces a larger and inherently more unstable medial malleolar fracture; as a result, fixation with two screws is preferred, one of which is directed perpendicular to the fracture

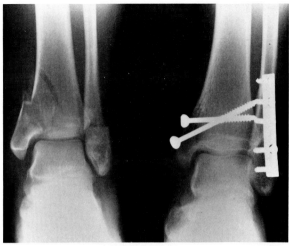

Fig. 18-26. Bimalleolar fracture produced by adduction. Note placement of medial malleolar screws; one at a right angle to the tibial cortex, the other perpendicular to the fracture line. Intramedullary fixation would have been preferable for the fibula.

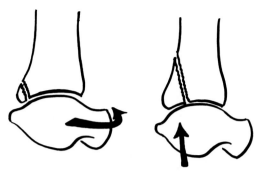

Fig. 18-27. Posterior marginal fractures produced by (*left*) ligamentous avulsion, and (*right*) vertical compression.

line and the other at a right angle to the tibial cortex (Fig. 18-26). The transverse lateral malleolar fracture is stabilized with an intramedullary device, after which the same postoperative regimen is followed as for external rotation injuries treated by open reduction and internal fixation. The end result is often worse than that following external rotation or abduction injuries because of the frequent articular surface comminution, which predisposes to post-traumatic arthritis.[81]

FRACTURES RESULTING PRIMARILY FROM VERTICAL COMPRESSION

As previously noted, vertical compression is often associated with other forces in the production of ankle fractures; however, compression is occasionally an isolated mechanism, and, depending on the position of the talus and the direction of the force, the posterior or anterior articular margins or the entire articular surface of the tibia may be fractured.

POSTERIOR MARGINAL FRACTURES

It should be understood that posterior marginal fractures are of two fundamental types: those without a significant element of vertical compression that include the tibial tubercle and occasionally a small portion of the articular surface, and those produced by compression of the talar dome, which usually involve a larger portion of the articular margin (Fig. 18-27). When abduction or external rotation forces are associated with vertical compres-

sion, the fractures are commonly confined to the more prominent posterolateral portion of the plafond; with adduction, the fragment is posteromedial. Posterior marginal fracture is not essential for posterior dislocation of the talus, but for talar displacement to occur without posterior marginal fracture there must be a tear of the posterior talofibular ligament.

Isolated posterior marginal fracture is a rare occurrence. According to Bonnin,[4] it is incurred by kicking a solid object with the ankle in either plantar flexion or neutral position. Patients with this injury often give a history of having been able to bear weight on the affected limb after the injury, and examination discloses tenderness and ecchymosis adjacent to the tendo Achillis. The fragment is held in place by the syndesmotic ligaments and posterior capsule; displacement is therefore rare, unless there is an associated fracture of the fibula (Fig. 18-28). A word of caution: before this diagnosis is made the proximal fibula should be carefully examined to exclude a Maisonneuve-type external rotation injury (see Fig. 18-3 and 18-17).

An undisplaced, isolated fracture of the posterior lip may be treated by application of a below-knee cast with the foot and ankle in neutral position. The cast may be removed for ranging exercises after a month, but weight bearing should be deferred for at least an additional month to allow further repair of the articular cartilage.

The treatment of displaced fractures varies with the size of the fragment. When a large segment is displaced, the posterior tibial socket loses its hold on the talus, favoring posterior subluxation. Most authors have stated that the fragment must involve between one fourth and one third of the articular surface to allow this instability. In McLaughlin's[55] series, failure to reduce fractures involving less than 10% of the articular surface was not associated

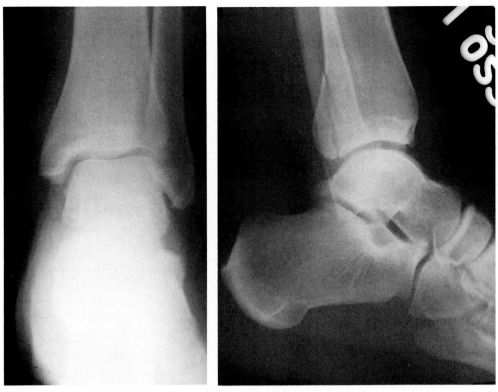

Fig. 18-28. Isolated fracture of the posterior lip of the tibia.

with posterior talar subluxation; with 10% to 25% of the articular surface involved, 20% of the unreduced fractures eventually had posterior subluxation; and with fragments of greater than 25%, 100% showed eventual subluxation and post-traumatic arthritis. He concluded that fractures involving over 25% of the articular surface should have open reduction and internal fixation. Nelson and Jensen[61] recommended open reduction and internal fixation for posterior marginal fractures involving one third or more of the articular surface. Their recommendation was apparently based on one patient in their series who obtained a "good result" following this method of treatment. No further documentation of this figure has been offered, although it is the figure upon which many orthopaedic surgeons base their decision for operative treatment. McDaniel and Wilson,[53] in their study of trimalleolar fractures, found a higher incidence of late degenerative changes in association with: (1) large posterior lip fragments, (2) inaccurate reduction, and (3) residual talar displacement. Anatomical reduction of the posterior lip was not achieved by closed reduction in any patient in their series. Denham's[19] observation that the strong ligamentous bond between the posterior lip fracture when the lateral malleolus is reduced has not been reliable in my experience, especially when the tibial fragment is large. Although there are insufficient data to permit definitive treatment recommendations, I prefer open reduction and internal fixation with two screws for fractures of the posterior margin involving over 25% of the articular surface.

When posterior marginal fracture is associated with fracture of the malleoli, the same guidelines for internal fixation of the posterior fragment apply; however, the presence of anteroposterior talar stability does not insure mediolateral stability. Once the posterior lip has been secured, the choice of treatment for the bimalleolar injury should be governed by the same indications that obtain for bimalleolar fractures alone.

ANTERIOR MARGINAL FRACTURES (TIBIAL PLAFOND INJURIES)

Fracture of the anterior margin of the tibia usually occurs as a crush of the anterior lip but may include a major fragment. The crush injuries usually occur when the dorsiflexed talus is forced against the anterior tibial margin, whereas large fragments are

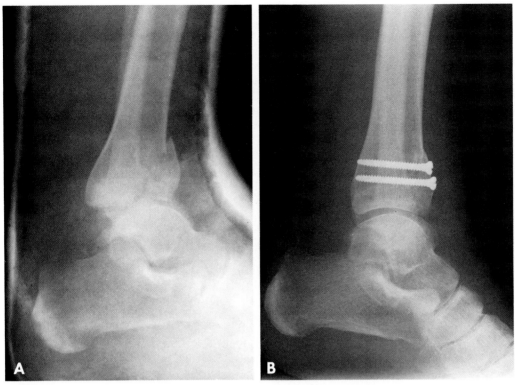

Fig. 18-29. (*A*) Fracture of the anterior lip of the tibia with a major fragment unsuccessfully reduced by closed methods. (*B*) Open reduction and internal fixation restored the contour of the tibial plafond.

more likely to result from a fall on the heel with the talus being driven forward and upward. Anterior marginal fractures occur as isolated injuries more often than those of the posterior margin, but may, when associated with adduction, include the anterior portion of the medial malleolus.

Both anterior and posterior marginal fractures are frequently comminuted, which makes anatomical reduction and secure fixation almost impossible. If the anterior margin has been crushed, prolonged casting is undesirable, since it increases the likelihood of a permanently stiff and painful ankle. Early motion will allow molding of the articular surface during healing and may be facilitated by skeletal traction applied through an os calcis pin. To prevent anterior subluxation of the talus, the traction should be exerted in a line slightly posterior to the long axis of the limb. It may be discontinued when the fracture site is no longer tender, which usually occurs within a month of injury. Range of motion exercises should be continued, but weight bearing is deferred for 3 months or longer.

If the anterior lip fracture includes displacement of a major fragment, the contour of the joint surface should be restored by open reduction and internal fixation (Fig. 18-29). Operation prevents anterior subluxation of the talus and permits removal of loose fragments of bone and cartilage from the joint. Because of the location of the anterior tibial vessels on the skeletal plane, these vessels may have been injured by the fracture and must be protected from further damage during operation.

When vertical compression drives the talus against the center of the plafond, the entire lower articular surface of the tibia may be comminuted. Anatomical reduction is impossible, although alignment of the joint can often be maintained by traction through an os calcis pin and early range of motion exercises. Traction may usually be discontinued after 3 or 4 weeks, and a cast applied until fracture healing occurs. Weight bearing is deferred for at least 3 months.

For further discussion of tibial plafond injuries, see Chapter 17.

Since fractures associated with compression damage the weight-bearing surface of the tibia, post-traumatic arthritis is a common sequel and ankle fusion a frequent end result.

OPEN FRACTURES

Open fractures of the ankle are usually produced by the internal pressure of displacing bone fragments rather than by the entry of an external object; however, proximity to the ground occasionally results in massive contamination of the wound.

As with other open fractures, treatment of the wound takes precedence over definitive fracture management. Since the fractures communicate with the joint, debridement and irrigation must be thorough enough to include not only the open fracture, but the joint and other fractures as well. Once the displacement has been reduced, there is usually sufficient skin for closure of the wound. Even when skin grafting is required, the wound should be closed, unless extensive contamination or a prolonged interval from injury to operation precludes creation of a clean wound—in which case the wound should be left open and closed 3 to 5 days later if infection has not occurred.

Routine tetanus prophylaxis is carried out, and systemic antibiotics are used as an adjunct to, but not a substitute for, thorough surgical cleansing of the wound. If the antibiotic is used early and in high doses, it should be discontinued after 48 hours to minimize cost, inconvenience, masking of infection, and the possibility of superinfection.

Topical antibiotics may also be useful in the prevention of infection.[30] The wound is irrigated at regular intervals during surgery with an antibiotic solution that provides broad-spectrum coverage. Pooled irrigant is removed by suction to minimize systemic absorption.

Under optimal circumstances, standard methods of internal fixation may be employed when the end result of the injury would otherwise be compromised. Where the risk of infection is high, malleolar fixation should be carried out with absorbable sutures.

INJURIES OF THE LIGAMENTS OF THE ANKLE

Ligamentous injuries are often grouped under the general heading of sprains; however, the term "sprained ankle" has the same order of diagnostic precision as a "swollen knee" or a "broken arm." For the purposes of this chapter, the term sprain will refer to a partial tear of a ligament. One therefore cannot sprain an ankle, but only specific ligaments. The term is not used for complete rupture of a ligament, since complete tears have more serious implications than those connoted by the term sprain.

Partial tears of ligaments may be divided clinically into those that are associated with tearing of a sufficient number of fibers to result in partial loss of the supporting function of the ligament, and those in which there is insufficient damage to interfere with function (*i.e.*, the joint remains stable). Ruptures may occur within the substance of a ligament, at its attachment to bone, or through the bone itself. The latter event is especially likely in osteopenic bone and often produces avulsion of a small fragment or shell of bone. The term sprain-fracture has been appropriately applied to these injuries.

The importance of ligamentous injuries is frequently unappreciated, and inadequate treatment justified by an off-hand "Oh, it's only a sprain." Since the sequelae of ligamentous injuries are often more serious than those of the more visible fracture, the tendency to equate visibility with severity must be resisted.

INJURIES OF THE LATERAL COLLATERAL LIGAMENTS

MECHANISM OF INJURY

Injury of the lateral ligaments follows forceful adduction of the foot. Such injuries are most common in the second decade of life, largely because of the greater physical activity levels during these years. Most adduction injuries occur with the ankle in plantar flexion, which initially stresses the anterior talofibular ligament. If this ligament ruptures and the force continues, the ankle is usually moving toward neutral dorsiflexion, so that stress is next applied to the calcaneofibular ligament, which may also tear. The posterior talofibular ligament is rarely injured because it is larger, stronger, and stressed only in forced dorsiflexion, which seldom occurs in adduction injuries. Since the anterior talofibular ligament blends with the capsule, capsular tears usually accompany tear of the ligament. Similarly, close association of the calcaneofibular ligament and the peroneal tendon sheath accounts for the frequent tear of the inner wall of the sheath seen with ruptures of this ligament.

Isolated injury of the anterior talofibular ligament is the most common lateral ligament injury, occurring much more often than combined rupture of the anterior talofibular and calcaneofibular ligaments, which is next in frequency. Isolated rupture of the calcaneofibular ligament is uncommon.[8]

Early histologic changes in injured ligaments are those of acute inflammation followed by scar formation. Very little change is seen in the healing response after 2 months; in fact, in Bröstrom's[11] series there was no evidence of reconstitution of the scar to normal ligamentous tissue as long as 40 years after injury.

CLINICAL FINDINGS

A history of adduction injury may be remembered, and roughly a third of the patients recall a previous sprain of the same ankle. Examination discloses swelling, tenderness, and ecchymosis, which are localized initially but later become diffuse. Indirect or stress pain is invariably present. With rupture of the anterior talofibular ligament, the plantar flexed talus may be displaced anteriorly, producing a positive anterior drawer sign (Fig. 18-30). If the calcaneofibular ligament is also torn, the degree of anterior displacement is increased. Within a few hours after injury, muscle spasm and swelling make signs of talar instability difficult to elicit without anesthesia.

RADIOGRAPHIC FINDINGS

Routine x-rays show only lateral soft-tissue swelling unless the ligamentous tear has avulsed its bone attachment. The severity of the injury may be further evaluated by stress films and arthrography. Stress films are taken with the foot in maximum adduction, and comparable views of the uninjured side are included for comparison. The study should include views with the ankles stressed in neutral position and in plantar flexion. Local or regional anesthesia may be necessary for an optimal study, especially if it is carried out more than a few hours after injury. The degree of talar tilt is measured as the angle subtended by lines drawn along the tibial plafond and the dome of the talus in the anteroposterior x-ray; however, interpretation of these measurements is sometimes difficult because of the wide range of normal values. Talar tilt of up to 25° has been reported in normal ankles with no history of injury,[63] and occasionally there is considerable variation between ankles in the same person. If only the anterior talofibular ligament is divided, talar tilt is usually increased in plantar flexion but not in the neutral position (Fig. 18-31). If both the anterior talofibular and calcaneofibular ligaments are torn, talar tilt is increased to a greater degree

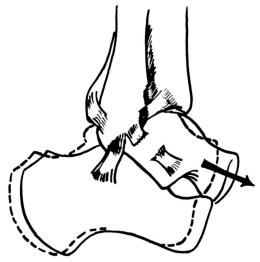

Fig. 18-30. A positive anterior drawer sign seen with rupture of the anterior talofibular ligament.

in plantar flexion and is also increased in the neutral position[46] (Fig. 18-32).

The talar instability resulting from rupture of the anterior talofibular ligament is sometimes more readily appreciated on a lateral stress film, with the foot held forward (anterior drawer test), than on either the adduction film or the clinical examination. For this reason, a lateral stress view should be included in the investigation of an unstable ankle.[29]

Arthrography is often useful in the evaluation of injuries to ankle ligaments.[9] It is performed by injecting 5 ml of a contrast medium after irrigating the ankle with saline to remove any blood from the joint. Injection should be made apart from the area of suspected ligamentous damage and within a week of injury; thereafter, capsular tears become sealed by clots or adhesions. In the normal arthrogram (Fig. 18-33), extra-articular leakage of dye into the tendon sheath of the flexor hallucis longus or flexor digitorum longus is seen in about 20% of cases. With abnormal arthrograms, the amount of leakage depends on the size of the tear, the amount of contrast material injected, and the time between injury and arthrogram. A tear of the anterior talofibular ligament is seen as an extravasation over the anterior portion of the lateral malleolus (Fig. 18-34). If the calcaneofibular ligament is also torn, the area of extravasation is usually larger, more posterior, and frequently extends into the peroneal tendon sheath (Fig. 18-35). Standard arthrography may be misleading in the diagnosis of calcaneofibular ligament injury when a large capsular tear

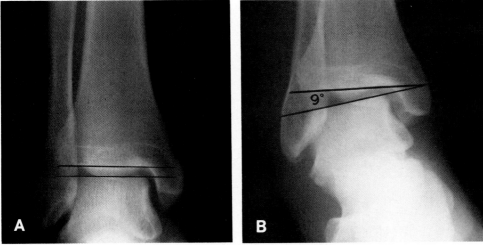

Fig. 18-31. Stress films of the lateral ligaments in (A) neutral and (B) plantar flexion in a patient with clinical evidence of a torn anterior talofibular ligament. Abnormal talar tilt in the neutral position was prevented by an intact calcaneofibular ligament.

accompanies a rupture of the anterior talofibular ligament. Dye escapes through the larger anterior capsular rent before it can be forced into the smaller hole in the peroneal tendon sheath. For this reason, direct injection of the dye into the sheath may be preferred.[3] No arthrographic findings diagnostic of rupture of the posterior talofibular ligament have been described. Rupture of the deltoid ligament allows leakage in the region of the medial malleolus, and rupture of the anterior tibiofibular ligament shows anterior extrusion of contrast material with no clear zone between it and the fibula.[9]

TREATMENT

The treatment of torn lateral ligaments is controversial, ranging from a "walk it out" philosophy to surgical repair, with immobilization occupying the middle ground.[1,4,10,27,67,72,77] Clearly no single approach serves best for all lesions; rather, treatment must be planned according to the severity of the injury and the needs of the patient. When the ankle is stable both clinically and radiographically, arthrography is not performed. An elastic bandage or taping may be used for comfort and ambulation continued (Fig. 18-36). With clinical evidence of more extensive injury, inversion stress films showing abnormal talar tilt in plantar flexion (but not in neutral), or arthrographic evidence of a tear of the anterior talofibular ligament, the ankle is immobilized in the neutral position for 3 to 4 weeks in a below-knee cast with weight bearing as pain and swelling permit. When clinical and radio-

graphic evidence suggest disruption of the anterior talofibular and calcaneofibular ligaments and capsule, I prefer to repair the ligaments surgically and immobilize the ankle in a below-knee cast for 3 to 4 weeks. The need for operative repair of these lesions is suggested by the difficulty in obtaining apposition of the torn ends of the ligaments by manipulation of the foot and ankle at surgery.[67,72,73] Ligaments allowed to heal by the formation of scar to fill the gap between their ends may become sufficiently elongated to permit talar instability, which predisposes to recurrent sprains.

INJURIES OF THE DELTOID LIGAMENT

MECHANISM OF INJURY

Injury of the deltoid ligament may be produced by either external rotation or abduction forces. It is more likely to follow rotational violence, since ligaments are more resistant to tension forces, which act parallel to the fibers, than to shear forces, which are exerted perpendicular to the fibers. Partial tears, involving the anterior fibers of the deltoid ligament, occur more often than complete ruptures.

CLINICAL FINDINGS

Tears of the deltoid ligament are manifest clinically by tenderness, swelling, and ecchymosis over the damaged portion of the ligament; complete tears are commonly accompanied by fracture of the fibula, injury to the syndesmotic ligaments, or both.

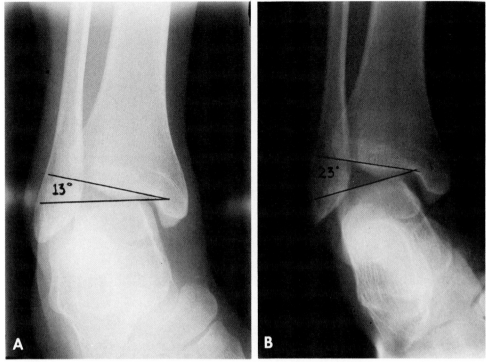

Fig. 18-32. Stress films of the lateral ligament in (*A*) neutral position and (*B*) plantar flexion in a patient with clinical evidence of a torn anterior talofibular and calcaneo-fibular ligaments (compare with Fig. 18-31).

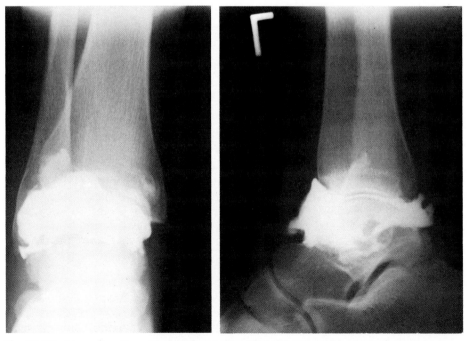

Fig. 18-33. Normal arthrogram of the ankle. The superior extension of dye into the tibiofibular area represents a synovial pouch, which may occur as a normal variant.

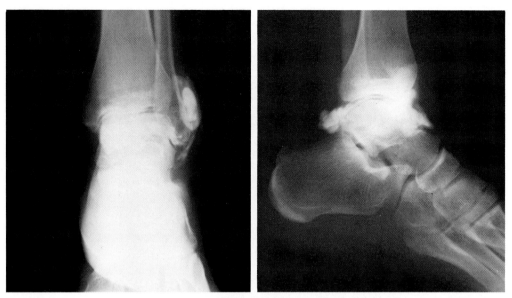

Fig. 18-34. Arthrogram showing a tear of the anterior talofibular ligament.

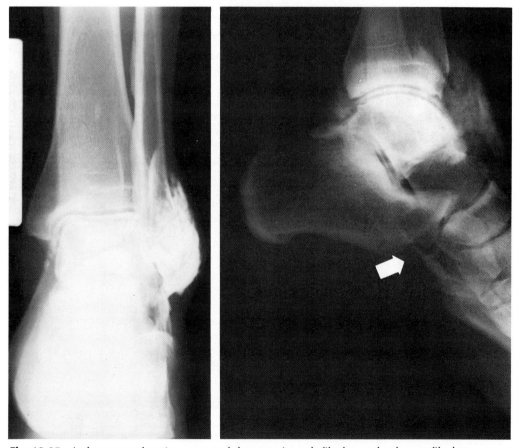

Fig. 18-35. Arthrogram showing a tear of the anterior talofibular and calcaneofibular ligaments.

RADIOGRAPHIC FINDINGS

The diagnosis of injury to the deltoid ligament may be inferred from an x-ray that shows widening of the clear space between the medial malleolus and the talus to greater than 4 mm on the mortise view.[28] Confirmation may be obtained by abduction–external rotation stress films or arthrography, but these examinations are usually unnecessary.

TREATMENT

There has been considerable controversy over the treatment for complete ruptures of the deltoid ligament. Surgical repair has been advocated by Braunstein and Wade,[6] and Dziob,[22] while Lauge-Hansen,[43] and Staples,[76] have favored closed treatment. In favor of operative repair are quicker and stronger ligamentous healing[14] and the opportunity to inspect and debride the joint. My preference, unless there are other indications for operation, is for closed treatment, since it has not been shown to be associated with a higher incidence of talar shift, recurrent injury, or subjective instability, and it avoids the risk of infection. Failure of closed reduction to correct lateral displacement of the talus may result from interposition of the deltoid ligament or the posterior tibial tendon, in which case operative repair is combined with removal of the interposed tissue. When operative treatment is performed, sutures are placed in the deep portion of the ligament before the fibula is reduced and tied after the fibula is fixed. If the fibula is stabilized first, it may be impossible to repair the deep fibers of the ligament.

INJURIES OF THE SYNDESMOTIC LIGAMENTS

MECHANISM OF INJURY

Broadly defined, diastasis means a separation of normally joined bony elements; however, the term is most commonly applied to injury of the inferior tibiofibular ligaments. It occurs in two forms: complete and partial. Complete diastasis occurs when the anterior and posterior tibiofibular and interosseous ligaments are torn and usually involves a strong abduction force. Partial diastasis more frequently accompanies external rotation violence and may involve either the anterior tibiofibular ligament or the anterior tibiofibular and interosseous ligaments. The posterior inferior tibiofibular ligament acts as a hinge upon which the fibula rotates outward; hence it is rarely torn in external rotation injuries. Fracture of the posterior tibial tubercle may occur as a result of compression by the externally rotating talus before the interosseous

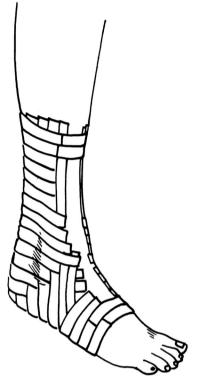

Fig. 18-36. Method of taping the ankle for a sprain of the anterior talofibular ligament.

ligament yields—a lesion that simulates the avulsion fracture of the posterior tubercle seen with abduction injuries (Fig. 18-37). If only the anterior tibiofibular ligament is torn, the tautness of the interosseous ligament snaps the lateral malleolus back into position as soon as the force is removed, so that diastasis is potential rather than real. If the interosseous ligament also tears, or if fracture of the fibula occurs, spontaneous reduction is less likely.

CLINICAL FINDINGS

The diagnosis of rupture of the anterior tibiofibular ligament in the absence of a fibular fracture rests on the presence of tenderness and swelling in the region of this ligament. These findings are often mistaken for a sprain of the anterior talofibular ligament because of its proximity. In the absence of direct trauma, fracture of the fibula above the tibial plafond (*i.e.*, above the fibular attachment of the tibiofibular ligament) indicates that the tibiofibular ligament is torn.

RADIOGRAPHIC FINDINGS

The diagnosis of diastasis often cannot be made from routine anteroposterior or mortise views because the variable depth of the peroneal groove prevents accurate assessment of tibiofibular overlap. The presence and extent of injury to the syndesmotic ligaments may be further evaluated by external rotation stress films of both ankles.

Abduction or abduction–external rotation injuries, in which all of the syndesmotic ligaments are torn, are frequently associated with wide separation of the tibia and fibula that is obvious on routine x-rays. According to Husfeldt,[37] diastasis is present when *la ligne claire* (the space between the medial cortex of the fibula and the posterior edge of the peroneal groove) is greater than 5.5 mm in the anteroposterior x-ray; unfortunately, it may also be present when this measurement is less than 5.5 mm.

TREATMENT

If the ringlike structure of the ankle mortise is remembered, it follows that if the other components of the ring are reduced by either open or closed methods, reduction of the syndesmosis is compelled; however, after several days, organization of clot and debris in the syndesmosis makes closed reduction more difficult, and open reduction and transsyndesmotic fixation may be necessary.

When the interosseus membrane is extensively torn, as often happens in the Maisonneuve fracture, marked fibular instability may be better managed by primary bolting of the syndesmosis (see Fig. 18-20).

DISLOCATIONS OF THE ANKLE

Since subluxations and dislocations of the ankle joint associated with malleolar fractures have already been discussed, it remains only to consider the displacements that follow extensive ligamentous and capsular damage without fracture. The talus may be dislocated at one, two, or all three of its articulations; however, I will consider only those that involve the ankle joint. Dislocation of the talus occurs as an isolated event, in association with fracture of the neck of the talus, or as an element in total extrusion of the talus.

ANTERIOR DISLOCATION

Isolated dislocation of the ankle may occur in either an anterior or a posterior direction. Medial or lateral dislocation is commonly associated with a fracture of the tibia or fibula. Anterior dislocation follows a force that results in posterior displacement of the tibia on the fixed foot. All ligamentous and capsular attachments from the tibia and fibula to the talus

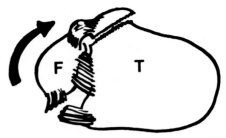

Fig. 18-37. Mechanism of fracture of the posterior tibial tubercle by external rotation.

are torn, with the exception, occasionally, of the posterior talofibular ligament. Clinically, the foot is usually slightly dorsiflexed and appears elongated anteriorly. The depressions on either side of the tendo Achillis are obliterated. The talus is prominent anteriorly, and the dorsalis pedis pulse may be absent. Motion of the ankle is limited and painful. Reduction should be prompt and is accomplished by traction in the long axis of the limb while applying posteriorly directed pressure to the anterior aspect of the foot. I prefer operative repair of the ruptured ligaments and capsule for those injuries in which operation is necessary to accomplish the reduction; however, Bonnin[4] states that surgical repair of the ligaments is unnecessary and recommends 8 weeks in plaster. If operative repair is carried out, less immobilization time is required.

POSTERIOR DISLOCATION

Posterior dislocation occurs more often than anterior displacment, but both are rare without fracture of the corresponding tibial margin. Posterior dislocation of the talus most often follows a blow to the posterior aspect of the tibia and results in plantar flexion of the ankle with apparent shortening of the foot. Reduction is carried out by exerting traction in the long axis of the limb and lifting the heel forward. Subsequent operative repair of the ligaments is again an individual decision.

COMPLICATIONS

NONUNION

Nonunion is most frequent in fractures of the medial malleolus; it occurs in 10% to 15% of patients treated by closed methods[47] (Fig. 18-38). It usually follows avulsion fractures in which the torn retinacular ligament and periosteum are drawn into the fracture site, where they prevent reduction and union. Nonunion at the level of the plafond is more

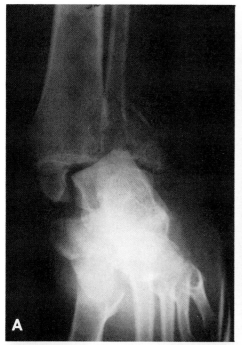

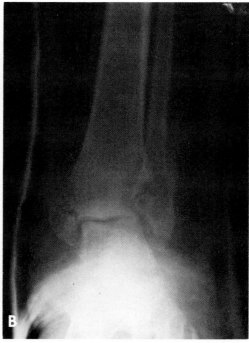

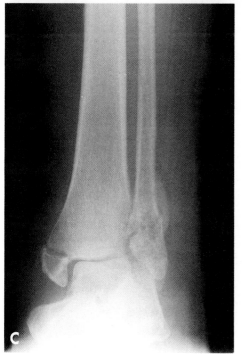

Fig. 18-38. (*A*) Avulsion fracture of the medial malleolus. (*B*) Failure of closed reduction. (*C*) Failure of bony union at 5 months.

commonly symptomatic than that below the plafond,[12,81] perhaps because a fibrous union at the joint line allows abnormal mediolateral talar movement that stresses the nonunion site. Occasionally bone union from osseous metaplasia of the inter-posed fibrous tissue develops as late as several years after injury.

If nonunion of the medial malleolus is sufficiently symptomatic to warrant treatment, union may be accomplished by electrical stimulation or by bone

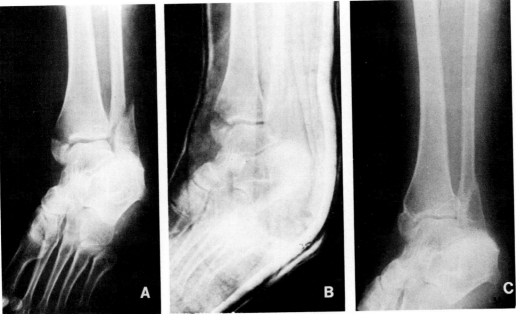

Fig. 18-39. (*A*) Avulsion fracture of the medial malleolus. (*B*) Failure of closed reduction. (*C*) Malunion with elongation 2 years after injury.

grafting; if undesirable deformity exists, interposed fibrous tissue may be removed and the malleolus repositioned with screw fixation.[7] Nonunion of a lateral or posterior malleolus is rare, although radiographic evidence of fibular union is extremely slow to appear.

MALUNION

Malunion (union with deformity) may occur at any of the malleolar fracture sites and is often responsible for late clinical deformity. At the medial malleolus, malunion usually results from elongation (Fig. 18-39); the lateral malleolus frequently unites in external rotation and may be shortened; and failure to reduce the posterior malleolus allows it to heal with superior displacement (Fig. 18-40). If the talus is shifted in the mortise, post-traumatic arthritis may be anticipated, and early reconstruction should be carried out by osteotomy through the fracture sites, repositioning of the malleoli and talus, and internal fixation. If talar displacement is not present, reconstruction is usually unnecessary; however, if symptoms warrant and arthritic changes have not developed, malleolar malunions may be reconstructed. While reconstruction is technically demanding and the results often unsatisfactory, it is presently the best alternative to ankle fusion[75] (Fig. 18-41). Reconstruction should not be attempted when post-traumatic arthritis is present.

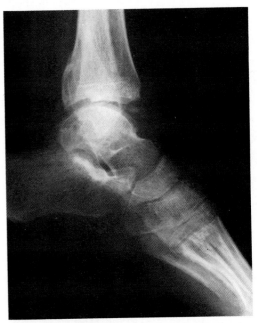

Fig. 18-40. Malunion of a posterior lip fracture. Unless reduced by operative methods, these fractures usually remain displaced superiorly.

INFECTION

Infection may follow either open fractures or the open treatment of closed fractures. In the latter

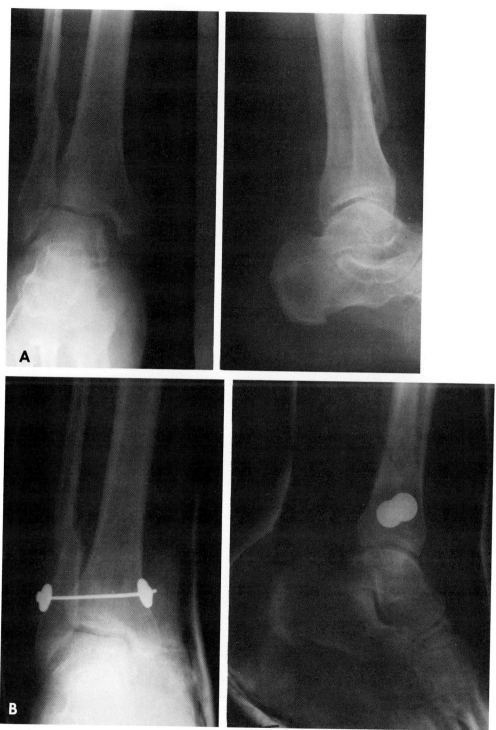

Fig. 18-41. Ankle reconstruction. (*A*) Five months after fracture of the fibula and tear of the deltoid (and interosseous) ligament. Note lateral displacement of the talus and the resulting tibiotalar incongruity. (*B*) Reconstruction by fibular osteotomy, removal of the interposed deltoid and interosseous ligaments, and bolting of the syndesmosis.

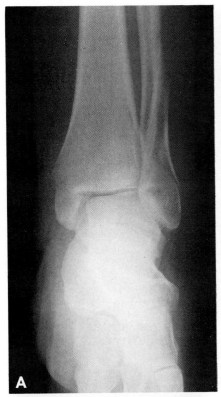

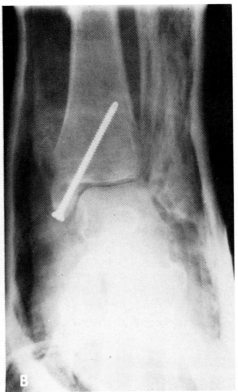

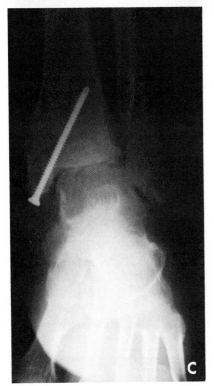

Fig. 18-42. (*A*) External rotation ankle fracture. (*B*) Failure to correct lateral shift of the talus with limited open reduction of only the medial mallelous. (*C*) Late result showing post-traumatic arthritis.

group the reported incidence varies from 1% to 18%.[12,26] Fortunately, such infections are usually superficial and respond readily to the usual measures for control of infection, namely, antibiotics and debridement. For resistant infections, hardware removal may be necessary.

POST-TRAUMATIC ARTHRITIS

Post-traumatic arthritis occurs in 20% to 40% of ankle fractures, regardless of the method of treatment.[12,49,79,81] It may also follow longstanding lateral ligament instability.[33] Predisposing factors are inaccurate reduction of the mortise, comminution of the plafond, and advanced age.[81] Patients often complain of aching in bad weather, starting pain and stiffness, and pain with excessive activity. Radiographic findings are joint narrowing (x-rays of the other ankle must be available for comparison), subchondral sclerosis, and osteophyte formation. These changes may occur within a few months of injury as a result of traumatically induced chemical changes in the articular cartilage, or later from joint incongruity (Fig. 18-42). The symptoms of post-traumatic arthritis are often minimal and controlled by reduction of weight-bearing activity, mild analgesics, and shoe modifications. Severe, persistent symptoms may be relieved by ankle fusion with surprisingly little loss of function.[51] In the older patient with minimal anatomical changes, ankle replacement may be an acceptable alternative to fusion.[25,62]

VASCULAR DAMAGE

Damage to the anterior or posterior tibial vessels may be inflicted either from injury or inadequate management after injury. Neither artery is essential to a healthy foot, but loss of either, in addition to other vascular effects of injury and treatment, may result in significant tissue death. The best treatment is prophylaxis; therefore, the possibility of vascular injury should be foremost in the mind of anyone dealing with trauma to the limbs. Constrictive dressings, traction, and unnecessary manipulation should be avoided in any limb with vascular insufficiency. Progressive vascular compromise demands prompt investigation, including angiography.

SUDECK'S ATROPHY

Sudeck's atrophy, a form of sympathetic dystrophy, may follow even minor injuries to the ankle and is characterized by rapidly developing osteoporosis

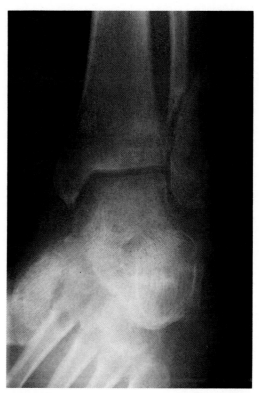

Fig. 18-43. Sudeck's atrophy following injury to the ankle.

distal to the injury, burning pain, and trophic changes in the foot (Fig. 18-43). Early restoration of normal function is often curative, but if this goal cannot be achieved or is ineffective, early sympathectomy should be considered.

SYNOSTOSIS

Ossification of the interosseous membrane may follow injuries to the syndesmosis (Fig. 18-44), although synostosis is relatively uncommon unless internal fixation of the syndesmosis has been carried out.[32] This complication eliminates much of the fibular "give" in normal ankle motion, so that patients sometimes complain of a wooden feeling in the ankle when walking. Since the condition is not disabling, excision of the ossified portion of the membrane is rarely necessary; however, in the occasional high performance athlete, excision of the mature synostosis may be beneficial.

OSTEOCHONDRAL FRACTURES

Osteochondral fractures of the talus may also complicate trauma to the ankle. They usually follow a

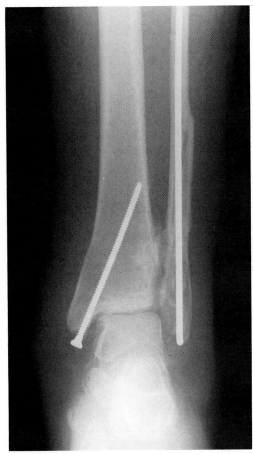

Fig. 18-44. Ossification of the interosseous membrane following a tear of the membrane.

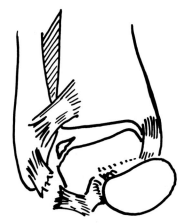

Fig. 18-45. Mechanism of production of osteochondral fracture of the talus.

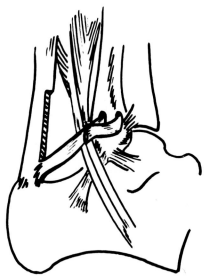

Fig. 18-46. Repair of recurrent dislocation of the peroneal tendons. (Redrawn from Jones, E.: Operative Treatment of Chronic Dislocation of Peroneal Tendons. J. Bone Joint Surg., **14:**574–576, 1932.)

sprain of the lateral ligaments wherein the lateral edge of the talus strikes the medial margin of the lateral malleolus, producing a fracture in the midportion of the lateral talar dome (Fig. 18-45). The lesion is seen less frequently on the medial aspect of the talus, where it probably represents an impaction fracture. Arthroscopy and polytomography may be useful in evaluating the location, orientation, and size of the fragment. The fragment may heal, become detached as a loose body in the joint, or remain in place without healing. It is frequently associated with persistent pain and swelling; if detached, it often produces locking and a feeling of instability. If a symptomatic undetached lesion does not heal after a period of plaster immobilization, the fragment should be excised and the defect in the talus drilled to facilitate cartilage repair. Osteotomy of the medial malleolus may be necessary to expose posteromedial talar lesions. The site of its origin may be covered with cartilage and

frequently defies identification. Since it is usually impossible to state whether necrosis of the bone in the fragment preceded or followed the fracture, the distinction between these lesions and those referred to as osteochondritis dissecans is unclear.

SUBLUXATION OF THE PERONEAL TENDONS

Recurrent anterior displacement of the peroneal tendons may complicate sprains of the lateral ligaments. The production of this lesion entails either rupture of the superior peroneal retinaculum or

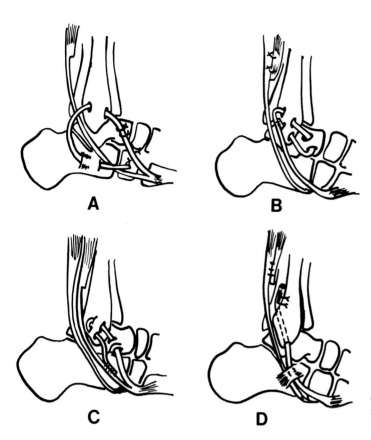

Fig. 18-47. Procedures for reconstruction of the lateral collateral ligament: (*A*) Chrisman, (*B*) Watson-Jones, (*C*) McLaughlin, (*D*) Evans.

stripping of the fibular periosteum by the retinaculum, which creates a redundant fold lateral to the fibula into which the tendons displace. Without the retinaculum to retain the tendons, recurrence is the rule. It may be recognized by a visible, and sometimes audible, anterior displacement of the tendons during dorsiflexion of the ankle. When recurrent, the condition is often associated with symptoms of peroneal irritation or a feeling of instability. If symptoms are unrelieved by immobilization of the plantar flexed and slightly inverted foot in a below-knee cast for 6 weeks, operative repair may be advisable. Many procedures have been recommended, most of which involve either construction of a restraining soft tissue loop or deepening of the peroneal groove on the posterior aspect of the lateral malleolus. I prefer the technique described by Jones,[39] wherein a lateral slip of the tendo Achillis is detached proximally, mobilized distally, and attached to the lateral malleolus just in front of the peroneal tendons (Fig. 18-46). Alternatively, if a redundant retinacular fold is found, it may be excised and the retinaculum reattached to a newly created groove in the posterior fibula.

TALAR INSTABILITY

A final complication of lateral collateral ligament injuries is talar instability resulting from elongation of the ligaments by scar formed in the healing process. The resulting loss of the supporting function of these ligaments predisposes to recurrent sprains, usually requiring progressively less trauma for their production. These episodes may prove disabling, especially in the athletically inclined person, in which case operation should be considered. Most techniques for reconstruction of the lateral ligaments employ the peroneus brevis tendon. The procedures recommended by McLaughlin[54] and Chrisman[13] use only one half of the tendon, whereas those of Watson-Jones[80] and Evans[24] require the entire tendon. These techniques are illustrated in Figure 18-47. Chrisman's technique provides the most anatomical reconstruction of both the anterior talofibular and calcaneofibular ligaments and is often preferred for that reason, although Evans' procedure has appealing simplicity.[70,74] Whichever technique is used, care must be taken to protect the sural nerve.

REFERENCES

1. Anderson, K. J., and Lecocq, J. F.: Operative Treatment of Injury to the Fibular Collateral Ligament of the Ankle. J. Bone Joint Surg., **36:**825–832, 1954.
2. Ashhurst, A. P. C., and Bromer, R. S.: Classification and Mechanism of Fractures of the Leg Bone Involving the Ankle. Arch. Surg., **4:**51–129, 1922.
3. Black, H. M.; Brand, R. L.; and Eichelberger, M. R.: An Improved Technique for the Evaluation of Ligamentous Injury in Severe Ankle Sprains. Am. J. Sports Med., **6:**276–282, 1978.
4. Bonnin, J. G.: Injuries to the Ankle. Darien, Connecticut, Hafner Publishing, 1970.
5. Bosworth, D. M.: Fracture-Dislocation of the Ankle with Fixed Displacement of the Fibula behind the Tibia. J. Bone Joint Surg., **29:**130–135, 1947.
6. Braunstein, P. W., and Wade, P. A.: Treatment of Unstable Fractures of the Ankle. Ann. Surg., **149:**217–226, 1956.
7. Brighton, C. T.; Black, J.; Friedenberg, Z. B.; Esterhai, J. L.; Day, L. J.; and Connolly, J. F.: A Multicenter Study of the Treatment of Non-union with Constant Direct Current. J. Bone Joint Surg., **63A:**2–13, 1981.
8. Bröstrom, L.: I. Anatomic Lesions in Recent Sprains. Acta Chir. Scand., **128:**483–495, 1964.
9. Bröstrom, L.; Lilijeahl, S. O.; and Lindvall, N.: II. Arthrographic Diagnosis of Recent Ligament Ruptures. Acta Chir. Scand., **129:**485–499, 1965.
10. Bröstrom, L.: III. Clinical Observations in Recent Ligament Ruptures. Acta Chir. Scand., **130:**560–569, 1966.
11. Bröstrom, L., and Sundelin, P.: IV. Histologic Changes in Recent and "Chronic" Ligament Ruptures. Acta Chir. Scand., **132:**248–253, 1966.
12. Burwell, H. N., and Charnley, A. D.: The Treatment of Displaced Fractures at the Ankle by Rigid Internal Fixation and Early Joint Movement. J. Bone Joint Surg., **47B:**634–660, 1965.
13. Chrisman, O. D., and Snook, G. A.: Reconstruction of Lateral Ligament Tears of the Ankle. An Experimental Study and Clinical Evaluation of Seven Patients Treated by a New Modification of the Elmslie Procedure. J. Bone Joint Surg., **51A:**904–912, 1969.
14. Clayton, M. L., and Weir, G. J., Jr.: Experimental Investigations of Ligamentous Healing. Am. J. Surg., **98:**373–378, 1959.
15. Coonrad, R. W.: Fracture-Dislocations of the Ankle Joint with Impaction Injury of the Lateral Weight-bearing Surface of the Tibia. J. Bone Joint Surg., **52A:**1337–1344, 1970.
16. Cooper, A. P.: On Dislocation of the Ankle Joints. *In* A Treatise on Dislocations and on Fractures of the Joints. London, Longman, Hurst, Reese, Orme and Brown; E. Cox and Son, 1822.
17. Cotton, F. J.: A New Type of Ankle Fracture. J.A.M.A., **64:**318–321, 1915.
18. David, J-P.: Mémoire sur les contre-coups dans les differentes parties du corps autre que la tête. Pris de l'academie royale de Chirurgie, 1771.
19. Denham, R. A.: Internal Fixation for Unstable Ankle Fractures. J. Bone Joint Surg., **46B:**206–211, 1964.
20. Destot, E.: Traumatismes du Pied et Rayons X, 2nd ed. Paris, Masson et Cie, 1937.
21. Dupuytren, G.: Of Fractures of the Lower Extremity of the Fibula, and Luxations of the Foot. [Reprinted in] Medical Classics, **4:**151–172, 1939.
22. Dziob, J. M.: Ligamentous Injuries about the Ankle Joint. Am. J. Surg., **91:**692–698, 1956.
23. Earle, H.: Simple, Succeeded by Compound Dislocations Forwards, of the Inferior Extremity of the Tibia, with Fracture of its Posterior Edge. Comminuted Fracture of the Fibula, Amputation of the Leg, and Death. Lancet, **2:**346–348, 1828–1829.
24. Evans, D. L.: Recurrent Instability of the Ankle: A Method of Surgical Treatment. Proc. R. Soc. Med., **46:**343–344, 1953.
25. Evanski, P. M., and Waugh, T. R.: Management of Arthritis of the Ankle. Clin. Orthop., **122:**110–115, 1977.
26. Eventov, I.; Salama, R.; Goodwin, D. R. A.; and Weissman, S. L.: An Evaluation of Surgical and Conservative Treatment of Fractures of the Ankle in 200 Patients. J. Trauma, **18:**271–275, 1978.
27. Freeman, M. A. R.: Treatment of Ruptures of the Lateral Ligament of the Ankle. J. Bone Joint Surg., **47B:**661–668, 1965.
28. Gaston, S., and McLaughlin, H. L.: Complex Fracture of the Lateral Malleolus. J. Trauma, **1:**69–78, 1961.
29. Glasgow, M.; Jackson, A.; and Jamieson, A. M.: Instability of the Ankle after Injury to the Lateral Ligament. J. Bone Joint Surg., **62B:**196–200, 1980.
30. Gingrass, R. P.; Close, A. S.; and Ellison, E. H.: The Effect of Various Topical and Parenteral Agents on the Prevention of Infection in Experimental Contaminated Wounds. J. Trauma, **4:**763–783, 1964.
31. Goergen, T. G.; Danzig, L. A.; Resnick, D.; and Owen, C. A.: Roentgenographic Evaluation of the Tibiotalar Joint. J. Bone Joint Surg., **59A:**874–877, 1977.
32. Grath, G.: Widening of the Ankle Mortise. A Clinical and Experimental Study. Acta Chir. Scand., [Suppl.] **263:**1–88, 1960.
33. Harrington, K. D.: Degenerative Arthritis of the Ankle Secondary to Longstanding Lateral Ligament Instability. J. Bone Joint Surg., **61A:**354–361, 1979.
34. Henderson, M. S.: Trimalleolar Fracture of the Ankle. Surg. Clin. North Am., **12:**867–872, 1932.
35. Hughes, J. L.; Weber, H.; Willenegger, H.; and Kuner, E. H.: Evaluation of Ankle Fractures. Clin. Orthop., **138:**111–119, 1979.
36. Huguier, P.-C.: Mémoire sur les luxations du pied considerées en général. Union Méd., Paris, **2:**120, 1848.
37. Husfeldt, E.: Significance of Roentgenography of Ankle Joint in Oblique Projection in Malleolar Fractures. Hospitalstid., **80:**788–797, 1937.
38. Inman, V. T.: The Joints of the Ankle. Baltimore, Williams & Wilkins, 1976.
39. Jones, E.: Operative Treatment of Chronic Dislocation of the Peroneal Tendons. J. Bone Joint Surg., **14:**574–576, 1932.
40. Klossner, O.: Late Results of Operative and Non-operative

Treatment of Severe Ankle Fractures. Acta Chir. Scand., [Suppl.] **293**:1–93, 1962.

41. Lane, W. A.: The Operative Treatment of Simple Fractures. Surg. Gynecol. Obstet., **8**:344–354, 1909.

42. Lauge-Hansen, N.: Fractures of the Ankle. II. Combined Experimental-Surgical and Experimental-Roentgenologic Investigations. Arch. Surg., **60**:957–985, 1950.

43. Lauge-Hansen, N.: "Ligamentous" Ankle Fractures: Diagnosis and Treatment. Acta Chir. Scand., **97**:544–550, 1949.

44. LeFort, L.: Note sur une variété non décrete de fracture verticale de la malléole externe par arrachement. Bull. Gen. Therap., **110**:193, 1886.

45. Leonard, M. H.: Injuries of the Lateral Ligaments of the Ankle: A Clinical and Experimental Study. J. Bone Joint Surg., **31A**:373–377, 1949.

46. LeRoy, L.: De la fracture marginale antérieure de la malléole externe. Paris, 1887.

47. Magnusson, R.: On the Late Results in Non-operated Cases of Malleolar Fractures. Acta Chir. Scand., [Suppl.] **90**:1–136, 1944.

48. Maisonneuve, J. G.: Recherches sur la fracture du perone. Arch. Gen. Med., **7**:165–187, 433–473, 1840.

49. Mast, J. W., and Teipner, W. A.: A Reproducible Approach to the Internal Fixation of Adult Ankle Fractures: Rationale, Technique, and Early Results. Orthop. Clin. North Am., **11**:661–679, 1980.

50. Mayer, P. J., and Evarts, C. M.: Fracture-Dislocation of the Ankle with Posterior Entrapment of the Fibula Behind the Tibia. J. Bone Joint Surg., **60A**:320–324, 1978.

51. Mazur, J. M.; Schwartz, E.; and Simon, S. R.: Ankle Arthrodesis. J. Bone Joint Surg., **61A**:354–361, 1979.

52. McCullough, C. J., and Burge, P. D.: Rotatory Stability of the Load-bearing Ankle. J. Bone Joint Surg., **62B**:460–464, 1980.

53. McDaniel, W. J., and Wilson, F. C.: Trimalleolar Fractures of the Ankle. An End Result Study. Clin. Orthop., **122**:37–45, 1977.

54. McLaughlin, H. L.: In Trauma. Philadelphia, W. B. Saunders, 1959.

55. McLaughlin, H. L., and Ryder, C. T., Jr.: Open Reduction and Internal Fixation for Fractures of the Tibia and Ankle. Surg. Clin. North Am., **29**:1523–1534, 1949.

56. Meyer, T. L., Jr., and Kumler, K. W.: A.S.I.F. Technique and Ankle Fractures. Clin. Orthop., **150**:211–216, 1980.

57. Mitchell, W. G.; Shaftan, G. W.; and Sclafani, J. J. A.: Mandatory Open Reduction: Its Role in Displaced Ankle Fractures. J. Trauma, **19**:602–615, 1979.

58. Müller, M. E.; Allgöwer, M.; and Willenegger, H.: Manual of Internal Fixation. New York, Springer-Verlag, 1970.

59. Neer, C. S. II: Injuries of the Ankle Joint: Evaluation. Conn. St Med. J., **17**:580–583, 1953.

60. Nélaton, A.: Eléments de pathologie chirurgicale, Vol. 3, 2nd ed, p. 296. Paris, Germer-Bailliere, 1874.

61. Nelson, M. C., and Jensen, N. K.: The Treatment of Trimalleolar Fractures of the Ankle. Surg. Gynecol. Obstet., **71**:509–514, 1942.

62. Newton, S. E.: An Artificial Ankle Joint. Clin. Orthop., **142**:141–145, 1979.

63. Olson, R. W.: Arthrography of the Ankle: Its Use in Evaluation of Ankle Sprains. Radiology, **92**:1439–1446, 1969.

64. Pankovich, A. M.: Maisonneuve Fracture of the Fibula. J. Bone Joint Surg., **58A**:337–342, 1976.

65. Pankovich, A.: Fractures of the Fibula Proximal to the Distal Tibio-fibular Syndesmosis. J. Bone Joint Surg., **60A**:221–229, 1978.

66. Pott, P.: Some Few General Remarks on Fractures and Dislocations. London, Hawes, Clarke, Collins, 1768.

67. Prins, J. G.: Diagnosis and Treatment of Injury to the Lateral Ligament of the Ankle. Acta Chir. Scand., [Suppl.] **486**:3–149, 1978.

68. Quigley, T. B.: Management of Ankle Injuries Sustained in Sports. J.A.M.A., **169**:1431–1434, 1959.

69. Ramsey, P. L., and Hamilton, W.: Changes in Tibiotalar Area of Contact Caused by Lateral Talar Shift. J. Bone Joint Surg., **58A**:356–357, 1976.

70. Rechtine, G. K.; McCarroll, J. R.; and Webster, D. A.: Reconstruction for Chronic Lateral Instability of the Ankle: A Review of Twenty-eight Surgical Patients. Orthop., **5**:45–50, 1982.

71. Rochet, V.: Du mécanisme du luxations doubles de l'astragale (énucleation). Rev. d'Orthop., **1**:269, 1890.

72. Ruth, C. J.: The Surgical Treatment of Injuries of the Fibular Collateral Ligaments of the Ankle. J. Bone Joint Surg., **43A**:229–239, 1961.

73. Savastano, A. A., and Lowe, E. B., Jr.: Ankle Sprains: Surgical Treatment for Recurrent Sprains. Am. J. Sports Med., **8**:208–211, 1980.

74. Silver, C. M., and Deutsch, S. D.: Evans' Repair of Lateral Instability of the Ankle. Orthop., **5**:51–56, 1982.

75. Speed, J. S., and Boyd, H. B.: Operative Reconstruction of Malunited Fractures about the Ankle Joint. J. Bone Joint Surg., **28**:270–286, 1936.

76. Staples, O. S.: Injuries to the Medial Ligaments of the Ankle. J. Bone Joint Surg., **42A**:1287–1307, 1960.

77. Staples, O. S.: Ruptures of the Fibular Collateral Ligaments of the Ankle. J. Bone Joint Surg., **57A**:101–107, 1975.

78. Tillaux, P.: Traité de chirurgie clinique, Vol. 2, p. 842. Paris, Asselin and Houzeau, 1848.

79. Vasli, S.: Operative Treatment of Ankle Fractures. Acta Chir. Scand., [Suppl.] **226**:1–74, 1957.

80. Watson-Jones, R.: Fractures and Joint Injuries, Vol. 2, 4th ed. Baltimore, Williams & Wilkins, 1955.

81. Wilson, F. C., and Skilbred, L. A.: Long-term Results in the Treatment of Displaced Bimalleolar Fractures. J. Bone Joint Surg., **48A**:1065, 1078, 1966.

82. Yablon, I. G.; Heller, F. G.; and Shouse, L.: The Key Role of the Lateral Malleolus in Displaced Fractures of the Ankle. J. Bone Joint Surg., **57A**:169–173, 1977.

19

Fractures and Dislocations of the Foot

James D. Heckman

Fractures in the foot vary in severity and location, depending on the direction and nature of the forces responsible for the injury. It is therefore necessary to consider not only the fractured bones, but also the direction of the forces that produced a given fracture. Without this knowledge, reduction of the fragments is more difficult and manipulation more traumatic to the surrounding soft tissues.

The preservation of the soft tissue structures is as important as the reduction of the fracture, particularly in the foot. One would experience a great deal of difficulty walking on scarred tissues, even if the bones had been anatomically reduced.

The foot (unlike the hand, which is designed essentially for grasping) is fundamentally a weight-bearing structure. It was strikingly described by Humphrey[400] in 1861:

> The human foot . . . affords a good illustration of animal mechanism, and . . . its form constitutes one of the great characteristics whereby man is distinguished from the lower [mammals]. As an instrument of support and . . . locomotion, it excels the foot of . . . any other animal. It evinces its excellence by enabling man to stand upright in a way that no . . . animal can do; and so efficiently does the foot accomplish this and perform the task of carrying the body, that the hand is set at liberty to minister to the will.

The foot consists of three morphologic functional segments, which develop in proximodistal order in the embryo: the tarsus, metatarsus, and phalanges. However, from an anatomical standpoint, the foot has the following three divisions: the hindfoot, comprised of the talus and the calcaneus; the midfoot, made up of the navicular, the cuboid, and the three cuneiforms; and the forefoot, with five metatarsals and 14 phalanges.

The incidence and severity of fractures and dislocations vary, depending on their location. In general, fractures involving joint surfaces carry a poorer prognosis than extra-articular fractures. In addition, one must always keep in mind, especially with the more severe fractures, possible complications to the circulatory status of the foot. Prolonged impairment of the blood flow can result in marked soft tissue loss.

ANATOMY

The foot is often considered by many as a simple appendage used in locomotion. Few physicians ever pause to think that it is well adapted to perform a variety of functions. Its accommodation to any surface irregularity, its versatility and speed of movements during running, jumping, and walking, and its behavior as if it were a ball-and-socket unit instead of a combination of 28 bones and 57 articulating surfaces make this structure a biomechanical marvel, which warrants more than just a passing thought. Fractures of the foot, therefore, require a more than casual knowledge of anatomy and some practical knowledge of biomechanics.

The skeletal, ligament, and muscle systems of the foot not only play an important functional role but are also involved in many of the problems encountered in dealing with fractures of this structure. Ignorance of the biomechanical and anatomical principles of the foot constitutes the greatest single handicap in the treatment of its fractures.

There are seven tarsal bones, two of which, the talus and the calcaneus, form the hindpart of the foot (Fig. 19-1). The navicular, cuboid, and three cuneiform bones form the midpart of the foot. The joints between the hindpart and the midpart of the foot, in addition to having individual names, are called the midtarsal joints, or Chopart's joint. Only the talus articulates with the tibia and the fibula. Its plantar surface rests on the calcaneus, which

makes the projection of the heel. The talus ends in front in a rounded head. Being directed somewhat medially as well as forward, this head tends to extend over the medial side of the distal end of the calcaneus, which has a projection there to support it, called the sustentaculum tali. The distal articular surfaces of these two bones are nearly on the same level and articulate at Chopart's joint with the navicular and the cuboid bones.

The forepart of the foot consists of the five metatarsals and the two phalanges of the great toe and the three phalanges for each of the lateral four

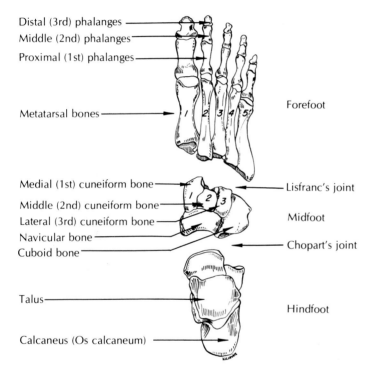

Fig. 19-1. Bones of the foot. Lisfranc's joint consists of the five tarsometatarsal joints. Chopart's joint consists of the talonavicular and calcaneocuboid joints.

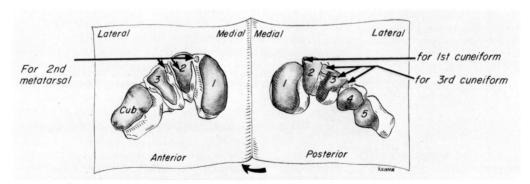

Fig. 19-2. Note the arching conformation of the tarsometatarsal articulations. There is no arching at the metatarsal head level. All metatarsal heads touch the underlying surface simultaneously in the standing position.

digits of the foot. The five tarsometatarsal articulations, collectively, are called Lisfranc's joint. Lisfranc's joint is an arcuate joint (Fig. 19-2). The arch formed by these structures lends stability to the foot. As the metatarsals extend distally to the metatarsophalangeal joints, they fan out. At the metatarsophalangeal level, all five metatarsal heads are on the same horizontal level. There is no metatarsal arch in the standing position. The weight

is not borne on the first and fifth metatarsal heads but is distributed among all five.

Looking first at the dorsal surface of the foot (Fig. 19-3), one perceives that the general contour of the tarsal portion of the foot is markedly convex from medial to lateral. There are no prominent bony points that make themselves evident above the general level. The structures underlying the skin, from superficial to deep (Fig. 19-4), are the

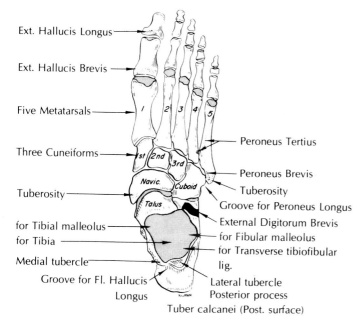

Fig. 19-3. In this dorsal view of the bones of the foot, note that at least three fifths of the entire surface of the talus is covered by articular cartilage.

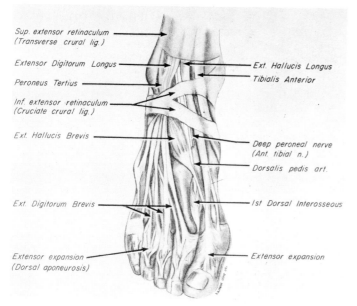

Fig. 19-4. Structures underlying the skin from medial to lateral at the level of the ankle are the tibialis anterior, extensor hallucis longus, extensor digitorum longus, and peroneus tertius tendons. Deep to these lie the deep branch of the peroneal nerve, and dorsalis pedis artery, and the short toe extensors.

inferior extensor retinaculum and, under it traversing from medial to lateral, the tibialis anterior, extensor hallucis longus, extensor digitorum longus, and peroneus tertius tendons.

At a slightly deeper level are located the deep branch of the peroneal nerve, the extensor hallucis brevis, and extensor digitorum brevis muscles, and the dorsalis pedis artery. This vessel (Fig. 19-5) arises from the anterior tibial artery and anasto-

moses with the lateral malleolar artery, which is frequently the terminal portion of the perforating branch of the peroneal artery. Figure 19-5 is diagrammatic, in order to simplify the anatomy of the dorsal arterial tree of the foot.

On the medial side of the foot (Fig. 19-6) underlying the skin and subcutaneous fat, the abductor hallucis originates from the plantar medial aspect of the calcaneus and inserts into the medial

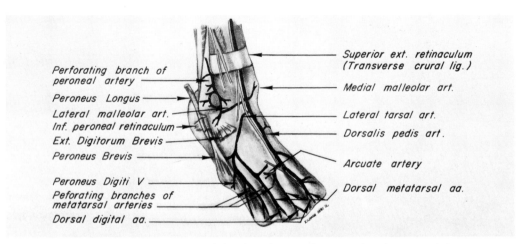

Fig. 19-5. Note the rich anastomosis of the dorsal arterial tree in this diagram of the arteries on the anterior aspect of the ankle and the dorsum of the foot.

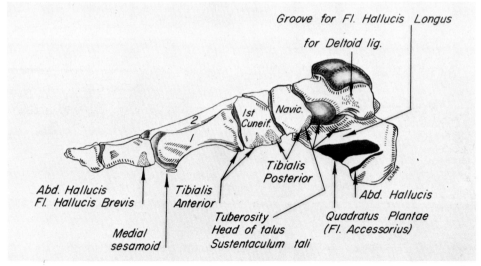

Fig. 19-6. Medial view of the bones of the foot. The abductor hallucis originates and inserts along the medial aspect of the foot from the plantar medial surface of the calcaneus to the medial aspect of the base of the proximal phalanx of the great toe. The tibialis posterior inserts on the plantar medial aspect of the navicular tubercle and the proximal edge of the first cuneiform. The tibialis anterior inserts on the plantar medial surface of first tarsometatarsal joint.

aspect of the base of the proximal phalanx of the great toe. The tibialis posterior tendon inserts at the plantar medial aspect of the navicular tubercle and the proximal edge of the first cuneiform before progressing plantarward to its ultimate insertions. The tibialis anterior tendon inserts at the plantar medial surface of the distal portion of the first cuneiform and the base of the first metatarsal and then progresses plantarward. The sustentaculum tali is seen to have a broad groove on its lower aspect. This is continuous behind with a groove on the medial and posteromedial surface of the talus for the flexor hallucis longus tendon.

The dorsolateral aspect of the foot, in addition to the extensor digitorum longus, the peroneus tertius tendon, and the extensor digitorum brevis muscle bellies, presents (Fig. 19-7) the peroneus brevis tendon, which inserts into the base of the fifth metatarsal, and the peroneus longus tendon, which dips into the plantar aspect of the foot in the groove between the cuboid and the fifth metatarsal (Fig. 19-8). Of the numerous ligamentous

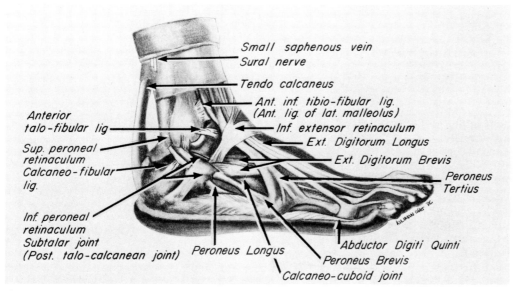

Fig. 19-7. Dorsolateral view of the foot. The peroneus brevis inserts into the base of the fifth metatarsal. The anterior talofibular ligament and calcaneofibular ligament are the principal stabilizing structures of the lateral aspect of the ankle joint.

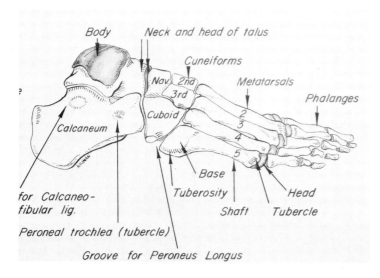

Fig. 19-8. Lateral view of the bones of the foot. A groove for the peroneus longus tendon is located between the cuboid and the base of the fifth metatarsal.

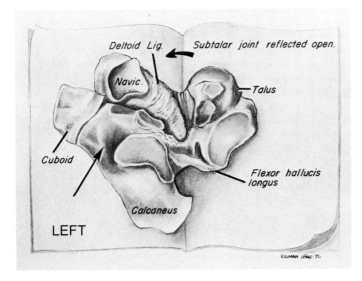

Fig. 19-9. The talocalcaneonavicular complex. The sinus tarsi is indicated by the straight arrow. (After Giannestras, N. J.: Foot Disorders: Medical and Surgical Management, 2nd ed. Philadelphia, Lea & Febiger, 1973.)

structures, the most important are the anterior talofibular ligament and the calcaneofibular ligament. Unrecognized rupture of either or both will lead to lateral instability of the ankle. Running parallel but plantar to the peroneal tendons is the sural nerve.

The sinus tarsi is the depression found on the lateral side of the tarsus and is distal to and on the same level as the lateral malleolus. On incision of the structures overlying the sinus tarsi—namely, the lateral portion of the inferior extensor retinaculum, the interosseous talocalcaneal ligament and reflection of the extensor digitorum brevis muscle belly distally—one exposes the lateral talocalcaneal, talonavicular, and calcaneocuboid articulations (Fig. 19-8). The distal surface of the talus articulates with the calcaneus and the navicular. The talocalcaneonavicular complex may be considered a ball-and-socket joint (Fig. 19-9). However, the socket, which is not rigid, moves around the ball. In fact, the malleable socket is exposed to constant changes and deformities, some of which may become pathologic.

The plantar fascia is a strong layer of white fibrous tissue whose thick central part is bound by thinner lateral portions. The central portion is attached to the medial calcaneal tubercle. As it progresses distally it divides into five sections, each extending into a toe and straddling the flexor tendons. The superficial layer of each section attaches to the deep skin fold between the toes and sole, while the deeper layer blends with the fibrous flexor sheath on each proximal phalanx and sends septa to the deep transverse ligament of the sole.

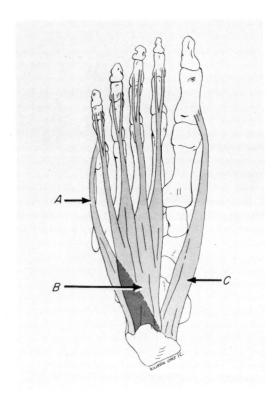

Fig. 19-10. The first subfascial layer consists of three muscles: (*A*) abductor digiti minimi, (*B*) flexor digitorum brevis, (*C*) abductor hallucis. (After Giannestras, N. J.: Foot Disorders: Medical and Surgical Management, 2nd ed. Philadelphia, Lea & Febiger, 1973.)

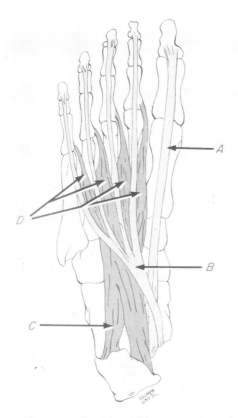

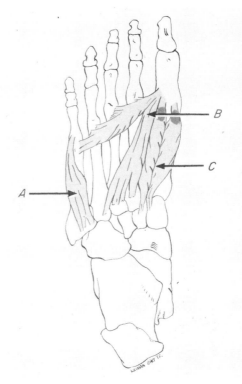

Fig. 19-11. The second subfascial layer consists of two tendons and two muscle groups: (*A*) tendon of the flexor hallucis longus, (*B*) tendon of the flexor digitorum longus, (*C*) quadratus plantae, and (*D*) lumbrical muscles. (After Giannestras, N. J.: Foot Disorders: Medical and Surgical Management, 2nd ed. Philadelphia, Lea & Febiger, 1973.)

Fig. 19-12. The third subfascial layer consists of three muscles: (*A*) flexor digiti minimi, (*B*) adductor hallucis, oblique and transverse heads, and (*C*) flexor hallucis brevis. (After Giannestras, N. J.: Foot Disorders: Medical and Surgical Management, 2nd ed. Philadelphia, Lea & Febiger, 1973.)

The plantar muscles in the sole of the foot are divided into four layers. The first two layers originate from the calcaneal tuberosity and the other two from the metatarsal shafts. The first subfascial layer (Fig. 19-10) consists (from lateral to medial) of the abductor digiti minimi, the flexor digitorum brevis, and the abductor hallucis. The muscles of the second subfascial layer (Fig. 19-11) are (from medial to lateral) the tendon of the flexor hallucis longus, the tendon of the flexor digitorum longus, the quadratus plantae, and the lumbrical muscles. In the third subfascial layer are (Fig. 19-12) the flexor digiti minimi, the adductor hallucis, and the flexor hallucis brevis. The flexor hallucis brevis splits into medial and lateral tendons (Fig. 19-13), which are inserted into the corresponding sides of the proximal phalanx of the great toe. A sesamoid bone is embedded into each tendon under the first

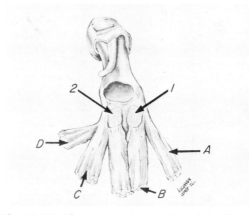

Fig. 19-13. The composite tendon of the flexor hallucis brevis: (*1*) medial sesamoid, (*2*) lateral sesamoid, (*A*) abductor hallucis, (*B*) flexor hallucis brevis, (*C*) oblique head of adductor hallucis, (*D*) transverse head of adductor hallucis. (After Giannestras, N. J.: Foot Disorders: Medical and Surgical Management, 2nd ed. Philadelphia, Lea & Febiger, 1973.)

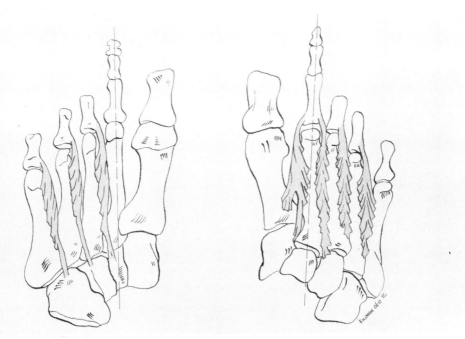

Fig. 19-14. Muscles of the fourth layer. The plantar interossei arise from only one metatarsal (*left*), but the dorsal interossei are bipinnate (*right*). (After Giannestras, N. J.: Foot Disorders: Medical and Surgical Management, 2nd ed. Philadelphia, Lea & Febiger, 1973.)

metatarsal head. The medial tendon and sesamoid are joined by the tendon of the abductor hallucis and the lateral tendon and sesamoid by the oblique and transverse heads of the adductor hallucis. The muscles of the fourth layer (Fig. 19-14) are the unipennate plantar and the bipennate dorsal interossei as well as the peroneus longus and tibialis posterior tendons.

The blood supply to the plantar aspect of the foot (Fig. 19-15) is furnished mainly by the posterior tibial artery. It divides into medial and lateral plantar branches. These, in turn, anastomose through the deep plantar arch with the arterial system on the dorsum of the foot.

The dorsal ligamentous structures of the tarsal and tarsometatarsal portions of the foot (Fig. 19-16) are numerous and extremely strong. In addition, they are reinforced by the long plantar ligament (Fig. 19-17) as well as the tibialis posterior and anterior tendons and the peroneus longus tendon on the plantar surface.

The nerve supply to the muscles of the plantar aspect of the foot as well as the principal portion of the sensory supply arise from the posterior tibial nerve. It splits into the medial and lateral plantar branches just as the posterior tibial nerve dips into

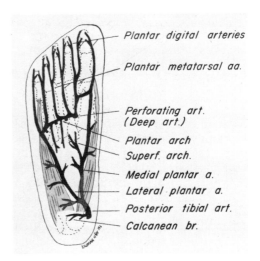

- Plantar digital arteries
- Plantar metatarsal aa.
- Perforating art. (Deep art.)
- Plantar arch
- Superf. arch.
- Medial plantar a.
- Lateral plantar a.
- Posterior tibial art.
- Calcanean br.

Fig. 19-15. The blood supply to the plantar aspect of the foot is furnished mainly by the posterior tibial artery. Note the extensive anastomoses.

the plantar medial aspect of the foot. The sensory supply to the dorsum of the foot is derived from the superficial branch of the common peroneal and the sural nerve (see Fig. 19-24).

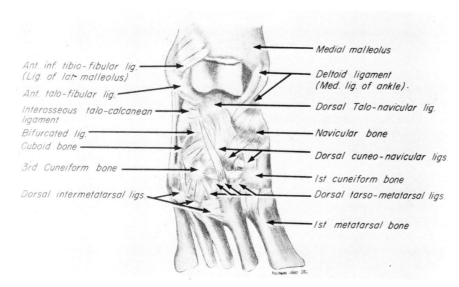

Fig. 19-16. The ligamentous support on the dorsum of the foot is extensive.

Ant. inf. tibio-fibular lig. (Lig. of lat. malleolus)
Ant. talo-fibular lig.
Interosseous talo-calcanean ligament
Bifurcated lig.
Cuboid bone
3rd Cuneiform bone
Dorsal intermetatarsal ligs.

Medial malleolus
Deltoid ligament (Med. lig. of ankle).
Dorsal Talo-navicular lig.
Navicular bone
Dorsal cuneo-navicular ligs.
1st cuneiform bone
Dorsal tarso-metatarsal ligs.
1st metatarsal bone

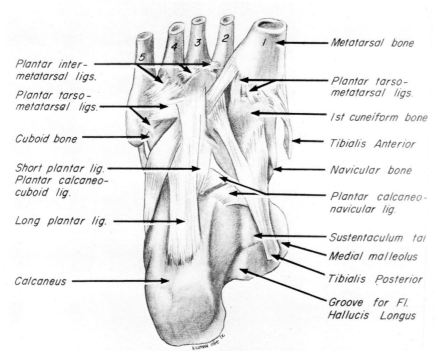

Plantar inter-metatarsal ligs.
Plantar tarso-metatarsal ligs.
Cuboid bone
Short plantar lig.
Plantar calcaneo-cuboid lig.
Long plantar lig.
Calcaneus

Metatarsal bone
Plantar tarso-metatarsal ligs.
1st cuneiform bone
Tibialis Anterior
Navicular bone
Plantar calcaneo-navicular lig.
Sustentaculum tal
Medial malleolus
Tibialis Posterior
Groove for Fl. Hallucis Longus

Fig. 19-17. The plantar ligamentous structures are reinforced by the tibialis anterior and posterior tendons as well as by the peroneus longus.

BIOMECHANICS

The structures and functions of the foot are just one segment of the integrated activities of the lower extremity responsible for gait. For efficient ambulation all components of the lower extremity must function properly. Weakness of musculature, loss of joint motion, and bony malalignment or destruction of soft tissue will each produce gait abnormalities. Alterations in gait, because of impairment of one function, will put excessive stress on the remaining structures to compensate for this deficiency. Thus, injury to any one component of this complex mechanism will result in excessive stress on the other components, and, with time, this excessive stress may lead to deterioration of the uninjured parts.

Much has been learned over the past two decades about the biomechanics of gait[1–3,6,7,15,18,19–24,29,31,34,38–42] and only a brief review is outlined here. An excellent, in-depth description of this subject is presented by Mann in Jahss's textbook *Disorders of the Foot*.[30] To emphasize the importance of foot function to normal gait, I will review some of the pertinent mechanical aspects of gait, emphasizing the foot's role in this process.

The main objective of gait (whether walking or running) is to move the body from one place to another in space. Such motion should ideally be accomplished efficiently, that is, by expending as little energy as possible. Energy expenditure is minimized by fluid motion, which avoids abrupt changes in direction. To move the body from point A to point B, energy (muscle contraction) must be expended to impart motion to the inert body at point A and energy must be absorbed at point B to arrest the body's momentum (inertia). To this end, the articulated skeleton of the foot acts as a rigid lever at push-off, allowing muscular contrac-

tion to propel the body forward, and at heel strike it becomes a flexible "shock absorber" to accommodate the impact of heel strike and allow maximal contact of the sole of the foot with the ground. This admittedly teleological assessment of foot function during gait can be used to understand and help physicians remember the important functions of the various foot components during the gait cycle.

The ankle joint is essentially a hinge joint, allowing only dorsiflexion and plantar flexion of the talus within the mortise. The talus normally does not rotate, invert, or evert appreciably within this mortise. Its axis of motion passes through the tips of the malleoli and thus lies about 25° externally rotated relative to the knee joint axis; it is also inclined slightly laterally (Fig. 19-18). The normal range of motion of the ankle joint (70°; 20° of dorsiflexion and 50° of plantar flexion) is critical, particularly during stance phase, to allow the body to "roll over" the foot, which at that phase is fixed to the ground. Limitation of this range of motion will impair progression of the normal gait. Indeed, given a normal range of motion of the ankle and other certain ideal circumstances (level ground,

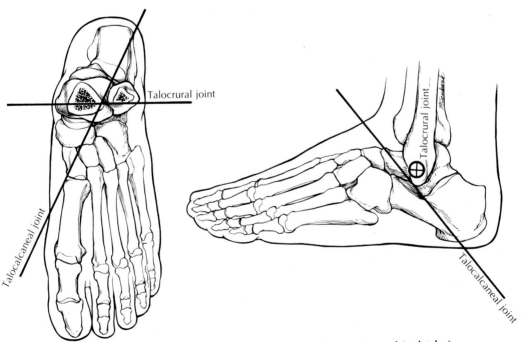

Fig. 19-18. The axes of rotation of the talocrural (ankle) and talocalcaneal (subtalar) joints as seen in the (*left*) dorsoplantar and (*right*) lateral projections. (After Isman, R. E., and Inman, V. T.: Anthropometric Studies of the Human Foot and Ankle. Bull. Prosthet. Res., **10–11**:105–107, 1969.)

exactly proper heel strike, correct shoe wear), the gait can closely approximate normal with little assistance from the foot itself.

However, it is rare (if not impossible) to meet these rigid criteria during normal walking, and thus the foot is depended on for much of the fine tuning of walking and running. Elimination of joint motion in the foot, destruction of the normal bony architecture, impairment of muscle function, and even disruption of the soft tissues will result in impairment of this critical function of the foot, resulting in increased stress on the more proximal limb structures.

The most important articulation of the foot is that between the talus and the calcaneus, the subtalar joint. This joint normally has 40° of motion, with an axis of rotation that passes through the medial dorsal navicular and the plantar lateral aspect of the calcaneus (see Fig. 19-18). Motion about this axis is best described as inversion and eversion from the neutral position, which, in a normal foot, is approximated by a straight line passing down the posterior aspect of the leg and bisecting the calcaneus. The total range of motion of this joint is quite variable, ranging from 10° to 65° with an average range of 40° ± 7°.[21]

When the capacity for inversion and eversion of the subtalar joint is added to ankle motion, a universal joint configuration is approximated.[50] At heel strike on uneven ground the subtalar joint can accommodate to allow the talus to be aligned correctly in the mortise, facilitating free ankle motion. Similarly, if the heel contacts the ground off center, either medially or laterally, the subtalar joint can accommodate this offset and allow normal ankle motion and then normal progression of gait. Loss of this accommodative ("shock absorber") function of the subtalar joint will cause the talus to bind in the ankle mortise, increasing sheer stress and decreasing efficiency of gait.

The heel pad also plays an important role in absorbing the shock of heel strike and helping to accommodate ankle motion.[4,47] The intricate arrangement of fat surrounded by firm fibrous septa that arise from the dermis and insert into the calcaneus (Fig. 19-19) buffers the impact of heel strike in a very efficient fashion. Damage to this hydraulic cushion cannot be repaired and can lead to impaired gait mechanics with significant pain on weight bearing.

Another important biomechanical consideration is the relationship between the alignment of the subtalar joint and the resulting configuration of the midtarsal joint. The midtarsal joint (also called Chopart's, or the transverse tarsal, joint) is the confluence of the talonavicular and calcaneocuboid joints. Normally this articulation allows a small amount of motion in both the sagittal and frontal planes. The degree of motion that can occur is determined to a large extent by the relative alignment of the calcaneus and the talus,[8,31] and others have shown that when the calcaneus is everted, the axes of the talonavicular and calcaneocuboid joints are parallel and thus motion can occur at the midtarsal joint. With the heel in inversion, however, the axes of the two joints are no longer parallel (Fig. 19-20), and motion at this joint is markedly restricted. From a mechanical point of view, this interrelationship improves the efficiency of gait: at heel strike the subtalar joint everts,

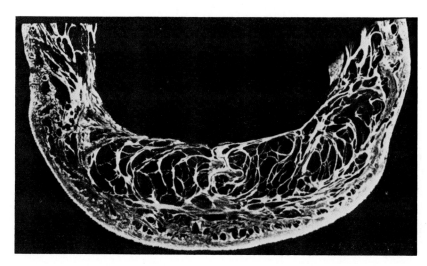

Fig. 19-19. Frontal section of the heel of an adult showing the fibrous septa arising from the dermis and inserting into the calcaneal periosteum. Contained within the septa are lobules of fat, creating a very effective hydraulic shock absorber. (Blechschmidt, E.: The Structure of the Calcaneal Padding. Foot Ankle, **2:**274, 1982.)

"unlocking" the midtarsal joint and creating a flexible midfoot to allow further accommodation of the foot to the ground and better absorption of the energy of impact. At push-off, the subtalar joint is inverted, "locking" the midtarsal joint to create a rigid lever at the midfoot to gain mechanical advantage for forward propulsion.

Between heel strike and push-off, the ankle joint dorsiflexes, allowing the body to move forward, and as this forward motion occurs, weight is transferred from the heel to the toes. During normal walking the vertical load applied to the foot is roughly equal to body weight, while during running the vertical load increases to two and a half times body weight. In addition to the vertical load, significant medial–lateral and forward–aft shear stresses occur as well.[30] The line of progression of the center of pressure as the foot moves from heel strike to toe-off is shown in Figure 19-21. From slightly lateral to the center of the heel it moves slightly more laterally in the midfoot, passing between the area of the first and second metatarsal heads and then under the great toe.[16] Proportionately, the weight is borne for a longer time on the metatarsal head area. During this phase the transverse metatarsal arch, which is seen only in the non-weight-bearing foot, is flat so that the weight is borne by all the metatarsals, with a higher concentration of pressure on the second and third metatarsal heads (Fig. 19-22).[7]

Also during gait, from about midstance to push-off, elevation of the longitudinal arch of the foot occurs. This is accomplished by a combination of factors: contraction of the extrinsic muscles (primarily the posterior tibial), intrinsic muscle contraction (flexor brevis), and passive dorsiflexion of the metatarsophalangeal joints. The dorsiflexion of the metatarsophalangeal joints places tension on the plantar fascia (which originates from the calcaneus and inserts into the bases of the proximal phalanges), creating a windlass effect to elevate the longitudinal arch[4,17] (Fig. 19-23). Elevation of the arch creates a stable lever arm, particularly when combined with locking of the midtarsal joint, for push-off.

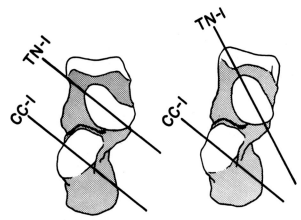

Fig. 19-20. Eversion of the heel (*left*) results in parallelism of the axes of motion of the calcaneocuboid (CC-1) and talonavicular (TN-1) joints, whereas inversion (*right*) produces divergence of these axes and restricts motion at the midtarsal joint. (Mann R., and Inman, V. T.: Phasic Activity of Intrinsic Muscles of the Foot. J. Bone Joint Surg., **46A**:476, 1964.)

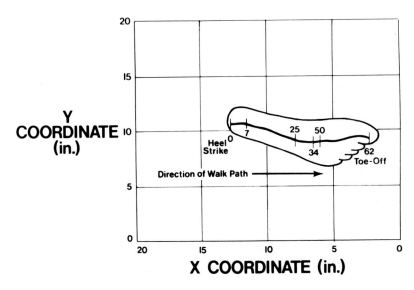

Fig. 19-21. The dark line on the sole indicates the line of progression of the center of pressure from heel strike to toe-off (62% of the normal walk cycle). Note that the greatest proportion of time is spent bearing weight on the metatarsal head area. (Jahss, M. H.: Disorders of the Foot, p. 49. Philadelphia, W. B. Saunders, 1982.)

This brief review of some of the pertinent aspects of foot biomechanics is presented to illustrate the important role of the foot in weight bearing. The foot serves as a flexible shock absorber during heel strike, converts to a relatively stable lever arm during push-off, provides a stable basis of support during stance, and generally greatly facilitates ambulation. Injury to part or all of this intricate mechanism will decrease its efficiency and result in increased stress in the more proximal links of the lower extremity. Restoration of these critical functions and preservation of the function of adjacent uninjured structures should be the goals of the surgeon who treats foot injuries.

EVALUATION OF FOOT INJURIES

HISTORY

As with any injury, a thorough evaluation must include, at a minimum, a complete history and physical examination combined with appropriate x-rays when indicated. Much can be learned from eliciting a thorough history of the injury. With regard to general information, the patient's age, vocation, and avocation and a review of his other activities of daily living will provide important background information. A careful review of past medical history will indicate previous foot problems, either static or progressive, which the physician must take into consideration when analyzing the presenting complaint. Certain systemic disorders must be identified (particularly diabetes and peripheral vascular disease), since they may substantially influence the progression or severity of the acute injury. Specific treatment methods may not be possible because of certain systemic disorders, or the goals of treatment may have to be modified because of the severity of some generalized medical conditions or because of the patient's avocational or vocational requirements.

Of great importance is definition of the mechanism of injury. Knowledge of the specific forces causing an injury will help the clinician to define the degree of injury to the structures in the foot, suspect the existence of certain systemic disease processes, and consider the possibility of injuries to other body structures. Certain mechanisms are known to cause specific injury patterns in the foot. For example, falling over a curb with the foot extremely plantar flexed (see Fig. 19-103) with the body's weight axially loaded on the equinus foot is known to produce injury to the tarsometatarsal joints. When the physician identifies a specific

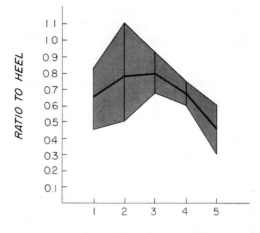

Fig. 19-22. Diagram of forces applied to the metatarsal heads during push-off. Note that the maximum load is applied on the second metatarsal head. (Collis, W. J. M., and Jayson, M. I. V.: Measurement of Pedal Pressures. An Illustration of a Method. Ann. Rheum. Dis. **31:**215, 1972.)

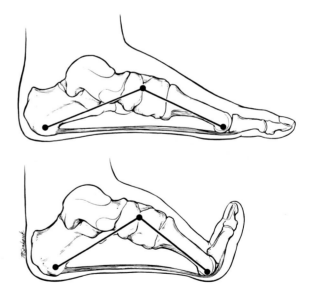

Fig. 19-23. The windlass effect of the plantar fascia (*top*). With dorsiflexion of the metatarsophalangeal joints (*bottom*), the longitudinal arch of the foot is elevated.

mechanism of injury such as this, he can direct his attention on physical examination to those structures that are most likely to be injured.

Eliciting a recent history of increasing jogging activity from 1 mile three times a week to 5 miles five times a week will make the alert clinician suspect that foot pain may be caused by a stress reaction. Discovering that the patient has stepped on a nail while wearing a tennis shoe should arouse concern about the possibility of a *Pseudomonas* infection in the bone or soft tissues. Knowing that the patient jumped from a height and landed on both heels should make the physician seek out a compression fracture of the lumbar spine, look for injuries elsewhere along the axis of applied force, and thoroughly evaluate both injured feet. Finally, knowing that a laceration of the foot was caused by a lawn mower blade should make the physician suspect the possibility of more extensive damage to the foot than is immediately apparent because of the large amount of energy imparted to the foot at the time of injury. These few examples of the mechanism of injury are presented to emphasize the importance of taking an adequate history in patients with foot injuries.

Patients with foot injuries will have a variety of specific complaints: pain, swelling, loss of function, decreased sensation, or deformity. The complaint should be recorded in the patient's own words to be used as a baseline for comparison as treatment progresses. Of particular importance are those symptoms that indicate the adequacy of neurovascular function. Complaints of increasing pain and decreasing sensation are of paramount importance in this regard and demand immediate attention.

PHYSICAL EXAMINATION

Following an adequate history, the injured part should be examined. An adequate examination cannot be done without removing the patient's shoes and socks! Examination begins with an inspection of the injured part and is aided greatly by comparison with the opposite, usually uninjured, extremity. Great variation in the configuration of the foot exists within the normal population; therefore, it is most helpful to compare the injured part with the opposite side to identify any deviation from normal in a particular patient. Inspection will identify *ecchymosis and swelling* as nonspecific signs of injury; *wounds,* indicating possible open fracture, dislocation, or soft tissue injury; *deformity* suggestive of fracture or dislocation; *pallor or cyanosis* indicative of impairment of circulation; and signs of pre-existing disease or deformity.

Gentle palpation, carefully done, will frequently elicit a discrete area of point tenderness—the best means of localizing the point of injury. Palpation may also reveal crepitus at the site of fracture. Palpation should be done gently and carefully because of the discomfort that it will cause the patient. Inspection and palpation will allow the clinician to recognize the point of maximal injury in most instances. Should any of these signs on inspection or palpation be positive, it will be necessary to obtain x-rays of the injured part to define specifically the extent and degree of injury.

Rarely, inspection and palpation of the injured part will be negative and will not enable the clinician to localize the complaint. In this circumstance, the injured part should be stressed to localize the point of injury. Stress should be carried out in a specific sequence of steps. First, the patient should be asked to move the injured part through an active range of motion without assistance and to identify specifically painful areas. If the patient cannot accomplish this, or if no pain is produced with active range of motion, the joints of the foot should be put through a gentle passive range of motion by the physician, again to elicit specific areas of pain. If neither active nor passive range of motion produces pain, a final stress test is weight bearing. The patient should be instructed, then and only then, to stand and walk on the injured part. If the patient passes through inspection, palpation, active range of motion, passive range of motion, and weight bearing without any abnormal signs, then the chances of significant injury are very remote.

All patients with injury of the foot should have a thorough assessment of neurovascular function. This should be accomplished early during the examination, before x-rays, to provide an adequate base line for adequate monitoring of these functions over time.

Impairment of sensation following injures to the foot usually occurs because of damage to peripheral nerves. The integrity of sensation to light touch and pin prick should be tested in the areas of distribution of the major peripheral nerves (Fig. 19-24). With the exception of the plantar surface of the great toe, the facility for two-point discrimination in the foot is much less than it is in the hand.[45,48]

The adequacy of circulation can be documented by critical assessment of the skin color, capillary filling in the nail beds and pulp, and palpation of peripheral pulses, remembering that the posterior tibial pulse is virtually always palpable unless there is excessive swelling in the region behind the medial malleolus or there is damage to the artery. The dorsalis pedis pulse is more variable, the artery being very small or absent in 12% of the population.[14] If pulses are not palpable, the Doppler flow meter technique should be used to confirm the

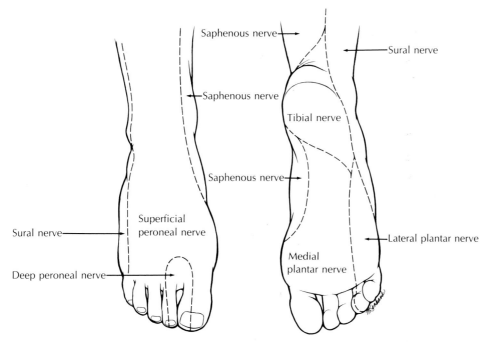

Fig. 19-24. The distribution of sensory nerves to the dorsal (*left*) and plantar (*right*) aspects of the foot.

integrity of the pedal circulation. Again, it is important to perform these assessments of neurovascular function early to establish a base line to which comparisons can be made as the patient's treatment progresses.

RADIOGRAPHIC EXAMINATION

Following a complete history and thorough physical examination, x-rays of the injured foot, taken in the appropriate projections, will enable the clinician to define the extent of osseous injury present. Because of the large number of relatively small bones in the foot and because these bones are frequently overlapped on many of the x-rays, it is sometimes difficult to visualize certain fracture lines. Inadequately exposed x-rays compound this problem and should never be accepted. Frequently, foot fractures are nondisplaced or only minimally displaced, further increasing the difficulty of x-ray diagnosis. Numerous accessory bones exist in the foot, and, in the adolescent, accessory ossification centers are common. These factors can often lead to errors both of underdiagnosis and overdiagnosis, and accurate interpretation of foot films requires considerable practice and experience. When doubt exists about the x-ray findings, or while awaiting radiographic consultation regarding a specific injury, if there is sufficient clinical evidence of injury (and in most instances such findings will have precipitated the x-ray evaluation in the first place), the foot should be splinted, elevated, and protected from weight bearing until a definitive diagnosis is reached.

Special views are often necessary to visualize adequately many of the fractures that can occur in the foot. These projections are described in the subsequent sections of this chapter under the specific fracture headings. In general, routine examination of an injured foot should include at least three basic views: anteroposterior, lateral, and oblique.[32]

Two x-ray views are rarely adequate to diagnose injuries of the foot. Oblique projections are often necessary to sort out the overlapping shadows of the numerous small bones.[36] Injuries of the hind part of the foot should be accompanied by routine anteroposterior, lateral, and mortise views of the ankle, both to help define the talus and to be certain that the ankle joint is not fractured as well. Because the total bone mass is much greater in the rearfoot than in the forefoot, the amount of x-ray exposure must be adjusted accordingly so that good-quality views will be obtained. As with all x-rays, poor processing of the film may produce streaks or other artifacts that may hide subtle but pertinent findings.

The foot contains many small accessory bones.[25,27,36,43,51] Their appearance on x-ray can lead to inappropriate diagnoses, and one should be aware of the commonly occurring accessory bones that may be misinterpreted. Shands and Wentz,[43] in a review of 850 children, found that 26% of those children over 8 years of age had at least one accessory bone, and they reported several other large series in adults in which the incidence of accessory bones ranged from 18% to 30%.

Figure 19-25, reproduced from Keats's Atlas,[25] illustrates the location of the more commonly ocurring accessory bones of the foot. A more extensive listing can be found in *Borderlands of the Normal and Early Pathologic in Skeletal Radiology* by Köhler and Zimmer.[27] The four most commonly occurring accessory bones are the os trigonum, the os tibiale externum (accessory navicular), the os peroneum, and the os vesalianum. Two accessory bones that Rogers and Campbell identify as frequently being mistaken for fractures are the os supratalare and the os supranaviculare.[36] In addi-tion to these accessory bones, a varying array of sesamoid bones are found on the plantar aspect of the forefoot. Figure 19-25 shows the location of sesamoids that have been reportd in the literature. Köhler and Zimmer[27] emphasize that the number and location of sesamoids are not always the same in the two feet of any one patient. Furthermore, failure of fusion of separate ossification centers often leads to persistent fragmentation of a sesa-moid, which can be incorrectly diagnosed as an acute fracture (see p. 1816).[373]

In general, it is possible to differentiate accessory bones, fragmented sesamoids, and atypically lo-cated sesamoids from fresh fractures by remem-bering that an accessory bone usually has an intact, smooth cortical surface around its entire circum-ference as opposed to the acute fracture, which has an irregular surface without a line of dense bone just beneath this surface. Comparison x-rays of the opposite foot are occasionally helpful in this situ-ation, as well as at other times when the physician is uncertain about the etiology of a suspicious

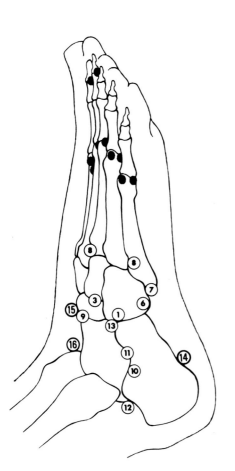
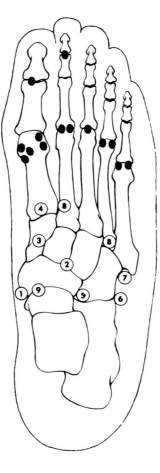

Fig. 19-25. Lateral (*left*) and an-teroposterior (*right*) drawings of the foot indicating the location of the commonly found acces-sory bones (*circles with num-bers*) and forefoot sesamoids (*shaded circles*). (1) Os tibiale externum, (2) processus uncina-tus, (3) os intercuneiforme, (4) pars peronea metatarsalia 1, (5) cuboides secundarium, (6) os peroneum, (7) os vesalianum, (8) os intermetatarseum, (9) os supratalare, (10) talus accesso-ries, (11) os sustentaculum, (12) os trigonum, (13) calcaneus se-cundarium, (14) os subcalcis, (15) os supranaviculare, (16) os talotibiale. (Keats, T. E., An Atlas of Normal Roentgen Variants That May Simulate Disease, 2nd ed., p. 371. Chicago, Year Book Medical Publishers, 1979.)

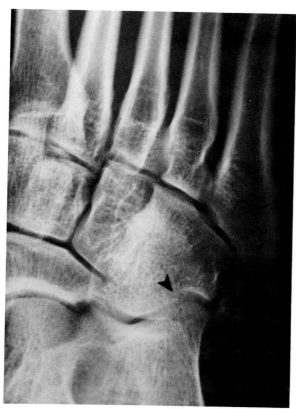

Fig. 19-26. Magnification view of the midfoot demonstrating a minimally displaced intra-articular fracture of the cuboid. This fracture was not seen on routine foot x-rays.

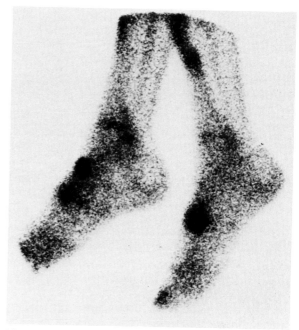

Fig. 19-27. [99m]Technetium bone scan of the feet in a 22-year-old cross-country runner with bilateral foot pain of 2 weeks' duration. Plain x-rays were normal, while the scan shows increased uptake in the base of the metatarsals bilaterally and in the navicular on the left, indicating stress reactions in these areas.

shadow on the x-ray. However, the accessory bones and sesamoids are not always bilaterally symmetrical.

Beyond the use of routine x-rays and special projections for specific fractures, certain other radiographic techniques are sometimes useful to diagnose fractures not apparent on the plain films, to define further the extent of injury, or to assess the progress of healing.

Magnification views (Fig. 19-26)[46] can be obtained with standard x-ray equipment, on occasion giving remarkably improved visualization of the bony architecture, including much better delineation of the cortical surface, or revealing the existence of an otherwise unrecognized fracture.[338]

Bone scanning techniques using [99m]technetium-labeled phosphorus complexes (Fig. 19-27) can be very helpful in the diagnosis of occult fractures, since increased uptake of this isotope can be seen as early as 24 hours after injury.[26,37] Stress fractures in the foot can be diagnosed by increased uptake

on the bone scan 2 to 3 weeks before conventional x-ray will demonstrate the fracture.[12,26,49]

Tomography is helpful in defining the degree of comminution of certain fractures, identifying joint incongruity resulting from fracture fragment displacement, isolating fractures that may be masked by overlapping shadows on the plain x-rays, and even assessing the degree of fracture healing in certain circumstances (Fig. 19-28). Polytomes (trispiral tomography) are more useful than regular tomograms for these purposes because "thin" sections, 1.5 to 2 mm apart, can be obtained.

Computed tomography (CT scanning) is as yet an incompletely defined modality in the evaluation of the acutely injured foot. It has been reported to aid in the late evaluation of patients with persistent symptoms following calcaneal fractures[277] (Fig. 19-29), but its role in the evaluation of acute foot injuries awaits further study.

Stress x-rays (Fig. 19-30) can on occasion be helpful in demonstrating the extent of ligamentous and other soft tissue injury to the foot. Stress x-rays can also be of particular importance following apparently satisfactory closed reduction of frac-

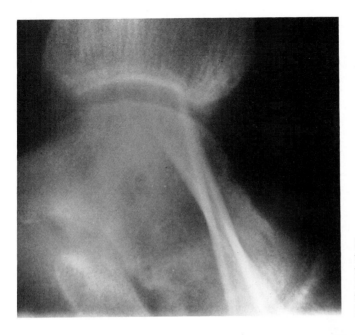

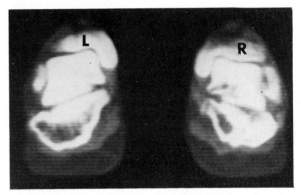

Fig. 19-28. Lateral tomogram of the talar neck taken 5 months after open reduction and internal fixation of a displaced fracture. Trabecular bridging, which was not apparent on routine x-rays, is evident, indicating fracture healing has occurred.

tures or dislocations in the foot. X-rays taken with gentle stress—perhaps just gravity—will sometimes show persistent or recurrent joint incongruity or osseous instability. Such signs of instability may at times dictate more aggressive treatment (see p. 1803).

These specialized techniques should be used judiciously to minimize the cost and amount of radiation exposure to the patient. Standard x-rays, properly taken and intelligently interpreted, remain the mainstay of radiographic diagnosis in foot trauma.

FRACTURES COMMON TO ALL PARTS OF THE FOOT

Several mechanisms or disease processes (stress, neuropathic changes, high-energy injury) can produce fractures in the foot that do not specifically occur in just one or two bones but may occur in any of the bones. Because the underlying mechanisms and disease processes are more important than the specific bone involved, these predisposing factors will be reviewed in this section, emphasizing the important underlying pathophysiology and outlining the general principles of care without focusing on any one particular bone of the foot.

STRESS REACTIONS AND FRACTURES

Although the problem of stress or march fractures among military personnel, especially recruits, has

Fig. 19-29. CT scan of the subtalar regions taken 8 months after fracture of the right calcaneus. Note widening of the right calcaneus and the incongruity of the subtalar joint.

been appreciated for many years, the recent worldwide increased interest in physical fitness, and particularly running, has produced a much larger number of symptomatic stress reactions in bone. Even though the second metatarsal was one of the first sites identified in the older literature as a focus for stress fractures and still remains a common location for this process, many bones of the foot have been found to be vulnerable to this injury. In a patient with foot pain and any recent history of increased or altered physical activity, the diagnosis of stress reaction must be considered. Running or athletic activity is certainly not the only cause of stress reactions. Any new mechanical stress applied

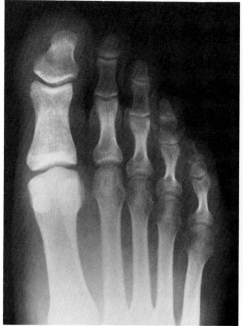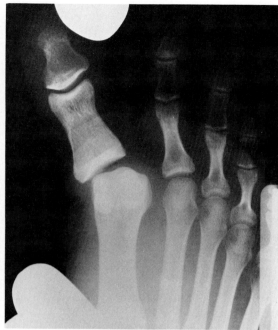

Fig. 19-30. Six weeks following abduction stress injury to the great toe metatarso-phalangeal joint, the routine anteroposterior x-ray appears normal (*left*). The patient complained of instability of the joint; stress x-rays confirmed persistent laxity of the lateral capsular structures (*right*).

to the foot can result in this problem, as demonstrated well by those patients who develop metatarsal stress fractures following Keller bunionectomy.[60]

Although most stress fractures in the foot occur in the second metatarsal and calcaneus (Fig. 19-31), the other bones are also vulnerable. In a series of 827 stress fractures in soldiers, Meurman[76] found 11% in the first metatarsal. The remaining three metatarsals were also represented, as well as the medial and lateral cuneiforms, the talus, and the lateral sesamoid. Hunter[66] and Torg and colleagues[87] identified stress fractures of the navicular as a significant problem in the athlete, and thus, the physician must be aware that this reaction can occur in any bone in the foot (see Fig. 19-27). Furthermore, Meurman found more than one stress fracture in ten of his patients, and Wilson and Katz[90] emphasized that bilateral stress fractures occur not uncommonly (in 27% of soldiers with calcaneal stress fractures).

The common underlying mechanism in all these reactions is excessive, repetitive stress applied to a bone that does not have the structural strength to withstand that stress.[57] If the stress continues to be applied over a long enough period, the bone, like any other mechanical structure, will fatigue and

break. The body attempts to prevent fatigue failure by remodeling the bone to strengthen it—specifically by adding trabeculae of new bone along the lines of stress. The process of new bone formation is slow, however, requiring up to 2 weeks to first resorb the old trabeculae and then to lay down more and stronger trabeculae along the new lines of stress. If excessive stress is applied before the new trabeculae are formed, the bone will fatigue and fail. In most of the long bones of the foot, oblique or transverse fracture lines occur through the shaft. In the primarily cancellous calcaneus, a characteristic compression fracture occurs, usually at the junction of the body and the tuberosity perpendicular to the normal bony trabeculae (see Fig. 19-31 *bottom*).

During the early stages of fatigue, the patient will develop mild to moderate pain and some localized swelling. He may try to disregard, "work-out" or "run through" the pain. Rarely will he see a physician at this early stage. At this point, within the first few days of symptoms, the physical findings are not very dramatic and fairly nonspecific, except that a discreet area of *point tenderness* can usually be identified on careful physical examination. X-ray evaluation at this stage is not helpful because the x-rays will appear normal. The only useful

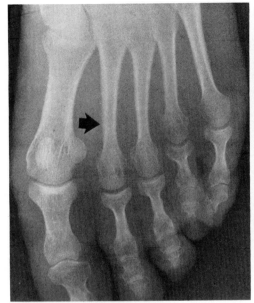
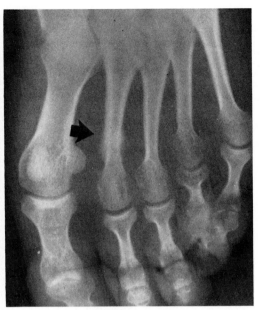
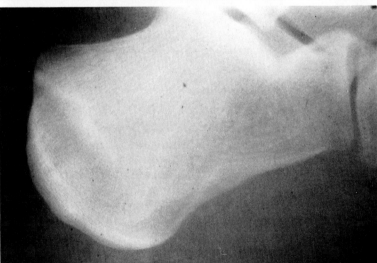

Fig. 19-31. A stress fracture of the metatarsal shaft. The patient noted pain in her foot after spring cleaning. Swelling and pain increased over the next 2 weeks. X-rays at that time were within normal limits. (*Top left*) Three weeks after onset of symptoms, a thin fracture line was noted in the second metatarsal shaft (*arrow*). (*Top right*) An x-ray at 4½ weeks demonstrated early callus formation. (*Bottom*) Stress fracture of the calcaneus with the characteristic compression of the cancellous tuberosity.

diagnostic modality is bone scanning,[12,49,63,85] which will demonstrate an area of increased radionucletide uptake as early as 2 days after the onset of symptoms.

Patients who present early will respond relatively quickly to treatment, which should include protection from stress until symptoms resolve (usually 1 to 2 weeks). Stress protection for the foot can be accomplished by elimination of the stressful activity and by protected ambulation with crutches or occasionally with a short-leg walking cast. X-rays repeated at 2 weeks may show periosteal new bone in the symptomatic area, but frequently, when treated early, these stress reactions may show little or no reactive bone on x-ray. When the symptoms have resolved, the patient may be allowed to return to his activities, but at a slower pace.

When the patient presents 2 weeks or more after the onset of symptoms, the findings on physical examination and x-rays frequently are more definitive. Often, at this stage, fatigue *fracture* of the bone will have occurred, resulting in significant pain, swelling, and tenderness and even occasionally in false motion at the fracture site. X-rays will show resorption, a transverse fracture line, trabecular condensation, or early periosteal new bone formation. Treatment at this stage is rest of the foot to allow normal healing of the fatigue fracture. Fortunately, in the foot, few of the fractures displace significantly and, if protected, will heal well. Torg and associates,[87] in a review of 15 navicular stress fractures, found it necessary to immobilize the foot in a cast and eliminate weight bearing to secure healing, while Van Hal and colleagues[382] found that stress fracture of the sesamoids frequently failed to heal with cast immobilization and required excision to allow the athlete to return to competition. Stress fracture of the base of the fifth metatarsal (Fig. 19-32) also may need a prolonged period without weight bearing to secure healing, and occasionally bone grafting has been found to be necessary to achieve union of stress fractures in this region. Generally, however, immobilization in a weight-bearing cast for stress fractures of other bones of the foot is adequate treatment. The immobilization should be continued until the fracture is nontender (usually 4 to 6 weeks), and then the patient may resume his activities but at a slower pace, only gradually regaining full activity.

NEUROPATHIC FRACTURES AND JOINT INJURIES

Charcot[53] in 1868 described rapidly progressive deterioration of weight-bearing joints not due to infection in patients with tabes dorsalis. Although tabes is no longer a commonly seen disorder, the same neuropathic condition occurs frequently in patients with diabetes mellitus and other, less common, diseases such as syringomyelia, peripheral nerve injury, leprosy, and congenital absence of pain. The common denominator in all these disorders is a significant decrease or complete absence of pain sensation combined with continued use of the insensitive limb. Because the peripheral neuropathy of diabetes so commonly affects the lower extremities, Charcot changes in the foot occur frequently in diabetic patients.

Although any injured joint in the foot may develop Charcot changes, it has been my experience that the most common area involved is the midfoot, with rapid deterioration of the talonavicular and calcaneocuboid joint or the tarsometatarsal joints. Collapse in this region results in loss of the normal longitudinal arch of the foot (Fig. 19-33). Newman[81] has identified six different conditions that affect the bones and joints of the patient with diabetic peripheral neuropathy: osteoporosis, new bone formation, bone loss, osteoarthropathy, pathologic fracture, spontaneous subluxations, and dis-

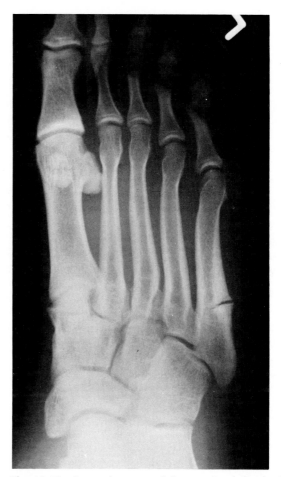

Fig. 19-32. Stress fracture of the proximal diaphysis of the fifth metatarsal.

locations. At times it is very difficult to distinguish these processes clinically or radiographically from infection, another common complication in the diabetic patient. Johnson,[67] in an extensive review of 118 cases, concluded that "the behavior of the bones and joints in neuroarthropathy can be explained on the basis of the usual responses of these tissues to trauma modified by the presence of decreased protective sensation" and not as a result of underlying bone weakness or impaired reparative response.

The usual initiating event is a fracture in or around a joint. Because of the lack of pain, the patient continues to stress (walk on) the fractured area. The normal healing response ensues with hematoma formation, and indeed the patient frequently first realizes something is wrong when he notes swelling and erythema of the foot. Continued ambulation creates excessive motion at the fracture

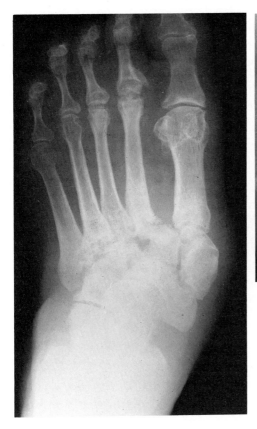 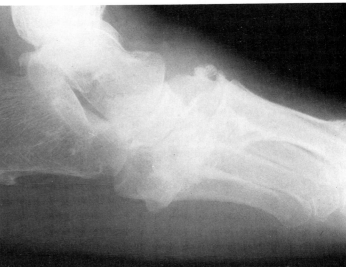

Fig. 19-33. Anteroposterior (*left*) and lateral (*right*) x-rays of the foot of a patient with adult onset diabetes mellitus of 10 years' duration. The patient noted spontaneous swelling and redness of the midfoot without specific injury. The x-rays show marked degeneration of the tarsometatarsal joints, flattening of the arch, and degeneration of several of the tarsal bones—all characteristic of Charcot changes.

site, which inhibits formation of bridging callus and completion of the normal healing process. Indeed, if a fracture is adequately immobilized and protected in the early stages following injury, it will usually heal. The instability created by failure of healing with continued use leads to rapid, severe degeneration of the bone and adjacent joints with subluxation or dislocation along with excessive new bone formation as the body attempts to heal the fracture. The deformity and instability that result produce persistent impairment of gait and the potential for the development of trophic ulcers over the displaced bony prominences.

Injuries to feet with neuropathic changes should be prevented by the use of proper footwear and protection of the foot from trauma and overuse. Treatment of early lesions should be the same as for injuries in patients with normal sensation, emphasizing adequate immobilization and rest of the foot until healing is complete. Even the most trivial injury must be taken seriously and protected until healed. At times it is very difficult to differentiate Charcot changes from infection because the patient frequently presents with swelling, local

redness, and warmth. If Charcot changes are suspected as the underlying cause, the patient should be placed on bed rest, with elevation and splinting of the foot, without immediate antibiotic treatment. The acute inflammation will resolve substantially over 2 to 3 days if the patient has Charcot arthropathy but will progress if infection is the underlying cause. Once the acute swelling has subsided, the foot should be placed in a cast until there is conclusive radiographic evidence of healing.

Often, patients with this disorder present late, after there has been significant displacement of bone fragments with frank dislocation of one or several joints. Little can be done to correct the deformity because of the degree of bony destruction that has occurred. The foot should be splinted and elevated until the soft tissue swelling subsides and then placed in a plaster cast, molded to correct the deformity passively as much as possible. Care must be taken when applying a plaster cast to insensitive feet, and the principles (minimal padding except over the toes, complete plaster coverage, early ambulation) of the total contact cast outlined by

Mooney and Wagner[80,88] for the management of diabetic foot ulcers should be followed closely. Warren[89] has indicated that as much as 6 months of cast immobilization may be required to allow consolidation of the unstable joint to a fibrous or bony union (Fig. 19-34). Once this is achieved, a specially molded shoe should be provided to relieve excessive weight bearing on any of the residual bony prominences.

In summary, in patients with neuropathic changes of the foot with impairment of pain sensation, injury may lead to rapidly progressive deterioration of the normal bony architecture because the patient fails to protect the injured part so that healing can occur. The potential for healing is retained, and aggressive early reduction and protection will usually result in union without deformity. Although most foot fractures can be treated by closed reduction and casting, if the surgeon deems that open reduction and internal fixation is the best way to achieve this end and there are no immediate contraindications (poor circulation, local infection), then surgical treatment should be undertaken. All foot injuries in these patients have the potential to develop Charcot changes and must be protected from stress until fully healed, since prevention of

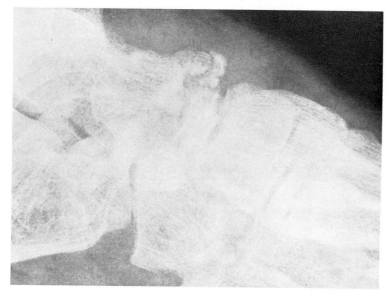

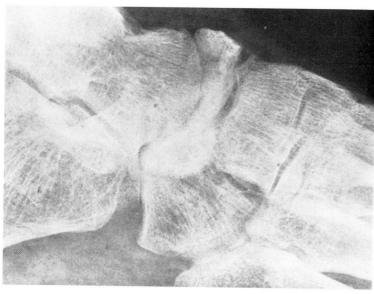

Fig. 19-34. Early disintegration of the navicular (*top*). After 6 months of walking-cast immobilization, the navicular is healed and the overall alignment of the foot is preserved (*bottom*). (Warren, G., Tarsal Bone Disintegration in Leprosy. J. Bone Joint Surg., **53B:**692, 1971.)

progressive deformity is the only satisfactory means of managing this difficult problem.

MULTIPLE (HIGH-ENERGY) INJURIES

Certain mechanisms of injury tend to produce multiple fractures, open injury, and substantial damage to the other soft tissues of the foot. These mechanisms, generally described as high-energy injuries, can be identified by taking an adequate history, identifying such mechanisms as falls from a height, motor vehicle wrecks, power lawnmower injuries, and high-velocity or close-range gunshot wounds, to name but a few.

Any time a violent force is applied to the foot, the degree of injury may be more extensive than is appreciated initially. Occasionally, the additional injury may be remote from the foot, as when a fall from a height produces a calcaneal fracture and, in addition, results in injury to the lumbar spine. As another example, when the foot strikes the firewall during a car wreck, it is well known that multiple proximal lower extremity injuries can occur as well as an injury to the foot. Within the foot, certain constellations of injuries are seen when specific forces are applied to it. Blows to the dorsum of the foot tend to result in multiple metatarsal fractures "across the board" (Fig. 19-35). Similarly, injuries to Lisfranc's joint or the midtarsal joint are often associated with compression fractures of the cuboid, while high-energy injuries to the rearfoot rarely result in isolated bony injury. A high index of suspicion will help the physician avoid overlooking such associated injuries either of parts remote from the foot or of adjacent pedal structures.

With high-energy injury, the likelihood of open fracture is significantly increased. Regardless of the mechanism of injury, all open wounds in the foot, as elsewhere, must be thoroughly debrided as soon after injury as is feasible. Complete surgical debridement of all contaminated and necrotic tissue remains the most important step in wound management, and it is even more critical in high-energy wounds because the degree of soft tissue damage is often much greater than the physician might suspect from initial inspection of the wound. Contaminated material can be driven deep into the soft tissues by high-velocity wounding implements such as a rotary lawn mower blade,[65,84] and extensive concussion of soft tissues from high-velocity missiles[74] can cause tissue death over a wide area. Often a single surgical debridement is insufficient. For this reason, these high-energy wounds should never be closed primarily, and repeat operative debridement should be undertaken frequently to ensure cleans-

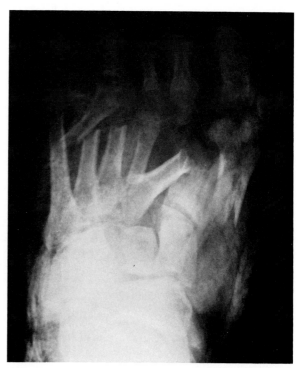

Fig. 19-35. Severe crushing injury of the forefoot resulting in multiple displaced metatarsal fractures. Primary concern must be given to the viability of the forefoot following injuries such as this.

ing of the wound. Tetanus prophylaxis must be provided, and a short-term "prophylatic" antibiotic (usually a cephalosporin) should be administered in the immediate postoperative period but should not be given for long periods to minimize the chance of a nosocomial superinfection.

Management of the osseous damage is often difficult in these injuries because of the multiplicity of fractures and dislocations combined with soft tissue injury. The basic objectives to be achieved with the severely injured foot are, in order:

Preserve circulation
Preserve sensation (particularly plantarly)
Maintain plantigrade position of the foot
Control infection
Preserve the plantar skin and fat pads
Preserve gross motion (dorsiflexion, plantarflexion, inversion, and eversion) both passively and actively
Achieve bony union
Preserve fine motion

In contrast to the management of most isolated fractures, bony union is a relatively low priority in the management of the severely mangled foot.

Local fusion or bone grafting can be accomplished late to secure union of the fractures, and the surgeon's initial attention must be directed to preserving the function of the soft tissues, since they are more difficult than bone to reconstruct or repair later.

Omer and Pomerantz[82] emphasized the importance of fasciotomy in the severely crushed foot. Excessive bleeding and edema formation in the closed spaces can produce compartment syndromes in the foot just as in the arm or leg. Early surgical decompression is the only effective means of preventing significant ischemic contractures of these muscles. Loeffler and Ballard[71] have described a utilitarian plantar incision beginning posterior to the medial malleolus, extending laterally and distally to the midline, and ending between the first and second metatarsal heads. All or any part of this incision can be used to gain access to all the compartments of the sole of the foot (Fig. 19-36). Omer and Pomerantz[82] have outlined a treatment

program for severe open injuries of the foot. It includes the following:

Multiple x-rays to delineate fully the extent of injury
Meticulous periodic circulatory assessment
Adequate and repeated debridement
Fasciotomy when indicated
Delayed wound closure 3 to 5 days after adequate debridement
Bulky compression dressing
Elevation
Internal fixation of unstable fractures at the time of wound closure
Static and dynamic splinting to prevent deformity (particularly equinus of the forefoot or ankle)
Early mobilization
Stable, underloaded weight bearing

With severe injuries, stabilization of the fractures and dislocations will facilitate management of the soft tissue wounds.[52,69] Although some authors

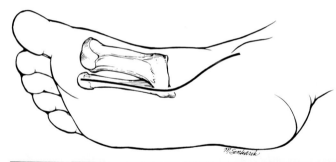

Fig. 19-36. (*Top*) Line drawing of the utilitarian incision used to gain access to the plantar compartments of the foot (after Loeffler and Ballard[71]). (*Bottom*) Following a closed crushing injury to the foot, surgical decompression was performed with the evacuation of over 200 ml of hematoma from the plantar compartments.

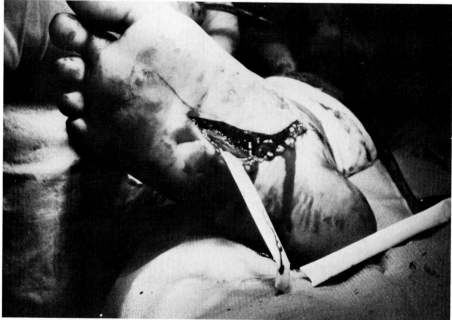

recommend fixation with multiple Kirschner wires,[82] others more recently have advocated the use of external fixation devices to secure stability in the severely injured foot. Kenzora and coauthors[68] recommended the use of the Hoffmann external fixation device for severe foot wounds to (1) stabilize major open fracture—dislocations, (2) maintain length where bone has been lost, (3) prevent contracture, (4) control joint position in highly comminuted articular injuries, and (5) provide unobstructed access and stability for soft tissue reconstruction (Fig. 19-37). They recommended that the device be used only temporarily until soft tissue healing has occurred and the bony architecture is stabilized sufficiently for casting. Maxwell and Hoopes[75] have advocated the use of local muscle flaps, pedicled myocutaneous flaps, and free myocutaneous flaps for soft tissue reconstruction, employing external fixation devices to maintain bony stability until soft tissue coverage is complete.

In the severely injured foot, multiple extensive reconstructive procedures may be necessary to achieve a viable sensate plantigrade foot, but despite the recent dramatic advances in prosthetic design, such a foot will still function better than any currently available prosthesis.

FRACTURES OF THE TALUS

The talus is one of the most important bones of the foot because it supports and distributes the body forces above it. It allows motion between the tibia and the foot and forms the important articulations with the calcaneus inferiorly (the subtalar joint) and the navicular anteriorly. Fractures of the talus are second in frequency among all tarsal fractures. The significance of these fractures rests on the function of the bone itself and on the fact that its blood supply is tenuous, since three fifths of the bone is covered by articular cartilage.[113] Fractures that damage the small area through which blood vessels enter the talar neck are particularly significant and can have catastrophic sequelae.

The mechanisms by which fractures of the talus occur reflect our mechanized age: a driver slams his foot on the brakes, trying to prevent an automobile accident; a pilot braces himself against the rudder controls as the plane crashes. Such suddenly applied forces cause the forefoot to be brought into hyperextension against overwhelming forces in the opposite direction. Fracture of the talar neck was so common after World War I that Anderson[93] referred to it as "aviator's astragalus." The types of

fracture that can occur are quite variable, and the methods of treatment also vary considerably. Each fracture of the talus should be treated individually, since no single method is satisfactory for all conditions.

This section of the chapter deals with fractures of the talar neck and talar processes. Total dislocation of the talus is described on page 1759.

ANATOMY

The body of the talus is covered superiorly by the trochlear articular surface, which carries the body weight to the foot. The surface is wider anteriorly than posteriorly (Fig. 19-38). Medially and laterally the articular cartilage extends plantarward to articulate with the medial and lateral malleoli, respectively. The inferior surface of the talar body is also composed largely of cartilage, which forms the articulation between the talus and the posterior facet of the calcaneus.

The neck of the talus, which is constricted inferiorly, laterally, and superiorly, is roughened by ligamentous attachments and vascular foramina. It deviates medially approximately 15° to 20° in the adult and is the area of the bone most vulnerable to fracture. The rounded head has continuous articular facets for the navicular anteriorly, the spring ligament inferiorly, the sustentaculum tali posteroinferiorly, and the deltoid ligament medially. The talus has no muscular or tendinous attachments. Its connection to adjacent structures is by articular capsule and synovial membrane only. Since the blood vessels must use these fascial structures to reach the talus, trauma associated with capsular tears may be complicated by avascular necrosis of the body of the talus.

There are two bony processes (posterior and lateral) of the talus, both of which are subject to fracture (Fig. 19-39). The posterior process is composed of medial and lateral tubercles separated by a groove for the tendon of the flexor hallucis longus (Fig. 19-40 *top*). The os trigonum, which is present in almost 50% of normal feet,[117] arises from a separate ossification center just posterior to the lateral tubercle of the posterior talar process and either fuses with the lateral tubercle or remains as a separate ossicle throughout life.

The lateral process of the talus (Fig. 19-40 *bottom*) is wedge shaped in the frontal plane. Its inferior medial surface forms the lateral third of the talar articulation with the posterior calcaneal facet, and its superolateral surface forms the articulation with the distal end of the fibula.

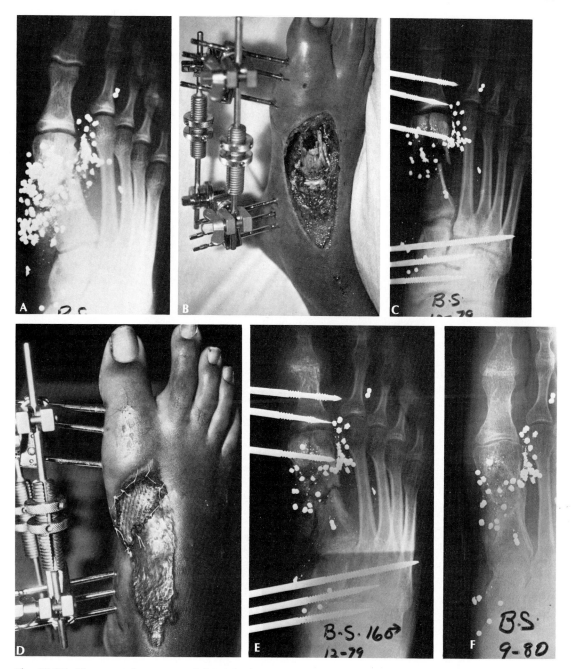

Fig. 19-37. The use of an external fixation device in the treatment of a close-range shotgun wound of the foot. (*A*) The initial x-ray. (*B, C*) After adequate initial debridement, the first ray is stabilized with the external fixation device. (*D*) A split-thickness skin graft is applied to achieve wound closure. (*E*) Cancellous bone graft bridges the bony defect. (*F*) One year after injury, adequate bony alignment and healing are seen. (Kenzora, J. E.; Edwards, C. C.; Browner, B. D.; et al: Acute Management of Major Trauma Involving the Foot and Ankle with Hoffmann External Fixation. Foot Ankle, **1:**355, 1981.)

BLOOD SUPPLY OF THE TALUS

Because avascular necrosis is a complication of certain fractures and dislocations of the talus, its blood supply has been studied in great detail by many investigators.[107,113,118,124,134,142,144,151,157] Approximately 60% of the surface is covered by articular cartilage,[113] and no muscles originate from or insert into the talus.[14,113] Thus, only a limited surface is available to provide adequate vascular perforation, and these relatively few vessels may be disrupted at the time of injury.

Although earlier investigators felt that the anterior tibial artery alone supplied the talus,[124,151] many studies have confirmed that branches of the posterior tibia and perforating peroneal arteries also contribute significantly. Wildenauer[157] was the first to describe the talar circulation fully and to identify the critical anastomotic sling of vessels in the tarsal sinus and tarsal canal, which lie beneath the neck of the talus.

The sinus tarsi is bounded by the calcaneus inferiorly, the body of the talus posteriorly, and the talar head and neck anteriorly. The tarsal canal, which is located medially, lies between the talus and calcaneus just behind and below the tip of the medial malleolus. Kelly and Sullivan[113] likened these two anatomical regions to a funnel: the tarsal sinus being the cone; the tarsal canal, the tube. The arteries (the artery to the sinus tarsi, an anastomotic loop between the perforating branch of the peroneal artery and a branch of the dorsalis pedis artery, and the artery of the canal, a branch of the posterior tibial artery) form an anastomotic sling inferior to the talus from which branches arise to enter the talar neck area (Fig. 19-41).

In an excellent study, Mulfinger and Trueta[134] summarized the studies of others and outlined the branches of the major extraosseous vessels that supply the talus. From the posterior tibial artery come the artery to the tarsal canal, which arises just proximal to the origin of the medial and lateral plantar arteries, and the deltoid branch, which supplies the medial surface of the body. From the anterior tibial (dorsalis pedis) artery come multiple branches to the dorsal talar neck and a branch to form the artery of the sinus tarsi. From the peroneal artery come branches to the posterior process and

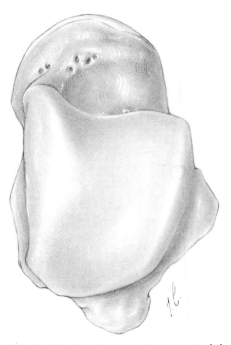

Fig. 19-38. On the superior aspect of the right talus, note the convergence of the sides of the trochlear surface in a posterior direction and vascular foramina on the neck. (After Giannestras, N. J.: Foot Disorders: Medical and Surgical Management, 2nd ed. Philadelphia, Lea & Febiger, 1973.)

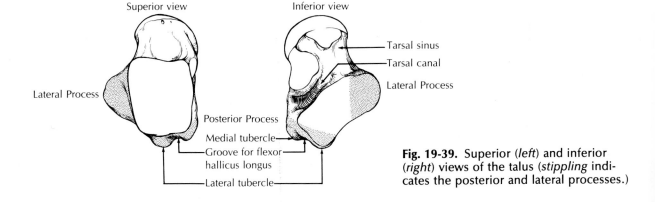

Superior view   Inferior view

Lateral Process

Tarsal sinus
Tarsal canal
Lateral Process

Posterior Process
Medial tubercle
Groove for flexor hallicus longus
Lateral tubercle

Fig. 19-39. Superior (*left*) and inferior (*right*) views of the talus (*stippling* indicates the posterior and lateral processes.)

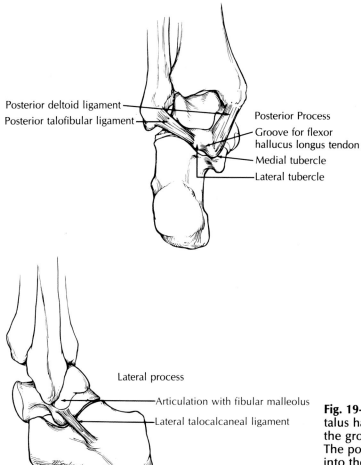

Posterior deltoid ligament
Posterior talofibular ligament

Posterior Process
Groove for flexor
hallucus longus tendon
Medial tubercle
Lateral tubercle

Lateral process
Articulation with fibular malleolus
Lateral talocalcaneal ligament

Fig. 19-40. (*Top*) The posterior process of the talus has two tubercles, which are separated by the groove for the flexor hallucis longus tendon. The posterior fibers of the deltoid ligament insert into the medial tubercle, and the posterior talofibular ligament inserts into the lateral tubercle. (*Bottom*) The lateral process of the talus.

a branch to form the artery of the sinus tarsi. In addition, Peterson and colleagues[144] emphasized the important contribution of many capsular and ligamentous vessels demonstrating "rich vascular connections" between the talus and the navicular, the calcaneus, and even the tibia through capsular and ligamentous vessels.

The talar head is thus nourished by branches of the dorsalis pedis and the artery of the tarsal sinus. The body receives most of its blood supply from the anastomotic sling in the tarsal canal and sinus with many branches of that sling entering the neck and coursing posterolaterally,[134] but the deltoid branches of the posterior tibial artery contribute significantly to the blood supply of its medial quarter, and branches of the peroneal artery make a minor contribution posteriorly in the region of the posterior process.

Peterson and Goldie[142] showed that nondisplaced fractures of the talar neck disrupt the intraosseous branches of the arteries of the tarsal sinus and tarsal canal, but the major vascular sling remains intact. With displaced fractures of the talar neck, branches from the dorsalis pedis artery to the talar neck as well as the artery to the tarsal canal and to the tarsal sinus (the major arterial supply to the talus) are ruptured. These findings confirm the clinical observation that the rate of avascular necrosis in talar neck fractures is directly related to the degree of fracture displacement.[96,110]

FRACTURES OF THE NECK OF THE TALUS

Coltart,[99] in a well-documented series, described 228 injuries of the talus and reported that fractures of the neck of the talus were second in frequency

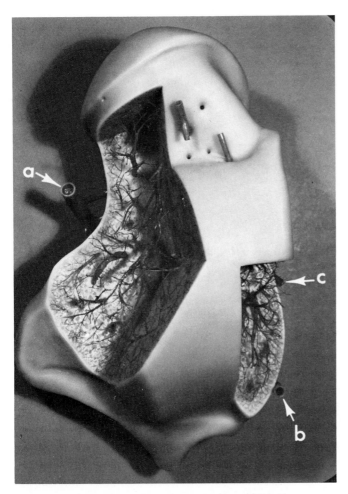

Fig. 19-41. The anastomotic sling of vessels that provides the blood supply to the body of the talus: laterally, the artery of the tarsal sinus (*a*); medially, the artery of the tarsal canal (*b*). Additional arteries enter dorsally through the neck and on the medial surface of the body (*c*). (Kelly, P. J., and Sullivan, C. R.: Blood Supply of the Talus. Clin. Orthop., **30:**38, 1963.)

to chip and avulsion fractures of this bone. Pennal[139] reported that 30% of talar fractures involved the neck. As consulting surgeon to the Royal Flying Corps, Anderson[93] coined the term *aviator's astragalus*. He reported on 18 cases of fracture and dislocation of the talus. Hawkins[110] in 1970 reviewed 57 fractures of the talar neck and developed a classification based on the degree of displacement of the proximal fragment. This classification has proved very helpful in predicting the long-term outcome of these fractures (see below). Several similar reviews of this subject[96,122,137,140,143] in recent years have provided a reasonably clear and consistent description of this injury.

MECHANISM OF INJURY

All authors concur that the most common mechanism of talar neck fracture is hyperdorsiflexion of the foot on the leg; only rarely will a direct blow to the dorsum of the foot produce this fracture.

Whereas Anderson and Coltart[93,99] both described "flying accidents" as the most common source of these fractures, with the sole of the foot resting on the rudder bar of the aircraft at the point of impact, today these fractures usually occur as a result of motor vehicle wrecks or falls from heights. In most cases, however, the force applied to the foot is one of hyperdorsiflexion.

Penny and Davis[140] have summarized well the progressive injuries to the talus that occur from this hyperdorsiflexion force:

With dorsiflexion, initially the posterior capsular ligaments of the subtalar joint rupture, the neck of the talus impacts against the leading anterior edge of the distal tibia, and a fracture line develops at this point and enters the nonarticular portion of the subtalar joint between the middle facet and the posterior facet. With a continuation of the dorsiflexion force, the calcaneus with the rest of the foot and including the head of the talus subluxes forward. If there is a concomitant inversion component to the force,

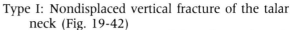

the foot may sublux or dislocate medially (if there is a concomitant eversion force, the foot dislocates laterally). If the force subsides at this moment, the foot recoils, the body of the talus tips into equinus and the fractured surface of the neck comes to ride on the upper surface of the os calcis. A continuation of the dorsiflexion force, however, produces further rupture of the posterior ankle capsular ligaments, the strong posterior talofibular ligament, and the superficial and posterior aspects of the deltoid ligament. . . . The body of the talus is then wedged posteriorly and medially out of the mortise and rotates around a horizontal and transverse axis so that the fracture surface faces upwards and laterally. This is a constant position for the body when there has been dislocation of the body out of the mortise occurring because of the direction of the posterior facet of the subtalar joint and because the talus pivots around the intact deep fibers of the deltoid ligament and flexor hallucis longus tendon. The body of the talus then comes to lie in the interval between the posterior aspect of the medial malleolus and the anterior aspect of the tendo achilles. It may be tightly jammed behind the medial malleolus, which is often concomitantly fractured, and the sustentaculum tali. The posterior tibial neurovascular structures almost invariably evade injury by this mechanism, lying anterior to and being protected by the flexor hallucis longus tendon.

CLASSIFICATION

The progressive displacement of the body of the talus produces one of three basic fracture configurations, which correlate with the three fracture types defined by Hawkins[110]:

Type I: Nondisplaced vertical fracture of the talar neck (Fig. 19-42)

Type II: Displaced fracture of the talar neck with subluxation or dislocation of the subtalar joint (the ankle joint remains aligned) (Fig. 19-43)

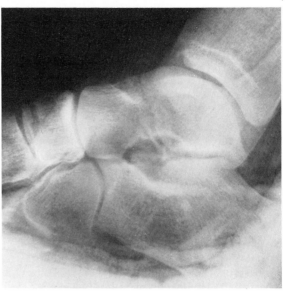

Fig. 19-42. Nondisplaced vertical fracture of the talar neck, Hawkins's type I.

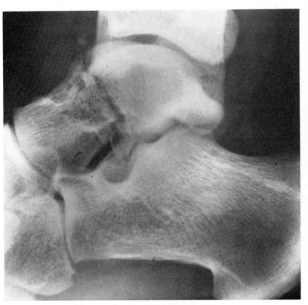

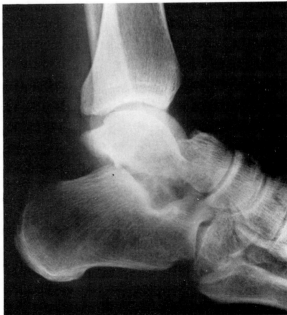

Fig. 19-43. Displaced Hawkins's type II fractures of the talar neck with subluxation (*left*) and dislocation (*right*) of the subtalar joint.

Type III: Displaced fracture of the talar neck with
dislocation of the body of the talus from both
the subtalar and ankle joints (Fig. 19-44)

Virtually all fractures of the talar neck fit into one
of these three types. Canale and Kelly[96] described
one patient in whom, in addition to the Hawkins's
type III configuration, the talar head was also
dislocated. Pantazopoulos and colleagues[137] treated
one patient with a talar neck fracture with dislocation of the head fragment; the body remained
reduced. These rare variants have been classified
as type IV.

SIGNS AND SYMPTOMS

The history is usually that of severe injury, repro-
ducing the rudder bar mechanism of an airplane
crash but more frequently seen following motor
vehicle wrecks or falls from heights. Males predominantly sustain this injury, and humans of any age
can be affected, although most are young adults.[106]
The patient will complain of intense pain in the
foot and ankle, and significant swelling will occur
even without displacement of the fracture. When
there is displacement of the fracture with concomitant subluxation or dislocation, the normal contours of the ankle and hindfoot are distorted. If
there is significant displacement of the body of the
talus, an open injury may result (21% in Hawkins's
series[110] and 16% in Canale and Kelly's series[96])
or the skin may be tented over the fragment and
be relatively ischemic because of the local tension
and swelling. Close attention must be given to the
skin in this situation with prompt reduction of the
displaced fragment to prevent slough and subsequent infection. Despite posteromedial displacement of the body with most type II injuries, the
posterior tibial neurovascular bundle is usually
spared;[140] however, close monitoring of the distal
neurovascular function is mandatory with this
injury.

In addition to the significant local soft tissue
injuries, fractures of both remote and adjacent
structures have been reported (64% in Hawkins's
series[110]). Of greatest significance is the high incidence (19%[96] to 28%[122]) of associated (usually
medial) malleolar fractures with this injury. Knowledge of this high frequency of associated ankle
fracture should alert the physician to search diligently for a talar neck fracture in patients with
medial malleolar fracture as the result of a hyperdorsiflexion injury.

RADIOGRAPHIC FINDINGS

Initial x-ray evaluation will demonstrate the fracture and the degree of displacement to facilitate

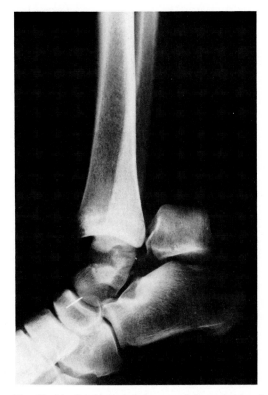

Fig. 19-44. Displaced fracture of the talar neck with
dislocation of both the subtalar and tibiotalar joints
(Hawkins's type III).

classification. Anteroposterior and oblique x-rays
of the ankle will demonstrate the alignment of the
talar body in the mortise, while the lateral x-ray
of the ankle and foot will best show the talar neck
fracture line and the alignment of the posterior
facet of the subtalar joint. Many of the minimally
displaced fractures assume a varus deformity at the
fracture site that cannot be appreciated on the
standard x-ray projections. Canale and Kelly[96] described the best x-ray technique to demonstrate the
entire talar neck in the anteroposterior direction.
With the ankle in maximum equinus, the foot is
placed on a cassette and pronated 15°, and the
x-ray tube is directed cephalad at a 75° angle from
the horizontal (Fig. 19-45). This projection is helpful in assessing the degree of initial displacement
and is a critical guide to the adequacy of reduction.

TREATMENT

Complications that can result from talar neck fracture include infection, delayed union or nonunion,
malunion, avascular necrosis of the body, and
osteoarthritis of the ankle and subtalar joints. Treatment should be designed to minimize these complications. Although some complications (most

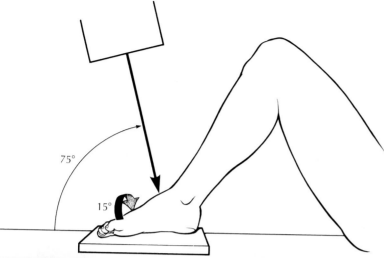

Fig. 19-45. (*Top*) The correct position of the foot for x-ray evaluation of the talar neck is shown. (*Bottom*) X-ray demonstrates the entire talar neck with anatomical reduction of the fracture.

Type I Fractures

Only those fractures in which there is *no* displacement of the fracture line and no incongruity of the subtalar joint should be designated as type I fractures. All authors agree that this type should be treated by below-the-knee cast immobilization for 8 to 12 weeks until clinical and x-ray signs of fracture healing are present.[95,96,99,104,110,114,139,143] Most authors recommend avoidance of weight bearing, especially during the first 4 to 6 weeks of treatment.

Type II Fractures

Displacement of the talar neck fracture (no matter how slight) with concomitant subluxation or dislocation of the posterior facet of the subtalar joint characterizes type II fractures. Persistent slight displacement will result in malunion (usually in varus), frequently producing an unacceptable result,[96,128] and reduction of the fracture should be achieved by closed or open means if necessary. Even moderate displacement of the fracture fragments may cause tenting of the skin and the possibility of skin necrosis. Prompt reduction of this fracture is critical to avoid skin slough and subsequent infection.

Closed Reduction. Closed reduction is accomplished by manipulation of the foot to "catch up with" the body fragment. Under adequate anesthesia, gentle traction is applied manually and the foot is flexed plantarward to bring the head fragment in proper relation to the body. Any varus or valgus malalignment should be corrected as well. With the foot held in equinus, lateral and anteroposterior x-rays of the talar neck should be taken

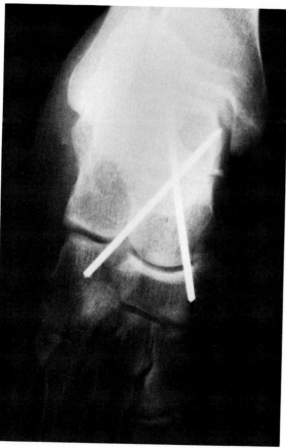

notably avascular necrosis) are predetermined by the degree and severity of the initial injury, all recent reviews of the subject conclude that the best results occur when prompt, perfectly anatomical reduction of the neck fracture is achieved and maintained.

to assess the adequacy of reduction. If an anatomical reduction has been achieved, the foot should be casted, still in equinus, in a short-leg non-weight-bearing cast. This position should be held for 1 month, and then with subsequent casts the foot can be brought out of equinus as long as the reduction is maintained. Non-weight-bearing cast immobilization is usually required for 3 months to achieve bony union.

Open Reduction. If reduction cannot be obtained and maintained by closed means (this occurs approximately 50% of the time), operative treatment is indicated, since it is imperative to achieve anatomical reduction of this fracture. Most authors recommend a longitudinal anteromedial incision over the talar neck just medial to the anterior tibial tendon. This allows direct access to the fracture site to visualize and manipulate both fragments. Penny and Davis[140] recommend an anterolateral approach that they believe lessens the chance of further damage to the blood supply of the talus and provides adequate exposure of the fracture. Once reduction is achieved and confirmed by x-rays, fixation can be achieved with two Kirschner wires driven across the fracture site parallel to the axis of the talar neck combined with a non-weight-bearing plaster cast (Fig. 19-46). The cast immobilization is continued for 8 to 12 weeks until the fracture is fully healed. Trillat and colleagues,[155] and more recently Lemaire and Bustin,[119] have recommended lag screw fixation to stabilize these talar neck fractures, and Penny and Davis recommend fracture fixation with AO cancellous screws.[140] These authors believe that this method provides more rigid fixation, facilitating union and minimizing the chance of late displacement of the fracture. They recommend closed reduction (or open reduction if necessary to achieve anatomical position) followed by lag screw fixation through a posterior approach (Fig. 19-47). In these small series of patients, good to excellent long-term results were achieved with this method.

Type III Fractures

In addition to talar neck fracture and subtalar dislocation, in Hawkins's type III injuries the talar body is dislocated from the ankle joint. In the vast majority of cases, the body fragment is wedged posteriorly and medially, rotating around the intact deep fibers of the deltoid ligament to lie in the soft tissues with the fracture surface pointing laterally and cephalad. A significant proportion (approximately 25%) of these injuries are open, and the

first step in management must be an adequate debridement of the open wound. Frequently with closed injuries, the displaced body will produce extreme tension on, and eventually necrosis of, the overlying skin, mandating prompt reduction. This is a true surgical emergency, since skin slough will produce disastrous consequences.

Even though most authors recommend an attempt at closed reduction initially, this is virtually impossible to achieve, and open reduction is usually required. A transverse Kirschner wire or Steinmann pin through the calcaneus attached to a traction bow can be used to apply traction to the calcaneus, increasing the space beneath the tibia to allow manual closed manipulation of the talar body back into position. This rarely provides enough space to allow reduction of the body, however, and the surgeon is forced to resort to open reduction.

Open reduction is achieved through either a posteromedial[140] or an anteromedial approach. Associated fracture of the medial malleolus facilitates reduction because the malleolus and attached deltoid ligament can be retracted distally, and, with a valgus stress, the ankle mortise can be opened to allow derotation and replacement of the body of the talus. Frequently the deep fibers of the deltoid ligament remain attached to the talar body. These fibers should not be released surgically because they may carry the only remaining arterial supply to the body. It is preferable to osteotomize the medial malleolus[140] and reflect it distally to facilitate reduction rather than cutting the intact deltoid ligament. Reduction is always difficult and will be facilitated by an adequate extensile exposure, use of the transverse calcaneal traction pin, and much patience.

Once reduction is achieved, internal fixation of the neck fracture with two large axial Kirschner wires or a lag screw will give stability to the fracture–dislocation complex (Fig. 19-48). With all open injuries and even in open reduction of closed injuries when extreme swelling exists, the skin should not be closed primarily. Delayed primary closure at 5 to 7 days will minimize the chance of a deep infection. Following open reduction and internal fixation, the foot should be splinted and elevated until the swelling subsides and then immobilized in a short-leg non-weight-bearing plaster cast.

AUTHOR'S PREFERRED TREATMENT

Type I fractures should be treated by closed methods. A short-leg non-weight-bearing cast with the foot in slight equinus is applied for the first month

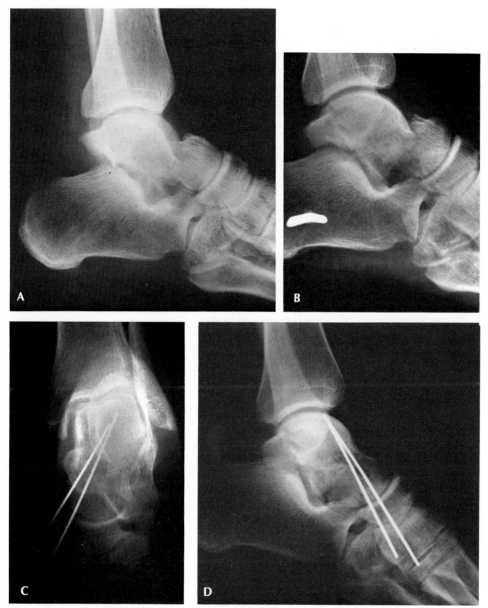

Fig. 19-46. (A) Type II talar neck fracture with dislocation of the subtalar joint. (B) Closed reduction was attempted with the aid of a transverse calcaneal traction pin, reducing the subtalar joint but failing to achieve *anatomical* reduction of the fracture. (C, D) After open reduction and fixation with two axial Kirschner wires, stable anatomical reduction of both the fracture and the joint has been accomplished.

and then replaced with a short-leg walking cast that is maintained for 2 more months or until there is x-ray evidence of healing. This sometimes requires tomograms in the lateral projection to demonstrate union across the fracture site. Once union

is achieved, active range of motion and progressive weight bearing as tolerated are instituted.

I believe it is imperative that all type II and type III fractures of the talar neck be reduced absolutely anatomically to achieve the best chance for bony

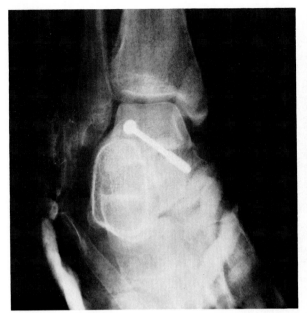 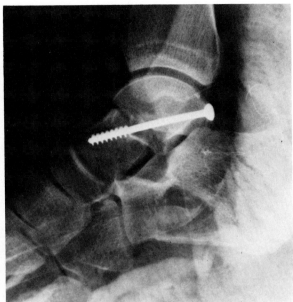

Fig. 19-47. Displaced fracture of the talar neck with mild comminution dorsally. (*Left*) Anteroposterior and (*right*) lateral views after reduction and fixation with a posterior-to-anterior compression screw. The small dorsal defect in the neck was produced by excision of the comminuted fragments.

union without deformity and to minimize the chances of avascular necrosis and late osteoarthritis of the ankle and subtalar joints. I will make one attempt under general or spinal anesthesia at closed reduction of a type II fracture. Once anatomical reduction is achieved, these fractures are usually stable and can be immobilized in a short-leg non-weight-bearing cast and treated as a type I injury. I have had no success reducing type III injuries closed and with these have proceeded immediately to an open reduction.

With persistently displaced type II and all type III fractures, I prefer prompt open reduction and rigid internal fixation of the fracture. I prefer an anteromedial surgical approach and will use a temporary transverse calcaneal traction wire to facilitate manipulation of the rear foot. If reduction still cannot be achieved, I will osteotomize the medial malleolus and reflect it distally, maintaining the remaining intact deltoid insertion to the talar body.

Rigid internal fixation using an AO cancellous screw has been most effective in achieving stable fixation of the fracture site once it is reduced. Because of the extreme swelling and tenuous blood supply to the skin, I prefer a delayed primary closure at 5 to 7 days rather than primary suture of wounds in this region.

With stable internal fixation, a short-leg non-weight-bearing cast provides adequate protection for soft tissue and bony healing. Usually by 3 months there is sufficient x-ray evidence of bony bridging to allow protected weight bearing. If signs of avascular necrosis of the talar body are present, then the patient is fitted with a patellar tendon–bearing double upright ankle–foot orthosis to protect the body of the talus from collapse until revascularization occurs (which may be as long as 2 years).

PROGNOSIS AND COMPLICATIONS

The several recent extensive reviews of fractures of the talar neck all emphasize multiple and frequent complications of this injury, often despite excellent reduction and stable fixation.[96,110,140,143] The frequency and severity of complications have been directly proportional to the degree of initial displacement, supporting the importance of Hawkins's classification. Although all reports endorse prompt anatomical reduction and adequate fixation, the damage incurred at the time of injury often cannot be corrected simply by reduction and fixation of the fracture–dislocation. For example, damage of the soft tissues (most notably skin laceration or necrosis and disruption of part or all of the blood supply to the talar body) and damage of the articular

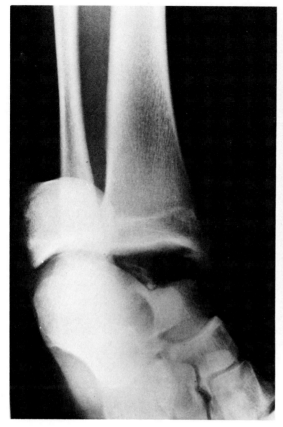

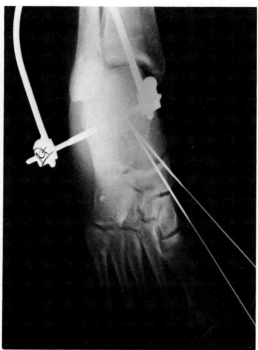

Fig. 19-48. (*Left*) Anteroposterior x-ray of type III talar neck fracture with lateral displacement of the talar body. (*Right*) After open reduction and internal fixation with two Kirschner wires. Note the transverse calcaneal traction pin used as a reduction aid.

cartilage of the subtalar and ankle joints occurs at the moment of injury and may not be fully corrected even by prompt reduction and fixation of the fracture–dislocation.

Skin Necrosis and Infection

Both closed and open injuries are prone to infection. The skin of the ankle and foot, particularly dorsally, is fragile and lacks a significant amount of protective subcutaneous tissue. Displacement of the talar fragments produces significant distortion of the soft tissues in the ankle region and often results in tenting of the skin, which may lead to necrosis and secondary infection. Infection, as a result of skin necrosis or an open wound, once established, tends to persist. This is attributed to the lack of blood supply to the talar body resulting from the injury. The body becomes a large sequestrum, harboring the residual infection.

The older literature is replete with reports of severe infections following this injury, and Syme in 1848[154] reported 11 deaths in 13 patients with open fracture–dislocations of the talus, all the result

of severe infection. He recommended a below-the-knee amputation as the appropriate treatment for this injury. The more recent literature[96,106,137] continues to report a significant risk of infection following displaced (primarily type III) talar neck fractures, and infection virtually guarantees a poor result.

The risk of infection secondary to skin necrosis with displaced closed fractures can be minimized, but not entirely eliminated, by *immediate* reduction of the displaced fragment to realign the ankle and improve skin circulation. With an open fracture–dislocation, an immediate, thorough surgical debridement is imperative. The wound should be left open and closed secondarily.

Persistent infection responds poorly to local debridement of sinus tracts and usually requires radical surgical debridement of the sequestered talar body. Talectomy alone in this situation leads to persistently poor results,[96,125] even if the infection ceases, and the best long-term results following extensive infection have been achieved with excision of the sequestered talus combined with tibio-calcaneal fusion.[96,137,139]

Delayed Union and Nonunion

Fracture healing is somewhat less of a problem than might be expected with this injury. Delayed union is common, but nonunion is *relatively* rare. In 13 patients with avascular necrosis following type II or type III injuries, Hawkins[110] found that union of the neck fracture occurred in all but was frequently delayed. Lorentzen and colleagues[122] reported only a 4% (5 of 123) incidence of nonunion in their series. Peterson and colleagues[143] defined delayed union as no evidence of fracture healing 6 months after the injury, and in their series 46 fractures, 6 delayed unions, but no nonunions occurred. Mindell and associates[129] reported three cases of delayed union in 40 fractures, all of which healed, although one required 18 months before solid bony union was present.

Delayed union can be anticipated with this fracture because of the relatively poor blood supply and the modest amount of periosteum present on the talar neck. Fracture healing occurs by endosteal callus formation in this situation. The fracture should be protected from weight-bearing stress until there is evidence of bridging callus, which will occur eventually in most instances. In the rare case of no evidence of healing 1 year following fracture, local corticocancellous bone grafting of the nonunion should be undertaken.[122]

Malunion

Many authors have stressed the importance of anatomical reduction of talar neck fractures:

> Following anatomical reduction of a vertical fracture dislocation of the talus, not complicated by avascular necrosis, a good or excellent result is the expected outcome.[110]

> The ability to obtain and maintain an anatomic reduction (closed or open) is the most important factor in predicting good results.[128]

> In the Type II fractures many poor results followed malunion.[96]

Hawkins identified the increased complication rate when the initial x-rays demonstrated any degree of fracture displacement and insisted that only nondisplaced fractures be classified as type I for this reason. Anatomical reduction is critical to obtain a good result. In a series of 46 patients, Peterson and co-workers[143] actually achieved better results in type III fractures than in type II fractures, and the critical variable was the adequacy of the initial reduction, with an "exact reduction" being achieved more frequently in patients with type III fractures.

Reduction must be achieved in both the frontal and sagittal planes. Residual dorsal displacement of the head fragment will limit ankle dorsiflexion and produce a painful gait.[96] More frequently, however, malunion in varus occurs. Canale and Kelly[96] found that 14 of 30 patients with type II fractures eventually healed in varus. This deformity resulted in excessive weight being borne on the lateral side of the foot, stressing the subtalar joint and producing a painful gait. Most patients in this group were treated initially by closed reduction and casting. Subsequent x-rays have shown inadequate reduction or loss of reduction in plaster leading to the malunion; thus any closed reduction that is less than anatomical should not be accepted and open reduction should be performed. Furthermore, after reduction the patient should be protected from weight bearing and followed closely with periodic x-rays until the fracture has healed.

Dorsal malunion was effectively treated in 3 cases by Canale and Kelly by dorsal talar beak resection, which allowed increased ankle dorsiflexion. However, five of their patients with very symptomatic varus malunion and subsequent degenerative arthritis of the subtalar joint required late triple arthrodesis.[96]

Avascular Necrosis

Avascular necrosis is but one of several complications that can produce poor results following talar neck fracture. It is often difficult to single out the one factor responsible for a poor result because usually more than one complication occurs, particularly with displaced fractures. Furthermore, there is not a direct, one-to-one correlation between the development of avascular necrosis and a poor result. Authors differ in their opinions on the role of avascular necrosis in producing long-term problems. Gillquist and colleagues[106] reported that "we could not find that avascular necrosis with deformity of the talus influenced to any substantial degree the end results after talar fracture." Although both Hawkins[110] and Canale and Kelly[96] believed that avascular necrosis was an important contributing factor in their patients with a poor result, only rarely did their patients request or require late reconstructive surgery specifically for this complication.

Avascular necrosis occurs rarely in type I fractures (0% to 13%), in 20% to 50% of type II fractures, and in 83% to 100% of type III fractures, producing an overall incidence of between 21% and 58% of all talar neck fractures and making it the most common complication of this injury.[96,110] The diagnosis of avascular necrosis is a radiographic one, with the talar body initially showing increased density compared to the surrounding bone (which is vascular and is undergoing disuse atrophy). Later there is partial or complete collapse of the subchondral bone, narrowing of the joint space, and occasionally fragmentation of the talar body.

The best radiographic indication of viability of the talar body is "Hawkins's sign," eloquently described by Hawkins[110] and confirmed as a valid sign by several subsequent authors:

The time to recognize the presence of avasclar necrosis is between the sixth and eighth week following the fracture–dislocation. By this time, if the patient has been nonweightbearing, disuse atrophy is evident by roentgenogram

in the bones of the foot and in the distal part of the tibia. An anteroposterior roentgenogram of the ankle, made with the foot out of the plaster cast, reveals the presence or absence of subchondral atrophy in the dome of the talus. Subchondral atrophy excludes the diagnosis of avascular necrosis[110] [Fig. 19-49].

More recently, bone scanning with the use of a pin hole collimator has been advocated by some[140] as an additional tool to aid in the diagnosis of avascular necrosis, although no series has yet been reported.

The extent of involvement of the talar body by avascular necrosis is variable and is directly related to the degree of vascular disruption that occurs at the time of injury.[118] With moderate displacement

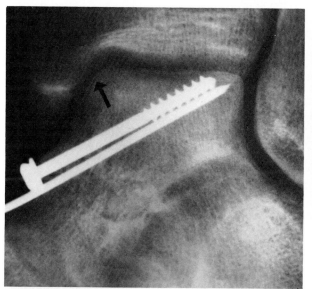
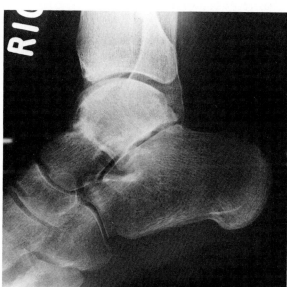
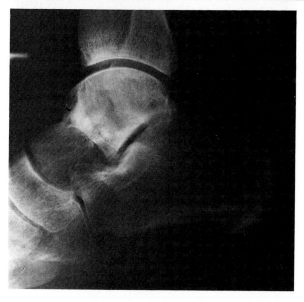

Fig. 19-49. (*Top left*) X-ray of the ankle taken 8 weeks following a talar neck fracture. Note the subchondral resorption of bone (*arrow*), indicative of vascularity of the talar body. (*Top right*) X-ray taken 16 weeks after another talar neck fracture. Note healing of the fracture but sclerosis of the body and no evidence of bony atrophy, both indicating avascularity. (*Bottom*) The same fracture as in *top right* 9 months later, showing creeping substitution of the avascular talar body.

of the body fragment, as usually occurs in type II injuries, some of the nutrient vessels may be uninjured, thus preserving part of the circulation and leading to only partial avascular necrosis. On the other hand, with most type III injuries, all the blood supply is destroyed, resulting in complete body necrosis.

Even though the major damage to the blood supply of the talar body may have occurred at the time of injury, it is felt to be important to achieve a prompt, accurate, and stable reduction of the talar neck fractures to minimize the adverse affects of avascular necrosis. Such treatment will facilitate union and subsequent revascularization. Because of the frequent complications of severe fracture–dislocation of the talus and because of the frequent association of avascular necrosis with these injuries, many authors have recommended radical primary (with 6 weeks of injury) surgical treatment to facilitate revascularization of the talus or to bypass its weight-bearing function. Primary triple arthrodesis,[125] total talectomy with tibiocalcaneal fusion,[147] talectomy,[95] subtalar arthrodesis,[115,116] and pantalar arthrodesis[396] have all been proposed as appropriate treatment for severe fracture-dislocation of the talus. Most recent extensive reviews, however, advocate a more conservative approach, with retention of the talar body fragment through anatomical reduction and fixation, and do not recommend a primary arthrodesis.[96,106,137]

All other factors being equal, the prognosis for a good or excellent result must be tempered by the discovery of Hawkins's sign of avascular necrosis on x-ray 6 or more weeks following fracture. Treatment at this stage should not be altered by that finding. The primary goal should always be anatomical union of the fracture, which will occur even in the face of avascular necrosis. The patient should be protected from weight-bearing until union is secure. When union has occurred, the body of the talus will still be avascular, since up to 36 months is required for complete creeping substitution of the body.[124,125] A dilemma is thus created: ideally, the talar dome should be protected from weight-bearing stress until it is fully revascularized, but practically no patient can be kept from bearing weight throughout the long time necessary for full revascularization to occur. Furthermore, some authors indicate that collapse may occur despite lack of weight bearing.[100]

Several authors recommend a pragmatic compromise solution: a patellar tendon–bearing brace. The brace will partially relieve the load on the talar dome while still allowing weight bearing. Use of

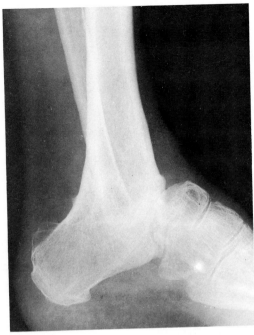

Fig. 19-50. Tibiocalcaneal fusion for severe fragmentation of the body of the talus 10 years after treatment. (Courtesy of Thomas A. Brady.) (After Giannestras, N. J.: Foot Disorders: Medical and Surgical Management, 2nd ed. Philadelphia, Lea & Febiger, 1973.)

the brace should be begun only after bony union has occurred and should be continued until reconstitution of the talar body is complete.

For patients with collapse of the talar dome secondary to avascular necrosis and symptomatic degenerative arthritis of the ankle joint, arthrodesis of this joint is indicated. Two methods, tibiocalcaneal arthrodesis and the Blair fusion,[94] have both been found effective. In their nine patients with persistent symptoms, Canale and Kelly[96] found that tibiocalcaneal fusion was superior to ankle fusion or talectomy. The technique of tibiocalcaneal fusion (Fig. 19-50) is described by Reckling.[147]

In 1943, Blair[94] described a technique of ankle fusion specifically designed to treat avascular necrosis of the talus (Fig. 19-51). He recommended excision of the avascular talar body and placement of a sliding corticocancellous graft from the anterior distal tibia into the residual, viable talar head and neck. Morris and colleagues[132] modified this procedure slightly and reported good results in ten patients in 1971. Dennis and Tullos reviewed seven cases in 1980[101] and advocated this procedure as a satisfactory reconstructive measure following se-

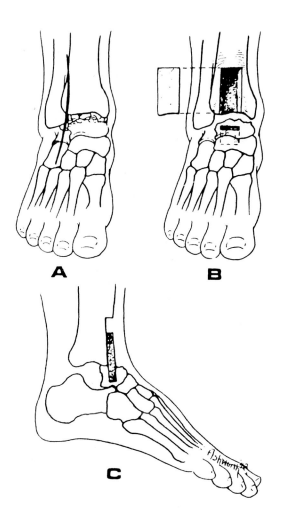

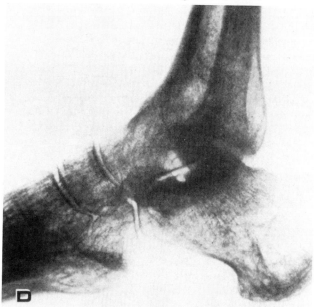

Fig. 19-51. Schematic drawing of the Blair-type fusion for the treatment of comminuted fractures and fracture–dislocations of the body of the talus. (*A*) Anterolateral incision. (*B*) Sliding graft from the distal, anterior surface of the tibia and a quadrilateral hole gouged in the neck of the talus. The sliding graft has been removed to permit a better view of the hole in the talar neck. (*C*) The sliding graft is embedded in the hole in the talar neck. Note the space left by removal of the talar body (*B* and *C*). (*D*) This x-ray shows healed fusion, 3½ years after the operation. (Blair, H. C.: Comminuted Fractures and Fracture Dislocations of the Body of the Astragalus: Operative Treatment. Am. J. Surg. **59**:38, 1943.)

vere talar injuries. They emphasized that the Blair fusion retains a normal appearance of the foot, minimizes shortening, and allows retention of some subtalar function. More recently, Lionberger and colleagues[121] recommended a modification of the Blair fusion technique that allows compression screw fixation of the fusion site. They reported good results in five patients.

In summary, avascular necrosis is a significant complication of talar neck fractures; however, there is not a direct relationship between the development of avascular necrosis and permanently disabling symptoms. As with other complications of this fracture, initially treatment should be directed at anatomical reduction and stable fixation. Weight bearing should be avoided only until fracture union has occurred, and then protected weight bearing can be allowed in a patellar tendon–bearing brace until the avascular body has reconstituted. Further surgical intervention should be directed by the

patient's symptoms, since no surgical procedure has been shown to enhance talar revascularization, and many patients with avascular necrosis are not sufficiently symptomatic to warrant further surgery. With collapse, degenerative changes, and severe ankle symptoms, either a Blair fusion or a tibio-calcaneal arthrodesis is indicated.

Post-Traumatic Arthritis

Post-traumatic arthritis of the ankle, the subtalar joint, or both joints has been identified by several investigators as as significant long-term complication of fractures of the talar neck. Although some degenerative changes occur secondary to avascular necrosis, osteoarthritis (particularly of the subtalar joint) has been identified in some patients without the radiographic stigmata of ischemic changes in the talar body. Certainly substantial damage to the articular surfaces can be anticipated to have occurred as a result of a fracture–dislocation of the talus, and even if avascular necrosis does not supervene, such injury will predispose to degenerative arthritic changes. Furthermore, the prolonged period of non-weight-bearing cast immobilization required for bony union will usually lead to significant arthrofibrosis and impaired nutrition of the articular cartilage. These three factors (the initial injury, avascular necrosis, and immobilization) thus combine to ensure a high incidence of arthritis in the peritalar joints.

Symptomatic post-traumatic arthritis should be treated by protected weight bearing (bracing) and anti-inflammatory medications. Care must be taken to localize the symptomatic joint accurately before arthrodesis is recommended. Frequently both the ankle and subtalar joints are involved,[96] and arthrodesis of one will only further stress the other, perhaps leading to increased pain despite a successful bony fusion. Preoperative injection of a local anesthetic into the presumed symptomatic joint should give virtually complete pain relief—a good indication for arthrodesis.

FRACTURES OF THE BODY OF THE TALUS

Fractures of the body of the talus differ from fractures of the talar neck in only minor ways. In particular, they occur much less frequently, with only rare reports in the literature describing injury to this part of the talus. The best review is by Sneppen and colleagues,[153] who emphasized the high complication rate following these fractures. Both avascular necrosis and arthritis of the ankle and subtalar joints occur often, resulting in disabling pain because of the critical functions of these articulations in gait.

MECHANISM OF INJURY AND CLASSIFICATION

The most common mechanism of injury resulting in fracture of the talar body is a fall from a height, producing an axial compression of the talus between the tibial plafond and the calcaneus. Associated fractures (particularly of the malleoli) occur frequently. A variety of fracture configurations have been identified:

1. Compression fracture of the talar dome with fracture limited to the superior articular surface of the talus and not involving the subtalar joint
2. Shearing fractures either in the sagittal or coronal plane
3. Fracture of the posterior process (see p. 1749)
4. Fracture of the lateral process (see p. 1746)
5. Crush fracture resulting in severe comminution and impaction of multiple fragments with involvement of both the ankle and subtalar joints

Occasionally the fracture is nondisplaced, but in most instances of talar body fracture there is significant displacement of the fragments with concurrent subluxation of the ankle or the subtalar joints. Careful inspection of the standard (anteroposterior, lateral, and mortise) x-rays of the ankle will demonstrate these fractures, and occasionally tomography will further define the extent of injury to the talus.

TREATMENT

Sneppen and colleagues[153] found a high complication rate in their review of 31 patients with fractures of the talar body. Most of these patients had been treated by closed reduction and prolonged casting. They concluded that more aggressive treatment is indicated for displaced fractures and recommended "exact reduction and stable fixation whenever possible." Open reduction should be performed for persistently displaced fragments that are large enough to accept fixation pins or screws. Some severe crush fractures may not be amenable to this technique, but most of the shear fractures can be reduced and internally fixed (Fig. 19-52). The fractures should generally be approached through an anteromedial ankle arthrotomy. Occasionally it may be necessary to osteotomize the medial malleolus to achieve adequate visualization of the fracture line. Once reduced, fixation should be secured with cancellous compression screws placed perpendicular to the fracture line.[354] If stable fixation is achieved, active range of motion of both the ankle and subtalar joints should be undertaken in the immediate postoperative period to decrease the likelihood of permanent joint stiffness and post-traumatic arthritis. Once motion is regained postoperatively, the fracture should be protected in a short-leg non-weight-bearing cast until bony union occurs.

PROGNOSIS AND COMPLICATIONS

A high incidence of avascular necrosis, malunion, and persistent arthritic symptoms characterizes the reports of these injuries in the older literature.[99,114,125,129] These problems may be minimized by anatomical reduction and internal fixation where feasible.[153] If avascular necrosis or degenerative arthritis develops, the principles of treatment as outlined for these sequelae after talar neck fractures should be followed (see p. 1740).

FRACTURE OF THE HEAD OF THE TALUS

Fracture of the talar head occurs rarely. The fracture line usually involves the articular surface of the

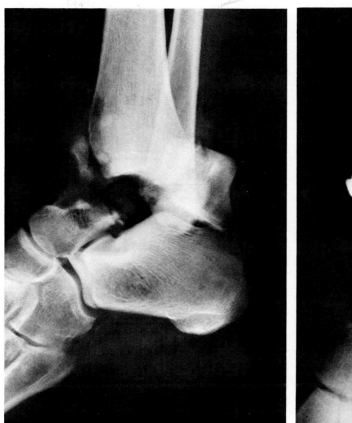 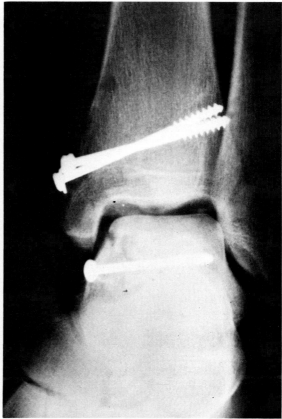

Fig. 19-52. (*Left*) Shear fracture of the talar body with dislocation of a large fragment of the body and comminuted fracture of the medial malleolus. (*Right*) After open reduction and screw fixation of the sagittal shear fracture of the talar body.

talar head, damaging the talonavicular articulation and frequently resulting in late talonavicular arthritis.

MECHANISM OF INJURY AND CLASSIFICATION

The fracture is most often described as a compression fracture of the head. Coltart[99] described six cases, four occurring as a result of flying accidents, and he felt that this was another form of "rudder bar" injury, with the foot being held in extreme plantarflexion and the force of impact transmitted along the longitudinal axis of the foot through the metatarsals and navicular, compressing the talar head. Comminution is not uncommon, with several fracture lines frequently passing through the head. The navicular may also fracture as a result of this longitudinal compressive force, further disrupting the talonavicular articulation.[95] Coltart[99] reported one case of talar head fracture associated with midtarsal joint dislocation, implicating abduction as well as longitudinal compression as the cause of this injury.

CLINICAL AND RADIOGRAPHIC FINDINGS

Physical examination will reveal localized tenderness and occasional crepitus over the fracture. Careful palpation of the calcaneocuboid joint should reveal tenderness if an abduction force has damaged this articulation as well. Occasionally only minimal swelling or ecchymosis occurs, and the significance of the injury can be easily overlooked. Anteroposterior, lateral, and oblique x-rays of the foot will demonstrate the fracture. Careful inspection of the nearby structures (navicular and calcaneocuboid joint) may reveal further injury.

TREATMENT

Nondisplaced fractures of the head of the talus should be treated by initial splinting, ice, and elevation followed by the application of a short-leg walking cast, molded well to preserve the longitudinal arch of the foot. Plaster immobilization is continued for 6 weeks, after which the patient's shoe should be fitted with a well-molded arch

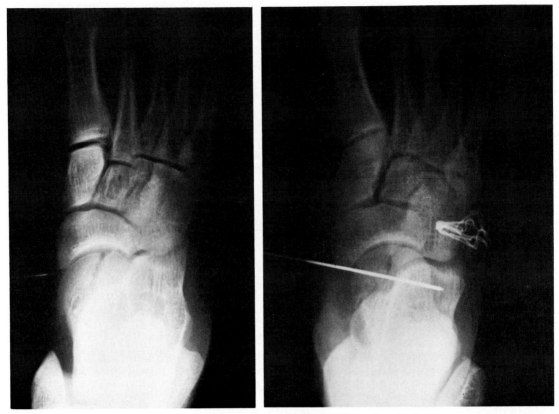

Fig. 19-53. (*Left*) Displaced fracture of the talar head. (*Right*) Closed reduction was inadequate, necessitating open reduction followed by Kirschner wire fixation.

support to splint the talonavicular joint for an additional 3 to 6 months.

Displaced fractures should be reduced to restore congruity of the talonavicular joint. Occasionally comminution is so severe that reduction cannot be accomplished, but small, free articular fragments should be excised and large fragments reduced and fixed to the talar neck with Kirschner wires (Fig. 19-53).

PROGNOSIS AND COMPLICATIONS

Healing proceeds uneventfully in most cases, and the major complication of this fracture is persistent talonavicular arthritis. Persistent pain at this joint can sometimes be decreased with a firm longitudinal arch support and a long steel shank in the shoe. If conservative methods fail, arthrodesis should be undertaken. Some authors recommend triple arthrodesis;[104] others, arthrodesis of the midtarsal joint.[95] I prefer the latter if injection of the midtarsal joint with lidocaine produces temporary but complete relief of the patient's pain.

FRACTURES OF THE TALAR PROCESSES

Two processes, the lateral and the posterior, project from the body of the talus and are prone to fracture either as an isolated event or in conjunction with other ankle or talar injuries. Fracture of either process has been reported only rarely, and significant confusion exists in the literature regarding the anatomical description, the mechanism of injury, the treatment, and the long-term results of these injuries.

FRACTURES OF THE LATERAL PROCESS OF THE TALUS

Since Dimon's description of this injury in 1961,[103] only about 50 cases of lateral process fracture have been reported in the English literature, but most authors agree that the fracture occurs more commonly than is suspected and is frequently overlooked. When the fracture extends into the subtalar joint, persistent pain and loss of motion of this articulation frequently occur. Nonunion is a frequent complication of displaced lateral process fractures. Prompt diagnosis of this fracture is important so that appropriate treatment can be instituted early to avoid some of the more serious long-term complications.

Anatomy

The lateral process of the talus (see Figs. 19-39 and 19-40) is a broad-based, wedge-shaped prominence of the lateral talar body with an articular surface dorsolaterally for the fibula and inferomedially for the anterior portion of the posterior calcaneal facet. The lateral talocalcaneal ligament originates from the tip of this process.

Mechanism of Injury and Classification

Most authors agree that fractures of the lateral process most frequently occur when the foot is dorsiflexed and inverted. A shearing stress is transmitted from the calcaneus to the lateral process, producing a fracture fragment of variable size. Occasionally the fragment is quite large and involves up to one third of the articular surface of the posterior talar facet. Hawkins[109] divided the fractures into three groups: (1) a nonarticular chip fracture, (2) a single large fragment involving both the talofibular articulation and the subtalar joint, and (3) a comminuted fracture involving both articulations. Displacement of the fracture fragment can occur, markedly increasing the chance of nonunion or malunion, with subsequent degenerative changes of the subtalar joint and pain in the region of the sinus tarsi.

Clinical and Radiographic Findings

Mukherjee and associates[133] reviewed 1500 sprains and fractures of the ankle region and found 13 cases of lateral process fracture. The mechanism of injury and the location of symptoms following fracture are both very similar to those of a simple inversion ankle sprain. The physical findings are also similar as well, with swelling and ecchymosis localized to the lateral aspect of the ankle. There is point tenderness over the lateral process just anterior and inferior to the tip of the lateral malleolus; however, the tenderness can be easily misinterpreted as a lateral ligament injury. Because of these similarities to lateral ankle sprains, the fracture is frequently overlooked at the time of the acute injury and only diagnosed later because of persistent symptoms.

Most of these fractures can be seen on standard x-rays of the ankle joint. Overlapping of the malleoli and the sustentaculum tali makes visualization somewhat difficult on the lateral view, but the fracture can be seen well on the mortise view because the process lies in the frontal plane in this projection (Fig. 19-54A). Confirmation of a suspected fracture of the lateral process and further definition of its size and the degree of articular involvement can be achieved with anteroposterior tomograms of the talus (Fig. 19-54B).

Treatment

The size of the fracture fragment and the degree of displacement appear to be the critical factors in determining treatment. As the size of the fragment increases, the likelihood of articular involvement (particularly of the subtalar joint) increases, and large fragments or extensive comminution of a large part of the lateral process require more aggressive treatment than small fractures of the tip of the process. Displacement is also a critical factor, particularly with large fragments. Unreduced, displaced fractures frequently do not unite, and if union does occur, a residual malalignment of the subtalar joint may produce persistent symptoms.[103,109,133]

Undisplaced fractures should be treated by cast immobilization for approximately 6 weeks. Most authors recommend avoiding weight bearing for at least the first 4 weeks of this treatment. Union will usually occur with a nondisplaced fracture, and a good prognosis can be anticipated. For displaced, large single fragments, Hawkins[109] recommended closed reduction followed by cast immobilization when satisfactory reduction could be achieved. Mukherjee and colleagues[133] recommend open reduction and fixation with Kirschner wires or a screw for all displaced fractures (Fig. 19-54C, D). For comminuted fragments both authors recommend primary surgical excision to avoid development of arthritic changes in the subtalar joint. The fracture is readily approached through a short incision over the sinus tarsi. Reduction must be absolutely accurate to restore the alignment of the posterior facet of the subtalar joint. Whenever possible, the fragment should be replaced and fixed because it is often very large, and removal may result in instability of the subtalar joint with persistent symptoms.

Prognosis and Complications

All reviews of this fracture[98,99,103,105,109,116,133,139,152] have been retrospective summaries of small series of cases. Many of the fractures presented late (months after the initial untreated injury) with persistent symptoms secondary to nonunion or

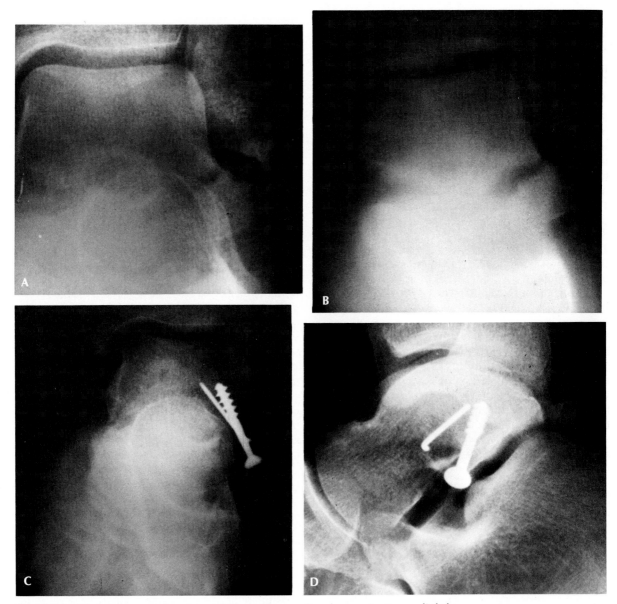

Fig. 19-54. (*A*) Anteroposterior x-ray of the ankle mortise demonstrating a slightly displaced large lateral-process fracture fragment. (*B*) Anteroposterior tomogram of the same fracture demonstrating extension of the fracture line into the subtalar joint. (*C, D*) Open reduction and internal fixation of the large single fragment with a Kirschner wire and cancellous screw.

degenerative changes of the subtalar joint. Those patients who did not develop these symptoms had nondisplaced fractures or had undergone early surgical reduction and fixation of single large fragments or excision of comminuted fracture fragments. In a series of 11 patients whom I have seen over the past 6 years, the best results have been

with closed treatment of nondisplaced fractures and open reduction and internal fixation of large single fragments. Comminuted, displaced fracture fragments should be excised primarily to allow early restoration of subtalar joint motion.

Regardless of the specific treatment employed, a surprisingly high proportion of patients who sustain a fracture of the lateral process of the talus will have persistent symptoms with pain in the subtalar joint that may require late subtalar arthrodesis.

FRACTURES OF THE POSTERIOR PROCESS OF THE TALUS

Anatomy

Foster* has accurately described the relatively complex anatomy of the posterior talar process in the following way: Two tubercles (the medial and lateral) compromise the posterior talar process. The tubercles are separated by the groove for the tendon of the flexor hallucis longus (see Figs. 19-39 and 19-40 *top*). The lateral tubercle is the larger of the two and projects more posteriorly. The length of this projection is variable, and it serves as the talar attachment for the posterior talofibular ligament. On the lateral x-ray, the lateral tubercle is seen in profile.

The medial tubercle projects medially and inferiorly from the groove for the flexor hallucis longus. It serves as the attachment for the posterior third of the deltoid ligament. The undersurface of the entire process (both tubercles) is composed of articular cartilage, forming the posterior 25% of the posterior articular facet of the subtalar joint. It is probable that most of this posterior process arises from a secondary ossification center that fuses with the talar body at about age 12.[123]

The os trigonum is a relatively frequently seen accessory bone of the foot found just posterior to the lateral tubercle of the posterior process. Burman and Lapidus[392] found a separate bone in 64 of 1000 feet examined by x-ray. They also described an elongated lateral tubercle as a "fused os trigonum" and reported this finding in an additional 429 of these 1000 feet, concluding that the os trigonum (fused or separate) occurred in almost 50% of all feet. They identified a significant degree of symmetry in the x-ray appearance of the configuration of the posterior talar process (or os trigonum) in the two feet of any one human, although McDougall[123] believed that the os trigonum may occur only in one foot. The os trigonum is round, oval, or triangular and of variable size. As with other accessory bones, its edges appear smooth, with dense cortical bone that helps to distinguish it radiographically from a fracture of the lateral tubercle.

Fractures of the Lateral Tubercle of the Posterior Process

Fracture of the lateral tubercle of the posterior process was first described by Cloquet in 1844 in

the French literature, and in 1882 Shepherd[150] described it in the English literature. Some authors[112,117] still refer to this injury as *Shepherd's fracture.*

Mechanism of Injury. Two mechanisms may be responsible for fracture of the lateral tubercle: avulsion or direct compression. Inversion of the ankle may produce the fracture as the posterior talofibular ligament avulses the tubercle.[116] A more commonly identified mechanism, however, has been compression of the lateral tubercle when the ankle is forced into extreme equinus.[108,111,116,123,126,146] The lateral tubercle is compressed between the calcaneus and the posterior lip of the tibia, resulting in fracture. Repetitive moderate trauma[123,156] may produce fracture of this tubercle, since several of the reported cases have occurred in athletes, particularly football and rugby players, who have developed subacute posterior ankle pain aggravated by the equinus posture of the kicking foot. Such fractures caused by this type of repetitive trauma may be another example of a stress fracture. Weinstein and Bonfiglio[156] postulated that fusion of the secondary ossification center with the body of the talus may be impeded by repetitive stress in the adolescent, leading to a persistent and painful pseudarthrosis.

Clinical and Radiographic Findings. Patients with fractures of the lateral tubercle of the posterior process, regardless of mechanism, present most frequently with "ankle sprain" symptoms. Posterolateral ankle tenderness can usually be elicited, and motion of both the ankle and subtalar joints will be painful. Active flexion of the great toe may also produce pain as the flexor hallucis longus moves over the fracture site. A lateral x-ray of the foot will best demonstrate the tubercle (Fig. 19-55 *top*). A comparison x-ray of the opposite foot will be helpful to show the configuration of the lateral tubercle and identify the existence of an os trigonum, which, when present, occurs bilaterally approximately 60% of the time; in 40% of the cases the patient will have only a unilateral free os trigonum.[392] There will usually be a definite fracture line with a rough, irregular surface, as opposed to the smooth, rounded cortical surface of the inconstant ossicle. At times, however, the x-ray findings will not be definitive because of the great variability of configuration of the posterior talar process, and close correlation with the clinical examination is important.

Treatment and Prognosis. Fracture of the lateral

---

* Foster, Robert. R.: Personal communication.

tubercle of the posterior talar process is most frequently nondisplaced or only minimally so, and when the physician suspects an acute fracture it should be treated initially in a short-leg cast or compressive dressing and protected from full weight bearing for from 4 to 6 weeks, when some x-ray signs of union should be seen.

Many reports in the literature describe ununited, persistently symptomatic fractures of this tubercle. This ununited fragment is at times very difficult to distinguish radiographically from the os trigonum because it assumes the same rounded and smooth appearance as the accessory bone. The symptoms caused by this ununited fracture are persistent pain in the ankle, particularly with strenuous physical activity, and limitation of ankle and subtalar joint motion. X-rays may show early degenerative articular changes in the area of the fragment (Fig. 19-55 *bottom*). Surgical excision of the ununited fragment through a posterolateral ankle arthrotomy usually relieves the pain and allows restoration of normal joint motion.[112,123,156]

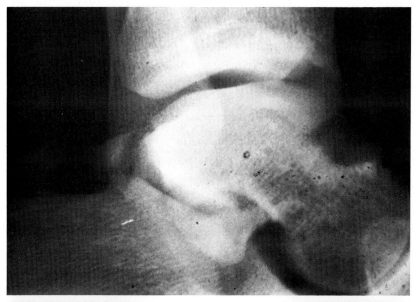

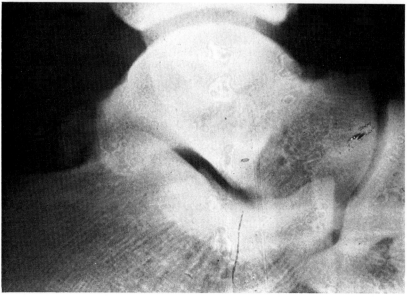

Fig. 19-55. (*Top*) Lateral view of the ankle showing a fresh fracture of the lateral tubercle of the posterior talar process. (*Bottom*) Lateral view of the same ankle 6 months after injury showing nonunion of the fracture and some early degenerative changes in the posterior portion of the subtalar joint. (Courtesy of Robert R. Foster, M.D.)

Fracture of the Medial Tubercle of the Posterior Process

Fracture of the medial tubercle of the posterior process of the talus is a rare injury. Cedell[97] described four cases in which pronation of the foot in the plantarflexed position resulted in avulsion of the tubercle by the fibers of the posterior portion of the deltoid ligament. All four patients were engaged in athletics and presented late after the injury with persistent medial ankle pain and swelling. The initial injury in each instance had been treated by a short period of rest and without plaster immobilization.

Visualization of this fracture is difficult on x-ray, but usually the fragment can be seen in the lateral projection (Fig. 19-56) and may be visualized as a small avulsion fleck off the medial wall of the talus in the anteroposterior projection.

I have had no experience in treating this fracture, but it seems prudent to immobilize the foot for 3 to 4 weeks to allow healing to occur. Cedell[97] surgically excised three persistently symptomatic ununited fragments with excellent results.

Fracture of the Entire Posterior Process

Fracture of the entire posterior process, involving both the medial and lateral tubercles, has not been reported in the literature. Foster* described the only case of which I am aware—a 20-year-old woman who sustained a displaced fracture as a result of an inversion force of the foot in a car wreck (Fig.

---
* Foster, Robert. R.: Personal communication.

19-57). The process was displaced and was compressing the posterior tibial neurovascular bundle; it thus required open reduction and fixation with two Kirschner wires. The fracture healed without residual symptoms.

DISLOCATIONS OF AND AROUND THE TALUS

Although subluxation or even complete dislocation of the talus, either at the subtalar or the ankle joint, occurs with certain talar fractures, on occasion subluxation or dislocation with minimal or no fracture can be seen. These joint injuries fall into two broad categories, subtalar dislocation and total talar dislocation. These two injury patterns will be reviewed next.

SUBTALAR DISLOCATION

Subtalar dislocation (also, and perhaps more appropriately, called peritalar dislocation)[159] is the simultaneous dislocation of the distal articulations of the talus at both the talocalcaneal and talonavicular joints. Although first described separately by Judcy[172] and Dufaurets[166] in 1811, only infrequent reviews of this injury have been presented in the literature, and most series are relatively small. Smith[187] found only seven cases (1.3%) in a review of 535 consecutive dislocations of all types, and Leitner[174] found 42 (1%) among 4215 acute dislocations. Fifteen percent of all talar injuries in Pennal's series[139] were subtalar disloca-

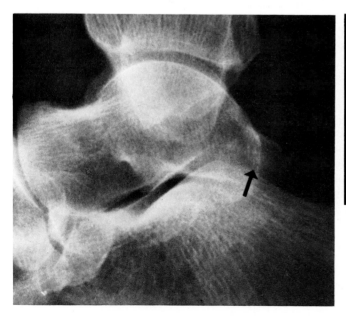

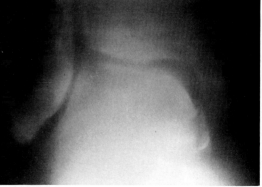

Fig. 19-56. (*Left*) Lateral view of the ankle demonstrating a moderately displaced fracture of the medial tubercle of the posterior process of the talus. (*Right*) The fragment can be visualized well on anteroposterior tomograms of the posterior portion of the talus.

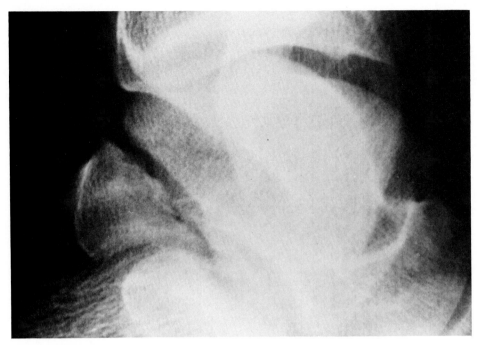

Fig. 19-57. Oblique view of the ankle mortise demonstrating fracture of the entire posterior process of the talus. (Courtesy of Robert R. Foster, M.D.)

tions. Most subtalar dislocations occur in males (6:1) of early adult age.

ANATOMY AND CLASSIFICATION

By definition, with this injury the tibiotalar joint is undisturbed. Subtalar dislocation can occur in any direction and always produces significant deformity. Most commonly (85%[164,168,171,178]) the foot is displaced medially with the calcaneus lying medially, the head of the talus prominent dorsolaterally, and the navicular medial and sometimes dorsal to the talar head and neck (Fig. 19-58). Less commonly (15%), lateral dislocation will occur. In this case, the calcaneus is displaced lateral to the talus, the talar head is prominent medially, and the navicular lies lateral to the talar neck (Fig. 19-59). Rare cases of anterior and posterior displacement of the foot following subtalar dislocation have also been reported,[168] but these usually have some degree of medial or lateral displacement as well and can be grouped with either the medial or lateral dislocation type. Distinction between medial and lateral subtalar dislocation is important because the method of reduction is different with each type and the long-term prognosis appears to be worse with the lateral dislocation. Main and Jowett[312] reported

a variant of this injury—the "swivel dislocation" of the midtarsal joint. This injury is discussed on page 1790.

MECHANISM OF INJURY

Inversion of the foot results in a medial subtalar dislocation, while eversion produces a lateral subtalar dislocation. The strong calcaneonavicular ligament resists disruption[162] and the inversion or eversion force is dissipated through the weaker talonavicular and talocalcaneal ligaments, disrupting these two joints and allowing displacement of the calcaneus, navicular, and all distal bones of the foot as a unit, either medially or laterally. With a medial subtalar dislocation the sustentaculum tali acts as a fulcrum about which the foot rotates to lever apart the talus and calcaneus, and in the lateral dislocation the foot pivots about the anterior process of the calcaneus, again causing the talus and calcaneus to separate.[188]

Although many of these dislocations result from a high-energy injury such as a fall from a height or a motor vehicle wreck, a significant number occur as the result of athletic injuries. Grantham[168] coined the term *basketball foot* to describe the medial dislocation, since four of his five patients sustained

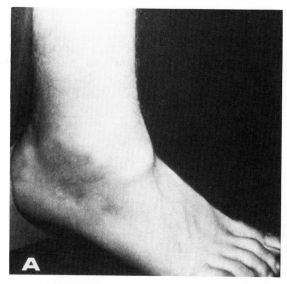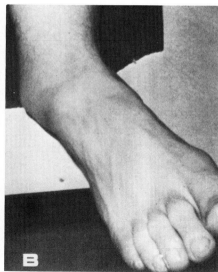

Fig. 19-58. In this medial subtalar dislocation, the head of the talus (*left*) is palpable on the dorsum of the foot. The heel (*right*) is displaced medially. (Buckingham, W. W., Jr.: Subtalar Dislocation of the Foot. J. Trauma, **13:**754, 1973.)

this injury in a fall on the basketball court. The greater incidence of medial dislocation would indicate that the forces required to produce it are less than those required to produce a lateral dislocation.

Frequently, associated fractures occur in the ankle and foot. Shearing osteochondral fractures from the dislocated articular surfaces of the talonavicular or talocalcaneal joint occur in up to 45% of patients and may be difficult to identify on routine x-rays even after reduction of the dislocation.[164] Other bones that are commonly fractured are both malleoli, the base of the fifth metatarsal, the cuboid, and the navicular tuberosity.[163]

SIGNS AND SYMPTOMS

As might be imagined, significant deformities are present in all cases of subtalar dislocation. The medial dislocation has been referred to as an "acquired clubfoot," while the lateral is described in the older literature as an "acquired flatfoot."[188] Because of the significant amount of displacement of the foot on the talus, and particularly with high-energy injuries, between 10% and 15% of these injuries will be open, and in all closed dislocations there will be significant distortion of the soft tissues and tenting of the skin over the prominent talar head. Significant swelling occurs soon after the injury, and this swelling may mask the bony deformity. Few instances of neurovascular compro-

mise have been reported despite the extreme distortion of the foot that can occur with this injury, but close, prompt evaluation of the distal neurovascular function remains imperative.

RADIOGRAPHIC FINDINGS

Standard anteroposterior, lateral, and oblique x-rays of the foot are difficult to obtain because of the distortion of the foot, and frequently inadequate x-rays are taken, leading to a delay or error in diagnosis. Often the physician has the initial clinical impression that an ankle injury is present, but ankle x-rays do not reveal the foot pathology.[169] On all x-ray views the talus lies in a normal relationship to the tibia and fibula, since the point of injury is distal to the ankle joint.[188]

The most helpful x-ray is an anteroposterior view of the foot showing the talonavicular dislocation. All reviews of this topic emphasize the importance of assessing the integrity of the talonavicular joint on the anteroposterior x-ray to be certain that the head of the talus articulates properly with the "cup" of the proximal navicular[159] (Figs. 19-60 and 19-61). In the lateral projection, close inspection will usually reveal the head of the talus lying superior to the navicular or cuboid in the medial subtalar dislocation, and the talar head will appear to be displaced inferiorly in a lateral subtalar dislocation.

TREATMENT

Closed Reduction

The keystone of treatment for all subtalar dislocations is prompt and gentle reduction under general or spinal anesthesia. All open injuries must be thoroughly debrided at the time of reduction, and the wound should be left open, with delayed primary closure anticipated in 3 to 5 days. Closed dislocations must be reduced promptly to minimize the chances of necrosis of the skin tented over the head of the talus. Promptness will facilitate reduction because it is accomplished more easily when there is less swelling. Several methods of closed reduction have been described in the literature[188] and share the following features:

1. General anesthesia to maximize muscular relaxation and minimize damage to the articular surfaces during manipulation
2. Knee flexion to relax the tension on the Achilles tendon, increasing the mobility of the calcaneus
3. Firm longitudinal manual foot traction with countertraction on the leg combined with initial accentuation of the deformity (inversion for medial and eversion for lateral dislocations), followed by:
   a. Reversal of the deformity (eversion for medial and inversion for lateral dislocations)
   b. Occasionally, direct digital pressure over the head of the talus tò aid in reduction following the application of traction

Closed reduction is usually accompanied by a satisfying snap or clunk as the joints reduce, and on clinical examination the adequacy of reduction is demonstrated by the normal alignment of the foot and normal, stable range of motion of the subtalar and midtarsal joints. X-rays will confirm the reduction, and these postreduction views should be inspected closely for small osteochondral fractures or other fractures that might have been missed on the initial x-rays of the distorted foot.

Following closed reduction, the dislocation is stable and should be immobilized initially in a short-leg posterior plaster splint. Internal fixation is unnecessary. Simple dislocations that are reduced readily by closed means and do not have associated fractures generally do very well. Immobilization for 3 to 4 weeks in a short-leg cast followed by a vigorous, active exercise program to regain subtalar and midtarsal joint motion will result in minimal long-term loss of function.[125,164] Only one case of habitual dislocation has been reported, which Larson[173] attributed to an inadequate period of

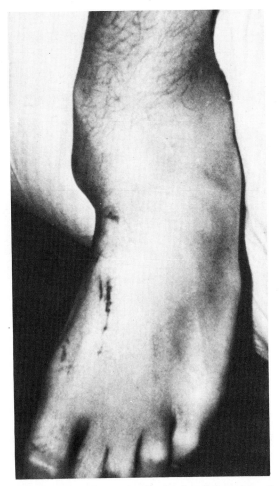

Fig. 19-59. In this lateral subtalar dislocation, the head of the talus is prominent medially, while the rest of the foot is dislocated laterally. (Buckingham, W. W., Jr.: Subtalar Dislocation of the Foot. J. Trauma, **13:**757, 1973.)

immobilization. On the other hand, prolonged immobilization of simple dislocations tends to lead to joint stiffness and impair long-term function.[163]

In approximately 10% of medial subtalar dislocations and 15% to 20% of lateral subtalar dislocations, closed reduction cannot be achieved.[170,171,174] Soft tissue interposition and bony blocks have been identified as factors preventing closed reduction. With medial subtalar dislocation the head of the talus may become trapped by the capsule of the talonavicular joint,[176] the transverse fibers of the cruciate–crural ligament,[159,174] or the extensor digitorum brevis muscle, creating a buttonhole effect that prevents reduction.

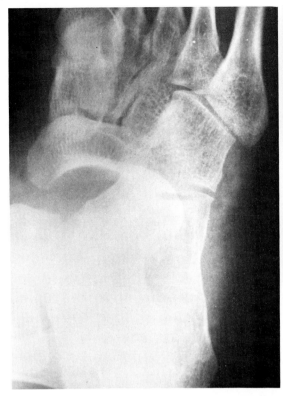

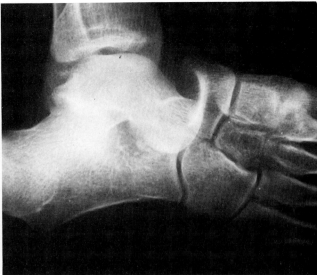

Fig. 19-60. (*Left*) Anteroposterior and (*right*) lateral x-rays of a medial subtalar dislocation. Note the dislocation of the talonavicular and subtalar joints while the normal alignment of the calcaneocuboid joint is maintained.

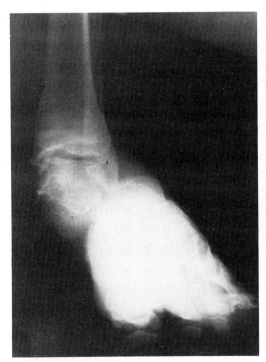

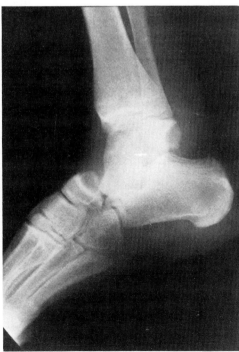

Fig. 19-61. X-ray of a lateral subtalar dislocation. The foot is displaced laterally in relationship to the talus. (Buckingham, W. W., Jr.: Subtalar Dislocation of the Foot. J. Trauma, **13**:758, 1973.)

Another common obstruction to closed reduction in medial dislocations is an impaction fracture of the articular surfaces of the talus and navicular. The extreme medial displacement of the foot at the moment of injury is immediately followed by a recoil of the foot toward the normal position, causing the lateral edge of the navicular to impinge on the medial side of the head of the talus. An impaction fracture is produced with the articular surfaces of the talus and navicular interlocked (Fig. 19-62). This interlocked fracture of the articular surfaces can sometimes be suspected on the anteroposterior x-ray.

With lateral subtalar dislocations, the most common obstruction to closed reduction is the interposed posterior tibial tendon[174,180] (Fig. 19-63) or an interlocked impaction fracture of the articular surfaces of the talus and navicular.

Open Reduction

When closed reduction of a medial subtalar dislocation cannot be accomplished, open reduction through a longitudinal anteromedial incision over the prominent head and neck of the talus should be carried out. This approach will allow access to all those structures that may be incarcerating the talar neck and also will allow visualization of an interlocked impaction fracture of the talar and navicular articular surfaces.

Once exposed, the talar head may be manipulated around the structure that is preventing reduction with the aid of a periosteal elevator, but on occasion partial or complete transection of the structure—particularly the extensor retinaculum—may be necessary to allow reduction.

With an irreducible lateral subtalar dislocation, a longitudinal incision placed more medially over the talar head should be made to allow access to the posterior tibial tendon as well as the talar head. Rarely, the posterior tibial tendon must be cut to allow reduction;[173] however, this should only be done as a last resort, and, of course, it should be repaired following reduction of the dislocation.

Disimpaction of the interlocked articular surfaces of the talus and navicular should be done carefully to avoid further articular cartilage damage. Shearing osteochondral fractures of either the subtalar or talonavicular joint surfaces may also act as a block to reduction.[176] Any small, loose articular fracture fragments should be removed, while large intraarticular fracture fragments of either the talonavicular or subtalar joints should be reduced and fixed with Kirschner wires to restore joint stability and congruity.

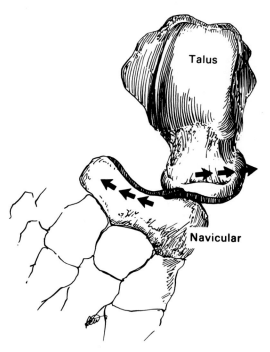

Fig. 19-62. Line drawing of a medial subtalar dislocation, irreducible by closed means because of interlocking of the articular surfaces of the talus and navicular. (Buckingham, W. W., Jr.: Subtalar Dislocation of the Foot. J. Trauma, **13**:759, 1973.)

Following removal of the obstruction to reduction, the reduction is inherently stable because of the configuration of the bony complex. There is no need for internal fixation. The reduced dislocation can be adequately immobilized in a short-leg cast for 3 to 4 weeks to allow soft tissue healing, and then the patient should begin an active assistive exercise program to regain strength and motion.

AUTHOR'S PREFERRED METHOD

Subtalar dislocation without fracture should be reduced closed whenever possible. Once reduced, the dislocation should be stable and should not recur. Therefore, I prefer a very short period of immobilization (3 weeks) to allow soft tissue healing. This should be followed by progressive weight bearing and active range of motion exercises for both the ankle and subtalar joints to restore motion, particularly subtalar motion. If an anatomical reduction cannot be achieved by closed means, then a prompt surgical reduction should be undertaken through a dorsal approach, usually over the prominent talar head. Small fracture fragments should be debrided from the joints, while large fragments

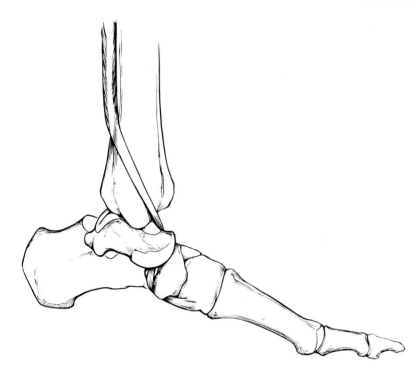

Fig. 19-63. Lateral subtalar dislocation with interposed posterior tibial tendon preventing closed reduction of the midtarsal joint. (After Leitner, B.: Obstacles to Reduction in Subtalar Dislocations. J. Bone Joint Surg., **36A**:299, 1954.)

should be anatomically reduced and rigidly fixed. Once the block to reduction is removed, the reduction again is usually stable; prolonged periods of immobilization should be avoided to prevent persistent joint stiffness.

PROGNOSIS AND COMPLICATIONS

Patients with simple, uncomplicated subtalar dislocations who undergo prompt reduction either by closed or open means generally do well with minimal symptoms at long-term follow-up. The only consistently abnormal finding in this group is limitation of subtalar joint motion, with the occasional associated symptoms of difficulty in walking on uneven ground and pain in the foot with weather change.[162,168,173,187]

Several complicating factors are known to decrease the likelihood of a good result:

1. Infection can occur either as a result of contamination of an open wound or secondary to skin necrosis and slough over the prominent talar head. This complication is best prevented by prompt reduction of the dislocation and adequate surgical debridement of any contaminated wound.

2. The mechanism of injury is an important factor in predicting the long-term results. The results are worse with the more violent mechanisms.

Simple inversion (the "basketball foot"[168]) rarely produces a dislocation with long-term morbidity, while more violent injuries such as those incurred in motor vehicle wrecks or during a fall from a height will more likely be associated with persistent symptoms. These violent injuries are more likely to produce associated fractures and more severe soft tissue injury, both of which decrease the chances of a good long-term result.[164]

3. Lateral subtalar dislocations tend to do worse than medial dislocations,[164,171] probably because the force required to produce dislocation in this direction is greater than that required for a medial dislocation. Another factor is the higher incidence of associated fractures and articular cartilage damage that occurs with lateral dislocation.

4. Associated fractures, either of the adjacent bones or osteochondral fractures of the dislocated joint surfaces themselves, increase the chance of a poor result (Fig. 19-64). Intra-articular fractures increase the likelihood of persistent arthritis,[178] while fractures of adjacent bones may require prolonged immobilization, which may result in persistent stiffness of the subtalar joint.

5. Finally, failure to diagnose a dislocation promptly will usually lead to a poor result. Even if the

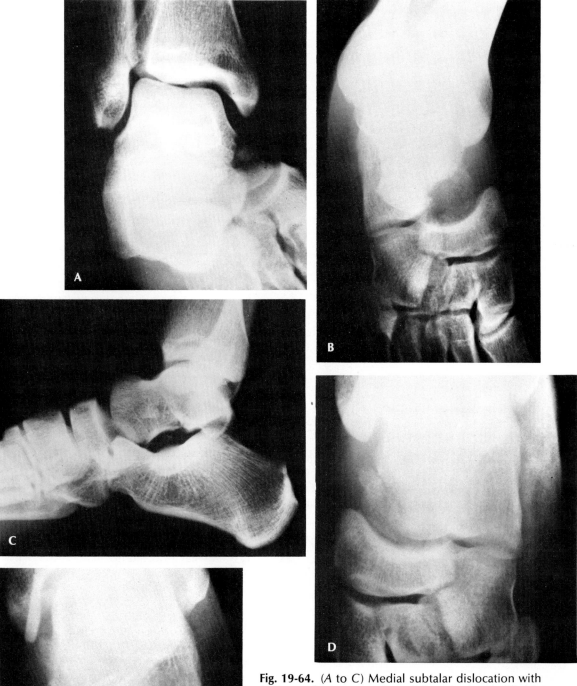

Fig. 19-64. (*A* to *C*) Medial subtalar dislocation with fracture of a large portion of the talar head. (*D*) After closed reduction, the persistent displacement of the talar head fragment necessitated open reduction and internal fixation to facilitate anatomical healing and early restoration of function (*E*).

early complication of skin necrosis is avoided, late reduction (attempted more than a month after dislocation) is difficult and usually must be combined with a triple arthrodesis to achieve a stable, plantigrade foot.

Avascular necrosis has been reported very rarely following this injury,[163,167,171] and most of the larger series do not include it as a complication. Because the talus is not disrupted from the ankle mortise, at least some of its blood supply remains intact. Recurrent dislocation is also a very infrequently reported complication[173] because of the intrinsic stability of the joints that have dislocated. Occasionally, subluxation occurs in plaster at a week or 10 days after reduction when the swelling subsides, but repeat closed reduction can be accomplished easily[171] and still lead to a good result.

TOTAL DISLOCATION OF THE TALUS

Total talar dislocation, which is a rare injury, in most reported cases has resulted from a continuation of the forces causing a subtalar dislocation. Extreme supination force first produces medial subtalar dislocation followed by total lateral talar dislocation, while extreme pronation force results in lateral subtalar dislocation, and, with further pronation, total medial talar dislocation is produced (Fig. 19-65).[175] Pinzur and Meyer[182] reported an exceedingly rare case of posterior dislocation of the talar body without fracture.

As expected, total dislocation of the talus is a devastating injury. Most are open injuries. Detenbeck and Kelly[165] reported the largest series (nine cases) in the literature and found an 89% incidence of persistent infection, all eventually requiring ta-

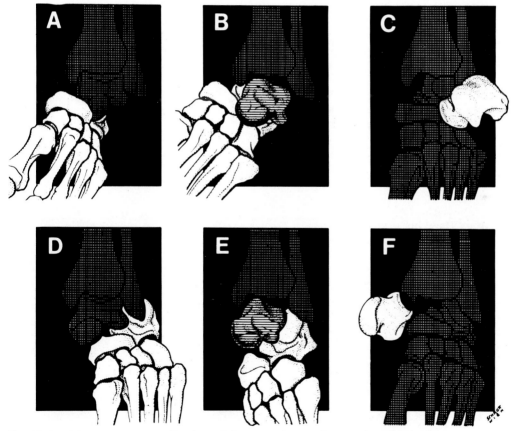

Fig. 19-65. More extreme application of the same forces that produced subtalar dislocation can result in total talar dislocation. Supination produces medial subtalar dislocation (*A*) followed by subluxation (*B*) and finally complete lateral dislocation of the talus (*C*). Pronation initially produces lateral subtalar dislocation (*D*), followed by talar subluxation (*E*) and eventually total medial dislocation of the talus (*F*). (Leitner, B.: The Mechanism of Total Dislocation of the Talus. J. Bone Joint Surg., **37A:**93, 1955.)

lectomy for control. Avascular necrosis is a common complication when infection is avoided, and degenerative arthritis of the ankle and subtalar joint is also a frequent late sequela of this injury.

TREATMENT AND PROGNOSIS

Initial treatment should be directed at the soft tissues with vigorous debridement of open wounds and release of skin tension by prompt reduction of the talus. Because of the high complication rate, some authors recommend primary excision of the talus and primary tibiocalcaneal arthrodesis.[165] Arthrodesis appears preferrable to talectomy alone, since most often simple talar excision results in a painful rearfoot. Other isolated reports[177,181,185] encourage reduction and preservation of the talus because occasionally infection can be avoided and the late complications of avascular necrosis and degenerative arthritis may be only minimally symptomatic or can be treated effectively by tibiotalar or even pantalar arthrodesis.

After a thorough initial debridement of any open wound, I believe that prompt reduction of the dislocated talus should be undertaken. Closed reduction may be tried in closed injuries with the aid of a transverse calcaneal pin for traction, but the chance of success is very slim. Open reduction can be accomplished through an anteromedial or anterolateral ankle arthrotomy. Occasionally reduction is unstable and requires Kirschner wire transfixion of the subtalar or talonavicular joints until soft tissue healing occurs. Cast immobilization for 6 weeks will allow capsular healing. Close inspection of the x-ray at 6 to 8 weeks should reveal the presence or absence of a "Hawkins's sign" (see p. 1741). If there is no evidence of subchondral resorption (as is most likely the case), early avascular necrosis should be suspected. The patient should be fitted with a patellar tendon–bearing ankle–foot orthosis to protect the talus from collapse until revascularization of the talar body is complete. Brace protection may be required for as long as 24 months. Should the patient's late symptoms warrant further treatment, arthrodesis of the symptomatic joint(s) should be undertaken.

FRACTURES OF THE CALCANEUS

The calcaneus (os calcis) is the tarsal bone most often fractured. Despite physicians' extensive experience with this injury, its major socioeconomic impact in regard to the time lost from work and recreation, and the attention given it for many years by surgeons throughout the world, there is still no method of treatment that yields consistently good results. Cave[206] pointed out that fracture of the calcaneus is one injury that has not increased in frequency with the advent of mechanized industry, automobile travel, or war. It has been a common, often disabling injury since humans assumed the erect posture and began to defy gravity.

ANATOMY

The articular surfaces of the calcaneus, the largest of the tarsal bones, are on its anterior half. The hindmost portion of the posterior half of the calcaneus is called the tuberosity. The Achilles tendon inserts into the posterior cortex of the tuberosity. On the plantar surface are two projections, the medial and lateral processes, which serve as the points of origin for the plantar fascia and the small muscles of the plantar surface of the foot. On the superior aspect are three articular surfaces (Fig. 19-66): the posterior, middle, and anterior facets. The posterior is the largest and is convex. The

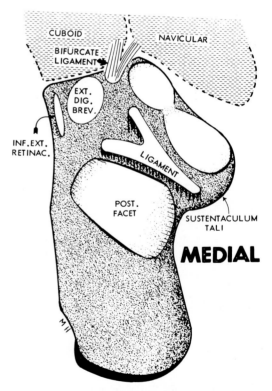

Fig. 19-66. The superior aspect of the left calcaneus. The anterior and sustentacular articular facets are illustrated but not labeled. (Harty, M.: Anatomic Considerations in Injuries of the Calcaneus. Orthop. Clin. North Am., 4:181, 1973.)

middle one, slightly concave, is situated on the sustentaculum tali. The anterior facet, also slightly concave, frequently is confluent with the middle one. Between the middle and posterior articular facets lies the interosseous sulcus (calcaneal groove), which opens broadly laterally and forms, with the talar sulcus, the sinus tarsi. The three calcaneal facets articulate with the corresponding talar facets to form the complex subtalar joint.

Along the flat lateral surface of the body of the calcaneus is a shallow groove for the peroneal tendons. The medial surface is concave and structurally stronger. From this surface projects a broad process, the sustentaculum tali, which projects toward the talus and contains the middle articular facet on its superior surface. On its undersurface is the broad groove for the tendon of the flexor hallucis longus. The anterior surface bears a somewhat saddle-shaped articular surface for the cuboid.

The calcaneus serves a dual purpose: it provides an elastic, firm support for the weight of the body and also functions as a springboard for locomotion.[231] It is the largest tarsal bone and forms the more vertical, shorter, and less yielding posterior limb of the longitudinal arch of the foot. Its anterior half supports the talus. The latter, in turn, carries the whole body load through the tibia.

The calcaneus has a very thin cortical shell, except at the posterior tuberosity; enclosed within the shell is a pattern of cancellous bone that reflects the static and dynamic stresses to which it is repeatedly subjected. Traction trabeculae radiate from the inferior cortex, while compression trabeculae converge to support the anterior and posterior facets (Fig. 19-67 *left*). Soeur and Remy[278] have designated this condensation of compact bone beneath the facets as the thalamic portion of the calcaneus. The neutral triangle of sparse trabeculae is the area through which the blood vessels traverse. Böhler's tuber joint angle is seen in the lateral x-ray projection.[199] It is the complement of the angle formed by two lines: a line drawn between the highest part of the anterior process and the highest part of the posterior articular surface and a line drawn between the same point on the posterior articular surface and the most superior point of the tuberosity (Fig. 19-67 *right*).[199] The tuber angle normally measures between 25° and 40°, with a very similar angle being found in the two calcanei of any normal individual.

The lateral process of the talus is wedge shaped in the lateral projection, with its apex pointed directly at the "crucial angle" as originally described by Gissane.[218,231] Axial compressive forces, with the talus acting as a bursting wedge, will disrupt the subtalar joint and distort the crucial angle (Fig. 19-67 *right*).

CLASSIFICATION

Fractures of the calcaneus have been classified in a variety of ways.[199,208,218,272,411] The primary importance of classification is to separate those fractures that tend to have a good prognosis from those that do poorly or require more aggressive treatment

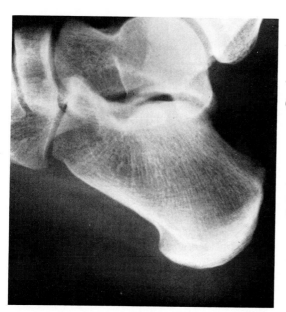

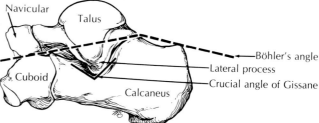

Fig. 19-67. (*Left*) Lateral x-ray of a normal calcaneus showing the trabecular pattern of bone converging superiorly to support the body weight. (*Right*) Line drawing of the lateral view of the calcaneus demonstrating Böhler's tuber angle (*dotted line*) and the crucial angle of Gissane.

to ensure a satisfactory outcome. Essex-Lopresti[218] was one of the first to emphasize the difference between extra-articular fractures, which tend to do well, and fractures involving the subtalar joint, which generally have a poorer prognosis. Various subtypes and configurations exist within each group of fractures.

Extra-articular fractures occur infrequently (25% to 30% of all calcaneal fractures[218,250]) and are divided anatomically into the following types: anterior process, tuberosity (beak or avulsion), medial process, sustentaculum tali, and body.

Intra-articular fractures (which comprise the remaining 70% to 75% of calcaneal fractures) can result in an infinite variety of patterns with varying degrees of fracture fragment displacement. For this reason, subdivision is sometimes difficult, and a review of the literature reveals a great variety of descriptions of fracture classification. Essex-Lopresti[218] identified two distinct fracture subtypes that occur with regularity: the tongue and the joint depression fractures. Some of the intra-articular fractures of the calcaneus are severely comminuted and defy any better description. Because the method of treatment may be modified by the configuration of the fracture fragments in the intra-articular type of injury, four general subtypes will be used in this description: nondisplaced, tongue, joint depression, and comminuted.

MECHANISM OF INJURY

Twisting forces cause many of the extra-articular calcaneal fractures, particularly fractures of the anterior process, the sustentaculum, and the medial process. Fracture of the tuberosity is most commonly caused by avulsive muscle forces as the triceps surae pulls loose a variably sized portion of the tuberosity. Direct blows, closed or open, can obviously result in fracture of any part of the calcaneus.

Falls from heights are responsible for the vast majority of intra-articular calcaneal fractures. Because the calcaneus is a relatively hollow structure, composed of cancellous bone enclosed in a thin cortical shell, any fall—even a short one—may result in fracture as the talus is driven downward into the calcaneus. In most large series of calcaneal fractures this mechanism is responsible for the fracture in 80% to 90% of cases. Simultaneous bilateral fractures of the calcaneus, of varying degrees of severity, occur 5% to 9% of the time with this mechanism.[246,247,272] When a person falls from a height, the compressive forces fracture not only the calcaneus but may produce a more proximal

injury as well. According to Cave,[206] 10% of calcaneal fractures are associated with compression fractures of the dorsal or lumbar spine and 26% are associated with other injuries of the lower extremities. Associated injuries occurred in 91 of 152 patients (60%) in a series of calcaneal fractures reviewed by Lance and associates[246,247] and in 70% of the 67 patients reviewed by Slatis and colleagues.[276]

RADIOGRAPHIC FINDINGS

Since the physician invariably depends on the radiographic findings to diagnose the location and degree of severity of calcaneal fractures, the foot, especially the heel, should be positioned accurately in order to obtain the proper x-rays. The initial x-ray examination of the patient who complains of rearfoot pain following an injury should consist of three views: dorsoplantar (anteroposterior), lateral, and axial calcaneal projection (Fig. 19-68). Most calcaneal fractures will be identified on at least one of these three views. The dorsoplantar view delineates the calcaneocuboid joint quite satisfactorily as well as demonstrating the amount of lateral spread of the calcaneus and any subluxation of the talonavicular joint.[235] The lateral view is excellent for demonstrating the tuber angle and the congruity of the posterior articular facet. The axial view best demonstrates the tuberosity, the body, the sustentaculotalar joint, and the posterior facet of the calcaneus. Slight adjustment in the inclination of the x-ray tube (usually between 15° and 40°) may be necessary to best demonstrate these different areas in the axial projection. An anteroposterior view of the ankle joint is useful, since if the lateral border of the calcaneus extends to the level of the tip of the lateral malleolus or beyond, this implies widening and spreading of the calcaneus. In addition, coincidental ankle fractures can be identified on this view.

Fractures of the calcaneus can be bilateral, and it is therefore advisable to obtain x-rays of both feet even if only one foot is thought to be injured. Even if no fracture is found, x-rays of the opposite calcaneus will be very helpful to compare with the injured foot. In addition, because of the high frequency of associated fractures, views of the ipsilateral ankle and the dorsolumbar spine should be obtained in all patients who have sustained a calcaneal fracture.

Special oblique views defining the subtalar joint are often very helpful to show the true extent of joint incongruity sustained in intra-articular calcaneal fractures. A variety of techniques has been

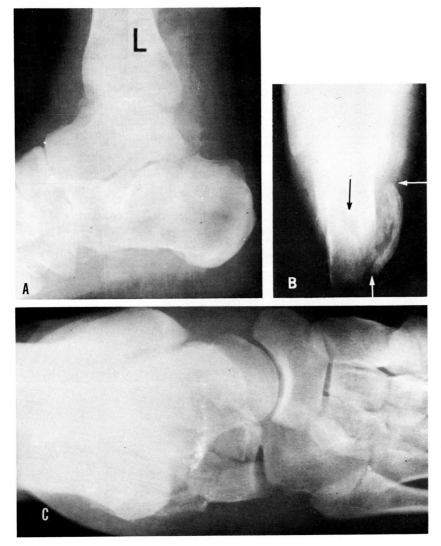

Fig. 19-68. (*A*) Lateral view showing joint depression type fracture of the calcaneus with decreased tuber angle. (*B*) Axial view of the calcaneus. The fracture line extends into the subtalar joint, and there is widening of the calcaneus. (*C*) Dorsoplantar x-ray of the foot showing extension of the calcaneal fracture into the calcaneocuboid joint.

described,[192,202,281,285,396] but the three oblique projections described by Isherwood[238] are relatively easily reproducible and yield much valuable information. The techniques of obtaining these x-rays are described below.

The Lateral Oblique Projection

The medial border of the foot is placed on the cassette, and the sole is inclined 45°. The x-ray tube is centered 2.5 cm below and 2.5 cm anterior to the lateral malleolus. This projection allows visualization of the anterior facet of the subtalar joint and the anterior calcaneal process (Fig. 19-69).

The Medial Oblique Axial Projection

The foot is passively dorsiflexed and inverted by the use of a broad strap around the forefoot, held by the seated patient. A 30° foam wedge is placed on the x-ray cassette, and the limb is internally rotated 60° until the foot rests on the wedge. The x-ray tube is centered 2.5 cm below and 2.5 cm anterior to the tip of the lateral malleolus and tilted 10° cephalad. This projection demonstrates both the middle and posterior facets and the tarsal canal. The interval between the calcaneus and the fibula in which the peroneal tendons lie can also be visualized (Fig. 19-70).

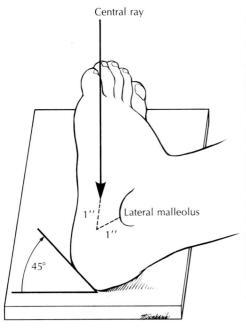

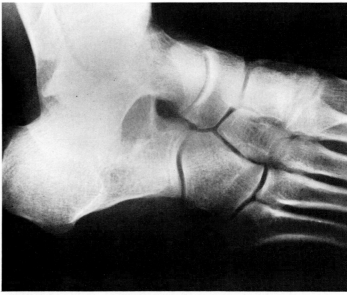

Fig. 19-69. (*Left*) The lateral oblique x-ray projection of the calcaneus is taken with the inner border of the foot placed on the film with the sole inclined 45°. The x-ray is centered 1 inch below and 1 inch anterior to the tip of the lateral malleolus. (*Right*) In this view the anterior process and facet can be visualized.

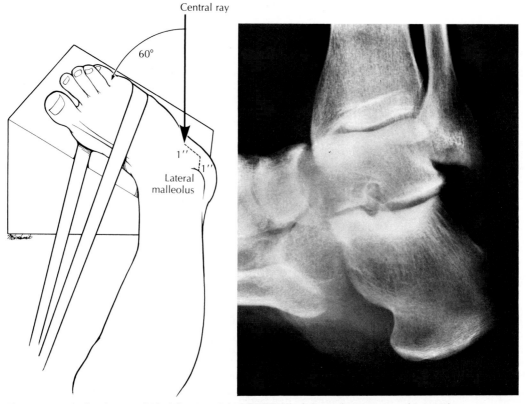

Fig. 19-70. (*Left*) The medial oblique axial projection of the calcaneus is taken with the foot passively dorsiflexed, inverted, and internally rotated 60°. The x-ray is tilted 10° cephalad and centered 1 inch anterior and 1 inch distal to the tip of the lateral malleolus. (*Right*) The middle and posterior facets are well delineated.

The Lateral Oblique Axial Projection

The foot is passively dorsiflexed and everted by the patient by means of the forefoot strap. The limb is externally rotated 60° to allow its lateral border to lie against the 30° foam wedge. The x-ray tube is centered 2.5 cm below the medial malleolus and tilted 10° cephalad. This view will throw the posterior facet into profile (Fig. 19-71).

Tomography

Tomography, particularly in the lateral projection, can also be helpful in delineating the subtalar articulation, and Smith and Staple[277] recently reported the usefulness of CT scanning in the evaluation of the subtalar joint and peroneal tendons in patients with healed calcaneal fractures with residual symptoms (see Fig. 19-29).

EXTRA-ARTICULAR FRACTURES OF THE CALCANEUS

FRACTURES OF THE ANTERIOR PROCESS

Classification and Mechanism of Injury

Two distinct fracture patterns involve the anteriormost portion of the calcaneus: avulsion fractures of the anterior process and compression fractures of the anterior calcaneus involving a variable portion of the calcaneocuboid joint.

Avulsion fracture of the anterior process is the more common of these two types of injuries, and in one large series of calcaneal fractures occurred in 15% of the patients.[204] This injury is seen more frequently in women and is an avulsion type of injury, occurring when the foot is adducted and plantarflexed and tension is placed on the bifurcate ligament. This ligament (see Fig. 19-66) connects the anterior process of the calcaneus to both the cuboid and navicular bones. Inversion stress of the foot will result in stretch of this ligament or avulsion fracture of the anterior process (Fig. 19-72). The extensor digitorum brevis originates from the anterior dorsal calcaneus, lateral to the bifurcate ligament, and Norfray and colleagues[260] have reported a series of avulsion fractures of the anterior and lateral portion of the calcaneus due to a similar inversion mechanism, which they attribute to avulsion of the origin of this muscle.

Hunt[236] described the compression fracture of the anterior calcaneal articular surface. The mechanism of injury in this relatively infrequent fracture pattern is forceful abduction of the forefoot with

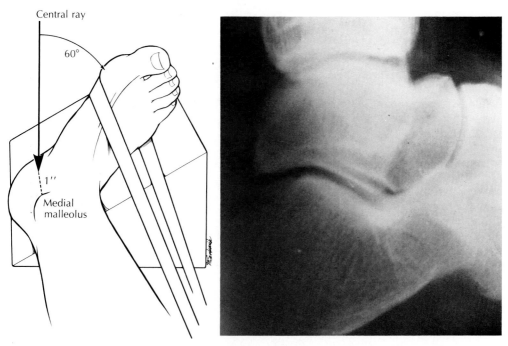

Fig. 19-71. (*Left*) The lateral oblique axial x-ray projection of the calcaneus is taken with the foot passively everted, dorsiflexed, and externally rotated 60°. The x-ray is tilted 10° cephalad and centered 1 inch below the tip of the medial malleolus. (*Right*) The posterior facet of the subtalar joint is well visualized.

compression of the calcaneocuboid joint. The anterior articular surface of the calcaneus is fractured, and a variably sized fragment can be displaced superiorly and posteriorly, resulting in significant joint incongruity (Fig. 19-73).

The avulsion fracture of the anterior process is usually small and does not involve the cuboid articulation, whereas the compression fracture fragment is larger and usually does involve the joint surface. It is important to distinguish between these two, since treatment may vary.

Signs and Symptoms

Pain and tenderness are located in the region of the sinus tarsi. Particularly with the avulsion type of fracture, the patient will give a history of inversion ankle injury, and, like the avulsion fracture of the base of the fifth matatarsal, this fracture may be overlooked unless the clinician has a high index of suspicion. The point of maximal tenderness will be 2 cm anterior and 1 cm inferior to the anterior talofibular ligament, which should help to distinguish this injury from a lateral ankle sprain.

Radiographic Findings

A lateral x-ray of the hind foot will best demonstrate the compression type fracture, while the lateral oblique projection most frequently will show the avulsion fracture of the anterior process. The amount of displacement will vary in either fracture. A small, inconsistent ossicle, the calcaneus secondarium (see Fig. 19-25), lies just adjacent to the anterior process and must not be confused with a fresh fracture. As with other accessory bones, it has a smooth, rounded contour as compared with a fresh fracture surface.

Treatment and Prognosis

A high index of suspicion, leading to early diagnosis of these fractures, is important. Avulsion fractures of the anterior process, when diagnosed early and immobilized in a short-leg cast for 4 weeks, heal well with little or no residual symptoms, although full recovery may take 6 to 9 months.[213] On the other hand, delay in diagnosis, combined with inadequate initial immobilization, tends to compromise the long-term results. With the rare compression type of fracture configuration, early diagnosis is also important, particularly to identify large, displaced articular fragments, which should be reduced and fixed to ensure congruity of the calcaneocuboid joint.[236] Degan and colleagues[213] reported seven patients with anterior process fractures who required late surgical excision because of persistent pain. Not all anterior process fractures heal, and not all nonunions are symptomatic;

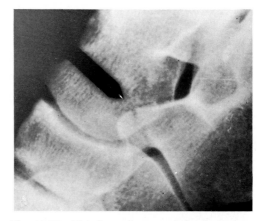

Fig. 19-72. This lateral x-ray of the foot shows a fracture of the anterior process (beak) of the calcaneus. (After Giannestras, N. J.: Foot Disorders: Medical and Surgical Management, 2nd ed. Philadelphia, Lea & Febiger, 1973.)

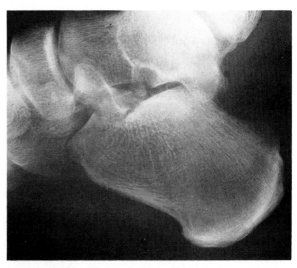

Fig. 19-73. Compression fracture of the anterior calcaneal articular surface with significant displacement of the fragment comprising the superior one third of the joint, producing incongruity of the calcaneocuboid articulation.

however, six of these seven patients had persistent ununited fragments, and late excision of the ununited fragment relieved symptoms in five of the seven patients.

FRACTURE OF THE TUBEROSITY

Classification and Mechanism of Injury

In a review of several large series of calcaneal fractures, fracture of the tuberosity was found to occur rarely.[218,246,247,272] Older classifications separated fractures of the tuberosity into at least two types—the so-called beak and avulsion fractures—depending on the portion of the tuberosity that was fractured. Earlier writers[218,272] believed that fracture of the more superior part of the tuberosity ("beak" fracture) was caused by direct trauma and that fracture of the more inferior part of the tuberosity (the "avulsion" fracture) was caused by a direct pull of the Achilles tendon. This concept prevailed because most anatomy textbooks indicate that the Achilles tendon does not insert into the uppermost portion of the tuberosity. Korn,[244] Lowy,[251] and others[252] have demonstrated, however, that the Achilles tendon in some people does insert into the uppermost portion of the tuberosity as well. Thus, avulsion can be the mechanism of fracture of all or any part of the tuberosity. Only rarely is direct trauma responsible for these fractures. The critical factor in management of any of these fractures is the degree of displacement of the fracture fragment.

Older people are prone to this injury (the average age in 11 reported cases[251,252,269] was 63 years). The usual mechanism of injury is a fall from a small height (off a curb or down stairs), and most authors postulate that the fragment is avulsed by a sudden pull of the Achilles tendon. In these elderly, usually female (8 of 11) patients, osteoporosis probably weakens the bone sufficiently to allow the avulsion fracture to occur.

Signs and Symptoms

Pain, swelling, and echymosis usually accompany the acute injury. Occasionally patients will present a few to several days after the injury complaining of a limp and particularly weakness with stair climbing. At this stage the patient may have a fairly typical calcaneal gait, finding it difficult to stand on tiptoe. Occasionally a displaced fragment will tent the relatively fragile skin posteriorly, potentially jeopardizing circulation to the area. A standard lateral x-ray will demonstrate fracture size and the degree of displacement (Fig. 19-74).

Treatment

The method of treatment is determined by the degree of displacement of the bony fragment. If the fracture is undisplaced, or only minimally so, closed treatment can be undertaken. The foot should be immobilized in slight (5° to 10°) equinus in a short-leg cast for 6 weeks. Partial weight bearing may be allowed as dictated by pain. X-rays should be repeated at 1 week to confirm maintenance of reduction of the fracture.

If the fragment is displaced, reduction and fixa-

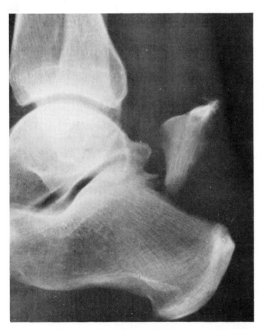
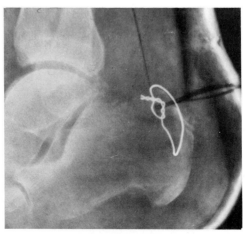

Fig. 19-74. (*Left*) Avulsion fracture of the superior portion of the calcaneal tuberosity. (*Right*) The fragment has been reduced and fixed with a cerclage wire, restoring the length of the Achilles tendon. The foot is immobilized in slight equinus in a short-leg cast.

tion should be undertaken to restore the Achilles tendon to its functional length. Open reduction can be achieved readily through a posterolateral surgical approach. Reduction of widely displaced fragments can be facilitated by the use of a bone hook. Fixation of the reduced fragment has been achieved in a variety of ways: cerclage wire around the fragment and through a transverse drill hole in the plantar portion of the tuberosity; axial Steinmann pin fixation, similar to the Essex-Lopresti technique (see p. 1779); or cancellous screw fixation. Regardless of the type of fixation, because of the great strength of the triceps surae, the fracture should be protected in a short-leg cast with the foot in 5° to 10° of equinus for 6 to 8 weeks until there is x-ray evidence of bony union. During the period of cast immobilization, the patient should avoid weight bearing or at most ambulate with a toe-touch gait on the affected limb.

FRACTURES OF THE MEDIAL CALCANEAL PROCESS

Anatomy and Mechanism of Injury

The medial process of the calcaneal tuberosity is a moderately large prominence seen well on the axial projection of the calcaneus (Fig. 19-75). It serves as the origin of the abductor hallucis and the medial portion of the flexor digitorum brevis and plantar fascia. Watson-Jones[411] called this injury a vertical fracture of the tuberosity and believed that it was caused by shearing forces produced from a fall on the heel when in a valgus position. Böhler[199] thought that it resulted from avulsion of the plantar fascia. The injury occurs rarely.

Clinical and Radiographic Findings

Localized pain and tenderness, swelling, ecchymosis, and limp characterize the acute findings in the patient with this injury. Joint range of motion is usually well preserved, although the physician may elicit pain on forced dorsiflexion of the ankle or toes. The axial x-ray best demonstrates the fracture and the degree of displacement. Usually a single fracture line separates the medial process from the body, but on occasion comminution may be present. Rarely is the fracture displaced greatly.

Treatment and Prognosis

Nondisplaced and minimally or moderately displaced fractures should be treated with rest for 4 weeks, either with a compression bandage applied to the foot and leg[204] or with well-molded short-leg walking plaster cast. Grossly displaced fragments should be reduced by closed manipulation and casted in a similar fashion until healed. Watson-

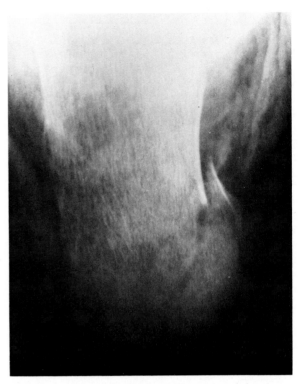

Fig. 19-75. Minimally displaced fracture of the medial process of the calcaneus.

Jones[411] indicated that "imperfect reduction" may result in persistent tenderness over the bony fragment, and he reported one malunion. Closed manipulation with medial–lateral compression of the heel by the palms of the hand should produce an adequate reduction that can be maintained by a short-leg cast applied with similar medial–lateral molding. Besides occasional thickening and tenderness of the heel (which are best treated by padding the heel and using custom-molded shoe inserts), no significant long-term complications have been reported to occur following this fracture.

FRACTURES OF THE SUSTENTACULUM TALI

Mechanism of Injury

Fracture of the sustentaculum tali is the result of two forces: landing on the heel combined with acute, severe inversion of the foot. As an isolated injury, it is uncommon. Lance and colleagues[246,247] reported only eight in 303 calcaneal fractures; Essex-Lopresti,[218] only one in 180 fractures.

Signs and Symptoms

The major portion of the swelling is on the medial aspect of the heel and the hind foot. Inversion of the foot produces acute pain just below the medial malleolus. It is for this reason that this fracture is mistaken by the uninitiated as a sprained ankle. Tenderness over the heel is minimial. The clue to possible fracture is the history of injury combined with pain just below the medial malleolus, which is often accentuated by passive hyperextension of the great toe. This motion increases the tension placed upon the flexor hallucis longus tendon as it passes under the sustentaculum, causing painful motion at the fracture site.

Radiographic Findings

An axial x-ray is necessary to demonstrate this lesion (Fig. 19-76). It must be taken precisely, and if there is any question of a fracture, a comparative x-ray of the opposite foot should be obtained. In addition, the special oblique calcaneal views as described on page 1763 should be obtained to rule out additional fractures of the calcaneus.

Treatment and Prognosis

Plaster immobilization is the treatment of choice for isolated nondisplaced fractures of the sustentaculum. All eight cases reported by Carey and colleagues[204] had satisfactory results after 6 weeks of plaster immobilization. Occasionally the axial view will show significant inferior displacement of the sustentacular fragment. According to Key and Conwell,[403] closed reduction should be attempted by inverting and plantarflexing the foot and then applying direct digital pressure to the sustentaculum at the medial border of the foot below the medial malleolus. Closed reduction should be followed by 6 weeks of plaster cast immobilization.

Rarely, nonunion of this fragment may occur, resulting in persistent pain with weight bearing. Careful surgical excision of the ununited fragment should be undertaken for persistent symptoms.

FRACTURE OF THE BODY NOT INVOLVING THE SUBTALAR JOINT

Anatomy and Classification

A very large number of calcaneal fractures (19.5% of the series by Rowe and colleagues[272]) involve the body of the calcaneus but do not communicate with the subtalar joint. Because the subtalar joint is spared, the prognosis for these injuries is better, and therefore most authors separate them from the intra-articular injuries. The mechanism of injury most frequently associated with fracture of the body is a fall from a height with the patient landing directly on the heel.

The configuration of the fracture varies greatly, and the only consistent feature is the sparing of the subtalar joint. Single fracture lines can occur, usu-

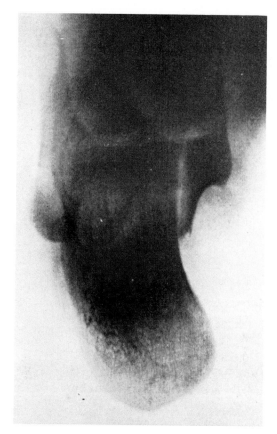

Fig. 19-76. Isolated fracture of the sustentaculum tali. (Warrick, C. K., and Bremner, A. E.: Fractures of the Calcaneum—with an Atlas Illustrating the Various Types of Fracture. J. Bone Joint Surg., 35B:38, 1953.)

ally running vertically or obliquely behind the posterior facet (Fig. 19-77), or significant comminution with a "cracked egg shell" appearance can be found. Even though the posterior articular facet is not involved, displacement can still occur, resulting in shortening and crushing of the body with widening on the axial projection and even significant reduction in Böhler's tuber angle. Thus, it is important to realize that the tuber angle can be decreased without a fracture line actually traversing the subtalar joint. Generally, these displaced non-articular calcaneal fractures widen the body and drive it superiorly. When the tuberosity is driven superiorly, the tuber angle will be decreased.

Signs and Symptoms

The symptoms following this fracture are usually more extreme than those occurring with the other extra-articular calcaneal fractures and are similar to those seen with intra-articular injuries. There is

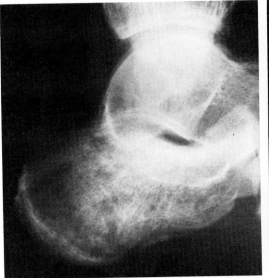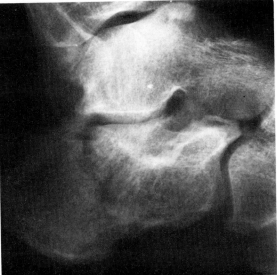

Fig. 19-77. (*Left*) A displaced fracture of the body of the calcaneus with decreased tuber angle but no involvement of the articular surface. (*Right*) The maintenance of joint congruity is seen well on the medial oblique axial view.

intense discomfort, with the inability to bear weight. Within an hour or two of injury, significant swelling and ecchymosis will usually occur. These findings will often be followed within the first 24 hours by skin blister formation over both sides of the heel. Any motion of the ankle or foot is painful. In this group of fractures, open injury occurs rarely.

Radiographic Findings

The fractures are usually visualized well on the standard lateral and axial calcaneal views; however, *it is imperative that the special oblique x-rays be obtained to be certain that there is no involvement of the subtalar joint.* An anteroposterior view is also necessary to evaluate the degree of involvement, if any, of the calcaneocuboid joint. A lateral x-ray of the opposite foot should be obtained to compare the measurement of Böhler's tuber angle. The degree of displacement, particularly the amount of widening of the heel on the axial projection and the change in Böhler's angle, should be assessed before treatment.

Treatment

As a rule, patients without subtalar involvement do well regardless of treatment, and many authors recommend minimal or no treatment for these fractures.[218,246,247,263,264,265,272] For nondisplaced and even most displaced fractures, initial treatment should consist of bed rest, elevation, and a bulky compression dressing for 48 to 72 hours to minimize

swelling and the formation of fracture blisters. As the swelling begins to subside, active range of motion exercises for the foot and ankle should be begun to prevent joint stiffness. Fracture union always occurs,[265] and after 4 to 6 weeks of toe-touch ambulation, the patient can usually begin to progressively bear more weight on the injured foot.

In certain circumstances, particularly with younger patients, two types of fracture displacement warrant an attempt to improve alignment: significant widening of the heel and decrease in the size of the tuber angle. Widening of the heel can lead to difficulty with shoe fitting and impingement on the lateral malleolus and peroneal tendons. Closed manipulative reduction, by medial–lateral compression of the calcaneus with the palms of the hands, will decrease the heel width. After the acute swelling has subsided, a well-molded plaster cast can aid in maintaining this reduction of heel width until bony union has occurred (at approximately 6 weeks). Cast removal should be followed by a period of intensive active range of motion exercises to restore joint motion. Such closed manipulation is easy to perform, and it should be attempted in all patients with significant residual widening following calcaneal fracture.

Restoration of Böhler's angle in extra-articular fractures has been advocated by some to minimize the relative lengthening of the Achilles tendon, which will occur if the tuberosity heals with cephalad displacement. Theoretically, this deformity can lead to weakness of plantarflexion. On the other hand, McLaughlin[253] stated that the calf muscles will contract and compensate for the deformity, allowing the patient to eventually regain push-off strength.

In certain young, active patients who have displaced extra-articular calcaneal fractures with flattening or reversal of the tuber angle, consideration should be given to restoring the tuber angle. This can be accomplished by traction. A threaded Kirschner wire or Steinmann pin is driven transversely through the upper portion of the tuberosity, and distal traction then applied to the wire will improve Böhler's angle. The wire should then be incorporated in a short-leg non-weight-bearing plaster cast and maintained for 4 weeks. The cast and pin are removed at 4 weeks, and active exercises are begun, with the patient protected from weight bearing until there is good evidence of fracture healing, usually 8 weeks after the time of fracture.

Author's Preferred Method

Fractures of the calcaneus that do not involve the subtalar joint should be treated by closed means. For the vast majority, I prefer to apply a compression dressing combined with bed rest and elevation to allow the initial swelling to subside. This is followed by a vigorous exercise program to restore ankle and subtalar joint motion. When significant widening of the calcaneus exists, I perform a closed reduction with manual compression of the calcaneus to decrease the chance of late peroneal tendon irritation. I do not make a vigorous attempt to restore Böhler's angle in these extra-articular fractures.

The patient must avoid weight bearing for 6 to 8 weeks, until the fracture heals. A reliable patient will be given crutches and instructed to continue active range of motion exercises at home. An unreliable patient should be protected in a short-leg non-weight-bearing cast until fracture healing has occurred, but before any patient's fracture is immobilized in a cast, he or she should maximize the active range of motion of both his ankle and subtalar joints.

Prognosis

Virtually all patients with nondisplaced, extra-articular fractures have a good result, and even those with displacement generally do well. Fracture union always occurs, and with early range of motion, joint stiffness is a minimal long-term problem. Aching pain with weather change can be expected to occur for from 12 to 18 months after the fracture.

INTRA-ARTICULAR FRACTURES OF THE CALCANEUS

Intra-articular fractures of the calcaneus comprise 60% of all tarsal injuries and 75% of all calcaneal fractures according to Cave.[206] The reader can readily realize that this will be the most common calcaneal fracture encountered.

Mechanism of Injury

This injury virtually always results from a fall from a height when the patient lands on his heels in such a manner that the entire body weight is absorbed by the calcaneus. The height of the fall does not have to be great. The patient can suffer an equally serious fracture of the calcaneus from a 4-foot fall as from a 10-foot fall. The injury depends on the location of the force of impact. Many investigators[190,218,243] of this type of fracture hypothesize that the lateral process of the talus acts as a wedge against the superior articular surface of the calcaneus (Fig. 19-78). Superimpose on this the weight and age of the patient, the mineral content of the bone, and the distance of the fall, and the resulting fracture will present varying degrees of widening and displacement. If the comminution of the articular surface is severe, degen-

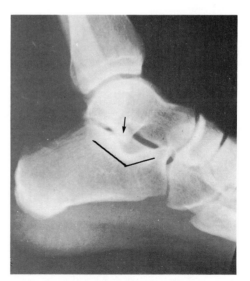

Fig. 19-78. On compressive loading, the lateral process of the talus acts like a driving wedge against the calcaneus, producing the fracture. The crucial angle, or Gissane's angle, is shown.

erative changes of the talocalcaneal joint can develop later. Widening of the bone produces lateral impingement on the fibula and possible entrapment of the peroneal tendons.

Classification

Although some intra-articular calcaneal fractures defy classification beyond a description of "comminuted," most demonstrate some basic fracture configurations that allow classification for treatment purposes. Because the vast majority of these fractures are produced by an axial compressive load applied to the heel, the major impact forces are vertical shearing or compression of the calcaneus as it is driven into the wedge-shaped lateral process of the talus. The point of impact on the calcaneus (medial or lateral side) and the position of the calcaneus relative to the talus (supination or pronation) are the major variables determining the particular configuration of fracture lines that develop.[281]

The calcaneus initially fractures into two main fragments, with the primary fracture line running from the plantar aspect dorsalward into the posterior facet of the subtalar joint when viewed from the side. On the axial projection, this primary fracture line runs obliquely from plantar–medial to dorsolateral (Fig. 19-79). Two main fracture fragments, an anteromedial and a posterolateral fragment, are produced.[218,281] As additional compression is applied, comminution occurs, with the formation of secondary fracture lines. Essex-Lopresti[218] identified two commonly occurring patterns of secondary fracture lines that produce two distinct fracture patterns (the tongue type and the joint depression type), each requiring different forms of treatment.

To understand the two patterns of fracture, exact knowledge of the architecture of the calcaneus is required. A strong subcortical strut extends along the lateral border of the posterior facet from the posterior to the anterior margin of the facet joint (see Fig. 19-78). Anteriorly, this cortical strut extends to the beak of the calcaneus and forms an obtuse angle. This is known as the "crucial angle," or Gissane's angle. Immediately above this angle is

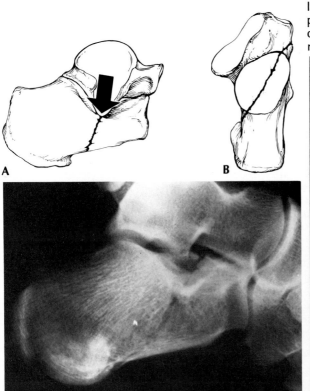

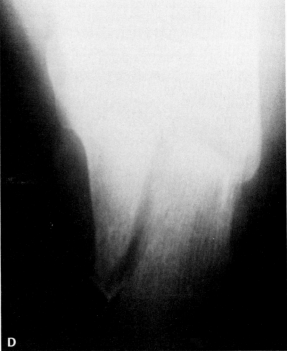

Fig. 19-79. The primary fracture line as seen in the lateral (*A*) and dorsal (*B*) views of the calcaneus, producing two main fracture fragments, anteromedial and posterolateral. Lateral (*C*) and axial (*D*) x-rays show the primary fracture line.

the wedge or spur of the lateral border of the talus. Axial views directly in line with the subtalar joint show the sustentaculum tali as a strong shelf on the medial border of the joint. The anterior facet of the subtalar joint is farther distal and superior to the posterior one. As a result of the downward driving force of the talar wedge, two basic intra-articular fracture patterns of the calcaneus result: the tongue type and the joint depression type. Treatment of the subtalar fracture centers around restoring the normal relationship between the crucial angle and the spur of the talus.

In the tongue type of fracture, the secondary fracture line extends directly posteriorly from the superiormost part of the primary fracture line (at the crucial angle), producing one large posterior, superior, and lateral fragment containing the majority of the posterior articular facet and the dorsal cortex of the tuberosity (Fig. 19-80). This fragment can be displaced because its anterior (articular) portion is driven plantarward and its posterior portion rocks dorsally, "like a seesaw, down at the front and up at the back."[218] Persistent displacement

of this fragment will result in incongruity of the posterior facet. Essex-Lopresti[218] pointed out that with extreme compression, the tongue fragment can be driven down into the body, coming to lie inside its lateral wall.

The other common configuration of the secondary fracture line was called the joint depression type by Essex-Lopresti.[218] It is seen more frequently than the tongue type. This fracture line also begins at the crucial angle and extends posteriorly, but it deviates dorsally to exit the bone just posterior to the articular facet, creating a fragment separate from the tuberosity—the thalamic portion[278]—containing the major portion of the posterior articular facet of the calcaneus (Fig. 19-81). This fragment displaces similarly to the tongue fragment because the anterior portion rotates plantarly and the posterior portion dorsally, resulting again in incongruity of the posterior facet joint as the calcaneal articular surface assumes a more vertical orientation.

Additional fracture lines frequently extend anteriorly to the calcaneocuboid joint as well as

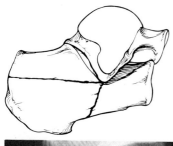 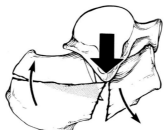

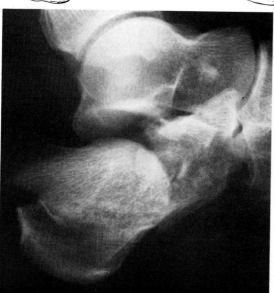

Fig. 19-80. (*Top left*) The secondary fracture line in the tongue type of fracture. (*Top right*) Displacement of the tongue-type fracture fragment producing incongruity of the subtalar joint. (*Bottom*) Lateral x-ray of a displaced tongue type fracture. Note the rotation of the posterior articular facet of the calcaneus.

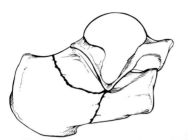 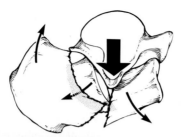

Fig. 19-81. (*Top left*) The secondary fracture line in the joint depression type of fracture. (*Top right*) Displacement of the joint depression fragment producing incongruity of the posterior facet. (*Bottom*) Lateral x-ray of a mildly displaced joint depression fracture. Note mild incongruity of the posterior subtalar joint.

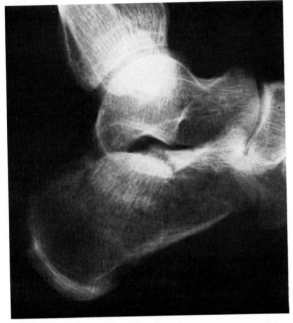

causing incongruity of this articulation. With a single primary fracture line, injury to the calcaneocuboid joint is unlikely, but with either the tongue or joint depression type of injury, extension to the anterior articulation is common and must be looked for on the anteroposterior x-ray of the foot.

The amount of comminution and the degree of displacement of the fracture fragments are directly related to the amount of energy applied to the calcaneus at the moment of impact. With the formation of secondary fracture lines and displacement of the fracture fragments, the body of the calcaneus is compressed and its vertical height is shortened. The body widens, particularly laterally, since the thalamic portion (joint depression or tongue fragment) is compressed inside the lateral wall of the body, resulting in a valgus appearance of the heel and a narrowing of the space between the lateral calcaneus and distal fibula where the peroneal tendons usually lie.

On the medial aspect, the most consistent deformity seen is overriding, medial displacement and persistent rotation of the anteromedial fracture fragment on the posterolateral fragment(s). McReynolds[254] emphasizes that this displacement is the most constant and critical deformity that must be corrected in the surgical management of these fractures.

Knowledge of the basic fracture configurations that occur in calcaneal fractures is helpful in the management of these injuries; however, on occasion comminution and fracture fragment displacement are so severe that, although it may be possible to identify a joint depression or a tongue fragment, the fracture is best designated simply as a comminuted fracture (Fig. 19-82).

With the above description of the basic fracture patterns, intra-articular fractures of the calcaneus can be divided into four separate types to be used as a guide to treatment: nondisplaced, tongue, joint depression, and comminuted.

Signs and Symptoms

As expected, the most common symptom is moderate to severe pain in the heel. Objectively, there is tenderness, swelling, and ecchymosis of the tissue surrounding the calcaneus. Watson-Jones[411] emphasized that ecchymosis extending onto the arch of the foot is pathognomonic of a calcaneal fracture. Blistering of the skin occurs frequently secondary to the severe soft tissue swelling that develops during the first 36 hours after fracture. The normal contour of the heel is distorted with widening and shortening, and a valgus deformity is not uncommon.

Because of the frequently violent mechanisms of injury in this fracture, compression fractures of the lumbar spine occur in 10% of patients,[206] and as many as 70% have associated lower extremity injuries.[276] These associated injuries may be so painful that the patient may not complain of heel pain initially, and all patients who have fallen from a height and sustained spinal or lower extremity injuries should be examined very carefully for calcaneal fractures.

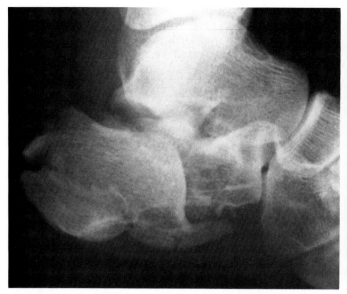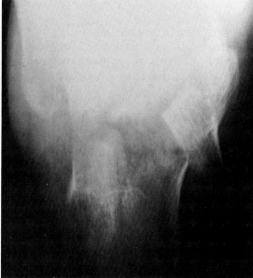

Fig. 19-82. A severely comminuted calcaneal fracture seen in the lateral (*Left*) and axial (*Right*) projections. Note extension of comminution into both the subtalar and calcaneocuboid joints.

Radiographic Findings

A complete radiographic evaluation will be necessary to adequately define the intra-articular fracture problem. A lateral view of the heel will demonstrate both the tongue and joint depression type of fracture patterns and, in particular, will allow the physician to distinguish any incongruity of the posterior facet of the subtalar joint resulting from displacement of one of these fragments. Böhler's tuber angle should be measured on this view and compared to the view of the opposite foot. Böhler[199] correctly pointed out that in the normal calcaneus, the angle may vary from 20° to 40°, and therefore a comparison x-ray of the uninjured foot is necessary to identify the exact degree of deformity on the injured side.[281] As pointed out previously, both Böhler's angle and the congruity of the posterior articular facet should be assessed. These are independent measurements, and an alteration in one does not necessarily imply an alteration in the other.

An axial view of the calcaneus will show the amount of widening of the heel, impingement of the lateral fragment on the peroneal space and the lateral malleolus, the degree of overriding of the superomedial fragment on the posterolateral fragment, and the degree of comminution and displacement of the subtalar fracture fragments. An anteroposterior view of the foot must be obtained to assess the calcaneocuboid and the talonavicular joints, since fracture lines will extend into the anterior body of the calcaneus, deforming the articulation, and severe displacement of calcaneal fractures may be associated with talonavicular subluxation.[280]

To assess fully the degree of joint involvement, the three oblique views described on pages 1763 and 1765 are also essential to complete the radiographic evaluation of these fractures.

Treatment

Cotton,[210] as early as 1908, wrote, "Ordinarily speaking, the man who breaks his heel bone is 'done', so far as his industrial future is concerned." Bankart,[195] 35 years later, wrote, "The results of treatment of crush fractures of the os calcis are rotten. . . . The best result that can be expected from a fracture of the os calcis involving the subastragaloid joint is a completely stiff but painless foot of good shape with a free movement of the ankle joint." Conn[208,209] wrote that fractures of the calcaneus are "serious and disabling injuries in which the end results continue to be incredibly bad." Although over the years this pessimism has diminished, the management of intra-articular, displaced fractures of the calcaneus continues to remain a problem. No ideal method of treatment has been proposed.

There is a great difference of opinion regarding

the treatment of these intra-articular fractures, and each method has its ardent proponents and opponents; there is no one method applicable to the treatment of all these fractures. There are essentially four basic methods of treatment: no reduction and early motion; closed reduction and fixation; open reduction and grafting or internal fixation; and primary arthrodesis. These basic approaches will be reviewed to give the reader some perspective on the difficulties encountered in the management of this fracture.

Treatment without Reduction. Goff[224] stated that as early as 1720 Petit and Desault advised rest until the fragments had consolidated as the ideal form of therapy for fractures of the calcaneus. McLaughlin,[253] Parkes,[263–265] Garcia and Parkes,[396] Lance and colleagues,[246,247] Rowe and colleagues,[272] and Lindsay and Dewar[250] have been ardent proponents of this method. They recommend elevation, compression, and early active motion for all intra-articular fractures. In addition, they have stated that, except in rare instances, this therapeutic regimen has led to satisfactory results. McLaughlin's logical presentation in his book[405] condenses his thoughts most succinctly: the fractures themselves vary greatly as to the amount of comminution, widening of the body, and displacement of the fragments. Furthermore, because of the excellent blood supply of the calcaneus, these fractures always heal, and therefore immobilization of the fracture by either internal or external means is unnecessary. In addition, attempts to maintain reduction of a comminuted intra-articular calcaneal fracture by external or internal means might be likened to "nailing a custard pie to the wall." Immobilization of the calcaneus by internal or external methods does not increase the chance of union, nor does it exert significant hold on the displaced fragments. According to the proponents of the early motion method, cast immobilization leads to scar tissue formation, which results in stiffness. The scar tissue decreases lymphatic and venous drainage, predisposing to chronic swelling. In addition, plaster immobilization decreases the normal pumping action of the calf muscle group, further reducing lymphatic and venous drainage. As a consequence, when the cast is removed, the leg is atrophied and the foot is stiff, swollen, and extremely painful. These factors result in 12 to 16 months of disability, regardless of the excellence of the postreduction x-rays.

The regimen recommended by McLaughlin[253] can be summarized as follows: After a complete x-ray examination has been made, sheet wadding or swathes are placed about the foot, between the toes and up to the level of the knee. An elastic bandage is then applied snugly. The foot of the bed is elevated. Ice bags are applied to both sides of the heel. The patient is kept in a recumbent position and after 24 hours is encouraged to move the foot and ankle, at first under the supervision of a physical therapist who has been instructed previously in this therapeutic regimen. The reasons for the initiation of this therapy are carefully explained to the patient by the orthopaedist, since the patient's cooperation is essential for success. These exercises are carried out hourly during the waking hours. Sufficient sedation is prescribed to alleviate as much of the pain as possible. After 3 to 5 days the pain begins to subside. The compression dressing is replaced with an elastic stocking. The patient is then allowed to dangle his or her legs briefly several times a day for the next 2 days. At the end of the first week, the patient is permitted to be ambulatory on crutches unless extenuating circumstances prevent ambulation. No weight bearing is permitted on the fractured foot. When nonambulatory, the patient is instructed to keep the feet elevated above waist level and continue the exercise program. Thus, pain and swelling subside rapidly, and motion of the foot and ankle is regained. Whirlpool therapy is also initiated.

After 10 to 14 days the patient is fitted with an oxford-style shoe that is well molded about the heel and has a built-in arch support. At the end of 3 weeks the patient is encouraged to rest the foot on the floor and to increase the amount of pressure as pain permits. Between 4 to 8 weeks after the injury the patient is usually bearing full weight, and, by the end of 12 weeks, if the patient is properly motivated, he or she is back at work. Some pain may persist for another 4 to 6 months. However, the patient is encouraged to continue full activity.

Lance and colleagues[246,247] and McLaughlin[253] reported that this form of treatment returned the patient to work in less than half the time of other methods. They recommended that an individually designed arch support be fitted in the shoe. There was no more impairment of push-off function than there was in fractures in which the tuber angle had been restored.

This method of treatment is perhaps best suited for the physician who has little experience with the treatment of intra-articular fractures of the calcaneus. It offers satisfactory results in the majority of patients and indeed may be the preferred method in certain circumstances.

Closed Reduction and Fixation.

Treatment with simple cast immobilization or with early motion and protected weight bearing does not always lead to satisfactory results, particularly in displaced intra-articular calcaneal fractures. Extensive radiographic and anatomical studies of these fractures by a number of surgeons from the 1930s until the present have led to a better understanding of the common patterns of injury that occur. This knowledge of the common forms of fracture displacement has been the basis for recommending more aggressive manipulative and surgical treatment of the displaced intra-articular fractures. The basic goal of this treatment is to restore the anatomical configuration of the fracture fragments, with emphasis placed on (1) restoring congruity of the subtalar joint, (2) restoring Böhler's angle, and (3) restoring the normal width of the calcaneus.

Many different techniques, devices, and "tricks" have been reported in the literature to be used in the closed reduction and fixation of calcaneal fractures. The common steps found in all these methods are disimpaction of the fracture fragments, reduction of the displaced fragments by manual manipulation or with percutaneous pins, and maintenance of reduction with plaster, pin traction, or a combination of pins and plaster. Several of these methods will be reviewed in detail.

Böhler's Method. Böhler's primary objective was to restore the tuber angle to normal and maintain this reduction until bony union occurred. His regimen[199] consisted of the insertion of a Steinmann pin or Kirschner wire transversely through the calcaneal tuberosity, as well as one through the midtibia. Traction and countertraction were then applied. Lateral compression of the calcaneus was achieved by the use of the Böhler clamp (Fig. 19-83) applied under the medial and lateral malleoli. The cast was applied with the pins incorporated in it, and the plaster was then molded well under the medial and lateral malleoli. The foot was held in a neutral position with the cast also well molded under the longitudinal arch. Initial immobilization was maintained for 4 weeks. At that time, the pins were removed and a well-molded short-leg cast was applied for 6 weeks. If the fracture appeared united (as almost invariably it did), a Blucher-type shoe with an individually fitted arch support was prescribed, and gradual full weight bearing was permitted.

Hermann's Method. Hermann[233] modified Böhler's method in 1937. On admission and after proper x-ray examination, the patient was taken promptly to surgery, and, under general or spinal anesthesia and with sterile technique, the foot was placed on a sandbag. A tightly rolled towel was placed on the medial side of the heel just below the medial malleolus. With a heavy wooden Cotton-type mallet, several blows were applied to the heel. The same procedure was carried out on the lateral side. This manuever overcame the widening of the calcaneus and also undoubtedly comminuted the

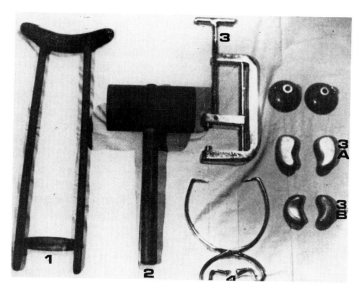

Fig. 19-83. Apparatus used in closed reduction of fractures of the calcaneus. (*1*) The crossbar of the sawed-off crutch is scooped out to fit the sole of the foot. (*2*) The Cotton-type wooden mallet weighs 7 lb. The broad face spreads the force of the blow and prevents contusion of the skin. (*3*) Böhler clamp; only the kidney-shaped lugs (*3A, 3B*) are used. (*4*) Ice tongs. (Aitken, A. P.: Fractures of the Os Calcis–Treatment by Closed Reduction. Clin. Orthop., **30**:70, 1963.)

fracture even more. Ice tongs were then clamped to the tuberosity of the calcaneus. With the knee flexed, downward traction was applied to the calcaneus, with counterpressure provided by the axillary portion of a crutch placed against the plantar surface of the foot at the level of the calcaneocuboid joint. Two small rolls of sheet wadding, one under each malleolus and parallel to the calcaneus, were then applied and held in position by more sheet wadding. The crutch and tongs were then removed, the heel was molded with the aid of a bone clamp to decrease its width, and a short-leg plaster cast was rapidly applied with the foot in equinus to relax the triceps surae muscles. The cast was molded very firmly under each malleolus. Two weeks after reduction the cast was changed and new pressure pads were applied under the malleoli, again with rather firm lateral pressure. Non-weight-bearing plaster immobilization was continued until fracture union occurred, usually in 10 to 12 weeks. The patient was then fitted with a brace, and weight bearing was begun.

Later, Hermann modified his technique by replacing the ice tongs with a Kirschner wire, driven transversely through the body of the calcaneus to effect traction. Giannestras[396] strongly advocated this modified Hermann technique for all displaced, articular fractures but particularly for the tongue type. Under general anesthesia, the patient is placed on the fracture table. Following adequate skin preparation, a 0.045-in diameter Kirschner wire is driven through the calcaneal tuberosity just distal to the superior cortical surface (Fig. 19-84A). Next, the knee is flexed over the knee support of the fracture table at an angle of approximately 70° to 80° in order to relax the triceps surae muscle group. Traction is exerted on the calcaneus through the Kirschner bow to reduce the fracture and reestablish the tuber angle. The heel is then palpated and carefully evaluated. In the normal foot, there is a finger breadth of space between each malleolus and the corresponding cortical surfaces of the calcaneus. In the typical comminuted fracture this space is obliterated. After adequate traction has been applied, lateral and axial x-rays are taken to determine whether the tuber angle has been reestablished, the body width is back within normal limits, and the posterior articular facet is disimpacted.

Several additional steps are carried out, depending on the position of the fragments. If the articular facet is not completely aligned, further traction is applied by exerting sufficient traction on the talocalcaneal interosseous ligament to actually disimpact and slightly separate the fragments (Fig. 19-84B). This step is carried out so that when traction is discontinued, the fragment will settle back into its original bed (Fig. 19-84C). If the width of the calcaneus is not reduced (Fig. 19-84E), compressive force is applied with a sterile Böhler clamp. However, instead of using the small metal pressure applicators, Hermann recommended use of two sterile oval blocks of wood, 10 cm long and 8 cm in circumference at their greatest width and tapering somewhat at each end. These are placed between the malleoli and the Kirschner wire. Careful but adequate compression is applied to reduce the width of the calcaneal body (Fig. 19-84F). Sterile dressings are then applied over the puncture incisions. The foot and leg are wrapped with a thin layer of sheet wadding. Two small rolls of sheet wadding of appropriate size are applied between the wire and the malleoli. The cast is applied about the foot and ankle, and mild compression is applied to the heel of the cast in the area overlying the rolls of sheet wadding. Traction is then released, and a long-leg cast is applied to extend to the midthigh with the foot in a neutral position and the knee in 35° of flexion. The wire is incorporated into the cast. At the end of 3 weeks, the cast and Kirschner wire are removed, and a new, well-molded, long-leg cast is applied for 1 to 3 weeks more, depending on the comminution of the fracture as well as its radiographic appearance when the first cast is removed.

The postreduction therapeutic regimen is just as important as the reduction and immobilization. The patient is instructed how to apply the pressure bandage after the cast is removed; a 3-inch elastic bandage is applied snugly before the patient gets out of bed. He is instructed in the performance of hourly active exercises of the foot, each one performed five times up to the maximum amount of pain tolerance. These are flexion and extension of the foot and ankle as well as eversion and inversion of the hind foot. For 4 weeks he also receives whirlpool therapy for the foot, 15 minutes daily.

No weight bearing is permitted until there is definite radiographic evidence of union. The patient is then fitted with a snug, heavy-duty elastic stocking that extends to the knee. He wears this during his waking hours. He also wears a well-fitted, rigid-shanked oxford shoe with a custom-fitted arch support.

Arnesen's Method. The principles of traction and manipulation to achieve reduction were employed by Arnesen[193] in an extension of the Böhler and Hermann methods. In addition to the transverse

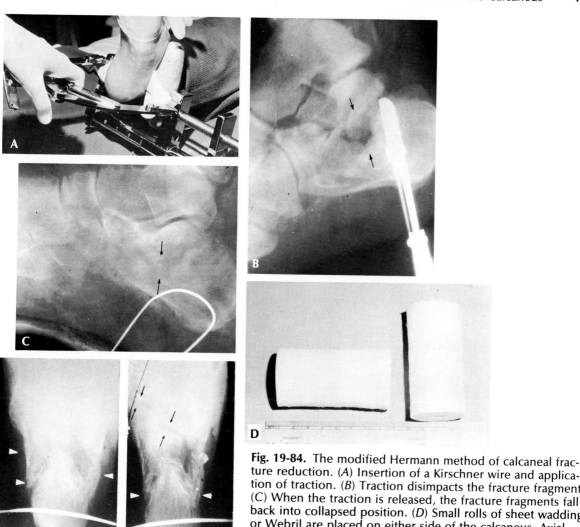

Fig. 19-84. The modified Hermann method of calcaneal fracture reduction. (*A*) Insertion of a Kirschner wire and application of traction. (*B*) Traction disimpacts the fracture fragments. (*C*) When the traction is released, the fracture fragments fall back into collapsed position. (*D*) Small rolls of sheet wadding or Webril are placed on either side of the calcaneus. Axial view before reduction (*E*) and after traction (*F*) and the application of medial–lateral compression, narrowing the heel and improving the alignment of the subtalar joint. (After Giannestras, N. J.: Foot Disorders: Medical and Surgical Management, 2nd ed. Philadelphia, Lea & Febiger, 1973.)

calcaneal traction pin, Arnesen placed a second wire transversely through the base of the metatarsals to apply traction in a line parallel to them These traction forces were combined with manual manipulation to achieve fracture reduction. Reduction was maintained by continued skeletal traction on the pins for 5 weeks, followed by another 5 to 7 weeks of non-weight-bearing plaster immobilization.

Essex-Lopresti's Method. Essex-Lopresti[218] was the first to clearly distinguish between the two most common types of displaced intra-articular calcaneal fractures: the tongue type and the joint depression type. He believed that this distinction was critical because a different method of treatment should be employed for each type: closed reduction with the aid of an axial percutaneous pin for the tongue type, and open reduction for the joint depression type. Although much controversy exists in the literature over the proper management of displaced intra-articular calcaneal fractures, significant support can be found for the Essex-Lopresti technique in tongue type fractures.[228] Although King[243] advocates a trial of this technique for joint depression

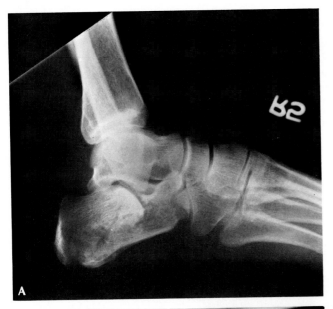

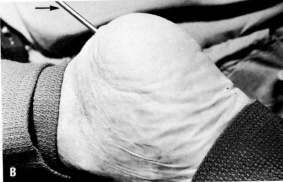

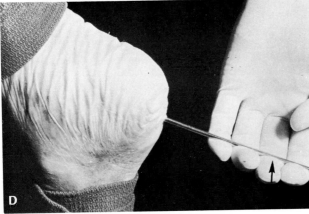

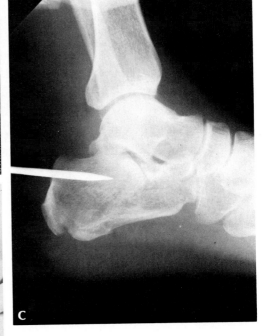

Fig. 19-85. (*A*) Tongue-type fracture of the calcaneus. (*B*) A heavy Steinmann pin is drilled into the tongue fragment in a longitudinal direction, angled to the lateral side. (*C*) X-ray showing proper placement of the pin before attempted reduction. (*D*) With the knee flexed 90°, a lifting force is applied to the free end of the pin.

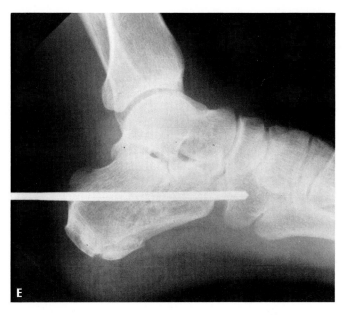

Fig. 19-85 (*Continued*). (*E*) After reduction the pin is drilled across the primary fracture line into the anterior portion of the calcaneus to maintain the reduction. If there is comminution of the anterior calcaneus, the pin should be driven into the cuboid.

fractures as well, most authors do not believe that this is an effective way to reduce joint depression injury.[218,228,278]

The Essex-Lopresti technique for tongue type fractures (Fig. 19-85*A*) is easy to perform, allows good reduction of the posterior articular facet, and provides a means of adequate fracture fixation when combined with a non-weight-bearing plaster cast. It is carried out as follows: The patient, properly anesthetized, is placed in the prone position on the table. Under sterile technique, a 1-cm incision is made over the displaced tuberosity of the calcaneus, just lateral to the insertion of the Achilles tendon (Fig. 19-85*B*). A heavy Steinmann pin is introduced into the tongue fragment in a longitudinal direction, angling slightly to the lateral side. X-rays are taken in both the lateral and axial planes at this time to determine the position of the pin. The pin should be well into the tongue fragment but not across the fracture site (Fig. 19-85*C*). The fracture is reduced by lifting upward on the pin until the knee is lifted off the table. With this maneuver, the facet fragment is reduced and brought up into position (Fig. 19-85*D*). At times there is an audible click as the fragment snaps back into place. At this point, the pin and foot are held in position by the assistant in preparation for reduction of the spreading of the calcaneus. King[243] recommends grasping the heel between the palms, which squeezes the displaced lateral wall into the fragment for added support. Axial x-rays are next obtained in order to determine whether accurate diminution

of the width of the calcaneus has taken place. The pin is then advanced across the fracture into the anterior fragment of the calcaneus (Fig. 19-85*E*). Essex-Lopresti recommended applying a slipper cast incorporating the pin for 2 weeks and maintaining the patient at absolute bed rest for 2 weeks. The theoretical advantage of the slipper cast is to allow early active range of motion of the subtalar joint. Some authors[243] believe that the slipper cast does not provide adequate stability and will allow collapse of the fracture. They recommend incorporation of the pin in a short-leg non-weight-bearing cast for 4 to 6 weeks. The pin is removed at 6 weeks, and the fracture is protected in another short-leg cast without weight bearing until clinically and radiographically healed—usually 10 to 12 weeks after fracture. Following healing, progressive weight bearing and active range of motion exercises of the ankle and subtalar joints are instituted.

Open Reduction. Techniques of closed or percutaneous pin manipulation described in the previous section are but a sample of a vast array of similar methods described in the literature to achieve reduction of displaced intra-articular calcaneal fractures without extensive surgical intervention. Often, however, particularly with a joint depression type of fracture, these closed methods have not been successful in restoring congruity of the subtalar joint or in producing a painless functional foot after the fracture has healed. Proponents of open reduction[191,228,232,255,256,257,262,278,287] correctly insist that direct manipulation of a joint depression fragment is the only means of achieving reduction of the posterior facet—an essential first step in restoring function of the subtalar joint.

Essex-Lopresti's Method. Essex-Lopresti[218] recommended an oblique lateral incision extending from the tip of the lateral malleolus anteriorly along the upper border of the calcaneus. With blunt dissection the depressed fragment is found rotated and displaced inside the lateral wall of the calcaneus. The fragment is elevated and rotated back into place and then transfixed with an axial pin placed through the tuberosity, just as in the technique used with the tongue type of fracture.

Palmer's Method. Palmer[262] described a technique of open reduction and bone grafting that gained extensive popularity after its publication in 1948. He credited Lenormant and Wilmoth[248] for the original description of this method. Maxfield[255,256] enthusiastically endorsed this technique and reviewed 40 patients so treated. Through a lateral, slightly curved incision beginning at the sinus tarsi and extending posteriorly to the calcaneal tuberosity, the peroneal tendons are identified, their sheath is opened, and the tendons are dislocated anteriorly to facilitate exposure. Care must be taken to protect the branches of the sural nerve. The foot is placed on a roll and inverted to expose the fracture site. Reduction is achieved by traction on the tuberosity and direct manipulation of the depressed fracture fragment. First, a transverse wire is placed through the tuberosity and traction is applied to disimpact the fragments. The central depressed fragment is then rotated upward to make the posterior facet surfaces congruent. A large bony defect is thus created inferior to the fragment, and the defect must be filled with an iliac crest bone graft to provide support for the articular fragment and prevent redisplacement when the traction is released. Postoperatively a short-leg non-weight-bearing cast is worn for 12 weeks.

Allan[191] endorsed open reduction and bone grafting for displaced intra-articular fractures, emphasizing the importance of restoring the step-off between the anteromedial and the posterolateral fragments (Fig. 19-86). Soeur and Remy[278] recommended a similar approach, emphasizing careful restoration of subtalar joint congruity. They recommended fixing the fracture fragments with multiple small Kirschner wires and did not recommend bone grafting. Hazlett[232] has recommended screw fixation of the reduced joint depression fragment to the anteromedial calcaneal fragment.

McReynolds's Method. A very different approach has been advocated by McReynolds for many years.[254] He contends that "the deformity of medial displacement, overriding, and rotation of the superomedial fragment is the most constant and significant deformity" in displaced intra-articular fractures of the calcaneus. He recommends a slightly oblique medial surgical approach, 5 to 7.5 cm long, in line with the long axis of the tuberosity. The rotated superomedial fragment is identified and rotated back into place and fixed with a special staple, restoring the integrity of the medial cortex. On occasion he finds it necessasry to manipulate separate lateral fragments of the subtalar articulation back into place with an elevator introduced through the fracture line of the medial cortex (Fig. 19-87).

● ● ●

The techniques of open reduction and fixation with or without bone grafting are technically demanding and often frustrating because of the extensive comminution that can be present. Before embarking on these approaches, the reader is encouraged to become very familiar with the original articles on the subject to minimize the complications and frustrations that may occur.

Primary Arthrodesis. Primary arthrodesis, that is, arthrodesis performed within 1 week after the injury, has been recommended by a number of investigators, the most ardent of whom have been Pennal and Yadav,[266] Harris,[229,230] Thompson,[279] Dick,[215] and Wilson.[290]

The technique described here was first reported by Hall and Pennal[226] in 1960. The procedure is performed 7 to 10 days after the fracture occurs, when the initial swelling and bleb formation have subsided. When the patient is admitted to the hospital, the foot and leg are elevated and kept at absolute rest. A firm pressure dressing and ice packs are applied and maintained until the patient is taken to surgery. The patient is in the prone position. A Steinmann pin is placed transversely through the posterosuperior part of the calcaneal tuberosity (Fig. 19-88). Another pin is placed transversely through the tibial shaft at the junction of the middle and distal thirds. Distraction is applied with the use of a Roger Anderson apparatus. This corrects any varus or valgus deformity, maintains accurate reduction, and permits subsequent visualization of the subtalar joint. Gallie's[220] posterior approach, lateral to the tendo calcaneus, is used. The articular surfaces of the calcaneus and talus are gouged out, and a trough 2 cm wide and 3 cm deep is cut across both bones. It is filled by two

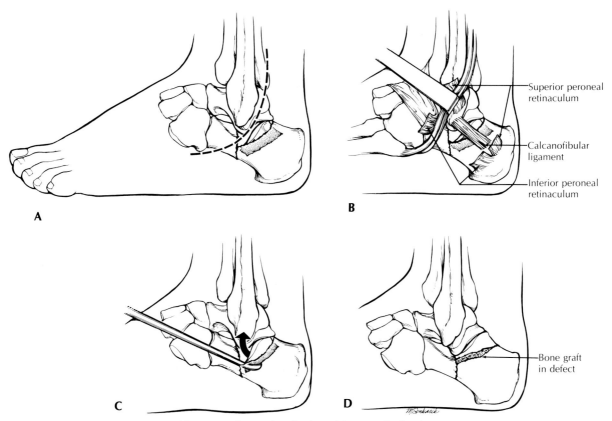

Fig. 19-86. Open reduction and bone grafting of a displaced intra-articular fracture of the calcaneus. (*A*) The posterolateral incision. (*B*) The peroneal tendons are retracted anteriorly after incision of the peroneal retinaculum. The calcaneofibular ligament is identified, detached distally, and reflected superiorly to expose the fracture. (*C*) The posterior facet is realigned with a periosteal elevator placed in the fracture site. (*D*) The defect created by replacing the facet is bone grafted. (From Allan, J. H.: The Open Reduction of Fractures of the Os Calcis. Ann. Surg., **141**:897, 1955.)

corticocancellous grafts placed vertically, cortex to cortex, with the cancellous surface of the grafts against the cancellous surfaces of the talus and the calcaneus. The lateral spreading of the calcaneus is corrected manually. X-rays are taken to check position of the calcaneus and the grafts; the tourniquet is released, and bleeding is controlled. The soft tissues are closed, and a cast extending from the toes to the knee is applied with the pins incorporated in the cast. The patient is permitted up on crutches within 1 week. At 4 to 6 weeks the cast is changed, and at 8 weeks a walking heel is applied. By 12 weeks union is usually solid; the cast is removed, and active full weight bearing is permitted. Pennal and Yadav[266] reported 75% excellent and very good results. Harris[230] wrote, "In all but insignificant fractures of the os calcis, fusion

of the subtalar joint will be necessary . . . The time-saving procedure is immediate reduction of the fracture by skeletal traction and compression, followed within 3 or 4 weeks by subtalar fusion by Gallie's technique."

Thompson[279] recommended primary triple arthrodesis of the talonavicular, talocalcaneal, and calcaneocuboid joints. He believed that this three-joint complex is a single unit in motion and, therefore, that fusion of the subtalar joint alone is insufficient, particularly since there is unrecognized damage to the other joints, especially the calcaneocuboid, in a majority of patients.

Author's Preferred Method

The many factors listed in the next section on prognosis undoubtedly influence the results of dis-

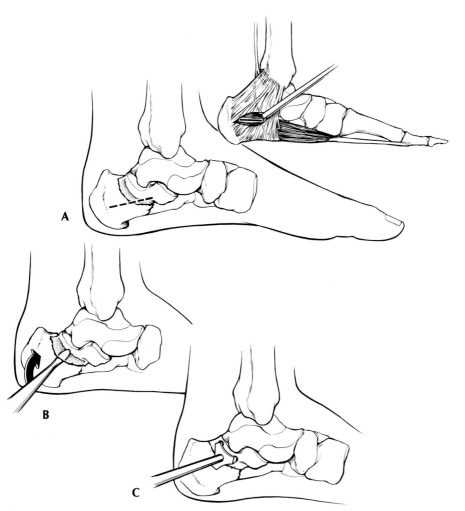

Fig. 19-87. McReynold's medial approach for open reduction and internal fixation of displaced intra-articular calcaneal fractures. (*A*) Medial longitudinal skin incision. Care is taken to protect the medial calcaneal nerve (*insert*). (*B*) Once the fracture site is exposed by denuding a portion of the medial cortical surface of the calcaneus, an elevator is inserted into the fracture site to mobilize the superomedial fragment and elevate any impacted, rotated articular fragments. The heel is then compressed to reduce its width, and the reduced medial wall is fixed (*C*) with a special staple placed in drill holes. (McReynolds, I. S.: The Case for Operative Treatment of Fractures of the Os Calcis. *In* Leach, R. E.; Hoaglund, F. T.; and Riseborough, E. J. (eds.): Controversies in Orthopaedic Surgery, p. 250. Philadelphia, W. B. Saunders, 1982.)

placed intra-articular calcaneal fractures. Many other, unknown variables are also important and await elucidation with further study. Because of the great variability in fracture patterns that leads to difficulty in classification and separation of fracture types, because of the great variety of techniques available for treatment, because of the prolonged recovery time occasionally needed for resumption of activities following this injury, and because of the lack

of prospective, controlled studies of the different treatment methods, it is very difficult to draw definitive conclusions about the results of treatment and recommend one specific treatment program for all displaced, intra-articular calcaneal fractures. Below is outlined my preferred method of treatment of these injuries.

All fractures are initially treated by strict bed rest, elevation, and a compression dressing until the

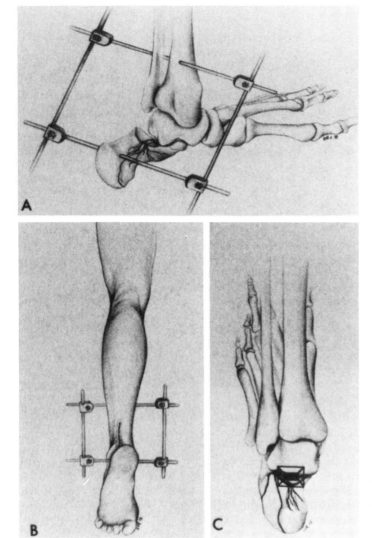

Fig. 19-88. Subtalar arthrodesis. (*A*) Placement of pins through the lower tibia and os calcis permits distraction of the subtalar joint, facilitating open reduction or arthrodesis. (*B*) With the patient prone, distraction is applied through the apparatus; the incision is made just lateral to the tendo Achillis. (*C*) A rectangular slot is cut in adjacent surfaces of the talus and os calcis into which corticocancellous slabs are inserted. (Pennal, G. F., and Yadav, M. P.: Operative Treatment of Comminuted Fractures of the Os Calcis. Orthop. Clin. North Am., 4:200, 1973.)

acute swelling has subsided. Sometimes this requires 5 to 6 days of hospitalization. Nondisplaced fractures and symmetrical joint depression fractures with a mild or moderate decrease in Böhler's tuber angle are treated by early mobilization, avoidance of weight bearing with crutches for approximately 6 weeks, and then progressive weight bearing. Displaced tongue-type fractures are treated by the method of Essex-Lopresti,[218] with the pin being left in place 6 weeks. I have used the slipper cast with good success in allowing early restitution of active ankle and subtalar motion. After the slipper cast is applied, a removable posterior plaster short-leg splint is also applied. The patient can remove the splint three times a day for joint exercises and then replace the foot in the splint when not exercising

for comfort and to prevent ankle equinus and loss of fracture reduction. Displaced joint depression fractures and severely comminuted fractures have been treated by closed reduction and early mobilization. Closed reduction is simply designed to compress the heel and minimize the residual excessive widening. Occasional attempts to use an "Essex-Lopresti" pin to manipulate a central depressed bone fragment have been uniformly unsuccessful in my hands.

Prognosis

In 1964 Lance and colleagues[247] reviewed 227 intra-articular calcaneal fractures treated over a 26-year period and concluded that the best treatment for all types of intra-articular fractures was a compression bandage and early active range of motion. Nonoperative treatment was employed in the majority of their patients, and although only 55% had excellent or good results at follow-up, these results were better than in the patients treated by a combination of operative measures. Lindsay and Dewar[250] reviewed 147 patients 8 years after they sustained displaced intra-articular fractures and found that 76% of the patients treated conservatively had good results while only 60% who underwent primary or late arthrodesis had good results. Of their conservatively treated patients, 81% without reduction had a good result while only 72% of those treated with closed reduction eventually had a good result. Thoren[281] reviewed 156 cases of fracture and concluded that with no or moderate displacement, early mobilization gave the best results, while in fractures with severe displacement of the posterior facet "an open reduction may give a better result, but in these cases early physiotherapy also can give sufficiently good results to warrant its use instead of the operative treatment." Parkes,[264,265] as well as many others, continues to advocate this treatment method.

Open reduction and fixation with or without grafting of the malaligned posterior facet of the subtalar joint can be supported by a number of retrospective reviews of these techniques. All 23 of the patients recorded by Palmer[262] returned to work 8 months after open reduction and bone grafting of the fracture. He reported only one "failure" secondary to loss of subtalar motion. Maxfield and McDermott[257] reported 68% excellent or good results with the technique in 19 patients. McReynolds,[254] using his medial approach, reported 64% good or excellent results in over 90 patients. Soeur and Remy,[278] using internal Kirschner wire fixation, reported that approximately 85% of their patients returned to work with minimal or no long-term problems. Reduction and fixation of tongue-type fractures using the Essex-Lopresti technique produced 80% good results in his hands and 83% in the small series so treated by Hammesfahr and Fleming.[228] Both reports indicated improved results when reduction of the displaced tongue fragment was achieved.

Primary (within 1 month of fracture) arthrodesis of the subtalar joint has been reported to have good results in from 51% to 100% of cases.[215,220,222,226,229,230,250,290] Primary triple arthrodesis was reported by Thompson[279] to produce excellent or good results in 53 of 56 patients with fractures.

This brief and very incomplete sampling of results reported in the treatment of intra-articular calcaneal fractures reflects the controversial nature of the problem. The numbers and percentages of success are generally not comparable, since there has been great inconsistency in defining results both anatomically and functionally. Some factors clearly are important determinants of outcome, however. They are discussed below.

Degree of Displacement. Nondisplaced intra-articular fractures fare better than displaced fractures. Early mobilization with protection from weight bearing until fracture union occurs will result in good function and early return to preinjury activity in the vast majority of these patients.[246]

The most crucial measure of displacement is the degree of congruity of the posterior articular facet. Thoren,[281] in an extensive review of the subject, found that the degree of subtalar incongruity (measured as none, moderate, or considerable) is more important than any other measurement, including the tuber angle, in determining the prognosis of these injuries. Hammesfahr and Fleming[228] also suggested that there is a positive correlation between the degree of facet reduction and a successful treatment outcome. Indeed, they emphasized that aggressive reduction of joint incongruity, combined with avoidance of weight bearing until fracture union occurs, can result in a good prognosis for intra-articular calcaneal fractures, contradicting the pessimism of early authors such as McLaughlin, Cotton, and others.[210,253]

Decreased Tuber Angle. It should be emphasized that a decreased tuber angle does not always correspond to incongruity of the posterior articular facet. The facet may be *symmetrically* depressed into the body of the calcaneus and not rotated, leading to a decrease in the tuber angle but not to facet incongruity. In these cases[221,228] good results can occur without surgical correction of the tuber angle. It has been previously argued[199,233] that if the tuber angle is not restored, the patient's gait will be impaired because of the relative shortening of the triceps surae; however, the more important factor appears to be incongruity of the subtalar joint. Persistent, severe decrease (0° or less) of the tuber angle has been associated with poor long-term results, while minor persistent changes in the angle do not always correlate with a bad outcome.[281]

Patient Age. Essex-Lopresti[218] recommended that patients over 50 years of age not be treated as aggressively as younger patients. Vestad[283] concluded that patients under the age of 50 had better results after open reduction and fixation, and he too recommended that most patients over 50 be treated with early mobilization.

Degree of Fracture Comminution. Occasionally (5% to 15%)[218,247] displaced intra-articular fractures are so severely comminuted that they are not amenable to surgical treatment. The fracture will unite, but the severe residual distortion virtually always produces persistent problems for the patient.

Premature Weight Bearing. Virtually all studies emphasize the importance of lack of weight bearing until fracture union occurs (6 to 12 weeks after injury). Certainly in those cases of reduction and fixation, early lack of weight bearing is important to prevent redisplacement of the fracture fragments, but it appears that all patients fare better if protected from weight bearing until fracture union occurs.

Manipulation and Surgical Treatment. In certain displaced intra-articular calcaneal fractures, operative intervention seems indicated. The most significant effect of operative intervention is seen with displaced, minimally comminuted, tongue-type fractures in which the tongue is reduced and the subtalar joint alignment is restored, whether by open or percutaneous pin techniques.[228] In joint depression fractures the positive effects of operative intervention are less well documented. Although Palmer[262] reported good to excellent results in over 80% of his patients so treated, other surgeons have reported less success.[257,283] The best results of open reduction and internal fixation are in those fractures with minimal comminution.[266]

The major complication of operative or pin fixation treatment has been infection of the operative site or pin tract infection. Infection in this region is particularly hard to manage and has been one of the major factors discouraging operative intervention. Proper, effective open reduction, internal fixation, and grafting demand a lucid understanding of the fracture patterns that can occur. As with any surgical procedure, the success rate will improve with the surgeon's experience. The results of surgical treatment of this fracture will not be very good if performed only rarely, and the surgeon should have extensive experience with the fracture before independently embarking on surgical treatment.

Complications

Fracture union is not a significant problem in the calcaneus. Most long-term complications result from malunion of the fracture fragments. Recovery is often slow. Regardless of the type of treatment, most authors recommend avoidance of weight bearing for 8 to 12 weeks following fracture. After weight bearing is begun, several months may be required to maximize recovery. Eighteen months was identified by Lindsay and Dewar[250] as the minimum time necessary before stabilization of the patient's symptoms occurs, and they found some patients at 10 years follow-up who were continuing to improve. Therefore, major surgical treatment of residual symptoms should be deferred until it is certain that the patient's rehabilitation has plateaued. Often, the working person can be returned to gainful employment despite some residual symptoms at 4 to 6 months after fracture with the use of an ankle–foot orthosis. A double upright patellar tendon–bearing (or calf lacer) brace with a free ankle joint and a cushioned heel will provide enough protection to allow a return to work. The orthosis must be worn only at work, however, so that strength and motion are not lost.

Other Problems: Sources of Pain. Many different factors are responsible for persistent long-term symptoms following a calcaneal fracture.[196,197,214,237,274,253] It is important to know the basic differential diagnosis of pain following calcaneal fractures so that appropriate therapy can be undertaken.

Subtalar Joint Pain. Limited motion secondary to scarring and post-traumatic arthritis can both result from calcaneal fractures (Fig. 19-89). These complications occur more frequently with displaced intra-articular fractures and less frequently when the displaced fractures are reduced after injury. Progressive degenerative arthritis of the subtalar joint presents as pain on weight bearing, is aggravated by inversion and eversion of the foot, and usually is referred to the region of the sinus tarsi. The source of pain can frequently be identified by injection of a local anesthetic agent into the joint. At times injection is difficult to perform because of the narrowing and distortion of the joint. The best access is through the area of the sinus tarsi, using x-ray control. If the injection relieves the patient's pain, the subtalar joint is its likely source. A further helpful diagnostic aid is immobilization in a short-leg walking cast for 2 to 3 weeks. If motion of the arthritic subtalar joint is the cause of the pain, plaster immobilization should give good relief. Definitive treatment can then be undertaken with an ankle–foot orthosis or a surgical arthrodesis of the arthritic joint(s). Some authors[215,220,226,230,241] have indicated that isolated subtalar arthrodesis—the Gallie procedure—is adequate treatment for this complication. Care must be taken, however, to be certain that symptoms are limited to the subtalar joint and that there is no significant degenerative arthritis of the calcaneocuboid or talonavicular joints. When these are involved, a triple arthrodesis should be performed.

Peroneal Tendonitis. A second cause of persistent pain is stenosing tenovaginitis of the peroneal tendons with or without frank dislocation of the tendons anteriorly. The tendons, at the time of fracture, are compressed against the fibula as the calcaneus widens and displaces laterally. Failure to restore the length and alignment of the calcaneus will result in permanent impingement on the tendons and the tip of the fibula itself. Relief of pain following injection of the peroneal tendon sheath with a local anesthetic confirms the diagnosis. A peroneal tenogram will demonstrate the impingement and compression of the tendons (Fig. 19-90). Symptoms of pain or instability (as a result of an anterior subluxation of the tendons) respond well to surgical excision of the excessive bone of the lateral calcaneus and rerouting of the tendons behind the malleolus.[214]

Bone Spur. A third source of pain is a plantar heel spur resulting from malunion of the fracture and disruption of the fat pad of the heel. The loss of the protective function of the heel fat pad results in excessive weight bearing directly on the bone, and any bony prominence can become painful with an overlying tender callus. Treatment should be conservative whenever possible with a pressure-relieving heel pad and cushioned heels in the shoe. Surgical excision of the bone spur should be undertaken only as a last resort.[253]

Arthritis of the Calcaneocuboid Joint. Degenerative

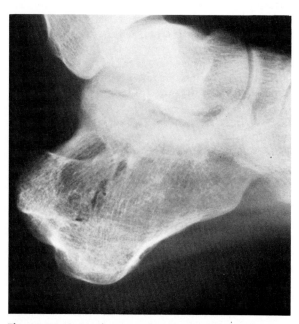

Fig. 19-89. Lateral x-ray of post-traumatic arthritis of the subtalar joint 2 years after an unreduced intra-articular tongue-type fracture of the calcaneus.

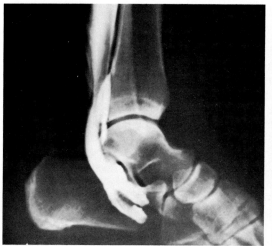 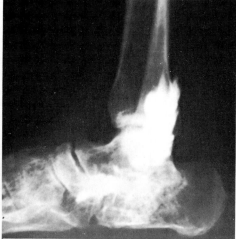

Fig. 19-90. (*Left*) Tendon sheaths of the peroneus longus and brevis tendons are well delineated in a normal foot. (*Right*) The tendons are trapped by the calcaneus, or the sheaths are scarred down. The tenogram is abnormal. (After Giannestras, N. J.: Foot Disorders: Medical and Surgical Management, 2nd ed. Philadelphia, Lea & Febiger, 1973.)

arthritis of the calcaneocuboid joint occasionally is the major source of pain following a calcaneal fracture. Disruption of this joint is usually associated with subluxation of the talonavicular joint as well. Injections of a local anesthetic will help pinpoint the source of pain. On occasion local steroid injections can give significant symptomatic relief. Surgical treatment should be a triple arthrodesis, even if the majority of the symptoms are limited to the calcaneocuboid joint, because of the high likelihood of occult subtalar and talonavicular arthritis.

Nerve Entrapment. Rarely, entrapment of the medial or lateral plantar branches of the posterior tibial nerve or the sural nerve laterally can result from soft tissue scarring following calcaneal fracture. Careful neurolysis may help if conservative measures do not work.

DISLOCATION OF THE CALCANEUS

Dislocation of the calcaneus from both the cuboid and talar articulations is exceedingly rare; only eight cases have been encountered in the literature.[204,227,284] Both violent trauma and moderate twisting forces have been described as causing the dislocation, in which the calcaneus is displaced primarily laterally (Fig. 19-91). In all but one case reported in the literature, stable reduction was achieved by closed means under anesthesia. Immobilization from 6 to 9 weeks in a short-leg cast allowed adequate healing and resulted in a stable, functional foot.

Viswanath and Shephard[284] reported on a patient with an irreducible calcaneal dislocation that required open reduction through a lateral incision. Persistent instability followed the open reduction, necessitating pin fixation across the calcaneocuboid joint. Although this patient at 2 years after injury had a residual varus deformity of the heel and a limp, other authors report no long-term sequelae following reduction of this dislocation.

INJURIES OF THE MIDTARSAL REGION

ANATOMY

The midpart of the foot is relatively rigid, with only a moderate amount of motion occurring through its joints. The lateral side of the midfoot is more stable than the medial side, which is more dynamic and mobile. The plantar ligaments, reinforced by multiple tendons inserting into the plantar aspect of the midfoot, secure the midfoot much more strongly than do the dorsal ligaments.[305] The primary articulation in this region is the midtarsal (Chopart's or transverse tarsal) joint, which is the integration of the motion of the talonavicular and calcaneocuboid joints. As described in the section on biomechanics, this joint is mobile when the heel is pronated and relatively fixed when the heel is supinated. The cuboid, extending to the fourth and fifth metatarsal bases, acts as a linkage across the three naviculocuneiform joints, allowing only minimal motion to occur. This configuration of multiple constrained joints minimizes susceptibility to injury, which is reflected in the small number of injuries reported to occur in this region. Furthermore, when injury does occur, more than one structure is frequently involved, and many fracture–dislocation patterns have been reported in the literature. Although isolated fractures, dislocations, and sprains can occur, the clinician must search carefully for associated injuries in the region whenever an apparently isolated injury is identified.

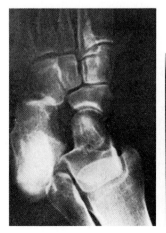
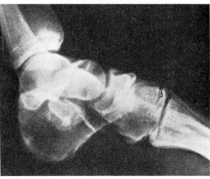

Fig. 19-91. (*Left*) Anteroposterior and (*right*) lateral x-rays of a dislocation of the calcaneus. (Viswanath, S. S., and Shephard, E.: Dislocation of the Calcaneum. Injury, 9:51, 1978.)

In this section, I will review injuries of the midtarsal joint and fractures of the navicular, the cuboid, and the cuneiforms.

RADIOGRAPHIC FINDINGS

X-ray evaluation of the region is often difficult because of overlap and superimposition of the bones.[318] It is important to obtain comparison x-rays of the opposite uninjured foot when injury of the midtarsal joint is suspected. Anteroposterior, lateral, and oblique views should be obtained, and each bone and its articulations (remember that all the bones in the midfoot articulate with at least four other bones[350]) should be inspected. On the anteroposterior projection, the navicular should overlap slightly the three cuneiforms to an equal degree. The alignment of the metatarsals should be checked to be certain there is no rotational malalignment or gap between them. In the lateral view the cuneiforms should be superimposed and lie in direct line with the navicular. The metatarsal shafts should be parallel, with the first metatarsal being the most dorsal.[318] Eichenholtz and Levine emphasize that frequently navicular body fractures are only seen on the lateral projection.[299] At times, when diagnosis is uncertain, tomography may aid in the diagnosis of injuries in the midtarsal region.

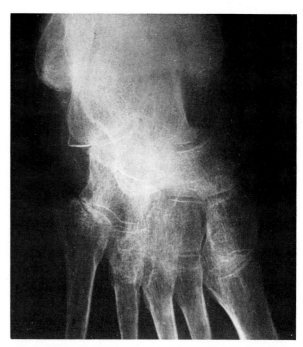

Fig. 19-92. Medial fracture–subluxation of the midtarsal joint. (Main, B. J. and Jowett, R. L.: Injuries of the Midtarsal Joint. J. Bone Joint Surg., **57B:**89, 1975.)

INJURIES OF THE MIDTARSAL JOINTS

CLASSIFICATION AND MECHANISM OF INJURY

Main and Jowett,[312] in an extensive review of 71 midtarsal joint injuries, identified five patterns of injury (which generally describe the direction in which the injury force is applied and the consequent direction of deformity, when present) based on the presumed mechanism of injury, the extent of injury, and the direction of displacement of the forefoot: medial, longitudinal, lateral, plantar, and crush. Within each group, sprains, fractures, dislocations, subluxations, or any combination of these injuries may be found.

Medial Stress Injury

Medial stress injuries were most commonly seen in the series by Main and Jowett (30%). Most were sprains of the midtarsal joint caused by inversion of the foot. In addition, fracture subluxation or dislocation of the joint may be found (Fig. 19-92). Hooper and McMaster[307] reported the only case of bilateral, recurrent midtarsal subluxation occurring after moderate injury with the forefoot subluxated in inversion and severe equinus at the midtarsal joint.

Seven cases of a variant of a medial subtalar dislocation (termed the *medial swivel dislocation*) were also found by Main and Jowett.[312] In this injury, a medially directed force dislocates the talonavicular joint, leaves the calcaneocuboid joint intact, and subluxates (but does not dislocate) the subtalar joint. The calcaneus does not invert as in a medial subtalar dislocation but apparently rotates on the interosseous talocalcaneal ligament, without tearing it (Fig. 19-93).

Longitudinal Stress Injury

Longitudinal forces were responsible for 41% of the midtarsal injuries reported by Main and Jowett.[312] Injuries of this type are usually severe, with a high incidence of associated fracture and significant residual displacement of the fracture fragments. In Main and Jowett's series of 24 displaced fractures, 18 patients had fair or poor results at long-term follow-up.

These injuries occur with the foot in varying degrees of plantarflexion, with the force being

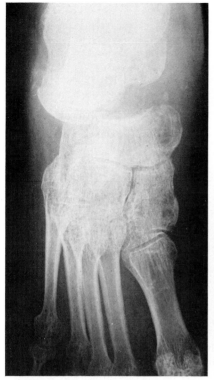
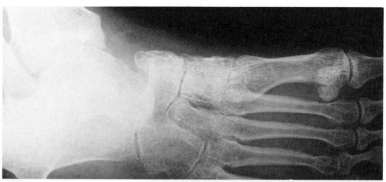
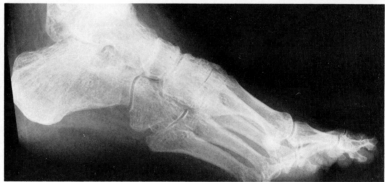

Fig. 19-93. Medial swivel dislocation of the midfoot. (*Left*) Anteroposterior view shows dislocation of the talonavicular joint and medial rotation of the calcaneus. (*Top right*) The calcaneocuboid joint remains intact. (*Bottom right*) Lateral view of the ankle shows rotational subluxation but not dislocation of the subtalar joint. (Main, B. J. and Jowett, R. L.: Injuries of the Midtarsal Joint. J. Bone Joint Surg., **57B**:90,1975.)

applied to the metatarsal heads and transmitted proximally along the rays to disrupt the midtarsal joint and fracture the cuboid or the navicular. With this mechanism, fractures tend to occur vertically through the navicular in line with the intercuneiform joints (Fig. 19-94).

Lateral Stress Injury

Lateral stress injuries occur less frequently (17%). The characteristic feature of these injuries is crushing of the cuboid or anterior calcaneus as the forefoot is driven laterally.[236] Avulsion fractures of the navicular tuberosity are seen frequently, and the navicular may subluxate laterally on the talar head.

Dewar and Evans[294] reported five such cases and emphasized that the injury is frequently misdiagnosed as an ankle sprain. They recommend early calcaneocuboid arthrodesis to restore midtarsal alignment and prevent persistent symptomatic subluxation and flat foot deformity. Stark,[320] on the other hand, presented one case treated effectively by closed reduction and casting. Hermel and Gershon-Cohen[304] presented five similar cases of cuboid fracture and appropriately applied the term *nutcracker fracture* to this injury. The mechanism of injury was similar in all cases, with crushing of the cuboid between the calcaneus and the bases of the fourth and fifth metatarsals (Fig. 19-95). Subluxation of the midtarsal joint was frequent, and four of the five patients sustained avulsion fractures of the navicular tuberosity.

Plantar Stress Injury

Plantarly directed forces applied to the forefoot on rare occasion (7%)[312] are responsible for disruption of the midtarsal joint, producing joint sprains with avulsion fractures of the dorsal lip of the navicular or talus or of the anterior process of the calcaneus. Pure dislocation without fracture, although very rare, usually occurs following this type of injury force, with plantar displacement of the navicular and cuboid.

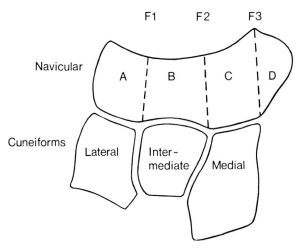

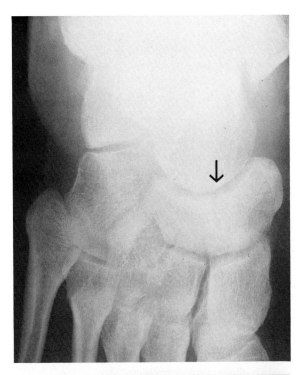

Fig. 19-94. (*Left*) With longitudinally applied stress, fracture of the navicular tends to occur (*dotted lines*) in line with the intercuneiform joints. (*Right*) Anteroposterior x-ray of midtarsal joint injury with navicular fracture between segments *B* and *C*. (Main, B. J. and Jowett, R. L.: Injuries of the Midtarsal Joint. J. Bone Joint Surg., **57B**:91, 1975.)

Crush Injury

Crushing is the final mechanism of injury described by Main and Jowett.[312] Open wounds are frequent with this type of injury, and inconstant fracture patterns, which are difficult to classify, occur.

TREATMENT AND PROGNOSIS

The most striking feature of injuries to the midtarsal joint is the frequent delay in accurate diagnosis. These injuries frequently masquerade as ankle sprains. Often an avulsion fracture of one of the bones is felt to be a trivial, isolated injury, and careful attention is not given to the entire joint complex. These oversights lead to incomplete diagnoses, inadequate treatment, and persistent problems.[294,312,317] The patterns of fracture, subluxation, and dislocation are variable and protean, but the classification presented by Main and Jowett[312] aids in the understanding of the commonly occurring mechanisms of injury. The clinician should be aware of the integrated function of this region of the foot and the frequently occurring combined injuries.

Initial treatment should be aimed at prompt restoration of the anatomy of the midtarsal joint by reduction of dislocations or subluxations and anatomical restoration of the bony architecture whenever possible. Nondisplaced fractures may be treated by short-leg plaster immobilization until healed—usually 4 to 6 weeks. Satisfactory closed

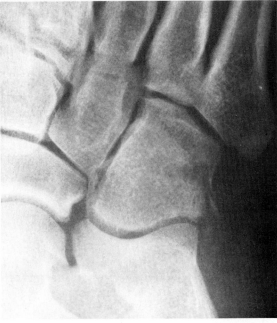

Fig. 19-95. Compression ("nutcracker") fracture of the cuboid secondary to lateral stress injury of the midtarsal joint.

reduction of fracture fragments is often difficult to achieve, and open reduction with Kirschner wire or screw fixation is often necessary.[298,303,312,314] Although many earlier authors recommended early local or triple arthrodesis because of the high likelihood of late degenerative changes, adequate initial reduction and fixation may well lead to an acceptable result, preserving the function of the midtarsal joint. Arthrodesis can be saved for the treatment of those patients with residual disability.[300]

Rarely, comminution is so extensive and the cancellous bone so severely crushed that reduction cannot be achieved. In this circumstance, arthrodesis, with an adequate amount of corticocancellous iliac bone graft, should be undertaken early to restore the longitudinal arch of the foot. On the medial side with fracture of the navicular and disruption of both the talonavicular and naviculocuneiform joints, both these articulations should be fused. For this Friedmann[301] recommended that a tibial cortical strut graft be placed in a slot from the talar neck to the first cuneiform. When there is severe crushing and comminution involving the calcaneocuboid articulation, this joint should be fused with cancellous iliac crest graft after the midtarsal joint is reduced to prevent a persistent pronation deformity.[294]

AUTHOR'S PREFERRED TREATMENT

Very frequently injuries of the midtarsal region are overlooked or the extent of injury is not appreciated. Closed reduction can usually be achieved under satisfactory anesthesia, frequently with the aid of a finger-trap traction device applied to the toes. It is most important to restore the normal midfoot alignment and maintain it to prevent persistent residual deformity. Maintenance of the reduction is difficult with plaster, and I prefer percutaneous pinning with multiple Kirschner wires. This percutaneous fixation is maintained for 6 weeks until soft tissue healing has occurred and early bony union is present. Only rarely have I performed a formal, primary arthrodesis. With severe crushing and comminution of one or more midtarsal bones, fibrous ankylosis or spontaneous bony fusion is frequently the result. For persistent late symptoms of pain and swelling, arthrodesis of the arthritic joint(s) is the best method of treatment.

ISOLATED INJURIES OF THE MIDFOOT

Specific, isolated injuries of parts of the midtarsal joint complex do occur, and these are reviewed here; however, diagnosis of an isolated injury should be made only after it is clear that no other part of this joint complex has been damaged.

TARSAL NAVICULAR FRACTURES

Three basic types of navicular fractures have been described with slight variation in the literature.[322,393,394,411] In the largest series reported in the literature, Eichenholtz and Levine[299] reviewed 66 cases and identified three types: cortical avulsion (47%), tuberosity (24%), and body (29%). For completeness, a fourth category—stress fracture—should be included.[62,87]

Cortical Avulsion Fractures

Cortical avulsion fractures (Fig. 19-96) occur as a result of a twisting force (usually eversion) applied to the foot. They occur more frequently in women. Both the talonavicular capsule and the anteriormost fibers of the deltoid ligament insert into the dorsal lip of the navicular, and excessive tension on either may avulse a variably sized fragment of bone. Most fragments do not involve a significant portion of the articular surface. It must be remembered that two accessory ossicles, the os supranaviculare and the os supratalare, can occur in this region (see Fig. 19-25).

Treatment of these avulsion fractures should be with initial splinting and then with a short-leg walking cast for 4 to 6 weeks. Persistent displacement of a fragment may result in a painful dorsal prominence irritated by shoe wear. If symptomatic,

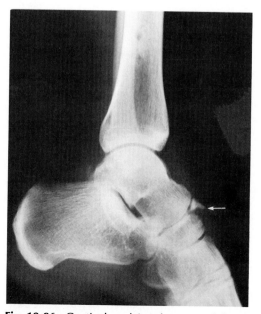

Fig. 19-96. Cortical avulsion fracture of the dorsal aspect of the navicular.

it should be excised; otherwise, it should be left alone. Large, displaced avulsion fractures comprising more than 20% to 25% of the articular surface should be reduced acutely and fixed with a Kirschner wire to restore the articular surface of the talonavicular joint.

Tuberosity Fractures

Acute eversion of the foot, resulting in increased tension on the posterior tibial tendon (or the anterior fibers of the deltoid ligament[299]), places an avulsion pull on the navicular tuberosity, producing this fracture. Rarely is the fragment displaced significantly. It should be remembered that often such an avulsion fracture is seen in conjunction with compression fractures of the cuboid,[294] and the clinician must be careful not to overlook these associated injuries.

Local tenderness, combined with pain on passive eversion or active inversion of the foot, are the characteristic signs of this fracture. The fracture is best identified (Fig. 19-97) on the anteroposterior and medial oblique x-rays of the foot in moderate equinus. The physician must rule out the possible presence of an accessory navicular (os tibiale externum), which can be confused with a fracture. The accessory navicular is frequently (64%)[43] bilateral and symmetrical with smooth, rounded edges, unlike the surface of a fresh fracture.

Treatment of avulsion fractures is with initial splinting and then a short-leg walking cast, well molded under the longitudinal arch with the foot in neutral position for 4 to 6 weeks. Occasionally nonunion occurs. If it remains asymptomatic, the nonunion is disregarded. If pain persists, excision of the fragment is carried out through a medial, slightly curved incision, convex dorsally, just above the tuberosity of the navicular. The ununited fragment is carefully shelled out of the posterior tibial tendon, the fracture surface of the tuberosity is freshened to bleeding bone, and the tendon is sutured to the bed under the same tension that existed before excision of the ununited fragment. Immobilization postoperatively in a short-leg cast is maintained for 4 to 6 weeks.

Body Fractures

Most fractures of the body of the navicular are associated with other injuries in the midtarsal joint, and these additional injuries must be identified and treated as well (see p. 1789). Isolated fractures of the navicular body have been reported to occur in variable patterns and from a variety of mechanisms. Vertical, or longitudinal, fractures usually occur in combination with other midtarsal joint injuries.[312] Transverse and oblique fractures occur rarely,[298,303] and crushing with extensive comminution may occur.[322]

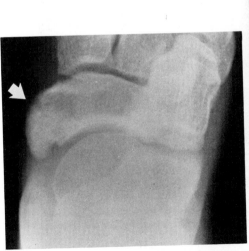
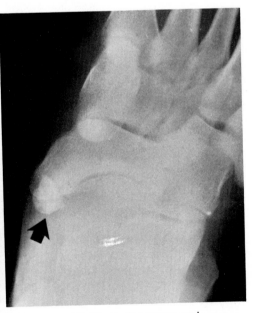

Fig. 19-97. (*Left*) Fracture of the navicular tuberosity. Note slight displacement and the sharp outline of the fracture surface. (*Right*) An accessory navicular with a smooth, rounded surface.

Anteroposterior, oblique, and lateral x-rays are needed to define these fractures, since occasionally they are seen only in one projection. Rarely, the navicular may be bipartite (bilaterally in 50% of the cases), with dorsolateral and inferomedial fragments.[321,291]

In undisplaced fractures of the navicular, comminuted or not, a snug below-the-knee walking cast should be worn for 6 weeks or until union is complete. The patient should then wear a well-molded longitudinal arch support as active weight bearing is resumed. If the fracture is displaced, closed treatment is of little or no value because even if reduction can be achieved, recurrent displacement of the fragments usually occurs.[299,303] Anatomical reduction is imperative for good joint function, and thus open reduction and fixation is usually indicated (Fig. 19-98). The fracture is approached through a dorsal longitudinal incision beginning at the talar neck and extending to the distal articular surface of the cuneiforms. The frag-

ments and both the talonavicular and naviculocuneiform articulations can thus be well visualized and anatomical reduction can be achieved. Large fragments are best fixed with screws, while smaller fragments are fixed with Kirschner wires. Postoperatively, the fracture is protected in a short-leg cast until union occurs, usually in 6 to 8 weeks.

Stress Fractures

Stress fractures of the navicular (Fig. 19-99), occurring primarily in young male athletes, have been reported with increasing frequency recently.[62,87] These fractures are very difficult to identify on plain x-rays, and bone scanning of the foot and tomography are frequently required to make the diagnosis. The fracture line is usually sagittally oriented in the middle third of the bone. It may be complete or incomplete.

Treatment for the fracture, when it is diagnosed early, is non-weight-bearing cast immobilization for 6 to 8 weeks or until tomography confirms

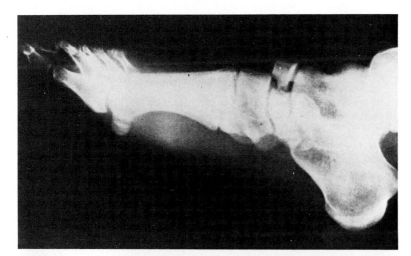

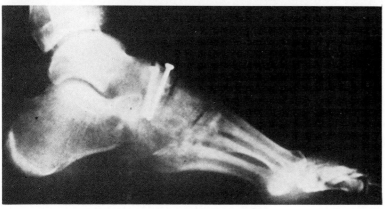

Fig. 19-98. (*Top*) Displaced fracture of the body of the navicular involving a significant portion of both the talonavicular and naviculocuneiform joints. (*Bottom*) Reduction secured by transfixion screw. (Greenberg, M. J., and Sheehan, J. J.: Vertical Fracture-Dislocation of the Tarsal Navicular. Orthopedics, **3**:254–255, 1980.)

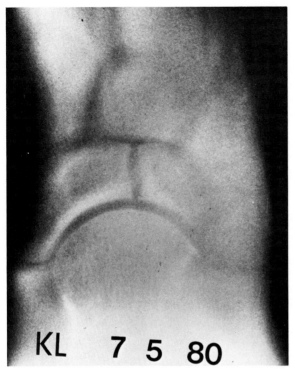

Fig. 19-99. Stress fracture of the navicular seen on a tomogram taken 5 months after the onset of symptoms in a 16-year-old runner. (Torg, J. S., et al.: Stress Fractures of the Tarsal Navicular. J. Bone Joint Surg., **64A**:704, 1982.)

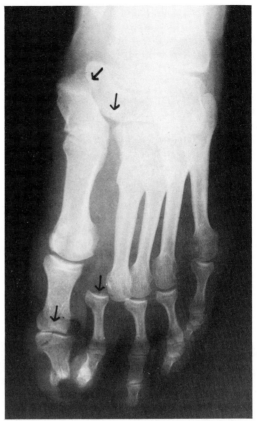

Fig. 19-100. Open dislocation of the medial cuneiform; note associated injuries of the first and second toes.

bony union. Delay in diagnosis or persistent weight bearing appears to lead to nonunion, delayed union, or fracture recurrence.[87] These complications can be difficult to treat and can lead to long-term disability and perhaps premature cessation of an athlete's career. A more complete description of this problem can be found on page 1720.

CUBOID INJURIES

The most frequent mechanism of cuboid injury is, as described, lateral subluxation of the midtarsal joint, which creates the "nutcracker fracture" described by Hermel and Gershon-Cohen.[304] When minimal impaction of the cuboid is present, conservative treatment with a short-leg walking cast is appropriate. Severe comminution and residual displacement may require calcaneocuboid arthrodesis to restore alignment of the foot and minimize late complications.[294] Drummond and Hastings[297] reported one case of total dislocation of the cuboid that required open reduction and pin fixation. The short-term result in this case was good.

CUNEIFORM INJURIES

Isolated fractures of the cuneiforms can obviously occur from direct blows. Other fractures, dislocations, and subluxations should make the physician suspect other injuries involving either the midtarsal or the tarsometatarsal joints (Fig. 19-100). Scattered reports of isolated cuneiform dislocations, subluxations, and fractures exist,[302,311,313,318,327] and occasionally cuneiform dislocation will occur as a variant of a tarsometatarsal dislocation.[292,306] Dislocation of a cuneiform usually requires open reduction, Kirschner wire fixation, and cast protection for 6 weeks to allow adequate ligamentous healing.

INJURIES OF THE TARSOMETATARSAL (LISFRANC'S) JOINTS

Injury of the tarsometatarsal joints has been reported by some to be very uncommon. Aitken and

Poulson[323] found only 16 cases in a review of approximately 82,500 fractures over a 15-year period. No series reported is very large, and thus it is difficult to draw definitive conclusions from the literature about the results of treatment. In my institution the injury is most frequently seen as the result of high-energy trauma and appears to be occurring more frequently. Early recognition is imperative, since significant long-term disability can result from inadequate treatment.

ANATOMY

The bony configuration as well as the ligaments and other supporting soft tissues provide intrinsic stability to these articulations. Normally there is slight motion across the tarsometatarsal joints. The fifth ray is the most mobile, with 10° to 20° of motion in dorsiflexion–plantarflexion at the fifth metatarsocuboid joint[337] and progressively less motion of the more medial joints except for the first metatarsocuneiform, which has approximately 20° of plantarflexion from the neutral position. Both the first and fifth metatarsals can abduct away from the midline of the foot as well.[338]

Intrinsic stability is provided primarily by the bony architecture. Two important considerations here are the recessed position of the base of the second metatarsal (Fig. 19-101 *top*) and the trapezoidal shape of the middle three metatarsal bases when viewed from end on (Fig. 19-101 *bottom*). The recessed base of the second metatarsal, locked between the medial and lateral cuneiforms, limits

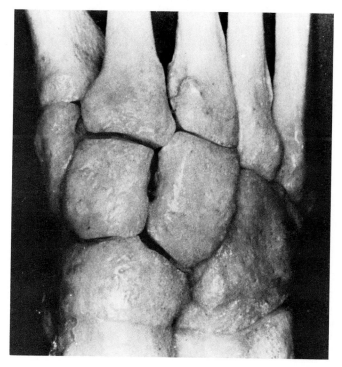

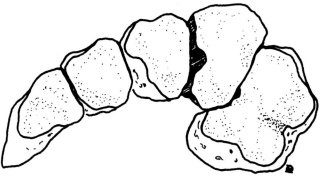

Fig. 19-101. Stability of the tarsometatarsal joint complex is created in part by the bony architecture. (*Top*) Seen from above, the second metatarsal base is recessed proximal to the bases of the other metatarsals. (*Bottom*) The trapezoidal shape of the three middle metatarsals in the frontal plane creates a "Roman arch" configuration. (From Lenczner, E. M.; Waddell, J. P.; and Graham, J. D.: Tarsal-Metatarsal. (Lisfranc) Dislocation. J. Trauma, **14**:1013, 1974.)

translation of the metatarsals in the frontal plane, while the trapezoidal shape of the metatarsal bases forms a "Roman arch" configuration, preventing plantar displacement of the bases.

All five metatarsal heads are held together by the strong transverse metatarsal ligaments, and the bases of the lateral four metatarsals are joined by firm ligaments as well. "Lisfranc's ligament"[340] is an especially large, strong structure extending between the medial cuneiform and the base of the second metatarsal, reinforcing the bony stability of the base of the second between the medial and lateral cuneiforms.

Even though the capsule of the medial cuneiform–first metatarsal joint is reinforced by ligaments, no ligament ties the first and second metatarsals together. This creates a relative weakness in the link between the first and the other metatarsals. Besides ligamentous and bony stability, the soft tissues of the plantar aspect of the foot (primarily the plantar fascia and the peroneus longus tendon) provide additional support. Conversely, the dorsal aspect of this articulation is not reinforced by structures of similar strength. The dorsalis pedis artery crosses Lisfranc's joint and dives deep between the bases of the first and second metatarsals to form the plantar arterial arch, making it suscep-

tible to damage at the time of injury or open reduction.

Because subtle subluxations may be hard to appreciate clinically and radiographically, it is important to understand the critical radiographic indicators of proper alignment of this articulation. Foster and Foster,[334] in a review of 200 normal foot x-rays, have shown that the most consistent relationship between the metatarsal bases and the tarsus is a straight, unbroken, parallel alignment of the medial edge of the base of the second metatarsal with the medial edge of the middle cuneiform on both anteroposterior and oblique projections of the foot (Fig. 19-102). Also, the medial aspect of the base of the fourth metatarsal is usually in line with the medial articular surface of the cuboid, although a step-off of 1 to 2 mm may occur in the normal foot. The position of the base of the fifth metatarsal is very variable and not very reliable as an indication of reduction. Frequently, however, there is a notch or change in the contour of the lateral margin of the articular surface, which indicates congruity with the lateral aspect of the cuboid. On the lateral projection of the normal foot, a metatarsal is never more dorsal than its respective tarsal bone but, on occasion, may be slightly plantar to the tarsal bone.

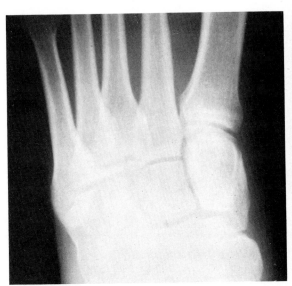 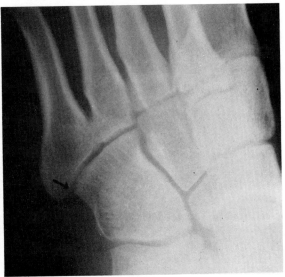

Fig. 19-102. Anteroposterior (*left*) and oblique (*right*) x-rays of a normal foot showing the normal bony relationships between the tarsus and the metatarsals: (1) The parallel alignment of the medial edge of the second metatarsal base and the medial edge of the second cuneiform, (2) alignment of the medial edge of the fourth metatarsal base with the medial surface of the cuboid, and (3) a notch in the base of the fifth metatarsal at the point of articulation with the lateral edge of the cuboid (*arrow*).

MECHANISMS OF INJURY

Because of the complicated arrangement of this articular complex, many different injury patterns may result from forces applied to it. The three most common mechanisms responsible for injury are twisting of the forefoot, axial loading of the fixed foot, and crushing.

Twisting can occur in equestrian accidents when the rider falls and the foot remains caught in the stirrup, forcefully abducting the forefoot on the tarsus. The entire forefoot is displaced laterally, fracturing the base of the second metatarsal. Impingement of the bases of the lateral metatarsals often produce a crushing or shear fracture of the cuboid bone as well. Wiley[346] identified the fractures of the base of the second metatarsal and the cuboid as pathognomonic signs of this abduction injury. In addition, fractures of the metatarsal necks may occur.

Axial loading of the fixed foot can occur in one of two ways: Extrinsic axial compression applied to the heel (Fig. 19-103 *top*) or extreme ankle equinus with axial loading of the body weight (Fig. 19-103 *bottom*). The first mechanism is seen when a heavy object falls on the heel of a kneeling patient or the patient forcibly kicks a fixed object or strikes the floor board of a car at impact. The second

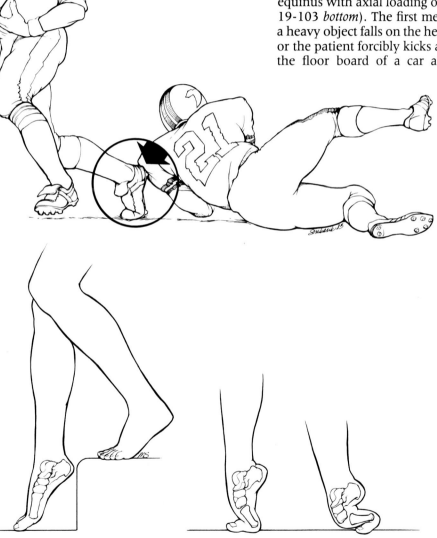

Fig. 19-103. (*Top*) An axial load applied directly to the heel, when the foot is fixed to the ground in equinus, can produce a tarsometatarsal injury. (*Bottom*) The common mechanism of Lisfranc's joint collapse when, with the ankle in extreme equinus, the body weight produces an axial load on the joint complex.

mechanism most commonly occurs from a missed step off a curb or other apparently trivial trauma. In both circumstances the toes are maximally hyperextended and a vertical load is applied to the metatarsals. The dorsal capsule of Lisfranc's joint, lacking sufficient muscular reinforcement, cannot support the load and collapses, resulting primarily in dorsal dislocation of the metatarsal bases. In most instances this is not associated with tarsal or metatarsal fractures.

If the axial load is applied between the first and second metatarsal heads, there will be diversion of the lesser metatarsals laterally and the first metatarsal medially. Occasionally the injury will disrupt the articulation between the navicular and the medial cuneiform rather than at the base of the first metatarsal. Navicular compression fractures may occur as well with this mechanism, since an axial load applied to the first metatarsal head may result in injury to any part of the ray.

Crushing of the midfoot will produce a great variety of injuries and is a common cause of Lisfranc's joint disruption. When the crushing force is applied dorsally, plantar dislocation of the metatarsal bases will occur; however, beyond this there are few specific injury patterns with this mechanism.[346]

CLASSIFICATION

The many different configurations of bone and joint injury of this articular complex have led to many attempts to classify them. A simplified classification was developed by Quénu and Küss,[344] who separated the injuries into three types (Fig. 19-104):

Homolateral: all five metatarsals displaced in the same direction
Isolated: one or two metatarsals displaced from the others
Divergent: displacement of the metatarsals in both the sagittal and coronal planes

Wiley[346] has stated simply that the injury is either direct (crushing), with a great variety of possible specific bone and joint injuries, or indirect (*i.e.,* abduction, plantar flexion).

The fact that the injury can be caused by many mechanisms, ranging in severity from crushing and high-velocity car crashes to the apparently trivial stepping off of a curb, should alert the clinician to look more diligently for injuries to Lisfranc's joint when evaluating the injured foot.

SIGNS AND SYMPTOMS

Suspicion of injury to Lisfranc's joint must be high whenever there is a history of foot injury, partic-

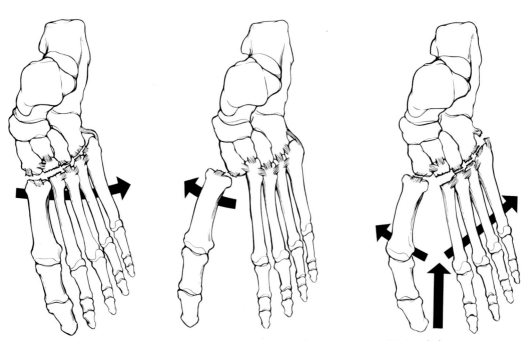

Fig. 19-104. The three commonly occurring patterns of tarsometatarsal joint dislocation: (*left*) homolateral, (*center*) isolated, and (*right*) divergent.

ularly with any of the mechanisms listed above. The degree of injury varies greatly. Cassebaum[327] pointed out that a simple sprain of Lisfranc's joint can be a "source of considerable disability." Sprain injuries without persistent subluxation or dislocation present as pain and swelling in the midfoot with point tenderness usually elicited somewhere along Lisfranc's joint. Another very helpful test for injury to this region is gentle passive supination and pronation of the forefoot with the hindfoot held fixed in the examiner's opposite hand. This maneuver will usually elicit pain if the tarsometatarsal joint has been injured. Anderson[391] points out that spontaneous reduction of dislocation at this level can occur. Thus, the clinical and x-ray appearance may be normal and the actual severity of injury easily overlooked.

With actual dislocation or fracture–dislocation there will be deformity as well. Because of the large amount of swelling that rapidly accompanies this injury, bony deformity is often hidden. The forefoot is usually shortened and wide; however, the specific deformity will depend on the direction of displacement of the bony parts.

The dorsalis pedis pulse may be diminished or absent because of compression or actual laceration. Although it has been inferred that gangrene of the forefoot can result from this arterial injury,[327] a review of the literature indicates that this occurs quite rarely; in the three cases of amputation reported by Gissane,[335] reduction was not carried out promptly and damage to the posterior tibial artery occurred as well. Careful evaluation of skin temperature and capillary filling in the toes should be a part of the initial assessment of any foot injury. Marginal circulation can be further evaluated and monitored with a Doppler flow meter.

RADIOGRAPHIC FINDINGS

Anteroposterior, oblique, and lateral x-rays of the foot are required to evaluate fully the extent of injury. Comparison of these films with comparable views of the opposite foot will be very helpful in diagnosis as well as evaluation of the adequacy of reduction.

On the anteroposterior projection (Fig. 19-105 *top left*), small fracture fragments in and around Lisfranc's joint should cause the physician to suspect significant injury in the area. Particularly common are fractures of the base of the second metatarsal either as a result of ligament avulsion or shearing of the proximal shaft, leaving the base reduced in the cuneiform mortise. Crush or shearing fractures

of the cuboid and, to a lesser degree, the navicular and medial cuneiform are also signs suggesting a Lisfranc's joint injury. Specific attention should be paid to the alignment of the medial aspect of the second metatarsal base and the middle cuneiform. These surfaces should form an unbroken, straight line. A similar unbroken straight line should extend from the medial surface of the cuboid to the medial side of the base of the fourth metatarsal.

The oblique x-ray (Fig. 19–105 *top right*) will "open up" the bases of the lateral metatarsals, which usually are overlapped on the anteroposterior view. Any significant displacement of one metatarsal in relation to the others may be more obvious in this view. Significant malalignment of the first tarsometatarsal joint will frequently be best seen on this view.

Laterally (Fig. 19-105 *bottom*), dorsal (or, less commonly, plantar) displacement of the metatarsal bases can be seen. Often what appears to be adequately reduced metatarsals on the anteroposterior view will show residual displacement on the lateral projection.

TREATMENT

As with any complicated injury with a wide spectrum of severity and variability in presentation, treatment methods will vary depending on the degree of soft tissue and other associated injury, the amount of displacement, and the configuration of the fractured or dislocated parts.

Sprains of this joint complex can occur and must be adequately protected and immobilized until soft tissue healing is complete. Although Cassebaum[327] recommended plaster immobilization for 3 to 5 weeks, I recommend that casting be maintained for 6 weeks to ensure complete ligament healing.

Subluxation or frank dislocation of Lisfranc's joint requires anatomical reduction. Although adequate function will sometimes be possible with an inadequately reduced joint, and although anatomical and near anatomical reduction does not always prevent the development of arthrosis, most authors[323,339,340,341,347,348] encourage restoration of the normal anatomical configuration of this joint to enhance the likelihood of normal appearance and function. In addition, although the actual number of instances of gangrene following this injury is very small[335,345] and is probably due to injury to other vessels in addition to the dorsalis pedis artery, grossly deformed joints should be reduced promptly to minimize stretching and compression of the vessels, to improve venous

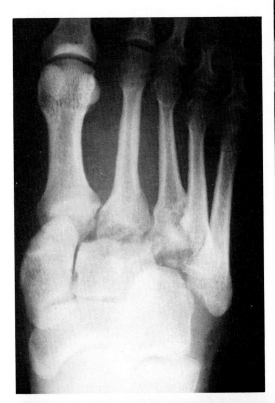

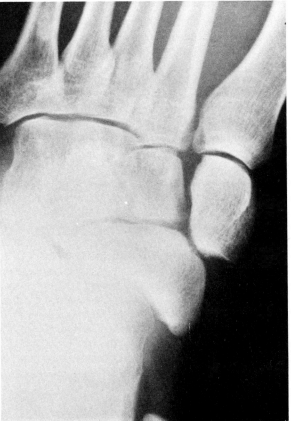

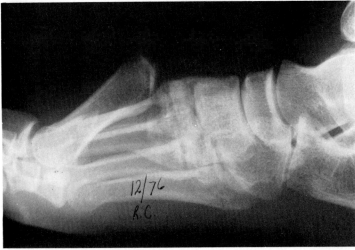

Fig. 19-105. (*Top left*) Anteroposterior x-ray of a homolateral Lisfranc's dislocation. Note the lateral displacement of the metatarsal bases in relation to the tarsus. (*Top right*) Oblique x-ray of a variant of Lisfranc's injury. Note medial displacement of the first metatarsal and medial cuneiform. The lateral metatarsals remain normally aligned. (*Bottom*) Lateral x-ray of a third injury showing dorsal displacement of the second metatarsal base.

return, and to decrease swelling. When the patient presents late, more than 24 hours after injury, with massive swelling of the foot, a 2- to 3-day period of splinting, strict bed rest, and elevation will help decrease the swelling before reduction.

Closed Reduction

Adequate reduction, regardless of the extent of displacement, can often be achieved by closed means. This is best accomplished under spinal or general anesthesia. Suspension of the toes in wire traps and the application of traction to the hindfoot, either manually or with a sling and weights across the ankle, will help to restore length to the shortened foot. This on occasion will be adequate to achieve reduction; however, further gentle manual manipulation of the metatarsal bases may be required to reduce them adequately. Following traction and manipulation, x-rays should be obtained in traction to confirm the adequacy of reduction (Fig. 19-106.). If the dislocation is well reduced on x-ray, the toe traction, which may be solely responsible for maintaining the reduction, should be released and the stability or reduction tested by gentle manipulation. If repeat x-rays show maintenance of perfect position, the reduction can be considered stable and treated with plaster cast immobilization alone; however, careful follow-up x-rays must be obtained periodically to confirm maintenance of the reduction.

Closed Reduction and Pin Fixation

If after release of traction and with gentle manipulation there is a loss of reduction, the dislocation should be considered unstable and the foot should be replaced in traction to proceed with rereduction and internal stabilization. The most frequently recommended method of fixation is percutaneous pinning with large (0.062-in) Kirschner wires. The position of placement of the wires is critical and depends on the number and direction of dislocations of the metatarsals involved (Fig. 19-107). The basic principle is to stabilize the metatarsal in a reduced position by fixing it to the tarsus. With an isolated metatarsal dislocation, one wire (or perhaps two wires if the first metatarsal is involved) should be placed through the shaft into the respective cuneiform or cuboid. With both the divergent and homolateral types of dislocation, two transfixion wires—one through the fifth metatarsal

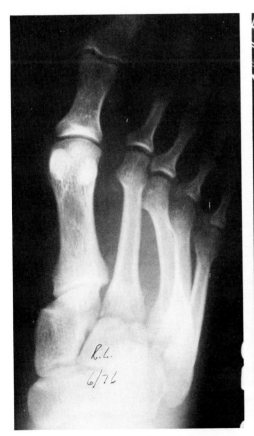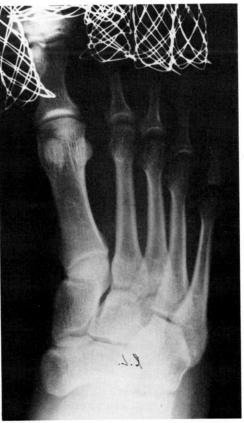

Fig. 19-106. (*Left*) Homolateral dislocation of the lateral three metatarsal bases. (*Right*) Reduction achieved with finger-trap traction.

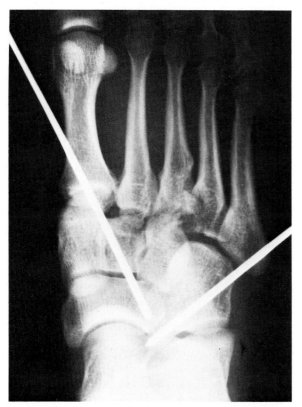

Fig. 19-107. An unstable divergent tarsometatarsal dislocation reduced and stabilized with two Steinmann pins.

base into the cuboid and one through the first metatarsal into the first cuneiform—will usually be sufficient. Oblique placement of the pins will provide a buttressing effect to prevent proximal migration of the metatarsals. If crushing of the cuboid has occurred, the lateral wire should be drilled into the calcaneus to ensure adequate purchase. It is usually not necessary with these types of injuries to pin the central three metatarsals, since they are tethered to the fifth metatarsal by intermetatarsal ligaments and will remain reduced as long as the fifth metatarsal is stabilized.

On occasion, particularly with crushing injuries and separation of individual metatarsals, it may be necessary to add additional pins to achieve adequate stability. The fixation pins should be left protruding percutaneously, with the exposed tip bent at a right angle to prevent migration.

Following stable closed reduction or closed reduction and pinning, the foot should be immobilized in a well-molded short-leg cast. Close observation of the neurovascular status is mandatory,

and the cast usually must be changed in a few days as the swelling subsides. Non-weight-bearing plaster immobilization and pin fixation are maintained for 6 to 8 weeks, after which the pins are removed and the patient is begun on a rehabilitation program that includes soaks, exercises, and progressive weight bearing in a shoe fitted with a properly contoured firm arch support. As long as 6 months of rehabilitation may be required before the patient's symptoms stabilize.

Open Reduction

Failure of closed reduction will necessitate open reduction. Several factors may lead to inadequate closed reduction:

Severe displacement of the metatarsal bases (especially seen in the crushing type of injury).

Entrapment of bony fragments in the joint. The most common example of this is a fragment of the base of the second metatarsal obstructing reduction.

Entrapment of soft tissue in a joint, especially the anterior tibial tendon interposed between the first and second metatarsals, the so-called complex dislocation[330,332] (Fig. 19-108).

Aitken and Poulson[323] have emphasized that "the key to reduction is the fracture-dislocation of the second metatarsal." This is the site where bony fragments are most likely to be incarcerated and where the entrapped anterior tibial tendon will be located. The primary surgical approach to the inadequately reduced Lisfranc's injury should be through a longitudinal incision on the dorsum of the foot just lateral to the extensor hallucis longus tendon. Care should be taken to avoid injury to the dorsalis pedis artery and the sensory branch of the deep peroneal nerve. Dissection will allow access to both the first and second metatarsal bases as well as their respective cuneiforms. The base of the second metatarsal is exposed, and the articulation of this bone is cleared of any loose bone fragments or interposed soft tissue. Once this is cleared, the second metatarsal can usually be reduced and the more lateral metatarsals will then fall into place. Aitken and Poulson[323] have recommended partial resection of the base of the second metatarsal if necessary to allow adequate reduction; however, this should only be done as a last resort. Through the same incision, the base of the first metatarsal should be reduced under direct vision. The reduced metatarsals can then be pinned to the tarsus with large percutaneous Kirschner

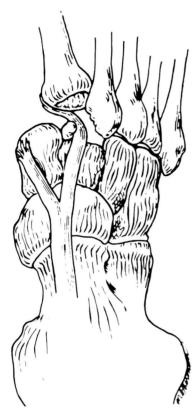

Fig. 19-108. Entrapment of the anterior tibial tendon in the interval between the fracture fragments of the second metatarsal base irreducible by closed means, requiring open reduction. (DeBenedetti, M. J.; Evanski, P. M.; and Waugh, T. R.: The Unreducible Lisfranc Fracture. Clin. Orthop., **136:**239, 1978.)

wires. The adequacy of reduction should be confirmed radiographically. On rare occasions, an additional longitudinal incision laterally, centered over the shaft of the fourth metatarsal, may be required to gain access to an irreducible lateral metatarsal dislocation.

Rarely,[306,332] the site of dislocation of the first ray extends not through the articulation between the first metatarsal and the medial cuneiform, but more proximally, between the medial cuneiform and the navicular. This diastasis may trap a portion of the anterior tibial tendon and block closed reduction. Open reduction through the same basic dorsomedial incision will allow access to this dislocation to remove the entrapped tendon.

After adequate open reduction and fixation with wires, the patient's postoperative immobilization and treatment should be the same as for closed treatment.

AUTHOR'S PREFERRED METHOD

Because I have seen several patients with persistent long-term problems after apparently trivial injuries to the tarsometatarsal joint, I am fairly aggressive in the management of these problems. Sprains and dislocations that can be reduced and remain stable are usually treated with 6 weeks of immobilization in a short-leg walking plaster cast.

Reduction is often easy to obtain, but frequently, when traction is released, there is significant, persistent subluxation of the joint. In these instances I repeat the closed reduction and place at least two 0.062-inch Kirschner wires percutaneously through the base of the unstable metatarsals into the tarsus. The pins are bent outside of the skin to prevent migration, and the foot is immobilized in a short-leg plaster cast. Weight-bearing is kept to a minimum during the first 4 weeks to prevent pin irritation and decrease the amount of stress on the unstable joint. The pins are usually removed at 6 weeks, when the patient is begun on a vigorous toe exercise program and progressive weight bearing.

If an anatomical reduction cannot be achieved by closed means, then I do an open reduction, usually through a longitudinal dorsal incision over the interval between the first and second rays. This incision provides adequate access to the base of the second metatarsal, the usual site of obstruction. Following open reduction the dislocation is again stabilized with percutaneous Kirschner wires, and the same postoperative regimen is carried out as for closed, percutaneous pinning.

PROGNOSIS

Substantial disagreement exists in the literature on the long-term effects of injury to Lisfranc's joint. In their classic paper, Aitken and Poulson[323] stated that both closed and open reduction of the dislocation yielded excellent results. However, even with "persistent dislocations" causing obvious deformity, the functional results were good. Post-traumatic arthritis and ankylosis of the tarsometatarsal joints were common but not a source of discomfort and disability in their patients.

Wilson[348] noted late radiographic signs of degenerative arthritis in all of his 22 patients, and "even cases with anatomic reduction by operation were not exempt." Residual stiffness of the foot was present in all but two of his patients. However, he noted that marked residual displacement led to significant persistent pain, whereas with anatomical or near-anatomical reduction, residual pain and functional impairment were less.

Wilppula[347] presented the most extensive long-term follow-up study of this injury with 26 patients folowed for 2 to 10 years (average 5 years). He found the following:

Some patients with persistent dislocations were able to work, although not in heavy occupations.

Slight residual separation (less than 5 mm) between the bases of the first and second metatarsals may be accepted, if the shape of the foot is otherwise good.

Arthrosis occurred in 15 of 26 patients, with the most severe changes occurring in patients with residual deformity.

In general, a good anatomical result meant a good functional result but did not guarantee a symptom-free foot.

The results of conservative (nonoperative) treatment were better when three or fewer metatarsals were dislocated or if the initial dislocation was so slight that the alignment as such could be considered good. In the case of more extensive dislocation, the results of open treatment were better.

Other concomitant fractures of the foot did not seem to influence the results.

COMPLICATIONS

The literature is very sparse regarding the management of residual pain in Lisfranc's joint following injury. Wilppula[347] noted that the symptoms following injury tend to "subside gradually during a period of several years." Because many patients were able to function well despite the development of arthrosis in the joint, there is no indication for arthrodesis in the primary management of this condition.

When a patient presents 6 weeks or more after injury with a persistently displaced dislocation, operative reduction is not indicated because the reduction is difficult and the results of operative intervention have not been good.[336] Before this 6-week point, open reduction and fixation should be tried.

For patients with significant residual symptoms (Fig. 19-109), partial stabilization of the joint can be achieved with a well-molded firm arch support and a long steel shank in the shoe. Should these measures fail to control symptoms adequately, arthrodesis of Lisfranc's joint as described by Compere and co-workers[329] should be considered.

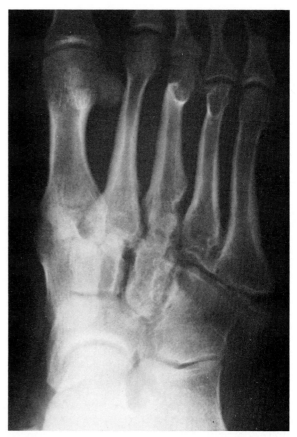

Fig. 19-109. Degenerative arthritis of the tarsometatarsal joint complex 5 years after fracture–dislocation. Moderate symptoms in this patient have necessitated the wearing of a well-molded firm arch support and a long steel shank in the shoe.

FRACTURES OF THE METATARSALS

Direct injury, particularly from a heavy object dropped on the forefoot, is the most common mechanism of fracture of the metatarsals. Such direct force can result in fracture of any metatarsal at any point. Indirect forces, particularly twisting the body with the toes fixed (as when a person catches the toe of the shoe in a narrow opening), will apply torque to the foot, producing fractures of the metatarsal shafts, particularly spiral fractures of the middle three metatarsals. Avulsion fractures, particularly the base of the fifth metatarsal, are common, and, as described previously, stress fractures occur commonly in the metatarsals, particularly at the second and third metatarsal necks and at the proximal portion of the shaft of the fifth.

FRACTURES OF THE METATARSAL SHAFT

ANATOMY AND MECHANISM OF INJURY

The first metatarsal, because of its important weight-bearing function, is much larger and stronger than the lesser metatarsals and is less frequently injured; however, if fractured, more aggressive treatment is needed to restore anatomical alignment and ensure preservation of this important weight-bearing function.

Direct blows to the forefoot may produce significant soft tissue injury as well as metatarsal fracture. The relatively fragile skin on the dorsum of the foot is particularly vulnerable to laceration and contusion. Extreme swelling of the entire foot usually occurs soon after these injuries. Occasionally, skin necrosis or slough may result from damage to the soft tissues. These complications can be minimized by eliciting the history of direct injury, monitoring the patient's circulatory status closely, and maintaining elevation of the injured part in the immediate postinjury period.

SIGNS AND SYMPTOMS

The patient complains of pain over the dorsum of the forefoot, which increases with dependency and weight bearing. The dorsum of the forefoot is swollen and ecchymotic. When the patient is seen within the first few hours, point tenderness is present over the fracture site; however, as swelling occurs, it becomes difficult to localize the tenderness. Plantar palpation of the head of the involved metatarsal shaft will produce pain and occasionally crepitus at the fracture site. Axial compression of the toe of the injured metatarsal will also elicit pain at the fracture site. Careful assessment of circulation and sensation of the toes is mandatory.

RADIOGRAPHIC FINDINGS

Standard anteroposterior, oblique, and lateral views of the foot should be obtained. Anderson[391] emphasizes the importance of achieving proper exposure for these views. Usually the x-ray is taken to view the entire foot, and the exposure is set to best show the tarsal bones. This leaves the forefoot overexposed and difficult to evaluate. In this case, the x-ray should be repeated to obtain the best exposure for viewing the details of the forefoot.

Although the anteroposterior and oblique views are used to identify the fractures, special attention must be paid to the lateral view as well. Although overlapping of the metatarsals makes interpretation difficult in this view, the most significant fracture displacements occur in the sagittal plane and can only be identified on the lateral x-ray. Significant plantar or dorsal displacement of a metatarsal fracture fragment will require reduction, and this displacement will be recognized only on a lateral view.

Careful inspection of the entire x-ray is important to avoid overlooking additional fractures. Particularly with crush injuries, multiple fractures will occur, and even with less violent mechanisms there is a high likelihood of multiple metatarsal fractures or a combination of fractures and proximal joint dislocations.

TREATMENT AND PROGNOSIS

Nondisplaced and minimally displaced metatarsal shaft and neck fractures can be treated with a short-leg walking cast worn for 2 to 4 weeks. Ambulation should be encouraged in the plaster as soon as tolerated by the patient. Johnson,[356] in an excellent review of 350 consecutive patients with forefoot fractures sustained in industrial accidents, concluded that "fractures of the forefoot have probably been overprotected and overtreated in the past." He found that early ambulation in an oversized, well-padded work shoe expedited union and significantly decreased time to return to work as compared to plaster immobilization. No significant late complications from minimally displaced or nondisplaced metatarsal fractures have been reported except for occasional reflex sympathetic dystrophy,[356] which seems to occur most often when the patient is immobilized in a non-weight-bearing cast. If walking cast treatment is chosen, the patient should be kept casted for as short a time as possible (2 to 3 weeks) and then encouraged to ambulate in a well-padded shoe.

With displaced metatarsal fractures, certain patterns of displacement may lead to significant residual symptoms if the fracture is not adequately reduced. On the other hand, substantial residual displacement in other planes can be accepted without the risk of long-term disability. Residual displacement of the shaft of the second, third, and fourth metatarsals in the frontal plane will not result in significant late complications. Fractures in this region heal despite significant separation of the fragments, and medial or lateral displacement or angulation will not result in significant long-term symptoms because these metatarsals lie deep in the foot musculature and are protected by the first and fifth metatarsals. Thus, fractures of the shafts of the second, third, and fourth metatarsals displaced in the frontal plane can be treated as nondisplaced fractures.

Displacement of any metatarsal fracture in the sagittal plane should be a cause for concern. Healing of the fracture with significant residual plantar displacement of the distal metatarsal fragment will increase the prominence of that metatarsal head, resulting in excessive loading on weight bearing, callus buildup, and pain in the region of the prominent head. Similarly, any significant dorsal bony prominence will be irritated by shoes and may result in a painful corn. Residual medial prominence of a fragment of the first metatarsal or lateral prominence of the fifth will also result in symptomatic shoe irritation.

These deformities should be avoided by achieving adequate reduction of the fracture initially. Closed methods (using traction and manipulation) in most instances will result in an adequate reduction (Fig. 19-110). The reduction is sometimes unstable after release of the traction, and closed percutaneous pinning should be undertaken in this instance.

If closed reduction fails, the surgeon may allow the fracture to heal in the malaligned position, planning to return at a later time to perform a corrective osteotomy or remove an offending bony prominence. However, it is best to proceed with open reduction of the fresh fracture. Open reduction (and stabilization with percutaneous wires) should be chosen unless other factors (severe swelling, multiple fractures, contaminated wounds, marginal or inadequate pedal circulation) increase the risk of greater complications.

Open reduction and internal fixation is also recommended by the Association for the Study of Internal Fixation (ASIF),[354] particularly for displaced fractures of the first and fifth metatarsal shaft (Fig. 19-111). The primary indication for this method of rigid internal fixation with plates and screws, in my mind, is a significantly displaced fracture of the shaft of the first metatarsal. The first metatarsal is infrequently fractured because of its size and strength. Because of its important weight-bearing function, inadequate reduction leading to malunion may produce more long-term disability than a malunion of equal degree of one of the lesser metatarsals.[355] The ASIF techniques for open reduction and internal fixation of diaphyseal fractures can be applied equally well to the foot using the small fragment set. A surgeon well versed in these techniques will be able to achieve adequate reduction and stabilization of the first metatarsal when all the proper indications for this exacting method are met.

One substantial advantage of open reduction and rigid internal fixation is the ability to begin early mobilization of adjacent joints in the immediate postoperative period. Although no one would now recommend the banjo splinting technique of immobilization that was used 40 years ago for these fractures,[403] immobilization in plaster, particularly when combined with multiple pinning, also can lead to stiffness of the foot. When rigid internal fixation is used, early active and passive range of motion can be instituted because the need for external stabilization with plaster is eliminated.

In all metatarsal shaft fractures, prolonged plaster and pin immobilization should be avoided. Pins can generally be removed at 3 to 4 weeks, when there are early clinical and radiographic signs of union. Weight bearing with plaster cast protection should be encouraged as soon after the injury as possible to minimize the degree of disuse osteoporosis and muscular atrophy in the foot and leg. Active motion of the toes should be carried out every day by the patient while immobilized, and, when the cast is removed, progressive weight bearing should be accompanied by an aggressive active range of motion exercise program for the entire foot.

FRACTURES OF THE METATARSAL HEAD

Occasionally, fracture of the metatarsal occurs through the head, producing a distal fragment that is wholly intra-articular and without capsular attachments. This seems to occur most often with "across-the-board" fractures of all the metatarsals, with the line of injury crossing the necks of the medial metatarsals and traversing the head of the shorter, lateral metatarsals. Because of the distal location of the fracture, the surgeon might suspect that aseptic necrosis would occur following this injury. As Smillie and others[350,352] point out, ischemia and subsequent fatigue fracture combine to produce progressive, irreversible deformity and osteochondritis dissecans (Frieberg's infraction) of the metatarsal head in adolescents.

All the metatarsal head fractures that I have treated have been the result of direct trauma and usually have been associated with proximal fractures of the medially adjacent metatarsals. All have been minimally displaced, usually angulated plantarly and laterally. Stable reduction has been achieved by gentle manual manipulation and traction. Reduction has been maintained by immobilization in a short-leg walking cast with a toe plate. No cases

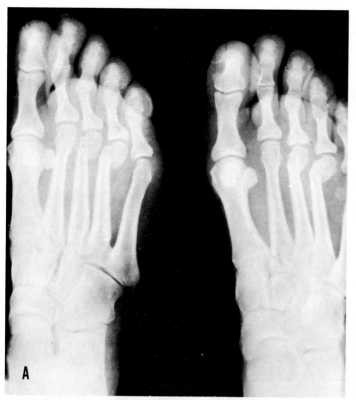

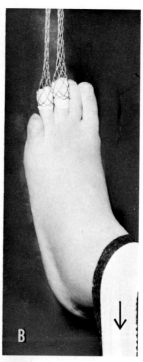

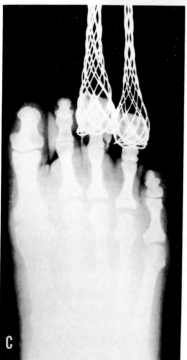

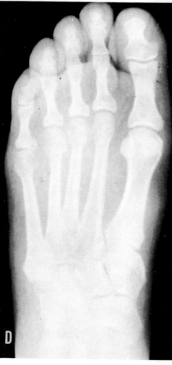

Fig. 19-110. (*A*) These displaced fractures of the metatarsals were treated with the closed method of reduction and Chinese finger-trap traction to each toe. (*B*) An early attempt at reduction and manipulation with use of Chinese finger traps on the toes and countertraction on the ankle resulted in satisfactory alignment. (*C*) Radiographic appearance of the same metatarsals with traction and countertraction applied. (*D*) The fractures united in excellent alignment. (From Giannestras, N. J.: Foot Disorders: Medical and Surgical Management, 2nd ed. Philadelphia, Lea & Febiger, 1973.)

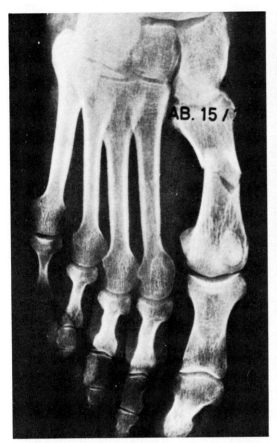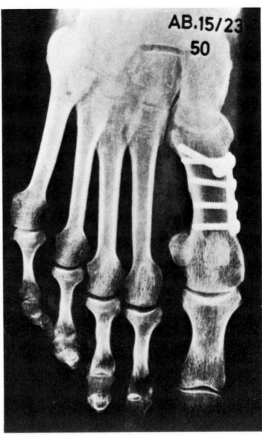

Fig. 19-111. (*Left*) Angulated fracture of the shaft of the first metatarsal treated by open reduction and rigid internal fixation. (*Right*) At 1 year the fracture is well healed. This method of treatment restores anatomical alignment and allows immediate postoperative active range of motion. (Heim, U., and Pfeiffer, K. M.: Small Fragment Set Manual, p. 250. New York, Springer-Verlag, 1974.)

of aseptic necrosis of the head have been noted in my patients (Fig. 19-112).

FRACTURES OF THE BASE OF THE FIFTH METATARSAL

Fracture of the base of the fifth metatarsal has been generally referred to as a "Jones fracture" after the original description of a fracture in this region personally sustained by Sir Robert Jones while dancing. He described a fracture "approximately three quarters of an inch from the fifth metatarsal base" (Fig. 19-113), occurring as he "trod on the outside of my foot, my heel at the moment being off the ground."[357] He subsequently treated five other patients in 1 month with similar fractures and reported these six cases in 1902. He concluded that an indirect mechanism ("cross-breaking strain

directed anteriorly to the metatarsal base and caused by body pressure on an inverted foot while the heel is raised") was responsible for causing the fracture. Because of the firm ligamentous attachments of the base of the fifth metatarsal to the cuboid and the fourth metatarsal, he believed that "it is obviously easier to break the bone than to dislocate it." He did not comment on treatment or the eventual outcome of the fracture except to state that in his case "the disability lasted several weeks."

CLASSIFICATION

Because of Sir Robert's eloquent description of his injury, all fractures of the base of the fifth metatarsal have come to be called Jones's fractures. Unfortunately, this has resulted in significant confusion in the management of these fractures because at least two distinct fracture patterns occur at the base

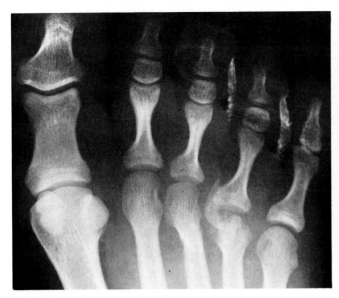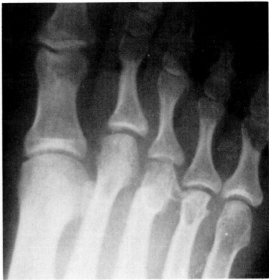

Fig. 19-112. (*Left*) Significantly displaced fracture of the articular surface of the fourth metatarsal head. This fracture was not diagnosed initially. (*Right*) When seen 1 year later, the patient was asymptomatic and had significant remodeling of the metatarsal head resulting in painless joint motion.

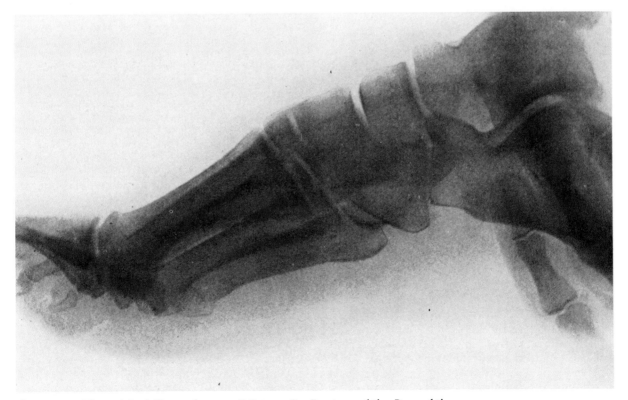

Fig. 19-113. The original "Jones fracture." (Jones, R.: Fracture of the Base of the Fifth Metatarsal by Indirect Violence. Ann. Surg., **35**:699, 1902.)

of the fifth metatarsal: avulsion fracture of a variably sized portion of the tuberosity (or styloid process) and transverse fracture of the proximal metatarsal diaphysis, within 1.5 cm. of the tuberosity. Two recent excellent reviews of fractures in this region[351,358] have defined these two different fractures, their mechanism, their clinical and radiographic appearance, and their treatment and prognosis.

AVULSION FRACTURE

The avulsion fracture of the base usually occurs indirectly. Sudden inversion of the foot, as when the person steps in a hole or lands on the lateral aspect of the foot when jumping, will produce avulsion of the bone as the peroneus brevis contracts to prevent further forefoot inversion. This mechanism can also produce lateral ankle ligament injury, and this fracture must be ruled out in patients complaining of lateral ankle pain following an inversion injury. Careful palpation over the base of the fifth metatarsal will elicit tenderness, and active eversion of the foot will be painful.

Anteroposterior, lateral, and oblique x-rays of the foot will show the avulsed fragment of bone (Fig. 19-114), which may vary in size from a small fleck to include virtually the entire tuberosity. Rarely is the articulation with the cuboid involved. Care must be taken to avoid confusion with two sesamoid bones, which can occur normally in this region. The first and more common is the os peroneum, a sesamoid lying within the tendon of the peroneus longus, which usually occurs bilaterally and was present in 15% of 1000 feet x-rayed by Dameron.[351] The other sesamoid in this region is the very rare os vesalianum, an ossicle within the peroneus brevis tendon lying just at the tip of the tuberosity (see Fig. 19-25). Both ossicles will have smooth, round surfaces with sclerotic subchondral bone, which should help to differentiate them from the avulsed fracture fragment. X-rays of the opposite foot will usually show symmetrical ossicles as well. The apophysis of the base of the fifth metatarsal fuses to the shaft by age 16 years,[351] and in persons over this age, failure of fusion of the apophysis should not be confused with a fresh fracture in this region.

Significant (greater than 1-cm) displacement of fracture surfaces can occur as the peroneus brevis retracts, pulling the avulsed fragment of bone proximally, yet the avulsion fracture generally produces few long-term complications, and, in most cases, symptomatic treatment alone is indicated. Splinting for a few days followed by 2 to 3 weeks of

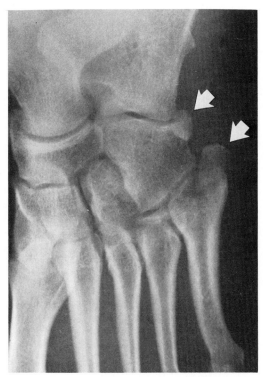

Fig. 19-114. Avulsion fracture of the base of the fifth metatarsal. The attachment of the peroneus brevis tendon has displaced the fragment proximally (*lower arrow*). This fracture is not to be confused with the sesamoid bone, which lies in the tendon of the peroneus longus (*upper arrow*). This sesamoid is *not* the same as the os vesalianum, an accessory bone that is occasionally seen at the base of the fifth metatarsal (but that is not present in this patient).

immobilization in a short-leg walking cast is usually adequate treatment. Several authors recommend an initial period of ice and elevation followed in a few days by taping with a Gibney boot to limit inversion, with progressive weight bearing in a shoe as tolerated. Most fractures unite and become asymptomatic within 4 to 6 weeks.

Significant displacement may result in nonunion; however, most nonunions are asymptomatic and require no further treatment because satisfactory stability is achieved by the fibrous tissue bridging the defect. Persistent symptomatic nonunion is best treated by excision of the fragment and suture of the peroneus brevis to the freshened distal fracture surface of the metatarsal base.

Gould and Trevino[353] reported three cases of entrapment of a branch of the sural nerve in the nonunion site that produced a positive Tinel's sign at the site of entrapment and persistent dysesthesias distally. All patients recovered well following excision of the ununited fragment of bone that was impinging on the nerve.

DIAPHYSEAL FRACTURE

Although the avulsion fracture causes few immediate or long-term problems, a fracture of the base of the diaphysis of the fifth metatarsal is a different clinical entity. Fracture in this area (Fig. 19-115) can be a product of direct or indirect forces or may be caused by repetitive stress.[351,358,362] The healing potential of this fracture is diminished, and the rate of fibrous union or subsequent "refracture" is high. Inadequate initial treatment may contribute to delayed or nonunion in this area, and thus the fracture must be distinguished from the less complicated, more proximal, avulsion fracture.

Because of the high frequency of delayed union (66.7%) in their series of young athletes (average age 20.3 years), Kavanaugh and associates[358] recommended surgical treatment in selected cases. Although they stated that treatment should be individualized depending on the patient's needs

and activity, they believed that surgical fixation was justified in the young, athletic adult. Displacement of the fracture fragments is usually not extreme, and fixation can be accomplished with a compression screw (Fig. 19-116). The authors recommended use of an AO malleolar screw, the threads of which should engage cortical bone to ensure adequate compression across the fracture site. This technique is also effective in securing union of refractures in this region.

Dameron[351] and Zelko and colleagues[362] have identified the high frequency of delayed union, nonunion, and "refracture" of the proximal diaphysis of the fifth metatarsal. They recommend treating these complications with a sliding bone graft; in all 12 of their patients, union occurred within at least 3 months, allowing full resumption of athletic activities.

AUTHOR'S PREFERRED TREATMENT

The small avulsion fractures of the base of the fifth metatarsal usually heal rapidly and rarely lead to persistent, disabling problems. I prefer to treat them

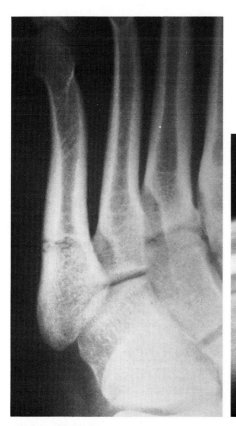
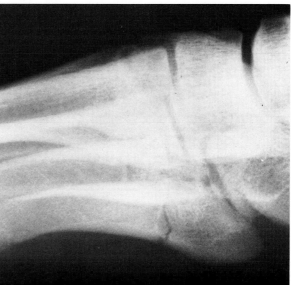

Fig. 19-115. Oblique (*left*) and lateral (*right*) x-rays of a diaphyseal fracture of the proximal fifth metatarsal.

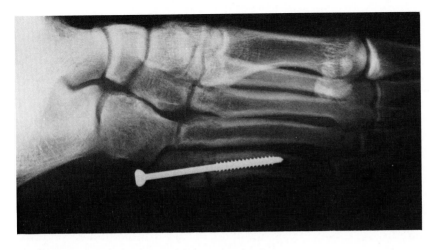

Fig. 19-116. Fracture of the proximal diaphysis of the fifth metatarsal in an athlete treated by compression screw fixation.

symptomatically using a short-leg walking cast or with a compression dressing, wooden-soled shoe, and crutches for 2 to 3 weeks, then allowing the patient to progress rapidly to full ambulation. On the other hand, a fracture of the proximal diaphysis (perhaps best named the "true Jones's fracture") tends to heal slowly and may not heal or may refracture when activity is resumed, particularly in the young athletic adult. I prefer a trial of 6 weeks of walking plaster immobilization initially in most of these patients, realizing that surgical intervention may be needed if the fracture fails to progress to union. I have not had any experience with AO screw fixation, having had good success with the sliding cortical graft. If the principles as outlined by the respective authors are followed, successful union should be achieved using either modality.

INJURIES OF THE METATARSOPHALANGEAL JOINTS

The metatarsophalangeal articulations are complex structures that are prone to sprains, subluxations, and dislocations. The sesamoids of the first ray may fracture in isolation or in combination with other injury to the first metatarsophalangeal joint. Although most of the injuries heal well, causing little long-term disability, occasionally symptoms will persist.

INJURIES OF THE FIRST METATARSOPHALANGEAL JOINT

The first metatarsophalangeal joint is a condylar articulation formed by the concave base of the proximal phalanx and the convex first metatarsal head. Motion occurs primarily in dorsiflexion (30°)

and plantarflexion (10°).[374] The joint capsule on both the medial and lateral sides is reinforced by strong collateral ligaments that restrain varus and valgus motion. Dorsally, the capsule is reinforced by the expanse of the extensor hallucis longus tendon; plantarly, there is a capsular thickening that is firmly attached to the base of the proximal phalanx and loosely attached to the metatarsal neck. This fibrous plate is very similar to the volar plate of the metacarpophalangeal joints of the hand. The plate (variously referred to as the plantar capsular ligament, plantar plate, and volar plate) blends laterally with the transverse metatarsal ligament. On its plantar surface the plate is reinforced by the tendons of the flexor hallucis longus and brevis. The flexor hallucis longus lies in the midline of the toe. Medial to it lies the conjoined tendon of the medial head of the flexor hallucis brevis and the abductor hallucis tendon, and laterally is the conjoined tendon of the lateral head of the flexor hallucis brevis and the adductor hallucis. Within the substance of each conjoined tendon lie the sesamoid bones, just proximal to the level of the metatarsophalangeal joint (see Fig. 19-13).

SPRAINS

Mechanism of Injury

Sprain injury of the first metatarsophalangeal joint has been reported with increasing frequency recently, particularly in athletics and ballet. The football injury has been called "turf toe" by Bowers and Martin.[364] They noted an increased frequency of problems with this joint in players competing on artificial playing surfaces in lightweight soccer-style shoes. Because of increased flexibility of the sole of the shoe, less protection is given to this joint. They found the common mechanism of injury to be forced hyperextension of the joint when the player's foot is in equinus and the toe is fixed to the ground. The extreme hyperextension produces temporary subluxation of the joint with stretching of the plantar capsule and plate. Rarely is there an associated fracture. The sprain, however, is very disabling, and Coker and colleagues[367] report more disability (missed practices and games) with sprain of this joint than with sprains of the ankle joint in a large series of college football players.

In ballet dancers, Sammarco and Miller[390] reported occasional hyperflexion injuries of the joint occurring primarily in male dancers. The dancer falls forward, "falling over" the extended toe, stretching and tearing the dorsal capsule as the body weight falls over the maximally extended great toe. Rarely, forceful abduction of the great toe will result in disruption of the lateral capsular ligament and avulsion of a small fragment of bone from the base of the proximal phalanx.

Signs and Symptoms

All sprain injuries of the first metatarsophalangeal joint will be painful and swollen. X-rays rarely show any bony abnormality except occasional capsular avulsion fractures.

Treatment

The joint remains stable but requires splinting to allow capsular healing. Taping the great toe to the second will provide some stability. Stiff-soled shoes also provide stability, and a spring steel insert has been designed for football shoes to protect the injured joint during healing and prevent recurrent injury.[367] Most injuries become painless after 2 to 3 weeks, but an additional 3 weeks may be needed for the patient to regain motion and return to dancing or competitive running. It has been found that early injection of steroids or lidocaine into the injured joint does not facilitate early return to competition, and this technique should be avoided.[366]

DISLOCATION

Mechanism of Injury

Although sprains of the first metatarsophalangeal joint are common, dislocation is relatively rare.[371,372] The joint is intrinsically stable and is supported by the strong capsular ligaments and extrinsic tendons, which prevent dislocation unless an extreme deforming force is applied to the joint. Thus, most dislocations result from high-energy injury such as automobile wrecks and are frequently associated with multiple injuries in the foot or elsewhere.[372]

Signs and Radiographic Findings

A simple dislocation is usually easily identified on physical examination. Most are dorsal dislocations with the proximal phalanx cocked up and displaced dorsally and proximally, producing a dorsal prominence and shortening of the toe. Tenting of the dorsal skin by the base of the proximal phalanx is common, occasionally producing impairment of capillary filling locally. Anteroposterior, lateral, and oblique x-rays of the forefoot will confirm the dislocation, demonstrating dorsal and proximal displacement of the base of the proximal phalanx on the metatarsal head. On the anteroposterior projection the base of the proximal phalanx will overlie the metatarsal head, producing a double density. Occasionally small avulsion fractures of the base of the proximal phalanx will be seen as well.

Rarely, fracture of the medial[369] or lateral[365] sesamoid will occur in addition to the dislocation. This is an important point to notice on the x-rays, since the degree of integrity of the sesamoids may affect the clinician's ability to achieve a satisfactory closed reduction of the dislocation.[372]

Treatment

Once diagnosed, dislocations should be reduced promptly to avoid circulatory compromise of the dorsal skin. Most dislocations reduce readily with application of gentle manual traction on the toe. If traction is ineffective, the block to reduction is usually the plantar lip of the proximal phalanx abutting against the dorsal edge of the metatarsal head. This block to reduction can be overcome by releasing all traction, accentuating the deformity by extremely hyperextending the proximal phalanx on the metatarsal head, and then applying direct thumb pressure to the base of the proximal phalanx dorsally, pushing it over the metatarsal head. Reduction will usually produce a satisfying clunk and be stable to moderate stress.

Crepitus on motion, gross instability on stress, residual joint incongruity, or intra-articular loose bodies on postreduction x-rays are all signs of an inadequate reduction. If these signs are not present, the joint should be considered adequately reduced and should be splinted in a short-leg walking cast with toe plate for 3 to 4 weeks to allow capsular healing to occur. Residual long-term complications from a simple, adequately reduced dislocation are uncommon.

If, following reduction, there is crepitus, gross instability, or x-ray evidence of joint incongruity or an intra-articular loose body, further treatment is indicated. Occasional reports in the literature[369,375] have indicated that fracture of a sesamoid with a loose fragment entrapped in the joint may produce any or all of these signs of an inadequate reduction. Should these findings persist after closed reduction, an arthrotomy should be performed to remove any intra-articular bony fragments and repair the disrupted plantar capsular structures.

Complex Dislocation

Occasionally, closed reduction of a dislocated first metatarsophalangeal joint cannot be achieved by traction or manipulation even under general anesthesia. This is a complex dislocation, very similar to the complex dislocation that occurs in the hand (see Chap. 6). The plantarly displaced first metatarsal head becomes entrapped by the medial and lateral tendons of the flexor hallucis brevis on either side. The plantar joint capsule remains attached to the base of the proximal phalanx, is displaced dorsal to the metatarsal head lying against the articular surface of the base of the proximal phalanx, and becomes entrapped between the base of the phalanx and the metatarsal head. Both collateral ligaments remain intact.[371] The metatarsal head is thus incarcerated by the transverse metatarsal ligament and plantar capsule dorsally, the lateral collateral ligament and the lateral tendon of the flexor hallucis brevis laterally, the medial collateral ligament, the adductor tendon and the medial tendon of the flexor hallucis brevis medially, and the fibers of the plantar aponeurosis plantarly. These structures act like a Chinese finger trap when traction is applied to the toe tightening around the metatarsal neck to prevent reduction. The flexor hallucis longus tendon usually lies on the lateral side of the metatarsal head as well.

The physician should suspect a complex dislocation of this joint when unfractured sesamoids are noted to be lying between the articular surfaces of the two bones on x-ray[376] (Fig. 19-117). The complex dislocation, irreducible by closed means, occurs because the "sesamoid mass" remains intact. Jahss[372] emphasizes that if sesamoid fracture occurs or if the intersesamoid ligament is disrupted, closed reduction of the dislocation can be achieved, and only when the sesamoid mass remains intact will the metatarsal head remain incarcerated and require surgical release.

The true complex dislocation requires open reduction. Most authors recommend a transverse plantar incision over the prominent metatarsal head.[371,380] The head lies in the subcutaneous tissue,

and care must be taken to avoid laceration of the displaced digital neurovascular bundles. Once the head is exposed, a periosteal elevator can be placed dorsal to the head to dislodge the entrapped plantar capsule, and then the proximal phalanx can be levered back into position using the elevator. Occasionally it will be necessary to release surgically a portion of the attachment of the plantar capsule to the transverse metatarsal ligament to allow the capsule to be removed from the joint.

Once reduced, as in the hand, the joint is stable. It should be splinted in a short-leg walking cast with toe plate for 3 weeks to allow capsular healing, and then the patient should begin an active range of motion exercise program.

FRACTURES OF THE SESAMOIDS

Mechanism of Injury

Sesamoid fractures can result from direct trauma, avulsion forces, or repetitive stress. The medial sesamoid is more frequently fractured than is the lateral, possibly because it bears more weight and thus is more vulnerable to the application of direct forces.[373] Excessive, repetitive stress of the flexor tendon complex, as in dancing and long distance running, is thought to be a cause of acute avulsion fractures or stress fractures of these bones.[382]

Signs and Radiographic Findings

Following acute injury, the patient will present with pain well localized over the fractured sesamoid, and with a stress fracture the patient will develop well-localized pain progressively over days or weeks. Tenderness can be elicited over the involved bone, and the pain can be accentuated by passive hyperextension of the metatarsophalangeal joint, which stretches the flexor hallucis brevis, in which lie the sesamoids.

Most fractures are transverse and will be seen best on anteroposterior and lateral x-rays (Fig. 19-118). Occasionally a tangential view of the sesamoids will reveal a small osteochondral or avulsion fracture. Care must be taken to differentiate fracture from failure of fusion of the multicentric centers of ossification of these bones. Partition is frequent, occurring in 8% to 33% of the population and 10 times more frequently in the medial than in the lateral sesamoid; in 85% of cases it is bilateral.[373]

Several features help to differentiate fractured from partitioned sesamoids:

Partition is present bilaterally in 85% of cases.
Fracture edges are rough and irregular, while a

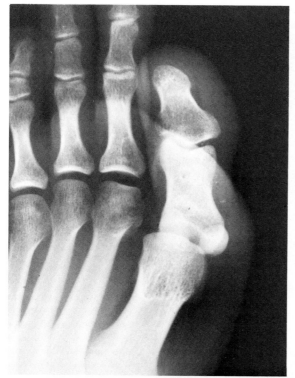

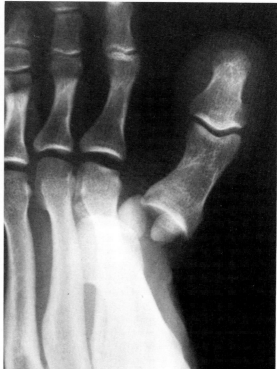

Fig. 19-117. Complex dorsal dislocation of the first metatarsophalangeal joint. Note the unfractured sesamoids lying between the metatarsal head and the base of the proximal phalanx.

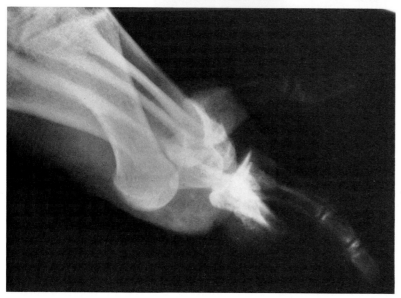

bipartite sesamoid will have smooth, sclerotic edges.

The partite sesamoid generally will be larger than the sum of the fractured fragments.

Evidence of callus formation 2 to 3 weeks after the onset of symptoms occurs only with the sesamoid fracture.

The line of fracture is usually transverse, except when the fracture is associated with dislocation of the first metatarsophalangeal joint, where either sesamoid characteristically will fracture longitudinally.

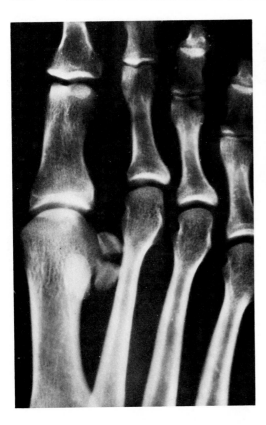

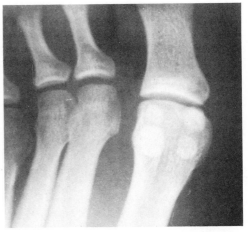

Fig. 19-118. (*Left*) Acute fracture of the lateral sesamoid. The edges of the fragments are sharp and without a subchondral bony rim. (*Right*) Bipartite sesamoids. The edges are rounded and smooth.

Treatment

Although earlier reports recommended surgical excision of the fractured sesamoid acutely,[378] most authors now agree that initial treatment should be conservative in an attempt to achieve healing of the fracture and preserve the important function of the sesamoids. Short-leg walking cast immobilization for 3 to 4 weeks should be employed for all fractures initially. Following cast removal, a stiff-soled shoe with a metatarsal pad may be needed for from 4 to 6 weeks. With extreme displacement of acute fracture fragments, or with some fragmented stress fractures, union will not occur with immobilization. For these patients who do not respond to conservative treatment and have persistent symptoms, excision of the involved sesamoid should be considered. Care must be taken to reconstruct the short flexor mechanism after excision of the bone fragments. The bone should be carefully shelled out of the tendon, and the tendon then repaired. The medial sesamoid should be approached from the medial aspect of the first ray, while the lateral sesamoid should be excised through a dorsal first web space incision as is done in the classic McBride bunionectomy. After excision and reconstruction of the tendon, the repair should be protected in a walking cast for 3 to 4 weeks.

INJURIES OF THE LESSER METATARSOPHALANGEAL JOINTS

Dislocation of the lesser toes occurs as the result of extreme medial or, more commonly, lateral displacement of the digit on the metatarsal head. This displacement occurs particularly when the bare foot is jammed into the leg of a piece of furniture. The base of the proximal phalanx is displaced dorsally and usually laterally, overriding the metatarsal head or neck (Fig. 19-119). Reduction is usually easily accomplished by applying manual traction to the toe or applying digital pressure directly distally to the base of the proximal phalanx, pushing it back into the reduced position.

Rao and Banzon[379] reported dorsal dislocation of the third and fourth metatarsophalangeal joints that could not be reduced by closed means. They described a complex dislocation in which the plantar capsule and deep transverse metatarsal ligament were entrapped between the base of the proximal

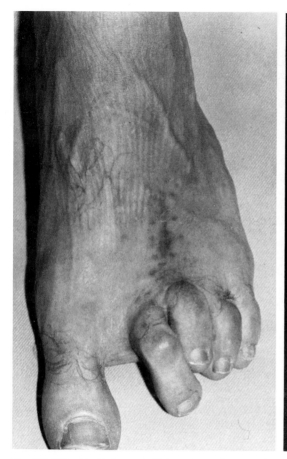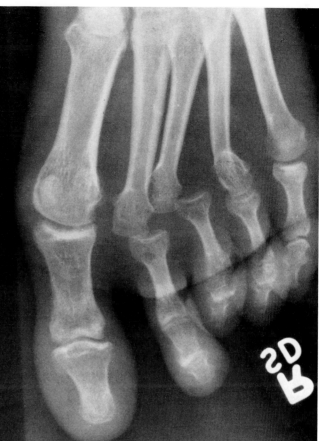

Fig. 19-119. (*Left*) Lateral dislocation of second and third metatarsophalangeal joints. The third toe is slightly rotated, and swelling is evident at the base of the toes. (*Right*) X-ray of the foot demonstrates unreduced dislocations of the second and third metatarsophalangeal joints.

phalanx and the dorsal aspect of the metatarsal head. The metatarsal head, displaced plantarly, was trapped between the flexor tendons laterally and the lumbrical tendons medially. Reduction was achieved by surgical division of the fibrocartilaginous plate and deep transverse metatarsal ligament through a dorsal approach. Murphy[377] reported a similar case occurring after a severe direct blow to the second toe.

English[370] described another cause of irreducible metatarsophalangeal dislocation—the "linked-toe dislocation of the metatarsal bone." He described two patients with multiple forefoot fractures and dislocations. Closed reduction of all injuries was accomplished except for dislocation of one metatarsal base and dislocation of the medially adjacent metatarsophalangeal joint. Only after open reduc-

tion of the metatarsal base could the neighboring metatarsophalangeal dislocation be reduced by simple manipulation. Reduction of the metatarsophalangeal joint was prevented by the proximal displacement of the adjacent metatarsal and the interosseous muscle, which arises from this metatarsal but inserts on the adjacent proximal phalanx. Once the metatarsal is reduced out to length, tension is released from the tendon of the interosseous muscle, facilitating reduction of the joint. This phenomenon must be remembered when dealing with multiple fractures in the same foot.

Persistent dislocations, discovered more than 3 weeks after injury, are difficult to reduce by closed means. If the patient develops a discrete, painful callus, the underlying metarsal head should be excised.

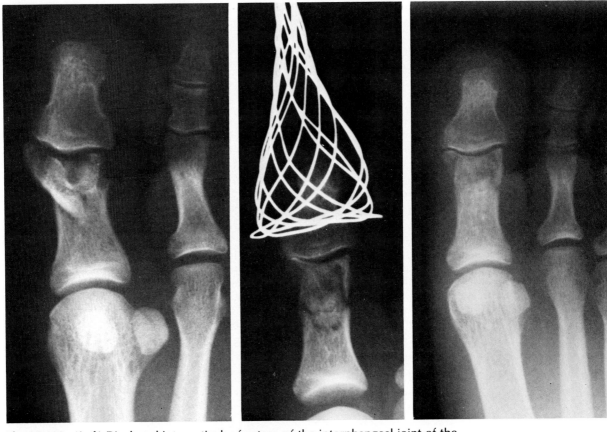

Fig. 19-120. (*Left*) Displaced intra-articular fracture of the interphangeal joint of the great toe. (*Center*) After the application of longitudinal traction, stable acceptable alignment is achieved. (*Right*) One year after injury the fracture is healed and the patient is asymptomatic.

INJURIES OF THE TOES

FRACTURES OF THE GREAT TOE

Mechanisms and Signs of Fracture

Two mechanisms are responsible for most hallux fractures: direct blows from objects being dropped on the unprotected foot and "stubbing" injuries as described by Jahss.[338] Most of these injuries can be prevented by use of proper protective footwear.

Patients have persistent pain after injury, frequently presenting 24 hours or more after the injury with significant swelling and a subungual hematoma. Rarely is there significant deformity, since most fractures are only minimally displaced. X-rays in the anteroposterior and oblique projections will demonstrate most fractures. On occasion, a lateral view will be required. This projection should be obtained with the lateral four toes pas-

sively dorsiflexed to avoid overlap with the hallux. Another method to achieve adequate x-ray visualization in the lateral projection is to use a dental x-ray film inserted between the first and second toes with the x-ray being directed laterally to obtain an isolated view of the great toe.

Treatment

All toe injuries are persistently painful and require adequate splinting and analgesic medication for 2 to 3 weeks. A nondisplaced fracture of the great toe may be adequately but minimally immobilized by adhesive plaster taping using the uninjured second toe as a splint. A hard-soled shoe or a postoperative wooden-soled shoe should be worn, and the patient should be given crutches to allow partial weight bearing as tolerated. If taping does not provide adequate pain relief, then the foot should be immobilized in a short-leg walking cast with a toe plate to provide firm support for the injured toe. After 10 to 14 days the cast can usually be replaced by a firm-soled shoe.

Displaced intra-articular fractures of the interphalangeal joint require reduction. Frequently this can be achieved by longitudinal traction applied through finger traps (Fig, 19-120). Once reduced, the fragments are frequently stable and the fracture can be treated by short-leg walking cast immobilization. If adequate reduction is not achieved by closed means, the interphalangeal joint should be opened through a midlateral incision and the fragments reduced and fixed with small diameter Kirschner wires. Occasionally displaced intra-articular fracture fragments do not heal, producing a painful subcutaneous mass or crepitus on joint motion (Fig. 19-121). These ununited, displaced fragments can be treated best by excision of the fragment and repair of the capsule and any attached collateral ligament.

DISLOCATIONS OF THE INTERPHALANGEAL JOINT

Dislocation or fracture–dislocation of the interphalangeal joint usually occurs when an axial load is applied to the end of the digit, as when the foot kicks a wall. Most dislocations are dorsal and can be reduced with digital block anesthesia and traction combined with gentle manipulation of the distal phalanx. Once reduced, the dislocation is usually stable and requires only 2 to 3 weeks of productive splinting to the second toe to allow soft tissue healing. Nelson and Uggen[389] reported one case of irreducible dislocation of the interphalangeal joint, and I have seen one case of dorsal fracture–dislocation of the interphalangeal joint that was irreducible by closed means (Fig. 19-122). In both cases the thickened plantar joint capsule (the plantar accessory ligament) was flipped into the joint, preventing closed reduction. Through a medial midline incision, open reduction of the displaced plantar capsule was accomplished, and the joint was found to reduce readily to a stable configuration.

INJURIES OF THE LESSER TOES

FRACTURES

Fractures of the lesser toes are quite common, resulting from direct blows or from striking the unprotected toe against a hard object (Fig. 19-123). As with the great toe, these injuries are quite painful and may cause significant impairment of function

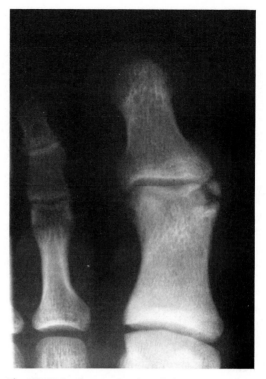

Fig. 19-121. One year after dislocation and spontaneous reduction of the great toe interphalangeal joint. A small avulsion fracture of the medial aspect of the proximal phalanx failed to heal and required surgical excision.

for 2 to 3 weeks until stabilized by fracture callus. Anterioposterior, oblique, and lateral forefoot x-rays (with the uninjured toes pulled dorsally) will adequately demonstrate the fracture. If significant displacement or angulation is present, these can be reduced by longitudinal manual traction or with wire finger traps. Usually, displaced fractures will be stable when reduced. Moderate degrees or persistent fracture angulation or displacement can be accepted on x-ray if the general, overall appearance of the toe is acceptable clinically. The toe should be splinted to the adjacent toe with adhesive tape after a gauze pad is placed in the web space to prevent skin maceration. Splinting with tape, combined with the use of a firm-soled shoe and adequate oral analgesics for 2 to 3 weeks, will allow healing in virtually all instances.[384]

DISLOCATIONS

Dislocation of the distal interphalangeal (DIP) or proximal interphalangeal (PIP) joints of the toes is rare. Manual reduction under digital block is easy

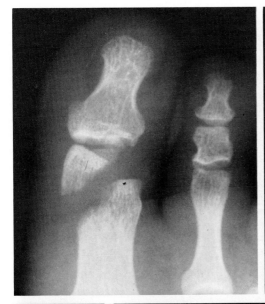

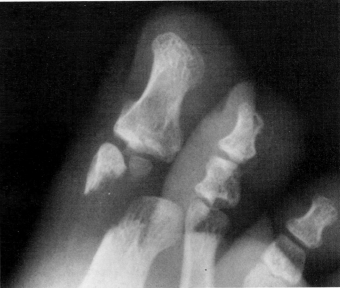

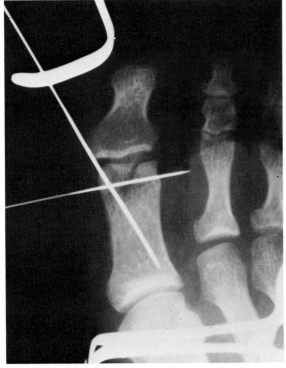

Fig. 19-122. (*Top left* and *Top right*) Displaced intra-articular fracture–dislocation of the interphalangeal joint of the great toe irreducible by closed means (note sesamoid interposed in the joint). (*Bottom*) After open reduction and fixation with Kirschner wires.

to accomplish and is usually stable. The toe should be splinted to the adjacent toe for 10 days to 2 weeks to allow capsular healing.

Jahss[387] reported an interesting series of ten patients with persistent, unreduced dislocation or recurrent dislocation of the proximal interphalangeal joint of the fifth toe following untreated ab-duction injury to that digit. The patients complained of deformity and toe irritation from shoes but no joint pain. The surgical treatment found most effective for these chronic problems was resection arthroplasty of the joint combined with syndactylization of the toe to the adjacent fourth toe.

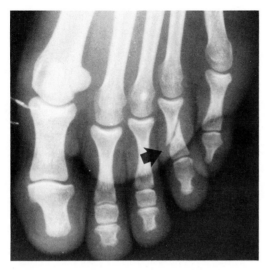

Fig. 19-123. A closed fracture of the shaft of the proximal phalanx. Taping to an adjacent toe is sufficient immobilization.

REFERENCES

Anatomy, Biomechanics, and Evaluation

1. Basmajian, J. V.: Weight-bearing by Ligaments and Muscles. Can. J. Surg., **4:**166–170, 1961.
2. Basmajian, J. V., and Bentzon, J. W.: An Electromyographic Study of Certain Muscles of the Leg and Foot in the Standing Position. Surg. Gynecol. Obstet., **98:**662–666, 1954.
3. Basmajian, J. V., and Stecko, G.: The Role of Muscles in Arch Support of the Foot. J. Bone Joint Surg., **45A:**1184–1190, 1963.
4. Blechschmidt, E.: The Structure of the Calcaneal Padding. Foot Ankle, **2:**260–283, 1982.
5. Bobechko, W. P., and Harris, W. R.: The Radiographic Density of Avascular Bone. J. Bone Joint Surg., **42B:**626–632, 1960.
6. Close, J. R.; Inman, V. T.; Poor, P. M.; and Todd, F. N.: The Function of the Subtalar Joint. Clin. Orthop., **50:**159–179, 1967.
7. Collis, W. J. M. F., and Jayson, M. I. V.: Measurement of Pedal Pressures. An Illustration of a Method. Ann. Rheum. Dis., **31:**215–217, 1972.
8. Elftman, H.: The Transverse Tarsal Joint and its Control. Clin. Orthop., **16:**41–45, 1960.
9. Frankel, V. H.: Biomechanics of the Musculoskeletal System. Introduction. Arch. Surg., **107:**405, 1973.
10. Genant, H. K.; Doi, K.; Mall, J. C.; and Sickles, E. A.: Direct Radiographic Magnification for Skeletal Radiology. Radiology, **123:**47–55, 1977.
11. Gertzbien, S. D., and Barrington, T. W.: Diagnosis of Occult Fractures and Dislocations. Clin. Orthop., **108:**105–109, 1975.
12. Geslian, G. E.; Thrall, J. H.; Espinosa, J. L.; and Older, R. A.: Early Detection of Stress Fractures using ⁹⁹ᵐTC-polyphosphate. Radiology, **121:**683–687, 1976.
13. Gordon, S. L.; Greer, R. B.; and Weidner, W. A.: Magnification Roentgenographic Technic in Orthopaedics. Clin. Orthop., **91:**169–173, 1973.
14. Goss, C. M. (ed.): Gray's Anatomy, 29th ed. Philadelphia, Lea & Febiger, 1973.
15. Gray, E. G., and Basmajian, J. V.: Electromyography and Cinematography of Leg and Foot ("Normal " and Flat) during Walking. Anat. Rec., **161:**1–15, 1968.
16. Grundy, M.; Tosh, P. A.; McLeish, R. D.; and Smidt, L.: An Investigation of the Centres of Pressure under the Foot while Walking. J. Bone Joint Surg., **57B:**98–103, 1975.
17. Hicks, J. H.: The Mechanics of the Foot. II. The Plantar Aponeurosis and the Arch. J. Anat., **88:**25–30, 1954.
18. Inman, V. T.: Human Locomotion. Can. Med. Assoc. J., **94:**1047–1054, 1966.
19. Inman, V. T.: Conservation of Energy in Ambulation. Arch. Phys. Med. Rehabil., **48:**484–488, 1967.
20. Inman, V. T.: The Influence of the Foot–Ankle Complex on the Proximal Skeletal Structures. Artif. Limbs, **13:**59–65, 1969.
21. Inman, V. T.: The Joints of the Ankle. Baltimore, Williams & Wilkins, 1976.
22. Inman, V. T.; Ralston, H. J.; and Todd, F.: Human Walking. Baltimore, Williams & Wilkins, 1981.
23. Isman, R. E., and Inman, V. T.: Anthropometric Studies of the Human Foot and Ankle. Bull. Prosthet. Res., **10–11:**97–129, 1969.
24. Jones, R. L.: The Human Foot. An Experimental Study of its Mechanics, and the Role of its Muscles and Ligaments in the Support of the Arch. Am. J. Anat., **68:**1–39, 1941.
25. Keats, T. E.: An Atlas of Normal Roentgen Variants That May Simulate Disease, 2nd ed. Chicago, Year Book Medical Publishers, 1979.
26. Kirchner, P. T., and Simon, M. A.: Current Concepts Review: Radioisotopic Evaluation of Skeletal Disease. J. Bone Joint Surg., **63A:**673–681, 1981.
27. Köhler, A., and Zimmer, E. A.: Borderlands of the Normal and Early Pathologic in Skeletal Roentgenology, 3rd ed. New York, Grune & Stratton, 1968.
28. Kuhns, J. G.: Changes in Elastic Adipose Tissue. J. Bone Joint Surg., **31A:**541–547, 1949.
29. Levens, A. S.; Inman, V. T.; and Blosser, J. A.: Transverse Rotation of the Segments of the Lower Extremity in Locomotion. J. Bone Joint Surg., **30A:**859–872, 1948.
30. Mann, R. A.: Biomechanics. In Jahss, M. H. (ed.): Disorders of the Foot, Vol. 1. Philadelphia. W. B. Saunders, 1982.
31. Mann, R., and Inman, V. T.: Phasic Activity of Intrinsic Muscles of the Foot. J. Bone Joint Surg., **46A:**469–481, 1964.
32. Merrill, V.: Atlas of Roentgenographic Positions and Standard Radiologic Procedures, Vol. I, 4th ed. St. Louis, C. V. Mosby, 1975.
33. Meschan, I.: Radiology of the Normal Foot. Semin. Roentgenol., **5:**327–340, 1970.
34. Milner, M.; Basmajian, J. V.; and Quanbury, A. O.: Multifactorial Analysis of Walking by Electromyography and Computer. Am. J. Phys. Med., **50:**235–258, 1971.

35. Prather, J. L.; Nusynowitz, M. L.; Snowdy, H. A.; et al: Scintigraphic Findings in Stress Fractures. J. Bone Joint Surg., **59A**:869–874, 1977.

36. Rogers, L. F., and Campbell, R. E.: Fractures and Dislocations of the Foot. Semin. Roentgenol., **13**:157–166, 1978.

37. Rosenthall, L.; Hill, R. O.; and Chuang, S.: Observation on the Use of ^{99m}TC-Phosphate Imaging in Peripheral Bone Trauma. Radiology, **119**:637–641, 1976.

38. Sammarco, G. J.; Burstein, A. H.; and Frankel, V. H.: Biomechanics of the Ankle: A Kinematic Study. Orthop. Clin. North Am., **4**:75–96, 1973.

39. Saunders, J. B. deC. M.; Inman, V. T.; and Eberhart, H. D.: The Major Determinants in Normal and Pathological Gait. J. Bone Joint Surg., **35A**:543–558, 1953.

40. Schwartz, R. P., and Heath, A. L.: The Definition of Human Locomotion on the Basis of Measurement. J. Bone Joint Surg., **29**:203–214, 1947.

41. Schwartz, R. P., and Heath, A. L.: The Oscillographic Recording and Quantitative Definition of Functional Disabilities of Human Locomotion. Arch. Phys. Med., **30**:568–578, 1949.

42. Schwartz, R. P.; Heath, A. L.; Morgan, D. W.; and Towns, R. C.: A Quantitative Analysis of Recorded Variables in the Walking Pattern of "Normal" Adults. J. Bone Joint Surg., **46A**:324–334, 1964.

43. Shands, A. R., Jr., and Wentz, I. J.: Congenital Anomalies, Accessory Bones, and Osteochondritis in the Feet of 850 Children. Surg. Clin. North Am., **33**:1643–1666, 1953.

44. Simon, S. R.; Mann, R. A.; Hagy, J. L.; and Larsen, L. J.: Role of the Posterior Calf Muscles in Normal Gait. J. Bone Joint Surg., **60A**:465–472, 1978.

45. Solomonow, M.; Lyman, J.; and Freedy, A.: Electrotactile Two-Point Discrimination as a Function of Frequency, Body Site, Laterality and Stimulation Codes. Ann. Biomed. Eng., **5**:47–60, 1977.

46. Takahashi, S., and Sakuma, S.: Magnification Radiography. New York, Springer-Verlag, 1975.

47. Tietze, A.: Concerning the Architectural Structure of the Connective Tissue in the Human Sole. Foot Ankle, **2**:252–259, 1982.

48. Weinstein, S.: Intensive and Extensive Aspects of Tactile Sensitivity as a Function of Body Part, Sex, and Laterality. *In* Kenshalo, D. R. (ed.): The Skin Senses, chap. 10, Springfield, IL., Charles C Thomas, 1968.

49. Wilcox, J. R.; Moniot, A. L.; and Green, J. P.: Bone Scanning in the Evaluation of Exercise-related Stress Injuries. Radiology, **123**:699–703, 1977.

50. Wright, D. G.; Desai, S. M.; and Henderson, W. H.: Action of the Subtalar and Ankle–Joint Complex during the Stance Phase of Walking. J. Bone Joint Surg., **46A**:361–382, 1964.

51. Zatzkin, H. R.: Trauma to the Foot. Semin. Roentgenol., **5**:419–435, 1970.

Fractures Common to All Parts of the Foot

52. Chapman, M. W.: The Use of Immediate Internal Fixation in Open Fractures. Orthop. Clin. North Am., **11**:579–591, 1980.

53. Charcot, J. M.: Sur Quelques Arthropathies qui Paraissent pendre d'une Lésion Cerveau ou de la Moelle Épiniere. Physiol. Norm. Pathol., **1**:161–178, 1868.

54. Clouse, M. E.; Gramm, H. F.; Legg, M.; and Flood, T.: Diabetic Osteoarthropathy. Clinical and Roentgenographic Observations in 90 cases. Am. J. Roentgenol. **121**:22–34, 1974.

55. Coventry, M. B., and Rothacker, G. W., Jr.: Bilateral Calcaneal Fracture in a Diabetic Patient. A Case Report. J. Bone Joint Surg., **61A**:462–464, 1979.

56. Darby, R. E.: Stress Fractures of the Os Calcis. J.A.M.A., **200**:1183–1184, 1967.

57. Devas, M.: Stress Fractures. Edinburgh, Churchill Livingstone, 1975.

58. Drez, D., Jr.; Young, J. C.; Johnston, R. D.; and Parker, W. D.: Metatarsal Stress Fractures. Am. J. Sports Med., **8**:123–125, 1980.

59. El-Khoury, G. Y., and Kathol, M. H.: Neuropathic Fractures in Patients with Diabetes Mellitus. Radiology, **134**:313–316, 1980.

60. Ford, L. T., and Gilula, L. A.: Stress Fractures of the Middle Metatarsals following the Keller Operation. J. Bone Joint Surg., **59A**:117–118, 1977.

61. Giesecke, S. B.; Dalinka, M. K.; and Kyle, G. C.: Lisfranc's Fracture–Dislocation: A Manifestation of Peripheral Neuropathy. Am. J. Roentgenol., **131**:139–141, 1978.

62. Goergen, T. G.; Venn-Watson, E. A.; Rossman, D. J.; et al: Tarsal Navicular Stress Fractures in Runners. Am. J. Roentgenol., **136**:201–203, 1981.

63. Grahame, R.; Saunders, A. S.; and Maisey, M.: The Use of Scintigraphy in the Diagnosis and Management of Traumatic Foot Lesions in Ballet Dancers. Rheumatol. Rehabil., **18**:235–238, 1979.

64. Hopson, C. N., and Perry, D. R.: Stress Fractures of the Calcaneus in Women Marine Recruits. Clin. Orthop., **128**:159–162, 1977.

65. Hulme, J. R., and Askew, A. R.: Rotary Lawn Mower Injuries. Injury, **5**:217–220, 1974.

66. Hunter, L. Y.: Stress Fracture of the Tarsal Navicular. Am. J. Sports Med., **9**:217–219, 1981.

67. Johnson, J. T. H.: Neuropathic Fractures and Joint Injuries. J. Bone Joint Surg., **49A**:1–30, 1967.

68. Kenzora, J. E.; Edwards, C. C.; Browner, B. D.; et al: Acute Management of Major Trauma involving the Foot and Ankle with Hoffmann External Fixation. Foot Ankle, **1**:348–361, 1981.

69. Ketenjian, A. Y., and Shelton, M. L.: Primary Internal Fixation of Open Fractures. A Retrospective Study of the use of Metallic Internal Fixation in Fresh Open Fractures. J. Trauma, **12**:756–763, 1972.

70. Korhonen, B. J.: Fractures in Myelodysplasia. Clin. Orthop., **79**:145–155, 1971.

71. Loeffler, R. D., Jr., and Ballard, A.: Plantar Fascial Spaces of the Foot and a Proposed Surgical Approach. Foot Ankle, **1**:11–14, 1980.

72. London, P. S.: Clinical Aspects of the Disruptive Effects of Road Accidents on the Human Body. Acta Orthop. Scand., **46**:460–474, 1975.

73. McBryde, A. M., Jr.: Stress Fractures in Runners. Orthopedics, **5**:913–928, 1982.

74. Madigan, R. R., and McMahan, C. J., Jr.: Power Lawn Mower Injuries. J. Tenn. Med. Assoc. **72:**653–655, 1979.

75. Maxwell, G. P., and Hoopes, J. E.: Management of Compound Injuries of the Lower Extremity. Plast. Reconstr. Surg., **63:**176–185, 1979.

76. Meurman, K. O. A.: Less Common Stress Fractures in the Foot. Br. J. Radiol., **54:**1–7, 1981.

77. Meurman, K. O. A., and Elfving, S.: Case Reports. Stress Fracture of the Cuneiform Bones. Br. J. Radiol., **53:**157–160, 1980.

78. Meurman, K. O. A., and Elfving, S: Stress Fracture in Soldiers: A Multifocal Bone Disorder. Radiology, **134:**483–487, 1980.

78. Miller, B.; Markheim, H. R.; and Towbin, M. N.: Multiple Stress Fractures in Rheumatoid Arthritis. J. Bone Joint Surg., **49A:**1408–1414, 1967.

80. Mooney, V., and Wagner, F. W., Jr.: Neurocirculatory Disorders of the Foot. Clin. Orthop., **122:**53–61, 1977.

81. Newman, J. H.: Non-infective Disease of the Diabetic Foot. J. Bone Joint Surg., **63B:**593–596, 1981.

82. Omer, G. E., Jr., and Pomerantz, G. M.: Initial Management of Severe Open Injuries and Traumatic Amputations of the Foot. Arch. Surg., **105:**696–698, 1972.

83. Orava, S.; Puranen, J.; and Ala-Ketola, L.: Stress Fractures caused by Physical Exercise. Acta Orthop. Scand., **49:**19–27, 1978.

84. Park, W. H., and DeMuth, W. E., Jr.: Wounding Capacity of Rotary Lawn Mowers. J. Trauma, **15:**36–38, 1975.

85. Saunders, A. J. S.; El Sayed, T. F.; Hilson, A. J. W.; et al: Stress Lesions of the Lower Leg and Foot. Clin. Radiol., **30:**649–651, 1979.

86. Scully, T. J., and Besterman, G.: Stress Fracture—a Preventable Training Injury. Milit. Med., **147:**285–287, 1982.

87. Torg, J. S.; Pavlov, H.; Cooley, L. H.; et al: Stress Fractures of the Tarsal Navicular. A Retrospective Review of Twenty-One Cases. J. Bone Joint Surg., **64A:**700–712, 1982.

88. Wagner, F. W., Jr.: The Dysvascular Foot: A System for Diagnosis and Treatment. Foot Ankle, **2:**64–122, 1981.

89. Warren, G.: Tarsal Bone Disintegration in Leprosy. J. Bone Joint Surg., **53B:**688–695, 1971.

90. Wilson, E. S., Jr., and Katz, F. N.: Stress Fractures. An Analysis of 250 Consecutive Cases. Radiology, **92:**481–486, 1969.

91. Worthen, B. M., and Yanklowitz, B. A. D.: The Pathophysiology and Treatment of Stress Fractures in Military Personnel. J. Am. Podiatry Assoc., **68:**317–325, 1978.

92. Yale, J.: A Statistical Analysis of 3,657 Consecutive Fatigue Fractures of the Distal Lower Extremities. J. Am. Podiatry Assoc., **66:**739–748, 1976.

Fractures of the Talus

93. Anderson, H. G.: The Medical and Surgical Aspects of Aviation. London, Oxford University Press, 1919.

94. Blair, H. C.: Comminuted Fractures and Fracture Dislocations of the Body of the Astragalus. Operative Treatment. Am. J. Surg., **59:**37–43, 1943.

95. Boyd, H. B., and Knight, R. A.: Fractures of the Astragalus. South. Med. J., **35:**160–167, 1942.

96. Canale, S. T., and Kelly, F. B., Jr.: Fractures of the Neck of the Talus. Long-term Evaluation of Seventy-One Cases. J. Bone Joint Surg., **60A:**143–156, 1978.

97. Cedell, C. A.: Rupture of the Posterior Talotibial Ligament with the Avulsion of a Bone Fragment from the Talus. Acta Orthop. Scand., **45:**454–461, 1974.

98. Cimmino, C. V.: Fracture of the Lateral Process of the Talus. Am. J. Roentgenol. **90:**1277–1280, 1963.

99. Coltart, W. D.: "Aviator's Astragalus." J. Bone Joint Surg., **34B:**545–566, 1952.

100. Cooper, A. P.: A Treatise on Dislocations, and on Fractures of the Joints, 2nd ed. Boston, Lilly, Wait, Carter, and Hendee, 1832.

101. Dennis, M. D., and Tullos, H. S.: Blair Tibiotalar Arthrodesis for Injuries to the Talus. J. Bone Joint Surg., **62A:**103–107, 1980.

102. DePalma, A. F.; Ahmad, I.; Flannery, G.; and Gandhi, O. P.: Aseptic Necrosis of the Talus. Revascularization after Bone Grafting. Clin. Orthop., **101:**232–235, 1974.

103. Dimon, J. H.: Isolated Displaced Fracture of the Posterior Facet of the Talus. J. Bone Joint Surg., **43A:**275–281, 1961.

104. Dunn, A. R.; Jacobs, B.; and Campbell, R. D., Jr.: Fractures of the Talus. J. Trauma, **6:**443–468, 1966.

105. Fjeldborg, O.: Fracture of the Lateral Process of the Talus. Supination–Dorsal Flexion Fracture. Acta Orthop. Scand., **39:**407–412, 1968.

106. Gillquist, J.; Oretorp, N.; Stenström, A.; et al: Late Results after Vertical Fracture of the Talus. Injury, **6:**173–179, 1974.

107. Haliburton, R. A.; Sullivan, C. R.; Kelly, P. J.; and Peterson, L. F. A.: The Extra-Osseous and Intra-Osseous Blood Supply of the Talus. J. Bone Joint Surg., **40A:**1115–1120, 1958.

108. Hamilton, W.G.: Stenosing Tenosynovitis of the Flexor Hallucis Longus Tendon and Posterior Impingement upon the Os Trigonum in Ballet Dancers. Foot Ankle, **3:**74–80, 1982.

109. Hawkins, L. G.: Fracture of the Lateral Process of the Talus. J. Bone Joint Surg., **47A:**1170–1175, 1965.

110. Hawkins, L. G.: Fractures of the Neck of the Talus. J. Bone Joint Surg., **52A:**991–1002, 1970.

111. Howse, A. J. G.: Posterior Block of the Ankle Joint in Dancers. Foot Ankle, **3:**81–84, 1982.

112. Ihle, C. L., and Cochran, R. M.: Fracture of the Fused Os Trigonum. Am. J. Sports Med., **10:**47–50, 1982.

113. Kelly, P. J., and Sullivan, C. R.: Blood Supply of the Talus. Clin. Orthop., **30:**37–44, 1963.

114. Kenwright, J., and Taylor, R. G.: Major Injuries of the Talus. J. Bone Joint Surg., **52B:**36–48, 1970.

115. Kleiger, B.: Fractures of the Talus. J. Bone Joint Surg., **30A:**735–744, 1948.

116. Kleiger, B., and Ahmed, M.: Injuries of the Talus and its Joints. Clin. Orthop., **121:**243–262, 1976.

117. Lapidus, P. W.: A Note on the Fracture of Os Trigonum. Report of a Case. Bull. Hosp. Joint Dis., **33:**150–154, 1972.

118. Larson, R. L.; Sullivan, C. R.; and Janes, J. M: Trauma, Surgery, and Circulation of the Talus—what are the Risks of Avascular Necrosis? J. Trauma, **1:**13–21, 1961.

119. Lemaire, R. G., and Bustin, W.: Screw Fixation of Fractures

of the Neck of the Talus using a Posterior Approach. J. Trauma, **20**:669–673, 1980.

120. Lieberg, O. U.; Henke, J. A.; and Bailey, R. W.; Avascular Necrosis of the Head of the Talus without Death of the Body: Report of an Unusual Case. J. Trauma, **15**:926–928, 1975.

121. Lionberger, D. R.; Bishop, J. O.; and Tullos, H. S.: The Modified Blair Fusion. Foot Ankle, **3**:60–62, 1982.

122. Lorentzen, J. E.; Christensen, S. B.; Krogsoe, O.; and Sneppen, O.: Fractures of the Neck of the Talus. Acta Orthop. Scand., **48**:115–120, 1977.

123. McDougall, A.: The Os Trigonum. J. Bone Joint Surg., **37B**:257–265, 1955.

124. McKeever, F. M.: Fracture of the Neck of the Astragalus. Arch. Surg., **46**:720–735, 1943.

125. McKeever, F. M.: Treatment of Complications of Fractures and Dislocations of the Talus. Clin. Orthop., **30**:45–52, 1963.

126. Milch, H.: Fracture of Processus Posticus Tali. Med. Rec., **154**:90–92, 1941.

127. Miller, O. E., and Baker, L. D.: Fracture and Fracture–Dislocation of the Astragalus. South. Med. J., **32**:125–136, 1939.

128. Miller, W. E.: Operative Intervention for Fracture of the Talus. *In* Bateman, J. E., and Trott, A. W. (eds.): Foot and Ankle, Chap. 8. New York, Brian C. Decker, 1980.

129. Mindell, E. R.; Cisek, E. E.; Kartalian, G.; and Dziob, J. M.: Late Results of Injuries to the Talus. J. Bone Joint Surg., **45A**:221–245, 1963.

130. Monkman, G. R.; Johnson, K. A.; and Duncan, D. M.: Fractures of the Neck of the Talus. Minn. Med., **58**:335–340, 1975.

131. Morris, H. D.: Aseptic Necrosis of the Talus following Injury. Orthop. Clin. North Am., **5**:177–189, 1974.

132. Morris, H. D.; Hand, W. L.; and Dunn, A. W.: The Modified Blair Fusion for Fractures of the Talus. J. Bone Joint Surg., **53A**:1289–1297, 1971.

133. Mukherjee, S. K.; Pringle, R. M.; and Baxter, A. D.: Fracture of the Lateral Process of the Talus. A Report of Thirteen Cases. J. Bone Joint Surg., **56B**:263–273, 1974.

134. Mulfinger, G. L., and Trueta, J.: The Blood Supply of the Talus. J. Bone Joint Surg., **52B**:160–167, 1970.

135. Nelson, T. L., and Gilbert, J. D.: Avascular Necrosis of Talus following Minor Ankle Trauma. Orthop. Rev., **10**:35–37, 1981.

136. O'Brien, E. T.: Injuries of the Talus. Am. Fam. Phys. **12**:95–105, 1975.

137. Pantazopoulos, T.; Galanos, P.; Vayanos, E.; et al: Fractures of the Neck of the Talus. Acta Orthop. Scand., **45**:296–306, 1974.

138. Pantazopoulos, T.; Kapetsis, P.; Soucacos, P.; and Gianakis, E.: Unusual Fracture–Dislocation of the Talus. Report of a Case. Clin. Orthop., **83**:232–234, 1972.

139. Pennal, G. F.: Fractures of the Talus. Clin. Orthop., **30**:53–63, 1963.

140. Penny, J. N., and Davis, L. A.: Fractures and Fracture–Dislocations of the Neck of the Talus. J. Trauma, **20**:1029–1037, 1980.

141. Percy, E. C.: Open Fracture of the Talus. Can. Med. Assoc. J., **101**:91–92, 1969.

142. Peterson, L., and Goldie, I. F.: The Arterial Supply of the Talus. A Study on the Relationship to Experimental Talar Fractures. Acta Orthop. Scand., **46**:1026–1034, 1975.

143. Peterson, L.; Goldie, I. F.; and Irstam, L.: Fracture of the Neck of the Talus. A Clinical Study. Acta Orthop. Scand., **48**:696–706, 1977.

144. Peterson, L.; Goldie, I. F.; and Lindell, D.: The Arterial Supply of the Talus. Acta Orthop. Scand., **45**:260–270, 1974.

145. Peterson, L.; Romanus, B.; and Dahlberg, E.: Fracture of the Collum Tali—an Experimental Study. J. Biomech., **9**:277–279, 1976.

146. Quirck, R.: Talar Compression Syndrome in Dancers. Foot Ankle, **3**:65–68, 1982.

147. Reckling, F. W.: Early Tibiocalcaneal Fusion in the Treatment of Severe Injuries of the Talus. J. Trauma, **12**:390–396, 1972.

148. Schrock, R. D.: Fractures of the Foot. Fractures and Dislocations of the Astragalus. A.A.O.S. Instructional Course Lectures **9**:361–368, 1952.

149. Schrock, R. D.; Johnson, H. F.; and Waters, C. H.: Fractures and Fracture–Dislocations of the Astragalus (Talus). J. Bone Joint Surg., **24**:560–573, 1942.

150. Shepherd, F. J.: A Hitherto Undescribed Fracture of the Astragalus. J. Anat. Physiol., **18**:79–81, 1882.

151. Sneed, W. L.: The Astragalus. A Case of Dislocation, Excision and Replacement. An Attempt to Demonstrate the Circulation in this Bone. J. Bone Joint Surg., **7**:384–399, 1925.

152. Sneppen, O., and Buhl, O.: Fracture of the Talus. A Study of its Genesis and Morphology based upon Cases with Associated Ankle Fracture. Acta Orthop. Scand., **45**:307–320, 1974.

153. Sneppen, O.; Christensen, S. B.; Krogsoe, O.; and Lorentzen, J.: Fracture of the Body of the Talus. Acta Orthop. Scand., **48**:317–324, 1977.

154. Syme, J.: Contributions to the Pathology and Practice of Surgery. Edinburgh, Sutherland & Knox, 1848.

155. Trillat, A.; Bousquet, G.; and Lapeyre, B.: Les Fractures–Séparations Totales du Col ou du Corps de l'Astragale. Intéret du Vissage par voie Posterieure. Rev. Chir. Orthop., **56**:529–536, 1970.

156. Weinstein, S. L., and Bonfiglio, M.: Unusual Accessory (Bipartite) Talus Simulating Fracture. A Case Report. J. Bone Joint Surg., **57A**:1161–1163, 1975.

157. Wildenauer, E.: Die Blutversorgung der Talus. Z. Anat., **115**:32, 1950.

Dislocations of and Around the Talus

158. Atsatt, R. F.: Subastragalar Dislocation of the Foot. Case Report. J. Bone Joint Surg., **13**:574–577, 1931.

159. Barber, J. R.; Bricker, J. D.; and Haliburton, R. A.: Peritalar Dislocation of the Foot. Can. J. Surg., **4**:205–210, 1961.

160. Bonnin, J. G.: Dislocations and Fracture–Dislocations of the Talus. Br. J. Surg., **28**:88–100, 1940.

161. Broca, P.: Mémoire sur les Luxations Sous-Astragaliennes. Mem. Soc. Chir. Paris, **3**:566–646, 1853.

162. Buckingham, W. W., Jr.: Subtalar Dislocation of the Foot. J. Trauma, **13**:753–765, 1973.

163. Christensen, S. B.; Lorentzen, J. E.; Krogsoe, O.; and

Sneppen, O.: Subtalar Dislocation. Acta Orthop. Scand., **48:**707–711, 1977.

164. DeLee, J. C., and Curtis, R.: Subtalar Dislocation of the Foot. J. Bone Joint Surg., **64A:**433–437, 1982.

165. Detenbeck, L. C., and Kelly, P. J.: Total Dislocation of the Talus. J. Bone Joint Surg., **51A:**283–288, 1969.

166. Dufaurets, M.: Luxation du Pied en Dehors, Compliquée de l'Issue de l'Astragale a travers la Capsule et les Tégumens Déchirés. J. Med. Chir. Phar., **22:**348–355, 1811.

167. Dunn, A. W.: Peritalar Dislocation. Orthop. Clin. North Am., **5:**7–18, 1974.

168. Grantham, S. A.: Medial Subtalar Dislocation: Five Cases with a Common Etiology. J. Trauma, **4:**845–849, 1964.

169. Gross, R. H.: Medial Peritalar Dislocation-associated Foot Injuries and Mechanism of Injury. J. Trauma, **15:**682–688, 1975.

170. Haliburton, R. A.; Barber, J. R.; and Fraser, R. L.: Further Experience with Peritalar Dislocation. Can. J. Surg., **10:**322–324, 1967.

171. Heppenstall, R. B.; Farahvar, H.; Balderston, R.; and Lotke, P.: Evaluation and Management of Subtalar Dislocations. J. Trauma, **20:**494–497, 1980.

172. Judcy, M.: Observation d'une Luxation Métatarsienne. Bull. Fac. Soc. Med. Paris, **11:**81–86, 1811.

173. Larson, H. W.: Subastragalar Dislocation (Luxatio Pedis sub Talo). A Follow-up Report of Eight Cases. Acta Chir. Scand., **113:**380–392, 1957.

174. Leitner, B.: Obstacles to Reduction in Subtalar Dislocations. J. Bone Joint Surg., **36A:**299–306, 1954.

175. Leitner, B.: The Mechanism of Total Dislocation of the Talus. J. Bone Joint Surg., **37A:**89–95, 1955.

176. Mac, S. S., and Kleiger, B.: The Early Complications of Subtalar Dislocations. Foot Ankle, **1:**270–274, 1981.

177. Mitchell, J. I.: Total Dislocation of the Astragalus. J. Bone Joint Surg., **18:**212–214, 1936.

178. Monson, S. T., and Ryan, J. R.: Subtalar Dislocation. J. Bone Joint Surg., **63A:**1156–1158, 1981.

179. Moore, B. H.: Subastragaloid Dislocation of the Foot. Surg. Gynecol. Obstet., **35:**788–792, 1922.

180. Mulroy, R. D.: The Tibialis Posterior Tendon as an Obstacle to Reduction of a Lateral Anterior Subtalar Dislocation. J. Bone Joint Surg., **37A:**859–863, 1955.

181. Newcomb, W. J., and Brav, E. A.: Complete Dislocation of the Talus. J. Bone Joint Surg., **30A:**872–874, 1948.

182. Pinzur, M. S., and Meyer, P. R., Jr.: Complete Posterior Dislocation of the Talus. Case Report and Discussion. Clin. Orthop., **131:**205–209, 1978.

183. Plewes, L. W., and McKelvey, K. G.: Subtalar Dislocation. J. Bone Joint Surg., **26:**585–588, 1944.

184. Segal, D., and Wasilewski, S.: Total Dislocation of the Talus. Case Report. J. Bone Joint Surg., **62A:**1370–1372, 1980.

185. Shahriaree, H.; Sajadi, K.; Silver, C. M.; and Moosavi, A.: Total Dislocation of the Talus: A Case Report of a Four-Year Follow-up. Orthop. Rev., **9:**65–68, 1980.

186. Shands, A. R., Jr.: The Incidence of Subastragaloid Dislocation of the Foot with a Report of One Case of the Inward Type. J. Bone Joint Surg., **10:**306–313, 1928.

187. Smith, H.: Subastragalar Dislocation. A Report of Seven Cases. J. Bone Joint Surg., **19:**373–380, 1937.

188. Straus, D. C.: Subtalus Dislocation of the Foot. Am. J. Surg., **30:**427–434, 1935.

189. Thomasen, E.: Luxation Pedis Subtalo. Acta Chir. Scand., **88:**115–131, 1943.

Fractures of the Calcaneus

190. Aitken, A. P.: Fractures of the Os Calcis—Treatment by Closed Reduction. Clin. Orthop., **30:**67–75, 1963.

191. Allan, J. H.: The Open Reduction of Fractures of the Os Calcis. Ann. Surg., **141:**890–900, 1955.

192. Anthonsen, W.: An Oblique Projection for Roentgen Examination of the Talo-Calcanean Joint, particularly regarding Intra-Articular Fracture of the Calcaneus. Acta Radiol., **24:**306–310, 1943.

193. Arnesen, A.: Treatment of Fracture of the Os Calcis with Traction and Manipulation. Acta Chir. Scand., **132:**566–573, 1966.

194. Backman, S., and Johnson, S. R.: Torsion of the Foot causing Fracture of the Anterior Calcaneal Process. Acta Chir. Scand., **105:**460–466, 1953.

195. Bankart, A. S. B.: Fractures of the Os Calcis. Lancet, **2:**175, 1942.

196. Barnard, L.: Non-Operative Treatment of Fractures of the Calcaneus. J. Bone Joint Surg., **45A:**865–867, 1963.

197. Barnard, L., and Odegard, J. K.: Conservative Approach in the Treatment of Fractures of the Calcaneus. J. Bone Joint Surg., **52A:**1689, 1970.

198. Bertelsen, A., and Hasner, E.: Primary Results of Treatment of Fracture of the Os Calcis by "Foot-Free Walking Bandage" and Early Movement. Acta Orthop. Scand., **21:**140–154, 1951.

199. Böhler, L.: Diagnosis, Pathology, and Treatment of Fractures of the Os Calcis. J. Bone Joint Surg., **13:**75–89, 1931.

200. Bradford, C. H., and Larsen, I.: Sprain-Fractures of the Anterior Lip of the Os Calcis. N. Engl. J. Med., **244:**970–972, 1951.

201. Brindley, H. H.: Fractures of the Os Calcis: A Review of 107 Fractures in 95 Patients. South. Med. J., **59:**843–847, 1966.

202. Brodén, B.: Roentgen Examination of the Subtaloid Joint in Fractures of the Calcaneus. Acta Radiol, **31:**85–91, 1949.

203. Calcaneal Fractures: Br. Med. J., **3:**310, 1973.

204. Carey, E. J.; Lance, E. M.; and Wade, P. A.: Extra-Articular Fractures of the Os Calcis. J. Trauma, **5:**362–372, 1965.

205. Carothers, R. G., and Lyons, J. F.: Early Mobilization in Treatment of Os Calcis Fractures. Am. J. Surg., **83:**279–280, 1952.

206. Cave, E. F.: Fracture of the Os Calcis—the Problem in General. Clin. Orthop., **30:**64–66, 1963.

207. Christopher, F.: Fracture of the Anterior Process of the Calcaneus. J. Bone Joint Surg., **8:**877–879, 1931.

208. Conn, H. R.: The Treatment of Fractures of the Os Calcis. J. Bone Joint Surg., **17:**392–405, 1935.

209. Conn, H. R.: Discussion of W. E. Gallie's Paper. J. Bone Joint Surg., **25:**736, 1943.

210. Cotton, F. J., and Wilson, L. T.: Fractures of the Os Calcis. Boston Med. Surg. J., **159:**559–565, 1908.

211. Crossan, E. T.: Fractures of the Tarsal Scaphoid and of the Os Calcis. Surg. Clin. North Am., **10**:1477–1487, 1930.

212. Dachtler, H. W.: Fractures of the Anterior Superior Portion of the Os Calcis due to Indirect Violence. Am. J. Roentgenol. **25**:629–631, 1931.

213. Degan, T. J.; Morrey, B. F.; and Braun, D. P.: Surgical Excision for Anterior-process Fractures of the Calcaneus. J. Bone Joint Surg., **64A**:519–524, 1982.

214. Deyerle, W. M.: Long term Follow-up of Fractures of the Os Calcis. Diagnostic Peroneal Synoviagram. Orthop. Clin. North Am., **4**:213–227, 1973.

215. Dick, I. L.: Primary Fusion of the Posterior Subtalar Joint in the Treatment of Fractures of the Calcaneum. J. Bone Joint Surg., **35B**:375–380, 1953.

216. Dodson, C. F., Jr.: Fractures of the Os Calcis. J. Ark. Med. Soc., **73**:319–322, 1977.

217. Essex-Lopresti, P.: Results of Reduction in Fractures of the Calcaneum. J. Bone Joint Surg., **33B**:284, 1951.

218. Essex-Lopresti, P.: The Mechanism, Reduction Technique, and Results in Fractures of the Os Calcis. Br. J. Surg., **39**:395–419, 1952.

219. Gage, J. R., and Premer, R.: Os Calcis Fractures. An Analysis of 37. Minn. Med., **54**:169–176, 1971.

220. Gallie, W. E.: Subastragalar Arthrodesis in Fractures of the Os Calcis. J. Bone Joint Surg., **25**:731–736, 1943.

221. Gaul, J. S., Jr., and Greenberg, B. G.: Calcaneus Fractures involving the Subtalar Joint: A Clinical and Statistical Survey of 98 Cases. South. Med. J., **59**:605–613, 1966.

222. Geckeler, E. O.: Comminuted Fractures of the Os Calcis. Arch. Surg., **61**:469–476, 1950.

223. Gellman, M.: Fractures of the Anterior Process of the Calcaneus. J. Bone Joint Surg., **33A**:382–386, 1951.

224. Goff, C. W.: Fresh Fracture of the Os Calcis. Arch. Surg., **36**:744–765, 1938.

225. Hall, M. C.: Complications at the Ankle and the Midtarsal Joints following Subtalar Arthrodesis by the Gallie Method: A Case Report. Clin. Orthop., **28**:207–209, 1963.

226. Hall, M. C., and Pennal, G. F.: Primary Subtalar Arthrodesis in the Treatment of Severe Fractures of the Calcaneum. J. Bone Joint Surg., **42B**:336–343, 1960.

227. Hamilton, A. R.: An Unusual Dislocation. Med. J. Aust., **1**:271, 1949.

228. Hammesfahr, R., and Fleming, L. L.: Calcaneal Fractures: A Good Prognosis. Foot Ankle, **2**:161–170, 1981.

229. Harris, R. I.: Fractures of the Os Calcis: Their Treatment by Tri-Radiate Traction and Subastragalar Fusion. Ann. Surg., **124**:1082–1100, 1946.

230. Harris, R. I.: Fractures of the Os Calcis: Treatment by Early Subtalar Arthrodesis. Clin. Orthop., **30**:100–110, 1963.

231. Harty, M.: Anatomic Considerations in Injuries of the Calcaneus. Orthop. Clin. North Am., **4**:179–183, 1973.

232. Hazlett, J. W.: Open Reduction of Fractures of the Calcaneum. Can. J. Surg., **12**:310–317, 1969.

233. Hermann, O. J.: Conservative Therapy for Fracture of the Os Calcis. J. Bone Joint Surg., **19**:709–718, 1937.

234. Hoaglund, F. T.: Fractures of the Os Calcis. Editor's Comment. *In* Leach, R. E.; Hoaglund, F. T.; and Riseborough, E. J. (eds.): Controversies in Orthopaedic Surgery, chap. 8. Philadelphia, W. B. Saunders, 1982.

235. Horn, C. E.: Fractures of the Calcaneus. Diagnosis and Treatment. Calif. Med., **108**:209–215, 1968.

236. Hunt, D. D.: Compression Fracture of the Anterior Articular Surface of the Calcaneus. J. Bone Joint Surg., **52A**:1637–1642, 1970.

237. Isbister, J. F.: Calcaneo-Fibular Abutment following Crush Fracture of the Calcaneus. J. Bone Joint Surg., **56B**:274–278, 1974.

238. Isherwood, I.: A Radiological Approach to the Subtalar Joint. J. Bone Joint Surg., **43B**:566–574, 1961.

239. Jaekle, R. F., and Clark, A. G.: Fractures of the Os Calcis. Surg. Gynecol. Obstet., **64**:663–672, 1937.

240. Johansson, J. E.; Harrison, J.; and Greenwood, F. A. H.: Subtalar Arthrodesis for Adult Traumatic Arthritis. Foot Ankle, **2**:294–298, 1982.

241. Kalamchi, A., and Evans, J. G.: Posterior Subtalar Fusion. A Preliminary Report on a Modified Gallie's Procedure. J. Bone Joint Surg., **59B**:287–289, 1977.

242. Kalish, S. R.: The Conservative and Surgical Treatment of Calcaneal Fractures. J. Am. Podiatry Assoc., **65**:912–926, 1975.

243. King, R. E.: Axial Pin Fixation of Fractures of the Os Calcis (Method of Essex-Lopresti). Orthop. Clin. North Am., **4**:185–188, 1973.

244. Korn, R.: Der Bruch Durch das Hintere obere Drittel des Fersenbeines. Arch. Orthop. Unfallchir., **41**:789, 1942.

245. Kovesdi, J. M., Jr.: Management of Fractures of the Os Calcis: A Literature Search. J. Am. Osteopath. Assoc., **75**:46–54, 1975.

246. Lance, E. M.; Carey, E. J., Jr.; and Wade, P. A.: Fractures of the Os Calcis: Treatment by Early Mobilization. Clin. Orthop., **30**:76–90, 1963.

247. Lance, E. M.; Carey, E. J. Jr.; and Wade, P. A.: Fractures of the Os Calcis: A Follow-up Study. J. Trauma, **4**:15–56, 1964.

248. Lenormant, C., and Wilmoth, P.: Les Fractures Sous-Thalamiques du Calcanéum. Leur Traitement par la Réduction a Ciel Ouvert et la Greffe Osteo-Periostique. J. Chir., **40**:1–25, 1932.

249. Leonard, M. H.: Treatment of Fractures of the Os Calcis. Arch. Surg., **75**:990–997, 1957.

250. Lindsay, W. R. N., and Dewar, F. P.: Fractures of the Os Calcis. Am. J. Surg., **95**:555–576, 1958.

251. Lowy, M.: Avulsion Fractures of the Calcaneus. J. Bone Joint Surg., **51B**:494–497, 1969.

252. Lyngstadaas, S.: Treatment of Avulsion Fractures of the Tuber Calcanei. Acta Chir. Scand., **137**:579–581, 1971.

253. McLaughlin, H. L.: Treatment of Late Complications after Os Calcis Fractures. Clin. Orthop., **30**:111–115, 1963.

254. McReynolds, I. S.: The Case for Operative Treatment of Fractures of the Os Calcis. *In* Leach, R. E.; Hoaglund, F. T.; and Riseborough, E. J. (eds.): Controversies in Orthopaedic Surgery, chap. 8. Philadelphia, W. B. Saunders, 1982.

255. Maxfield, J. E.: Os Calcis Fractures. Treatment by Open Reduction. Clin. Orthop., **30**:91–99, 1963.

256. Maxfield, J. E.: Treatment of Calcaneal Fractures by Open Reduction. J. Bone Joint Surg., **45A**:868–871, 1963.
257. Maxfield, J. E., and McDermott, F. J.: Experiences with the Palmer Open Reduction of Fractures of the Calcaneus. J. Bone Joint Surg., **37A**:99–106, 1955.
258. Nade, S., and Monahan, P. R. W.: Fractures of the Calcaneum: A Study of the Long-term Prognosis. Injury, **4**:200–207, 1973.
259. Noble, J., and McQuillan, W. M.: Early Posterior Subtalar Fusion in the Treatment of Fractures of the Os Calcis. J. Bone Joint Surg., **61B**:90–93, 1979.
260. Norfray, J. F.; Rogers, L. F.; Adamo, G. P.; et al: Common Calcaneal Avulsion Fracture. Am. J. Roentgenol, **134**:119–123, 1980.
261. O'Connell, F.; Mital, M. A.; and Rowe, C. R.: Evaluation of Modern Management of Fractures of the Os Calcis. Clin. Orthop., **83**:214–223, 1972.
262. Palmer, I.: The Mechanism and Treatment of Fractures of the Calcaneus. J. Bone Joint Surg., **30A**:2–8, 1948.
263. Parkes, J. C., II: The Nonreductive Treatment for Fractures of the Os Calcis. Orthop. Clin. North Am., **4**:193–195, 1973.
264. Parkes, J. C., II: Injuries of the Hindfoot. Clin. Orthop., **122**:28–36, 1977.
265. Parkes, J. C., II: The Conservative Management of Fractures of the Os Calcis. In Leach, R. E.; Hoaglund, F. T.; and Riseborough, E. J. (eds.): Controversies in Orthopaedic Surgery, chap. 8. Philadelphia, W. B. Saunders, 1982.
266. Pennal, G. F., and Yadav, M. P.: Operative Treatment of Comminuted Fractures of the Os Calcis. Orthop. Clin. North Am., **4**:197–211, 1973.
267. Piatt, A. D.: Fracture of the Promontory of the Calcaneus. Radiology, **67**:386–390, 1956.
268. Pridie, K. H.: A New Method of Treatment for Severe Fractures of the Os Calcis. A Preliminary Report. Surg. Gynecol. Obstet., **82**:671–675, 1946.
269. Protheroe, K.: Avulsion Fractures of the Calcaneus. J. Bone Joint Surg., **51B**:118–122, 1969.
270. Reich, R. S.: Editorial: Fractures of the Calcaneus. Milit. Med., **140**:491–492, 1975.
271. Rothberg, A. S.: Avulsion Fracture of the Os Calcis. J. Bone Joint Surg., **21**:218–220, 1939.
272. Rowe, C. R.; Sakellarides, H. T.; Freeman, P. A.; and Sorbie, C.: Fractures of the Os Calcis. A Long-term Follow-up Study of 146 Patients. J.A.M.A., **184**:920–923, 1963.
273. Salama, R.; Benamara, A.; and Weissman, S. L.: Functional Treatment of Intra-Articular Fractures of the Calcaneus. Clin. Orthop., **115**:236–240, 1976.
274. Schottstaedt, E. R.: Symposium: Treatment of Fractures of the calcaneus. J. Bone Joint Surg., **45A**:863–864, 1963.
275. Shannon, F. T., and Murray, A. M.: Os Calcis Fractures Treated by Non-Weight Bearing Exercises: A Review of 65 Patients. J. R. Coll. Surg. Edinb., **23**:355–361, 1978.
276. Slatis, P.; Kiviluoto, O.; Santavirta, S.; and Laasonen, E. M.: Fractures of the Calcaneum. J. Trauma, **19**:939–943, 1979.
277. Smith, R., and Staple, T.: CAT Scan Evaluation of the Hindfoot—an Anatomical and Clinical Study. Foot Ankle, **2**:346, 1982.
278. Soeur, R., and Remy, R.: Fractures of the Calcaneus with Displacement of the Thalamic Portion. J. Bone Joint Surg., **57B**:413–421, 1975.
279. Thompson, K. R.: Treatment of Comminuted Fractures of the Calcaneus by Triple Arthrodesis. Orthop. Clin. North Am., **4**:189–191, 1973.
280. Thompson, K. R., and Friesen, C. M.: Treatment of Comminuted Fractures of the Calcaneus by Primary Triple Arthrodesis. J. Bone Joint Surg., **41A**:1423–1436, 1959.
281. Thoren, O.: Os Calcis Fractures. Acta Orthop. Scand. (Suppl.) **70**:1–116, 1964.
282. Trickey, E. L.: Treatment of Fractures of the Calcaneus. J. Bone Joint Surg., **57B**:411, 1975.
283. Vestad, E.: Fractures of the Calcaneum. Open Reduction and Bone Grafting. Acta Chir. Scand., **134**:617–625, 1968.
284. Viswanath, S. S., and Shephard, E.: Dislocation of the Calcaneum. Injury, **9**:50–52, 1977.
285. Warrick, C. K., and Bremner, A. E.: Fractures of the Calcaneum—with an Atlas Illustrating the Various Types of Fracture. J. Bone Joint Surg., **35B**:33–45, 1953.
286. Wells, C.: Fractures of the Heel Bones in Early and Prehistoric Times. Practitioner, **217**:294–298, 1976.
287. Whittaker, A. H.: Treatment of Fractures of the Os Calcis by Open Reduction and Internal Fixation. Am. J. Surg., **74**:687–696, 1947.
288. Widén, A.: Fractures of the Calcaneus: A Clinical Study with Special Reference to the Technique and Results of Open Reduction. Acta Chir. Scand. (Suppl.) **188**:1–119, 1954.
289. Wilson, D. W.: Functional Capacity Following Fractures of the Os Calcis. Can. Med. Assoc. J., **95**:908–911, 1966.
290. Wilson, P. D.: Treatment of Fractures of the Os Calcis by Arthrodesis of the Subastragalar Joint. J.A.M.A., **89**:1676–1683, 1927.

Injuries of the Midtarsal Region

291. Brailsford, J. F.: The Radiology of Bones and Joints, 5th ed. London, Churchill, 1953.
292. Brown, D. C., and McFarland, G. B., Jr.: Dislocation of the Medial Cuneiform Bone in Tarsometatarsal Fracture-dislocation. A Case Report. J. Bone Joint Surg., **57A**:858–859, 1975.
293. Day, A. J.: The Treatment of Injuries to the Tarsal Navicular. J. Bone Joint Surg., **29**:359–366, 1947.
294. Dewar, F. P., and Evans, D. C.: Occult Fracture–subluxation of the Midtarsal Joint. J. Bone Joint Surg., **50B**:386–388, 1968.
295. Dick, I. L.: Impacted Fracture–dislocation of the Tarsal Navicular. Proc. R. Soc. Med., **35**:760, 1941.
296. Dixon, J. H.: Letter to the Editor: Isolated Dislocation of the Tarsal Navicular. Injury, **10**:251, 1979.
297. Drummond, D. S., and Hastings, D. E.: Total Dislocation of the Cuboid Bone. J. Bone Joint Surg., **51B**:716–718, 1969.
298. Eftekhar, N. M.; Lyddon, D. W.; and Stevens, J.: An Unusual Fracture–Dislocation of the Tarsal Navicular. J. Bone Joint Surg., **51A**:577–581, 1969.

299. Eichenholtz, S. N., and Levine, D. B.: Fractures of the Tarsal Navicular Bone. Clin. Orthop., **34**:142–157, 1964.

300. Fogel, G. R.; Katoh, Y.; Rand, J. A.; and Chao, E. Y. S.: Talonavicular Arthrodesis for Isolated Arthrosis—9.5-Year Results and Gait Analysis. Foot Ankle, **3**:105–113, 1982.

301. Friedmann, E.: Key Graft Fixation in Mid-Tarsal Fracture Dislocation. Am. J. Surg., **96**:81–83, 1958.

302. Gopal-Krishnan, S.: Dislocation of Medial Cuneiform in Injuries of Tarsometatarsal Joints. Int. Surg., **58**:805–806, 1973.

303. Greenberg, M. J., and Sheehan, J. J.: Vertical Fracture Dislocation of the Tarsal Navicular. Orthopedics, **3**:254–255, 1980.

304. Hermel, M. B., and Gershon-Cohen, J.: The Nutcracker Fracture of the Cuboid by Indirect Violence. Radiology, **60**:850–854, 1953.

305. Hillegass, R. C.: Injuries to the Midfoot. A Major Cause of Industrial Morbidity. *In* Bateman, J. E. (ed.): Foot Science, Chap. 21. Philadelphia, W. B. Saunders, 1976.

306. Holstein, A., and Joldersma, R. D.: Dislocation of First Cuneiform in Tarso-Metatarsal Fracture–Dislocation. J. Bone Joint Surg., **32A**:419–421, 1950.

307. Hooper, G., and McMaster, M. J.: Recurrent Bilateral Mid-Tarsal Subluxations. A Case Report. J. Bone Joint Surg., **61A**:617–619, 1979.

308. Kleiger, B.: The Mechanism and the Roentgenographic Evaluation of Fracture of the Tarsal Bones. Clin. Orthop., **30**:10–19, 1963.

309. Lehman, E. P., and Eskeles, I. H.: Fracture of Tarsal Scaphoid: With Notes on the Mechanism. J. Bone Joint Surg., **10**:108–113, 1928.

310. London, P. S.: A Special View for Mid-Tarsal Fracture–Subluxation. Injury, **5**:65–66, 1973.

311. McGlinchey, J. J.: Dislocation of the Intermediate Cuneiform Bone. Injury, **12**:501–502, 1980.

312. Main, B. J., and Jowett, R. L.: Injuries of the Midtarsal Joint. J. Bone Joint Surg., **57B**:89–97, 1975.

313. Marymont, J. H., Jr.; Mills, G. Q.; and Merritt, W. D., III.: Fracture of the Lateral Cuneiform Bone in the Absence of Severe Direct Trauma. Diagnosis by Radionuclide Bone Scan. Am. J. Sports Med., **8**:135–136, 1980.

314. Nadeau, P., and Templeton, J.: Vertical Fracture Dislocation of the Tarsal Navicular. J. Trauma, **16**:669–671, 1976.

315. O'Rahilly, R.: A Survey of Carpal and Tarsal Anomalies. J. Bone Joint Surg., **35A**:626–642, 1953.

316. Penhallow, D. P.: An Unusual Fracture–Dislocation of the Tarsal Scaphoid with Dislocation of the Cuboid. J. Bone Joint Surg., **19**:517–519, 1937.

317. Ross, P. M., and Mitchell, D. C.: Dislocation of the Talonavicular Joint: Case Report. J. Trauma, **16**:397–401, 1976.

318. Schiller, M. G., and Ray, R. D.: Isolated Dislocation of the Medial Cuneiform Bone—a Rare Injury of the Tarsus. A Case Report. J. Bone Joint Surg., **52A**:1632–1636, 1970.

319. Seymour, N.: The Late Results of Naviculo-Cuneiform Fusion. J. Bone Joint Surg., **49B**:558–559, 1967.

320. Stark, W. A.: Occult Fracture-Subluxation of the Midtarsal Joint. Clin. Orthop., **93**:291–292, 1973.

321. Wiley, J. J., and Brown, D. E.: The Bipartite Tarsal Scaphoid. J. Bone Joint Surg., **63B**:583–586, 1981.

322. Wilson, P. D.: Fractures and Dislocations of the Tarsal Bones. South. Med. J., **26**:833–845, 1933.

Injuries of the Tarsometatarsal (Lisfranc's) Joint

323. Aitken, A. P., and Poulson, D.: Dislocations of the Tarso-Metatarsal Joint. J. Bone Joint Surg., **45A**:246–260, 1963.

324. Ashhurst, A. P. C.: Divergent Dislocation of the Metatarsus. Ann. Surg., **83**:132–136, 1926.

325. Blair, W. F.: Irreducible Tarsometatarsal Fracture–Dislocation. J. Trauma, **21**:988–990, 1981.

326. Cain, P. R., and Seligson, D.: Lisfranc's Fracture–Dislocation with Intercuneiform Dislocation: Presentation of Two Cases and a Plan for Treatment. Foot Ankle, **2**:156–160, 1981.

327. Cassebaum, W. H.: Lisfranc Fracture–Dislocations. Clin. Orthop., **30**:116–129, 1963.

328. Collett, H. S.; Hood, T. K.; and Andrews, R. E.: Tarso-Metatarsal Fracture Dislocations. Surg. Gynecol. Obstet., **106**:623–626, 1958.

329. Compere, E. L.; Banks, S. W.; and Compere, C. L.: Pictorial Handbook of Fracture Treatment, 5th ed. Chicago, Year Book Medical Publishers, 1963.

330. DeBenedetti, M. J.; Evanski, P. M.; and Waugh, T. R.: The Unreducible Lisfranc Fracture. Case Report and Literature Review. Clin. Orthop., **136**:238–240, 1978.

331. Del Sel, J. M.: The Surgical Treatment of Tarso-Metatarsal Fracture–Dislocations. J. Bone Joint Surg., **37B**:203–207, 1955.

332. Denton, J. R.: A Complex Lisfranc Fracture–Dislocation. J. Trauma, **20**:526–529, 1980.

333. Easton, E. R.: Two Rare Dislocations of the Metatarsals at Lisfranc's Joint. J. Bone Joint Surg., **20**:1053–1056, 1938.

334. Foster, S. C., and Foster, R. R.: Lisfranc's Tarsometatarsal Fracture–Dislocation. Radiology, **120**:79–83, 1976.

335. Gissane, W.: A Dangerous Type of Fracture of the Foot. J. Bone Joint Surg., **33B**:535–538, 1951.

336. Hardcastle, P. H.; Reschauer, R.; Kutscha-Lissberg, E.; and Schoffmann, W.: Injuries to the Tarsometatarsal Joint. J. Bone Joint Surg., **64B**:349–356, 1982.

337. Hicks, J. H.: The Mechanics of the Foot. I. The Joints. J. Anat., **87**:345–357, 1953.

338. Jahss, M. H.: Disorders of the Anterior Tarsus and Lisfranc's Joint. *In* Jahss, M. H. (ed.): Disorders of the Foot, vol. 1, chap. 25. Philadelphia, W. B. Saunders, 1982.

339. Jeffreys, T. E.: Lisfranc's Fracture–Dislocation: A Clinical and Experimental Study of Tarso-Metatarsal Dislocations and Fracture–Dislocations. J. Bone Joint Surg., **45B**:546–551, 1963.

340. Latourette, G.; Perry, J.; Patzakis, M. J.; et al: Fractures and Dislocations of the Tarsometatarsal Joint. *In* Bateman, J. E., and Trott, A. W. (eds.): The Foot and Ankle, chap. 7. New York, Brian C. Decker, 1980.

341. Lenczner, E. M.; Waddell, J. P.; and Graham, J. D.: Tarsal–Metatarsal (Lisfranc) Dislocation. J. Trauma, **14**:1012–1020, 1974.

342. Norfray, J. F.; Geline, R. A.; Steinberg, R. I.; et al: Subtleties

of Lisfranc Fracture–Dislocations. Am. J. Roentgenol., **137:**1151–1156, 1981.

343. O'Regan, D. J.: Lisfranc Dislocations. J. Med. Soc. N.J., **66:**575–577, 1969.

344. Quénu, E., and Küss, G.: Étude sur les Luxations du Métatarse (Luxations Métatarso-Tarsiennes) du Diastasis entre le 1. et le 2. Métatarsien. Rev. Chir. Paris, **39:**281–336, 720–791, 1093–1134, 1909.

345. Turco, V. J.: Diastasis of First and Second Tarso-Metatarsal Rays: A Cause of Pain in the Foot. Bull. N.Y. Acad. Med., **49:**222–225, 1973.

346. Wiley, J. J.: The Mechanism of Tarsometatarsal Joint Injuries. J. Bone Joint Surg., **53B:**474–482, 1971.

347. Wilppula, E.: Tarsometatarsal Fracture–Dislocation. Late Results in 26 Patients. Acta Orthop. Scand., **44:**335–345, 1973.

348. Wilson, D. W.: Injuries of the Tarsometatarsal Joints. Etiology, Classification and Results of Treatment. J. Bone Joint Surg., **54B:**677–686, 1972.

Fractures of the Metatarsals

349. Angevine, C. D.; Atwater, E. C.; and Jacox, R. F.: Fender–Kicker Syndrome. Arthritis Rheum., **16:**102–105, 1973.

350. Campbell, W. C.: Infraction of the Head of the Second and Third Metatarsal Bones: Report of Cases. Am. J. Orthop. Surg., **15:**721–724, 1917.

351. Dameron, T. B., Jr.: Fractures and Anatomical Variations of the Proximal Portion of the Fifth Metatarsal. J. Bone Joint Surg., **57A:**788–792, 1975.

352. Gauthier, G., and Elbaz, R.: Frieberg's Infraction: A Subchondral Bone Fatigue Fracture. A New Surgical Treatment. Clin. Orthop., **142:**93–95, 1979.

353. Gould, N., and Trevino, S.: Sural Nerve Entrapment by Avulsion Fracture of the Base of the Fifth Metatarsal Bone. Foot Ankle, **2:**153–155, 1981.

354. Heim, U., and Pfeiffer, K. M.: Small Fragment Set Manual. New York, Springer-Verlag, 1974.

355. Irwin, C. G.: Fractures of the Metatarsals. Proc. R. Soc. Med., **31:**789–793, 1938.

356. Johnson, V. S.: Treatment of Fractures of the Forefoot in Industry. In Bateman, J. E. (ed.): Foot Science, chap. 20. Philadelphia, W. B. Saunders, 1976.

357. Jones, R.: Fracture of the Base of the Fifth Metatarsal Bone by Indirect Violence. Ann. Surg., **35:**697–700, 1902.

358. Kavanaugh, J. H.; Brower, T. D.; and Mann, R. V.: The Jones Fracture Revisited. J. Bone Joint Surg., **60A:**776–782, 1978.

359. Smillie, I. S.: Osteochondritis Dissecans: Loose Bodies in Joints. Edinburgh, E & S Livingstone, 1960.

360. Stewart, I. M.: Jones's Fracture: Fracture of Base of Fifth Metatarsal. Clin. Orthop., **16:**190–198, 1960.

361. Whiteside, J. A.; Fleagle, S. B.; and Kalenak, A.: Fractures and Refractures in Intercollegiate Athletes. An Eleven-Year Experience. Am. J. Sports Med., **9:**369–377, 1981.

362. Zelko, R. R.; Torg, J. S.; and Rachun, A.: Proximal Diaphyseal Fractures of the Fifth Metatarsal—Treatment of the Fractures and their Complications in Athletes. Am. J. Sports Med., **7:**95–101, 1979.

Injuries of the Metatarsophalangeal Joint

363. Barnett, J. C.; Crespo, A.; and Daniels, V. C.: Intra-Articular Accessory Sesamoid Dislocation of the Great Toe. Report of Case. J. Fla. Med. Assoc., **66:**613–615, 1979.

364. Bowers, K. D., Jr., and Martin, R. B.: Turf-Toe: A Shoe-Surface related Football Injury. Med. Sci. Sports, **8:**81–83, 1976.

365. Brown, T. I. S.: Avulsion Fracture of the Fibular Sesamoid in Association with Dorsal Dislocation of the Metatarsophalangeal Joint of the Hallux: Report of a Case and Review of the Literature. Clin. Orthop., **149:**229–231, 1980.

366. Coker, T. P., Jr., and Arnold, J. A.: Sports Injuries to the Foot and Ankle. In Jahss, M. H. (ed.): Disorders of the foot, vol. II, chap. 57. Philadelphia, W. B. Saunders, 1982.

367. Coker, T. P.; Arnold, J. A.; and Weber, D. L.: Traumatic Lesions of the Metatarsophalangeal Joint of the Great Toe in Athletes. J. Ark. Med. Soc., **74:**309–317, 1978.

368. Daniel, W. L.; Beck, E. L.; Duggar, G. E.; and Bennett, A. J.: Traumatic Dislocation of the First Metatarsophalangeal Joint. A case report. J. Am. Podiatry Assoc., **66:**97–100, 1976.

369. DeLuca, F. N., and Kenmore, P. I.: Bilateral Dorsal Dislocations of the Metatarsophalangeal Joints of the Great Toes with a Loose Body in One of the Metatarsophalangeal Joints. J. Trauma, **15:**737–739, 1975.

370. English, T. A.: Dislocations of the Metatarsal Bone and Adjacent Toe. J. Bone Joint Surg., **46B:**700–704, 1964.

371. Giannikas, A. C.; Papachristou, G.; Papavasiliou, N.; et al: Dorsal Dislocation of the First Metatarsophalangeal Joint. Report of Four Cases. J. Bone Joint Surg., **57B:**384–386, 1975.

372. Jahss, M. H.: Traumatic Dislocations of the First Metatarsophalangeal Joint. Foot Ankle, **1:**15–21, 1980.

373. Jahss, M. H.: The Sesamoids of the Hallux. Clin. Orthop., **157:**88–97, 1981.

374. Kelikian, H.: The Hallux. In Jahss, M. H. (ed.): Disorders of the Foot, vol. 1, chap. 22. Philadelphia, W. B. Saunders, 1982.

375. Konkel, K. F., and Muehlstein, J. H.: Unusual Fracture–Dislocation of the Great Toe: Case Report. J. Trauma, **15:**733–736, 1975.

376. McKinley, L. M., and Davis, G. L.: Locked Dislocation of the Great Toe. J. La. State Med. Soc., **127:**389–390, 1975.

377. Murphy, J. L.: Isolated Dorsal Dislocation of the Second Metatarsophalangeal Joint. Foot Ankle, **1:**30–32, 1980.

378. Parra, G.: Stress Fractures of the Sesamoids of the Foot. Clin. Orthop., **18:**281–285, 1960.

379. Rao, J. P., and Banzon, M. T.: Irreducible Dislocation of the Metatarsophalangeal Joints of the Foot. Clin. Orthop., **145:**224–226, 1979.

380. Salamon, P. B.; Gelberman, R. H.; and Huffer, J. M.: Dorsal Dislocation of the Metatarsophalangeal Joint of the Great Toe. J. Bone Joint Surg., **56A:**1073–1075, 1974.

381. Sammarco, G. J.: The Foot and Ankle in Classical Ballet and Modern Dance. In Jahss, M. H. (ed.): Disorders of the Foot, Vol. II, Chap. 59. Philadelphia, W. B. Saunders, 1982.

382. Van Hal, M. E.; Keene, J. S.; Lange, T. A.; and Clancy, W. G., Jr.: Stress Fractures of the Great Toe Sesamoids. Am. J. Sports Med., **10**:122–128, 1982.

383. Zinman, H.; Keret, D.; and Reis, N. D.: Fracture of the Medial Sesamoid Bone of the Hallux. J. Trauma, **21**:581–582, 1981.

Injuries of the Toes

384. Cobey, J. C.: Treatment of Undisplaced Toe Fractures with a Metatarsal Bar made from Tongue Blades. Clin. Orthop., **103**:56, 1974.

385. Dobas, D. C., and Slavitt, J. A.: Impact Fractures of the Lesser Digits. A Clinical Description with a Case History. J. Am. Podiatry Assoc., **67**:571–573, 1977.

386. Howland, W. J.: Pseudo-Dislocation of the Proximal Interphalangeal Joint of the Fifth Toe. Am. J. Roentgenol. **103**:653–657, 1968.

387. Jahss, M. H.: Chronic and Recurrent Dislocations of the Fifth Toe. Foot Ankle, **1**:275–278, 1981.

388. Jahss, M. H.: Stubbing Injuries to the Hallux. Foot Ankle, **1**:327–332, 1981.

389. Nelson, T. L., and Uggen, W.: Irreducible Dorsal Dislocation of the Interphalangeal Joint of the Great Toe. Clin. Orthop., **157**:110–112, 1981.

390. Sammarco, G. J., and Miller, E. H.: Forefoot Conditions in Dancers. II. Foot Ankle, **3**:93–98, 1982.

General

391. Anderson, L. D.: Injuries of the Forefoot. Clin. Orthop., **122**:18–27, 1977.

392. Burman, M. S., and Lapidus, P. W.: The Functional Disturbances caused by the Inconstant Bones and Sesamoids of the Foot. Arch. Surg., **22**:936–975, 1931.

393. Cave, E. F. (ed.): Fractures and Other Injuries. Chicago, Year Book Medical Publishers, 1958.

394. Davis, F. J.; Fry, L. R.; Lippert, F. G.; et al: The Patellar Tendon-bearing Brace: Report of 16 Patients. J. Trauma, **14**:216–221, 1974.

395. DePalma, A. F.: The Management of Fractures and Dislocations: An Atlas, 2nd ed. Philadelphia, W. B. Saunders, 1970.

396. Garcia, A., and Parkes, J. C.: Fractures of the Foot. *In* Giannestras, N. J. (ed.): Foot Disorders: Medical and Surgical Management, 2nd ed., chap. 18. Philadelphia, Lea & Febiger, 1973.

397. Geckeler, E. O.: Dislocations and Fracture–Dislocations of the Foot: Transfixion with Kirschner Wires. Surgery, **25**:730–733, 1949.

398. Heck, C. V.: Fractures of the Bones of the Foot (except the Talus). Surg. Clin. North Am., **45**:103–117, 1965.

399. Henderson, M. S.: Fractures of the Bones of the Foot (except the OS Calcis). Surg. Gynecol. Obstet., **64**:454–457, 1937.

400. Humphrey, G. M.: The Human Foot And The Human Hand. London, MacMillan, 1861.

401. Inman, V. T.: UC-BL Dual-Axis Ankle-control System and UC-BL Shoe Insert: Biomechanical Considerations. Bull. Prosthet. Res., **10–11**:130–145, 1969.

402. Jahss, M. H.: Unusual Diagnostic Problems of the Foot. Clin. Orthop., **85**:42–49, 1972.

403. Key, J. A., and Conwell, H. E.: The Management of Fractures, Dislocations, and Sprains, 4th ed. St. Louis, C. V. Mosby, 1946.

404. Lapidus, P. W., and Guidotti, F. P.: Letter to the Editor: Immediate Mobilization and Swimming Pool Exercises in some Fractures of Foot and Ankle Bones. Clin. Orthop., **56**:197–206, 1968.

405. McLaughlin, H. L.: Trauma. Philadelphia, W. B. Saunders, 1959.

406. Micheli, L. J.: Thromboembolic Complications of Cast Immobilization for Injuries of the Lower Extremities. Clin. Orthop., **108**:191–195, 1975.

407. Morrison, G. M.: Fractures of the Bones of the Feet. Am. J. Surg., **38**:721–726, 1937.

408. Rubin, G.: The Patellar–tendon-bearing (PTB) Orthosis. Bull. Hosp. Joint Dis., **33**:155–173, 1972.

409. Turco, V. J.: Injuries to the Ankle and Foot in Athletics. Orthop. Clin. North Am., **8**:669–682, 1977.

410. Urquhart, D. R.: Injuries to the Foot. Physiotherapy, **53**:127–130, 1967.

411. Wilson, J. N. (ed.): Watson-Jones Fractures and Joint Injuries, 5th ed. Edinburgh, Churchill Livingstone, 1976.

Volumes 1 and 2
Index

3